KELLY'S
ENCYCLOPEDIA
OF
MEDICAL SOURCES

ENCYCLOPEDIA

OF

MEDICAL SOURCES

By

EMERSON CROSBY KELLY

M.D., F.A.C.S.

Associate Professor of Surgery, Albany Medical College
Attending Surgeon, Albany Hospital
Editor, Medical Classics

BALTIMORE

THE WILLIAMS & WILKINS COMPANY

1948

PREFACE

Several years ago it was my good fortune to assist my chief in the writing of a *Surgical Diagnosis*. After the book had left the press, it was discovered that we had put McBurney's point in the wrong place. A search showed that we had put it where about fifty per cent of surgical books put it, that is, a third of the distance along a line drawn from the anterior superior spine to the umbilicus. McBurney placed it "very exactly between an inch and a half and two inches from the anterior spinous process of the ilium on a straight line drawn from that process to the umbilicus." If we are going to use this point in diagnosis and in writings, we certainly should place it where McBurney did.

A few years later there appeared in *Surgery* an article in which Homans' sign was said to be negative. There was neither footnote nor reference and a considerable time was spent in finding just what Homans' sign is and where the original paper is to be found. I wondered how many other pieces of medical information are incorrectly used, how much time is spent in finding original descriptions and how incorrect are the titles of articles and volume numbers with pagination which have crept into the literature.

Accordingly, for some time I have kept a list of references to medical eponyms and original work. No attempt has been made to pin down the first description of any condition because someone, in due time, comes forward with an earlier paper and reference. Priority is an irritating and troublesome study. A search for the earliest *or* best article has been conducted and great care has been exercised in copying the correct title with exact reference. I believe that about ninety-five per cent of the papers listed have been consulted in the original. In some cases the references of an earlier worker have had to be accepted and credit given.

Many useful references have been found in *Textbook of Surgery* by Homans, *History of Medicine* by Garrison and *Medical Bibliography* by Garrison and Morton.

I am grateful to many people who have made my work easier and, above all, have made it a pleasure. I am indebted to Miss Marion F. Dondale and Miss Helen A. Fraser of the Albany Medical College Library; to Miss Maude E. Nesbit and Miss Heath Babcock and their staff of the New York State Medical Library; to Dr. Archibald Malloch and Miss Janet Doe of the New York Academy of Medicine. Dr. Judson Gilbert of Schenectady has been helpful with his suggestions and enthusiasm. Mr. Gordon Mestler of Rochester, N. Y. has given aid.

Above all I am grateful to my wife for her encouragement and forbearance and for tending to her knitting on many a long evening.

EMERSON CROSBY KELLY, M.D.

A

Aagren, Gunnar. Stockholm biochemist.
Isolated the hormone, secretin, in crystalline form.
Ueber die pharmakodynamischen Wirkungen und chemischen Eigenschaften des Secretins. Skand. Arch. f. Physiol., Leipzig, 70: 10–87, 1934
The behavior of crystallized secretin when digested with proteolytic enzymes with E. Hammarsten, J. Physiol., 90: 330–334, Aug. 1937
See also E. Hammarsten

Aaron, Charles Dettie. Detroit physician. 1866–
SIGN—pain in epigastrium on pressure over McBurney's point in appendicitis; also pyloric spasm observable under fluoroscope by pressure at same point.
A sign indicative of chronic appendicitis. J. A. M. A., 60: 350–351, Feb. 1, 1913
Chronic appendicitis, pyloro-spasm and duodenal ulcer. Ibid., 64: 1845 (only), May 29, 1915

Abadie, Charles. Paris ophthalmologist. 1842–1932
SIGN—spasm of levator palpebrae superioris muscle, in exophthalmic goiter.
Spasms des muscles de l'oeil. In his: *Traité des maladies des yeux.* 1877. Vol. 2, pp. 458–459

Abadie, Joseph Louis Irénee Jean. French surgeon. 1873–
OPERATION—excision of tongue.
Technique de l'ablation des cancers du plancher de la bouche. Bull. Soc. Chir. Paris, n. s., 36: 920–927, 1910

Abba, Francesco. Turin bacteriologist. 1862–
SOLUTION—basal phenolphthalein peptone, for isolating B. coli communis from water.
Ueber ein Verfahren, den Bacillus coli communis schnell und sicher aus dem Wasser zu isolieren. Zbl. Bakt., 19: 13–15, Jan. 18, 1896

Abbé, Ernest Carl. German physicist. 1840–1905
CONDENSOR or ILLUMINATOR—
COUNTING CELL—for blood corpuscles.
Ueber neue Mikroskope. S. B. jena. Ges. f. Med. u. Naturw., pp. 107–128, 1886
Developed oil immersion and compensating ocular. Ibid.

Abbe, Robert. New York surgeon. 1851–1928
OPERATION—obliterative aneurysmorrhaphy, by suture of internal wall of sac.
Aneurysmorrhaphy: personal experience with modern method of treating aneurysm. Ann. Surg., 48: 10–14, July 1908
OPERATION—for tic douloureux; intracranial excision of a portion of second and third branches from gasserian ganglion.
The surgical treatment of inveterate tic douloureux. New York M. J., 50: 121–123, Aug. 3, 1889
Simplified operation for intracranial resection of the trigeminal in inveterate neuralgias. Trans. Amer. Surg. Ass., 21: 117–123, 1903
RINGS—catgut rings for supporting ends of intestine to be sutured together.
Intestinal anastomosis. M. News, 54: 589–592, June 1, 1889
Intestinal anastomosis and suturing. Med. Rec., 41: 365–370, 1892
STRING METHOD—treatment of esophageal stricture by passing a string up through it from below, through a gastric fistula, and then cutting the stricture so a bougie may be passed.
A new and safe method of cutting esophageal strictures. Med. Rec., 43: 225–226, Feb. 25, 1893
Pioneer in radium therapy in America. *Radium*

and radio-activity. Yale M. J., 10: 433–447, June 1904
Performed intraspinal section of spinal posterior Roots. Dec. 31, 1888, at suggestion of C. L. Dana, q. v.
A contribution to the surgery of the spine. M. Rec., 35: 149–152, Feb. 9, 1889
Gave experimental proof that beta rays rather than gamma rays from radium are the effective force in cell destruction.
Radium Beta rays: the efficient factor in repressive action on vital cells. M. Rec., 86: 909–913, Nov. 28, 1914

Abbott, Alexander Crever. Philadelphia bacteriologist. 1860–1935
AGAR—glycerol infusion; culture medium. In his: *The principles of bacteriology.* Philadelphia, Lea, 1899 5 ed., p. 102
AGAR—milk; culture medium. Ibid , p. 114
SOLUTION—bile peptone, for enrichment of typhoid bacilli. Ibid., 10 ed., 1921, p. 521
STAINING METHOD—for spores. Ibid., 1892, pp. 134–135

Abbott, Edville Gerhardt. Portland, Me. surgeon. 1871–1938
METHOD or TREATMENT—of scoliosis.
Simple, rapid and complete reduction of deformity in fixed lateral curvature of the spine. New York M. J., 93: 1217–1219, June 24, 1911
Correction of lateral curvature of the spine; a simple and rapid method for obtaining complete correction. Ibid., 95: 833–847, Apr. 27, 1912

Abbott, Frank. American dentist
PASTE—prepared from arsenous acid, morphine and creosote, used to kill nerve of tooth.
Dental pathology and practice. Phila., 1896, 240 pp.

Abbott, J. See L. Shattuck

Abbott, Maude Elizabeth. Montreal physician. 1869–1940
Wrote important works on malformations of heart.
Congenital cardiac disease.
In: *Modern medicine.* Osler. Philadelphia and New York, 4: 323–425, 1908
Atlas of congenital cardiac disease. New York, Amer. Heart Ass., 1936. 62 pp.

Abbott, William Osler. Philadelphia physician. 1902–1943
TUBE—Miller-Abbott or Abbott-Rawson, for intestinal deflation.
For 1934 paper, see T. G. Miller
Intubation studies of the human small intestine. III. A technique for the collection of pure intestinal secretion and for the study of intestinal absorption with T. G. Miller, J. A. M. A., 106: 16–18, Jan. 4, 1936
A tube for use in the postoperative care of gastro-enterostomy cases with A. J. Rawson, Ibid., 108: 1873–1874, May 29, 1937
Intubation studies of the human small intestine. X. A nonsurgical method of treating, localizing and diagnosing the nature of obstructing lesions with C. G. Johnston, S. G. O., 66: 691–697, Apr. 1938
A tube for use in the postoperative care of gastro-enterostomy patients—a correction with A. J. Rawson, J. A. M. A., 112: 2414 (only), June 10, 1939
See also T. G. Miller

Abderhalden, Emil. Halle physiologist. 1877–
REACTION or TEST or DIALYSIS or SERUM—a serum reaction based on the fact that when a foreign

protein gets into the blood the body reacts by elaborating a ferment which causes disintegration of the protein.

Die Diagnose der Schwangerschaft mittels der optischen Methode und dem Dialysierverfahren. Z. phys. Chem., 77: 249–258, 1912

Weitere Beitrage zur biologischen Feststellung der Schwangerschaft. Ibid., 81: 90–98, 1912

Schutzfermente des tierischen Organismus: ein Beitrag zur Kenntnis der Abmehrmassregeln des tierischen Organismus gegen körper-. blut- und zellfremde Stoffe. Berlin, Springer, 1912. 110 pp.

(Same) English trans. by J. O. Gavronsky and W. E. Lanchester. London, Bale, 1914. 242 pp.

REACTION—for cystine.
Familiäre Cystindiathese. Z. phys. Chem., 38: 558–561, 1903

REACTION—for glutamic acid.
Ueber die bei der Isolierung der Monoaminosäuren mit Hilfe der Estermethode entstehenden Verluste with A. Weil, Z. phys. Chem., 74: 445–471, 1911

REACTION—for pyrrolidonecarboxylic acid.
Versuche über Veresterung von Monoaminosäuren mittels Jodäthyl. Trennung der Pyrrolidoncarbonsäure von der Glutaminsäure. Z. phys. Chem., 78: 115–127, 1912

Weitere Beitrag zur Kenntnis der Glutaminsäure und der Pyrrolidoncarbonsäure with K. Kautzsch, Ibid, 78: 333–343, 1912

REAGENT—for determining amino-acids in urine.
Der Abbau der Peptide im Organismus with P. Bergell, Z. phys. Chem., 39: 9–11, 1903

Ueber das Auftreten von Monoaminosäuren im Harn von Kanischen nach Phosphorvergiftung. Ibid., 464–466

SERUM, CANCER SERUM—blood serum from an animal which has been injected with cancer fluid and has thus developed protective ferments; has been used in treating patients with cancer. See reaction

TEST—for proteins and their decomposition products.
Ueber die Verwendung von Triketohydrindenhydrat zum Nachweis von Eiweissstoffen und deren Abbaustufen with H. Schmidt, Z. phys. Chem., 72: 37–43, 1911

Einige Beobachtungen und Versuche mit Triketohydrindenhydrat. (Ruhemann). Ibid., 85: 143–147, 1913
Isolated norleucine. Garrison

Neuere Ergebnisse auf dem Gebiete der Fermentforschung, ihre Anwendung auf die klinische Diagnostik, insbesondere zur Diagnose der Schwagnerschaft with A. Weil, Verh. Ges. dtsch. Naturf., 34, 2 Teil, 2 Hälfte, 478, 1913

Abe, Minoru. Japanese physician
Noted that ingestion of fructose by dogs with mild diabetes did not cause abnormal increase in blood sugar
The availability of fructose in the body of normal and diabetic animals. J. Biochem., 19: 69–110, Jan. 1934

Abe, Nakao. Japanese bacteriologist
MEDIUM—for gonococci.
Ueber die Kultur der Gonokokken. Zbl. Bakt., Orig., 1 Abt., 44: 705–709, 1907

Abel, John Jacob. Baltimore physiologist. 1857–1938
METHOD—of obtaining amino-acids directly from blood, by vivi diffusion.

On the removal of diffusible substances from the circulating blood by means of dialysis with L. G. Rowntree and B. B. Turner, Trans. Ass. Amer. Phys., 28: 51–54, 1913
Isolated epinephrin.
On the blood-pressure-raising constituent of the suprarenal capsule. Johns Hopk Hosp. Bull., 8: 151–157, July 1897
Further observations on the chemical nature of the active principle of the suprarenal capsule. Ibid., 9: 215–218, Sept.–Oct. 1898
Made pharmacological studies of phthaleins which led to use of phenolsulphonephthalein as a function test in renal disease.
On the pharmacological action of some phthaleins and their derivatives, with especial reference to their behavior as purgatives with L. G. Rowntree, J. Pharmacol., 1: 231–264, Aug. 1909
Isolated bufagin.
The poisons of the tropical toad, Bufo agua; a preliminary communication with D. I Macht, J. A. M. A., 56: 1531–1535, May 27, 1911
Two crystalline pharmacological agents obtained from the tropical toad, Bufo agua with D. I. Macht, J. Pharmacol., 3: 319–377, 1911–12
Devised method of plasmaphaeresis.
Plasma removal with return of corpuscles (plasmaphaeresis). Ibid., 5: 625–641, July 1914
Obtained insulin in crystalline form.
Crystalline insulin. Proc. Nat. Acad. Sci., 12: 132–136, Feb. 1926
Also, with E. M. K. Geiling, C. A. Rouiller, F. K. Bell and O. Wintersteiner. J. Pharmacol., 31: 65–85, May 1927

Abelin, Isaak. Bern physiologist. 1883–
Described serologic antibodies against hormones (against thyroxine).
Ueber das Vorkommen einer jodhaltigen, antithyroxinartig wirkenden Substanz in der Schilddrüse. Biochem. Z., 286: 160–181, 1936

Abelin, J. German physician
REACTION—for arsphenamine in urine. *Ueber eine neue Methode das Salvarsan nachzuweisen.* Munch. med. Wschr., 58: 1002–1003, May 9, 1911
REACTION—for neoarsphenamine in urine.
Ueber das Verhalten des Neosalvarsans und des Salvarsans im Organismus. Arch. exp. Path. Pharmak., 75: 317–332, 1914
See also M. Perelstein

Abernethy, John. English surgeon. 1764–1831
FASCIA—sheet of areolar tissue over external iliac artery.
OPERATION—for ligation of external iliac artery.
In his: *Surgical observations.* London, 1809 pp. 234–292. (Same), 1817, Vol 1, pp. 254–315
SARCOMA—fatty tumor found principally on trunk.
Ibid., Vol. 2, pp. 27–30

Abrahams, Robert. New York physician. 1864–1935.
SIGN—dullness over acromion process in early pulmonary tuberculosis.
Auscultation at the acromion process: its significance in apical disease. Arch. of Diagnosis, 6: 111–113, Apr. 1913

Abrahamson, Emanuel M. Brooklyn physician 1897–

REAGENT—tungstic acid, for precipitating proteins from blood.
A stable solution of tungstic acid. Amer. J. Clin. Path., Tech. Suppl., 4: 75–77, 1940

Abram, John Hill. Liverpool physician
TEST—for lead in urine; modification of von Jaksch test.
Three cases of lead poisoning; with a note on a simple method for the detection of lead in organic fluids. Lancet, 1: 164–165, Jan. 16, 1897

Abrami, P.
See G. F. I. Widal

Abrams, Albert. San Francisco physician. 1863–1924
REFLEX—contraction of myocardium, with reduction in area of cardiac dullness, which results when skin of precordial region is irritated; observed with fluoroscope.
The clinical value of the heart reflex. Med. Rec., 59: 10–12, Jan. 5, 1901
REFLEX—contraction of lung following stimulation of chest wall. *Some cardiorespiratory phenomena revealed by the Röntgen rays.* Amer. Med., 5: 11–15, Jan. 3, 1903
TREATMENT—of angina pectoris by percussing seventh cervical spine.
Spondylotherapy, physio-therapy of the spine based on a study of clinical physiology. San Francisco, 1912. 3. ed. 673 pp.

Abramson, David Irvin. Cincinnati physician. 1905–
METHOD—of determining blood flow in man.
Plethysmographic studies of peripheral blood flow in man. I. Criteria for obtaining accurate plethysmographic data with H. Zazeela and J. Marrus, Amer. Heart J., 17: 194–205, Jan. 1939

Abt, A. F.
See C. J. Farmer

Abt, Georges. French physician
SOLUTION—yeast autolysate, culture medium for colon-typhoid group.
Culture et conservation des microbes sur les milieux a la levure autolysée with G. Blanc, C. R. Soc. Biol., Paris, 84: 452–453. Mar. 5, 1921

Achalme, Pierre Jean. French physician. 1866–
BACILLUS—
Examen bactériologique d'un cas de rhumatisme articulaire aigu; mort de rhumatisme cérébrale. C. R. Soc. Biol., 9 s., 3: 651–656, 1891

Achard, Emile Charles. French physician. 1860–1941
SYNDROME—
Le virilisme pilaire et son association à l'insuffisance glycolytique (Diabète des femmes à barbe) with J. Thiers, Bull. Acad. Med. Paris, 86: 51–66, July 19, 1921
TEST—for kidney function.
Diagnostic de la perméabilité rénale with J. Castaigne, Bull. Soc. méd. Hôp. Paris, 14: 637–651, Apr. 30, 1897
L'exploration clinique des fonctions rénales par la glycosurie phloridzique with V. Delamare, Ibid., 16: 379–395, Apr. 7, 1899
L'examen clinique des fonctions rénales par l'élimination provoquée with J. Castaigne, Oeuvre méd. chir., Paris, Masson, 1900. 40 pp.
Coined term paratyphoid fever.

Infections paratyphoïdiques with R. Bensaude, Bull. Soc. méd. Hôp. Paris, 13: 820–833, Nov. 27, 1896

Achilles
REFLEX—takes name from Achilles tendon.

Achúcarro, Nicolás. Spanish scientist. 1881–1918
METHOD—tannin, for neuroglia.
Nuevo método para le estudio de la neuroglia y del tejido conjuntivo. Bol. Soc. Espan. Biol., Madrid, 1: 139–141, Oct. 1911

Ackermann, Conrad Theodor. German physician. 1825–1896
ANGLE—at base of skull, characteristic of kyphosis, encephalocele and hydrocephalus.
Die Schädeldifformität bei der Encephalocele congenita. Halle, Niemeyer, 1882. 79 pp.

Ackermann, Dankwart. Heidelberg physiologist
REACTION—for guanidine.
Nachweis von Guanidin. Z. phys. Chem., 47: 366–367, 1906

d'Acosta, José. Jesuit missionary. 1539–1600
DISEASE—mountain sickness; described after his travels in Peru in 1590.
Efecto estrano que haze en ciertas tierras de Indias el aire, o viento que corre. Forms Lib. 3, ch. 9 of his: *Historia natural y moral de las Indias.* Sevilla, Juan de Léon, 1590

Acree, Solomon Farley. American chemist. 1875–
REACTION—for proteins.
On the detection of formaldehyde in milk. Preliminary contribution. J. Bio. Chem., 2: 145–148, 1906
A formaldehyde color test for proteids. Amer. Chem. J., 37: 604–619, 1907

Acrel, Olof of. Swedish surgeon. 1717–1806
GANGLION—on extensor tendons of wrist.
Historia tumorum rariorum circa carpum et in vola manus obvenientium, qui, simillimi licet facie, qua indolem tamen et sanandi methodum prorsus discrepant. Comment. phys. Soc. reg. scient. Gotting., (1779), Vol. 2, 1780

Adachi, Kiyohisa. Japanese physician
STAIN—for flagella of spirocheta morsus Muris.
Flagellum of the microorganism of rat-bite fever. J. exp. M., 33: 647–651, May 1, 1921

Adair, F. L. See M. E. Davis

Adair, Frank Earl. New York surgeon. 1887–
Described plasma cell mastitis.
Plasma cell mastitis—a lesion simulating mammary carcinoma: a clinical and pathologic study with a report of ten cases. Arch. Surg., 26: 735–749, May 1933.
See also B. J. Lee

Adam, A. See H. Chaoul

Adami, John George. Montreal pathologist. 1862–1926
THEORY—for explanation of heredity, resembling Ehrlich's side-chain t. of immunity.
An address on theories of inheritance, with special reference to the inheritance of acquired conditions in man. Brit. med. J., 1: 1317–1323, June 1, 1901
See also C. S. Roy

Adamkiewicz, Albert. Vienna pathologist. 1850–1921
DEMILINE OF—crescent-shaped cells beneath the neurilemma of medullated nerve-fibers.
Die Nervenkörperchen. Ein neuer, bisher unbekannter morphologischer Bestandtheil der peripherischen Ner-

ven. S. B. Akad. Wiss. Wien., 91, 3 Abth., 274–284, Mar. 19, 1885
STAIN—safranine for myelin.
Neue Rückenmarkstinctionen. I. Ergebnisse am normalen Gewebe. Ibid., 89, 3 Abth., 245–265, Apr. 3, 1884
SERUM—obtained from cancer tissue, a supposed alexin, used hypodermically for cancer.
Untersuchungen über den Krebs und das Princip seiner Behandlung. Wien, Braumüller, 1893. 134 pp.
TEST—for proteins.
Farbenreactionen des Albumin. Arch. f. exp. Path., 3: 412–426, Apr. 1875
Adams, James Alexander. Glasgow surgeon. 1857–1930
OPERATION—shortening of round ligaments of uterus for displacement.
A new operation for uterine displacements. Glasgow M. J., 17: 437–446, 1882
Adams, John. English physician. 1806–1877
Distinguished between hypertrophy and carcinoma of prostate.
The anatomy and diseases of the prostate gland. London, Longmans, 1851
Adams, M. See R. M. Wilder
Adams, Robert. Dublin physician. 1791–1875
SYNDROME—Stokes-Adams s. or disease; bradycardia and transient vertigo as a sign of fatty or fibrous myocarditis.
Cases of diseases of the heart, accompanied with pathological observations. Dublin Hosp. Rep., 4:353–453, 1827 Also: Medical classics, 3: 633–696, Feb. 1939
Also: F. A. Willius and T. E. Keys' Cardiac classics. St. Louis, Mosby, 1941, pp. 397–399
Wrote important paper on rheumatic gout.
Treatise on rheumatic gout, or chronic arthritis, of all the joints. London, Churchill, 1857. 362 pp.
Adams, W. L. See I. H. Einsel
Adams, Sir William. London ophthalmologist. 1783–1827
OPERATION—excision of a wedge-shaped piece from eyelid for relief of ectropion.
Practical observations on ectropium, or eversion of the eye-lids. . . . London, Callow, 1812
Adams, William. English surgeon. 1820–1900
KNIFE, SAW—for osteotomy.
OPERATION—subcutaneous intracapsular division of neck of femur for ankylosis of hip.
A new operation for bony anchylosis of the hip joint, with malposition of the limb, by subcutaneous division of the neck of the thigh-bone. London, Churchill, 1871
OPERATION—subcutaneous division of palmar fascia at various points for Dupuytren's contraction.
Observations on contraction of the fingers. . . . London, Churchill, 1879
OPERATION—crushing projecting portion of deflected nasal septum with forceps and inserting splint.
. In, W. S. Watson: *Diseases of the nose.* . . . London, 1875. 472 pp. pp. 305–307
Adamson, Horatio George. London dermatologist
TECHNIC—Kienböck-Adamson; epilating doses of low voltage roentgen irradiation.
A simplified method of x ray application for the cure of ringworm of the scalp; Kienböck's method. Lancet, 1: 1378–1380, May 15, 1909

Addis, Thomas. San Francisco physician. 1881–
COUNT—of urinary sediments, to determine type of renal pathology.
A clinical classification of Bright's disease. J. A. M. A., 85: 163–167, July 18, 1925
The number of formed elements in urinary sediment of normal individuals J. Clin. Invest., 2: 409–415, June 1926
TECHNIC—concentration test of urine; after patient is on a dry diet for twenty-four hours, specific gravity of urine is determined.
A test of the capacity of the kidney to produce a urine of high specific gravity with M. C. Shevky, Arch. Intern. Med., 30: 559–562, Nov. 1922
Made important study of renal function.
Renal function and the amount of functioning tissue: the ratio; urea in one hour's urine/urea in 100 c.c. of blood, after giving urea and water. Arch. Intern. Med., 30: 378–385, Sept. 1922
See also R. L. Wilbur
Addison, Sir Christopher. English anatomist. 1869–
PLANES—used as landmarks in topography of thorax and abdomen.
LINE—transpyloric.
POINT—midepigastric.
On the topographical anatomy of abdominal viscera in man, especially the gastrointestinal canal. J. Anat. and Physiol., 33: 565–586, July 1899
Addison, Thomas. English physician. 1793–1860
ANEMIA—pernicious of Addison-Biermer; idiopathic anemia.
On the constitutional and local effects of disease of the suprarenal capsules. London, Highley, 1855. 43 pp.
Also: Collected writings. London, New Sydenham Soc., 1868. pp. 209–239
Also: In German. Klassiker der Med., No. 20. Leipzig, 1912
Also: In *A clinical study of Addison s disease.* By L. G. Rowntree and A. M. Snell. Mayo Clinic Monographs. Phila., Saunders, 1931. pp. 30–53
Also: Medical classics, 2: 244–280, Nov. 1937
DISEASE or SYNDROME—chronic suprarenal insufficiency usually due to tuberculosis of suprarenal capsules.
(First announcement) *Anemia—disease of the suprarenal capsules.* London M. Gaz., 48: 517–518, 1849
(First paper) *On the constitutional and local effects of disease of the suprarenal capsules.* London, Highley, 1855. 43 pp. See ANEMIA
KELOID—morphea.
On the keloid of Alibert, or on true keloid. Med.-chir. Trans., 37: 27–47, 1854
Also in: Collected writings. London, New Sydenham Soc., 1868. pp. 165–185
Employed static electricity in treatment of spasmodic and convulsive diseases.
On the influence of electricity as a remedy in certain convulsive and spasmodic diseases with G. Bird and W. Gull, Guy's Hosp. Rep., 2: 493–507, 1837
Made important observations on blood.
Experimental and practical researches on inflammation and on the origin and nature of tubercle of the lungs. London, Churchill, 1843
Described xanthoma diabeticorum.
On a certain affection of the skin, vitiligoidea—a.

plana, b. tuberosa, with remarks with W. Gull, Guy's Hosp. Rep., 7: 265–276, 1851
See also R. Bright, J. Morgan

Adie, William John. English physician. 1886–
SYNDROME—
Pseudo-Argyll Robertson pupils with absent tendon reflexes; a benign disorder simulating tabes dorsalis.
Brit. Med. J., 1; 928–930, May 30, 1931

Adler, Alexander. Budapest surgeon
METHOD—of mammaplasty.
Über einen Fall von selten grosser Gynäkomastie. Plastische Operation. Zbl. Chir., 64: 889–893, Apr. 10, 1937

Adler, Aldred. Vienna psychiatrist, 1870–1937
Made important contributions to psychiatry.
Studie über Minderwertigkeit von Organen. Berlin, Wien, Urban & Schwarzenberg, 1907
Ueber den nervösen Charakter . . . Wiesbaden, Bergmann, 1912. 195 pp.
Organ inferiority and its psychial compensation. Washington, Nerv. & Ment. Dis. Pub. Co., 1917
The neurotic constitution. . . . New York, Moffat, 1917. 456 pp.

Adler, L. See F. Hitschman

Adler, Oskar. Czecho-Slovak physician. 1879–
TEST—benzidin, for blood.
Ueber das Verhalten gewisser organischer Verbindungen gegenüber Blut mit besonderer Berücksichtigung des Nachweises von Blut with R. Adler, Z. phys. Chem., 141: 59–67, 1904

Adler, Rudolf. Carlsbad chemist. 1882–
TEST—for nitrite in urine.
Ueber eine Reaktion im Harn bei der Behandlung mit Resorcin with O. Adler, Z. phys. Chem., 41: 206–209, 1904

Aldersberg, David. Vienna physician.
TEST—for bilirubin and urobilin in feces.
Ueber den Nachweis von Bilirubin und Urobilin in den Fäzes mit Trichloress'gsäure with O. Porges, Biochem. Z., 150: 348–349, Aug. 14, 1924

Adrian, Edgar Douglas. English physiologist. 1889–
Awarded Nobel prize in 1932, with C. S. Sherrington for work on physiology of nervous system.
The electric response of denervated muscle with D. R. Owen, J. Physiol., 55: 326–331, Nov. 18, 1921
The all-or-nothing response of sensory nerve fibers with A. Forbes, Ibid., 56: 301–330, July 21, 1922

Adson, Alfred Washington. Rochester, Minn. surgeon. 1887–
MANEUVER—to test pressure by scalenus anticus.
SYNDROME—
Cervical rib: a new method of anterior approach for relief of symptoms by division of the scalenus anticus. with J. R. Coffey, Ann. Surg., 85: 839–857, June 1927
OPERATION—complete excision of parotid gland.
Preservation of the facial nerve in the radical treatment of parotid tumors with W. O. Ott, Arch. Surg., 6: 739–746, May 1923
OPERATION—
The surgical treatment of glossopharyngeal neuralgia. Arch. Neurol. Psychiat., 12: 487–506, Nov. 1924
OPERATION—
Treatment of Raynaud's disease by lumbar ramisection and ganglionectomy and perivascular sympa-

thetic neurectomy of the common iliacs with G. E. Brown, J. A. M. A., 84: 1908–1910, June 25, 1925
OPERATION—
The surgical indications for sympathetic ganglionectomy and trunk resection in the treatment of chronic arthritis, with L. G. Rowntree, S. G. O., 50: 204–215, Jan. 1930
Reported sympathectomy for relief of Hirschsprung's disease.
The results of sympathectomy in the treatment of peripheral vascular diseases, Hirschsprung's disease, and cord bladder. Ann. Int. Med., 6: 1044–1068, Feb. 1933
See also W. McK. Craig

Aeby, Christopher Theodor. Swiss anatomist. 1835–1885
PLANE—through nasion and basion, perpendicular to median plane of cranium.
Eine neue Methode zur Bestimmung der Schädelform von Menschen und Säugethieren. Braunschweig, 1863
Die Schädelformen des Menschen und der Affen. Eine morphologische Studie. Leipzig, Vogel, 1867. 132 pp.

Afanasyeff, Mikhail Ivanovich. Russian bacteriologist. 1850–1910
BACILLUS—found in expectoration of whooping cough and pathogenic for dogs.
Lektsii po klinicheskoi mikroskopii i bakteriologii. St. Petersburg, 1896. 154 pp.

Agababow, Alexander Grigoryevich. Kasan scientist.
CILIARY PLEXUS—
O nervnikh okonchaniakh v tsiliarnom tiele u mlekopitayushtshikh i chelevieka. (on nerve endings in ciliary bodies in mammals).
Kazan, V. M. Klyuchnikoff, 1893
Die Innervation des Ciliarkörpers. Anat. Anz., 8: 551–561, July 8, 1893
METHOD—for staining elastic tissue.
Untersuchungen über die Natur der Zonula ciliaris. Arch. mikr. Anat., 50: 566–588, 1897

Agatston, Sigmund Arthur. New York ophthalmologist. 1879–1945
OPERATION—
Muscle retroplacement in the correction of squint. Simplified technic. Report of cases and results. Amer. J. Ophth., 7: 361–364, May 1924

Aglietti, Francesco. Italian physician. 1757–1836
Published early periodical devoted to history of medicine.
Giornale per servire alla storia ragionata della medicina di questa secolo. Venice, 1783–95

Agnew, Cornelius Rea. American ophthalmologist. 1830–1888
OPERATION—
A method of operating for divergent squint. Trans. Amer. Ophth. Soc., pp. 31–34, 1866

Agnew, David Hayes. Philadelphia surgeon. 1818–1892
OPERATION—for syndactylism.
In his: *Principles and practice of surgery.* Philadelphia, Lippincott, 1883. 3 vols. vol. 3, pp. 371–372
SLING or SPLINT—for fracture of metacarpus. Ibid., Ed., 1878. vol. 1, p. 919
SPLINT—for fracture of patella. Ibid., p. 974

Agote, Luis. Argentina surgeon. 1869–
Transfused citrated blood.
Nuevo procedimiento para la transfusion del sangre.
An. Inst. Mod. de Clin. Med., Buenos Aires, 1:
25–30, 1914–5
Agramonte, A. See W. Reed
Agulhon, Henri. French physician
REAGENT—for testing for reducing substances.
*Recherche colorimétrique de l'alcool en présence de
l'acétone. Réactions colorées de certains groupements
organiques en présence d'acides minéraux et de bichro-
mate de potassium.* Bull. Soc. Chim. biol. Paris, s.
4, 9: 881–885, Sept. 20—Oct. 5, 1911
Ahlfeld, Joh. Friedrich. Leipzig obstetrician. 1843–
1929
METHOD—of expressing placenta.
Ueber bimanuelle Placentarexpression. Schmidt's
Jahrb. d. . . . Gesamm. Med., 174: 43–45, 1877
Abwartende Methode oder Credé'scher Handgriff?
Leipzig, Grunow, 1888. 36 pp.
SIGN—spasms of portion of the uterine wall after
the third month of gestation.
Beobachtungen über die Dauer der Schwangerschaft.
Mschr. f. Geburtsch., 34: 180–225; 266–305, 1869
Airy, Sir George Biddell. English scientist. 1801–
Described astigmatism and fitted cylindrical lenses
for the condition.
*On a peculiar defect in the eye and a mode of correcting
it.* Cambridge Philos. Trans., 2: 267–271, 1827
Aitkin, John. Edinburgh surgeon. ?–1790
OPERATION—double pelviotomy for narrow pelvis.
Principles of midwifery, or puerperal medicine.
Edinburgh, 1784; 2 ed., 1785. 216 pp.
Akatsu, Seinai. New York physician
BOUILLON—basal ascitic fluid, for studying fer-
mentation by bacteria.
*The influence of carbohydrates on the cultivation of
spirochetes.* J. Exper. Med., 25: 375–380 (376), Mar.
1917
Akerman, Nils. Stockholm surgeon
OPERATION—
Zur Behandlung dislozierter Zygomatikusfrakturen.
Acta chir. Scandinav., 80: 359–364, Feb. 28, 1938
Akimoto, C. See I. Otaki
Alanson, Edward. English surgeon, 1747–1823
AMPUTATION—circular amputation with stump
shaped like a hollow cone.
*Practical observation on amputation and the after-
treatment, to which is added an account of the amputa-
tion above the ancle with a flap.* London, Johnson, 1
ed., 1779; 2 ed., 1782. 296 pp.
Albaran y Dominguez, Joaquin. Paris and Cuba
urologist. 1860–1912
GLANDS—in bladder, subtrigonal. In his: *Les tumeurs
de la vessie.* Paris, Steinheil, 1892. pp. 78–79
OPERATION—
Technique de la néphropexie. Pr. méd., 14: 253–256,
Apr. 21, 1906
TEST—polyuria t. for renal inadequacy.
*Exploration des functions rénales. Étude medico-chi-
rurgical.* Paris, Masson, 1905. 604 pp.
TUBULE—in cervical part of prostate.
*Contribution a l'étude de l'anatomie macroscopique de
la prostate hypertrophiée* with B. Motz, Ann. d.
malad. d. organes genito-urinaires, 20: 769–817, 1902

Systematized use of cystoscopy and catheterization
of ureters.
Étude sur le rein des urinaires. Paris, 1889. 184 pp.
*Médicine operatoire des voies urinaires: anatomie nor-
male et anatomie pathologique chirurgicale.* Paris,
Masson, 1909. 991 pp.
Made a cystoscopic diagnosis of ectopic vaginal
ureter.
*Uretère surnuméraire ouvert dans la vulve et dans le
vagin.* Gaz. d. hôp., 70: 743, 1897
Albee, Fred Houdlett. New York surgeon. 1876–1945
OPERATION—for production of surgical ankylosis
of hip.
*Arthritis deformans of the hip: a preliminary report
of a new operation.* J. A. M. A., 50: 1977–1980, June
13, 1908
OPERATION—spinal fusion.
*Transplantation of a portion of the tibia into the spine
for Pott's disease. A preliminary report.* J. A. M. A.,
57: 885–886, Sept. 9, 1911
*A report of bone transplantation and osteoplasty in
the treatment of Pott's disease of the spine.* New York
M. J., 95: 469–475, Mar. 9, 1912
*The bone-graft operation for tuberculosis of the spine:
twenty years' experience.* J. A. M. A., 94: 1467–1471,
May 10, 1930
OPERATION—
*Synthetic transplantation of tissues to form new finger
with restored function of hand.* Ann. Surg., 69: 379–
383, Apr. 1919
BONE MILL—
The improved Albee bone mill. Amer. J. Surg., 39:
657–660, Mar. 1938
OPERATION—for slipping patella; a wedge-shaped
tibial graft is used to prevent patella from slipping
laterally.
*The bone graft wedge in the treatment of habitual dis-
location of the patella.* M. Rec., 88; 257–259, Aug. 14,
1915
Also: *Orthopedic and reconstruction surgery, indus-
trial and civilian.* Phila., Saunders, 1919. 1138 pp.
(pp. 624–630)
SAW—for cutting bone grafts. Ibid., p. 177
OPERATION—fixation of fracture of neck of femur
by bone graft.
*The bone graft peg in the treatment of fractures of neck
femur: author's technic.* Ann. Surg., 62: 85–91; 125,
July 1915
*Late end-results in ununited fracture of neck of femur
treated by the bone peg or the reconstruction operation.*
J. Bone and Joint Surg., 10: 124–143, Jan. 1928
Albers-Schönberg, Heinrich Ernst. Hamburg sur-
geon. 1865–1921
DISEASE—marmorization of bones; osteosclerosis
fragilis generalisata; marmorknochen.
Röntgenbilder einer seltenen Knochenerkrankung.
Fort. a. d. Geb. d. Röntgenstr., 7: 158–159, 1903–04
*Ein seltene, bisher nicht bekannte Strukturanomalie
des Skelettes.* Ibid., 23: 174–177, 1915
Invented the compression diaphragm for intensify-
ing the object by cutting out secondary rays.
Die Röntgen-Technik. Hamburg, Gräfe and Sillem,
1903
Albert, Eduard. Vienna surgeon. 1841–1900
DISEASE—achillobursitis.

Achillodynie. Wien. med. Presse, 34: 41–43, Jan. 8, 1893
Zur Klinik der Krankheiten der Schnensheiden und Schleimbeutel. Wien. med. Wschr., 20: 1248–1251, Nov. 5; 1303–1305, Nov. 19, 1870
OPERATION—joint excision for flail-joint of knee.
Ueber Gelenksresektionen bei Caries. Wien Klin., 9: 85–100, 1883
Introduced arthrodesis.
Einige Fälle von kunstlicher Ankylosebildung an paralytischen Gliedmassen. Wien. med. Presse, 23: 725–728, 1882
Albert, Henry. Iowa City physician. 1878–1930
BROTH—blood veal infusion.
The pathogenicity of Bacillus influenzae for laboratory animals with Sarah R. Kelman, J. Infect. Dis., 25: 433–443 (434), Dec. 1919
STAIN—
A new stain for diphtheria bacilli. J. A. M. A., 74: 28, Jan. 3, 1920
Modification of stain for diphtheria bacilli. Ibid., 76: 240, Jan. 22, 1921
See also Mary J. Erickson
Albertini, Ippolito Francisco. Italian physician. 1662–1746
TREATMENT—complete rest and little food in aneurysm of aorta.
Animadversiones super quibusdam difficilis respirationis vitiis, a laesa cordis et praecordiorum structura pendentibus. Bologna, 1748
Albini, Guiseppe. Italian physiologist. 1827–1911
NODULES—remains of fetal structures, sometimes seen on free edge of auriculo-ventricular valves of infants.
Lezioni di embriologia nell'universita di Napoli, in un corso straordinario nell'anno 1867. pp. 144. In Army Medical Library
Albright, Fuller. Boston physician. 1900–
FORMULA or SOLUTION—irrigation fluid for urinary lithiasis.
Nonsurgical aspects of the kidney stone problem with H. W. Sulkowitch and R. Clute, J. A. M. A., 113: 2049–2053, Dec. 2, 1939
SYNDROME—
Syndrome characterized by osteitis fibrosa disseminata, areas of pigmentation and endocrine dysfunction, with precocious puberty in females: report of five cases with A. M. Butler, A. O. Hampton and P. Smith, New Engl. J. Med., 216: 727–746, Apr. 29, 1937
See also W. Bauer, H. F. Klinefelter
Albright, H. L. See H. M. Clute
Aldenburg, H. See C. Wren
Aldor, Ludwig von. Karlsbad physician
TEST—for albumoses in urine.
Ueber den Nachweis der Albumosen im Harn und über die enterogene Albumosurie. Berl. klin. Wschr., 36: 764–767; 785–787, Aug. 28, 1899
Aldrich, Charles Anderson. Chicago pediatrician. 1888–
TEST—in phlegmasia alba dolens and occult edema.
The intradermal salt solution test. II. Its prognostic value in "nephritis" with generalized edema with W. B. McClure, J. A. M. A., 82: 1425–1428, May 3, 1924
See also W. B. McClure

Aldrich, Martha. Rochester, Minn. scientist
METHOD—for determination of bile salts.
Studies in the metabolism of the bile. I. Quantitative Pettenkofer test applicable to the determination of bile acids in blood with M. S. Bledsoe, J. Biol. Chem., 77: 510–537, May 1928
Aldrich, Robert Henry. Boston surgeon. 1902–
DYE MIXTURE—for treatment of burns.
The role of infection in burns. The theory and treatment with special reference to gentian violet. New Engl. J. Med., 208: 299–309, Feb. 9, 1933
Treatment of burns with a compound of anilin dyes. Ibid., 217: 911–914, Dec. 2, 1937
Aldrich, Thomas Bell. American physiologist. 1861–
Isolated adrenaline in crystalline form.
A preliminary report on the active principle of the suprarenal gland. Amer. J. Physiol., 5: 457–461, 1901
See also O. Kamm
Alexander, G. L. See J. H. Biggart
Alexander, John. Ann Arbor, Mich. surgeon. 1891–
OPERATION—
Multiple intercostal neurectomy for pulmonary tuberculosis. Amer. Rev. Tuberc., 20: 637–684, Nov. 1929
OPERATION—
Supraperiosteal and subcostal pneumonolysis with filling of pectoral muscles. Arch. Surg., 28: 538–547, Mar. 1934
Alexander, Samuel. New York surgeon. 1859–1910
OPERATION—prostatectomy by median suprapubic and median perineal incision.
Prostatectomy. N. Y. Med. J., 63: 171–176, Feb. 8, 1896
Alexander, William. Liverpool surgeon. 1844–1919
OPERATION—Alexander-Adam's o.; shortening of round ligaments of uterus for displacement.
A new method of treating inveterate and troublesome displacements of the uterus. Med. Times and Gaz., 1: 327–328, Apr. 1, 1882
The treatments of backward displacements of the uterus and of prolapsus uteri by the new method of shortening the round ligaments. London, Churchill, 1884. 71 pp.
The operations of ventrofixation or ventrosuspension of the uterus and shortening the round ligaments. A study and a comparison. S. G. O., 7: 408–413, Oct. 1908
OPERATION—ligation of vertebral arteries for cure or relief of epilepsy.
The treatment of epilepsy. Edinburgh, Pentland, 1889. 220 pp.
Alferow, Serge. Charkow, Russia, scientist
SILVER SALT—
Nouveaux procédés pour les imprégnations a l'argent. Arch. Phys., 1: 694–697, 1874
Alford, L. B. See E. L. Opie
Algeri, G. See V. Marchi
Alibert, Jean Louis. French physician. 1768–1837
DISEASE—mycosis fungoides (pian fungoide).
Pian fungoide, framboesia mycoides (mycosis fungoides). In his: *Description des maladies de la peau.* Paris, 1806. p. 157, pl. 36
ALIBERT'S MENTAGRA—sycosis barbae. Ibid.: Paris, Wahlen, 1825. 2 vols. vol. 2, p. 214
Described keloid (cancroide).

Note sur la keloide. J. univ. d. sci. méd., Paris, 2: 207–216, 1816

Keloide; kelis. In his: *Monogr. d. dermat.,* Paris, 2 ed., 2: 195–212, 1835

Introduced terms "syphilides", "dermatoses", "dermatolysis".

Monographie des dermatoses, ou précis théorique et pratique des maladies de la peau. Paris, Dagnac, 1832. 2 vols., 528 pp.; 705 pp.

Allan, D. M. See W. R. Bloor

Allarton, George. London surgeon

OPERATION—median lithotomy.

Lithotomy simplified, or a new method of operating for stone in the bladder, to which is appended an interesting and unique case of Cesarian section. London, Ash & Flint, 1854. 80 pp.

Allbutt, Sir Thomas Clifford. English physician. 1836–1925

THEORY—mechanical, of cardiac pain in coronary occlusion.

In: *Diseases of the arteries including angina pectoris.* New York, Macmillan Co., 1915. vol. 2, p. 368 et seq.

Described joint symptoms in locomotor ataxia.

Remarks on a case of locomotor ataxy with hydroarthrosis. St. George's Hosp. Rep., 4: 259–260, 1869

Investigated visceral neuroses.

On visceral neuroses, being the Gulstonnian lectures on neuralgia of the stomach and allied disorders, delivered at the Royal College of Physicians in March, 1884. London, Churchill, 1884. 103 pp.

Observed effect of strain in producing heart disease.

The effects of overwork and strain on the heart and great blood-vessels. St. George's Hosp. Rep., 5: 23–53, 1871

Over-stress of the heart.

In: *System of medicine.* (Allbutt and Rolleston) London, 1909 6: 418–492

Allen, Alfred Henry. American chemist. 1846–1904

TEST—for phenol.

The distinctive tests for carbolic acid, cresylic acid, and creasote. Pharm. J., 9: 234–236, Sept. 21, 1878

TEST—for glucose in urine.

Chemistry of urine; a practical guide to the analytical examination of diabetic, albuminous, and gouty urine. London, Churchill, 1895. 212 pp.

Allen, Arthur Wilburn. Boston surgeon. 1887–

OPERATION—

A method of re-establishing continuity between the bile ducts and the gastro-intestinal tract. Ann. Surg., 121: 412–424, Apr. 1945

See also J. C. White

Allen, C. W. See R. Matas

Allen, Charles. Irish dentist

Printed first English book on dentistry, anonymously.

The operation for the teeth. Dublin, 1686

Reprinted under Allen's name as *Curious observations* ... Dublin, 1687

Reprinted by British Dental Association in 1924.

Allen, Clyde I. Detroit surgeon. 1893–

Did important work on carcinoma of the lung.

Primary carcinoma of the lung with a report of a case treated by operation with F. J. Smith, S. G. O., 55: 151–161, Aug. 1932

Allen, Duff Shederic. St. Louis surgeon. 1895–

OPERATION—

Intracardiac surgery—a new method: preliminary report with E. A. Graham, J. A. M. A., 79: 1028–1030, Sept. 23, 1922

Allen, Edgar. St. Louis scientist. 1892–

Isolated active principle ovarian hormone (oestrin).

An ovarian hormone: preliminary report on its localization, extraction and partial purification, and action in test animals with E. A. Doisy, J. A. M. A., 81: 819–821, Sept. 8, 1923

TEST—for recognition of the estrus hormone.

The induction of a sexually mature condition in immature females by injection of the ovarian follicular hormone with E. A. Doisy, Amer. J. Physiol., 69: 577–588, 1924

Allen, Edgar Van Nuys. Rochester, Minn. physician. 1900–

Developed arteriography.

Arteriography: a roentgenographic study of the peripheral arteries of living subjects following their injections with a radiopaque substance with J. D. Camp, J. A. M. A., 104: 618–624, Feb. 23, 1935

Allen, F. H. Jr. See C. D. May

Allen, F. N. See R. M. Wilder

Allen, Frederick Madison. New York physician. 1879–

DIET or TREATMENT—for diabetes by certain days of fasting, followed by a restricted diet; called also starvation treatment.

Studies concerning diabetes. J. A. M. A., 63: 939–943, Sept. 12, 1914

The treatment of diabetes. Boston M. and S. J., 1: 241–247, Feb. 18, 1915

Total dietary regulation in the treatment of diabetes with E. Stillman and R. Fitz, Monog. Rockefeller Inst. M. Research, No. 11, N. Y., 1919

DIET—for hypertension; salt and water restriction.

Arterial hypertension. J. A. M. A., 74: 652–655, Mar. 6, 1920

PARADOXIC LAW—the more sugar that is given to a normal individual, the more that is utilized.

Studies concerning glycosuria and diabetes. Boston, Leonard, 1913. 1179 pp.

TREATMENT—cooling of traumatized and potentially infected limbs.

Local asphyxia and temperature changes in relation to gangrene and other surgical problems. Trans. Ass. Amer. Phys., 52: 189–194, 1937

Resistance of peripheral tissues to asphyxia at various temperatures. S. G. O., 67: 746–751, Dec. 1938

Allen, Harvey Stuart. Chicago surgeon. 1906–

Introduced aseptic pressure dressings in local burn therapy.

The treatment of patients with severe burns with S. L. Koch, S. G. O., 74: 914–924, May 1942

Allen, Joseph Garrott. Chicago surgeon. 1912–

MODIFICATION—of the Quick test for prothrombin.

Use of serial dilutions in determination of prothrombin by the one stage technic with O. C. Julian and L. R. Dragstedt, Arch. Surg., 41: 873–878, Oct. 1940

See also L. R. Dragstedt

Allen, J. H. See C. S. O'Brien

Allen, Jesse Hall. Philadelphia surgeon. 1868–

OPERATION—
A two stage operation for fistula-in-ano with B.
Haskell, S. G. O., 58: 651–654, Mar. 1934
Allen, Willard Myson. Rochester, Minn. physician.
1904–
Proved that progestin is necessary for the conserva-
tion of early pregnancy.
*Physiology of the corpus luteum: III. Normal growth
and implantation of embryos after very early ablation
of the ovaries, under the influence of extracts of the
corpus luteum* with G. W. Corner, Amer. J. Physiol.,
88: 340–346, Mar. 1929
Prepared the hormone progesterone in crystalline
form.
Crystalline progestin with O. Wintersteiner, Science,
80: 190–191, Aug. 24, 1934
See also O. Wintersteiner
Allerhand, J. Vienna
STAIN—iron, for myelin.
*Eine neue Methode zur Färbung des Centralnerven-
systems.* Neurol. Zbl., 16: 727–733, Aug. 15, 1897
Allers, R. See S. Frankel
Allingham, Herbert William. English surgeon.
1862–1904
OPERATION—inguinal colotomy by incision parallel
with and one-half inch above Poupart's ligament.
*Inguinal colotomy, its advantages over the lumbar
operation, with special reference to a method for pre-
venting feces passing below the artificial anus.* Brit.
med. J., 2: 874–878, Oct. 22, 1887
*Colotomy, inguinal, lumbar, and transverse, for cancer
or stricture with ulceration of the large intestine.*
London, Baillière, 1892. 199 pp.
Allingham, William. English surgeon. 1829–1908
OPERATION—excision of rectum by an incision into
the ischiorectal fossae, about the rectum and extending backward to the coccyx.
ULCER—fissure of anus.
*Fistula, hemorrhoids, painful ulcer, stricture, pro-
lapsus, and other diseases of the rectum, their diagnosis
and treatment.* London, Churchill, 1871. 239 pp.
Same, 7 ed., 1901
Allis, Oscar Huntington. Philadelphia surgeon.
1836–1931
CLAMP
*Acupressure forceps: an instrument for the instan-
taneous arrest of hemorrhage during surgical opera-
tions.* Med. News, 43: 233–235, Sept. 1, 1883
INHALER—an apparatus for administering ether by
the drop method.
*Some remarks upon the relative strength of chloroform
and ether, with hints upon their use as anesthetics.*
Philadelphia M. Times, 5: 145–149, Dec. 5, 1874
REDUCTION—of dislocations of the hip.
*The mechanism and reduction of dislocations of the
hip.* Med. Bull. Phila., 20: 41–46, Feb. 1898
SIGN—relaxation of the fascia between the crest of
the ilium and the greater trochanter, a sign of frac-
ture of the neck of the femur.
*The fascia lata; its use in standing at rest; its value in
the diagnosis of fracture of the neck of the femur.*
Philadelphia M. Times, 6: 579–581, Sept. 2, 1876
Allison, Nathaniel. St. Louis surgeon. 1876–1932
ATROPHY—of bone due to disuse.
Bone atrophy: a clinical study of the changes in bone

which result from nonuse with B. Brooks, Arch. Surg.,
5: 499–526, Nov. 1922
OPERATION—alcohol injection of nerves leading to
selected muscle groups in treatment of spastic
paralysis.
*Muscle group isolation and nerve anastomosis in the
treatment of the paralyses of the extremities* with S. I.
Schwab, Amer. J. Orthop., 8: 95–124, Aug. 1910
Almour, R. See S. J. Kopetzky
Almquist, Herman James. California poultry
husbandman. 1903–
METHOD—of extracting vitamin K from alfalfa leaf.
Purification of the antihemorrhagic vitamin. J. Biol.
Chem., 114: 241–245, May 1936
Further studies on the antihemorrhagic vitamin. Ibid.,
120: 635–640, Sept. 1937
Almy, Thomas Pattison. New York physician. 1915–
METHOD—
Treatment of diabetic acidosis and diabetic coma
with Katharine Swift and E. Tolstoi, J. A. M. A.,
129: 863–868, Nov. 24, 1945
Aloy, Jules-Francois. Toulouse physician
REACTION—for morphine.
*Précipitation de quelques alcaloides par le nitrate
d'uranium. Réaction de la morphine.* Bull. Soc. Chim.
Biol. Paris, 29: 610–611, 1903
REAGENT—for alkaloids.
Ibid.
REACTION—for strychnine and formaldehyde.
*Transformations provoquées par la lumière solaire en
présence de composés uraniques.* Ibid., 37: 1135,
1925
*Transformations provoquées par la lumiàre en présence
de composés uraniques. Réactions caractéristiques de la
strychnine, de la morphine, de la codéine et du formol*
with A. Valdiguie and R. Aloy, Ibid., 39: 792–795,
1926
REAGENT—for testing for phenols.
Sur un réactif des corps à fonction phénol with F.
Laprade, Ibid., 33: 860–861, 1905
Alpert, F. See M. Nonne
Alt, A. See J. Tillmans
Altemeier, William Arthur. Cincinnati surgeon.
1910–
PROCEDURE—
*The rapid identification of the Clostridium welchii in
accidental wounds.* S. G. O., 78: 411–414, Apr. 1944
Althaus, Julius. London dermatologist. 1831–1900
CREAM—for syphilis; metallic mercury, 1 part;
lanolin, 4 parts; carbolic oil, 2 %, 5 parts.
Syphilis of the nervous system. London, Longmans,
Green, 1890. 35 pp. (p. 23–26)
Altimas, G. T. See J. R. Goodall
Altmann, Richard. German histologist. 1852–1900
SOLUTION—aniline acid fuchsin.
In his: *Die Elementarorganismen und ihre Bezie-
hungen zu den Zellen.* Leipzig, Veit, 1890. 145 pp.
p. 28
Altschule, M. D. See D. R. Gilligan
Alvarez, E. Pinerua. See Pinerua
Alvarez, J. G. See P. de la Camara
Alvarez, Walter Clement. Rochester, Minn. physi-
cian. 1884–
Called attention to a type of patient in whom psychic

factors cause profound changes in the secretion and
motility of the digestive tract.
Peristalsis in health and disease. Amer. J. Roent., 8:
1–12, Jan. 1921
Ways in which emotion can affect the digestive tract
J. A. M. A., 92: 1231–1237, Apr. 13, 1929
DIET—smooth for duodenal ulcer.
In his: *The mechanics of the digestive tract.* New York,
Hoeber, 1922, p. 111; 2 ed., 1928, pp. 327–329
See also C. Gianturco
Alzheimer, Alois. German neurologist. 1864–1915
DISEASE or SCLEROSIS—a presenile condition
marked by symptoms of progressive mental weak-
ness and characterized pathologically by hyaline
degeneration of smaller cerebral blood vessels.
Ueber eine eigenartige Erkrankung der Hirnrinde.
Zbl. Nervenheilk., 30: 177–179, Mar. 1, 1907
Also: Allg. Z. f. Psychiat., 64: 146–148, 1907
METHOD—light-green-acid, for neuroglia changes.
MODIFICATION—of Mallory's phosphomolybdic
acid hematoxylin stain for neurolgia changes.
MODIFICATION—of Mann's eosin-methyl blue stain
for neuroglia changes.
STAINS—for granules in neuroglia cells.
*Beiträge ur Kenntnis der pathologischen Neuroglia
und ihrer Beziehungen zu den Abbausorgängen im
Nervengewebe.*
In: *Histologische und histopathologische Arbeiten
über die Grosshirnrinde.* Herausgegeben von F.
Nissl und H. Alzheimer Jena, Fischer, 1909–10. Vol.
3, pp. 401–562
Amann, Jules. Lausanne pharmacist
TEST—for phenol in urine.
*Un nouveau procédé de dosage clinique des phénols de
l'urine.* Rev. med. Suisse Romande, 16: 657–661,
Nov. 20, 1896
TEST—for indican in urine.
*Une nouvelle méthode de recherche de l'indogène (indi-
can) dans l'urine.* Ibid., 17: 448–450, 1897
Ambard, Leo. Paris physician. 1876–
COEFFICIENT or CONSTANT or FORMULA—
for findings the urea index in kidney disease.
Lois numériques de la sécrétion de l'urée. J. Physiol.
Path. gén., 12: 209–219, Mar. 1910
*Rapports entre le taux de l'urée dans le sang et l'élimi-
nation de l'urée dans l'urine.* C. R. Soc. Biol., Paris,
2: 411–413, Nov. 19, 1910
*Rapports de la quantité et du taux de l'urée dans l'urine,
la concentration de l'urée du sang étant constante.*
Ibid., 2: 506–508, Dec. 3, 1910
LAW—of urea excretion.
*Les lois numériques de la secrétion rénale de l'urée et
du chlorure de sodium* with A. Weill, J. Physiol.
Path. gén., 14: 753–765, July 1912
LAWS—governing the rate of excretion of sodium
chloride.
Ibid.
Ambrunjanz, G. Russian surgeon
OPERATION—for cardiospasm.
In: Nov. chir. Arch., 19: 501–503, 1929 (Russisch)
Also, Abstr.: *Ueber eine Modifikation der Hellerschen
Operation beim Kardiospasmus.* Zentralorgan f. d.
Ges. Chirurg. und ihre Grenzgebiete, 50: 747, 1930
Amerlinck, A. See N. Goormaghtigh
Amesbury, Joseph. London surgeon. 1795–

SPLINT—
*Observations on the nature and treatment of fractures of
the upper third of the thigh-bone and of fractures of
long standing; shewing that fractures of the neck of the
femur and others which occur in the upper third of this
bone, admit of being united, so as to restore the natural
powers of the limb.* London, Underwood, 1828. 315 pp.
Amici, Giovanni Battista. Italian physician. 1786–
1863
DISK or LINE or STRIA—a membrane supposed to
separate the disks of sarcous matter in striated
muscles; same as membrane of Krause or Dobie's
lines.
Constructed the first microscope with achromatic
lenses.
Put forth the idea of water-immersion for improved
achromatic lenses of the compound microscope.
De microscopj catadiottrici memoria. Modena, 1818
Same, in French: Ann. de chim. et phys., Paris,
13: 384–410, 1820
Amman, Jan Coenraad. Dutch. 1669–1730
METHOD—of instructing deaf-mutes.
*Dissertatio de loquela, qua non solum vox humana, et
loquendi artificium ex originibus suis erruunter....*
Amstelaedami, Wolters, 1700
Ammann, Paul. German physician. 1634–1690
Wrote important book on lethal wounds.
*Praxis vulnerum lethalium. Sex decadibus historiarum
rariorum.* Francofurti, 1690. 483 pp.
Ammon, Frederich August von. German physician.
1799–1861
FILAMENTS OF—fine hairs, or cilia, on the inner
surface of the ciliary body of the eye.
OPERATION—blepharoplasty by a flap from the
cheek.
OPERATION—dacryocystotomy.
FISSURE—a pear-shaped aperture in the sclera at an
early fetal period.
*Klinische Darstellungen der Krankheiten und Bild-
ungsfehler des menschlichen Auges, der Augenlider
und der Thränenwerkzeuge nach eigenen Beobachtungen und Untersuchungen.* Berlin, Reimer, 1838–
1847. 4 pts. in 1 vol. 190 pp.
Amoss, Harold Lindsay. Durham, N. C. pathologist.
1886–
METHOD—of immunization of horses against the
meningococcus.
*A method for the rapid preparation of antimeningitis
serum* with Martha Wollstein, J. exp. Med., 23:
403–417, Mar. 1916
See also J. H. Kastle
Amussat, Jean Zuléma. French surgeon. 1796–1856
OPERATION—lumbar colotomy by an incision across
the outer border of the quadratus lumborum.
*Mémoire sur la possibilité d'établir un anus artificiel
dans la région lombaire sans pénétrer dans le péritonie.*
Paris, Baillière, 1839
OPERATION—proctoplasty by dissection and mobilization of the rectal pouch to the proper site.
*Histoire d'une opération d'anus artificiel pratiqué
avec succès par un nouveau procédé, dans un cas
d'absence congénitale de l'anus; suivie de quelques
réflexions sur les obturations du rectum.* Gaz. méd.
de Paris, 3: 753–758, Nov. 28, 1835
Anderodias. See G. Dubreuil

Andersch, Carl Samuel. German anatomist. 1732–1777
GANGLION—the petrous ganglion; the petrous portion of the glosso-pharyngeal g.
Tractatio anatomico-physiologica de nervis humani corporis aliquibus, quam editit Ernst. Ph. Andersch. Regiomonti, Fasch, 1797. 2 parts, 178 pp.; 187 pp.
Andersen, E. See J. S. Thannhauser
Anderson, F. O. See J. R. Goodall
Anderson, H. H. See A. C. Reed
Anderson, James. London pathologist. 1891–
METHOD—
A rapid method of ripening haematoxylin with hypochlorite. J. Path. Bact., 26: 303 (only), Apr. 1923
STAIN—alum-carmine for nervous system.
Alum carmine for counter-staining Weigert—Pal preparations. Ibid., 29: 117 (only), Jan. 1926
STAIN—for neuroglia.
Modification of Victoria blue method of Anglade and Morel for neuroglia fibers in frozen sections. Ibid., 26: 431–432, July 1923
Anderson, James Stirling. English physician
Distinguished types of Corynebacterium diphtheriae.
On the existance of two forms of diphtheria bacillus—B. diphtheriae gravis and B. diphtheriae mitis—and a new medium for their differentiation and for the bacteriological diagnosis of diphtheria with F. C. Happold, J. W. McLeod and J. G. Thomson, J. Path. Bact., 34: 667–681, Sept. 1931
Anderson, John. London scientist. 1880–
STAIN—for myelin.
How to stain the nervous system. Edinburgh, Livingstone, 1929. pp. 139, pp. 54–56; 72–74
Anderson, John F. American physician. 1873–
DERMACENTER ANDERSONI (VENUSTUS), wood tick responsible for Rocky Mountain spotted fever.
Spotted fever (tick fever) of the Rocky Mountains; a new disease. U. S. Pub. Health & Marine Hospt Service Hyg. Lab. Bull., No. 14, 1903. 50 pp.
METHOD—
A method of producing tetanus toxin with J. P. Leake, J. med. Res., 33: 239–241, Nov. 1915
TEST—of Anderson and Goldberger, for typhus fever; the patient's blood is injected into the peritoneal cavity of guinea pigs, when, if the disease is typhus, a typical temperature curve will be obtained.
Typhus fever. Its etiology and the methods of its prevention. Pub. Health Rep., Wash., 30: 1303–1311, Apr. 30, 1915
Inoculated monkeys with measles.
Experimental measles in the monkey; a preliminary note with J. Goldberger, Ibid., 36: 847–848, June 9, 1911
(Same) *A supplemental note.*
Ibid., 36: 887–893, June 16, 1911
Anderson, L. A. P. See C. S. Swaminath
Anderson, Patrick. Scottish physician.
PILL—compound gamboge pill.
De colica spasmodica flatulenta. Edinburgh, 1765
Anderson, Roger. Seattle, Wash. surgeon. 1891–
METHOD—
An automatic method of treatment for fractures of the tibia and the fibula. S. G. O., 58: 639–646, Mar. 1934
SPLINT—the well-leg, counter extension s.

New method for treating fractures, utilizing the well leg for countertraction. Ibid., 54: 207–219, Feb. 1932
The well-leg countertraction method; details of technique. Amer. J. Surg., 18: 36–50, Oct. 1932
Andrade, Eduardo Penny. Florida bacteriologist. 1872–1906
INDICATOR—decolorized acid fuchsin.
Influence of glycerin in differentiating certain bacteria. J. med. Res., 14: 551–553, Apr. 1906
Andral, Gabriel. Paris physician. 1797–1876
DECUBITUS or SIGN—in the early stage of pleurisy, the patient tends to lie on the sound side.
Clinique médicale, ou choix d'observations recueillies à la clinique de M. Lerminier. Paris, Gabon, 1823–1827. 5 vols.
(Same) *Diseases of the chest.* . . . Trans. by D. Spillan, Phila., Haswell, Barrington & Haswell, 1838. 299 pp. p. 360; 397
Same. 1843, 408 pp.
First to urge a chemical examination of the blood in morbid conditions. (Garrison)
Essai d'hématologie pathologique. Paris, Fortin, Masson & Cie, 1843. 186 pp.
(Same) *An essay on the blood in disease.* Trans. by J. F. Meigs and A. Stillé, Phila., Lea & Blanchard, 1844
Andre, Charles. French physician
Noted relation between high atmospheric temperatures and heat conditions.
Influence de l'altitude sur la température. Lyon, 1888. 123 pp.
André, or Andry, Nicholas. Paris physician. 1658–1742 Coined term orthopedics.
L'orthopédie ou l'art de prevenir et de corriger dans les enfants, les difformités du corps. Paris, La Veuve Alix, 1741. 2 vols.
Same, in English. London, Millar, 1743. 2 vols.
Andresen, Albert Frederick Ruger. Brooklyn physician. 1885–
DIET—modification of the Lenhartz diet for gastric ulcer.
The treatment of gastric hemorrhage. J. A. M. A., 89: 1397–1402, Oct. 22, 1927
Andrew, R. H. See F. Fenger
Andrewes, Christopher Howard. London physician. 1896–
TEST—for uremia.
An unexplained diazo-colour-reaction in uremic sera. Lancet, 1: 590–591, Mar. 22, 1924
See also W. Smith
Andrewes, Sir Frederick William. London pathologist. 1859–1932
Described Bacillus alkalescens, a cause of dysentery in man.
Dysentery bacilli: the differentiation of the true dysentery bacilli from allied species. Lancet, 194: 560–563, Apr. 20, 1918
Andrews, Edmund. Chicago physician. 1824–1904
OXYGEN MIXTURES—
The oxygen mixture, a new anesthetic combination. Chicago M. Exam., 9: 656–661, Nov. 1868
Liquid nitrous oxide as an anesthetic. Ibid., 13: 34–36, 1872
OPERATION—
A new method of valvular gastrostomy with a mucous

membrane lining with E. W. Andrews, J. A. M. A., 22: 734–737, May 19, 1894

Andrews, Edmund. Chicago surgeon. 1892–
OPERATION—for hernia.
A method of herniotomy utilizing only white fascia. Ann. Surg., 80: 225–238, Aug. 1924
The closure of large femoral and inguino-femoral defects the result of destruction or relaxation of Poupart's ligament. S. G. O., 39: 754–759, Dec. 1924
Further experiences with purely fascial herniotomy. Ann. Surg., 88: 874–878, Nov. 1928

Andrews, Edward Wyllys. Chicago surgeon. 1856–1927
OPERATION—for hydrocele, by complete eversion of the tunica vaginalis, (wrong-side-out).
The "bottle operation" method for the radical cure of hydrocele. Ann. Surg., 46: 915–918, Dec. 1907
OPERATION—for inguinal hernia.
Imbrication or lap joint method: a plastic operation for hernia. Chicago M. Record, 9: 67–77, Aug. 1895
OPERATION—colohepatopexy or colon substitution: to prevent reformation of adhesions between liver and stomach, the colon and omentum are sutured between these two structures.
Colohepatopexy or colon substitution: a new operation for perigastric adhesions after gallstone operations. J. A. M. A., 45: 819–821, Sept. 16, 1905
OPERATION—use of glass tube to drain ventricle in hydrocephalus.
An improved technique in brain surgery. Glass tubes versus gold or platinum for subdural drainage of the lateral ventricles in internal hydrocephalus. Trans. Amer. Surg. Ass., 29: 111–126, 1911

Andrews, Justin Meredith. Baltimore zoologist. 1902–
MEDIUM—serum-saline-citrate, for cultivation of intestinal protozoa.
Cultivation of trichomonas, thermal death-point, anaerobic conditions, attempts at sterilization. J. Parasit., 12: 148–157, Mar. 1926

Andriezen, W. Lloyd. English pathologist
MODIFICATION—of Golgi's bichromate and silver nitrate method, for nerve tissue.
A modified Golgi's method for the study of the human brain. Brit. med. J., 1: 909 (only), Apr. 28, 1894

Andry, See Nicholas André

Andry-Thomas, M. French neurologist
EVIDENCE—of recovery of nerve conduction after injury.
La sensibilité douloureuse de la peau à la piqûre et au pincement dans la période de restauration des nerfs sectionnés aprés suture ou greffe. Rev. neurol., 1: 311–313, 1916

Anduyned. See I. Barraquer

Anel, Dominique. Toulouse surgeon. 1679–1730
OPERATION—dilatation of the lacrimal duct by a probe, followed by an astrigent injection.
PROBE—used in dilating the lacrimal duct.
SYRINGE—a delicate syringe for treatment of lacrimal passages.
Nouvelle méthode de guérir les fistules lacrimales, ou recueil de différentes pièces pour et contre, et en faveur de la même méthode nouvellement inventée. Turin, Zappatte, 1713. 158 pp.

Anglade, Dominique. French neurologist. 1867–

METHOD—Victoria blue for neuroglia.
Sur un nouveau procédé de coloration de la névroglie with Ch. Morel, Rev. neurol., 9: 157–158, Feb. 15, 1901

Angle, Edward Hartley. St. Louis dentist. 1855–1930
CLASSIFICATION—of various types of malocclusion.
Notes on orthodontia. Trans. 9th Internat. Congr. Med., Washington, 5: 565–585, 1887
Treatment of malocclusion of the teeth. Angle's system. Philadelphia, White Dental Mfg. Co., 1887; 7 ed., 1907
The Angle system of regulation and retention of the teeth.... Philadelphia, White, 4 ed., 1895. 112 pp.

Anglesey, Marquis of. French gentleman. 1768–1854
LEG—a form of jointed artificial leg; made originally for the Marquis.

Angström, Anders Jonas. Swedish physicist. 1814–1879
LAW—the wave lengths of light absorbed by a substance are the same as those given off by it when luminous.
UNIT—employed for measuring wave-lengths of light.
Optiske Undersökningar.
Presented to the Stockholm Academy in 1853

Anichkov, Nikolay Nikolaevich. Russian physician. 1885–
Produced arteriosclerosis by feeding cholesterol-rich diet.
Ueber experimentelle Cholesterinsteatose und ihre Bedeutung für die Entstehung einiger pathologische Prozesse with S. S. Chalatow, Zbl. f. allg. Path. u. path. Anat., 24: 1–9, 1913

Annandale, Thomas. Scottish surgeon. 1838–1907
OPERATION—fixation of displaced cartilages of the knee-joint by sutures.
An operation for displaced semilunar cartilage. Brit. M. J., 1: 779 (only), Apr. 18, 1885
An address on internal derangements of the knee-joint and their treatment by operation. Ibid., 1: 319–321, Feb. 12, 1887
Reported recovery after operation on an acoustic neuroma.
On intracranial surgery. Edinburgh M. J., 39: 898–910, Apr. 1894

Anrep, B. von. Würzburg pharmacologist
Introduced cocaine as an anesthetic.
Ueber die physiologische Wirkung des Cocain. Arch. Physiol., 21: 38–77, 1880
See also T. Weyl

Ansbacher, Stefan. German-American chemist. 1905–
Reparted synthesis of a vitamin K compound, 2-methyl-1, 4-naphtoquinone.
Simple compounds with vitamin K activity with E. Fernholz, J. Amer. Chem. Soc., 61: 1924–1925, July 1939

Anson, Mortimer L. Princeton, N. J. physiologist. 1901–
METHOD—for determination of digestive activity.
The estimation of pepsin with hemoglobin with A. E. Mirsky, J. gen. Physiol., 16: 59–63, Sept. 20, 1932

Anstie, Francis Edward. English physician. 1833–1874
RULE or LIMIT—used in connection with life insurance examination: the maximum amount of alcohol which can be taken by an adult without injury

is 1½ oz. daily, equivalent to about 3 oz. of whiskey or gin or 5 glasses of beer.

Stimulants and narcotics, their mutual relations; with special researches on the action of alcohol, ether, and chloroform on the vital organism. Phila., Lindsay and Blakiston, 1865. 414 pp.

Anton, Bernhard. German physician

Demonstrated B. typhosus in gall-bladder in cases of typhoid.

Untersuchungen über Typhus abdominalis with G. Futterer, Munch. med. Wschr., 35: 315–318, 1888

Anton, Pros German neurologist

OPERATION—for hydrocephalus, by puncture of the corpus callosum.

Balkenstich bei Hydrozephalien, Tumoren und bei Epilepsie with von Bramann, Munch. med. Wschr., 55: 1673–1677, Aug. 11, 1908

Antyllus. Greek physician. about 350 A.D.

OPERATION—ligation of an artery on both sides of an aneurysm, followed by evacuation of the contents through an incision.

See Antylli, veteris chirurgi. By P. Nicolaides. Halis Magdeb., (1709)

Aoki, Y. See R. Kanenko

Apathy, Stefan. Hungarian scientist

STAIN—of nervous tissue, with methylene blue.

Erfahrungen in der Behandlung des Nervensystems für histologische Zwecke. Z. wiss. Mik., 9: 15–37, 1892

STAIN—gold chloride.

Ueber die Muskelfasern von Ascaris, nebst Bemerkungen über die von Lumbricus und Hirudo. Ibid., 10: 319–361 (349), 1893

Apelt, Friedrich. German physician. 1877–1911

REACTION—see Nonne—Apelt r.

Apert, Eugène. Paris pediatrician. 1868–1940

SYNDROME—a congenital malformation consisting of a pointed shape of the top of the head and syndactylia of the four extremities: called also acrosphenosyndactylia.

Nouvelle observation d'acrocéphalosyndactylie with Tixier, Huc and Kermorgant, Bull. Soc. méd. Hôp. Paris, 3 s., 47: 1672–1675, Dec. 7, 1923

Apostoli, Georges. French physician. 1847–1900

TREATMENT—of uterine disease with electricity: the positive pole is inserted into the uterus and the negative pole is applied externally.

Sur une nouvelle application de l'électricité aux accouchements. Ann. de gynec., 15: 327–337, May 1881

Sur un nouveau traitement de la métrite chronique et en particulier de l'endométrite par la galvano-caustique chimique intrautérine. Paris, Doin, 1887. 68 pp.

Same, in English. Detroit, Davis, 1888. 119 pp.

Aran, Francois-Amilcar. French physician. 1817–1861

DISEASE—of Aran and Duchenne; myelopathic or progressive muscular atrophy.

Recherches sur une maladie non encore décrite du systeme musculaire (atrophie musculaire progressive). Arch. gén. de méd., Paris, 4 s., 24: 4–35, Sept.; 172–214, Oct. 1850

Arana, Guillermo Bosch. Buenos Aires surgeon. 1885–1939

OPERATION—

Phalangization of the first metacarpal. S. G. O., 40: 859–862, June 1925

Arangues, Mario Esteban. Spanish ophthalmologist

OPERATION—for ptosis.

Tratamiento del blefaroptosis: juicio critico de los procedimientos empleados y descripción de una operación original. Pediat. espan., 9: 246–254, Aug. 20, 1920

Aranzi (Arantius), Julius Caesar. Italian physician. 1530–1589

BODY—the tubercle of fibrocartilage at the tip of the aortic and pulmonary semilunar valves.

De humano foetu liber tertio editus, ac recognitus. . . . Venetiis, Brechtonum, 1587. 301 pp.

CANAL or DUCT—the ductus venosus. Ibid.

NODULE—same as body.

LIGAMENT (1)—one of the arched ligaments which connect the diaphragm with the lowest ribs and the first lumbar vertebra; same as arcuate ligament. Ibid.

LIGAMENT (2)—the inferior pubic ligament. Ibid.

VENTRICLE—the lower end of the fourth ventricle. Ibid.

Archibald, R. M. See R. A. Phillips

Arganaraz, Raul. Paraguay otolaryngologist. 1884–

OPERATION—dacryostomy.

Trepanación y cateterismo lácrimonasal. Sem. mèd., B. Air., 38: pt. 2, 249–256, 1931

The treatment of chronic dacryocystitis and lacrimonasal fistulization: author's procedure. Transl. by W. H. Crisp, Amer. J. Ophth., 15: 1117–1120, Dec. 1932

Argyll Robertson, Douglas. See D. A. Robertson

Arloing, Saturnin. French physician. 1846–1911

Introduced sero-agglutination of tubercle bacilli in diagnosis.

Sur l'obtention de cultures et d'émulsions homogènes du bacille de la tuberculose humaine en milieu liquide et "sur une variété mobile de ce bacille". C. R. Acad. Sci., Paris, 126: 1319–1321, May 9, 1898

Agglutination du bacille de la tuberculose vraie. Ibid., 1398–1400, May 16, 1898

Arlt, Benno R. German surgeon

OPERATION—to form a new thumb.

Daumenplastic. Wien. klin. Wschr., 30: 15–16, Jan. 4, 1917

Arlt, Carol Ferdinand. Vienna ophthalmologist. 1812–1887

OPERATION—transplantation of the ciliary bulbs for cure of distichiasis.

RECESS or SINUS—in lower part of lacrymal sac.

TRACHOMA—granular conjunctivitis.

Die Pflege der Augen in gesunden und kranken Zustande, . . . Prag. Gerzabek, 1846. 152 pp.

Die Krankheiten des Auges für praktische Aerzte geschildert. Prag, Credner & Kleinbub, 1854–6. 3 vols.

Armand-Delille, Paul Felix. French scientist. 1874–

MEDIUM—164, for cultivation of Koch's bacilli.

Culture du bacille de Koch en milieu chimiquement défini (2) with A. Mayer, G. Schaeffer and E. Terroine, C. R. Soc. Biol., Paris, 74: 272–274, Feb. 8, 1913

SOLUTION—104. Ibid.

SOLUTION—118. Ibid.

Armani. Italian chemist

TEST—for caffeine.

Réactions colorées de la caféine with Barboni, Repert

de pharm., 22: 514 (only), Nov. 1910. Also: Soc. chim. Italiana, 1910

Armentano, L. See A. Szent-Györgyi

Armstrong, A. R. See E. J. King

Armstrong, Charles. Washington, D. C., U. S. Public Health Service, surgeon. 1886–
Isolated and described the virus of benign lymphocytic choriomeningitis.
Experimental lymphocytic choriomeningitis of monkeys and mice produced by a virus encountered in studies of the 1933 St. Louis encephalitis epidemic with R. D. Lillie, Pub. Health Rep., 49: 1019–1027, Aug. 31, 1934.
See also R. S. Mackenfuss

Armstrong, George. London physician. 1735–1781
Described congenital hypertrophic stenosis of the pylorus.
An account of the diseases most incident to children: to which is added an essay on nursing. London, Caddell, 1771, 2 ed., 188 pp.
Also: new ed., London, 1783. Ch. 4, p. 42

Arneth, Joseph. German physician. 1873–
COUNT or FORMULA—leukocytic; classification of polymorphonuclear leukocytes into five groups, depending on number of lobes.
Die neutrophilen weissen Blutkörperchen bei Infektions-Krankheiten. Jena, Fischer, 1904. 200 pp. p. 37, plate 8
"Toxische" Leukozytenveränderungen, Hämogramm und qualitative Blutlehre. Dtsch. med. Wschr., 55: 1667 (only), Oct. 4, 1929
THEORY—of differentiation of neutrophilic myelocyte into neutrophil. See COUNT, 1904

Arnett, John Hancock. Philadelphia physician. 1889–
Reported use of ephedrine in amytal poisoning.
Ephedrine and picrotoxin used successfully in amytal poisoning. J. A. M. A., 100: 1593 (only), May 20, 1933

Arnold, Carl. Hannover chemist
TEST—for hydrogen peroxide.
Die qualitativen Reaktionen des Wasserstoffsuperoxyds und deren Anwendbarkeit bei Gegenwart von Milch with C. Mentzel, Z. Untersuch. Nahr.-u. Genussw., 6: 305–309, Apr. 1, 1903

Arnold, Friedrich. German anatomist. 1803–1890
CANAL—a passage in the petrous portion of the temporal bone for the auricular branch of the pneumogastric nerve.
Ueber den Ohrknoten. Eine anatomischphysiologische Abhandlung. Heidelberg, Winter, 1828. 54 pp.
Also, transl.: Rep. gén. d'anat. et physiol. path., Paris, 8: 1–31, 1829
GANGLION—same as otic or auricular ganglion. Ibid.
LIGAMENT—the suspensory l. connecting the incus with the roof of the middle ear. Ibid.
FOLD—a slip of mucous membrane sometimes found at the junction of the nasal duct with the lacrimal sac; same as Beraud's valve.
Anatomische und physiologische Untersuchungen über das Auge des Menschen. Heidelberg, 1832
MEMBRANE—pigmented layer of iris. Ibid.
BUNDLE or FASCICULUS—the frontal tract of the crusta cerebri.
Bemerkungen über den Bau des Hirns und Rücken-

marks, nebst Beiträgen zur Physiologie des zehnten und eilften Hirnnerven.... Zürich, Höhr, 1838. 218 pp.
CONVOLUTION—the inferior posterior convolution of the cerebrum. Ibid.
NERVE OF—auricular branch of the vagus. Ibid.
OPERCULUM—that of the island of Reil. Ibid.

Arnold, George. Liverpool scientist
METHOD—orange, of plasma staining.
The prophase in the ovigenesis and the spermatogenesis of Planaria lactea O. F. M. (Dendrocoelum lacteum Oerst.) Arch. Zellforsch., 3: 431–448 (434), Oct. 5, 1909
TECHNIC—chrome osmium.
The rôle of the chondriosomes in the cells of the guinea-pig's pancreas. Ibid., 8: 256–271, May 29, 1912

Arnold, Julius. Heidelberg physician. 1835–1915
STAINING—intra-vitum.
Ueber vitale und supravitale Granulafärbung der Nirenepithelien. Anat. Anz., 21: 417–425, July 12, 1902
MALFORMATION—spina bifida and cranium bifidum.
Myelocyste, Transposition von Gewebskeimen und Sympodie. Beitr. path. Anat., 16: 1–28, 1894
BODIES—small pieces of erythrocytes in the blood.
Ueber die Herkunft der Blutplättchen. Zbl. f. allg. Path. u. path. Anat., 8: 289–294, May 1, 1897

Arnold, R. C. See J. F. Mahoney

Arnold, Vinzenz. Lemberg physician
REACTION—for proteins, based on the Morner reaction for cystein.
Eine Farbenreaktion von Eiweisskörpern mit Nitroprussidnatrium. Z. phys. Chem., 70: 300–309, 1911
Ueber dem Cysteingehalt tierischen Organe. Ibid., 314–325
TEST—for acetoacetic acid in urine.
Eine neue Reaction zum Nachweis der Acetessigsäure im Harn. Wien. klin. Wschr., 12: 541–544, 1899
TEST—for nephrorosein in urine.
Ueber das Vorkommen eines dem Urorosein nahestehenden Farbstoffes in gewissen pathologischen Harnen. Z. phys. Chem., 61: 240–243, 1909

Arnott, James. English physician
DILATOR—a distensible cylinder of oiled silk for urethral strictures.
A treatise on stricture of the urethra, containing an account of improved methods of treatment, with an appendix noticing the application of a new instrument to the treatment of enlarged prostate gland, gleet, fistula, and other diseases of the urethra, esophagus, and rectum. London, Burgess and Hill, 1819. 183 pp.
ANESTHESIA—local a. produced by a freezing mixture of ice and salt.
On the remedial agency of a local anesthetic or benumbing temperature, in various painful and inflammatory diseases. London, Churchill, 1851. 54 pp.

Arnstein, C. German scientist
SOLUTION—of methylene blue.
Die Methylenblaufärbung als histologische Methode. Anat. Anz. 2: 125–135, Mar. 1, 1887

Arny, Henry Vinecome. New York pharmacist. 1868–
SOLUTIONS—standard colorimetric s.
Standard colored fluids and some official colorimetric

tests with A. Taub, J. Amer. Pharm. Ass., 12: 839–849, 1923
TEST—
 Lactic acid tests with M. C. Dimler, Ibid., 18: 459–462, 1929

Aron, E. See A. G. Weiss

Aron, Max. Strasbourg physician
TEST—urinary-suprarenal test for cancer.
 Présence, dans l'urine des sujets atteints de tumeur maligne, d'un principe doué d'une action sur la corticosurrénale. C. R. Acad. Sci., Paris, 197: 1702–1704, 1933
 Essai d'une méthode histologique de diagnostic du cancer. C. R. Soc. Biol., Paris, 115: 403–406, 1934
 Presénce d'un principe spécifique dans l'urine des individus atteints de cancer. Application à un procédé de diagnostic du cancer et essai d'interprétation de la nature de ce principe. Pr. méd., 42: 833–836, May 23, 1934

Aronson, Hans. German bacteriologist. 1865–1919
AGAR—fuchsin sulphite, for diagnosis of cholera.
 Eine neue Methode der bakteriologischen Choleradiagnose. Dtsch. med. Wschr., 41: 1027–1029, Aug. 26, 1915
SERUM—an antistreptococcus serum.
 Die Grundlagen und Aussichten der Blutserumtherapie. Berlin. Klinik, 5: Hft. 63, 1–42, 1893
STAIN—gallein, for myelin.
 Ueber die Anwendung des Gallein zur Färbung des Centralnervensystems. Z. med. Wiss., 28: 577–579, Aug. 2, 1890

Arreguine, Victor. Argentina physician. 1894–
TEST—for acetoacetic acid in urine.
 La formación de la B-metil umbeliferona como reacción del ácido aceto-acético y sus ésteres with E. D. Garcia, Ann. Soc. quim. argentina, 7: 424–432, Nov. 1919

Arrhenius, Svante August. German chemist, 1859–1927
THEORY—of electrolytic dissociation.
 Ueber die Dissociation der in Wasser gelösten Stoffe. Z. phys. Chem., 1: 631–648, 1887

Arrigoni, P. See G. Moretti

Arrilaga, Francisco C. Argentine physician
Described "Ayerza's disease, to which he gave the name.
 Cardiacos negros. Buenos Ayres, Thesis No. 2536, 1912

Arris, Edward. English surgeon. ?–1675
The Arris and Gale lectureship at the Royal College of Surgeons of England was established by a bequest of £510 in 1646.

Arruga, Dr. Barcelona ophthalmologist
OPERATION—dacryostomy.
 Ueber eine Verbesserung der Totischen Operation. Klin. Mbl. Augenheilk., 81: 280–285, Aug.–Sept. 1928

d'Arsonval, Jacques-Arsène. French physicist. 1851–1940
CURRENT—used therapeutically to stimulate metabolism.
 Récherches d'électrothérapie: la voltaisation sinusoidale. Arch. Physiol. norm. path., 5 s., 4: 69–80, 1892
DIFFERENTIAL AIR CALORIMETER—
 Calorimètre différential enregistreur. C. R. Soc. Biol., Paris, 8 s., 3: 104–105, Mar. 6, 1886

FATHER OF ELECTROTHERAPY.

Arthaud, G. French biologist
REAGENT—for uric acid.
 Sur un procédé de dosage de l'acide urique with Butte, C. R. Soc. Biol., Paris, 1: 625–627, 1889

Arthur, Grace. Minnesota psychologist. 1883–
TESTS—for intelligence.
 An attempt to sort children with specific reading disability from other non-readers. Jour. Applied Psychol., 11: 4–263, Aug. 1927
 A point scale for performance tests. N. Y., Commonwealth Fund. Vols. 1 & 2 Vol. 2, rev. ed., 1943

Arthus, Nicholas Maurice. French bacteriologist 1862–1945
PHENOMENON—susceptibility to repeated injections of serum, with localized destruction of tissue at site of injection.
 Injections répétées de sérum du cheval chez le lapin. C. R. Soc. Biol., Paris, 55: 817–820, June 16, 1903
 De l'anaphylaxie à l'immunité, protéotoxies: envenimations: anaphylaxie: immunité: sérums antivenimeux. Paris, Masson 1921
 Also, transl. by H. E. Sigerist Bull. Hist. Med., 14: 366–390, Oct. 1943
 Also: Baltimore, Johns Hopk. Press, 1943. 26 pp.
METHOD or TEST—for demonstration of action of trypsin.
 Recherches sur la trypsine with A. Huber, Arch. de Physiol., 6: 622–630, 1894
 Established importance of calcium content of blood in clotting.
 Nouvelle théorie chimique de la coagulation du sang with C. Pagès, J. de Physiol., 2: 739–746, 1890

Arzt, Leopold. German physician. 1883–
SYMMETRICAL TYLOMA OF—
 Ueber Berufserkrankungen bei Melkern. Wien. klin. Wschr., 37: 630 (only), June 19, 1924

Asch, Morris J. American laryngologist. 1833–1902
OPERATION—for correction of deflection of the nasal septum.
SPLINT—for nose.
 A new operation for deviation of the nasal septum, with a report of cases. New York M. J., 52: 675–677; 693, Dec. 20, 1890

Ascherson, Ferdinand Moritz. German physician 1798–1879
Wrote on congenital fistulae of neck.
 De fistulis colli congenitis adjecta fissuarum branchialium in mammalibus avibusque historia succinta. Berlin, Jonas, 1832. 22 pp.
 Same, in English. Manchester, Irwin, 1848
MEMBRANE—the covering of casein inclosing the milk-globules.
 Pharmaceutische Botanik in Tabellen-Form.... Berlin, Schuppel, 1831. 82 pp.
VESICLES—formed by shaking together oil and liquid albumin. Ibid.

Aschheim, Selmar. Berlin gynecologist. 1878–
REACTION—for pregnancy.
 Das Hormon des Hypophysenvorderlappens with B. Zondek, Klin. Wschr., 7: 831–835, Apr. 29, 1928
 Die Schwangerschaftsdiagnose aus dem Harn durch Nachweis des Hypophysenvorderlappenhormons with B. Zondek, Ibid., 1404–1411; 1453–1457, July 1928
 Ueber Luteincystenbildung im Ovarium bei Blasenmole und Chorionepithelioma malignum. Die Ent-

stehung dieser Luteincysten durch Wirkung des Hypophysenvorderlappeninkret. Zbl. Gynäk., 52: 602–609, Mar. 10, 1928
Pregnancy tests. J. A. M. A., 104: 1324–1329, Apr. 13, 1935
Foreign letters. Simplified method of Aschheim-Zondek's test for pregnancy. J. A. M. A., 129: 1040 (only), Dec. 8, 1945

Aschner, Bernhard. Austrian gynecologist. 1883–
PHENOMENON or REFLEX or TEST—oculacardia reflex: slowing of pulse brought about by pressure on eyeball, a result of vagus irritability.
Ueber einen bisher noch nicht beschriebenen reflex vom Auge auf Kreislauf und Atmung. Verschwinden des Radialispulses bei Druck auf das Auge. Wien. klin. Wschr., 21: 1529–1530, Oct. 29, 1908
TEST—
Ueber brustartige Erscheinungen (Hyperämie und Hämorrhagie am weiblichen Genitale) nach subkutaner Injektion von Ovarial- oder Placentrarextrakt. Arch. Gynaek., 99: 534–540, 1913

Aschoff, Karl Albert Ludwig. Berlin pathologist. 1866–1942
BODIES or NODULES—rheumatic nodules in myocardium.
Zur Myocarditisfrage. Verh. dtsch. path. Ges., 8: 46–53, 1904
Also, English transl. by F. A. Willius In: F. A. Willius and T. E. Keys' *Cardiac Classics*, St. Louis, Mosby, 1941. pp. 733–739
NODE—of Aschoff and Tawara; at base of interauricular septum, forming beginning of auricular-ventricular bundle of His.
Die heutige Lehre von den pathologisch-anatomischen Grundlagen der Herzschwäche. Krittische Bemerkungen auf Grund einiger Untersuchungen with S. Tawara Jena, Fischer, 1906. 79 pp.
SINUSES— outpouchings of mucosa of gall bladder into external layers of its wall; called also Rokitansky s.
Bemerkungen zur pathologischen Anatomie der Cholelithiasis und Cholecystitis. Verh. dtsch. path. Ges., 9: 41–48, 1905
THEORY—enterogenous, of origin of appendicitis.
Die Wurmfortsatzentzündung. Jena, G. Fischer, 1908
Demonstrated cholesterol in epithelial cells of mucous membrane of gall bladder.
Zur Frage der Cholesterinbildung in der Gallenblase. Münch. med. Wschr., 3: 1847–1848, Sept. 18, 1906
Coined first term reticulo-endothelial system.
Das retikulo-endotheliale System und seine Beziehungen zur Gellenfarbstoffbindung. Münch. med. Wschr., 69: 1352–1356, Sept. 15, 1922

Ascoli, Alberto. Italian veterinarian. 1877–
REACTION or TEST—a blood-serum test to confirm the diagnosis of malignant tumors, syphilis, typhoid, etc.
La precipitina del carbonchio ematico. Pathologica, Genova, 3: 101, 1910–11
Diagnosi biologica del carbonchio ematico with E. Valenti, Clin. vet., Milano, 33, sez. prat.: 329–335, 1910
Die specifische Meiostagminreaktion. Münch. med. Wschr., 57: 62–63, Jan. 11, 1910
Die Präzipitindiagnose bei Milzbrand. Zbl. f. Bakt., 1 Abt., 58, Orig.: 63–70, 1911
Allgemeine Betrachtungen zur Serodiagnose bösartiger

Geschwülste. Seuchenbekämpfung. Wien. 6: 81–84, 1929

Ascoli, Giulio. Pavia pathologist
STAIN—for nerve fibers.
Dell' anatomia e della minuta struttura del sistema simpatico degli irudinei. Boll. Soc. med. chir., Pavia, pp. 177–198, 1911

Aselli, Caspar. Italian anatomist. 1581–1626
Discovered the lacteal vessels.
De lactibus seu lacteis venis, quarto vasorum mesaraicorum genere, novo invento, dissertatio. . . . Mediolani, Bidellum, 1627. 79 pp.
PANCREAS—an assemblage of lymphatic glands at the root of the mesentery. Ibid.

Ashburn, Percy Moreau. U. S. Army surgeon, Manila. 1872–1940
Demonstrated that a virus in the circulating blood is the causative agent of dengue fever.
Experimental investigations regarding the etiology of dengue fever, with a general consideration of the disease with C. F. Craig, Philippine J. Sci., Sec.B, 2:93–151, May 1907
Also: J. Infect. Dis., 4: 440–475, 1907

Ashby, H. See G. A. Wright
Ashby, S. F. English scientist
BASAL SOLUTION—
Some observations on "nitrification." J. Agric. Sci., 2: 52–67, Jan. 1907

Ashhurst, Astley Paston Cooper. American surgeon. 1876–1932
POSITION—of flexion for fractures of lower end of humerus.
An anatomical and surgical study of fractures of the lower end of the humerus. Philadelphia, 1918. pp. 89–90

Askanazy, Max. Königsberg pathologist. 1865–1940
Called attention to a relationship between the parathyroid glands and decalcification of skeleton in a case of osteitis fibrosa.
Ueber Ostitis deformans ohne osteides Gewebe. Arb. a. d. path. Anat. Inst., Tubingen, Leipzig, 4: 398–422, 1904
HYPERPLASTIC PANMYELOPATHY OF—Ibid.
Reported association of amyloidosis with multiple myeloma.
Ueber knötchenförmige lokale Amyloidbildung in der Darmmuskulatur. Verh. dtsch. Path. Ges., 7: 32–34, 1904

Askanazy, S.
Proposed Diuretin as a remedy for anginal pain.
Klinisches über Diuretin. Dtsch. Arch. f. klin. Med., 56: 209–230, 1895

Asmacher, Fr. Düsseldorf pharmacologist
REACTION—for histamine.
Ueber eine Farbreaktion des Histamins und Schwermetallkomplexsalze des Methylimidazols. Biochem. Z., 284: 339–342, 1936

Assman, Georg. Leipzig physician
METHOD—for preparing blood films.
Ueber eine neue Methode der Blut- und Gewebsfärbung mit dem eosinsauren Methylenblau. Münch. med. Wschr., 53: 1350–1351, July 10, 1906

Assmann, Herbert. German pathologist. 1882–
THEORY—new bone formation in osteoblastic carcinoma metastases is of the nature of a foreign body or "defense" reaction to a foreign tissue.
Zum Verständnis der Knochenneubildung bei der

osteoplastischen Karzinose. Arch. f. path. Anat., 188: 32–44, Apr. 6, 1907

Asthoewer, Hermann. Dortmund physician
INCISION—for approach to diaphragmatic hernia, suggested in 1894.

Die Aufklappung des Rippenbogens zur Erleichterung operativer Eingriffe im Hypochondrium und Zwerchfellkuppelraum. Zbl. f. Chir., 30: 1257–1259, Nov. 14, 1903

Atchley, D. W. See J. W. Ferrebee

Atkins, John. British naval surgeon. 1685–1757
Recognized African trypanosomiasis (sleeping sickness).

The navy surgeon: or a practical system of surgery. London, Ward and Chandler, 1734. pp. 364–367

Also: *The navy surgeon . . . and physical observations on the coast of Guiney.* London, Hodges, 1742

Atkinson, Edward. Leeds surgeon. 1830–1905
Reported case of rupture of normal spleen (case is of doubtful authenticity).

Death from idiopathic rupture of spleen. Brit. M. J., 2: 403–404, Sept. 26, 1874

Atlee, W(ashington) Lemuel. Philadelphia surgeon. 1808–1878
OPERATION—
Case of successful operation for vesico-vaginal fistula. Amer. J. med. Sci., 39: 67–82, Jan. 1860

Atwater, Wilbur Olin. American scientist. 1844–1907
Studied the balance of nutrition.

A digest of metabolism experiments in which the balance of income and outgo was determined. Rev. ed. with C. F. Langworthy, U. S. Dept. Agric. Off. Exper. Stations, No. 45, 1897. 434 pp.

RESPIRATION CALORIMETER—
Description of a new respiration calorimeter and experiments on the conservation of energy in the human body with E. B. Rosa, Ibid., No. 63, 1899. 94 pp.

RESPIRATION CALORIMETER—
A respiration calorimeter, with appliances for the direct determination of oxygen with F. G. Benedict, Washington, Carnegie Inst., 1905. 193 pp.

Aub, Joseph Charles. Boston physician. 1890–
TREATMENT—
Lead poisoning with L. T. Fairhall, A. S. Minot and P. Reznikoff, Medicine, 4: 1–250, Feb.–May, 1925
Wrote important work on calcium and phosphcrus.
Calcium and phosphorus metabolism. Harvey Lectures, s. 24, pp. 151–174, 1928–29
See also W. Bauer

Aubert, Hermann. German physician. 1826–1892
Described dark adaptation.
Physiologie der Netzhaut. Breslau, Morgenstern, 1865. 394 pp.
PHENOMENON—when the head is turned toward one side a vertical line appears to incline toward the other side; an optical illusion. (Dorland Med. Dict.) Ibid.

Aubry, Pierre Ernst Marie. French chemist
REAGENT and TEST—for bismuth in urine.
Recherche du bismuth dans l'urine. J. Pharm. Chim., Paris, 25: 15–18, 1922

Auchincloss, Hugh. New York surgeon. 1878–
OPERATION—a modification of the Kondolean o. for elephantiasis.
A new operation for elephantiasis. Puerto Rico J. Pub. Health, 6: 149–150, Dec. 1930

Auenbrugger, Leopold Joseph. Austrian physician. 1722–1809
The inventor of percussion as a diagnostic procedure.
SIGN—a bulging of the epigastrium due to extensive pericardial effusion.
Inventum novum ex percussione thoracis humani ut signo abstrusos interni pectoris morbus detegendi. Vindobonae, Trattner, 1761
Also, trans. by J. Forbes in: *Epoch-making contributions to medicine. . . . By C. N. B. Camac, Phila., Saunders, 1909. pp. 125–147*
Also, facsimile of original publication, Vienna, 1922
Also, trans. by J. Forbes, Baltimore, Johns Hopkins Press, 1936. 31 pp.
Same, with introduction by H. E. Sigerist, Bull. Inst. Hist. Med., 4: 373–403, May 1936
Also, trans. by J. Forbes in: F. A. Willius and T. E. Keys' Cardiac classics. St. Louis, Mosby, 1941. pp. 193–213

Auer, Clara Meltzer. See S. J. Meltzer
Auer, John. American physiologist. 1875–
PHENOMENON—
Local autoinoculation of the sensitized organism with foreign protein as a cause of abnormal reactions. J. Exp. Med., 32: 427–444, Oct. 1, 1920
Described physiological reactions leading to fatal anaphylactic shock.
The physiology of the immediate reaction of anaphylaxis in the guinea-pig with P. A. Lewis, Ibid., 12: 151–173, 1910
See also S. J. Meltzer

Auerbach, Leopold. German anatomist. 1828–1897
GANGLION and PLEXUS—of sympathetic nerves between the circular and longitudinal muscular coats of intestine.
Ueber einen Plexus myentericus, einen bisher unbekannten Ganglio-nervösen Apparet im Darmkanal der Wirbelthiere. Breslau, 1862
Ueber einen Plexus gangliosus myogastricus. Carlsbad, 1863

Aufricht, Gustave. New York City surgeon. 1894–
PROCEDURE—
Combined nasal plastic and chin plastic: correction of microgenia by osteocartilaginous transplant from large hump nose. Amer. J. Surg., 25: 292–296, Aug. 1934
A few hints and surgical details in rhinoplasty. Laryngoscope, 53: 317–335, May 1943

Aujeszky, Aladar. Budapest pathologist. 1869–1933
DISEASE—pseudohydrophobia; an infectious bulbar paralysis observed in Hungary and Brazil, where it is called the "scratching pest" (peste de cocar). Dorland.
Ueber eine neue Infektionskrankheit bei Haustieren. Zbl. f. Bakt., 1 Abt., 32: 535–357, Sept. 5, 1902
STAIN—for spores.
Eine einfache Sporenfärbungsmethode. Ibid., 23: 329–331, Feb. 27, 1898

Auspitz, Heinrich. Vienna physician. 1835–1886
DERMATOSIS—granuloma fungoides.
Ein Fall von Granuloma fungoides (Mykosis fungoides Alibert). Viertelj. Dermat. u. Syph., Wien, n. F., 12: 123–143, 1885
SIGN—the bleeding points disclosed by removing the scale of psoriasis.
Ueber das Verhältniss der Oberhaut zur Papillarschicht insbesondere bei pathologischen Zuständen der

Haut. Arch. f. Dermat. u. Syph., 2: 24–58 (54), 1870

Austrian, Charles Robert. Baltimore physician. 1885–

REACTION—ophthalmic, for typhoid fever, by use of antigen prepared from mixed culture of large number of different strains of typhoid bacilli.
Observations of the typhoidin reaction with A. L. Bloomfield, Arch. Intern. Med., 17: 663–669, May 1916
See also Florence R. Sabin

Autenrieth, Johann Heinrich Ferdinand von. Tübingen physician. 1772–1835
PUSTULE or EXANTHEM—
Versuche für die praktische Heilkunde aus den klinischen Anstalten von Tübingen. Bd. 1, Hft. 1 u. 2, viii, 9–506 pp. 8° Tübingen, J. G. Cotta, 1807 (DSG)

Autenrieth, Wilhelm. Freiburg chemist. 1863–
TEST—for detection and estimation of potassium in urine.
Ueber eine einfache Methode der Bestimmung des Kaliums im Harn with R. Bernheim, Z. Phys. Chem., 37: 29–39, 1902
TEST—for cholesterol.
Ueber kolorimetrische Bestimmungsmethoden: Die Bestimmung des Gesamtcholesterins im Blut und in Organen with A. Funk, Münch. med. Wschr., 69: 1243–1248, June 10, 1913

Aveling, James Hobson. London physician. 1828–1892
APPARATUS—
On immediate transfusion. Trans. Obstet. Soc. London, 6: 126–136, 1864

Avellis, Georg. German laryngologist. 1864–1916
SYNDROME—recurrent paralysis of soft palate.
Klinische Beiträge zur halbseitigen Kehlkopflähmung. Berl. Klinik, 40: 1–26, 1891

Averill, Charles. London surgeon
TABLE—
Description of a new operating table, in use at Cheltenham Casualty Hospital, by Charles Averill, Surgeon to the Institution. London Med. Gaz., 5: 52–54, Oct. 10, 1829

Avery, John Waite. American surgeon. 1868–
EVACUATOR—
The Avery evacuator: a preliminary report. New York M. J., 91: 78–79, Jan. 8, 1910

Avery, Oswald Theodore. American physician. 1877–
MEDIUM—oleate agar, for influenza bacilli.
A selective medium for B. influenza; oleate-hemoglobin agar. J. A. M. A., 71: 2050–2051, Dec. 21, 1918
METHOD—
Determination of types of pneumococcus in lobar pneumonia: a rapid cultural method. Ibid., 70: 17–19, Jan. 5, 1918
BROTH—dextrose-blood.
Acute lobar pneumonia: prevention and serum treatment with H. T. Chickering, R. Cole and A. R. Dochez, Rockefeller Inst. Mon., No. 7, p. 19, Oct. 16, 1917
METHOD—mouse, for typing pneumococci. Ibid., p. 23
See also A. R. Dochez, M. Heidelberger

Axenfeld, David. German physiologist. 1848–1912
TEST and REACTION—for albumin in urine.
Ueber eine neue Eiweissreaction. Zbl. med. Wiss., 23: 209–211, Mar. 28, 1885

Axenfeld, Karl Theodor Paul Polykarpus. German ophthalmologist. 1867–1930
CONJUNCTIVITIS—a form due to the diplococcus of Morax and Axenfeld.
DIPLOCOCCUS—of Morax and Axenfeld.
Ueber die chronische Diplobacillenconjunctivitis. Zbl. f. Bakt., 21: 1–9, Jan. 9, 1897
Beiträge zur Aetiologie der Bindehautentzündungen. Ueber chronische Diplobacillenconjunctivitis. Ber. d. Ophth. Gesellsch. Heidelberg, 1896, Rostock, 25: 140–155, 1897

Axhausen, Georg. Berlin surgeon. 1877–
OPERATION—transposition of nipple.
Ueber Mammaplastik. Med. Klin., 22: 1437–1440, Sept. 17, 1926
THEORY—carcinoma cells secrete a substance which stimulates osteogenesis.
Histologische Studien über die Ursachen und den Ablauf des Knochenumbaus im osteoplastischen Karzinom. Arch. f. path. Anat., 195: 358–462, 1909

Ayer, James Bourne. Boston neurologist. 1882–
Used term "aseptic meningitis" for meningeal reaction following an aseptic irritation as exhibited by the presence of lymphocytes, macrophages, plasma cells and fibroblasts in the subarachnoid space.
A pathological study of experimental meningitis from subarachnoid inoculation. Rockefeller Inst. Mon., 12: 26–44, Mar. 25, 1920
Introduced cisterna puncture.
Puncture of the cisterna magna. Arch. Neurol. & Psychiat., 4: 529–541, Nov. 1920
MANOMETER—water, for determining spinal fluid pressure. Ibid.
See also W. G. Denis, G. L. Tobey, Jr.

Ayers, S. Henry. American scientist. 1893–
AGAR—fuchsin sulphite; for cultivation of colon-aerogenes group.
A synthetic medium for the direct enumeration of organisms of the colon-aerogenes group with P. Rupp, J. Bact., 3: 433–436, Sept. 1918
SOLUTION—basal sodium ammonium phosphate; to study acid and alkali production by bacteria.
Simultaneous acid and alkaline bacterial fermentation from dextrose and the salts of organic acids respectively with P. Rupp, J. Infect. Dis., 23: 188–216, Aug. 1918
SOLUTION—yeast infusion peptone; culture medium.
Extracts of pure dry yeast for culture media with P. Rupp, J. Bact., 5: 89–98, Jan. 1920

Ayerza, Abel. Buenos Aires physician. 1861–1918
DISEASE and SYNDROME—erythremia with sclerosis of pulmonary artery. By Luis Ayerza
Maladie d'Ayerza, sclerosa secondine de l'artere pulmonaire (cardioques noirs). Semana méd., 32: 43–44, Jan. 1925
Consideraciones sobre la denominación de la "enferma-dad de Ayerza." Présna méd. argent., Buenos-Aires, 12: 92–93, June 20, 1925
Also: Semana méd., 32: pt. 2, pp. 386–388, 1925

Ayres, Daniel. Brooklyn surgeon. 1822–
TABLE—
Dr. Daniel Ayres' operating table. Amer. Med. Gaz., N. Y., 9: 241–243, Apr. 1858
OPERATION—
Congenital exstrophy of the urinary bladder, complicated with prolapsus uteri following pregnancy: successfully

treated by a new plastic operation. Ibid., 10: 81–89, 1859
Ayrton, R. See E. G. D. Murray
Ayscough, James. English physician
Used test-reading of print at a distance.
A short account of the eye and nature of vision, ... London, (n.d.) (1752) 26 pp.
Azoulay, Léon. Paris physician
METHOD—osmic acid for myelin.
Coloration de la myéline des tissus nerveux et de la

graisse par l'acide osmique et le tanin ou ses analogues. Anat. Anz., 10 : 25–28, Sept. 10, 1894
PROCESS—ammonium vanadate, for nerve tissue.
Préparations du système nerveux colorées par deux méthodes nouvelles: 1° acide osmique et tannin; 2° vanadate d'ammoniaque et tannin. Bull. Soc. anat. Paris, 5 s., 69 : 924–926, Dec. 1894
Aztec
EAR—lacking the lobule and appearing as if the whole ear were pushed forward and downward.

B

Babcock, William Wayne. Philadelphia surgeon. 1872–
OPERATION—cholecystograstrostomy for peptic ulcer.
The control of hyperchlorhydria and its consequences by cholecystogastrostomy. M. Rec., 98: 476–477, Sept. 18, 1920
Cholecystogastrostomy and cholecystoduodenostomy. Amer. J. Obstet. Gynec., 1: 854–859, Apr. 1921
OPERATION—for varicose veins.
A new operation for the extirpation of varicose veins of the leg. New York M. J., 86: 153–156, July 27, 1907
A modified extractor for the removal of varicose veins of the leg. J. A. M. A., 55: 210 (only). July 16, 1910
OPERATION—
The single stage operation for pulsion diverticulum of the esophagus with C. Jackson, S. G. O., 53: 667–669, Nov. 1931
OPERATION—removal of duct papilloma through a curved areolar incision.
A simple operation for the discharging nipple. Surgery, 4: 914–916, Dec. 1938
OPERATION—
Advancement of the receding lower jaw. Ann. Surg., 106: 1105–1108, Dec. 1937
OPERATION—for inguinal hernia.
The ideal in herniorrhaphy. A new method efficient for direct and indirect inguinal hernia. S. G. O., 45: 534–540, Oct. 1927
OPERATION—for incisional hernia.
Interdigitation in the repair of large ventral hernias with observations on lipectomy. S. G. O., 40: 852–857, June 1925
OPERATION—for spina bifida.
Spina bifida and its surgical treatment, with a description of an efficient osteoplastic operation. Monthly Cyclo. and Med. Bull., 4: 257–268, May 1911
OPERATION—for relief of aortic aneurysm.
Operative decompression of aortic aneurysm by carotidjugular anastomosis. Surg. Clin. N. Amer., 9: 1031–1041, Oct. 1929
Babès, Victor. Budapest bacteriologist. 1854–1926
BODIES—Babès-Ernst b. or corpuscles or metachromatic granules, seen in protoplasm of bacteria and staining deeply with anilin dyes.
Ueber isolirt färbbare Antheile von Bacterien. Z. f. Hyg., 5: 173–190, 1888
REACTION—mallein, for diagnosis of glanders.
Observations sur la morve: diagnostic de la morve . . . substances chimiques produites par le bacille de la morve. Arch. de Med. exper. et d'Anat. path., Paris, 3 : 619–645, 1891

STAIN—anilin-safranin.
Ueber einige Färbungsmethoden, besonders für krankhafte Gewebe, mittelst Safranin und deren Resultate. Arch. mik. Anat., 19 : 356–365, 1883
Ueber Safraninlösung mit Anilinöl. Z. wiss. Mikr., 4 : 470–471, 1887
Babington, Benjamin. London physician.1794–1866
Invented the "glottiscope",—crude, obsolete, but a forerunner of present instruments.
(No title) Report to Hunterian Society, Mar. 18, 1829, London M. Gaz., 3 : 555 (only), 1829
Babinski, Joseph Francois Felix. Paris physician. 1857–1932
REFLEX or PHENOMENON or SIGN—extension of toes instead of flexion on stimulating sole of foot; indicates organic, as distinguished from hysteric, hemiplegia.
Sur le réflexe cutane plantaire dans certaines affections organiques du système nerveux central. C. R. Soc. Biol., 3 : 207–208, 1896
Du phénomène des orteils et de sa valour sémiologique. Sem. Med., 18: 321–322, 1898
SYNDROME—
Lésion bulbaire unilatérale: thérmo-asymétrie et vasoasymétrie; hémianesthésie alterne à forme syringomyélique. Rev. neurol., 14: 1177–1182, Dec. 30, 1906
SYNDROME—the association of cardiac and arterial disorders with chronic or late syphilitic manifestations.
Des troubles pupillaires dans les anévrismes de l'aorte. Bull. Soc. méd. Hôp. Paris, 18: 1121–1124, Nov. 8, 1901
BABINSKI-NAGEOTTE SYNDROME—Horner's syndrome and dysphagia with contralateral hemiplegia, etc.
Hémiasynergie, latéropulsion et myosis bulbaires avec hémianesthésie et hémiplégie croisées. with J. Nageotte, Rev. neurol., 10: 358–365, Apr. 30, 1902
Described the pupillary reflex.
Sur la paralysie du mouvement associé de l'abaissement des yeux. Rev. neurol., 7 : 525–527, 1900
Described syndrome of pituitary tumor with acromegalia.
Tumeur du corps pituitaire sans acromégalie et avec arrêt de développement des organes génitaux. Ibid., 8: 531–533, June 15, 1900
Baccelli, Guido. Rome physician. 1832–1916
METHOD—treatment of tetanus by injections of carbolic acid.
Ein neuer Fall von Tetanus, behandelt und geheilt nach der Baccelli'schen Methode. By Prof. G. Galli (Baccelli's assistant) Med. Woch., Berlin, 7: 271–272, June 18; 292–294, July 2, 1906

METHOD or OPERATION—introduction of a wire thread into sac of an aneurysm.
Di un nuovo methodo di cura per taluni aneurismi dell'aorta. Lezione clinica. Roma, 1877. 67 pp.
MIXTURE—containing quinin sulphate, used by injection in malaria.
La infezione malarica with E. Marchiafava, G. internaz. d. sc. med., Napoli, n. s. 11: 919–924, 1889
Also: Trans. X Internat. Med. Congr., Berlin, 1890
SIGN—pectoriloquie aphonique, a sign of pleural effusion.
Sulla transmissione dei suoni attraverso i liquidi endopleurici di differente natura. Arch. Med., Chir. ed Igiena. Roma, 1875
Introduced injection of corrosive sublimate in treatment of syphilis.
Le iniezioni endovenose di sublimato corrosivo in un caso di sifloma della lingua e in una stenosi bronchiale. Gaz. med. di Roma, 19: 289–293, 1893

Bach, A. German chemist
Discovered, with Chodat, oxygenase and peroxidase, the enzymes of autoxidation in plants. (Garrison)
Ueber den gegenwärtigen Stand der Lehre von den pflanzlichen Oxydationsfermenten with R. Chodat, Biochem. Zbl., 1: 417–421, May 15: 457–461, June 1, 1903

Bach, Hugo. German physician. 1859–
LAMP—mercury vapor arc in quartz, air cooled.
Anleitung und Indikation für Bestrahlungen mit der Quarzlampe. Künstliche Höhensonne. Würzb. Anhandl. a. d. Gesamtgeb. d. prakt. Med., 15: Hft. 1–2, 1915
Also: Würzburg, 1915. 41 pp.
Ultraviolet light, by means of the Alpine sun lamp; treatment and indications. Transl. by M. E. Jutte, N. Y., Hoeber, 1916. 114 pp.

Bachman, George William. San Juan, P. R. parasitologist. 1890–
TEST—for diagnosis of trichinosis by acid hydrolyzed extracts of larvae of Trichinella spiralis.
An intradermal reaction in experimental trichiniasis. J. Prevent. Med., 2: 169–173, Mar. 1928; 2: 513–523, Nov. 1928

Bachmann, Fritz. German bacteriologist
BROTH—indicator extract; culture medium.
Beitrag zur Kenntnis obligat anaërober Bakterien. Zbl. f. Bakt., 2 Abt., 36: 1–41, Dec. 14, 1912

Bacz, Z. M. See W. B. Cannon

Bade, Peter. Hannover surgeon
OPERATION—for slipping patella; the entire patellar ligament is transplanted medially and drawn distally to a lower level.
Die habituelle Luxation der Patella. Z. orthop. Chir., 11: 451–488, 1903

Badham, Charles. London physician. 1780–1845
Coined term bronchitis.
Observations on the inflammatory affections of the mucous membrane of the bronchiae. London, Callow, 1808. 133 pp.

Badham, John. English physician
Wrote an important description of infantile paralysis.
Paralysis in childhood. Four remarkable cases of suddenly induced paralysis in the extremities, occurring in childhood, without any apparent cerebral or cerebrospinal lesion. London M. Gaz., 17: 215–217, 1835

Baecchi, Brunetto. Parma physician
TEST—for sperm.

Su di una nuova reazione dello sperma. Arch. Farmacol. sper., 14: 491–500, 1913
REAGENT—for blood
Nuova reazione chimica del sangue. Arch. int. med. leg. de Belgique, 4: 163–169, May 1913

Baehr, G. See also N. E. Brill, L. Loewe, H. Plotz

Bälz, Erwin O. E. von. German physician. 1849–1913
DISEASE—painless papules of the mucous membrane of the lips: cheilitis glandularis.
Über Erkrankungen der Schleimdrüsen des Mundes. By P. G. Unna, Mschr. f. pr. Dermat., 11: 317–321, Oct. 1, 1890

Baer, Benjamin Franklin. Philadelphia surgeon. 1846–1920
OPERATION—
Supravaginal hysterectomy without ligature of the cervix, in operation for uterine fibroids: a new method. Amer. J. Obstet., 26: 489–504, Oct. 1892

Baer, Karl Ernst von. Russian anatomist. 1792–1876
Discovered the mammalian ovum and the chorda dorsalis or notochord.
Established the real identity of the Graffian follicles.
LAW—the more specialized forms and structures arise from the more general, and by a gradual change.
VESICLE—the ovule.
CAVITY—the segmentation cavity of the blastoderm.
De ovi mammalium et hominis genesi. Epistolam ad Academiam Imperialem Scientiarum Petropolitanam. Lipsiae, Vossii, 1827. 40 pp.
(Same) Z. organ. Physik., 2: 125–193, 1828
(Same) Original in facsimile, 1931
Established modern theory of germ layers.
Ueber Entwickelungsgeschichte der Thiere: Beobachtung und Reflexion. Königsberg, Bornträger, 1828. 271 pp.
Classified animals into four groups.
Histoire du développement des animaux. Répert. gén. d'anat. et physiol., 8: 42–103, et seq., 1829

Baer, William Stevenson. Baltimore surgeon. 1872–1931
TREATMENT—
The treatment of chronic osteomyelitis with the maggot (larvae of the blowfly). J. Bone and Joint Surg., 13: 438–475, July 1931

Baerensprung, Friedrich Wilhelm Felix von. Berlin physician. 1822–1864
DISEASE or ERYTHRASMA—eczema marginatum affecting the thighs.
Ueber die Folge und dem Verlauf epidermischer Krankheiten. Halle, Schmidt, 1854. 64 pp.
Showed that herpes zoster is due to a lesion of the spinal ganglia.
Die Gürtelkrankheit. Ann. d. Char.-Krankenh . . . zu Berl., 9: 2 Hft., 40, 1861
Neue Beobachtungen über Herpes. Ibid., 10: 1 Heft., 37, 1862; 11: 2 Hft., 96, 1863

Bäumler, Christian. English physician. 1836–1933
Described three cases of pericarditis epistenocardia, but probably did not recognize its significance.
Cases of partial and general idiopathic pericarditis. Trans. Clin. Soc. London, 5: 8–22, 1872

Baeyer, Adolf. Münich chemist.
TEST—for glucose.
Ueber die Beziehungen der Zimmtsäure zu der Indigogruppe. Ber. dtsch. chem. Ges., 13: 2254–2263, 1880

TEST—for acetone.
Darstellung von Indigblau aus Orthonitrobenzaldehyd.
with V. Drewsen, Ibid., 15: 2856–2865, Nov. 27, 1882
Ueber die Einwirkung des Caro'schen Reagens auf Ketone with V. Villiger, Ibid., 33: 124–126, 1900
Baginsky, S. Polish chemist
REACTION—for adrenaline.
Sur la détection histochimique de l'adrénaline. Bull. histol. appli. physiol. . . . , 5: 129–130, Mar. 1928
Baglivi, Giorgio. Italian physician. 1668–1706
The first to distinguish between smooth and striped muscle. 1700 (Garrison)
Opera omnia medico-practica et anatomica.—Lugduni, Anisson and Posuel, 1710
Also: Norimbergae, Stein et Raspe, 1751
Bahrenberg, Louis Peter Henry. Cleveland physician. 1873–1940
TECHNIC—for cancer cells, by centrifuging aspirated fluid and sectioning sedimented cells.
On the diagnostic results of the microscopical examination of the ascitic fluid in two cases of carcinoma involving the peritoneum. Cleveland med. Gaz., 11: 274–278, Mar. 1896
Bailey, Garland Howard. Baltimore physician. 1890–
METHOD—
Hemolytic antibodies for sheep and ox erythrocytes in infectious mononucleosis with S. Raffel, J. Clin. Invest., 14: 228–244, Mar. 1935
Bailey, Harold Capron. New York obstetrician. 1879–1929
Called attention to shock occurring soon after delivery in eclampsia.
Shock in eclampsia. Amer. J. Obstet., 64: 260–270, Aug. 1911
Bailey, O. T. See F. D. Ingraham
Bailey, Percival. American surgeon. 1892–
With H. Cushing, applied name medulloblastoma.
Medulloblastoma cerebelli: a common type of midcerebellar glioma in childhood with H. Cushing, Arch. Neurol. Psychiat., 14: 192–224, Aug. 1925
A classification of the tumors of the glioma group on a histogenetic basis with a correlated study of prognosis with H. Cushing, Phila., Lippincott, 1926
HEAD REST—
Head rest for exposure of the cerebellum. J. A. M. A., 98: 1643 (only), May 7, 1932
METHOD—of staining neuroglia.
A new principle applied to the staining of the fibrillary neuroglia. J. Med. Res., 44: 73–77, Sept. 1923
STAIN—acid violet, for hypophysis.
Cytological observations on the pars buccalis of the hypophysis cerebri of man, normal and pathological. Ibid., 42: 349–381 (353), June–Sept. 1921
See also H. W. Cushing
Bailey, Sadie F. Pittsburgh
AGAR—hormone; culture medium.
"Hormone" mediums. Simple method of preparation and value of hormone blood agar for preserving pneumococci and streptococci. J. Infect. Dis., 36: 340–342, Mar. 1925
AGAR—phenol red lead acetate; for differentiation of colon-typhoid-dysentery group.
A modification of the Kligler lead acetate medium with G. R. Lacy, J. Bact., 13: 183–189, Mar. 1927
Baillarger, Jules Gabriel Francois. French physician. 1809–1890

LAYER or LINE or STRIA or STRIATIONS or STRIPE—of cerebral cortex.
Recherches sur la structure de la couche corticale des circonvolutions du cerveau. Mém. Acad. roy. d. méd., 8: 149–183, 1840
De la structure de la couche corticale des circonvolutions du cerveau. Ann. med. psychol., 1: 1–3, 1855
Baillie, Matthew. English physician. 1761–1823
Described hepatization of lungs in pneumonia.
The morbid anatomy of some of the most important parts of the human body. London, Johnson and Nicol, 1793. p. 52
Described transposition of viscera.
Of a remarkable transposition of the viscera. Philos. Trans., London, 78: 483–489, 1788
Also in: F. A. Willius and T. E. Keys' Cardiac classics, pp. 257–262, 1941
Bainbridge, Francis Arthur. English physiologist. 1874–1921
Showed that cardiac reflex action is produced by inhibition of vagus tone and excitation of accelerator nerves.
On some cardiac reflexes. J. Physiol., 48: 332–340, 1914
Bainbridge, William Seaman. New York surgeon. 1870–1947
TABLE—
The evolution of the operating table. New York M. J., 94: 909–918, Nov. 4, 1911
The evolution of the operating table; additional data. Ibid., 95: 57–58, Jan. 13, 1912
Baker, Albert Rufus. Cleveland ophthalmologist. 1858–1911
OPERATION—for keratoplasty.
Some remarks on transplantation of the cornea and allied subjects. Amer. J. Ophth., 6: 1–10, Jan. 1889
Baker, D. D. See J. R. Veal
Baker, Sir George. Devonshire physician. 1722–1809
Discovered Devonshire colic, due to cider-drinking, was a lead poisoning.
An essay concerning the cause of the endemial colic of Devonshire. London, 1767
An inquiry concerning the cause of the endemial colic of Devonshire. Paper read June 29, 1767. M. Trans., Coll. Phys., London, 1: 175–256, 1785
Baker, Henry. English physician. 1698–1774
One of the pioneers of experimental morphology, supplemented Trembley's work on polyps. (Garrison)
An attempt towards a natural history of the polype. London, Dodsley, 1743. 218 pp.
Baker, Henry A. Boston surgeon
VELUM—an obturator used in cleft-palate.
An appliance for congenital cleft palate. Dental Cosmos, 23: 178–186, Apr. 1881
An improved appliance in the physiological treatment of cleft palate. Boston Med. & Surg. J., 110: 127–130; 134, Feb. 7, 1884
Baker, J. P. See S. Weiss
Baker, Lenox Dial. Durham, N. C. surgeon. 1901–
MODIFICATION—of Nicola operation on shoulder.
Nicola operation: simplified technic. J. Bone Joint Surg., 22: 118–119, Jan. 1940
Baker, William Morrant. London surgeon. 1839–1896
CYST—hernia of the synovial membrane of a joint through an opening in its capsule.

On the formation of synovial cysts in the leg in connection with disease of the knee-joint. St. Bartholomew's Hosp. Rep., 13: 245–261, 1877
Also: Medical Classics, 5: 785–804, May 1941
The formation of abnormal synovial cysts in connection with the joints. St. Bartholomew's Hosp. Rep., 21: 177–190, 1885
Also: Medical Classics, 5: 805–820, May 1941
TUBES—tracheotomy.
On the use of flexible tracheotomy tubes. Med.-Chir. Trans., 60: 71–84, 1877
Described
Erythema serpens. St. Barth. Hosp. Rep., 9: 198–211, 1873

Bakeš, J. German surgeon
DILATORS—for sphincter of Oddi.
Zur drainagelosen Gallenchirurgie und der methodischen Dilatation der Papille. Zbl. Chir., 55: 1858–1868, July 28, 1928

Balard, Antoine Jérome. Montpellier pharmacologist. 1802–1876
Discovered bromine. (Balard called it muride. Gay-Lussac named it bromide).
Mémoire sur une substance particulière contenue dans l'eau de la mer. Ann. Chir. et Phys., 32: 337–381, 1826
Discovered amyl nitrite.
Mémoire sur l'alcool amylique. C. R. Acad. Sci., 19: 634–641, 1844

Balbiani, Édouard Gérard. French physician. 1823–1899
Balbiana—a genus of Sarcosporidia.
*Leçons sur les sporozoaires. . . . *Paris, Doin, 1884. 184 pp.

Baldwin, Aslett. London surgeon
OPERATION—
The radical cure of femoral hernia. Lancet, 2: 150–152, July 21, 1906

Baldwin, Helen. New York physician. 1865–
METHOD—for quantitation determination of oxalic acid in urine.
An experimental study of oxaluria, with special reference to its fermentative origin. J. exp. Med., 5: 27–46, Oct. 1, 1900

Baldwin, James Fairchild. Columbus, Ohio gynecologist. 1850–1936
OPERATION—
The formation of an artificial vagina by intestinal transplantation. Ann. Surg., 40: 398–403, Sept. 1904
Also: Amer. J. Obstet., 56: 636–640, Nov. 1907

Baldwin, Walter Isaac. San Francisco surgeon. 1885–1926
OPERATION—arthrodesis of wrist.
Orthopaedic surgery of the hand and wrist.
In: Jones' *Orthopedic surgery of war injuries.* London, 1921. Vol. 1, pp. 239–282, (249–251)

Baldwin, Wesley Manning. American anatomist. 1881–
Described histology of ampulla of Vater.
The pancreatic ducts in man, together with a study of the microscopical structure of the minor duodenal papilla. Anat. Rec., 5: 197–228, May 1911

Baldy, John Montgomery. Philadelphia gynecologist. 1860–1934
OPERATION—of Baldy-Webster, for retroversion of uterus by shortening of round ligaments.

Retrodisplacements of the uterus and their treatment. New York M. J., 78: 167–169, July 25, 1903
Operation for retrodisplacement of the uterus. J. A. M. A., 56: 481–484, Feb. 18, 1911

Balfour, Donald Church. Rochester, Minn. surgeon. 1882–
OPERATION—resection of sigmoid colon.
A method of anastomosis between sigmoid and rectum. Ann. Surg., 51: 239–241, Feb. 1910
OPERATION—modification of Billroth II gastric resection.
Restoration of gastro-intestinal continuity by means of anticolic gastrojejunostomy following partial gastrectomy for cancer of the pyloric end of the stomach. S. G. O., 25: 473–477, Nov. 1917

Balfour, George William. English physician. 1823–1903
TEST—of death by searching for possible movements of cardiac muscle.
Clinical lectures on diseases of the heart and aorta. London, Churchill, 1876
TREATMENT—
On the treatment of aneurism by iodide of potassium. Edinburgh M. J., 14: 33–47, July 1868; 15: 47–65, July 1869

Balfour, John Hutton. Edinburgh surgeon. 1808–1884
DISEASE—chloroma.
Case of peculiar disease of the skull and dura mater. Edinburgh M. & S. J., 43: 319–325, Apr. 1, 1835

Ball, Sir Charles Bent. Irish surgeon. 1851–1916
OPERATION—iliac colotomy in the left linea semilunaris.
The rectum and anus; their diseases and treatment. London, Cassell, 1887. 410 pp. pp. 363–371
OPERATION—for rectal prolapse; colopexy. Ibid., pp. 212–215
OPERATION—cutting of the sensory nerve trunks of the anus for relief of pruritis ani. Ibid.
OPERATION—
The radical cure of hernia by torsion of the sac. Brit. M. J., 2: 461–462, Sept. 6, 1884

Ball, Isaac. New York physician
Wrote second book on physiology published in the New World.
An analytical view of the animal economy calculated for the students of medicine, as well as private gentlemen, interspersed with many allegories, and moral reflections, drawn from the subject, to awaken the mind to an elevated sense of the great author of nature. New York, Hunt, 1808. 2 ed. 90 pp.

Ball, Robert P. New York roentgenologist. 1902–
TECHNIC—of roentgen pelvicephalography, depending essentially on a volumetric comparison of fetal head and birth canal.
Roentgen pelvimetry and fetal cephalometry: a new technic with S. S. Marchbanks, Radiology, 24: 77–84, Jan. 1935

Ballance, Sir Charles Alfred. English surgeon. 1856–1936
OPERATION—of ventricular drainage.
Some experiences in intracranial surgery. Trans. Amer. Surg. Ass., 24: 160–174, 1906
OPERATION—on facial nerve.
The operative treatment of facial palsy by the introduction of nerve grafts into the fallopian canal and by

other *intratemporal methods* with A. B. Duel, Arch. Otol., 15: 1–70, Jan. 1932
SCALE—of measurements of size of arteries; useful in banding.
A treatise on the ligation of the great arteries in continuity, with observations on the nature, progress and treatment of aneurism with W. Edmunds, London, Macmillan, 1891. 596 pp.
SIGN—in splenic rupture: non-shifting dullness in the left flank caused by clotting of blood in the left gutter.
On splenectomy for rupture without external wound: with remarks on the symptoms produced by the removal of the organ. Practitioner, 60: 347–358, Apr. 1898

Ballenger, Edgar Garrison. Atlanta, Ga. urologist. 1877–1945
OPERATION—for hydronephrosis.
Conservation of the hydronephrotic kidney with H. P. McDonald, J. Urol., 47: 203–208, Mar. 1942
TREATMENT—
Suction treatment for undescended testicles with O. F. Elder and H. P. McDonald, South. Surg., 4: 297–304, Oct. 1935

Ballingall, Sir George. English surgeon. 1780–1855
DISEASE—mycetoma.
Practical observations on fever, dysentery, and liver complaints, as they occur amongst the European troops in India; with introductory remarks on the disadvantages of selecting boys for Indian military service. Edinburgh. Brown & Constable, 1818. 248 pp.

Balloni, Antonio. Torino pathologist
TEST—for albumin in urine.
Methodo pratico per la ricerca qualitativa dell' albumina nelle urine. Minerva Med., 1: 259–260, Feb. 24, 1935

Ballonius, Gulielmus. French physician. 1538–1616
Applied name rheumatism.
Opuscula medica, de arthritide, de calculo et urinarum hypostasi.
In: *Quibus omnibus Galeni et veterum authoritas contra I. Fernelium defenditur. Item libellus vere aureus de rheumatismo et pleuritide dorsali, qui duo affectus ab antiquis non sat abunde fuerunt explicati et definiti.* Editore Jacobo Thevart, Paris, Quesnel, 1643. 300 pp.

Balme, Paul Jean. French physician. 1857–
COUGH—present in the recumbent position, due to obstruction of the nasopharynx.
De l'hypertrophie des amygdales (palatines, pharyngée, linguale). Paris, 1888. 158 pp.

Baló, József. Budapest neurologist
DISEASE—
Leukoenkephalitis periaxialis concentricaról. Magy. orv. arch., Budapest, 28: 108–124, 1927
Encephalitis periaxialis concentrica. Arch. Neur. Psychiat., Chicago, 19: 242–264, Feb. 1928

Balser, W. German physician
NECROSIS—fatty necrosis with gangrenous pancreatitis.
Ueber Fettnekrose, eine zuweilen tödliche Krankheit des Menschen. Arch. f. path. Anat. u. Physiol., 90: 520–535, Dec. 1, 1882
Ueber multiple Pankreas- und Fettnekrose. Verh. d. XI Cong. f. inn. Med., pp. 450–461, 1892

Balsum-of-Peru
"From El Salvadore." The early Spanish in South America so jealously guarded the product that every ounce of it had to pass through their customs in Peru. The name it thus acquired is still used. Natural History, 53: 137, Mar. 1944

Balzer, Félix. Paris physician. 1849–1929
Suggested bismuth in treatment of syphilis.
Expériences sur la toxicité du bismuth. C. R. Soc. Biol., 9 s., 1: 537–544, 1889

Bamberger, Eugen. Vienna physician. 1858–1921
DISEASE—Bamberger—Marie d.; hypertrophic pulmonary osteoarthropathy.
(Report before a medical society, no title). Wien. klin. Wschr., 2: 226, Mar. 14, 1889
Ueber Knochenveränderungen bei chronischen Lungen- und Herzkrankheiten. Z. klin. Med., 18: 193–217, 1891

Bamberger, H. See G. Seiffert

Bamberger, Heinrich. Austrian physician. 1822–1888
ALBUMINURIA—hematogenic, during the later periods of severe anemia. (Dorland)
Ueber Morbus Brighti und seine Beziehungen zu anderen Krankheiten. Samml. klin. Vortr., Leipz., No. 173, Inn. Med., No. 581, pp. 1533–1568, 1879
DISEASE—chronic polyserositis.
Ueber zwei seltene Herzaffektionen mit Bezugnahme auf die Theorie des ersten Herztons. Wien. med. Wschr., 22: 1–4, Jan. 6; 25–28, Jan. 13, 1872
DISEASE—saltatory spasm.
Saltatorischer Reflexkrampf, eine merkwürdige Form von Spinal-Irritation. Wien. med. Wschr., 9: 49–53, Jan. 22: 65–67, Jan. 29, 1859

Bancroft, Edward Nathaniel. English physician
Noted transmission of yaws by flies.
Essay on the natural history of Guiana. London, 1769. p. 385

Bancroft, Frederic Wolcott. New York surgeon. 1880–
OPERATION—exclusion of pylorus and removal of pyloric mucous membrane.
A modification of the Devine operation of pyloric exclusion for duodenal ulcer. Amer. J. Surg., 16: 223–230, May 1932
Demonstrated the value of a high protein diet in increasing the number of blood platelets.
Evaluation of blood clotting factors in surgical diseases, with special reference to thrombosis and embolism and certain bleeding conditions with I. N. Kugelmass and M. Stanley-Brown. Ann. Surg., 90: 161–189, Aug. 1929
CLOTTING INDEX—
Postoperative thrombosis and embolism with Margaret Stanley-Brown and S. Chargaff, Ann. Surg., 106: 868–879, Nov. 1937
See also A. J. Quick

Bancroft, Joseph. English physician. 1836–1894
Discovered Filaria bancrofti.
Cases of filarious disease. Trans. Path. Soc. Lond., 29: 406–419, 1878

Bandl, Ludwig. German obstetrician. 1842–1892
RING—contraction r.; a thickening of the uterus during labor, just above the internal os, and marking the lower limit of the contractile portion of the uterus.

Ruptur der Gebärmutter und ihre Mechanik. Wien, 1875

Ueber das Verhalten des Uterus und Cervix in der Schwangerschaft und während der Geburt. Stuttgart, 1876

Bandler, Clarence Garfield. New York surgeon. 1880–
OPERATION—
Circumcision. Amer. J. Surg., 6: 455–457, Apr. 1929

Banerjee, Prabodh. Calcutta, India, surgeon
OPERATION—
Intraperitoneal herniorrhaphy in inguinal hernia. S. G. O., 54: 706–711, Apr. 1932

Bang, Bernhard Laurits Frederik. Copenhagen physician. 1848–1932
BACILLUS—B. abortus or abortion bacillus.
DISEASE—caused by B. abortus.
Die Aetiologie des Seuchenhaften („infectiösen") *Verwerfens.* Dtsch. Z. Thiermed., 1: 241–278, 1897
METHOD—for prevention of spread of bovine tuberculosis by isolation of affected cows and by removal of calves of affected cows as soon as they are born and feeding them with milk of healthy cows. (Dorland)
Kampen mod Tuberkulosen hos Kvaeget. Maanedsskr. f. Drylaeger, 11, 1900

Bang, Ivar Christian. Swedish physical chemist. 1869–1918
METHOD—for estimation of quantities of sugar, albumin, urea, etc., in blood by examination of a few drops collected on blotting-paper.
Eine neue Methode zur Zuckerbestimmung. Lund, Ohlsson, 1911. 10 pp.
METHOD—for determination of glucose in urine.
Zur Methodik der Zuckerbestimmung. Biochem. Z., 2: 271–290, 1907
TEST—for albumoses in urine.
Eine neue Methode zum Nachweis der Albumosen im Harn. Dtsch. med. Wschr., 24: 17–18, Jan. 13, 1898
METHOD—for determination of residual nitrogen.
Blodets halt av restkväve under fysiologiska och patologiska förhållanden. Allm. sven. läkartidn., Stockholm, 13: 485–487, May 16, 1916

Banister, J. B. See A. H. McIndoe

Bankart, Arthur Sydney Blundell. London surgeon. 1879–
OPERATION—
Recurrent or habitual dislocation of the shoulder-joint. Brit. M. J., 2: 1132–1133, Dec. 15, 1923
The pathology and treatment of recurrent dislocation of the shoulder-joint. Brit. J. Surg., 26: 23–29, July 1938

Banks, B. M. See J. Fine

Banks, Henry Stanley. English physician
TREATMENT—sulphonamide, of meningococcal meningitis.
Chemotherapy of meningococcal meningitis: review of 147 consecutive cases. Lancet, 2: 921–927, Oct. 28, 1939

Banks, N. P. See L. Shattuck

Bannerman, R. G. See W. Cramer

Bannister, Henry Martyn. Chicago physician. 1844–1920
DISEASE—
Acute angioneurotic edema. J. Nerv. and Ment. Dis., 21: 627–631, Oct. 1894

Banti, Guido. Florence physician. 1852–1925

DISEASE—a form of splenic anemia attended with cirrhosis of liver, hypertrophy of spleen and ascites. First mentioned in: *Dell' anemia splenica.* Firenze, succ. Le Monier, 1882. 70 pp. and in: Pubbl. d. r. Inst. di studi sup.—in Fierenze, Sez. di med. e. chir., 9: 53–122, 1883
First described in: *La splenomegalia con cirrosi del fegato.* Sperimentale. Commun. e Rev., pp. 447–452, 1894
Also, in French: Semaine méd., 14: 318, 1894
Also, in English: Med. Weekly, Paris, 2: 364–365, 1894
Also, in German: Beitr. Path. Anat., 24: 21–33, 1898
Also, in Italian and English: Med. Classics, 1: 901–927, June 1937

Banting, Frederick Grant. Canadian physician. 1891–1941
Awarded Nobel prize in 1923, with J. J. R. MacLeod.
Isolated insulin for treating diabetes.
First report: *The internal secretion of the pancreas* with C. H. Best and J. J. R. MacLeod, Amer. J. Physiol., 59: 479, 1922
The internal secretion of the pancreas with C. H. Best, J. Lab. clin. Med., 7: 251–266, Feb. 1922
Pancreatic extracts in the treatment of diabetes mellitus. Canadian M. Ass., J., 12: 141–146, Mar. 1922
Insulin. Internat. Clinics. s 34, 4: 288–292, 1924
See also J. J. R. MacLeod

Banting, William. English physician. 1797–1878
CURE or DIET or TREATMENT—of corpulence, called banting or bantingism, by food poor in saccharine, farinaceous or oily matter but rich in nitrogenous material.
Letter on corpulence, addressed to the public. London, Harrison, 1863. 21 pp. 2. ed., 1863, 32 pp.

Banyer, Henry. English physician. fl. 1739
OINTMENT—for chronic eczema.
Pharmacopoeia pauperum; or the hospital dispensatory;— London, Warner; 1721. 2 ed.

Banzhaf, Edwin J. New York physician
METHOD—of purification and concentration of antidiphtheritic serum.
The further separation of antitoxin from its associated proteins in horse serum. (Society report) Med. Rec., 75: 581–582, Apr. 3, 1909

Baptist, Margaret. See W. K. Cuyler

Baraban, Leon Dominique. French physician. 1850–1905
CORPUSCLES or TUBULES—psorospermia.
Sur un cas de tubes psorospermiques observés chez l'homme with G. Saint-Remy, C. R. Soc. Biol., Paris, 10 s., 1: 201–202, Mar. 3, 1894

Barach, Alvan Leroy. New York physician. 1895–
Introduced therapeutic use of helium.
Use of helium as a new therapeutic gas. Proc. Soc. Exp. Biol., 32: 462–464. Dec. 1934
The use of helium in the treatment of asthma and obstructive lesions in the larynx and trachea. Ann. Int. M., 9: 739–765, Dec. 1935
APPARATUS—
A simple apparatus for administering oxygen. J. A. M. A., 78: 334–335, Feb. 4, 1922
CHAMBER—
An oxygen chamber simplified in design and operation. Ibid., 97: 390–391, Aug. 8, 1931
MASK—injector meter m. for oxygen inhalation.
Inhalational therapy equipment. By Mr. M. Eckman

and A. L. Barach, Mod. Hosp., 52: 78–84, Feb. 1939

TENT—
A portable oxygen tent with C. A. L. Binger, J. A. M. A., 85: 190–192, July 18, 1925
A new oxygen tent. Ibid., 87: 1213–1214, Oct. 9, 1926
See also R. L. Levy

Bárány, Robert. Vienna otologist. 1876–1936
Awarded Nobel prize in 1914.
Coined term "vestibular nystagmus."
SYMPTOM—in disturbances of equilibrium of the vestibular apparatus, the direction of fall is influenced by changing the position of the patient's head.
SYMPTOM or TEST—called also caloric test: if the normal ear is irrigated with hot water (110°–120°F.), a rotary nystagmus is developed toward the side of the irrigated ear; with cold water, a rotary nystagmus is developed away from the irrigated side; there is no nystagmus if the labyrinth is diseased.
Untersuchungen über den vom Vestibularapparat des Ohres reflektorisch ausgelösten rythmischen Nystagmus und seine Begleiterscheinugen. (Ein Beitrag zur Physiologie und Pathologie des Bogengangapparates). Mschr. Ohrenheilk., 40: 193–297, 1906; 41: 477–526, 1907
Also: Berlin, Coblenz, 1906. 107 pp.
Ueber die vom Ohrlabyrinth ausgelöste Gegenrollung der Augen bei Normalhörenden. Arch. f. Ohrenheilk, 58: 1–30, 1906
SYNDROME—unilateral deafness, vertigo, and pain in occipital region.
Vestibularapparat und Zentralnervensystem. Med. Klin., Berlin, 7: 1818–1821, 1911

Barasty, P. See P. Duval

Barber, Helene. See Florence Hulton-Frankel

Barber, Marshall Albert. American bacteriologist. 1868–
TECHNIC—"single cell."
On heredity in certain micro-organisms. Kansas Univ. Sci. Bull., 4: 3–48 (41), Mar. 1907
The rate of multiplication of Bacillus coli at different temperatures. J. infect. Dis., 5: 380–400, Oct. 20, 1908
See also C. A. Kofoid

Barberio, Michele. Naples pathologist. 1862–
TEST—for indican in urine.
Nuovo metodo per la ricerca dell' indicano nelle urine. Policlinico, 18: 517–519, Apr. 23, 1911

Barboni. See Armani

Barborka, Clifford Joseph. Rochester, Minn. physician. 1893–
Described insulin atrophy.
Fatty atrophy from injections of insulin: report of two cases. J. A. M. A., 87: 1646–1647, Nov. 13, 1926

Barbour, Alexander Hugh Freeland. Scottish obstetrician. 1856–1927
RING—retraction r. of uterus.
The anatomy of labor as studied in frozen sections, and its bearing on clinical work. Edinburgh, Johnston, 1889. 85 pp.

Barbour, Henry Gray. American physician. 1886–1943
METHOD—for determination of specific gravity of body fluids.
Blood specific gravity: its significance and a new method for its determination with W. F. Hamilton, Amer. J. Physiol., 69: 654–661, Aug. 1924
The falling drop method for determining specific gravity with W. F. Hamilton, J. Biol. Chem., 69: 625–640, Aug. 1926
The falling drop method for determining specific gravity. Some clinical applications with W. F. Hamilton, J. A. M. A., 88: 91–94, Jan. 8, 1927

Barcroft, Joseph. English physician. 1872–1947
OXYGEN CHAMBER—
The flow of oxygen through the pulmonary epithelium with A. Cook, H. Hartridge, T. R. Parsons and W. Parsons, J. Physiol., 53: 450–472, May 18, 1920
THEORY—
Observations upon the size of the spleen with J. G. Stephens, J. Physiol., 64: 1–22, Oct. 5, 1927
The blood in the spleen pulp with L. T. Poole, Ibid., pp. 23–29
See also T. Lewis, Stoke

Bard, Louis. Lyon physician. 1857–1930
SYNDROME—of Bard and Pic: "syndrome pancreatico-biliaire;" typical symptoms of cancer of the head of the pancreas are painless jaundice, distended gall bladder, cachexia and loss of weight.
Contribution à l'étude clinique et anatomo-pathologique du cancer primitif du pancréas with A. Pic, Rev. de méd., 8: 257–282; 363–405, 1888

Bard, Philip. Boston scientist. 1898–
Demonstrated a rage center in cats just posterior to the stalk of the pituitary.
A diencephalic mechanism for the expression of rage with special reference to the sympathetic nervous system. Amer. J. Physiol., 84: 490–515, 1928

Bard, Samuel. American physician. 1742–1821
Wrote early American contribution to medical ethics.
A discourse upon the duties of a physician, with some sentiments on the usefulness and necessity of a public hospital. New York, Robertson, 1769. 18 pp.
Described diphtheria.
An enquiry into the nature, cause, and cure of the angina suffocativa or sore throat distemper. New York, Insley and Car. 1771

Bardach, Bruno. Vienna chemist
TEST—for proteins.
Eine neue Reaktion des Eiweisses. Z. phys. Chem., 54: 355–358, Jan 28, 1908
TEST—for mercury in urine.
Zum Nachweis von Quecksilber im Harn. Z. anal. Chem., 40: 534–537, 1901

Bardeen, Charles Russell. American anatomist. 1871–1935
DISK—primitive: the embryonic structure which develops into the intervertebral ligament.
Development of the limbs, body-wall and back in man with W. H. Lewis, Amer. J. Anat., 1: 1–36, Nov. 7, 1901

Bardenheuer, Bernhard. German surgeon. 1839–1913
EXTENSION—for fractured limbs.
Die permanente Extensionsbehandlung. Die subacutanen und complicirten Fracturen und Luxationen der Extremitäten und ihre Folgen. Stuttgart, Enke, 1889. 810 pp.
OPERATION—interilio-abdominal amputation.
Exarticulatio femoris im Sacroiliacalgelenk. Verh. dtsch. Ges. Chir., 26: 1; 130, 1897
Abstr.: Zbl. Chir., 24: 132–134, 1897

OPERATION—for slipping patella.
  Ueber Kapselverengerung bei Gelenkaffektionen. (Brief report) Ibid., 27: 1027 (only), 1900
RESECTION—of sacroiliac joint.
  Ueber die Resektion der Synchondrosis Sacro-iliaca wegen Tuberkulose. Abstr. by Krecke: Zbl. Chir., 26: 1329 (only). Dec. 16, 1899
SPLENOPEXY—
  Ueber Splenopexis bei Wandermilz. Article is by Dr. Plucker, the patient was on the service of Dr. Bardenheuer. Ibid., 22: 905–907, Oct. 5, 1895
Bardet, Georges. French physician.
SYNDROME—of Bardet and Biedl: same as Frölich's s.
  Sur un syndrome d'obesité congénitale avec polydactylie et rétinite pigmentaire. Thesis de Paris, 1920
Bardsley, Sir James Lomax. Manchester physician. 1801–1876
Introduced emetin as a remedy for dysentery (amoebiasis). 1829
  Hospital facts and observations. London, Burgess & Hill, 1830. p. 149
Barfoed, Christen Thomsen. Swedish physician. 1815–1899
TEST and REAGENT—for glucose.
  Ueber die Nachweisung des Traubenzuckers neben Dextrin und verwandten Körpern. Z. anal. Chem., 12: 27–37, 1873
Bargen, Jacob Arnold. Rochester, Minn. physician. 1894–
BACILLUS or ORGANISM—specific in ulcerative colitis.
  Experimental studies on the etiology of chronic ulcerative colitis: preliminary report. J. A. M. A., 83: 332–336, Aug. 2, 1924
  The etiology of chronic ulcerative colitis: experimental studies with suggestions for a more rational form of treatment. Arch. intern. Med., 36: 818–829, Dec. 15, 1925
  Changing conceptions of chronic ulcerative colitis. J. A. M. A., 91: 1176–1181, Oct. 20, 1928
SERUM—
  Serum treatment for chronic ulcerative colitis with E. C. Rosenow and G. F. C. Fasting, Arch. intern. Med., 46: 1039–1047, Dec. 1930
TECHNIC—for recovery of Diplostreptococcus from case of ulcerative colitis.
  The management of colitis. New York, Nat. Med. Book Co., 1935 p. 233
  Suggested term "regional ileitis."
  Regional migratory chronic ulcerative colitis with H. M. Weber, S. G. O., 50: 964–972, June 1930
  See also P. W. Brown, F. W. Rankin
Barger, George. English scientist. 1878–1939
Isolated histamine from ergot.
  The presence in ergot and physiological activity of B-imidazolylethylamine with H. H. Dale, Abstr.: J. Physiol., 40: xxxviii–xxxix, 1910
  Also: Proc. Chem. Soc., 26: 128, 1910
Isolated histamine from animal intestinal mucosa.
  B-iminazolylethylamine, a depressor constituent of intestinal mucosa with H. H. Dale, J. Physiol., 41: 499–503, 1911
REACTION—thiocrome r. for vitamin Bi.
  A crystalline fluorescent dehydrogenation product from vitamin Bi with F. Bergel and A. R. Todd, Nature, 136: 259 (only), Aug. 17, 1935

Isolated ergotoxine.
  An active alkaloid from ergot with F. H. Carr and H. H. Dale, Brit. med. J., 2: 1792 (only), Dec. 22, 1906
Barillot, E. See P. Chastaing
Barkan, Otto. San Francisco ophthalmologist. 1887–
OPERATION—goniotomy.
  A new operation for chronic glaucoma: restoration of physiological function by opening Schlemm's canal under direct magnified vision. Amer. J. Ophth., 19: 951–966, Nov. 1936
  Recent advances in the surgery of chronic glaucoma. Ibid., 20: 1237–1245, Dec. 1937
Barker, Arthur Edward James. London surgeon
FORMULA—for spinal anesthesia.
  A report on clinical experiences with spinal analgesia in 100 cases, and some reflections on the procedure. Brit. med. J., 1: 665–674, Mar. 23, 1907
  A second report on clinical experiences with spinal analgesia: with a second series of one hundred cases. Ibid., 1: 244–249, Feb. 1, 1908
Barker, N. W. See N. M. Keith
Barker, Samuel Booth. Memphis, Tenn. physiologist. 1912–
METHOD—
  The direct colorimetric determination of urea in blood and urine. J. Biol. Chem., 152: 453–463, Feb. 1944
Barkow, Hans Carl Leopold. German anatomist. 1798–1873
LIGAMENT—the anterior and posterior l. of the elbow-joint.
  Syndesmologie, oder die Lehre von den Bändern, durch welche die Knochen des menschlichen Körpers zum Gerippe vereint werden. Breslau, Aderholz, 1841. 121 pp.
Barlow, Orpheus William. Albany physician. 1897–
TECHNIC—tranquilizing, in use of sedative.
  Comparative potentiating effects of certain therapeutic agents on sodium evipal hypnosis with D. R. Climenko and E. Homburger, Proc. Soc. Exper. Biol. & Med., 49: 11–13, Jan. 1942
Barlow, Sir Thomas. London physician. 1845–1945
DISEASE—infantile scurvy.
  On subcutaneous nodules connected with fibrous structures, occurring in children the subjects of rheumatism and chorea. Trans. Int. M. Cong., 4: 116–128, 1881
  On cases described as "acute rickets" which are probably a combination of scurvy and rickets, the scurvy being an essential, and the rickets a variable, element. Med.-Chir. Trans., London, 66: 159–219, 1883
  Notes on rheumatism and its allies in childhood. Brit. M. J., 2: 509–514, Sept. 15, 1883
Described subphrenic abscess in children.
  Perforation of the stomach, with obscure thoracic symptoms. London M. Gaz., 1: 13–16, 1845
Described non-suppurative encephalitis.
  On a case of early disseminated myelitis occurring in the exanthem stage of measles and fatal on the eleventh day of that disease with F. G. Penrose, Med.-Chir. Trans., London, 70: 77–91, 1887
Barnard, H. See L. E. Hill
Barnard, Joseph Edwin. English scientist
ORGANISM—of Gye and Barnard, of cancer.
  The microscopical examination of filterable viruses associated with malignant new growths. Lancet, 2: 117–123, July 18, 1925

Barnard, William George. London physician. 1892–
CARCINOMA—oat-celled.
The nature of the "oat-celled sarcoma" of the mediasti-
num. J. Path. Bact., 29: 241–244, July 1926
Barnes, Algernon S., Jr. St. Louis physician. 1831–
METHOD—
Method of demonstrating living trichinae. Amer.
month. micros. J., 14: 104 (only), Apr. 1893
Barnes, Robert. English obstetrician. 1817–1907
BAG or DILATOR—a rubber bag for dilating the
cervix uteri.
The physiology and treatment of placenta praevia;
being the Lettsomian lectures on midwifery for 1857.
London, Churchill, 1858. 208 pp.
CURVE—the segment of a circle whose center is the
promontory of the sacrum, the concavity looking
dorsad. (Dorland)
On the mechanism of labour, more especially with
reference to Naegele's obliquity and the influence of the
lumbo-sacral curve. Trans. Obstet. Soc. London,
1883, 25: 258–290, 1884
Barnett, B. See R. G. MacFarlane
Barney, James Dellinger. Boston urologist. 1878–
SIGN—of ureteral calculus.
A tender point one inch downward from McBurney's
point, on right or left side of abdomen. A point in the
clinical diagnosis of ureteral calculus. Ann. Surg.,
107: 636–639, 1938
See also H. W. Sulkowitch
Baronio, Giuseppe. Italian surgeon. 1759–1811
Pioneer in experimental surgery on animals.
Degli innesti animali. Milan, 1804. 78 pp.
Opuscoli di fisica animale e chirurgia. Milano, Pirola,
n. d. 82 pp. In D.S.G.
Barr, David Preswick. St. Louis physician. 1889–
Reported proved case of hyperparathyroidism and
coined the term.
Hyperparathyroidism. J. A. M. A., 92: 951–952,
Mar. 23, 1929
Barraquer, Ignacio. Spanish ophthalmologist
TECHNIC—in incipient cataract.
Un procédé d'extrême douceur pour l'extraction "in
toto" de la cataracte with Anduyned, Clin. Ophthal.,
Paris, 22: 329–333, 1917
Also: Siglo med., 64: 266, Apr. 21, 1917 et seq.
Barre, J. A. See G. Guillain
Barrenscheen, Hermann Karl. Austrian biochemist.
1887–
TEST—for bismuth in urine.
Zum Nachweis kleinster Wismutmengen im Harn
with Margarete Frey, Mikrochemie, pp. 1–5, Sept.
3, 1929
Barret, Harvey Park. American bacteriologist. 1885–
MEDIUM—for cultivation of amoebae of cold-blooded
vertebrates.
Cultivation of Endoamoeba ranarum with N. M. Smith,
Ann. trop. Med., 20: 85–88, Fen. 1926
METHOD—for cultivation of Balantidium coli.
Cultivation of Balantidium coli with N. Yarbrough,
Amer. J. Trop. Med., 1: 161–164, May 1921
Barret, John Frederick. London chemist
TEST—for acetone in urine.
A simple micro-test for acetone in urine. Biochem. J.,
30: 888–889, May 1936
TEST—for nitrogen retention in blood.
A simple test for gross nitrogen retention in the blood.
Lancet, 1: 84, Jan. 11, 1936

Barrett, Normal Rupert. English surgeon. 1903–
METHOD or INCISION—for diaphragmatic hernia.
The pathology, diagnosis, and treatment of congenital
diaphragmatic hernia in infants with C. E. W.
Wheaton, Brit. J. Surg., 21: 420–433, Jan. 1934
Barringer, Benjamin Stockwell. New York urol-
ogist. 1878–
METHOD or OPERATION—removal of papilloma
of bladder by an endotherm snare and insertion of
gold radon seeds into base of tumor.
The past and present in genito-urinary carcinoma:
bladder, prostate, testicle, penis. Amer. J. Surg., 23:
438–441, Mar. 1934
Barrón, E. S. Guzmán. Peru-American physician.
1898–
TEST—
Bilirubinemia. Medicine, 10: 77–133, Feb. 1931
See also G. A. Harrop
Barrow, A(lbert) Boyce. London surgeon
OPERATION—for pharyngeal diverticula.
A case of esophageal pouch successfully treated by
excision. Lancet, 1: 928–929, Apr. 8, 1905
Barrows, E. See A. W. Ulin
Barry, G. London scientist
Isolated from tar pure compounds which are capable
of inducing malignant disease.
The production of cancer by pure hydrocarbons. Part
III with J. W. Cook, G. A. D. Haslewood, C. L.
Hewett, I. Hieger & E. L. Kennaway, Proc. Roy.
Soc., ser. B., 117: 318–350, Apr. 1, 1935
Barry, Martin. English biologist. 1802–1855
Observed union of spermatozoön with ovum.
RETINACULA—set of filaments within the graafian
follicles.
Early stages of the ovum of the mammalia and other
vertebrata. Philos. Trans., London, pp. 301–341,
1838
Researches in embryology. London, Taylor, 1839
Barsiekow, Max. German bacteriologist
MEDIUM or SOLUTION—basal salt pepton, cul-
ture medium for differentiation of colon typhoid
group.
Beiträge zur Differentialdiagnose des Typhusbacillus.
Wien. klin. Rund., 15: 823–825, Nov. 2, 1901
Bartel, Julius. Vienna pathologist
MODIFICATION—of Wiegert's method of nerve
staining.
Zur Technik der Gliafärbung. A. wiss. Mikr., 21:
18–22, 1904
Bartelink, D. L. German physician
Described tomography.
Röntgenschnitte. Fort. a. d. Geb. d. Röntgenstrahl.,
47: 399–407, 1933
Barth, Jean Baptiste (père). German physician.
1806–1877
HERNIA—beneath a persistent vitelline duct.
Observations et réflexions sur quelques cas de hernies
inguinales et crurales. Strasbourg, 1836. 49 pp.
Barthe de Sandfort, Edmond French physician
Introduced ambrine (paraffin-resin solution) in
treatment of burns.
La kéritherapie (nouvelle balnéation thermocireuse).
J. de Méd. Int., Paris, 17: 211–214, 1913
Barthel, Chr. Stockholm bacteriologist
SOLUTION—albumin; culture medium.
Obligat anaërobe Bakterien in Milch und Molkerei-
produkten. Zbl. f. Bakt., 2 Abt., 26: 1–47, 1910

Barthélemy, P. Toussaint. French dermatologist. 1850–1906
DISEASE—acnitis.
De l'acnitis ou d'une variété spéciale de folliculites et périfolliculites généralisées et disséminées. Ann. Dermat. et Syphil., 22: 1–38, Jan. 25, 1891
Étude sur le dermagraphisme ou dermoneurose toxivasomotrice. Paris, 1893

Barthez, Paul-Joseph. French physician. 1734–1806
Introduced term "vital principle" (vitalis agens) to denote the cause of the phenomena in the living body. (Garrison)
Oratio academica de principio vitali hominis:— Monspelii, Rochard, 1773. 28 pp.

Bartholinus, Caspar. Danish anatomist. 1654–1738
GLANDS—vulvovaginal.
Exercitationes miscellaneae varii argumenti in primis anatomici. Lugd. Bat., ex. off. Hackiana, 1675. 151 pp.

Bartholinus, Thomas. Danish anatomist. 1616–1680
ANUS—aditus ad aqualductum cerebri.
CANAL—the duct of Bartholin's gland.
DUCT—the larger of the sublingual ducts.
FORAMEN—obturator foramen.
Described the adrenal medulla.
Anatomia,—Lugd. Bat., Hackium, 1651. 576 pp.
Claimed discovery of intestinal lymphatics and their connection with the thoracic duct. (Garrison)
De lacteis thoracicis in homine brutisque nuperrimé observatis, historia anatomica. Hafniae, Martzan, 1652. 71 pp.

Bartle, H. J. See B. B. V. Lyon

Bartlett, Edwin I. San Francisco surgeon. 1883–
TECHNIC—of suprahyoid neck dissection.
Neck dissections with C. L. Callander, Surg. Clin. No. Amer., 6: 481–504, Apr. 1926

Bartlett, Elisha. American physician. 1804–1855
Made clear differentiation between typhoid and typhus fevers.
The history, diagnosis and treatment of typhoid and of typhus fever, with an essay on the diagnosis of bilious remittent and of yellow fever. Phila., Lea & Blanchard, 1842. 393 pp.

Bartlett, R. M. See F. A. Collier

Bartlett, Ralph W. American scientist
METHOD—of treatment of congenital dislocation of hip.
Mechanism for reducing congenitally dislocated hips. J. med. Res., 10: 440–448, Dec. 1903

Bartlett, Willard. St. Louis surgeon. 1868–
FILIGREE—of silver-wire.
An improved filigree for the repair of large defects in the abdominal wall. Ann. Surg., 38: 47–62, July 1903

Bartley, Elias Hudson. American physician. 1849–
METHOD—for determination of uric acid.
Medical chemistry. Philadelphia, 1904

Barton, A. L.
BACILLUS—Bartonella or Bartonia bacilliformis, the blood parasite causing Oroya fever.
Descripción de elementos endo-globulares hallados en las enfermos de fiebre verrucosa. Crón. Méd., Lima, 26: 7–10, 1909

Barton, John Rhea. American surgeon. 1794–1871
FRACTURE—of the distal end of the radius.
Views and treatment of an important injury of the wrist. Med. Exam., Phila., 1: 365–368, Nov. 7, 1838

OPERATION—for ankylosis of knee, by removinga V shaped piece.
On the treatment of anchylosis, by the formation of artificial joints. N. Amer. Med. & Surg. J., 3: 279–292, 1826
Also: Phila., Harding, 1827. 17 pp.

Baruch, Simon. New York physician. 1840–1921
LAW—when the temperature of water used in a bath is above or below that of the skin, the effect is stimulating: when both temperatures are the same, the effect is sedative.
The principles and practice of hydrotherapy. N. Y., Wood, 1898. 435 pp.
SIGN—of typhoid fever: resistance of the temperature in the rectum to a bath of 65°F. for 15 minutes.
The treatment of typhoid fever. Trans. N. Y. Med. Soc., pp. 90–103, 1889

Barwell, Richard. London surgeon. 1826–1916
OPERATION—osteotomy for genu valgum by division of the tibia.
A treatise on diseases of the joints. Phila., Blanchard & Lea, 1861. 463 pp.
Also: London, Hardwicke, 1865. 469 pp.
OPERATION—excision of cancer of tongue by use of two ecraseurs.
A lecture on cancer of the tongue and its removal. Brit. M. J., 1: 697–698, Mar. 30, 1899

von Basch, Samuel Siegfried Karl. Vienna scientist. 1837–1905
Invented a sphygmomanometer and made scientific blood pressure measurements.
Die volumetrische Bestimmung des Blutdrucks am Menschen. Med. Jahrb., 6, 1876
Also: Wien, Ueberreuter, 1876. 30 pp.
Ueber die Messung des Blutdrucks am Menschen. Z. Klin. Med., 2: 79–96, 1881
Ein Metall-Sphygmomanometer. Wien. Med. Wschr., 33: 673–675, 1883

von Basedow, Karl Adolf. Merseburg physician. 1799–1854
DISEASE—exophthalmic goiter.
TRIAD—Merseburg t.: goiter, exophthalmos and tachycardia, the three cardinal symptoms of Basedow's disease.
Exophthalmos durch Hypertrophie des Zellgewebes in der Augenhöhle. Wschr. f. d. ges. Heilk., Berlin, 6: 197–204, Mar. 28: 220–228, Apr. 4, 1840

Baseilhac, Jean. See Frère Côme

Basham, William Richard. English physician. 1804–1877
MIXTURE—liquor ferri et ammonii acetatis.
In his: *Renal diseases.* London, Churchill, 1870. 244 pp.

Bashford, Ernest Francis. London physician. 1873–1923
Showed that animals once successfully inoculated against cancer are resistant to a second inoculation.
Scientific report on the investigations of the Imperial Cancer Research Fund. 5th Scient. Rep., p. 29, 1912

Bass, Charles Cassedy. American physician. 1875–
CHAMBER—blood counting c. of Bass and Johns.
Practical clinical laboratory diagnosis with F. M. Johns, N. Y., Rebman, 1917. 178 pp.
METHOD—of centrifugation for concentration of Malarial parasites.

A method of concentrating malaria plasmodia for diagnostic and other purposes with F. M. Johns, Amer. J. Trop. Dis., 3: 298–303, Nov. 1915
METHOD—for culture of plasmodia of malaria in vitro.
The cultivation of malarial plasmodia (Plasmodium Vivax and Plasmodium Falciparum) in vitro with F. M. Johns, J. Exp. Med., 16: 567–579, Oct. 1912
TEST—for typhoid fever.
A quick macroscopic typhoid agglutination test with J. A. Watkins, Arch. intern. Med., 6: 717–729, Dec. 1910

Basset, Antoine. French surgeon. 1882–
OPERATION—total vulvectomy.
L'epithélioma primitif du clitoris; son retentissement ganglionnaire et son traitement opératoire. Paris, Thèses, 1912. Steinheil, 131 pp.

Bassi, Agostino. Italian physician. 1773–1856
Found the pathogenic organism (Botrytis Bassiana) of silkworm disease, or muscardine. 1837 (Garrison)
Founder of the doctrine of pathogenic micro-organisms. (L. T. Morton)
Del mal del segno calcinaccio o muscardino, malattia che affige i bachi da seta e sul modo di liberarne le bigattaje anche le piu infestate. Lodi, Orcesi, 1835–36. 2 vols.

Bassini, Edoardo. Italian surgeon. 1846–1924
OPERATION—for inguinal hernia.
Nuovo metodo per la cura radicale dell'ernia inguinale. Padova, Prosperini, 1889. 106 pp.
Ueber die Behandlung des Leistenbruches. Arch. f. klin. Chir., 40: 429–476, 1890
OPERATION—for femoral hernia.
Nuovo metodo operativo per la cura radicale dell'ernia crurale. Padova, Draghi, 1893
Neue Operations-Methode zur Radicalbehandlung der Schenkelhernie. Arch. f. klin. Chir., 47: 1–25, 1894
OPERATION—modification of Hahn's nephropexy.
Un caso di rene mobile fissato col mezzo dell'operazione cruenta. Ann. Univ. di Med., Milano, 261: 281–286, 1882

Bastedo, Walter Arthur. New York physician. 1873–
SIGN or TEST—
The dilatation test for chronic appendicitis. Amer. J. Med. Sci., 142: 11–14, July 1911

Bastian, Henry Charlton. London neurologist. 1837–1915
LAW—loss of all reflexes in total obstruction of the conducting paths of the cord, high up. Stedman
On the symptomatology of total transverse lesions of the spinal cord; with special reference to the condition of the various reflexes. Med.-chir. Trans., 73: 151–217, 1890
Also: Proc. Roy. Med. and Surg. Soc., London, 2: 69–75, 1890
Described word blindness.
On the various forms of loss of speech in cerebral disease. Brit. and For. Med.-chir. Rev., London, 43: 209–236, 1869
Also: pp. 470–492.
On the different kinds of aphasia, with special reference to their classification and ultimate pathology. Brit. med. J., 2: 931–936, 1887
A treatise on aphasia and other speech defects. London, Lewis, 1898. 366 pp.

Bataillon, E. French physician

STAIN—borax methylene blue, for gonads.
Observations sur les phenomènes karyokinétiques dans les cellules du blastoderme des Téléostéens with R. Koehler, C. R. Soc. Biol., Paris, 117: 521–524, Oct. 16, 1893

Batchelder, A. P. See K. F. Meyer

Bate, John Throckmorton, Jr. Louisville, Ky. surgeon. 1897–
FASCIA STRIPPER—
Instrument for subcutaneous removal of fascia lata strips for suture purposes. Ann. Surg., 95: 313–314, Feb. 1932

Bateman, Thomas. English physician. 1778–1821
DISEASE—mulluscum contagiosum.
Delineations of cutaneous diseases exhibiting the characteristic appearances of the principal genera and species comprised in the classification of the late Dr. Willan; and completing the series of engravings begun by that author. (Atlas of 72 colored plates), London, Longman, 1817
HERPES IRIS—
Ibid., Plate 52
PURPURA SENILIS—
Ibid., Plate 30
Described lichen urticatus.
A practical synopsis of cutaneous diseases. London, 1813. 2 ed.

Bates, Uri C. Seattle surgeon. 1875–
OPERATION—
New operation for the cure of indirect inguinal hernia. J. A. M. A., 60: 2032–3033, June 28, 1913

Bates, William Horatio. American surgeon
OPERATION—
On the necessity of sufficiently extended urethral incisions for the permanent cure of strictures of the urethra. New York M. J., 25: 5–13, Jan. 1877

Bateson, William. American physician. 1861–1926
Noted phenomena of linkage of chromosomes.
Further experiments on inheritance in sweet peas and stocks with R. C. Punnett, Proc. roy. Soc., s. B., 77: 236–238, 1906

Batko, J. See A. Krokiewicz

Batson, Oscar Vivian. Philadelphia anatomist. 1894–
TECHNIC—of injection of vertebral veins.
The function of the vertebral veins and their role in the spread of metastases. Ann, Surg., 112: 138–149, July 1940

Batten, Frederick Eustace. British neurologist. 1865–1918
DISEASE—Batten-Mayou d.; juvenile amaurotic idiocy.
Cerebral degeneration with symmetrical changes in the maculae in two members of a family. Trans. Ophthal. Soc. U. King., 23: 386–390, 1903
TYPE—
Two cases of myotonia atrophica, showing a peculiar distribution of muscular atrophy with H. P. Gibb, Proc. R. Soc. Med., 2: neur. sect., 32, 1908–09
Myotonia atrophica with H. P. Gibb, Brain, 32: 187–205, Aug. 1909
See also J. S. R. Russell

Battey, Robert. Augusta, Ga. gynecologist. 1828–1895
OPERATION—normal ovariotomy, or the induction of menopause by oöphorectomy.

First communication: J. Gynecol. Soc., Boston, 7: 331-335, 1872

Normal ovariotomy—case. Atlanta M. & S. J., 10: 321-329, Sept. 1872

Also: Trans. Med. Ass. Georgia, 24: 36-69, 1873

Battle, William Henry. London surgeon. 1855-1936

INCISION—for abdominal section, a vertical incision of the rectus sheaths with retraction of the rectus inward; called also Kammerer or Jaboulay or Lennander i.

Modified incision for removal of vermiform appendix. Brief note. Brit. M. J., 2: 1360, Nov. 30, 1895

A case of incision for removal of appendix, arranged for the certain prevention of hernia. Brief note. Trans. Clin. Soc., 29: 227, 1896

A contribution to the surgical treatment of diseases of the appendix vermiform. Brit. M. J., 1: 965-967, Apr. 17, 1897

OPERATION—for femoral hernia.

A clinical lecture on femoral hernia. Lancet, 1: 302-305, Feb. 2, 1901

The radical cure of femoral hernia. Edinburgh M. J., 23: 489-496, June 1908

SIGN—in fracture of posterior cranial fossa, blood accumulates beneath deep fascia, produces discoloration in line of posterior auricular artery and first appears near tip of mastoid.

Three lectures on some points relating to injuries to the head. Brit. M. J., 2: 75-81, July 12, 1890

Baudelocque, Jean Louis, Sr. French obstetrician. 1746-1810

Invented a pelvimeter.

DIAMETER or LINE—the external conjugate diameter of pelvis.

L'art des accouchements. Paris, Méquignon, 1781. 2 vols.

Baudelocque, Louis Auguste, Jr. French obstetrician. 1800-1864

OPERATION—extraperitoneal cesarian section.

Nouveau moyen pour délivrer les femmes contre faites à terme et en travail, substitué à l'operation appelée césarienne;—— Paris, 1824. 30 pp.

Opération césarienne. Élytrotomie ou section du vagin, précédée, or non, de la ligature, ou de la compression de l'artère iliaque interne. Paris, l'auteur, 1844. 26 pp.

Baudisch, O. See Elizabeth Dyer

Baudouin, A. See H. Claude, F. Levy

Baudouin, F. Tours physician

REACTION—for bile in urine.

Un nouveau réactif des pigments biliaires dans l'urine. Semaine méd., 22: 398-399, Dec. 3, 1902

Bauer, C. P. See A. E. Kanter

Bauer, J. H. See A. Stokes

Bauer, Julius. Düsseldorf physician

TEST—for differentiation of cow's milk and human milk.

Ueber eine Reaktion zur Unterscheidung von Kuh- und Frauenmilch. Mschr. Kinderheilk., 11: 474-475, 1913

TEST—modification of Wassermann t.

Simplification de la technique du sérodiagnostic de la syphilis. Semainé med., 28: 429-430, Sept. 2, 1908

Bauer, Karl Heinrich. Göttingen surgeon. 1890-

Described the "Magenstrasse."

Ueber das Wesen der Magenstrasse. Arch. f. klin. Chir., 124: 567-659, June 23, 1923

HYPOTHESIS—of inheritance of blood groups.

Zur Lösung des Problems der Blutgruppenvererbung. Klin. Wschr., 7: 1588-1592, Aug. 19, 1928

Bauer, R. See R. Fontaine

Bauer, Richard. Vienna physician

TEST—of liver function; depends on the detection of galactose in urine after peroral administration of 30 Gm. of galactose, which is not eliminated by normal livers.

Ueber die Assimilation von Galaktose und Milchzucker beim Gesunden und Kranken. Wien. med. Wschr., 56: 20-23, Jan. 1, 1906

Weitere Untersuchungen über alimentäre Galaktosurie. Ibid., 2532-2546, Dec. 22, 1906

Bauer, Walter. Boston surgeon. 1898-

DISEASE—(see Fuller Albright)

A case of osteitis fibrosa cystica (osteomalacia?) with evidence of hyperactivity of the parathyroid bodies. Metabolic study II with F. Albright and J. C. Aub, J. Clin. Invest., 8: 229-248, Feb. 20, 1930

Bauhin, Caspar. Swiss anatomist. 1560-1624

GLANDS—mixed glands near the tip of the tongue; same as Nuck's, Nuhm's or Blondin's g.

VALVE—ileocecal v.

De humani corporis—Basel, 1588

Baum, Fritz. German ophthalmologist

OPHTHALMOFUNDOSKOP—

"Ophthalmo-Fundoskop". Ein neues Instrument zur Untersuchung des Augenhintergrundes in bisher nicht erzielten Vergrösserungen bei reflexlosem Bilde. Klin. Mbl. Augenheilk., 47: 161-164, Aug. 18, 1909

Baumann, Eugen. Freiburg i. B. physician. 1846-1896

Introduced trional and tetronal.

Ueber die Beziehungen zwischen chemischer Constitution und physiologischer Wirkung bei einigen Sulfonen with A. Kast, Z. phys. Chem., 14: 52-74, 1890

Demonstrated iodine in thyroid gland.

Ueber das normale Vorkommen von Jod im Tierkörper. Ibid., 21: 319-330; 481-493, 1895; 22: 1-17, 1896

TEST—for free acids in gastric juice.

COEFFICIENT—the ration of ethereal to total sulphates in urine.

Ueber die synthetischen Processe im Thierkörper. Berlin, Hirschwald, 1878. 31 pp.

Introduced sulphonal.

Ueber Disulfone. Ber. dtsch. chem. Ges., 19: 2808-2814, 1886

Baumé, Antoine. French chemist. 1728-1805

SCALE—a hydrometer s. for determining the specific gravity of liquids.

Éléments de pharmacie théorique et pratique;—— Paris, Samson, 1769. 2 ed. 1017 pp.

Baumgarten, Paul Clemens von. German pathologist. 1848-1928

STAINING—for bacillus of leprosy.

Ueber Untersuchungsmethoden zur Unterscheidung von Lepra- und Tuberkelbacillen. Z. wiss. Mikro., 1: 367-371, 1884

STAIN—carmine and aniline blue, for cartilage and nerve centers.

Beiträge zur Entwicklungsgeschichte der Gehörknöchelchen. Arch. mikr. Anat., 40: 512-530, 1892

SYNDROME—of Cruveilhier-Baumgarten; dilated veins in abdominal wall, patent umbilical vein, caput Medusa and loud venous murmur at umbilicus.

E. L. Armstrong et al.

*Ueber Vollständiges Offenbleiben der Vena Umbili-
calis; zugleich ein Beitrag zur Frage des Morbus
Bantii.* Baumgarten Arbeiten, 1908, 6
Arb. a. d. Geb. d. path. Anat. . . . Inst. zu Tübing,
Leipzig, 6: 93–110, 1907
Baumgartner, Leona. See Alice C. Evans
Baunscheidt, Carl. Swiss inventor
TREATMENT—of chronic rheumatism, etc., by
acupuncture.
Der Braunscheidtismus. Bonn, Whittmann, 1857. 5
Aufl.
Bausch, Johannes Laurentius.
Famous patient suffering with trigeminal neuralgia.
See Johannes Michael Fehr.
Baxter, Henry. Glasgow physician
MODIFICATION—of the tryptophan reaction for
the early diagnosis of meningeal tuberculosis.
*The tryptophane reaction as an aid to the early diagno-
sis of meningeal tuberculosis.* Edinburgh M. J., 44:
663–668, Oct. 1937
Bayer, Gustav. Innsbrück physician. 1879–
REACTION—for adrenaline.
*Methoden zur Verschärfung von Adrenalin und
Brenzcatechinreaktionen.* Biochem. J., 20: 178–188,
1909
Bayle, Antoine Laurant Jessé. French physician.
1799–1858
DISEASE—dementia paralytica or general paralysis
of the insane.
Recherches sur les maladies mentales. Paris Thesis,
1822. 109 pp.
Bayle, Gaspard Laurent. French physician. 1774–
1816
Described the coarse characters of the tubercle and
its identity with the pulmonary, granular and other
varieties of tuberculosis, in 1803. Formed a basis for
Laennec's work in 1819.
GRANULATION—gray tubercular nodules of the
lung that have undergone fibroid degeneration.
Recherches sur la phthisie pulmonaire. Paris, Gabon,
1810. 439 pp.
Also, transl. by Barrow. Liverpool, Longman, 1815.
479 pp.
Bayles, Theodore Bevier. Boston physician. 1911–
YARDSTICK—
*A yardstick for rheumatoid arthritis applied to pa-
tients receiving gold-salt therapy* with M. G. Hall,
New Engl. J. Med., 228: 418–421, Apr. 1, 1943
Bayliss, Sir William Maddock. English physician.
1860–1924
Described peristalsis of the intestines as a reflex
through the intrinsic ganglia.
The movements and innervation of the small intestine
with E. H. Starling, J. Physiol., 24: 99–143, May
11, 1899
*The movements and the innervation of the large intes-
tine* with E. H. Starling, Ibid., 26: 107–118, Dec. 31,
1900
Demonstrated cause and mechanism of pancreatic
secretion (secretin).
*Preliminary communication on the causation of the
so-called "peripheral reflex secretion" of the pancreas*
with E. H. Starling, Lancet, 1: 813 (only), Mar. 22,
1902
The mechanism of pancreatic secretion with E. H.
Starling, J. Physiol., 28: 325–353, 1902

Developed theory of chemical control of the body by
means of hormones.
The chemical regulation of the secretory process with
E. H. Starling, Proc. Roy. Soc. London, 73: 310–322,
Mar. 21, 1904
Described the role of capillaries in wound shock.
Intravenous injection in wound shock. London and
New York, Longmans, Green, 1918. 172 pp.
Bayne-Jones, Stanhope. American pathologist. 1888–
TEST—flocculation, for titration of toxins and anti-
toxins.
*The titration of diphtheria toxin and antitoxin by
Ramon's flocculation method.* J. Immunol., 9: 481–
504, Nov. 1924
Baynton, Thomas. English physician. 1761–1820
OPERATION—application of adhesive straps and a
bandage to indolent leg ulcers.
*Descriptive account of a new method of treating old
ulcers of the legs.* London, Robinson, 1797. 115 pp.
TREATMENT—
*An account of a successful method of treating diseases
of the spine.* London, Longman, 1813
Bayon, Henry Peter G. English physician
Produced cancer by injection of tar.
*Epithelial proliferation induced by the injection of gas-
works tar.* Lancet, 2: 1579, 1912
Bayrac, Henri Pierre. French physician
TEST—for uric acid in urine.
Étude du rapport de l'azote de l'urée à l'azote total.
Lyon, 1887. 59 pp.
Bazin, Antoine Pierre Ernest. French dermatologist.
1807–1878
Brought order out of chaos in the field of parasitol-
ogy in dermatology (Goodman).
Reported favorable influence of an acute infection on
mycosis fungoides.
DISEASE—buccal psoriasis.
DISEASE—erythema induratum.
Described acne varioliformis.
De l'acné varioliforme. Paris, Brière, 1851. 24 pp.
*Leçons théoriques et cliniques sur les affections cu-
tanées parasitaires.* Paris, Chamerot & Delahaye,
1858. 236 pp.
Leçons sur la scrofule. . . . Paris, 1861 2 éd. p. 145;
501
Beach, A. See C. S. Venable
Beach, M. V. English surgeon
OPERATION—
*Inguinal hernia: a new operation with special applica-
tion to the services.* Brit. J. Surg., 32: 499–504, Apr.
1945
Beacon, Dean N. Denver, Col. physician
METHOD—
*A modification of Goodpasture's technic for the peroxi-
dase reaction in blood smears.* J. Lab. clin. Med., 11:
1092–1093, Aug. 1926
Béal, Raymond. French ophthalmologist
TYPE—
*Sur une forme particulière de conjonctivite aigue avec
follicules.* Ann. d'Ocul., 137: 1–33, Jan. 1907
Beale, Lionel Smith. London scientist. 1828–1896
CELLS—of ganglia; bipolar c.
*On the anatomy of nerve-fibers and cells, and the ulti-
mate distribution of nerve-fibers.* Abstr.: Quart. J.
Micr. Soc., n.s.3: 97–109, 1863
*On the structure of the so-called apolar, unipolar, and
bipolar nerve-cells of the frog.* Ibid., pp. 302–307

New observations upon the structure and formation of certain nervous centers—London, Churchill, 1864. 31 pp.
Beall, D. See E. G. L. Bywaters
Bean, W. B. See T. D. Spies
Beard, George Miller. New York physician. 1839–1883
DISEASE—neurasthenia or nervous exhaustion.
Neurasthenia or nervous exhaustion. Boston M. & S. J., 80: 217–221, Apr. 29, 1869
Neurasthenia (nerve exhaustion); with remarks on treatment. St. Louis M. & S. J., 1879
Also: New York, Wood, 1879. 20 pp.
A practical treatise on nervous exhaustion (neurasthenia); its symptoms, nature, sequences, treatment. New York, Wood, 1880. 198 pp.
TREATMENT—of cancer.
A new method of treating malignant tumors by electrolyzing the base. Arch. Electrol. & Neurol., 1: 74–89, May 1874
Beardsley, Hezekiah. Connecticut physician. 1748–1790
Described case of "schirrosity of pylorus."
Congenital hypertrophic stenosis of the pylorus.
Cases and observations by the Medical Society of New Haven County in the State of Connecticut. New Haven, Meigs, 1788. pp. 81–84
also reprinted by W. Osler in: Arch. Pediat., 20: 355–357, 1903
Beatson, George Thomas. Glasgow surgeon. 1848–1933
OPERATION—ovariotomy in cases of inoperable cancer of the breast, on the theory that lack of the internal secretion of the ovary will produce atrophy of the tumor.
On the treatment of inoperable cancer of the mamma; suggestions for a new method of treatment, with illustrative cases. Lancet, 2: 104–107; 162–165, 1896
The treatment of cancer of the breast by oöphorectomy and thyroid extract. Brit. med. J., 2: 1145–1148, 1901
Beatty, W. See P. A. T. Levene
Beau, Joseph Honoré Simon. French physician. 1806–1865
DISEASE or SYNDROME—cardiac insufficiency, asystolia.
Recherches d'anatomie pathologique sur une forme particulière de dilatation et d'hypertrophie du coeur. Arch. gén. de méd., 2 s., 10: 428–447, Apr. 1836
LINES—transverse lines on the finger nails seen after wasting diseases.
Note sur certains caractères de séméiologie rétrospective présentés par les ongles. Ibid., 4 s., 11: 447–458, Aug. 1846
Beaulieu, Jacques de or Frere Jacques. 1651–1714
"A strolling incisor". Garrison
Introduced the lateral operation for stone in 1697.
Beaumé, Lucien. French physician. 1865–
SIGN—sternalgia or pain beneath the sternum in angina pectoris.
Contribution à l'étude des myocardites; évolution; étiologie; pathogénie. Paris, 1892. 88 pp.
Beaumont, William. American physician. 1785–1853
First to study digestion and movements of the stomach in situ.
A case of wounded stomach. (Erroneously reported over name of J. Lovell.) M. Recorder, Phila., 8: 14–19; 840, 1825

Further experiments on the case of Alexis San Martin who was wounded in the stomach by a load of duck shot, detailed in the Recorder for Jan. 1825. M. Recorder, 9: 94–97, 1826
Experiments and observations on the gastric juice and the physiology of digestion. Plattsburgh, Allen, 1833. 280 pp.
Also: Facsimile of ed. of 1833, Cambridge, Harvard Univ. Press, 1929
Beauperthuys, Louis Daniel. Guadeloupe physician. 1803–1871
Advanced theory of mosquito transmission of yellow fever.
TREATMENT—of leprosy with bichloride of mercury.
Travaux scientifiques. Gaceta oficial di Cumana, 57, 1854
Also: Bordeaux, Berlier, 1891
Becher, E. See C. F. W. Ludwig
Becher, Friedrich Erwin. Halle physician. 1890–
TEST—for kidney insufficiency.
Die Diazo- und Urochromogenreaktion im Blutfiltrat bei Niereninsufficienz, ihre Erklärung und klinische Bedeutung. Dtsch. Arch. klin. Med., 148: 10–18, July 1925
*Studien über das Verhalten der Xanthoproteinreaktion im entweissten Blut unter normalen und pathologischen Verhältnisse; II Mitteilung. Die Xanthroproteinkolorimeterwerte bei Krankheiten,*with Elfriede Herrmann, Ibid., 152: 82–98, July 1926
Becher, Wolf. German physician. 1862–1906
Introduced a solution of lead into the stomach of a guinea-pig, making it opaque to x-rays, and showing the possibility of radiological diagnosis of gastric disease. Garrison and Morton.
Zue Abwendung des Röntgenschen Verfahrens in der Medicin. Dtsch. ed. Wschr., 22: 202, 1896
Bechterew, Vladimir Mikhailowich von. Russian neurologist. 1857–1927
LAYER—of fibers in cerebral cortex between Baillarger's layer and tangential fibers: called also Kaes-Bechterew line.
Zur Frage über die äusseren Associationsfasern der Hirnrinde. Neurol. Zbl., 10: 682–684, July 16, 1891
NUCLEUS—origin of fibers of median and vestibular roots of auditory nerve; called also nucleus angularis and nucleus vestibuli.
(Origin and course of striae medullares s. acousticae.) Med. Obozr., Mosk., 37: 470–478, 1892
(Tracts of the spinal cord and brain; —) St. Petersburg, Rikker, 1892. 2 ed. 390 pp.
Die Functionen der Nervencentra with Weinberg, Jena, 1908. 2 ed., 1909
DISEASE—spondylitis deformans.
Oderevenielost pozvonochnika s iskrevleniyem yevo kak osobaya forma zabolievaniya. Wrach. St. Petersburg, 13: 899–902, 1892
Steifigkeit der Wirbelsäule und ihre Verkrümmung als besondere Erkrankungsform. Neurol. Zbl., 12: 426–434, 1893
REFLEX—dilatation of pupil on exposure to light, seen in tabes and general paralysis.
Die Bedeutung der pathologischen-anatomischen Veränderungen in der progressiven Paralyse der Irren bezüglich des Auftretens apoplectoider und epipleptoider Anfälle. Arch. f. Psychiat., 14: 552–567, 1883
Beck, Alfred. Kiel surgeon
APPARATUS—for direct blood transfusion.

Die Methodik der Bluttransfusion und die Vermeidung ihrer Gefahren. Ergebn. inn. Med. u. Kinderh., 30: 150–220, 1926

Beck, Carl. American surgeon. 1856–1911
OPERATION—
On the use of the temporal fascia to cover in cranial defects. Ann. Surg., 44: 170–174, Aug. 1906
OPERATION—gastrostomy.
Demonstration of specimens illustrating a method of formation of a prethoracic esophagus with A. Carrel, Illinois M. J., 7: 463–464, May 1905
OPERATION—
A new operation for balanic hypospadias. New York M. J., 67: 147–148, Jan. 29, 1898
OPERATION—reconstruction of finger.
The crippled hand and arm. Phila., Lippincott, 1925
OPERATION—
A new operation for inguinal hernia. Med. News, 75: 359–360, Sept. 16, 1899

Beck, Claude Schaeffer. Cleveland surgeon. 1894–
METHOD—of controlling ventricular fibrillation.
The control of the heart beat by the surgeon with special reference to ventricular fibrillation occurring during operation with F. R. Mautz, Ann. Surg., 106: 525–537, Oct. 1937
OPERATION—increasing blood supply to heart in coronary sclerosis by grafting on a piece of skeletal muscle.
The development of a new blood supply to the heart by operation. Ann. Surg., 102: 801–813, Nov. 1935
OPERATION—cardio-omentopexy.
The production of a collateral circulation to the heart. I. An. experimental study with V. L. Tichy, Amer. Heart J., 10: 849–873, 1935
Further data on the establishment of a new blood supply to the heart by operation. J. Thoracic Surg., 5: 604–611, Aug. 1936
TECHNIC—
Wounds of the heart. The technic of suture. Arch. Surg., 13: 205–227, Aug. 1926
See also E. C. Cutler

Beck, Emil G. Chicago surgeon. 1866–1932
PASTE—bismuth subnitrate, 1 part, and vaseline. 2 parts.
Fistulous tracts, tuberculous sinuses and abscess cavities. A new method of diagnosis and treatment by bismuth paste. J. A. M. A., 50: 868–872, Mar. 14, 1908
Some practical points in the application of the bismuth paste in chronic suppurative diseases. S. G. O., 9: 255–258, Aug. 1909
Bismuth paste in chronic suppurations. St. Louis, Mosby, 1910

Beck, M. See B. Proskauer

Beck, Theodric Romeyn. Albany physician. 1791–1855
Wrote on forensic medicine.
Elements of medical jurisprudence. Albany, Websters and Skinners, 1823. 2 vols. (and many subsequent editions)

Beck, Walter. Breslau surgeon
Advocated use of prostigmin as a prophylactic against post-operative abdominal distension.
Zur Prophylaxe nach gynaekologischen Operation mit Prostigmin. Munch. med. Wschr., 79: 389–390, Mar. 4, 1932

Becker, Ernst. German physician

Described aspiration of stomach content as a cause of bronchopneumonia.
Beiträge zur Geschichte der Aspirationspneumonie. Göttengen, Schmidt, 1887. 75 pp.

Becker, Georg. German physician
Used salvarsan in treatment of anthrax.
Die bakteriologische Blutuntersuchung beim Milzbrand des Menschen. Dtsch. Z. Chir., 112: 265–283, 1911

Becker, Otto Heinrich Enoch. German ophthalmologist. 1828–1890
TEST—for astigmatism.
Zur Anatomie der gesunden und kranken Linse. Wiesbaden, Bergmann, 1883
Experimented on traumatic aortic insufficiency. (Homans)
Ueber die sichtbaren Erscheinungen der Blutbewegung in der menschlichen Netzhaut. Arch. f. Ophth., 18: 206–296, 1872

Becker, Wesley C. Chicago scientist
AGAR—defibrinated blood, to isolate certain cocci.
The necessity of a standard blood-agar plate for the determination of hemolysis by streptococci. J. infect. Dis., 19: 754–759, Dec. 1916

Beckers, W. German scientist
REACTION—for apomorphine.
Ueber neue Erkennungsreaktionen für Apomorphin with L. Grimbert and A. Leclère, Suddeut. Apoth. Z., 55: 198, 1915

Beckman, Harry. Milwaukee physician. 1892–
TECHNIC—intraspinal injection of 25 per cent magnesium sulphate (7 cc.) in tetanus.
Treatment in general practice. Phila., Saunders, 1930. pp. 220–221
Same, 1942. p. 265

Béclard, Pierre Augustin. French surgeon. 1785–1825
Excised the parotid gland.
Extirpation de la parotide, pratiquée à hôpital de la Pitié. Arch. gén. de méd., 4: 60–66, 1824
HERNIA—femoral h. through the saphenous opening.
Élémens d'anatomie générale. . . . . Paris, Bechet, 1827. 2 ed.

Béclère, Antoine. Paris physician. 1856–1939
Reported successful radio-therapy of a pituitary adenoma, 1901
The radio-therapeutic treatment of tumors of the hypophysis, gigantism and acromegaly. Arch. Roent. Ray, London, 14: 142–150, Oct. 1909

Becquerel, Antoine Henri. French physicist. 1852–1908
RAYS—emitted from uranium.
Sur les radiations émises par phosphorescence. C. R. Acad. Sci., Paris, 122: 420–421, Feb 24, 1896
Action physiologique des rayons du radium with P. Curie, Ibid., 132: 1289–1291, June 3, 1901

Beddard, Arthur Philip. London physiologist
TESTS—for indigo and methylene blue in urine.
Blue urine. Guy's Hosp. Rep., 56: 127–130, 1903
TREATMENT—
A suggestion for treatment in delayed chloroform poisoning. Lancet, 1: 782–783, Mar. 14, 1908

Beddoes, Thomas. English physician. 1760–1808
Founder of aërotherapy or pneumotherapy.
Considerations on the medical use, and on the production of factitious airs with J. Watt, Bristol, Johnson, 1794
See also J. Watt

Bedell, Arthur Joseph. Albany ophthalmologist. 1879–
Made important studies of fundus oculi.
Photographs of the fundus oculi; a photographic study of normal and pathological changes seen with the ophthalmoscope. Phila., Davis, 1929. 317 pp. 95 pl.

Bednar, Alois. Vienna physician. 1816–1888
APHTHAE—two ulcers occurring on the hard palate of cachectic infants.
Die Krankheiten der Neugebornen und Säuglinge vom clinischen und pathologisch-anatomischen Standpunkte. Wien, Gerold, 1850–53

Beer, Edwin. New York surgeon. 1876–1938
OPERATION—transurethral fulguration of bladder tumors.
Removal of neoplasms of the urinary bladder. A new method of employing high-frequency (Oudin) current through a catheterizing cystoscope. J. A. M. A., 54: 1768–1769, May 28, 1910

Beer, Georg Joseph. German ophthalmologist. 1763–1818
Introduced iridectomy (1798).
KNIFE—used in operations for cataract and for excision of staphyloma of cornea.
OPERATION—a flap method for cataract.
Methode den grauen Staar sammt der Kapsel auszuziehen. Nebst einigen andern wesentlichen Verbesserungen der Staaroperation überhaupt. Wien, Schaumburg, 17:9. 60 pp.

Begbie, James. Scottish physician. 1798–1869
DISEASE—exophthalmic goiter; same as Graves' disease.
Anemia and its consequences; enlargement of the thyroid gland and eyeballs. Anemia and goitre, are they related? Month. J. Med. Sci., 9: 495–508, Feb. 1849
DISEASE—hysteric chorea; same as Bergeron's disease.
Remarks on rheumatism and chorea; their relation and treatment. Ibid., 7: 740–754, Apr. 1847

Begg, C. L. See O. S. Lowsley

Behan, Richard Joseph. Pittsburgh surgeon. 1879–
INCISION—for radical mastectomy.
Cancer, with special reference to cancer of the breast. St. Louis, Mosby, 1938. 844 pp. pp. 507–508

Behla, Robert Franz. German physician. 1850–
BODIES—found in cancer and thought by the discoverer to be the parasite causing the disease.
Die pflanzenparasitäre Ursache de Krebses und die Krebsprophylaxe. Berlin, Schoetz, 1903. 48 pp.

Behre, J. A. See S. R. Benedict

Behrend, Moses. Philadelphia surgeon. 1877–
MODIFICATION—
A modified Whipple operation for carcinoma at the ampulla of Vater. Amer. J. Surg., 72: 599–603, Oct. 1946

Behrens, Charles August. Michigan bacteriologist. 1885–
AGAR—blood cell; culture medium for Trypanosoma brucei.
An attenuated culture of Trypanosoma brucei. J. infect. Dis., 15: 24–62, July 1914

Behrens, Rudolph August. German physician. ?–1747
Described purpura hemorrhagica.
Observationum de morbo maculoso haemorrhagico et noxiis nonnulis mytulis perscripta. Brunsvigae, 1735

Behring, Emil Adolf von. German bacteriologist. 1854–1917
Awarded first Nogel prize in 1901.
Successfully elaborated antitoxins against diphtheria and tetanus.
METHOD—of inoculation against diphtheria.
SERUM—against diphtheria.
Ueber die Zustanderkommen der Diphtherie-Immunität und der Tetanus-Immunität bei Thieren with S. Kitasato, Dtsch. med. Wschr., 16: 1113–1114; 1145–1148, 1890
Zur Behandlung diphtheriekranker Menschen mit Diphtherieheilserum. Ibid., 19: 389–392; 415–418, 1893
Die Geschichte der Diphtheria. Leipzig, Thieme, 1893. 208 pp.
TUBERCULIN—an extract of tubercle bacilli used for protective inoculation against tuberculosis.
Tuberkulosebekämpfung. Marburg, Elwert, 1903. 34 pp.

Beigel, Hermann. German physician. 1830–1879
DISEASE—tricharrhexis nodosa.
Ueber Auftreibung und Bersten der Haare, eine eigenthümliche Erkrangkung des Haarschaftes. S. B. math. naturwiss. Class., 17: 612–617, 1855
The human hair: its structure, growth, diseases and their treatment. London, Renshaw, 1869. 152 pp.

Beijerinck, Martinus Willem. Dutch bacteriologist. 1851–1931
SOLUTION—basal phosphate. Akad. d. Wissensch. zu Amsterdam, Mar. 30, 1901, Verslagen, 633; May 25, 1901, Verslagen, 8.
Also: *Ueber oligonitrophile Mikroben.* Zbl. f. Bakt., 2 Abt., 7: 561–582, Aug. 10, 1901
SOLUTION—ammonium chloride.
Bildung und Verbrauch von Stickoxydul durch Bakterien with D. C. J. Minkman, Ibid., 25: 30–63, 1910
Studied mosaic disease of tobacco plant, caused by a filtrable virus.
Ueber ein Contagium vivum fluidum als Ursache der Fleckenkrankheit der Tabaksblätter. Verhand. d. k Akad. van Wetensch. te Amsterdam, Sect. 2, Deel 6, No. 5, 1898

Belchier, John. London surgeon. 1706–1785
Experimented on staining bones of fowls by feeding madder-soaked bran.
An account of the bones of animals being changed to a red colour by aliment only. Philos. Trans., 1735–1736, 39: 287–288; 299–300, 1738

Belfield, William Thomas. Chicago surgeon. 1856–1929
OPERATION—vasotomy.
Diseases of the urinary and male sexual organs. New York, Wood, 1884. 351 pp.
TREATMENT—
Pus tubes in the male and their treatment by injections through the vas deferens. Amer. J. Dermat. & Genit.-Urin. Dis., 11: 11–12, Jan. 1907
Same. Med. Rec., 71: 731–732, May 4, 1907

Belieres, Louis. French chemist
TEST—for bile pigments and indoxyl in icteric urine.
Recherche de l'indoxyle dans les urines ictériques. J. Pharm. Chim., Paris, 7 s., 8: 429–430, 1913

Bell, Benjamin. Scottish surgeon. 1749–1806
Differentiated gonorrhea from syphilis.
Treatise on gonorrhoea virulenta and lues venerea.

Edinburgh, Watson and Mudie, 1793. 2 vols.
Classified ulcers.
A treatise on the theory and management of ulcers.
Edinburgh, Elliot, 1778

Bell, Sir Charles. English surgeon. 1774–1842
LAW—anterior roots of spinal nerves are motor, posterior are sensory.
An idea of a new anatomy of the brain, submitted for the observation of the author's friends. London, Strahan & Preston, 1811. 36 pp.
Also: Baltimore M. & Phil. Lycaeum, 4: 305–318, 1811
Also: *The nervous system of the human body.* Washington, Green, 1833. p. 8
Also: Klassiker d. Med., Vol. 13 Leipzig. Barth, 1911
Also: Medical Classics, 1: 105–120, Oct. 1936
NERVE—the external respiratory nerve.
On the nerves; giving an account of some experiments on their structure and functions, which lead to a new arrangement of the system. Phil. Trans., 111: 398–424, 1821
Also: *The nervous system of the human body.* Washington, Green, 1833. p. 39
Also: Medical Classics, 1: 123–150, Oct. 1936
PALSY or PARALYSIS—facial paralysis. See Nerve.
Also: *On the nerves of the face, being a second paper on that subject.* Phil. Trans., 119: 317–330, 1829
Also: *The nervous system of the human body.* Washington, Green, 1833. p. 59
Also: Medical Classics, 1: 155–169, Oct. 1936
PHENOMENON or SIGN—an outward and upward rolling of the eyeball on an attempt to close the eye, occurring on the affected side in peripheral facial (Bell's) palsy.
On the motions of the eye, an illustration of the uses of the muscles and nerves of the orbit. Phil. Trans., 113: 166–186, 1923
Also: *The nervous system of the human body.* Washington, Green, 1833. p. 101
Also: Medical Classics, 1: 173–190, Oct. 1936
OPERATION—extraperitoneal cesarean section.
(No title) In: *Institutes of Surgery,* vol. 2, p. 227 (only), 1838

Bell, Elexious Thompson. Minneapolis anatomist. 1880–
TEST—
On the differential staining of fats. J. Path. Bact., 19: 105–113, July 1914

Bell, F. Gordon. Scottish surgeon
TUMOR—derived from adult seminal tubules: has slow growth and high cure rate.
Tumours of the testicle; the teratoid group. Brit. J. Surg., 13: 7–38, July 1925
(Same) *The spermatocytoma group.* Ibid., 282–301, Oct. 1925

Bell, F. K. See J. J. Abel

Bell, I. R. See S. Gelfan

Bell, John. Scottish anatomist. 1763–1820
Ligated the gluteal artery.
On wounds of the arteries; of the aneurism which forms over the wounded artery; with general instructions and rules of conduct of the operations on great aneurisms. Principles of surgery. Vol. 1, Discourse 9, pp. 404–428 (417–426), 1801

Bell, L. M. See H. M. Clute

Bell, Luther Vose. Somerville, Mass. physician. 1806–1862
DISEASE or MANIA or DELIRIUM—a suddenly appearing and severe delirium lasting only a short time and ending usually in death.
On a form of disease resembling some advanced stages of mania and fever, but so contra-distinguished from any ordinarily observed or described combination of symptoms, as to render it probable that it may be an overlooked and hitherto unrecorded malady. Amer. J. Insanity, 6: 97–127, Oct. 1849

Bell, Richard D. Boston chemist
METHOD—of Bell and Doisy, for determination of phosphorus content of blood plasma.
Rapid calorimetric methods for determination of phosphorous in urine and blood with E. A. Doisy, J. biol. Chem., 44: 55–67, Oct. 1920
See also E. A. Doisy

Bell, William Blair. Liverpool gynecologist. 1871–1936
Used an extract of posterior lobe of pituitary gland on a parturient woman.
The pituitary body and the therapeutic value of the infundibular extract in shock, uterine atony, and intestinal paresis. Brit. M. J., 2: 1609–1613, Dec. 4, 1909
Advocated use of lead in cancer.
The influence of saturine compounds on cell-growth, with special reference to the treatment of malignant neoplasms. A preliminary communication. Lancet, 2: 1005–1009, Nov. 11, 1922

Bellerby, C. W. See A. S. Parkes

Bellini, Lorenzo. Italian anatomist. 1643–1704
DUCTS—the excretory ducts of the kidney.
TUBES—the connecting tubes of the kidney.
Exercitatio anatomica de structura et usu renum. Florentiae, Stellae, 1662. 28 pp.
LIGAMENT—a band from the capsule of the hip joint to the trochanter major.
Opera omnia. Venetiis, Hertz, 1732. 2 ed.

Belloc, Hippolyte. French physician
CANNULA or SOUND or TUBE—a curved instrument for plugging the posterior nares for nosebleed.
Traité pratique de la phthisie laryngée, de la laryngite chronique et des maladies de la voix. By A. Trousseau and H. Belloc, Paris, Baillière, 1837
Also, in German: Quedlinb. & Leipz., 1838

Belloste, Augustin. French surgeon. 1654–1730
PILL—containing mercury.
SOLUTION—of mercurous nitrate.
Traité du mercure. Paris, 1738. 131 pp.

Belsey, R. H. R. See E. G. L. Bywaters, E. D. Churchill

Benario, J. Frankfurt a. M. physician
FIXING—of blood films.
Ueber die morphologischen Bestandtheile des Blutes und ihre diagnostische Verwerthung. Z. f. ärztl. Landpraxis, 3: 197; 243, 1894

Bence Jones, Henry. See H. B. Jones

Benda, Carl. German physician. 1857–1933
METHOD—alizarin.
Die Mitochondria. Ergebn. Anat., 12: 743–781 (752), 1902
METHOD—rapid, of myelin staining.
Markscheidenfärbung der peripherischen Nerven. Berl. klin. Wschr., 40: 748–749, Aug. 10, 1903

METHOD—of staining, with light green.
Neue Mittheilungen über die Entwickelung der Genitaldrüsen und über die Metamorphose der Samenzellen (Histiogenese der Spermatozoen). Verh. physiol. Ges. Berlin, Dec. 11, 1891, in: Arch. f. Anat. & Physiol., (Physiol.), pp. 549–552, 1891
METHOD—of staining of nerve tissue (neuroglia).
Erfahrungen über Neurolgliafärbungen und eine neue Färbungsmethode. Neurol. Zbl., 19: 786–798, Sept. 1, 1900
STAIN—iron haematoxylin.
"Über die Spermatogenese der Säugethiere." Verh. physiol. Ges. Berlin, Nov. 27, 1885, Feb. 12, 1886, in: Arch. f. Anat. & Physiol., (Physiol.), pp. 186–187; 386–388, 1886
Bendien, S. G. T. Dutch physician
TEST—for malignancy.
Haemagglutinegehalte van het bloedserum bij carcinoompatiënten. Ned. Tijdschr. Geneesk., 70: pt. 1, 2856–2858, June 26, 1926
Spezifische Veränderungen des Blutserums; ein Beitrag zur serologischen Diagnose von Krebs und Tuberkulose. Jena, Fischer, 1931. 99 pp.
Bends, Jacob Christian. Belgian ophthalmologist. 1812–1858
Described the infectious forms of granular conjunctivitis.
Quelques considérations sur la nature de l'ophthalmie dite militaire, par rapport à son apparition dans l'armée danoise depuis 1851. Ann. d'ocul., Brux., 33: 164–176, 1855
Benecke, Dr. German physician
STAIN—for fibrils.
Ueber eine Modification des Weigert'schen Fibrinfärbeverfahrens. Verh. d. Anat. Ges., 7: 165–168, 1893 in: Anat. Anz., 8: 165–168, 1893
Benedek, Ladislaus. Hungarian physician
METHOD—
(Cerebro-spinalfluid oxydase reaction) with J. Thurzó, Orv. hetil., 70: 1375–1377, 1926
Über eine neue Oxydationsreaktion des Liquor cerebrospinalis. Klin. Wschr., 6: 356–357, Feb. 19, 1927
REACTION—
Tuschreaktion des Liquor cerebrospinalis. (Vorläufige Mitteilung) with E. von Thurzó, Münch. med. Wschr., 76: 411–412, Mar. 8, 1929
Beneden, Edouard van. Belgian anatomist. 1846–1910
Described segmentation of mammalian ovum.
La maturation de l'oeuf, la fécondation et les premières phases du développement embryonnaire des mammifères. Bull. Acad. roy. de sci. de Belgique, 2 s., 40: 686–736, 1875
Discovered the centrosome.
Contributions à l'etude de la vésicle germinative et du premier noyau embryonnaire. Ibid., 41: 38–85, 1876
Benedick, Arthur Jerome. New York physician. 1888–
SOLUTION—phenolphthalein sucrose, for detection of cholera vibrio.
A simplified bacterial technique for detecting cholera carriers. Amer. J. Pub. Health, 1: 906–909, Dec. 1911
Benedict, Francis Gano. American biochemist. 1870–
APPARATUS—for study of output of carbon dioxide and consumption of oxygen.
A portable respiration apparatus for clinical use. Boston M. & S. J., 178: 667–678, May 16, 1918

APPARATUS—helmet respiration a.
A helmet for use in clinical studies of gaseous metabolism. New Engl. J. Med., 203: 150–158, July 24, 1930
METHOD—
The determination of creatine and creatinine with V. C. Myers, Amer. J. Physiol., 18: 397–405, May 1, 1907
Studied the influence of inanition on metabolism.
The influence of inanition on metabolism. Washington, Carnegie Inst., Pub. No. 77, 1907
Made, with Joslin, extensive studies on metabolism.
Metabolism in diabetes mellitus. Ibid., No. 136, 1910
See also W. O. Atwater, J. A. Harris
Benedict, Stanley Rossiter. American physiologic chemist. 1884–1936
METHOD—for determination of total blood sugars.
The analysis of whole blood: II. The determination of sugar and of saccharoids (non-fermentable copper-reducing substances). J. biol. Chem., 92: 141–159, June 1931
METHOD—
Note on the determination of amino-acid nitrogen in urine with J. R. Murlin, Ibid., 16: 385–388, Dec. 1913
METHOD—
A modification of the molybdic method for the determination of inorganic phosphorus in serum with Ruth C. Theis, Ibid., 61: 63–66, Aug. 1924
METHOD—for preparation of creatinine.
Studies in creatine and creatinine metabolism. I. The preparation of creatine and creatinine from urine. Ibid., 18: 183–190, July 1914
REACTION—for creatinine.
Some applications of a new color reaction for creatinine with J. A. Behre, Ibid., 114: 515–532, June 1936
REAGENT—of Benedict-Hopkins-Cole.
A note on the preparation of glyoxylic acid as a reagent. Ibid., 6: 51–52, Mar. 1909
REAGENT—for sulphur.
The estimation of total sulphur in urine. Ibid., 363–371, Aug. 1909
REAGENTS—for uric acid.
On the colorimetric estimation of uric acid in urine. Ibid., 20: 619–627, 1915
The determination of uric acid in urine. Ibid., 51: 187–207, Mar. 1922
A method for the direct determination of uric acid in urine with Elizabeth Franke, Ibid., 52: 387–391, 1922
SOLUTION—for examination of sugar.
The detection and estimation of reducing sugars. Ibid., 3: 101–107, 1907
A reagent for the detection of reducing sugars. Ibid., 5: 485–487, 1909
TEST—for acetate.
Methods for the detection of acetate, cyanide, and lithium. Amer. Chem. J., 32: 480–483, 1904
TEST—for blood phosphate.
See method for phosphorus, 1924
TEST—for phenols in blood.
The colorimetric determination of phenols in the blood. J. biol. Chem., 36: 95–98, Oct. 1918
See also J. C. Bock, R. C. Lewis, T. P. Nash, Jr., Ruth C. Theis
Benedikt, Moriz. Austrian physician. 1835–1920
SYNDROME—paralysis of the parts supplied by the

oculomotor nerve of one side, with paresis and tremor of the upper extremity on the other. (Dorland)
Tremblement avec paralysie croisée du moteur oculaire commun. Bull. méd., Paris, 3: 547–548, May 1, 1889

Beneke, Rudolf Caesar. German pathologist. 1861–
Applied term "chorio-angioma" to benign tumors of placenta.
Ein Fall von Chorionangion. Verh. dtsch. path. Ges., 2: 407–419, 1900

Bengen, M. F. Frankfort chemist
TEST—for pasteurized milk.
Ueber den Nachweis der Dauerpasteurisierung. Z. Untersuch. Lebensm., 66: 126–136, July–Aug. 1933

Bengis, Robert Oliver. Amer chemist. 1890–
AGAR—glucose ammonium phosphate; for cultivation of B. coli.
The production and collection of B. coli in quantity on synthetic media. J. infect. Dis., 18: 391–396, Apr. 1916

Béniqué, Pierre Jules. French physician. 1806–1851
SOUND—a lead or tin sound, having a wide curve, for dilating urethral strictures.
De la rétention d'urine et d'une nouvelle méthode pour introduire les bougies et les sondes dans la vessie; comment peut-ou prévenir les rétrécissements de l'uretre? Paris, Méquignon-Marvis, 1838. 260 pp.

Benivieni, Antonio. Florentine surgeon. 1443–1502
"He appears as a founder of pathology before Morgagni." Garrison
De abditis nonnullis ac mirandis morborum et sanationum causis. Florentiae, Giunta, 1507
also: Basileae, 1528

Benjamin, B. See I. M. Tarlov

Benjamin, Charles Emile. Leiden physician. 1873–
Made early study of parathyroid tumors.
Ueber die Glandulae parathyreoideae (Epithelkörperchen). Beutr. path. Anat., 31: 143–182, 1902

Bennet, James Henry. English surgeon. 1816–1891
Differentiated between benign and malignant uterine tumors.
A practical treatise on inflammation, ulceration and induration of the neck of the uterus. London, Churchill, 1845

Bennett, Alexander Hughes. London surgeon. 1848–1901
Described clinical localization and operative removal of a brain tumor.
A case of cerebral tumour. By A. H. Bennett
The surgical treatment. By R. J. Godlee. Med. chir. Trans., 68: 242–275, 1885

Bennett, Edward Hallaran. Irish surgeon. 1837–1907
FRACTURE—of the first metacarpal bone with dislocation of the carpo-metacarpal joint.
On fracture of the metacarpal bone of the thumb. Brit. M. J., 2: 12–13, July 3, 1886

Bennett, George Eli. Baltimore surgeon. 1885–
METHOD—of lengthening quadriceps tendon.
Lengthening of the quadriceps tendon. J. Bone & Joint Surg., 20: 279–316, Apr. 1922
OPERATION—for recurrent dislocation of shoulder.
The use of fascia for the reinforcement of relaxed joints. Arch. Surg., 13: 655–666, Nov. 1926
OPERATION—for stabilization of knee joint. Ibid.

Bennett, John Hughes. English physician. 1812–1875
DISEASE—leukemia.
Case of hypertrophy of the spleen and liver, in which

death took place from suppuration of the blood. Edinburgh M. & S. J., 64: 413–423, 1845
Discovered the parasite of aspergillosis.
On the parasitic vegetable structures found growing in living animals. Trans. Roy. Soc. Edinb., 15: 2 pt., 277–294, 1844
Described benefits of cod-liver oil.
Treatise on the oleum jecoris aselli, or cod liver oil. Edinburgh, Maclachlan, Stewart, 1841

Bennett, Sir William Henry. English surgeon. 1852–1931
OPERATION—for varicocele by partial excision of the pampiniform plexus.
On varicocele; a practical treatise. London, Longmans, 1891. 105 pp.

Bennhold, Hermann. Hamburg physician.
STAIN—
Eine spezifische Amyloidfärbung mit Kongorot. Münch. med. Wschr., 2: 1537–1538, Nov. 3, 1922

Benoit. See A. E. Deléarde

Bensaude, R. See E. C. Achard

Bensley, Robert Russell. American-Canadian biologist. 1867–
CELLS—"neck chief cells" of stomach.
The histology and physiology of the gastric glands. Royal Canad. Inst., Toronto, Proc., 1: 11–16, Feb. 1897
The structure of the mammalian gastric glands. Quart. J. micr. Sci., 41: 361–389, Nov. 1898
STAIN—acid fuchsin and methyl green.
Studies on the pancreas of the guinea pig. Amer. J. Anat., 12: 297–388 (308). Nov. 1911
STAIN—for pancreas, with neutral red. Ibid.

Benthsáth, A. See A. Szent-Györgyi

Béraneck, Edmund. Swiss bacteriologist. 1859–1920
TUBERCULIN—
Tuberculin; the rationale of its use; its possibilities and limitations. Edinburgh M. J., n.s. 12: 101–113, 1914

Bérard, Auguste. French surgeon. 1802–1846
Wrote classic work on parotid tumors.
Maladies de la glande parotide et de la région parotidienne; opérations que ces maladies réclament. Paris, Germer-Baillière, 1841. 314 pp.

Béraud, Brúno Jean Jacques. French surgeon. 1825–1865
LIGAMENT—suspensory 1. of the pericardium, extending to the third and fourth vertebrae.
VALVE—a slip of mucous membrane sometimes found at junction of nasal duct with lacrimal sac. (Dorland)
Atlas complet d'anatomie chirurgicale topographique. Paris, Baillière, 1862–65. 109 pp.

Bercovitz, Zaccharias. New York gynecologist. 1895–
METHOD or PUPILLARY REACTION—for early diagnosis of pregnancy.
Studies on the pupillary reactions of pregnant and nonpregnant women and their practical application to the diagnosis of pregnancy as a simple procedure. Amer. J. Obstet. Gynaec., 19: 767–778, June 1930
MODIFICATION—
Modified technic for making Wright's blood stain. J. Lab. clin. Med., 19: 438 (only), Jan. 1934

Berens, Conrad. New York ophthalmologist. 1889–
METHOD—of testing for deficiencies in color vision.
Group color vision tests with L. Stein, J. A. M. A., 113: 1563–1564, Oct. 21, 1939

Béres, T. See A. Szent-Györgyi

Berg, Albert Ashton. New York surgeon. 1872–
OPERATION—for regional ileitis: resection of ileum,
closure of both ends of divided ileum and implanting
proximal terminus of ileum by a side-to-side anastomosis at the transverse colon.
*An operative procedure for right-sided ulcerative
ileocolitis.* Ann. Surg., 104: 1019–1023, Dec. 1936
Right-sided (regional) colitis. By B. B. Crohn and A.
A. Berg, J. A. M. A., 110: 32–37, Jan. 1, 1938

Berg, Fredrik Theodor. Swedish physician. 1806–
1887
Discovered Oidium albicans in thrush.
Torsk i mikroskopiskt anatomiskt hänseende. Hygiea,
Stockholm, 3: 541–550, 1841

Berg, R. See F. J. Cotton

Bergeim, Olaf. American chemist. 1888–
APPARATUS—for determination of intragastric con-
ductance and temperature.
*Gastric response to foods. I. The determination and
significance of intragastric conductance.* Amer. J.
Physiol., 45: 1–11, Dec. 1, 1917
MODIFICATION—of Herter-Foster method of quan-
titative determination of indole in feces.
The determination of fecal indole. J. biol. Chem., 32:
17–22, Oct. 1917
See also J. O. Halverson

Bergel, F. See A. R. Todd

Bergell, P. See E. Abderhalden, G. Barger

Berger, Emile. Austrian physician. 1855–1926
SIGN—an irregular-shaped pupil in tabes dorsalis.
Die Sehstörungen bei Tabes dorsalis——Wiesbaden,
Bergmann, 1889. 114 pp.

Berger, Louis. Brooklyn surgeon. 1894–
CRUSHER—
Instrument for crushing the spur of a colostomy.
Am. J. Surg., 58: 152–154, Oct. 1942

Berger, Oskar. Breslau physician. 1844–1885
PARESTHESIA—of one or both legs, in young
persons, accompanied by weakness, but without
objective symptoms. (Dorland)
Ueber eine eigentümliche Form von Paraesthesie.
Bresl. ärztl. Z., 1: 60–61, Apr. 12, 1879

Berger, Paul. French surgeon. 1845–1908
OPERATION—interscapulothoracic amputation.
*Amputation du membre supérieur dans la contiguité
du tronc (désarticulation de l'omoplate).* Bull. Soc.
Chir. Paris, 9: 656, 1883
*L'amputation du membre supérieur dans la contiguité
du tronc (amputation interscapulo-thoracique).* Paris,
Masson, 1887. 371 pp.

Bergeron, Étienne Jules. French physician. 1817–
1900
DISEASE—of Bergeron-Henoch, hysteric chorea.
Named by R. Berland in honor of his professor in:
*Traitement par le tartre stibié d'une forme de chorée
dite électrique.* Poitiers, 1880
Described ulcero-membranous stomatitis.
*Note sur l'emploi du chlorate de potasse dans le traite-
ment de la stomatite ulcéreuse.* Rec. de mém. de Méd.
Mil., Paris, 2 s., 16: 1–46, 1855

Bergman, P. G. See R. A. A. Tigerstedt

Bergmann, Ernst von. Russian surgeon. 1836–1907
Successfully treated pulsion diverticulum of
esophagus.
Ueber den Oesophagusdivertikel und seine Behandlung.
Arch. klin. Chir., 43: 1–30, 1892
FIBER—from glia cells of cerebellum.

Die chirurgische Behandlung von Hirnkrankheiten.
Berlin, Hirschwald, 1888
OPERATION—radical mastoidectomy.
Krankenvorstellung; Geheilter Hirnabszess. Berl.
klin. Wschr., 25: 1054–1056, 1888

Bergmann, Gustav von. Berlin physician. 1878–
SYNDROME—
*Das "epiphrenale syndrom," seine Beziehung zur
Angina pectoris und zum Kardiospasmus.* Dtsch.
med. Wschr., 58: 605–609, Apr. 15, 1932
TEST—bilirubin elimination.
*Zur funktionellen Pathologie der Leber insbesondere
der Alkohol-Ätiologie der Cirrhose.* Klin. Wschr., 6:
776–780, Apr. 23, 1927

Bergonié, Jean. French physician. 1857–1925
LAW—of irradiation.
*Interprétation de quelques résultats de la radiothérapie
et essai de fixation d'une technique rationelle* with L.
Tribondeau, C. R. Acad. Sci., Paris, 143: 983–985,
Dec. 10, 1906

Berherian, D. A. Beirut, Syria physician
METHOD—of staining.
A method of staining hair and epithelial scales. Arch.
Dermat. & Syphl, 36: 1171–1175, Dec. 1937

Berkley, Henry Johns. Baltimore physician. 1860–
1940
MODIFICATION—of Golgi's bichromate and silver
nitrate method.
*Studies on the lesions produced by the action of certain
poisons on the cortical nerve cell.* Johns Hopk. Hosp.
Rep., 6: 1–108, 1897
STAIN—rapid method for myelin.
*Die Osmium-Kupfer-Hämatoxylin-Färbung. Eine
schnelle Weigert-Methode.* Neurol. Zbl , 11: 270–272,
May 1, 1892

Berkow, Samuel Gordon. Perth Amboy, N. J.
Physician. 1899–
METHOD—
*A method of estimating the extensiveness of lesions
(burns and scalds) based on surface area proportions.*
Arch. Surg., 8: 138–148, Jan. 1924

Berlin, D. D. See H. L. Blumgart, C. G. Mixter

Berlin, Rudolf. German ophthalmologist. 1833–1897
DISEASE—traumatic edema of the retina.
Zur sogenannten Commotio retinae. Klin. Mbl. Augen-
heilk., 11: 42–78, 1873
Made important contribution to cytoarchitecture of
the cerebral cortex.
Beitrage zur Strukturlehre der Grosshirnwindungen.
Erlangen, Junge, 1858. 27 pp.
Suggested term "dyslexia."
Eine besondere Art der Wortblindheit. Wiesbaden,
Bergmann, 1887

Berman, Louis. New York chemist. 1893–
TEST—for iron in blood.
*A rapid method for the determination of iron in small
quantities of blood.* J. biol. Chem., 35: 231–236, Aug.
1918
*The determination of hemoglobin by the acid hematin
method.* Arch. intern. Med., 24: 553–556, Nov. 1919

Berman, Nathan. New Haven bacteriologist. 1893–
SOLUTION—peptone, for studying bacteria.
SOLUTION—trypsinized casein; culture medium.
*Bacterial nutrition: Further studies on the utilization
of protein and non-protein nitrogen* with L. F. Rettger,
J. Bact., 3: 367–388, July 1918
The influence of carbohydrate on the nitrogen metab-

olism of bacteria with L. F. Rettger, Ibid., 389–402, July 1918

Berman, S. See B. E. Greenberg

Bernard, A. See L. Tixier

Bernard, Claude. French physiologist. 1813–1878
CANAL—a supplementary pancreatic duct: same as Sanatorini's duct.
Remarques d'anatomie comparée sur le pancréas. C. R. Soc. Biol., 1: 117–119, 1849
LAYER—glandular layer of cells which line the acini of the pancreas. Ibid.
PUNCTURE—of floor of fourth ventricle causing diabetes.
Chiens rendus diabétiques. Ibid., 1849, 1: 60, 1850
SYNDROME—mitosis, ptosis, exophthalmos, and anhidrosis caused by paralysis of cervical sympathetic: same as Horner's s.
Des phénomènes oculo-pupillaires produits par la section du nerf sympathique cervical; ils sont indépendants des phénomènes vasculaires calorifiques de la tête. C. R. Acad. Sci., 55: 381–388, Sept. 1, 1862
Discovered production of glycogen by liver; isolated glycogen.
De l'origine du sucre dans l'économie animale. Arch. gén. de méd., 3 s., 18: 303–319, *1848*
Also, with English trans.; Med. Classics, 3: 552–580, Jan. 1939
De suc pancréatique et de son rôle dans les phénomènes de la digestion. C. R. Soc. Biol., 1848, 1: 99–115, 1850
Also, with English trans.: Med. Classics, 3: 581–617, Jan. 1939
Sur le mécanisme de la formation du surre dans le foie. C. R. Acad. Sci., (Mémoires), 41: 461–469, 1855
Nouvelles recherches expérimentales sur les phénomènes glycogéniques du foie. Ibid., 44: 1325–1331, 1857
Initiated study of endocrinology by originating idea of an internal secretion.
Remarques sur la sécrétion du sucre dans le foie, faites à l'occasion de la communication de M. Lehmann. Ibid., 40: 589–592, 1855
Showed that tryptophan is a by-product of pancreatic digestion and not a true constituent of pancreatic juice.
Mémoire sur le pancréas et sur le rôle du suc pancréatique dans les phénomènes digestifs, particulièrement dans la digestion des matières grasses neutres. Paris, Baillière, 1856. 190 pp.
Made observations of pharmacology of cyanates, regarding them as a muscle poison which abolished muscular activity.
Leçons sur les effets des substances toxiques et médicamenteuses. Paris, Baillière, 1857. 488 pp. pp. 354–385
Discovered vasoconstrictor and vasodilator nerves.
De l'influence de deux ordres de nerfs qui déterminent les variations de couleur du sang veineux dans les organes glandulaires. C. R. Acad. Sci., 47: 245–253; 393–400, 1858
Studied "paralytic secretions" occasioned by section of glandular nerves.
Du rôle des actions réflexes paralysantes dans le phénomène des sécrétions. J. de l'anat. et de la physiol., 1: 507–513, 1864
Did important work on diabetes, showing that there is primarily an excess of sugar in the blood, followed by an excess in the urine. (L. T. Morton)

Leçons sur la diabète et la glycogénèse animals. Paris, Baillière, 1877. 576 pp.

Bernays, Augustus Charles. St. Louis surgeon. 1854–1907
OPERATION—
A new surgical operation for the treatment of cancer of the stomach. Ann. Surg., 6: 449–464, Dec. 1887

Bernhardt, Martin. Berlin neurologist. 1844–1915
DISEASE or PARESTHESIA or PARALYSIS or SIGN or SYNDROME—numbness and paresthesia, with pain on motion in that part of the thigh supplied by the external cutaneous nerve; called also Bernhardt-Roth syndrome.
Neuropathologische Beobachtungen. Dtsch. Arch. f. klin. Med., 22: 362–393, 1878
Ueber isolirt im Gebiete des N. cutaneus femoris externus vorkommende Parästhesien. Nuerol. Zbl., 14: 242–244, Mar. 15, 1895
FORM—of progressive muscular atrophy.
Weiterer Beitrage zur Lehre von den hereditären und familiären Erkrankungen des Nervensystems. Ueber die spinal-neuritische Form der progressiven Muskelatrophie. Arch. f. path. Anat. u. Physiol., 133: 259–294, Aug. 3, 1893

Bernheim, Alice Rheinstein. New York physician. 1883–
TEST—icterus index, of liver function.
The icterus index (a quantitative estimation of bilirubinemia): an aid in diagnosis and prognosis. J. A. M. A., 82: 291–295, Jan. 26, 1924

Bernheim, Bertram Moses. Baltimore surgeon. 1880–
OPERATION—direct, arteriovenous blood transfusion.
Blood transfusion, hemorrhage and the anemias. Phila., Lippincott, 1917. 259 pp. pp. 97–108

Bernheim, Hippolyte-Marie. Nancy physician. 1840–1919
Wrote on hypnotism.
De la suggestion dans l'état hypnotique et dans l'état de veille. Paris, Doin, 1884. 110 pp.
Hypnotisme, suggestion, psychothérapie. Paris, Doin, 1891. 518 pp.
Described relation of typhoid fever to gall bladder disease.
Ictère. Dict. Encycl. Sci. Méd., 15: 432, 1889

Bernheim, R. See W. Autenrieth

Bernheim, Stefan. Austrian ophthalmologist. 1861–1918
FIBER—from optic tract to Luy's body.
Ueber die Entwickelung und den Verlauf der Markfasern im Chiasma nervorum opticorum des Menschen. Wiesbaden, Bergmann, 1889. 61 pp.

Bernou, André-Edouard-Maurice. French physician. 1889–
TREATMENT—oleothorax in pulmonary tuberculosis.
Therapeutic oleothorax. Bull. Acad. Méd. Paris, 87: 457–461, Apr. 25, 1922

Bernstein, Felix. German physician. 1878–
HYPOTHESIS—concerning mode of inheritance of blood groups.
Ergebnisse einer biostatischen zusammenfassenden Betrachtung über die erblichen Blutstruckturen des Menschen. Klin. Wschr., 3: 1495–1497, Aug. 12, 1924
Zusammenfassende Betrachtungen über die erblichen

Blutstrukturen des Mensschen. Z. f. ind. Abst.-u.
Vererbungslehre, 37: 237–270, 1925
Bernstein, Julius. Swiss physiologist. 1839–1917
THEORY—changes in surface tension are a control-
ling factor in development of the energy of muscular
contraction.
*Untersuchungen zur Thermodynamik der bioelektri-
schen Ströme.* Arch. f. d. ges. Physiol., Bonn. 92:
521–562, 1902; 122: 129–195; 24: 462–468, 1908
Bernthsen, August. German biochemist. 1855–
SOLUTION—of methylene violet.
Studien in der Methylenblaugruppe. Ann. Chim.,
230: 73–136; 137–211, 1885
Berry, G. P. See T. M. Rivers
Bert, Paul. French physician. 1830–1886
THEORY—caisson disease is due to injury to tissues
by nitrogen bubbles liberated too quickly from the
blood.
*Recherches expérimentales sur l'influence que les
changements dans la pression barométrique exercent
sue les phénomènes de la vie.* C. R. Acad. Sci., 73:
213–216; 503–507, 1871
Communication sur les effets de l'air comprimé. Bull.
Soc. Méd. de l'Yonne, 1872, 13: pt. 2, 48–55, 1873
Proved that high altitude symptoms are due to im-
perfect oxygenation of the blood.
*La pression barométrique; recherches de physiologie
expérimentale.* Paris, Masson, 1878. 1168 pp.
Berthelot, Albert-Charles-Marie. French bacte-
riologist. 1881–
SOLUTION—vegetable infusion, a culture medium.
*Sur l'emploi du bouillon de legumes comme milieu de
culture.* C. R. Soc. Biol., 80: 131–132, Feb. 3, 1917
Berthelot, Pierre Eugene Marcellin. French pharm-
acologist. 1827–1907
TEST—for carbon monoxide.
Sur une réaction de l'oxyde de carbone. C. R. Acad.
Sci., 112: 597, 1895
Devised a method for liquefying gases.
*Sur un procédé simple et sans danger pour démontrer
la liquéfaction des gaz et celle de l'acide carbonique en
particulier.* Ibid., 30: 666–667, May 27, 1850
Showed that bacteria acting in clay soils are able to
fix nitrogen (L. T. Morton)
*Fixation de l'azote par la terre végétable nue ou avec
le concours des légumineuses.* Rev. scient., Paris, 43:
450–454, 1889
Berthold, Arnold Adolf. German physician. 1803–
1861
Injected and transplanted tissue into capons, with
production of secondary male characteristics of
comb growth; proved existence of an internal secretion.
Transplantation der Hoden. Arch. Anat., Physiol. u.
wiss. Med., pp. 42–46, 1849
Berthollet, Claude Louis. French chemist. 1748–
1822
LAW—if two salts in solution, by double decomposition, can produce a salt less soluble than either,
such a salt will be produced.
Recherches sur les lois da l'affinité. Paris, Baudonin,
1801
Same: *Researches into the laws of chemicai affinity.*
Transl. by M. Farrel, Baltimore, Nicklin, 1809.
212 pp.
Bertie, Elizabeth. See C. J. Watson

Bertillon, Alphonse. French criminologist. 1853–
1914
SYSTEM—the recorded measurement and description
of criminals for future identification.
*Les signalements anthropométriques, méthode nouvelle
de détermination de l'identité individuelle.* Paris,
Masson, 1886. 31 pp.
Bertin, Exipère Joseph. French anatomist. 1712–1781
BONES or OSSICLES—the sphenoturbinal bones,
partly closing the sphenoidal sinuses.
*Traité d'ostéologie suivi de trois mémoires de M.
Herissant, sur différens points d'ostéologie.* Paris,
Méquignon, 1783. 4 vols.
Bertolus, G. See J. B. A. Chauveau
Bertrand, Gabriel. French scientist. 1867–
METHOD—for determination of glucose in urine.
Le dosage des sucres réducteurs. Bull. Soc. Chim. biol.
Paris, 35: 1285–1299, 1906
REAGENT—for alkaloids.
L'acide silicotungstique comme réactif des alcaloides.
C. R. Acad. Sci., 128: 742–745, Mar. 20, 1899
Bertrandi, Giovanni Ambrogio Maria. Italian
surgeon. 1723–1765
SUTURE—a continuous suture passing back and
forth.
Trattato delle operazioni di chirurgia. Nizza, Floteront,
1763
Berven, Elis G. E. Stockholm surgeon. 1885–
TONSIL APPLICATOR—for radium treatment.
*Malignant tumors of the tonsil: a clinical study with
special reference to radiological treatment.* Acta radiol.,
supp. 11: 1–285, 1931
Berze, Josef. Vienna psychiatrist
TREATMENT—
Die Insulin-Chok-Behandlung der Schizophrenie.
Wien. med. Wschr., 82: 1365–1369, Dec. 2, 1933
Berzelius, Johan Jacob. Swedish chemist. 1779–1848
Isolated biliverdin; confused it with chlorophyll.
Lehrbuch der Chemie. Dresden, Arnold, 1825–31.
4 vols.
Besnier, Ernest. French dermatologist. 1831–1909
DISEASE—benign sarcoid; Besnier—Boeck—Schau-
mann d.
*Lupus pernio de la face: synovites fongueuses (scrofu-
lotuberculeuses), symétriques des extrémités supérieures.*
Ann. de dermat. & Syph., 2 s., 10: 333–336, 1889
RHEUMATISM—chronic arthrosynovitis.
Rheumatisme. Dict. encyclopéd. des sci. méd.,
Paris, 3 s., 4: 446–819, 1876
Besredka, Alexandre. French physician. 1870–1940
ANTIVIRUS—
*De l'anaphylaxie et de l'anti-anaphylaxie vis-à-vis du
serum de cheval* with Edna Steinhardt, Ann. Inst.
Pasteur, 21: 117–127; 384–391, 1907
Anaphylaxie et antianaphylaxie; bases expérimentales.
Paris, Masson, 1917. 146 pp.
Also, in English: London, Heinemann, 1919. 143 pp.
SOLUTION—egg stomach digest, a culture medium.
Le bouillon a l'oeuf with F. Jupille, Ann. Inst. Pas-
teur, 27: 1009–1017, Nov. 25, 1913
VACCINE—
Immunisation locale; pansements spécifiques. Paris,
Masson, 1925. 251 pp.
Besson, Albert. French bacteriologist. 1868–
AGAR—basal litmus.

Technique microbiologique et serotherapique. Paris, Baillière, 1920. p. 59

AGAR—phosphate infusion, a culture medium. Ibid., p. 41

BOUILLON—serum, a culture medium. Ibid., p. 31

MEDIUM—citrated blood. Ibid., p. 34

SOLUTION—glucose infusion; for differentiation of colon-typhoid group.

Variations dans la réduction du rouge-neutre par les microbes; utilisaiion pour le diagnostic with A. Ranque, Ch. Senez, C. R. Soc. Biol., 81: 928–930, Oct. 26, 1918

Best, Charles Herbert. Toronto physiologist. 1899– Discovered an enzyme which specifically inactivates histamine.

The inactivation of histamine with E. W. McHenry, J. Physiol., 70: 349–372, Dec. 4, 1930

Histamine with E. W. McHenry, Physiol. Rev., 11: 372–477, Oct. 1931

See also F. G. Banting

Best, F. Dresden physician

STAIN—carmin, for glycogen.

Ueber Karminfärbung des Glykogens und der Kerne. Z. wiss. Mikr., 23: 319–322, Nov. 15, 1906

Best, Rollin Russell. Omaha surgeon. 1897–

PHYSIOLOGIC FLUSH or TREATMENT—

Cholangiographic demonstration of the remaining common duct stone and its non-operative management. S. G. O., 66: 1040–1046, June 1938

Physiologic biliary flush in the management of biliary tract disease. Southwest. Med., 23: 396–399, Dec. 1939

Besta, Carlo. Italian neurologist. 1876–

METHOD—of staining nerve tissue.

Sull'apparato reticolare interno (apparato del Golgi) della cellula nervosa. Anat. Anz., 36: 476–486 (477), May 21, 1910

STAIN—tin, for myelin.

Sulla struttura della guaina mielinica delle fibre nervose periferiche. Riv. Sperim. Freniatr., 31: 569–583, 1905

Bethe, Albrecht. Strassburg physician. 1872–

METHOD—for staining nerve fibers with methylene blue.

Studien über das Centralnervensystem von Carcinus Maenas nebst Angaben über ein neues Verfahren der Methylenblaufixation. Die Fixation von Methylenblaupräparaten. Chemische Vorbemerkungen. Arch. mikr. Anat., 44: 579–622, 1895

STAIN—molybdenum—toluidine for neurofibrils.

Das Molybdänverfahren zur Darstellung der Neurofibrillen und Golginetze im Centralnervensystem. A. wiss. Mikr., 17: 13–35, May 1, 1900

Bethencourt, Jacques de. French physician Coined term venereal disease to replace Morbus Gallicus or French disease.

Nova penitentialis quadragesima, nec non purgatorium in morbum Gallicum sive Venereum. Paris, 1527 Trad. par A. Fournier, Paris, Masson et fils, 1871. 94 pp.

Bethune, Normal. Montreal surgeon. 1890–

PROCEDURE—lobectomy.

Pleural poudrage; a new technic for the deliberate production of pleural adhesions as a preliminary to lobectomy. J. Thoracic Surg., 4: 251–261, Feb. 1935

Bettencourt, Rodriques. French physician. 1853–1933 Transplanted thyroid into a myxedematous patient with striking improvement.

(Un cas de myxedème traité par la greffe hypodermique du corps thyroide du mouton.) with J. A. Serrano, Prog. méd., 12: 170–171, Aug. 30, 1890

Bettendorff, Anton Joseph Hubert Maria. German chemist. 1839–

TEST—for arsenic.

Ein Reagens auf Arsen und Bereitung arsenfreier Salzsäure. Z. Chem., 5: 492–494, 1870

Bettinger, Julius. German physician. 1802–1887 Demonstrated the experimental inoculability of syphilis. Articles were published anonymously by "Palatinus", read before the Society of Physicians of the Palatinate in Sept. 1855. Published without title in Aerztl. Intell.-Blatt, München. 3: 426–428, Aug. 29, 1856

Bettman, Adalbert Goodman. Portland, Ore. surgeon. 1883–

GAUZE—for healing areas.

A simpler technic for promoting epithelization and protecting skin grafts. J. A. M. A., 97: 1879–1881, Dec. 19, 1931

TREATMENT—of burns with tannic acid and silver nitrate.

The tannic acid-silver nitrate treatment of burns. A method of minimizing shock and toxemia and shortening convalescence. Northwest Med., 34: 46–51, Feb. 1935

Betz, Wladimir Aleksandrovich. Russian anatomist. 1834–1894

CELL AREA—same as psychomotor area.

CELLS—giant pyramidal cells of motor area.

Anatomischer Nachweis zweier Gehirncentra. Zbl. med. Wiss., 12: 578–580; 595–599, 1874

Ueber die feiner Structur der Gehirnrinde des Menschen. Ibid., 19: 193–195; 209–213; 231–234, 1881

Beurmann, Charles Lucien de. French physician. 1851–1923

DISEASE—of Beurmann-Gougerot: disseminated gummatous sporotrichosis.

Sporotrichoses with H. Gougerot, Presse méd., 15: 481–484, July 31, 1907

Les sporotrichoses with H. Gougerot, Paris, Alcan, 1912. 852 pp.

Beuttner, Oskar. German gynecologist. 1866–1929

METHOD—removal of adnexa uteri with preservation of a portion of ovaries and transverse cuneiform excision of fundusuteri.

Die transversale fundale Keilexzision des Uterus—— Stuttgart, Enke, 1911. 67 pp.

Bevan, Arthur Dean. American surgeon. 1860–1943

INCISION—for exposing the gall bladder.

On the surgical anatomy of the bile ducts and a new incision of their exposure. Ann. Surg., 30: 15–27, July 1899

INCISION—for splenectomy.

Surgical technic of splenectomy with presentation of new incision. Ibid., 88: 347–354, Sept. 1928

OPERATION—

Pulsion diverticulum of the esophagus—Cure by the Sippy-Bevan operation. Surg. Clin. Chicago, 1: 449–457, June 1917

OPERATION—for slipping patella by imbrication of the vastus internus.
Dislocation of patellae. Surg. Clin. N. Amer., 4: 929–935, Oct. 1920
OPERATION—for "sliding hernia."
Sliding hernias of the ascending colon and cecum, the descending colon and sigmoid, and of the bladder. Ann. Surg., 92: 754–760, Oct. 1930
OPERATION—for undescended testicle.
Operation for undescended testicle and congenital inguinal hernia. J. A. M. A., 33: 773–777, Sept. 23, 1899
The surgical treatment of undescended testicle. Ibid., 41: 718–724, Sept. 19, 1903
The operation for undescended testis. A further study and report. Ann. Surg., 90: 847–863, Nov. 1929
Described acquired type of diaphragmatic hernia.
Diaphragmatic hernia. Arch. Surg., 1: 23–37, July 1920

Bevan, E. J. See C. F. Cross

Bevan-Lewis, W. See W. B. Lewis

Beyea, Henry Dorrance. Philadelphia surgeon. 1867–1924
OPERATION—gastroplication.
The elevation of the stomach in gastroptosis by the surgical plication of the gastrohepatic and gastrophrenic ligaments; an original operation. Philadelphia M. J., 1: 257–262, Feb. 7, 1903

Bezançon, Fernand. French physician. 1868–
AGAR—glycerol egg yolk; for cultivation of tubercle bacilli.
Culture du bacille tuberculeux sur le "jaune d'oeuf gélose." C. R. Soc. Biol., 55: 603–604, May 9, 1903
AGAR—serum placenta; culture medium.
Précis de microbiologie clinique. Paris, Masson, 1920. p. 119

Bezold, Albert von. German physiologist. 1836–1868
GANGLION—a series of ganglion cells in the interauricular septum.
Demonstrated the accelerator nerves of the heart and their origin in the spinal cord, 1862. (Garrison)
Untersuchungen über die Innervation des Herzens. Leipzig, Englemann, 1863. 328 pp. pp. 191–232

Bezold, Friedrich von. Munich aurist. 1842–1908
ABSCESS—mastoiditis abscess in the neck.
MASTOIDITIS—a form in which pus has escaped into the neck.
PERFORATION—of inner surface of mastoid bone.
SIGN—of mastoiditis: an inflammatory swelling below the apex of the mastoid process.
Die Corrosionsanatomie des Ohres mit Rücksicht auf die Otiatrik. Mschr. Ohrenheilk., 11: 121–127, Oct. 1877
Erkrankungen des Warzentheiles. Arch. f. Ohrenheilk., 13: 26–68, Nov. 6, 1877
TEST—for audition.
TRIAD—retarded bone conduction, lessened perception of deep tones and negative Rinne's sign, indicating otosclerosis. (Dorland)
Ueber die funktionelle Prüfung des menschlichen Gehörorgans. Wiesbaden, Bergmann, 1897–1900. 3 vols.

Bial, Manfred. Berlin physician. 1869–
REAGENT and TESTS—for pentoses in urine.
Die Diagnose der Pentosurie. Dtsch. med. Wschr., 28: 253–254, Apr. 10, 1902
Bemerkungen zu der Arbeit von F. Sachs: "Farbenre-

aktionen der Pentosen." Biochem. Z., 3: 323–325, 1907

Bialocour, F. See H. Strauss

Bianchi, Giovanni Battista. Italian anatomist. 1681–1761
NODULE—the corpora arantii, of heart.
SYNDROME—a sensory aphasic s. (Dorland)
Opera anatomico-practica. Augustae Taurinorum, (1715). 51 pp.

Biasotti, A. See B. A. Houssay

Bichat, Marie Francois Xavier. French physiologist. 1771–1802
CANAL—the arachnoid canal, transmitting the venae magnae Galeni.
FISSURE—between the fornix and upper surface of cerebellum.
FORAMEN—from subarachnoid space to third ventricle.
LIGAMENT—lower part of posterior sacroiliac l.
MEMBRANE—a subendothelial fibroelastic layer in intima of an artery.
TUNIC—the intima of a blood vessel.
Traité d'anatomie descriptive. Paris, Gabon, 1801–03. 5 vols.
Anatomie générale, appliquée a la physiologie et a la médicine. Paris, Brosson et al., 1802. 2 vols.
Also, in English: Boston, Cummings and Hilliard, 1813. 259 pp.
Founder of scientific histology and pathologic anatomy.
Traité des membranes en général et de diverses membranes en particulier. Paris, Richard et al., 1799–1800

Bickel, Adolf. Berlin physician. 1875–
Early recognized importance of bile and pancreatic juice in preventing formation of peptic ulcer.
Beobachtungen an Hunden mit extirpiertem Duodenum. Berl. klin. Wschr., 46: 1201–1202, June 28, 1909

Bickel, Verne Tillman. Lamar, Mo. surgeon. 1902–
REACTION—of Bickel and French, for alcohols.
Alpha-naphthylisocyanate as a reagent for alcohols. J. Amer. Chem. Soc., 48: 747–751, Mar. 1926

Bickfalvi, Karl. Klausenburg physiologist
PEPSIN—
Beitrag zur Verwendung der Magenverdauung als Isolationsmethode. Zbl. med. Wiss., 21: 833–836, Nov. 17, 1883

Bickford, Reginald G. London surgeon
METHOD—for removal of cast.
A rapid and painless method of removing plaster casts. Brit. M. J., 1: 539–540, Mar. 30, 1940

Bickham, Warren Stone. New York surgeon. 1861–
OPERATION—of Matas-Bickham.
Operation for the radical cure of arteriovenous aneurysms, with preservation of circulation in artery and vein.
In his: *Textbook of operative surgery.* Philadelphia, Saunders, 1924. Vol. 2, pp. 70–72

Bidder, Friedrich Heinrich. German anatomist. 1810–1894
GANGLION—in auricular septum.
Die Selbstständigkeit des sympathischen Nervensystems durch anatomische Untersuchungen nachgewiesen with A. W. Volkmann, Leipzig, Breitkopf und Härtel, 1842. 88 pp.
Ueber functionell verschiedene und räumlich getrennte

Nervencentra im Froschnerzen. Arch. f. Anat., Physiol. u. wissen. Med., Berlin, pp. 163–177, 1852
ORGAN—nuptial excrescence.
Vergleichend-anatomische und histologische Untersuchungen über die männlichen Geschlechts- und Harnwerkzeuge der nackten Amphibien. Dorpat, Karow, 1846. 74 pp.
Recorded observation of psychic secretion of gastric juice, and proved the gastric juice always contains hydrochloric acid in excess.
Die Verdauungssäfte und der Stoffwechsel. Eine physiologisch-chemische Untersuchung with C. Schmidt, Mittau u. Leipzig, Reyher, 1852, 413 pp.
Biedermann, Dr. St. Gallen surgeon
ESOPHAGOSCOPE—
Das Broncho- und Oesophagoteleskop. Schweiz. med. Wschr., 19: 382 (only), Apr. 9, 1938
Biedert, Philipp. Berlin physician. 1847–1916
METHOD—for staining tubercle bacilli in sputum.
Ein Verfahren, den Nachweis vereinzelter Tuberkelbacillen zu sichern, nebst Bemerkungen über die Färbbarkeit der Bacillen und Aetiologie der Tuberkulose. Berl. klin. Wschr., pp. 713–717, Oct. 18; 742–744, Oct. 25, 1886
MIXTURE—a food for young infants; cream, 4 fl. oz.; water, 10 fl. oz.; milk-sugar, ½ oz.
Die Kinderernährung im Säuglingsalter. Stuttgart, Enke, 1880. 392 pp.
Biedl, Arthur. Prag physician. 1869–1933
SYNDROME—Laurence-Moon-Biedl; adiposcgenital (Frählich's) dystrophy with atypical retinitis pigmentosa, mental retardation, and skeletal abnormalities, usually polydactylism and syndactylism.
Geschwisterpaar mit adiposo-genitaler Dystrophie. Dtsch. med. Wschr., 48: 1630, 1922
Showed that adrenal cortex is essential for life.
Innere Sekretion. Berlin, Wien, Urban und Schwarzenburg, 1910
Also, English transl., 1912
Also, in German, 2 ed., 1913; 4 ed., 1922
Bieling, Richard Franz Ludwig. German physician. 1888–
AGAR—glucose blood, for differentiation of streptococci from pneumococci.
Methoden zur Differenzierung der Streptokokken und Pneumokokken. Zbl. Bakt., 86: 257–266, June 11, 1921
REAGENT and TEST—for viability of tissues.
Untersuchungen über die intramolekulare Atmung von Mikroorganismen. Klin. Wschr., 2: 1317–1318, July 9, 1923
Bielschowsky, Max. Berlin neurobiologist
CLASSIFICATION—
Neoblastic tumors of the sympathetic nervous system. In: *Cytology and cellular pathology of the nervous system.* Ed. by W. Penfield, New York, Hoeber, 1932
METHOD—impregnation m. for material embedded in paraffin or cellcidin.
METHOD—for demonstrating nonmyelinated nerve fibers.
Die Silberimprägnation der Neurofibrillen. J. Psychol. Neurol., Lpz., 3: 169–189, 1904
Die Darstellung der Axenzylinder peripherischer Nervenfasern und der Axenzylinder zentraler markhaltiger Nervenfasern. Ibid., 4: 227–231, 1904–05
METHOD—for neurofibrils in sections.

Eine Modifikation meines Silberimprägnationsverfahrens zur Darstellung der Neurofibrillen. Ibid., 12: 135–137, 1908–09
Bien, G. E. See V. E. Levine
Bier, Karl Gustav August. Berlin surgeon. 1861–
ANESTHESIA—vein a.
Ueber einen neuen Weg Localanästhesie an den Gliedmassen zu erzengen. Arch. klin. Chir., 86: 1007–1016, 1908
Also: Verh. dtsch. Ges. Chir., 37: 2 Teil, 204–213, 1908
Ueber Venenanästhesie. Berl. klin. Wschr., 46: 477–489, 1909
AMPUTATION—osteoplastic a. of leg.
Ueber Amputationen und Exartikulationen. Samml. klin. Vortr., n. F., No. 264, (Chir., No. 78, p. 1439–1474, 1900
HYPEREMIA or TREATMENT—induction of venous congestion by applying a rubber band to proximal part of a limb. First proposed for chronic infections, in 1904 Bier used it in acute infections.
Ueber ein neues Verfahren der konservativen Behandlung von Gelenktuberkulose. 31. Cong. Dtsch. Gesell. f. Chir., June 1892; reviewed in Zbl. Chir., 19: 57, 1892
Behandlung chirurgischer Tuberkulsose der Gliedmassen mit Stauungshyperämie. Wien. med. Bl., 16: 207–209, Apr. 13; 219–221, Apr. 20; 244–246, May 4; 258–260, May 11; 267–268, May 18, 1893
Also: Festschr. z. Fr. von Esmarch, Kiel & Leipzig, 1893. pp. 53–85
Hyperämie als Heilmittel. 1 ed., 1893. Also: 2 ed., Leipzig, Vogel, 1903. 220 pp.
Bier's hyperemic treatment. By W. Myer and V. Schmieden, Philadelphia, Saunders, 1909
Introduced spinal anesthesia with cocaine.
Versuch über Cocainisirung des Rückenmarkes. Dtsch. Z. f. Chir., 51: 361–369, Apr. 1899
Bemerkungen zur Cocainisierung des Rückenmarkes. Münch. med. Wschr., 47: 1226 (only), Sept. 4, 1900
Biermer, Anton. Zurich physician. 1827–1892
ANEMIA—pernicious or Addison-Biermer-Ehrlich a. First announced in 1868, in Versammlung deutscher Naturforscher und Ärzt in Dresden. Siehe Tageblatt, 1868, No. 8, IX Sekt., S. 173
. . . über eine . . . eigentümliche Form von progressiver, perniziöser Anämie. . . . Correspond. f. Schweizer. Aerzte, 2: 15–17, Jan. 1, 1872
SIGN or CHANGE OF SOUND—a change of percussion sound on change of patient's position, encountered in pneumothrax.
Krankheiten der Bronchien und des Lungen-Parenchymus. Handb. spec. Path. u. Therap., 5: 531–822, 1865–7
Biernacki, Edmond Adolfovich. Polish physician. 1866–1912
SIGN—analgesia of ulnar nerve in paretic dementia. In: Gaz. lekarska, No. 2, 1894
Analgesie des Ulnarisstammes als Tabessymptom. Neurol. Zbl. 13: 242–246, Apr. 1, 1894
Abstr.: Ibid., 456–457, June 15, 1894
Bielsalski, Konrad. German orthopedic surgeon. 1868–1930
OPERATION—of Biesalski-Mayer; transplantation of long peroneal tendon.

Die physiologische Sehnenverpflanzung with L. Mayer, Berlin, Springer, 1916
The physiological method of tendon transplantation. By L. Mayer (New York), S. G. O., 22: 182–197, Feb. 1916

Biett, Laurent Théodore. Paris physician. 1781–1840
DISEASE—lupus erythematoides migrans.
In: *Abrégé pratique des maladies de la peau.* By P. L. A. Cazenave and H. E. Schedel, (Biett's pupils), Paris, 1828. p. 11; 415

Bigelow, G. H. See A. W. Sellards
Bigelow, Henry Jacob. Boston surgeon. 1818–1890
LIGAMENT—iliofemoral or Y or Moses Gunn 1.
The mechanism of dislocation and fracture of the hip, with the reduction of the dislocations by the flexion method. Phila., Lea, 1869. 150 pp. pp. 17–20
METHOD—of reduction of dislocation of the hip. Ibid.
OPERATION—litholapaxy; crushing of a calculus by a special kind of lithotrite and removal of fragments by another apparatus.
Lithotrity by a single operation. Amer. J. M. Sci., 75: 117–134, Jan. 1878
SEPTUM—the calcar femorale, a vertical lamina of strong tissue on front of lesser trochanter, serving to strengthen neck of femur.
The true neck of the femur; its structure and pathology. Boston M. & S. J., 92: 1–5; 29–33, Jan. 7 & 14, 1875
First in America to excise the hip-joint. (Garrison)
Resection of the head of the femur. Amer. J. M. Sci., 24: 90, July 1852
Wrote early works on ether anesthesia.
Insensibility during surgical operations produced by inhalation. Boston Med. & Surg. J., 35: 309–317; 379–382, 1846
Ether and chloroform: a compendium of their history and discovery. Boston, Clapp, 1848

Biggart, John Henry. Scottish physician
Produced diabetes insipidus in dogs by injury to hypothalamus.
Experimental diabetes insipidus with G. L. Alexander, J. Path. and Bact., Edinburgh, 48: 405–425, 1939

Bijlon. See D. Bylon
Bilharz, Theodor. German helminthologist. 1825–1862
BILHARZIA—a genus of flukes or trematodes.
Ein Beitrag zur Helminthographia humana.... Z. wiss. Zool., 4: 53, 1852
Distomum haematobium und sein Verhältniss zu gewissen pathologischen Veränderungen der menschlichen Harnorgane. Wien. med. Wschr., 6: 49–52; 65–68, 1856

Bilinski, Josef. German chemist
TEST—for sugar in urine.
Eine einfache und genaue Methode zur Zuckerbestimmung im Harn. Mschr. Chem. u. ver. Teile. Wiss., 26: 133–141, 1905

Billard, Charles Michel. French physician. 1800–1832
Wrote early work on pediatrics.
Traité des maladies des enfans nouveau-nés et à la mammelle. Paris, Bailliere, 1828. 1 vol. and atlas

Billings, Frank. Chicago physician. 1854–1932
Developed, with E. C. Rosenow, doctrine of focal infection from bacteria of streptococcus-pneumococcus group via teeth, tonsils and other portals.
Chronic focal infections and their etiologic relations to

arthritis and nephritis. Arch. intern. Med., 9: 484–498, Apr. 15, 1912
Focal infections. New York, Appleton, 1916. 166 pp.
Billings, Frank Seaver. American physician. 1845–1912
SWINE-PLAGUE OF—
Swine plague, with especial reference to the porcine pests of the world. Lincoln, Neb., 1888. 414 pp.
Billings, William Chester. U. S. Public Health Surgeon. 1872–1939
TECHNIC—for discovery of specific organism, Necator Americanus, of hookworm disease.
Some points about hookworm disease, its diagnosis and treatment with J. C. Hickey, J. A. M. A., 67: 1908–1912, Dec. 23, 1916
Billroth, Theodor. Vienna surgeon. 1829–1894
OPERATION—resection of stomach, pylorectomy; Billroth I.
Offenes Schreiben an Herrn Dr. L. Wittelshöfer. Wien. med. Wschr., 31: 162–165, 1881
Ueber einen neuen Fall von gelungener Resektion des carcinomatösen Pylorus. Mitgetheilt von Dr. Anton Wölfler (Billroth's assistant). Ibid., 1427
Gastro-Enterostomie, by A. Wölfler, Zbl. f. Chir., 8: 705–708, Nov. 21, 1881
OPERATION—pylorectomy; Billroth II. After resection both stomach and duodenum are closed and a typical gastrojejunostomy (anterior in Billroth's original technic) is performed. First reported by von Hacker at 14. Cong. Deut. Gesell. f. Chir., Berlin, Apr. 10, 1885
Zur Casuistik und Statistik der Magenresektionen und Gastroenterostomieen. Arch. f. klin. Chir., 32: 616, 1885
DISEASE—spurious meningocele or cephalohydrocele traumatica.
Ein Fall von Meningocele spuria cum fixtula ventriculi cerebri. Arch. f. klin. Chir., 3: 398–412, 1862
DISEASE—malignant lymphoma.
Neue Beobachtungen über die feinere Structur pathologische veränderter Lymphdrüsen. Arch. f. path. Anat., 21: 423–443, 1861
DISEASE—spurious traumatic meningitis.
Ueber akute Meningitis serosa und akutes Hirnödem nach chirurgischen Operationen. Wien. med. Wschr., 19: 1–4; 17–29, Jan. 2 and 6, 1869
Resected the esophagus.
Ueber die Resection des Oesophagus. Arch. f. klin. Chir., 13: 65–69, 1872
OPERATION—excision of tongue.
Osteoplastische Resectionen des Unterkiefers nach eigener Methode. Arch. f. klin. Chir., 2: 651–657, 1862
Resected the larynx.
Ueber die erste am Menschen Th. Billroth ausgeführte Kehlkopf-Exstirpation und die Anwendung eines Künstlichen Kehlkopfes, by C. Gussenbauer, Verh. dtsch. Ges. f. Chir., 3, Hft. 2: 76–89, 1874
Also: Arch. f. klin. Chir., 17: 343–356, 1874
Performed abdominal resection of tumor of bladder.
Exstirpation eines Harnblasenmyoms nach vorausgehenden tiefen und hohen Blasenschnitt, by C. Gussenbauer, Ibid., 18: 411–423, 1875
Binder, Karl. Tübingen chemist
REACTION—for oxygen.
Ueber eine neue scharfe Reaktion auf elementaren Sauerstoff with R. E. Weinland, Ber. dtsch. chem. Ges., 46: 255–260, Feb. 8, 1913

Binet, Alfred. French physiologist. 1857–1911
TEST—of mental capacity.
La mésure du développement de l'intelligence chez les jeunes enfants with Th. Simon, Paris, Coneslant, 1911
Same, in English, Baltimore, Williams & Wilkins, 1916. 336 pp.
Binetti, M. See J. Thomas
Bing, Albert. Austrian otologist. 1844–1922
SIGN—entotic s. of disease of malleus or incus.
Vorlesungen über Ohrenheilkunde. Wien, Braumüller, 1890. 286 pp.
Binger, C. A. L. See A. L. Barach, W. B. Cannon
Bingman, D. L. C. See F. A. Coller
Binkley, S. B. See E. A. Doisy and R. W. McKee
Binnie, John Fairbairn. American surgeon. 1863–1936
TREATMENT—of snapping hip.
Snapping hip (hauche a ressort; schnellende hufte). Ann. Surg., 58: 59–66, July 1913
Binz, Karl. German pharmacologist. 1832–1913
TEST—for quinine in urine.
Vorlesungen über Pharmakologie. Berlin, Hitschwald, 188(5)–86
Birch, C. L. See E. L. Boyden
Bircher, Heinrich. Swiss surgeon. 1850–1923
OPERATION—to reduce the size of a dilated stomach.
Neue Beiträge zur operativen Behandlung der Magenerweiterung. Correspond. f. Schweizer Aerzte, Basel, 24: 553–563, 1894
Bircher, Mat Edwin. Zurich physician
DIET—raw.
Der Einfluss der fruktovegetabilen und vorwiegend rohen Ernährungsweise auf die Viskosität des Blutes, auf dessen Hämoglobingehalt und auf den Blutdruck. Münch. med. Wschr., 75: 1628–1629, Sept. 21, 1928
Birch-Hirschfeld, Arthur. Königsberg physician. 1871–
PHOTOMETER—
Ueber Nachtblindheit im Kriege. Arch. f. Ophth., 92: 273–340, Dec. 13, 1917
Birch-Hirschfeld, Felix Victor. German pathologist. 1842–1899
STAINING METHOD—for amyloid.
Lehrbuch der pathologischen Anatomie. Leipzig, Vogel, 1882. 2 ed.
Bird, Golding. English physician. 1814–1854
FORMULA—the last two figures expressive of the specific gravity of urine nearly represent the number of grains of solids in each ounce.
Observations on urinary concretions and deposits. . . . London, Churchill, 1842. 58 pp.
Same, 5 ed. 1857. pp. 59
TREATMENT—of bed sores by mild galvanic currents.
Lectures on electricity and galvanism in their physiological and therapeutical relations. London, Longmans, 1849. 212 pp.
See also T. Addison
Bird, Samuel Dougan. Australian physician. 1833–1904
SIGN—a definite zone of dulness with absence of respiratory sounds in hydatid disease of lungs.
On hydatids of the lung; their diagnosis, prognosis, and treatment, and observations on their relations to pulmonary consumption, and other diseases of the chest. Melbourne, Mullen, 1874. 44 pp.

Birkett, John. English surgeon. 1815–1904
HERNIA—inguino-properitoneal.
Description of a case of intra-parietal inguinal hernia, with references to cases which were probably of a similar kind. Guy's Hosp. Rep., 7: 270–291, 1861
Birkhaug. Konrad Elias. Rochester, N. Y. bacteriologist. 1892–
TREATMENT—of erysipelas with antitoxin.
Erysipelas. V. Observations on the etiology and treatment with erysipelas antistreptococcic serum. J. A. M. A., 86: 1411–1417, May 8, 1926
Birt, C. English physician
TEST—for diagnosis of syphilis.
A simple modification of Wassermann's reaction. Jour. R. A. M. C., London, 15: 415–421, Oct. 1910
Bisbini, B. Italian physician
TEST—for lactic acid in stomach contents.
La ricerca qualitativa dell'acido lattico nel succo gastrico. Rinasc. med., 3: 514–516, Dec. 1, 1926
Bischoff, Theodor Ludwig Wilhelm von. German anatomist. 1807–1882
CROWN—the inner layer formed from the duplication of the epithelial capsule of the ovum.
Beiträge zur Lehre von den Eyhüllen des menschlichen Fötus. Bonn, Marcus, 1834. 112 pp.
Entwickelungsgeschichte des Kaninchen-Eies. Braunschweig, Vieweg, 1842
Proved that fibrin of blood is the toxic element and advised use of defibrinated blood.
Beiträge zur Lehre von dem Blute und der Transfusion desselben. Arch. f. anat. Physiol. u. wiss. Med., pp. 347–372, 1835
Demonstrated presence of free CO_2 and oxygen in blood.
Commentatio de novis quibusdam experimentis chemico-physiologicis ad illustrandam doctrinam de respiratione institutis. Heidelbergae, Mohr. 1837. 42 pp.
Bishop, C. See O. S. Lowsley
Bishop, Edward Stanmore. Manchester surgeon. 1848–1912
CLAMP—for intestinal resection.
On methods of occlusion in enterectomy, with description of a new clamp for that purpose. Brit. M. J., 2: 867–869, Nov. 3, 1883
SUTURE—
Enterorraphy. Med. Chronicle, 2: 448–459, Sept. 1885
Bishop, Eliot. Brooklyn obstetrician. 1880–
METHOD—of Pomeroy and Bishop, of tubal sterilization.
A simple method of tubal sterilization with W. F. Nelms, New York State J. M., 30: 214–216, Feb. 15, 1930
Operative methods of sterilization in the female. Amer. J. Obst. & Gynec., 34: 505–507, Sept. 1937
Bishop, Francis W. Rochester, N. Y. scientist
Introduced the luminous heat cabinet for fever therapy.
A comparison of three electrical methods of producing artificial hyperthermia with Emmy Lehman and S. L. Warren, J. A. M. A., 104: 910–915, Mar. 16, 1935
Bishop, George Holman. American physiologist. 1889–
APPARATUS—
An apparatus for microdissection. Amer. Nat., 54: 381–384, July–Aug. 1921
Bishop, K. S. See H. M. Evans

Bishop, Louis Faugeres. American physician. 1864–1941
SPHYGMOSCOPE—for measuring blood pressure, especially diastolic.
In his: *Heart disease, biood-pressure and the Nauheim-Schott treatment.* New York, Treat, 1911. 3 ed., pp. 106–108
Biskra—a town in Africa
BUTTON—see Leischmaniasis cutis.
Bissell, J. Dougal. New York gynecologist. 1864–1935
OPERATION—for uterine prolapse and cystocele, by excision of a section of the round and broad ligaments for uterine retroversion.
A vaginal hysterectomy technique for the cure of prolapse of the uterus when the removal of the uterus is necessitated; with special reference to lapping of the vaginal fascia in all forms of vaginal prolapse. Trans. Amer. Gynes. Soc., 43: 157–169, 1918
Vaginal prolapse. S. G. O., 28: 138–145, Feb. 1919
Fascia lapping as applied to the tissues of the vaginal wall—a misnomer. Ibid., 48: 549–550, Apr. 1929
Bitot, Pierre A. Bordeaux physician. 1822–1888
SPOTS—on the cornea; called also xerosis corneae; an indication of vitamin deficiency.
Mémoire sur une lésion conjonctivale non encore décrite, coincidant avec l'héméralopie. Gaz. hebd. de méd. et de chir., 10: 284–288, May 1, 1863
Bitter, Ludwig. Kiel physician. 1882–
AGAR—china blue malachite green; for diagnosis of typhoid fever.
Zur Methodik des Typhusbakteriennachweises in Stuhl und Urin. Zbl. f. Bakt., 59: 469–478, July 15, 1911
Bittner, John Joseph. Bar Harbor, Maine scientist. 1904–
Demonstrated that mammary carcinoma is transmitted in mice from mother to their offspring through milk.
Some possible effects of nursing on the mammary gland tumor incidence in mice. Science, 84: 162 (only), Aug. 14, 1936
Also: Amer. J. clin. Path., 7: 430–435, Sept. 1937
Bittó, Béla von. German chemist
REACTION—for creatinine.
Ueber eine Reaction der Aldehyde und Ketone mit arom. Nitroverbindungen. Ann. Chem., 269: 377–382, 1892
Bizzozero, Giulio. Italian physician. 1846–1901
CORPUSCLES—the blood platelets. Coined term blood platelets.
Su di un nuovo elemento morfologico del sangue dei mammiferi e della sua importanza nella trombosi e nella coagulazione. Osservatore, Torino, 17: 785–787; 18: 97–99, 1882
Ueber einen neuen Formbestandtheil des Blutes und dessen Rolle bei der Thrombose und der Blutgerinnung. Arch. f. path. Anat., 90: 261–332, Nov. 8, 1882
STAIN—for blood.
Sulla produzione dei globuli rossi del sangue. I. Sulla produzione dei globuli rossi negli uccelli with A. A. Torre, Arch. Sci. med., 4: 388–412, 1880
Bjeloussow, A. K. Charkof anatomist
MASS—gum arabic, for histologic injections.
Eine neue Methode von Injection anatomischer Praeparate vermittelst kalter Masse. Arch. Anat. Phys. Anat., pp. 379–384, 1885

Bjerrum, Jamik Peterson. Denmark ophthalmologist. 1851–1926
SCOTOMA—
Vejledning i anvendelsen af øjespejlet. Kjøbenhavn, Priors, 1890. 84 pp.
Black, Douglas Andrew Kilgour. Scottish physician
FORMULA—in burns, give plasma in cc. equal to 1000 times the product of the difference of 5 less 500 divided by the per centage of hemoglobin.
Treatment of burn shock with plasma and serum. Brit. M. J., 2: 693–697, Nov. 23, 1940
Black, Greene Vardiman. Chicago physician, 1836–1915
Wrote early report on pathologic histology of dental fluorosis (mottled enamel).
Mottled teeth: an endemic developmental imperfection of the teeth, heretofore unknown in the literature of dentistry with F. S. McKay, Dental Cosmos, 58: 129–156, Feb. 1916
Black, Joseph. Scottish chemist. 1728–1799
Discovered carbon dioxide.
Defined "specific heat", "capacity for heat", and "latent heat".
Dissertatio de humore acido a cibis ortu, et magnesia alba. Edinburgi, Hamilton and Balfour, 1754
Black, Otis Fisher. American chemist. 1867–1933
TEST—
The detection and quantitative determination of b-oxybutyric acid in the urine. J. Biol. Chem., 5: 207–210, Oct. 1908
Blackadder, H. Howe. Edinburgh surgeon
Described lumbricoid worms in the appendix vermiformis.
Notices of certain accidents and diseased structures of the caput cecum coli and its appendage. Edinburgh M. & S. J., 22: 18–23, July 1824
Blackall, John. English physician. 1771–1860
Investigated albumen in urine.
Observations on the nature and cure of dropsies, and particularly on the presence of the coagulable part of the blood in dropsical urine; . . . London, Longman, 1813
Blackberg, Solon Nathaniel. American physician. 1897–
TEST—for melanin.
Melanuria with J. O. Wanger, J. A. M. A., 100: 334–336, Feb. 4, 1933
See also G. F. Laidlaw
Blackfan, K. D. See W. E. Dandy, C. D. May
Blackley, Charles Harrison. English homeopath. 1820–1900
Gave early experimental demonstration of pollen hypersensitiveness.
Experimental researches on the causes and nature of catarrhus aestivus (hay-fever or hay-asthma). London, Baillière, 1873. 202 pp.
Hay fever: its causes, treatment and effective prevention; experimental researches. London, Baillière, 1880. 2 ed.
Blades Brian Brewer. St. Louis surgeon, 1906–
OPERATION—one-stage lobectomy.
Individual ligation technique for lower lobe lobectomy with E. M. Kent, Jr. J. Thoracic Surg., 10:84–101, Oct. 1940
Blaes, Gérard. Dutch anatomist. 1626–1682
DUCT—of parotid gland.
Observata anatomica in homine, simia, equo, vitulo,

ove, testudine, echino, glire, serpente, ardea, variisque animalibus aliis; accedunt extraordinaria in homine reperta, proxim medicam aeque ac anatomen illustrantia. Lugd. Bat. et Amstelodami, Gaasbeeck, 1674
Anatome animalium. Amstelodami, a Someren, 1681

Biagden, Sir Charles. English surgeon. 1748–1820
Demonstrated the importance of perspiration in maintenance of constant body temperature.
Experiments and observations in an heated room. Philos. Trans., 65: 111–123; 484–494, 1775

Blair, Vilray Papin. American surgeon. 1871–
METHOD—of skin grafting.
The use and uses of large split skin grafts of intermediate thickness with J. B. Brown, S. G. O., 49: 82–97, July 1929
OPERATION—radical excision of tongue.
Operation for advanced carcinoma of the tongue or floor of the mouth. Ibid., 30: 149–153, Feb. 1920
OPERATION—for facial paralysis.
Notes on the operative correction of facial palsy. South. M. J., 19: 116–120, Feb. 1926
OPERATION—of Blair and Mirault, for single harelip.
Mirault operation for single harelip with J. B. Brown, S. G. O., 51: 81–98, July 1930
OPERATION—
The correction of scrotal hypospadias and of epispadias with J. B. Brown and W. J. Hamm, Ibid., 57: 646–653, Nov. 1933

Blair, W. M. See W. F. Taylor

Blaizot, L. See C. J. H. Nicolle

Blake, Clarence John. Boston otologist. 1843–1919
DISKS—of paper.
Application of paper dressings in treatment of perforations of the membrana tympani. Trans. Internat. Otol. Cong., New York, 1876

Blake, Edward Thomas. English physician. 1842–1905
CINGULA ATHLETICA—a ring of dilated blood vessels running around the waist which he declared was "a pathognomonic sign of hypertrophic emphysema when it occurs in the gouty." (Rolleston)
Constipation and some associated disorders, including recent observations on intestinal innervation and the venous hearts; with sections on venous stasis of abdomen, piles, fissure, pruritis ani, rupture and corpulency. London, Glaisher, 1900. 286 pp.

Blake, Eugene Maurice. New Haven, Conn. ophthalmologist. 1882–
HOLDER—
A conjunctival flap holder for cataract sutures. Amer. J. Ophth., 17: 529–530, June 1934

Blake, Francis Gilman. American physician. 1887–
METHOD—
Methods for the determination of pneumococcus types. J. exp. Med., 26: 67–80, July 1917

Blake, Joseph Augustus. American surgeon. 1864–1937
METHOD—of traction for supracondylar fracture.
La suspension avec extension dans le traitement des fractures des membres. Arch. d. méd. et pharm. mil., Paris, 66: 289–313, 1916
Traitement des fractures des membres ou moyen de la suspension et de la traction with K. Bulkley, Pr. méd., 25: 653–659, Nov. 19, 1917
The treatment of fractures of the extremities by means of suspension and traction with K. Bulkley, S. G. O., 26: 245–258, Mar. 1918

OPERATION—for hernia, by a vertical overlapping of tissue.
Umbilical hernia. Ann. Surg., 39: 1003–1006, June 1904

Blakemore, Arthur Hendley. New York surgeon. 1897–
OPERATION—
Electrothermic coagulation of aortic aneurysms with B. G. King, J. A. M. A., 111: 1821–1827, Nov. 12, 1938
TUBES—
The severed primary artery in the war wounded: a nonsuture method of bridging arterial defects with J. W. Lord, Jr. and P. L. Stefko, Surgery, 12: 488–508, Sept. 1942
A nonsuture method of blood vessel anastomosis: experimental and clinical study with J. W. Lord, Jr., J. A. M. A., 127: 685–691, Mar. 24: 748–753, Mar. 31, 1945

Blalock, Alfred. Baltimore surgeon. 1899–
CRUSHER—see G. W. Duncan
OPERATION—
The surgical treatment of malformations of the heart in which there is pulmonary stenosis or pulmonary atresia with Helen B. Taussig, J. A. M. A., 128: 189–202, May 19, 1945
TECHNIC—
The treatment of myasthenia gravis by removal of the thymus gland: preliminary report with A. McG. Harvey, F. R. Ford and J. L. Lilienthal, Jr., Ibid., 117: 1529–1533, Nov. 1, 1941
See also G. W. Duncan, E. G. Nyström, K. L. Pickrell

Blanc, G. See G. Abt

Blanchard, Evelyn Lyman. Los Angeles scientist. 1909–
TEST—dark adaptation for vitamin A.
Measurement of vitamin A status of young adults by the dark adaptation technic with H. A. Harper, Arch. Int. M., 66: 661–669, Sept. 1940

Blankaart or Blancard, Stephan. Dutch physician. 1650–1702
Wrote Greek and Latin lexica, published in Amsterdam in 1679; translated into English in 1684, it became the first medical dictionary to appear in Great Britain. (Garrison)
Physical dictionary in which all the terms relating either to anatomy, chirurgery, pharmacy, or chemistry are very accurately explained. London, Crouch, 1684. 302 pp.

Blandin, Phillippe Frédéric. French surgeon. 1798–1842
GLAND—mixed glands near tip of tongue.
Traité d'anatomie topographique. . . . Paris, Méquignon, 1826. 2 ed., 1834

Bland-Sutton, Sir John. London surgeon. 1855–1936
Reported torsion of fallopian tube.
Remarks on salpingitis and some of its effects. Lancet, 2: 1146–1148; 1206–1209, 1890

Blane, Sir Gilbert. English physician. 1749–1834
Introduced use of lemons and limes in British navy to prevent scurvy.
Observations on the diseases incident to seamen. London, Cooper, 1785. 502 pp.

Blanke, E. See K. H. Slotta

Blankenhorn, Marion Arthur. Cleveland physician. 1885–

TEST—qualitative, for bile pigments, bile salts and urobilin in blood plasma.
The bile content of the blood in pernicious anemia.
Arch. intern. Med., 19 : 344–353, Mar. 1917
See also T. D. Spies

Blaskovics, Laszlo de. Budapest physician. 1869–
OPERATION—for ptosis.
A new operation for ptosis with shortening of the levator and tarsus. Arch. Ophth., 52 : 563–573, Nov. 1923
Treatment of ptosis: the formation of a fold in the eyelid and resection of the levator and tarsus. Ibid., 1 : 672–680, June 1929

Blaud, Pierre. French physician. 1774–1858
PILL—of ferrous sulfate and potassium carbonate.
Pilules anti-chlorotiques. Bull. gén. de Thérap., 2 : 154–155, 1832
Memoire sur les maladies chlorotiques, et sur un mode de traitement spécifique dans ces affections. Rev. méd. franc. et étrang., Paris, 1 : 337–367, 1832

Bledsoe, M. S. See Martha Aldrich

Blegny, Nicholas de. French surgeon. 1652–1722
Wrote important work on medico-legal relations of surgery.
La doctrine des rapports de chirurgie. Lyons, Amaulry, 1684
Founded the first medical journal. Garrison
Nouvelles decouvertes sur toutes les parties de la médécine. Paris, 1679–81

Blendermann, Hermann Ludwig. Berlin chemist. 1858–
TEST—for hydroxy acid in urine.
Beiträge zur Kenntniss der Bildung und Zersetzung des Tyrosins im Organismus. Z. phys. Chem., 6 : 234–262, 1882

Blessig, Robert. German physician. 1830–1878
GROOVE—a tract in the embryonic eye corresponding in position with the future ora serrata.
De retinae textura disquisitiones microscopicae. (Dorpat), Schünmanni et Mattieseni, 1855. 86 pp.

Bleuler, Paul Eugen. Swiss neurologist. 1857–1939
Introduced concept "schizophrenia."
Dementia praecox oder Gruppe der Schizophrenien. Leipzig, Deuticke, 1911. 420 pp.

Bliss, Eleanor A. See P. H. Long

Blix, C. See P. J. Wising

Blix, Magnus Gustav. Upsala physician. 1849–1904
HOT TUBE OF—to determine thermal points on skin.
Experimentelle Briträge zur Lösung der Frage über die specifische Energie der Hautnerven. Z. Biologie, 20 : 141–156, 1884; 21 : 145–160, 1885

Bloch, Bruno. Swiss physician. 1878–1933
DISEASE—incontinentia pigmenti.
Eigentümliche, bisher nicht beschriebene Pigmentaffektion (Incontinentia pigmenti). Abstr. in: Schweiz. med. Wschr., 7 : 404–405, May 1, 1926
REACTION—"dopa", for melanoblasts.
Chemische Untersuchungen über das spezifische pigmentbildende Ferment der Haut, die Dopaoxydase. Z. phys. Chem., 98 : 226–254, Feb. 28, 1917
Der Nachweis der Oxydase in den Zellen des myeloischen Systems durch 3,4-Dioxyphenylalanin with S. N. Peck, Folia haemat., 41 : 166–173, May 1930

Bloch, M. H. Danzig surgeon
Suggested repair of wounds of heart. (No title) In discussion : Verh. dtsch. Ges. Chir., 11 Cong., Berlin, part 1, 108–109, 1882

Bloch, P. See H. A. Danlos

Blocq, Paul Oscar. French physician. 1860–1896
DISEASE—astasia-abasia.
Sur une affection caractérisee par de l'astasie et de l'abasie. Arch. d. neurol., 15 : 24–51; 187–211, 1888

Blonde, P. See E. Chabrol

Blondlot, Prosper René. French physicist. 1849–
RAY—n-rays.
Rayons N; recueil des communications faites à l'Académie des sciences, avec des notes complémentaires et une instruction pour la confection des écrans phosphorescents. Paris, Gauthier-Villars, 1904. 78 pp.

Bloodgood, Joseph Colt. Baltimore surgeon. 1866–1935
OPERATION—for inguinal hernia; a flap of the anterior layer of rectus sheath is sutured to Poupart's ligament.
The transplantation of the rectus muscle in certain cases of inguinal hernia in which the conjoined tendon is obliterated. Johns Hopk. Hosp. Bull., 9 : 96–100, May 1918
The transplantation of the rectus muscle or its sheath for cure of inguinal hernia when the conjoined tendon is obliterated. The transplantation of the sartorius muscle for the cure of recurrent hernia when Poupart's ligament has been destroyed. Ann. Surg., 70 : 81–88, July 1919
THEORY—of causation of chronic mastitis. Described "senile parenchymatous hypertrophy" of breast.
Senile parenchymatous hypertrophy of female breast; its relation to cyst formation and carcinoma. S. G. O., 3 : 721–730, Dec. 1906
Chronic cystic mastitis of the diffuse, non-encapsulated, cystic adenomatous type: (shotty breast). Ann. Surg., 90 : 886–903, Nov. 1929
Described blue-dome cyst of breast.
The pathology of chronic cystic mastitis of the female breast; with special consideration of the blue-domed cyst. Arch. Surg., 3 : 445–542, Nov. 1921

Bloomfield, A. L. See C. R. Austrian, L. G. Rowntree

Bloor, Walter Ray. American biochemist. 1877–
METHOD—determination of cholesterol.
Studies on blood fat. II. Fat absorption and the blood lipoids. J. Biol. Chem., 23 : 317–326 (320–321), Nov. 1915
METHOD—of determination of cholesterol esters.
The separate determination of cholesterol and cholesterol esters in small amounts of blood with A. Knudson. Ibid., 27 : 107–112, Oct. 1916
METHOD—calorimetric, for determination of cholesterol in blood plasma.
The determination of cholesterol in blood. Ibid., 24 : 227–231, Mar. 1916; 29 : 437–445, Apr. 1917
Determination of fatty acids (and cholesterol) in small amounts of blood plasma with K. F. Pelkan and D. M. Allan, Ibid., 52 : 191–205, May 1922
METHOD—
A method for the determination of fat in small amounts of blood. Ibid., 17 : 377–384, Apr. 1914
METHOD—for determination of phosphatides of blood.
A method for the determination of "lecithin" in small amounts of blood. Ibid., 22 : 133–149, Aug. 1915
METHOD—for determination of phosphates.
Methods for the determination of phosphoric acid in small amounts of blood. Ibid., 36 : 33–48, Oct. 1918

Bloxam, Charles Loudon. London chemist. 1832–1887
REACTION—for strychnine.
Die Farbenreaction des Strychnins. Chem. News, 55: 155, 1891

Blum, F. Frankfurt a M. physician
TEST—adrenaline glycosuria in suprarenal disease.
Ueber Nebennierendiabetes. Dtsch. Arch. f. klin. Med., 71: 146–167, Oct. 30, 1901

Blum, P. See H. Gongerot

Blum, Paul. Strasbourg physician. 1878–1933
Among the first to report the clinical benefits derived from histidine for peptic ulcer.
Orientation nouvelle de la pathogénie de l'ulcère expérimental gastrique et de la therapeutique de l'ulcère humain. Bull. gén. de Thérap., 184: 253–260, June 1933

Blume, H. See A. O. Gettler

Blumenau, Leonid Vasilyevich. Russian neurologist. 1862–1932
NUCLEUS—the lateral portion of the cuneate nucleus.
Mozg chelovieka.... (The human brain). S.-Peterburg, Buze, 1907–1910 Parts 1–3. 312 pp.

Blumenbach, Johann Friedrich. Göttingen physiologist. 1752–1840
CLASSIFICATION—of sub-divisions of human race.
De generis humani varietate nativa. Gottingae, Vandenhoeck, 1776. 100 pp. 2 ed.
CLIVUS, PLANE or SLOPE—the bony surface sloping down from the pituitary fossa.
PROCESS—the uncinate process.
Collectio craniorum diversarum gentium illustrata. Gottingae, Dieterich, 1790–1820

Blumenthal, Ferdinand. Berlin physician. 1870–
TEST—for acetone in urine.
Ueber Entstehung von Aceton aus Eiweiss. Dtsch. Med. Wschr., 27: 6–7, Jan. 3, 1901
TEST—for hippuric acid in urine.
Zur Methode der Hippursäurebestimmung. Z. klin. Med., 40: 339–343, 1900
TEST—for pentoses in urine; a modified Bial test.
Fermentwirkung in Krebsorganen. (Brief note) Münch. med. Wschr., 57: 547, Mar. 8, 1910

Blumer, George. American physician. 1858–1940
SHELF—carcinomatous metastasis in cul-de-sac of Douglas, felt as a firm posterior ridge on digital rectal examination.
The rectal shelf: a neglected rectal sign of value in the diagnosis and prognosis of obscure malignant and inflammatory disease within the abdomen. Albany M. Ann., 30: 361–366, May 1909
The significance of metastatic malignant growths in the rectum with special reference to the diagnosis of carcinoma of the stomach. Ibid., 57: 123–126, Dec. 1938
See also W. S. Thayer

Blumgart, Herrman Ludwig. Boston physician. 1895–
OPERATION or TREATMENT—of angina pectoris by thyroidectomy.
Congestive heart failure and angina pectoris; the therapeutic effect of thyroidectomy on patients without clinical or pathologic evidence of thyroid toxicity with S. A. Levine and D. D. Berlin, Arch. intern. Med., 51: 866–877, June 1933
See also J. R. Campbell, Jr., C. G. Mixter

Blundell, James. English obstetrician. 1790–1878
Rediscovered blood transfusion.
Experiments on the transfusion of blood by the syringe. Med.-chir. Trans., London, 9: 56–82, 1918
Observations on transfusion of blood. With a description of his gravitator. Lancet, 2: 321–324, June 13, 1829

Blunt, T. P. See A. H. Downes

Blyth, Alexander Wynter. English physician. 1846–1921
TEST—for lead in drinking-water.
A manual of practical chemistry: the analysis of foods and the detection of poisons. London, Griffin, 1879. 468 pp.

Boari, Achille. Italian surgeon
BUTTON—a device analogous to the Murphy button for ureterocystostomy.
Chirurgia dell'uretere,... Roma, 1900. 444 pp.

Boas, Friedrich. German physician
SOLUTION—basal ammonium chloride.
Untersuchungen über Säurewirkung und Bildung löslicher Stärke bei Schimmelpilzen. Zbl. f. Bakt., 2 Abt., 56: 7–11, Apr. 22, 1922

Boas, Ismar Isidor. Berlin physician. 1858–1938
BACILLUS—of Boas-Kaufmann, found in stomach in carcinoma of that organ; called also Boas-Oppler b.
Diagnostik und Therapie der Magenkrankheiten nach dem heutigen Stande der Wissenschaft bearbeitet. Leipzig, Thieme, 1890–93. 2 vols.
REAGENT and TEST—for blood.
Die Phenolphthalinprobe als Reagens auf okkulte Blutungen des Magendarmkanals. Dtsch. med. Wschr., 37: 62–64, Jan. 12, 1911
Beitrag zur Methodik und Technik der okkulten Blutuntersuchungen des Magendarmkanals. Berl. klin. Wschr., 50: 154–157, Jan. 27, 1913
TEST—for free HCl in gastric juice.
Ueber das Troppaeolinpapier als Reagens auf freie Salzsäure im Mageninhalt. Dtsch. med. Wschr., 13: 852–854, Sept. 29, 1887
Ein neues Reagens für den Nachweis freier Salzsäure im Mageninhalt. Zbl. klin. Med., 9: 817–821, Nov. 10, 1888
TEST—for lactic acid in gastric juice.
Eine neue Methode der qualitativen und quantitativen Milchsäurebestimmung im Mageninhalt. Dtsch. med. Wschr., 19: 940–943, Sept. 28, 1893
SIGN—lactic acid in gastric juice in certain cases of carcinoma of stomach. Ibid.
TEST MEAL—see E. A. Ewald

Boas, Johan Erik Vesti. Berlin physician. 1855–1936
METHOD—of withdrawing bile and pancreatic juice from empty stomach.
TEST—for gastric motility: chlorophyl t.
Ueber Darmsaftgewinnung beim Menschen. Zbl. f. klin. Med., 10: 97–99, Feb. 9, 1889
Ueber Dünndarmverdauung beim Menschen und deren Beziehungen zur Magenverdauung. Ibid., 17: 155–177, 1890
See also C. A. Ewald

Boas, Kurt (Walter Ferdinand). Freiburg medical student. 1890–
REACTION—for adrenaline.
Zur Methodik des Adrenalinnachweises. Zbl. Physiol., 22: 825–826, Mar. 20, 1909

Bobbs, John Stough. Indianapolis surgeon. 1809–1870

OPERATION—cholecystotoy for removal of gall
stones.
Case of lithotomy of the gall-bladder. Trans. Indiana M.
Soc., 18: 68-73, 1868
Bochdalek, Victor. Prague anatomist. 1801–1883
GANGLION—a swelling at junction of superior and
middle dental nerves.
*Neue Untersuchungen der Nerven des Ober- und
Unterkiefers.* 1855
Bochicchio, A. Rome
TEST—for salicylic acid in milk.
*Nuovo metodo per la ricerca dell'acido salicilico nel
latte.* G. soc. ital. d'igiene, 24: 291–295, June 30,
1902
Bock, A. V. See L. J. Henderson
Bock, August Carl. German anatomist. 1872–1833
GANGLION—carotid g.
NERVE—glosso-pharyngeal n.
Tabulae chirurgico-anatomicae. . . . Leipzig, Voss,
1833. 75 pp.
Bock, H. Eisleben physician
TEST—blood coagulation t. for cancer.
*Ueber die Bedeutung der Blutgerinnungsvalenz für
Krebsdiagnose* with C. Rausche, Dtsch. med. Wschr.,
52: 2025–2026, Nov. 26, 1926
Also: Zbl. f. Chir., 53: 1440, 1926
Bock, Joseph Carl. American chemist. 1884–
APPARATUS—for determination of total nitrogen in
urine.
*An examination of the Folin-Farmer method for the
colorimetric estimation of nitrogen* with S. R. Benedict,
J. biol. Chem., 20: 47–59, Jan. 1915
CALORIMETER—
A new form of calorimeter with S. R. Benedict,
Ibid., 33: xix (only), 1918; 35: 227–230, Aug. 1918
TEST—
The estimation of amino-acid nitrogen in blood. Ibid.,
28: 357–368, Jan. 1917
Bockhart, Max. German physician
IMPETIGO—epidemic abscesses produced by pyo-
genic bacteria, in contrast to contagious impetigo.
*Ueber die Aetiologie und Therapie der Impetigo, des
Furunkels und der Sykosis.* Mschr. prakt. Dermat.,
6: 450-471, May 15, 1887
Bodansky, Aaron. American biochemist. 1896–1941
UNIT—for measuring blood phosphatase.
*Deviation from the "Beer Law" in the Kuttner-Cohen
method for determination of phosphorus* with Lois
Hallman and R. Bonoff, Proc. Soc. exp. Biol., N. Y.,
28: 762-763, Apr. 1931
*Experimental factors influencing blood phosphatase
values* with H. L. Jaffe and J. P. Chandler, J. biol.
Chem., 97: lxvi-lxvii, July 1932
*Phosphatase studies. I. The determination of inorganic
phosphate, Beer's law and interfering substances in
the Kuttner-Lichtenstein method* with Lois F. Hallman
and R. Bonoff, Ibid., 99: 197-206, Dec. 1932
*Phosphatase studies: II. Determination of serum phos-
phatase. Factors influencing the accuracy of the determination.* Ibid., 101: 93-104, June 1933
Bodian, David. American anatomist. 1910–
METHOD—
*A new method for staining nerve fibers and nerve end-
ings in mounted paraffin sections.* Anat. Rec., 65:
89-97, Apr. 25, 1936
*The staining of paraffin sections of nervous tissues with
activated protargol: the role of fixatives.* Ibid., 69: 153-
162, Sept. 1937

Bodington, George. English physician. 1799–1882
One of the first to advocate scientific open air treat-
ment of pulmonary tuberculosis.
*An essay on the treatment and cure of pulmonary con-
sumption.* London, Longmans, 1840
Boeck, C. W. See D. C. Danielssen
Boeck, Caesar Peter Moeller. Norwegian derma-
tologist. 1845–1917
DISEASE—of Besnier-Boeck-Schaumann.
Multipelt benignt hud-sarkoid. Norsk. Mag. f. Laege-
vidensk., 60: 1321–1334, 1899
Multiple benign sarkoid of the skin. J. Cut. and Genito-
Urin. Dis., 17: 543-550, Dec. 1899
TREATMENT—of lupus vulgaris.
Trans.: *The nature of lupus erythematosus.* London,
New Sydenham Soc., 1900. p. 286
Boeck, J. Leiden physician
MODIFICATION—of Bielschowsky's method of
staining nerve tissue.
*Die motorische Endplatte bei den höheren Vertebraten,
ihre Entwickelung, Form und Zusammenhang mit
der Muskelfaser.* Anat. Anz., 35: 193–226, Oct. 28,
1910
Boeck, Karl Wilhelm. Norwegian leprologist. 1808–
1875
SCABIES—called also Norwegian itch.
Om den spedalske sygdom. Elephantiasis graecorum.
Norsk. Mag. f. Laegevidensk., 4: 1–73; 127–216,
1842
See D. C. Denielssen
Boeck, William Charles. Baltimore scientist. 1894–
MEDIUM—Locke-egg-serum.
The cultivation of Endamoeba histolytica with J.
Drbohlav, Amer. J. Hyg., 5: 371-407, July 1925
Also: Proc. Nat. Acad. Sci., Washington, 11: 235-
238, 1925
SOLUTION—glucose serum: culture medium.
Chilomastix mesnili and a method for its culture.
J. exp. Med., 33: 147-175, Feb. 1921
STAIN—iodine protozoan.
*Technique of fecal examination for protozoan infec-
tions.* Bull. Hyg. Lab., 133: 62-74, Oct. 1923
Böhler, Lorenz. Vienna orthopedist. 1885–
METHOD—of pin traction for fractures.
Technik der Knochenbruchbehandlung. Wien, Maud-
rich, 1929
Also, English transl. from 4 ed. by W. Hey Groves,
London, Wright, 1935
*Diagnosis, pathology and treatment of fractures of the
os calcis.* J. Bone and Joint Surg., 13: 75-89, Jan.
1931
*Entstehung, Erkennung, und Behandlung der Fersen-
beinbrueche.* Wien, Maudrich, 1933
OPERATION—for slipping patella.
*Ein Fall von doppelseitiger habitueller Patellarluxa-
tion. Zugleich ein Beitrage zur Mechanik und Statik
des Kniegelenkes.* Z. orthop. Chir., 38: 303-310, 1918
Bönniger, Dr. German physician
TEST—for lactic acid in gastric contents.
Zum Nachweis der Milchsäure im Magensaft. Dtsch.
med. Wschr., 28: 738-739, 1902
Boerhaave, Hermann. Dutch physician. 1668–1738
GLANDS—sweat glands.
Gave course of lectures on ophthalmology, 1708.
Introduced idea of "affinity" between chemical
substances.
Proved that smallpox is spread exclusively by con-
tagion.

Described rupture of esophagus, 1724.

Institutiones medicae in usus annuae exercitationis domesticos digestae. Lugduni Batavorum, J. van der Linden, 1708

Opera anatomica et chirurgica. . . . Leyden 1725. 2 vols.

Elementa chemiae. Leyden, 1732

Opera omnia medica. Venetiis, apud L. Basilium, 1742

Boerner, Fred. Philadelphia bacteriologist. 1889–

Procedure—

Determination of the phagocytic power of whole blood or plasma-leukocyte mixtures for clinical or experimental purposes. Description of an improved method, with representative findings with S. Mudd, Amer.J. med. Sci., 189: 22–35, Jan. 1935

TECHNIC—

A simplified complement fixation technic for the serological diagnosis of syphilis with Marguerite Lukens, Amer. J. clin. Path., (tech. suppl.), 9: 13–23, Jan. 1939

Simplified microscopic and macroscopic flocculation tests for the diagnosis of syphilis with C. A. Jones and Marguerite Lukens, Ibid., 10: 141–151, Nov. 1940

Börnstein, E. German scientist

REACTION—for saccharin.

Zur Erkennung des Benzoësäure-Sulfinids (Fahberg's "Saccharin") in Nahrungsmitteln. Z. anal. Chem., 27: 165–168, 1888

Böttcher, Arthur. German anatomist. 1831–1889

CELLS—of the cochlea.

Observationes microscopicae de ratione qua nervus cochleae mammalium terminatur. (Dorpat), Schunmanni et Mattieseni, 1856. 62 pp.

Boez, L. See A. Borrel

Bogen, Emil. Cincinnati physician. 1896–

INDICATOR—for rough location of pH range.

A universal indicator for hydrogen ion concentration. J. A. M. A., 89: 199 (only), July 16, 1927

Bogojawlensky, N. F. Russian surgeon

OPERATION—hypophysectomy.

Intrakranialer Weg zur Hypophysis cerebri durch die vordere Schädelgrube. Zbl. Chir., 39: 209–212, Feb. 17, 1912

Bogomoloff, Timofei Vasilgevich Ivanovich. St. Petersburg physician. 1844–

REACTION—for urobilin.

(On the relation of the coloring matter of biliary acids to the pigments of urine and excreta.) Sanktpeterburg, Trei, 1871. 53 pp.

Zur Harnfarbstofflehre. Z. med. Wiss., 13: 210–214, 1875

TEST—for albumin.

Carminsäure als differentielles Reagens für verschiedene Eiweissarten with N. J. Wassilieff, St. Petersburg. med. Wschr., 14: 294–296, Aug. 2, 1897

Bogros, Annet Jean. French anatomist. 1786–1823

SPACE—in lower abdominal wall where external iliac artery can be found without opening peritoneum.

Essai sur l'anatomie chirurgicale de la région iliaque, et description d'un nouveau procédé pour faire la ligature des artères épigastrique et iliaque externe. Paris, 1823. 29 pp.

Bohn, Johann. Leipzig physiologist. 1640–1718

Experimented upon the decapitated frog (1686) in an entirely modern manner, declaring the reflex phenomena to be entirely material and mechanical,

as against the current view of "vital spirits" in the nerve-fluid. Garrison

Circulus anatomico-physiologicus. . . . Leipzig, Gleditsch, 1686. 479 pp.

Wrote treatise on lethal wounds.

De renuntiatione vulnerum seu vulnerum lethalium examen. Leipzig, Gleditsch, 1689. 400 pp.

Bohr, Christian. Swedish physician. 1855–1911

Studied exchange of gases in respiration.

Ueber die Lungenathmung. Skand. Arch. Physiol., 2: 236–268, 1891

EFFECT—of CO_2 on dissociation curve of hemoglobin.

Ueber einen in biologischer Beziehung wichtigen Einfluss, den die Kohlensäurespannung des Blutes auf dessen Sauerstoffbindung übt. Ibid., 16: 402–412, 1904

Boivin, Marie Anne Victoire Gillain. French physician. 1773–1841

Described hydatidiform mole.

Nouvelles recherches sur l'origine, la nature et le traitement de la môle vésiculaire ou grossesse hydatique. Paris, Méquignon, 1827

Bokarius, Nikolai Sergieyevich. Russian physician! 1869–

REAGENT—for sperm.

(Micro-chemical reactions of semen). Vestnik obsh. hig., sudeb. 1 prakt. med., St. Petersb., 43, pt. 2: 1–22, 1906

Boldyreff, W. Russian physiologist

NEUTRALIZATION MECHANISM—See below: Quart. J. exp. Physiol., 8: 1–12, Apr. 4, 1914

OIL TEST BREAKFAST—

Der Übertritt des natürlichen Gemisches aus Pankreasaft, Darmsaft und Galle in den Magen. Arch. ges. Physiol., 121: 13–53, Dec. 30, 1907

Über die Gewinnung des Pankreassaftes bei menschen zu diagnostischen Zwecken. Ibid., 140: 436–462, May 31, 1911

Caused gastric ulcers by preventing regurgitation of duodenal juice through pylorus.

Ueber den Uebergang der natürlichen Mischung des Pankreas-, des Darmsaftes und der Galle in den Magen. Die Bedingungen und wahrscheinliche Bedeutung dieser Erscheinung. Zbl. Physiol., 28: 457–460, Oct. 22, 1904

(The self-regulation of the acidity of the contents of the stomach.) Trans. 11th Pirogoff's Cong. of Phys., St. Petersburg, 1910

The self-regulation of the acidity of the gastric contents and the real acidity of the gastric juice. Quart. J. exp. Physiol., 8: 1–12, Apr. 4, 1914

Boll, Franz Christian. Rome physician. 1849–1879

Discovered a light sensitive substance in the retina.

Sull'anatomia e fisiologia della retina. Firenze, Loescher, 1877

Same. Preuss. Akad. d. Wiss., 41: 783–787, 1876

Bolland, A. Krakau scientist

TEST—for blood in presence of iron.

Zur Kenntnis der Guajakreaktion. Z. anal. Chem., 46: 621–643, 1907

Bolliger, Adolph. Sydney scientist

REACTIONS—for creatinine.

On a new reaction for the determination of creatinine. J. Proc. Roy. Soc. N. S. Wales, 69: 224–227, 1935

The reaction of creatinine with 1, 3, 5-trinitrobenzol, 2, 4, 6-trinitrotoluol, and 2, 4, 6-trinitrobenzoic acid. Ibid., 70: 211–217, 1936

The colorimetric determination of creatinine in urine

and blood with 3,5-dinitrobenzoic acid. M. J. Australia, 2: 818–821, Dec. 12, 1936

Bollinger, Otto von. Munich physician. 1843–1909
Discovered ray fungus (actinomycosis) in cattle in 1876. Garrison
Ueber eine neue Pitzkrankheit beim Rinde. Z. med. Wiss., 15: 481–485, July 7, 1877

Bolthazard, V. See M. S. Curie

Bolton, Joseph Shaw. English physiologist. 1867–
MODIFICATION—formaldehyde, of Golgi's bichromate and silver nitrate method.
On the chrome-silver impregnation of formalin-hardened brain. Lancet, 1: 218–219, Jan. 22, 1898
STAIN—for myelin.
On the nature of the Weigert-Pal method. J. Anat. and Physiol., 32: 247–266, Jan. 1898

Bolton, Meade. Baltimore pathologist
METHOD—preparation of potatoes for test-tube cultures.
A method of preparing potatoes for bacterial cultures. Med. News, 1: 318 (only), Mar. 19, 1887

Boltz, Oswald Herman. New York physician. 1895–
REACTION—
Studies on the cerebro-spinal fluid with an acetic anhydride-sulphuric acid test. State Hosp. Q., Utica, 8: 198–208, Feb. 1923
Also: Amer. J. Psychiat., n. s., 3: 111–119, July 1923

Bonain, Adolphe. French physician. 1869–
LIQUID or MIXTURE—for anesthetizing the tympanic membrane in paracentesis.
Note au sujet de l'anesthesique local employé en otorhino-laryngologie sous la denomination liquide de Bonain. Ann. d. mal. de l'oreille, du larynx, Paris, 33: 216–221, 1907

Bonanto, Mary V. See J. T. Freund

Bonazzi, Augusto. Wooster, Ohio scientist
MODIFICATION—of Gerlach and Vogel's basal solution.
Studies on Azotobacter chroococcum Beij. J. Bact., 6: 331–369, May 1921

Bond, Charles John. Leicester surgeon.
TEST—for radio-sensitive substances.
A color test for radio-sensitive substances. Brit. M. J., 2: 637, Oct. 8, 1927

Bondi, Samuel. Vienna chemist
TEST—for acetoacetic acid in urine.
Ueber die Einwirkung von freiem Jod auf Azetseeigsäure und deren Nachweis im Harn. Wien. klin. Wschr., 19: 37–39, Jan. 11, 1906

Bondy, Gustav. Vienna otologist
OPERATION—mastoidectomy.
Totalaufmeisselung mit Erhaltung von Trommelfell und Gehörknöchelchen. Mschr. Ohrenheilk., 44: 15–23, 1910

Bonet, Théophilus. Swiss physician. 1620–1689
Made a collection of all the postmortem examinations performed during the 16th and 17th centuries. Garrison
Sepulchretum, sive anatomia practica ex cadaveribus morbo denatis. Genevae, Chouët, 1679. 1706 pp.

Bonfils, Émile Adolphe. French physician
DISEASE—same as Hodgkin's d.
Quelques réflexions sur un cas d'hypertrophie ganglionnaire générale; avec fistules lymphatiques et avec cachexie, sans leucémie. Rec. d. trav. Soc. méd. d'obs. de Paris, 1: 157, 1857–8
Same. Clermont, Huet, n. d. 25 pp.

Bonham, C. D. See R. T. Frank

Boni, Icilio. Italian pathologist. 1869–
METHOD—of capsule staining.
Methode zur Darstellung einer "Kapsel" bei allen Bakterienarten. Zbl. Bakt., 28: 705–707, Dec. 8, 1900

Bonjean, Joseph. French physician
ERGOTIN—a purified extract of ergot.
Histoire physiologique, chimique, toxicologique et médicale du seigle ergoté. Paris, Crochard, 1842 36 pp.
Practical treatise of the use of ergotine. Paris and London, Germer-Baillière, 1862. 16 pp.

Bonnet, Amédée. French surgeon. 1802–1858
CAPSULE—the posterior part of the sheath of the eyeball.
Traité des sections tendineuses et musculaires dans le strabisme, la myopie, la disposition à la fatigue des yeux, le bégaiement, les pieds bots, etc. Paris, Germer-Baillière, 1841. 664 pp.
SIGN—in sciatica, pain is induced by adduction of thigh.
Traité des maladies des articulations. 1845. 2 vols.

Bonnet, Frederic. Worcester, Mass. chemist. 1878–
TEST—for formaldehyde.
A colorimetric method for the detection and estimation of formaldehyde. J. Amer. Chem. Soc., 27: 601–605, 1905

Bonnet, P. See A. Lararjet

Bonney, Victor. London physician. 1872–
STAIN—triple, for plasma.
Eine neue und sehr schnelle Dreifach-Färbung. Arch. f. path. Anat. u. Physiol., 193: 547–549, Sept. 4, 1908

Bonnier, Pierre. French physician. 1861–1918
SYNDROME—vertigo, pallor and various aural and ocular disturbances: due to lesion of Deiter's nucleus or of vestibular tracts related thereto.
Vertige. Paris, Rueff, (1893). 208 pp.
Un nouveau syndrome bulbaire. Pr. méd., 11: 174–177, Feb. 18, 1903
Un syndrome bulbaire: autopsie. Ibid., 861–863, Dec. 16, 1903

Bonoff, R. See A. Bodansky

Bonomo, Giovanni Cosimo. Italian physician. ?–1696
Discovered the parasitic nature of scabies, gave first good description of itch mite and made a drawing of it. "Letter" to Redi, 1687
Epistola che contiene osservazioni intorno a'pellicelli del corpo umano, fatte . . . e da lui con altre osservazioni scritte in una lettera all'illustrissimo Francesco Redi. Firenze, Martini, 1687. 16 pp.
Trans. in part: Philos. Trans., London, 22: 1296–1299, 1702
Photostatic copy of "Letter" is given by J. E. Lane: Arch. Dermat. and Syph., 18: 1–25, July 1928

Bontius, Jacobus. Dutch physician. 1592–1631
Described beri-beri from East Indian cases, and tropical dysentery in Java.
De medicina Indorum. Leyden, Hackium, 1642. pp. 115–120
Also, in English. London, 1769

Booher, James Mathew. Chicago physician. 1879–
LUNGMOTOR—
Demonstration of the lungmotor. Dent. Summary, 36: 948–952, Nov. 1916

Bookman, Milton Ralph. New York surgeon. 1884–

OPERATION—gastrostomy.
An improved gastrostomy. S. G. O., 21: 132-133, July 1915
Booth, James Arthur. New York physician. 1856-1935
OPERATION—use of an aluminum plate to cover a cranial defect.
Report of a case of tumor of the left frontal lobe of the cerebrum; operation; recovery with B. F. Curtis, Ann. Surg., 17: 127-139, Feb. 1893
Boothby, Walter Meredith. Rochester, Minn. surgeon. 1880-
APPARATUS—of Boothby and Cotton. See F. J. Cotton
APPARATUS—for determination of respiratory exchange.
Laboratory manual of the technic of basic metabolic rate determination with Irene Sandiford, Philadelphia, Saunders, 1920. p. 35 et seq.
MASK—B.L.B., of Boothby-Lovelace-Bulbulian.
Design and construction of the masks for the oxygen inhalation apparatus by A. H. Bulbulian, Proc. Staff Meet. Mayo Clinic, 13: 654-656, Oct. 12, 1938
One hundred per cent oxygen: indications for its use and methods of its administration with E. W. Mayo and W. R. Lovelace, J. A. M. A., 113: 477-482, Aug. 5, 1939
Introduced glycine (glycocoll) in treatment of myasthenia gravis.
Myasthenia gravis: preliminary report on the effect of treatment with glycine. Proc. Staff Meet., Mayo Clinic, 7: 557-562, 1932
See also F. J. Cotton, H. S. Plummer
Borchardt, Leo. Königsberg chemist. 1879-
TEST—for levulose and sucrose in urine.
Ueber die diabetische Lävulosurie und den qualitativen Nachweis der Lävulose im Harn. Z. phys. Chem., 55: 241-259, 1908
Bordet, Jules Jean Baptiste Vincent, Belgian bacteriologist. 1870-
Awarded Nobel prize in 1919.
BACILLUS—B. pertussis, etiologic agent of whooping cough; Bordet-Gengou b.
Le microbe de la coqueluche with O. Gengou, Ann. Inst. Pasteur, 20: 731-741, 1906
Note complémentaire sur le microbe de la coqueluche with O. Gengou, Ibid., 21: 720-726, 1907
BLOOD AGAR—for B. Pertussis. Ibid.
ANTIGEN—
Recherches sur la coagulation du sang et les serums anticoagulants with O. Gengou, Ibid., 15: 129-144, Mar. 1901
METHOD—for preparation of an antigen, an alcoholic extract of the acetone-insoluble lipoids of calf- or beef-heart tissue.
L'antigène syphilitique de l'Institut Pasteur de Bruxelles with G. Ruelens, C. R. Soc. Biol., 82: 880-883, Feb. 22, 1919
PHENOMENON—of Bordet-Gengou; complement fixation.
Les sérums hémolytiques, leurs antitoxines et les théories des sérums cytolytiques. Ann. Inst. Pastuer, 14: 257-296, 1900
Sur l'existence de substances sensibilisatrices dans la plupart des sérums antimicrobiens with O. Gengou, Ibid., 15: 289-302, 1901

Sur le mode d'action des sérums cytoliques et sur l'unité de l'alexine. Ibid., 303-318
PHENOMENON or TEST—serum test for human blood: called also biologic or precipitin or Uhlenhuth's t.
Sur l'agglutination et la dissolution des globules rouges par le sérum d'animaux injectés de sang défibriné. Ibid., 12: 688-695, Oct. 1898
Agglutination et dissolution des globules rouges par le sérum. Ibid., 13: 273-297, Apr. 1899
Discovered bacterial hemolysis, 1898. Ibid.
Studied properties of sera of immunized animals.
Contribution à l'étude du sérum chez les animaux vaccinés. Ann. Soc. Sci. méd. nat. Brux., 4: 455-530, 1895
Borelli, Giovanni Alfonso. Neapolitan mathematician. 1608-1679
THEORY—neurogenic t. of heart's action, heat being attributed to action of extrinsic and intrinsic nerves.
He treated locomotion, respiration, and digestion (the grinding and crushing action of the stomach) as purely mechanical processes. Garrison
De motu animalium. Romae, Bernabo, 1680-81
Born, Gustav. Breslau anatomist. 1851-1900
METHOD—of grafting embryonic parts.
Ueber Verwachsungsversuche mit Amphibienlarven. Arch. Ent. Mech. Org., 4: 349-465, Dec. 31, 1896
Bornholm disease. Danish Island. See E. Sylvest
Boroschek, L. See J. Rudisch
Borovsky, Peter Fokich. Russian physician. 1863-1932
Described the protozoon later named Leishmania tropica.
(On sart sore.) Voenno Med. Zur., St. Petersburg, 76: 925-941, 1898
Also, English transl. by C. A. Hoare: Trans. Roy. Soc. Trop. Med. and Hyg., London, 32: 78-90, 1938
Borowskaja, D. P. Moscow
MODIFICATION—of Lange colloidal gold test.
Zur Methodik der Goldsolbereitung. Z. Immun. Forsch., 82: 178-182, May 8, 1934
Borrel, Amédée. French physician. 1867-1936
SOLUTION—glycerol asparagin, for cultivation of tubercle bacilli.
Milieu synthétique pour la culture du Bacille tuberculeux with A. de Coulon, L. Boez and J. Quimaud, C. R. Soc. Biol., 86: 388-390 (389), Feb. 10, 1922
Borrmann, Robert. German physician. 1870-
TYPES—of carcinoma.
In F. Henke and O. Lubarsch: *Handbuch der speziellen pathologischen Anatomie und Histologie.* Berlin, Springer, 1926. Vol. 4, pt. 1, p. 865
Bose, Heinrich. German surgeon. 1840-1900
HOOKS—small hooks used in tracheotomy.
OPERATION—a method of performing tracheotomy.
Die Verengerung und Verschliessung des Kehlkopfes, als complication weiter abwarts gelegener Luftfisteln. Giessen, Keller, 1865. 160 pp.
Bose, P. K. Calcutta, India physician
REACTION—for reducing carbohydrates.
Ein neuer empfindlicher Nachweis reduzierender Kohlenhydrate. Z. anal. Chem., 87: 110-114, 1932
Bossi, Luigi Maria. Genoa gynecologist. 1859-1919
DILATOR—for cervix uteri.
Sulla provocazione artificiale del parto e sul parto forzato col mezzo della dilatazione meccanica del collo

uterino. Ann. di Ostet. e Ginec., Milano, 14: 881-828, Dec. 1892

Bostock, John. English physician. 1773-1846
CATARRH—hay-fever.
Case of a periodical affection of the eyes and chest. Med.-chir. Trans., 10: 161-165, 1819
Of the catarrhus aestivus, or summer catarrh. Ibid., 14: 437-446, 1828

Bostroem, Eugen Waldemar. Jena physician. 1850-1928
METHOD—of staining actinomyces.
Untersuchungen über die Aktinomykose des Menschen. Beitr. path. Anat., 9: 1-240, 1890

Bosworth, David Marsh. New York surgeon. 1897-
OPERATION—for stabilization of knee joint.
Use of fascia lata to stabilize the knee in cases of ruptured crucial ligaments with B. M. Bosworth, J. Bone and Joint Surg., 18: 178-179, Jan. 1936
OPERATION—
An operation for meniscectomy of the knee. Ibid., 19: 1113-1116, Oct. 1937

Bosworth, Francke Huntington. New York rhinologist. 1843-1925
SAW—for removal of septal spurs.
Deformities of the nasal septum. A new operation for their correction, with an analysis of its results in 166 cases, as throwing new light on the pathology of diseases of the upper air-tract and their relation to the so-called nasal reflexes. Med. Rec., 31: 115-122, Jan. 29, 1887

Botallus, Leonardus. Italian physician. 1530-?
LIGAMENT—the persistent remains of ductus arteriosus.
FORAMEN—connects the auricles of the fetal heart; foramen ovale.
Opera omnia, medica et chirurgica. . . . Ludg. Bat. 1660. 800 pp.

Botelho, C.
AGAR—lacto-phenol peptone; for isolation of members of colon-typhoid group.
Sur un nouveau milieu de culture indiquant rapidement la présence de bacilles du groupe typhique dans un milieu bactériologiquement impur. C. R. Soc. Biol., 80: 435-437, May 5, 1917

Bottini, Enrico. Italian surgeon. 1837-1903
CAUTERY—
La galvano-caustica nella pratica chirurgica. Novara, Merati, 1873. 125 pp.
OPERATION—for prostatic hypertrophy by making a channel through the prostate with the galvano-cautery.
Di un nuovo cauterizzatore ed incisore termo-galvanico contro le iscurie da ipertrofia prostatica. Galvani, Bologna, 2: 437-452, 1874
Ueber radicale Behandlung der auf Hypertrophie der Prostata beruhenden Ischuria. Verh. d. X internat. med. Cong., 1890, 3, 7. Abth., 90-97, 1891

Bouchard, A. See J. M. Charcot

Bouchard, Charles Jacques. French physician. 1837-1915
DISEASE—dilatation of stomach from inefficiency of gastric muscles.
Du rôle pathigenique de la dilatation de l'estomac et des relations cliniques de cette maladie avec divers accidents morbides. Bull. Soc. méd. Hôp. Paris, 3 s., 1: 226, 1884
Called attention to autointoxication.

Leçons sur les auto-intoxications dans les maladies . . . Paris, Savy, 1887. 348 pp.
Called attention to diseases caused by diminished nutrition.
Maladies par ralentissement de la nutrition. . . . Paris, Savy, 1882. 412 pp.
See also M. S. Curie

Bouchardat, Apollinaire. French physician. 1806-1886
TREATMENT—of diabetes by use of a diet that excludes substances rich in carbohydrates, as sugar, milk, etc.
De la glycosurie ou diabète sucré; son traitement hygiénique. . . . Paris, Germer-Baillière, 1875. 336 pp.
See also E. M. Peligot

Bouchut, Jean Antoine Eugène. French physician. 1818-1891
RESPIRATION—seen in children with bronchopneumonia, in which inspiration is shorter than expiration.
Études sur la pneumonie des nouveau-nés et enfants à la mamelle. Paris, 1843. 33 pp.
TUBES—for use in intubation of larynx.
D'une nouvelle méthode de traitement du croup par le tubage du larynx. Bull. Acad. Méd. Paris, 23: 1160-1162, 1857
Described neurasthenia.
De l'état nerveux aigu et chronique ou nervosisme. Paris, Baillière, 1860

Bouckaert, J. J. See C. Heymans

Bougard, Jean Joseph. Belgian physician. 1815-1884
PASTE—a caustic cancer p.
Sur la guérison du canrer; caustiques et opérations sanglantes. J. de méd., chir. et pharmacol., Brux., 46, 1868
Also: Bruxelles, Manceaux, 1868. 32 pp.

Bouillaud, Jean Baptiste. French physician. 1796-1881
DISEASE—endocarditis, rheumatic form.
LAW OF COINCIDENCE or SYNDROME—coincidence of pericarditis and endocarditis in the rule in acute articular rheumatism, and their non-coincidence is the rule in chronic articular rheumatism.
SIGN—retraction in precordial region in adherent pericarditis.
Traité clinique des maladies du coeur, précédé de recherches nouvelles sur l'anatomie et la physiologie de cet organe. Paris, Baillière, 1835. 2 vols.
Also, abstr., English transl. by E. Hauser in: F. A. Willius and T. E. Keys' Cardiac classics. St. Louis, Mosby, 1941. pp. 446-455
Nouvelles recherches sur le rheumatisme articulaire aigu en général et spécialement sur la loi de coincidence de la péricardite et de l'endocardite avec cette maladie, ainse que un la formule des émissions sanguines coup sur coup dans son traitement. Paris, Baillière, 1836. 162 pp.
Also, in English: Philadelphia, Haswell et al., 1837. 64 pp.
Described venous obstruction and dropsy.
Observations sur l'état des veines dans les infiltrations des membres. J. de Physiol. exp. et path., Paris, 3: 89-93, 1823
Pointed out that aphasia is correlated with a lesion in the anterior lobes of the brain. Garrison
Recherches cliniques propres à démontrer que la perte

de la parole correspond à la lésion des lobules antéri-eurs du cerveau, et à confirmer l'opinion de M. Gall, sur le siège de l'organe du language articulé. Arch. gen. de méd., 8: 25–45, 1825

Bouilly, Vincent Georges. French gynecologist. 1848–1903
OPERATION—excision of a part of mucous membrane of neck of uterus for atresia of cervix.
Affections chirurgicales de l'uterus. Chir. d. org. genito-urin., Paris, pp. 669–719, 1888

Bouin, Paul. French anatomist. 1870–
FLUID—fixing f. for histologic work.
Phénomenes cytologiques anormaux dans l'histogenese et l'atrophie expérimentale du tube séminifère. Nancy, 1897. p. 19

Bouma, Jac. Utrecht physiologist
REAGENT—for indican in urine.
Ueber die Bestimmung des Harnindicans als Indi-goroth mittelst Isatinsalzsäure. Z. phys. Chem., 32: 82–93, 1901

Bourceau, Dr. Tours
TEST—for albumin in urine.
Un nouveau réactif des albumines urinaires. C. R. Soc. Biol , 40: 317–318, 1897

Bourdillon, Robert Benedict. English scientist
Isolated "calciferol" for irradiated ergosterol.
The absorption spectrum of vitamin D, with others, Proc. Roy. Soc. Lond., S. B., 104: 561–583, 1929
The quantitative estimation of vitamin D by radiog-raphy, with others, London H. M. Stationery Office, 1931, Med. Res. Council Spec. Report, No 158

Bourget, Louis. Swiss chemist. 1856–1913
TEST—for iodids in urine and saliva.
Manuel de chimie clinique. . . . Paris, Rueff, 1891. 147 pp.

Bourguet, Julien. French otolaryngologist. 1877–
OPERATION—dacryostomy.
Le traitement de la dacryocystite par la méthode de Dupuy-Dutemps et Bourguet; résultats opératoires d'après 790 cas. Bull. Soc. chir. Paris, 20: 43–52, Jan. 20, 1928

Bourneville, Désiré-Magloire. French physician. 1840–1909
DISEASE—epiloia; tuberous sclerosis; Bourneville-Brissaud d.
Contribution a l'étude de l'idiotie; idiotie et épilepsie hémiplégique. Arch. Neurol., 1: 81–91, 1880
Recognized cretinism and myxedema as the same condition.
Note sur un cas de crétinisme avec myxoedème: (ca-chexie pachydermique) with H. d'Olier, Prog. méd., Paris, 8: 709–711, Aug. 28, 1880

Bourquelot, Émile. French pharmacologist. 1851–1921
Worked on synthesis of glucosides.
La synthèse des glucosides par les ferments. J. Pharm. Chim., Paris, 7 s., 8: 337–359, 1913

Bousseau. Paris surgeon
Described separation of epiphysis of upper end of femur.
Disjonction épiphysaire traumatique de la tête du fémur et des épines iliaques antérieures. Mort; autopsie. Bull. Soc. Anat. Paris, 42: 283–286, Apr. 1867

Boussingault, Jean Baptiste Joseph Dieudonné. Paris physician. 1802–1887
Suggested use of iodized salt for prevention of goiter.

Mémoire sur les salines iodifères des Andes. Ann Chim. (Phys.), 54: 163–177, 1833
Made one of the first endemicological studies in the goitrous regions of the Andes in 1831. Ibid. Analyzed foods.
Analyses comparées des alimens consommés et des produits rendu par une vache laitière. Ibid., 71: 113–136, 1839

Bouveret, Léon. French physician. 1850–1926
DISEASE or SYNDROME—paroxysmal tachycardia.
De la tachycardie essentielle paroxystique. Rev. d. méd. Paris, 9: 753–837, 1889

Boveri, Theodor. German physician. 1862–1915
FLUID—for fixation; picro-acetic acid. In his: Zellen-Studien, 1: 11, 1887
Defined splitting of chromosomes as a definite act of reproduction.
Die Vorgänge der Befruchtung und Zelltheilung in ihrer Beziehung der Vererbungsfrage. Verh. München. anthrop. Ges., pp. 27–39, 1888

Bowditch, Henry Ingersol. Boston physician. 1808–1892
Described pleuritic effusions.
On pleuritic effusions, and the necessity of paracen-tesis for their removal. Amer. J. M. Sci., 23: 320–350, Apr. 1852

Bowditch, Henry Pickering. Boston physiologist. 1840–1911
LAW—nerves cannot be tired out by stimulation.
Note on the nature of nerve-force. J. Physiol., 6: 133–135, 1885
Ueber den Nachweis der Unermüdlichkeit des Säuge-thiernerven. Arch. f. Anat. u. Physiol., Physiol. Abt., Leipzig, 505–508, 1890
LAW—any stimulus that will produce a contraction of heart muscle will cause as powerful a pulsation as the most powerful stimulus.
Ueber die Eigenthümlichkeiten der Reizbarkeit, welche die Muskelfasern des Herzens zeigen. Beitr. d. k. sächs. Ges. d. Wiss., 23: 652–689, 1871
Also: Arb. a. d. Physiol. Anst. zu Leipzig, 1871, 6: 139–176, 1872
STAIRCASE EFFECT or TREPPE—the phenomenon of gradual increase in extent of muscular contrac-tion following rapidly repeated stimulation. Ibid.

Bowen, Arthur. Los Angeles surgeon. 1899–
CUP—
Bowen speculum cup. Amer. J. Surg., 42: 435–436, Nov. 1938

Bowen, John Templeton. Boston dermatologist. 1857–1941
DISEASE—precancerous dermatosis.
Precancerous dermatoses: a study of two cases of chronic atypical epithelial proliferation. J. Cutan. Dis., 30: 241–255, May 1912
Precancerous dermatoses: a sixth case of a type re-cently described. Ibid., 33: 787–802, Dec. 1915

Bowie, Donald James. Montreal physician. 1887–
STAIN—for pepsinogen granules.
A method for staining the pepsinogen granules in gastric glands. Anat. Rec., 64: 357–367, Feb. 25, 1936

Bowman, D. E. See J. P. Visscher

Bowman, Sir William Paget. English ophthalmol-ogist. 1816–1892
CAPSULE—globular dilatation which forms the beginning of a uriniferous tubule within the kidney.

On the structure and use of the malpighian bodies of the kidneys with observations on the circulation through the gland. Philos. Trans., Part 1, 57–80, 1842
Also: Med. Classics, 5: 258–291, Dec. 1940
THEORY—of urinary secretion: in the glomeruli, water and inorganic salts are produced, while urea and related bodies are eliminated by the epithelial cells in the convoluted tubes. Ibid.
MEMBRANE or LAYER or LAMINA—the uppermost layer of the corneal stroma.
TUBES—formed artificially between the lamellae of the cornea in process of injection.
MUSCLE—the ciliary muscle.
Lectures. Lond. med. Gaz., 40: 743–753, Oct. 29; 826–835, Nov. 12, 1847
Lectures on the parts concerned in the operations on the eye, and on the structure of the retina; to which are added, a paper on the viterous humor; and also a few cases of ophthalmic disease. London, Longman, 1849. 143 pp.
Also: Collected papers, 2: 95–224, 1892
Also: Med. Classics, 5: 292–336, Dec. 1940
OPERATION—
Observations on artificial pupil, with a description of a new method of operating in certain cases. Med. Times & Gaz., n.s., 4: 11–14; 33–35, 1852
PROBE—for use on the nasal ducts.
On the treatment of lacrimal obstructions. Ophth. Hosp. Rep., 1: 10–20, 1857
Discovered and described striated flat plates which make up striated muscle fibers.
On the minute structure and movements of voluntary muscle. Philos. Trans., 130: 457–501, 1840
Additional note on the contraction of voluntary muscle in the living body. Ibid., 131: 69–72, 1841
Wrote classical work on glaucoma, and was the first Englishman to take up iridectomy for that disease.
Glaucomatous affections and their treatment by iridectomy. Brit. med. J., 2: 377–382, 1862
Boyce, Frederick Fitzherbert. New Orleans physician. 1903–
MODIFICATION—of Quick's test
Studies of hepatic function by the Quick hippuric acid test. 1. Biliary and hepatic disease with Elizabeth M. McFetridge, Arch. Surg., 37: 401–426, Sept. 1938
TEST—of serum volume.
A serum volume test for the hemorrhagic diathesis in jaundice with Elizabeth M. McFetridge, J. Lab. clin. Med., 23: 202–212, Nov. 1937
Boyce, Rubert William. Liverpool pathologist. 1863–1911
TEST—for copper in tissue.
On a green leucocytosis in oysters associated with the presence of copper in the leucocytes with W. A. Herdman, Proc. roy. Soc., 1897, 62: 30–38, 1898
Boyd, Eldon Mathews. Kingston, Canada pharmacologist. 1907–
PROCEDURE—extraction of lipids at room temperature.
The extraction of blood lipids. J. biol. Chem., 114: 223–234, May 1936
Boyd, Harold Buhalts. Memphis, Tenn. surgeon. 1904–
TECHNIC—of onlay bone graft with fixation by vitallium screws.
Congenital pseudoarthrosis: treatment by dual bone

grafts. J. Bone and Joint Surg., 23: 497–515, July 1941
See also J. S. Speed
Boyd, L. J. See K. Lange
Boyd, T. C. English physician
SOLUTION—hydrolyzed meat: culture medium.
Preparation of a bacteriological nutrient medium by means of mineral acid. Ind. J. med. Res., 5: 408–412, Oct. 1917
Boyden, Edward Allen. American anatomist. 1886–
DEVICE—standard Rehfuss tube transformed into an electrode.
Reaction of gall bladder to stimulation of gastrointestinal tract. II. Response to faradic excitation of stomach, small intestine and cecum, by Carroll L. Birch and E. A. Boyden, Amer. J. Physiol., 92: 301–316, Mar. 1, 1930
Localized pain accompanying faradic excitation of the stomach and duodenum with L. G. Rigler, Proc. Soc. exp. Biol., N. Y., 31: 655–656, Mar. 1934
Localization of pain accompanying faradic excitation of stomach and duodenum in healthy individuals with L. G. Rigler, J. clin. Invest., 13: 833–851, Nov. 1934
MEAL—used with Graham-Cole method of visualizing human gall bladder to study rate of emptying.
The effect of natural foods on the distension of the gallbladder, with a note on the change in pattern of the mucosa as it passes from distension to collapse. Anat. Rec., 30: 333–334, Aug. 1925
A study of the behavior of the human gall bladder in response to the ingestion of food: together with some observations on the mechanism of the expulsion of bile in experimental animals. Ibid., 33: 201–255, Aug. 25, 1926
SPHINCTERS OF—
The phylogeny of the sphincter choledochus. Abstr.: Anat. Rec., (suppl.), 64: 7 (only), 1936
Boyer, Baron Alexis de. French surgeon. 1757–1833
BURSA—beneath the hyoid bone.
CYST—of subhyoid bursa.
Traité complet d'anatomie, ou description de toutes les parties du corps humain. Paris, Migneret, 1803–09. 4 vols.
SPLINT—
Lecons sur les maladies des os. . . . Paris, Migneret, 1803. 2 vols.
Also: Trans. by J. Hartshorne, Phila., Humphreys, 1905. 368 pp.
Boyer, Louis. French physician
BROTH—bone infusion; culture medium.
Nouveau bouillon de culture particulièrement favorable au développement du Streptocoque pyogène. C. R. Soc. Biol., 81: 229–231, Mar. 9, 1918
See also S. Costa
Boyksen, Diedrich Otto. Hamburg physician. 1891–
TEST—skin, for diagnosis of cancer.
Zur Intrakutanreaktion bei Karzinom. Zbl. Chir., 51: 894–896, Apr. 26, 1924
Biochemische Reaktionen bei Carcinom. Z. Krebsforsch., 23: 110–127, Mar. 20, 1926
Boyle, Robert. English physicist. 1627–1691
Experimented with intravenous medication, to animals. See R. Lower
Made experiments with flames and animals in vacuo (1660), demonstrating that air is necessary for life as well as for combustion. Garrison
Nova experimenta physico-mechanica de vi aeris

elastica et ejusdem effectibus. Roterodami, Leers, 1669

Early investigator of blood specific gravity; showed that both serum and whole blood are heavier than water.

Memoirs for the natural history of human blood, especially the spirit of that liquor. London, Smith, 1683 Also: *The physiological works of the Hon. Robert Boyle.* By Peter Shaw, London, 1725

Boylston, Zabdiel. American physician. 1680-1766 Inoculated for the smallpox, at Boston, June 26, 1721.
An historical account of the small-pox inoculated in New England. London, Chandler, 1726

Boys, F. See E. P. Lehman

Bozeman, Nathan. American surgeon. 1825-1905 CATHETER—a double-current uterine c.
SPECULUM—a bivalve s.
SUTURE—a form of button-suture.
Urethro-vaginal and vesico-vaginal fistules; remarks upon their peculiarities and complications; their classification and treatment; modifications of the button suture; report of cases successfully treated. North Amer. M.-Chir. Rev., Phila., 1857 Also: Montgomery, Bartlett and Winibish, 1857. 59 pp.

OPERATION—hysterocystocleisis.
TREATMENT—of pyelitis, complicating vesical and fecal fistula in women.
The gradual preparatory treatment of the complications of urinary and fecal fistulae in women. Trans. Internat. Med. Cong., Washington, 2: 514-558, 1887
Chronic pyelitis: successfully treated by kolpo-ureterocystotomy. Amer. J. med. Sci., 95: 255-265; 368-376, 1888
Successfully removed a pancreatic cyst.
Removal of a cyst of the pancreas weighing twenty and one-half pounds. Report in: Proc. New York Path. Soc., New York M. Rec., 21: 46-47, 1882

Bozsan, Eugene John. New York surgeon. 1889–
OPERATION—drilling through neck of femur in fracture to promote bony healing, no fixation being used but leg being placed in Whitman's abduction spica.
A new treatment of intracapsular fractures of the neck of the femur and Legg-Calvé-Perthes disease. Technique. J. Bone and Joint Surg., 16: 75-87, Jan. 1934

Bozzini, Philipp. Mainz physician. 1773-1809 Invented "light conductor" speculum, utilizing illumination and reflection by mirrors.
Der Lichtleiter. Weimar, 1807

Bozzolo, Camillo. Italian physician. 1845-1920 Introduced thymol as a hookworm vermifuge.
L'anchilostomiasi e l'anemia che ne conseguita (anchilostomanemia). Giorn. internaz. d. Sci. Med., Napoli, n. s. 1: 1054-1069; 1245-1253, 1879

Bozzolo, G. See G. A. Brossa

Braasch, William Frederick. Rochester, Minn. urologist. 1878–
INSTRUMENT—for prostatic resection.
Median bar excisor. J. A. M. A., 70: 758-759, Mar. 16, 1918

Brackett, Elliott Gray. Boston surgeon. 1860–
OPERATION—
Treatment of old ununited fracture of the neck of the femur by transplantation of the head of the femur to the

trochanter. Boston M. and S. J., 177: 351-353. Sept. 13, 1917
Fractures of neck of femur. Operation of transplantation of femoral head to trochanter. Report of cases showing result eight years after operation. Ibid., 192: 1118-1120, June 4, 1925
OPERATION—
A study of the different approaches to the hip-joint, with special reference to the operations for curved trochanteric osteotomy and for arthrodesis. Ibid., 166 235-242, Feb. 15, 1912

Bradford, Edward Hickling. Boston surgeon. 1848-1926
FRAME—for restraint of a child in a recumbent position.
A treatise on orthopedic surgery with R. W. Lovett, New York, Wood, 1890. p. 55

Bradley, B. See J. B. Cleland

Bradley, H. C. See L. B. Mendel

Bradshaw, Thomas Robert. Liverpool physician. 1857-1927
TEST—for myelopathic albumiose in urine.
ALBUMOSURIA—same as Bence Jones' proteinsuria.
The recognition of myelopathic albumose in the urine. Brit. med. J., 2: 1442-1444, Nov. 24, 1906

Bradwell, Stephen. English physician
Author of first book on First Aid.
Helps for suddain accidents endangering life. . . . London, Purfoot, 1633. 127 pp.

Bragg, Sir William. See R. W. Paul

Brahdy, B. See T. Brehme

Brahmachari, Upendraneth. Calcutta physician
LEISHMANOID—
Chemotherapy of antimonial compounds in kala-azar infection; dermal leishmanoid with positive flagellate culture from the peripheral blood. (III. N. S.) Calcutta Med. J., 21: 401-404, 1925-27

Braid, James. Scottish surgeon. 1795-1860
BRAIDISM or hypnotism—coined term hypnotism or neuro-hypnotism.
Neurypnology, or, the rationale of nervous sleep considered in relation with animal magnetism. London, Churchill, 1843. 265 pp.
STRABISMUS—turning of eyes simultaneously upward and inward; a means of inducing the hypnotic state.
Observations on trance: or human hybernation. London, Churchill, 1850. 72 pp.

Braille, Louis. Paris teacher of blind. 1809-1852
SYSTEM—of reading by blind.
Procédé pour écrire au moyen des points. Paris, 1837

Brain, R. T. London physician
TEST—
A new test of renal function with H. D. Kay, Quart. J. Med., 22: 203-216, Jan. 1929

Bramann, von. See P. Anton

Bramigk, Fritz. Jena physician
SOLUTION—peptic digest; culture medium.
Peptonselbstbereitung. Zbl. f. Bakt., 86: 427-432, June 28, 1921

Branca, Albert. French physician. 1868-1929
SOLUTION—sublimate formol, for fixing histologic specimens.
Recherches sur la cicatrisation épithéliale (épithéliums cylindriques stratifiés) la trachée et sa cicatrisation. J. Anat., Paris, 35: 767-807, 1899

Branch, Hira Edmund. Detroit surgeon. 1907–
TREATMENT—of burns with gentian violet and
silver nitrate.
*Extensive burns; treatment with silver nitrate and
methyl rosaniline.* Arch. Surg., 35: 478–485, Sept.
1937

Brand, A. F. See H. Eagle

Brand, Ernst. German physician. 1827–1897
TREATMENT or BATH—for fever.
Die Hydrotherapie des Typhus. Stettin, Von der
Nahmer, 1861. 309 pp.
*Answeisung für die Krankenwarter bei der Behand-
lung des Typhus mit Bädern. (Anhang zu "Die
Heilung des Typhus.")* Berlin, Hirschwald, 1868.
15 pp.

Brandes Max August Ludwig. Dortmund surgeon.
1881–
OPERATION—
Zur operativen Therapie des Hallux valgus. Zbl.
Chir., 56: 2434–2440, Sept. 28, 1929

Brandt, Thure. Swedish gynecologist. 1809–1895
METHOD or TREATMENT—of disease of fallopian
tubes by pressing out their contents into uterus by
massage. Invented system of uterine gymnastics for
prolapse.
*Nouvelle méthode gymnastique et magnétique pour le
traitement des maladies des organes du bassin et
principalement des affections utérines.* Stockholm,
Fritze, 1868. 86 pp.
*Die Bewegungscur als Heilmittel gegen weibliche
sogenannte Unterleibsleiden und Prolapsen.* Stockholm, 1880. 111 pp. 2 ed.

Brandt-Rehberg, P. Copenhagen physiologist
TEST—of kidney function; creatinine clearance.
*Über die Bestimmung der Menge des Glomerulusfil-
trats mittels Kreatinin als Nierenfunktionsprüfung,
nebst einigen Bemerkungen über die Theorien der
Harnbereitung.* Zbl. inn. Med., 50: 367–377, Apr. 13,
1929

Branham, H. H. American physician
BRADYCARDIAC REACTION—closure of fistula
of an arteriovenous aneurysm results in decrease in
pulse, rise in diastolic and in mean arterial pressure
and decrease in venous pressure.
*Aneurismal varix of the femoral artery and vein fol-
lowing a gunshot wound.* Internat. J. Surg., 3: 250–
251, Nov. 1890

Branower, William. New York anesthetist. 1881–
RESPIRATOR—
*Artificial respiration by an apparatus which permits
measured and controlled volumes and pressures.* J.
Thoracic Surg., 5: 377–385, Apr. 1936
Clinical application of studies in resuscitation. New
York State J. Med., 39: 2094–2099, Nov. 15, 1939

Brashear, Walter. Maryland surgeon. 1776–1860
First in United States to amputate at hip joint.
(no title). Trans. Kentucky med. Soc., 1852, 2:
265, 1853

Bratton, Andrew Calvin. Baltimore pharmacologist.
1912–
TEST—for sulfanilamide.
*A new coupling component for sulfanilamide deter,
mination* with E. K. Marshall, Jr. J. Biol. Chem.-
128: 537–550, May 1939
See also E. K. Marshall, Jr.

Brauer, Ludolph. German physician. 1865–
METHOD—production of artificial pneumothorax by

injection of nitrogen for treatment of tuberculosis c
lung. Advocated collapse therapy by extrapleura
thoracoplasty.
*Die Behandlung der einseitigen Lungenphthisis m
künstlichem Pneumothorax (nach Murphy).* Abstr.
Münch. med. Wschr., 53: 338–339, Feb. 13, 1906.
Ueber Pneumothorax. Marburg, Elwert, 1906. 40 pp
Ueber Lungenchirurgie. Assoc. franc. de chir., Proc.
verb., Paris, 21 Cong., pp. 569–574, 1908, Verh
ges. dtsch. Naturf. u. Aerzte, 80 Versamml., pt. 2
166–186, 1909
OPERATION—cardiolysis for adhesive pericarditis
*Ueber chronisch adhäsive Mediastinoper kardilis un
deren Behandlung.* Münch. med. Wschr., 49: 1072
1032, 1902

Braun, C. D. German chemist
REACTION—for picric acid.
*Ueber die Umwandlung der Pikrinsäure in Pikro
minsäure und über die Nachweisung des Trauben
zuckers.* Z. anal. Chem., 4: 185–188, 1865

Braun, Georg. Prague ophthalmologist. 1876–
HEMIKINESIMETER—
Ein neues Hemikinesimeter. Kln. Mbl. Augenheilk.
87: 441–450, Oct. 23, 1931

Braun, Gustav August. Austrian gynecologist. 1829–
1911
HOOK— *Ueber das technische Verfahren bei vernachläs
sigten Querlagen und über Decapitationsinstrumente
Wien. med. Wschr., 11: 713–716, 1861

Braun, Heinrich Freidrich Wilhelm. German sur
geon. 1862–1934
Synthesized novocaine or procaine; isolated by Alfre
Einhorn and used clinically by Braun. Did importan
work on local anesthesia.
*Ueber Infiltrationsanästhesie und regionäre Anästhesie
Samml. klin. Vortr., n.F., Leipzig. No. 228, Chir
No. 67, pp. 1177–1192, 1898
*Ueber einige neue örtliche Anesthetica (Stovain
Alypin, Novocain).* Dtsch. med. Wschr., 31: 1667–
1671, 1905
*Die Lokalanästhesie, ihre wissenschaftliche Grundla
gen und praktische Anwendung.* Leipzig, Barth, 190
Also, trans. by P. Shields, Phila. and New York
Lea and Febiger, 1914
OPERATION—ligation of ileocolic vein to preven
extension of pylephlebitis complicating appendicitis
*Die Unterbindung der Vena ileocolica bei mesenterialer
Pyämie nach Appendicitis.* Beitr. klin. Chir., 86
314–326, 1913

Braun, Ludwig. German physician. 1867–1936
Employed cinematograph to record cardiac changes
during all phases of heart contraction. Garrison and
Morton
Ueber Herzbewegung und Herzstoss. Jena, Fischer,
1898

Braun, Wilhelm. German surgeon
SKIN GRAFT—buried Reverdin grafts.
*Ueber Hautpfropfungen (mit Krankenvorstellung).
Dtsch. med. Wschr., 47: 369 (only), Mar. 31, 1921

Braune, Christian Wilhelm. German anatomist.
1831–1892
CANAL—uterine cavity and the vagina after the os is
fully dilated in labor.
*Die Lage des Uterus und Fetus am Ende der Schwang-
erschaft nach Durchschnitten an gefrornen Cadavern,
Leipzig, Veit, 1872. 4 l., 4 pl. fol.
Studied human locomotion.

Die Bewegungen des Kniegelenkes with O. Fischer, Abh. sachs. Ges. (Akad.) Wiss., Leipzig, 17: 78–150, 1891

Der Gang des Menschen with O. Fischer, Ibid., 21: 153–322, 1895

Braunschwig, H. See Hieronymus Brunschwig

Bravais, L. F. French physician

EPILEPSY—localized e.; same as Jacksonian e.

Recherches sur les symptômes et le traitement de l'épilepsie hémiplégique. Paris Thèse, No. 118, 1827. 46 pp.

Bravo, Francisco

Wrote first medical book published in the new world, in Mexico City. Garrison

Opera medicinalia. Mexico, Ocharts, 1570. 2 vols. 304 pp.

Described typhus fever.

De morbo tabardete vulgariter dicto. Ibid., ff. 1–90

Braxton Hicks.—see Hicks

Breck, L. W. See F. A. Lowe

Breda, Achille. Padua dermatologist. 1850–1933

DISEASE—yaws or frambesia Brasiliana.

Beitrag zum klinischen und bacteriologischen Studium der brasilianischen Framboesie oder "Boubas". Arch. f. Dermat, u. Syph., 33: 3–28, 1895

Breh, F. Detroit scientist

METHOD—

The determination of potassium in blood serum with O. H. Gaebler, J. biol. Chem., 87: 81–89, May 1930

Brehme, Th. Heidelberg physician

METHOD—for determination of sugar in blood.

Zur Frage der Milchsäurebestimmung in kleinen Blutwengen, Modifikation der Clausenschen Methode. with B. Brahdy, Biochem. Z., 175: 348–356, Aug. 30, 1926

Brehmer, Gustav Adolf Robert Herrmann. German physician. 1826–1899

Founder, in 1859, of first sanitorium for pulmonary tuberculosis.

Demonstrated that pulmonary tuberculosis is curable.

Die Therapie der chronischen Lungenschwindsucht. Wiesbaden, Bergmann, 1887

Breisky, August. German gynecologist. 1832–1889

DISEASE—kraurosis vulvae.

Die Krankheiten der Vagina. Hand. d. allg. u. spec. Chir., 4: 1–156, 1879

Also in: Pitha and Billroth's *Chirurgie* Stuttgart, 1879

Also, in English: Encycl. Obst. and Gynec., New York, Wood, 1887

Ueber Kraurosis vulvae, eine wenig beachtete Form von Hautatrophie am Pudendum muliebre. Z. Heilkunde, 6: 69–80, 1885

Die Krankheiten der Vagina. Stuttgart, Enke, 1886. 230 pp.

Breithaupt. German physician

Described osteoperiostitis of metatarsal bones: same as Busquet's disease or march foot.

Zur Pathologie des menschlichen Fusses. Med. Zeitung, Berlin, 24: 169–175, 1855

Bremer, Ludwig. St. Louis physician. 1844–1914

MIXTURE—methylen blue and eosin.

Ueber das Paranuclearkörperchen der gekernten Erythrocyten, nebst Bemerkungen über den Bau der Erythrocyten im Allgemeinen. Arch. mik. Anat., 45: 433–450 (446), 1895

TEST—for diabetic blood.

An improved method of diagnosticating diabetes from a drop of blood. New York Med. J., 63: 301–303, Mar. 7, 1896

Brenizer, Addison Gorgas. Charlotte, N. C. urologist. 1883–

MODIFICATION—

Ureteral transplantations; modifications of methods. Amer. J. Surg., 28: 210–233, May 1935

Brenn, Lena. See J. H. Brown

Brennemann, Joseph. Chicago pediatrician. 1872–

SYNDROME—abdominal pain with mesenteric and retroperitoneal lymphadenitis and infections of the upper respiratory tract.

"The abdominal pain of throat infections in children," and appendicitis. J. A. M. A., 89: 2183–2186, Dec. 24, 1927

Brenner, Alexander. German surgeon. 1859–1936

OPERATION—for hernia

Zur Radikaloperation der Leistenhernien. Zb. Chir., 25: 1017–1023, Oct. 15, 1898

Brenner, Fritz. German physician. 1877–

TUMOR—of ovary; oophoroma folliculare; characterized by slow growth, does not give rise to specific symptomatology and microscopically resembles metastatic epithelioma.

Das Oophoroma folliculare. Frankfurt. Z. f. Path., 1: 150–171, 1907

Brenner, Rudolf. German physician. 1821–1884

FORMULA—of cathode or anode in auditory meatus.

Untersuchungen und Beobachtungen auf dem Gebiete der Elektrotherapie. Leipzig, Giesecke u. Devrient, 1868–69. 2 vols.

Breschet, Gilbert. French anatomist. 1784–1845

CANAL—of the diploë.

SINUS—sphenoparietal s.

VEINS—of the diploë.

Essai sur les veines de rachis. In his: *Thèses présentées et soutenues publiquement le 28. avril 1819.* 288 pp.

Breton, M. See L. C. A. Calmette

Bretonneau, Pierre Fidèle. French physician. 1778–1862

ANGINA, DISEASE or DIPHTHERIA. Originated term diphtheria. Performed successful tracheotomy, July 1, 1825.

Des inflammations spéciales du tissu maqueux, et en particulier de la diphthérite, ou inflammation pelliculaire, connue sous le nom de croup, d'angine maligne, d'angine gangréneuse, etc. Paris, Crevot, 1826. 540 pp.

Also: New Sydenham Soc., London, 1859

Also, trans. by M. Nülle. Berlin, 1827

In 1813, distinguished "dothiénenterite" as a separate disease. (Osler) Wrote important monograph on the contagion of "dothienenteritis" or typhoid fever.

Notice sur la contagion de la dothinentérie. Arch. gén. de méd., Paris, 21: 57–78, 1829

Breuer, Josef. German physician. 1842–1925

Discovered the "unconscious mind." Garrison and Morton

Studien über Hysterie with S. Freud, Leipzig, Wien, Deuticke, 1893

Breus, Carl. Austrian obstetrician. 1852–1914

MOLE—a malformation of ovum consisting of tuberous subchorional hematoma of the decidua; hematomole.

Das tuberöse subchoriale Hämatom der Decidua; eine typische Form der Molenschwangershaft. Leipzig Deuticke, 1892. 32 pp.

CLASSIFICATION—of pelvic deformities.
Die pathologischen Beckenformen with A. Kolisko, Leipzig, Deuticke, 1900–04
Brewer, G. See W. F. Hamilton
Brewer, George Emerson. New York surgeon. 1861–1939
OPERATION—transfusion of blood by paraffine coated glass cannulae.
Direct blood transfusion by means of paraffine coated glass tubes with N. B. Leggett, S. G. O., 9: 293–295, Sept. 1909
Brezin, David. American surgeon. 1912–
OINTMENT—sulfathiazole, cod liver oil and lanolin; an agent to stimulate healing.
Pilonidal cyst. Report of a new procedure for operation and treatment. Amer. J. Surg., 59: 18–24, Jan. 1943
Bricheteau, Isidore. French physician. 1789–1861
Described pneumopericardium.
Observation d'hydropneumopéricarde accompagnée d'un bruit de fluctuation perceptible a l'oreille. Arch. gén. de méd., 4 s., 4: 334–339, 1844
Brickner, Richard Max. New York neurologist, 1896–
PHENOMENON—
Oscillopsia: a new symptom commonly occurring in multiple sclerosis. Arch. Neurol. Psychiat., 36: 586–589, Sept. 1936
SIGN—
Brickner's sign of diminished oculo-auricular associated movement. In C. A. McKendree's *Neurological Examination.* Philadelphia, Saunders, 1928. p. 191
Brickner, Walter M. New York surgeon. 1876–1930
SIGN—of bursitis of shoulder; pain referred to anterior deltoid region on gently pressing the circumflex nerve against the inner aspect of humerus.
Shoulder disability (stiff and painful shoulder). Amer. J. Surg., 26: 196–204, June 1912
Bricq, R. See A. Vernes
Bridges, C. B. See T. H. Morgan
Bridges, J. W. See R. M. Yerkes
Brieger, Ludwig. Berlin physician. 1849–1909
BACILLUS—B. cavicidus. Isolated and named toxins, typhotoxine and tetanine.
Ueber ein neues Krämpfe verursachendes Ptomain. Ber. dtsch. chem. Ges., 19: 3119–3121, Dec. 9,1886
Ueber Ptomaine. Verhandl. d. Cong. f. innere Med., Wiesb., 5: 83–91, 1886
Ueber Ptomaine. Berlin, Hirschwald, 1885–86. 3 vols.
Briggs, Alfred Poyneer. St. Louis biochemist. 1888–
MODIFICATION—of the Bell-Doisy method for determination of phosphorus content of blood plasma.
A modification of the Bell-Doisy phosphate method. J. biol. Chem., 53: 13–16, July 1922
Briggs, James Emmons. American surgeon. 1869–1942
BAG—
A method of controlling the bleeding after suprapubic prostatectomy. New England Med. Gaz., Boston, 41: 391–393, 1906
Bright, Richard. English physician. 1789–1858
DISEASE—any one of a group of kidney diseases attended with albuminuria and nephritis.
BLINDNESS or EYE—dimness or complete loss of sight without a lesion of the retina or optic disk; seen in uremia.

GRANULATIONS—those of a large white kidney.
Cases illustrative of some of the appearances observable on the examination of diseases terminating in dropsical effusion. In his: *Reports of medical cases selected with a view of illustrating the symptoms and cure of disease by a reference to morbid anatomy.* Guy's Hosp. Rep., 1: 1–74, 1827
Also: London, Longman, 1827. pp. 229
Also: London, Milford, 1927. 172 pp.
Cases and observations, illustrative of renal disease accompanied with the secretion of albuminous urine. Guy's Hosp. Rep., 1: 338–400, 1836
Described pancreatic diabetes and pancreatic steatorrhoea.
Cases and observations connected with disease of the pancreas and duodenum. Med.-Chir. Trans., London, 18: 1–56, 1832–33
Described unilateral (Jacksonian) epilepsy.
Fatal epilepsy, from suppuration between the dura mater and arachnoid in consequence of blood having been effused in that situation. Guy's Hosp. Rep., 1: 36–40, 1836
Described post-mortem findings in a case of congenitally short esophagus.
Account of a remarkable misplacement of the stomach. Ibid., 598–603
Described acute yellow atrophy of liver.
Observations on jaundice. Ibid., 604–637
Described status lymphaticus.
Observations on abdominal tumors. Ibid., 3: 401–460 (437), 1838
Wrote important description of appendicitis.
Inflammations of the cecum and appendix vermiformis: In: *Elements of the practice of medicine* with T: Addison, London, Longman, 1839. Vol. 1, p. 498
Brill, Isidor Cherniac. Portland, Oregon physician. 1888–
TEST BREAKFAST—
The effect of a normal meal upon the blood sugar level in health and in certain conditions of disease. J. Lab. clin. Med., 8: 727–731, Aug. 1923
Brill, Nathan Edwin. New York physician. 1860–1925
DISEASE—a form of typhus fever.
An acute infectious disease of unknown origin: a clinical study based on 221 cases. Amer. J. Med. Sci., 139: 484–502, Apr. 1910
Described giant follicular hyperplasia in spleen and lymph nodes; called Brill-Symmers disease.
Generalized giant lymph follicle hyperplasia of lymph nodes and spleen: a hitherto undescribed type with G. Baehr and N. Rosenthal, J. A. M. A., 84: 668–671, Feb. 28, 1925
Brines, Osborne Allen. Detroit biochemist. 1893–
APPARATUS—for transfusion of blood; modified Unger a.
The transfusion of unmodified blood. Arch. Surg., 7 306–320, Sept. 1923; 12: 124–139; 140–150, Jan. 1926; 16: 1080–1088, May 1928
Brinkhous, K. M. See E. D. Warner
Brinton, William. English physician. 1823–1867
DISEASE—linitis plastica.
The diseases of the stomach, with an introduction on its anatomy and physiology. London, Churchill, 1859 406 pp. pp. 310–331

Brion, Albert. German physician. 1876–
DISEASE—paratyphus.
  Ueber eine Erkrankung mit dem Befund eines
  typhusähnlichen Bakteriums im Blute (Paratyphus)
  with H. Kayser, Münch. med. Wschr., 49: 611–615,
  Apr. 15, 1902
Briquet, Paul. French physician. 1796–1881
ATAXIA—a hysteric condition with anesthesia of the
  skin of the legs.
  Traité clinique et thérapeutique de l'hystérie. Paris,
  Baillière, 1859. 724 pp. p. 297
SYNDROME—shortness of breath and aphonia de-
  pendent on hysteric paralysis of diaphragm. Ibid.,
  p. 475
GANGRENE—of lung in bronchiectasis.
  Mémoir sur un mode de gangrène du poumon, dé-
  pendant de la mortification des extrémités dilatées de
  bronches. Arch. gén. de méd., Paris, 3 s., 11: 5–23,
  May 1841
Brissand, E. See G. F. I. Widal
Brissaud, P. Edouard. French physician. 1852–1909
DISEASE—habit spasm, or chorea variabilis.
  La chorée variable des dégenérés. Rev. neurol., 4: 417–
  431, July 30, 1896
INFANTILISM—dysthyroidal infantilism.
  L'infantilisme vrai. N. iconog. de la Salpêtriere,
  Paris, 20: 1–17, 1907
SYNDROME—in hemiplegia due to pontine lesions,
  occasionally the paralysis is of spasmodic type.
  Recherches anatomo-pathologiques et physiologiques
  sur la contracture permanente des hémiplégiques.
  (Paris), Versailles, 1880. 206 pp.
  L'hémispasme facial alterne with J.-A. Sicard, Pr.
  méd., 16: 234–236, Apr. 11, 1908
Brisseau, Michel. French physician. 1676–1743
Demonstrated true nature and location of cataract.
  Traité de la cataracte et du glaucoma. Paris, d'Houry,
  1709
  also, facsimile: 1921
Brittingham, Harold Hixon. Boston physician.
1894–
TEST—dumb-bell swinging for myocardial function.
  Cardia functional tests with P. D. White, J. A. M. A.,
  79: 1901–1904, Dec. 2, 1922
Broadbent, Sir John Francis Harpin. English
physician. 1865–
SIGN—same as Walter Broadbent s.
SIGN—of adherent pericarditis; no visible epigastric
  movements because of adhesions to diaphragm.
  Adherent pericardium. London, Baillière et al., 1895.
  126 pp.
Broadbent, Walter. English physician
SIGN—of pericardial adhesion; retraction on left side
  of back near eleventh and twelfth ribs.
  An unpublished physical sign. Lancet, 2: 200–201,
  July 27, 1895
Broadbent, Sir William Henry. English physician.
1835–1907
APOPLEXY—cerebral hemorrhage beginning outside
  ventricle and progressing until it enters the ven-
  tricle.
  On ingravescent apoplexy. Abstr.: Proc. roy. Med. and
  Chir. Soc., London, 8: 103–108, May 23, 1876
SIGN—of aneurysm of left ventricle: pulsation of
  lateral wall of thorax with systole of ventricle.
  The pulse. London, Cassell, 1890
  Heart disease with special reference to prognosis and

treatment. London, Baillière, Tindall and Cox, 1897
  Also: New York, William Wood, 1897
  Also, Chapt. 17, in: F. A. Willius and T. E. Keys'
  Cardiac classics, St. Louis, Mosby, 1941. pp. 712–
  715
SIGN—same as Walter Broadbent's.
  Adherent pericardium. Trans. Med. Soc. London, 21:
  109–122, Jan. 10, 1898
Broca, Pierre Paul. French surgeon. 1824–1880
AMNESIA—inability to remember spoken words.
ANGLE—basillar a. or basiopic a., that between the
  nasobacilar line and Meissner's horizontal.
APHASIA—ataxic a.
AREA—for speech; gray matter between middle ol-
  factory root and peduncle of callosum.
CENTER—speech c.
CONVOLUTION—inferior or third left frontal con-
  volution; speech center.
FISSURE—surrounding the third left frontal convolu-
  tion.
REGION—same as convolution.
SPACE—the central part of the anterior olfactory lobe.
  Perte de la parole; ramollissement chronique et destruc-
  tion partielle du lobe antérieur gauche du cerveau.
  Bull. Soc. d'anthrop. de Paris, 2: 235–238, 1861
  Remarques sur le siège de la faculté du langage articulé,
  suivies d'une observation d'aphémie (perte de la parole).
  Bull. Soc. anat. de Paris, 36: 330–357; 398, Aug.
  1861
POUCH—pudendal sac or sac dartoique de la femme.
  De l'etranglement dans les hernies abdominales, et des
  affections qui peuvent le simuler. Paris, Martinet,
  1853. 182 pp.
Brocq, Louis Anne Jean. French dermatologist.
1856–1928
DISEASE—parakeratosis psoriasiformis.
  Les parapsoriasis. Ann. de dermat. et de syph.,
  Paris, 4 s., 3: 313–315; 433–468, 1902
  See J. B. E. Vidal
Broden, A. Belgian physician
METHOD—of concentration of Trypanosoma Gam-
  biense.
  Diagnostic de la maladie du sommeil. Ann. Soc. Belge.
  d. med. Trop., 1: 1–38, Nov. 1920
Broders, Albert Compton. Rochester, Minn. path-
ologist. 1885–
INDEX—of malignancy.
  Squamous-cell epithelioma of the lip: a study of five
  hundred and thirty-seven cases. J. A. M. A., 74: 656–
  664, Mar. 6, 1920
  Squamous-cell epithelioma of the skin. Ann. Surg., 73:
  141–160, 1921
  Epithelioma of the genito-urinary organs. Ibid., 75:
  574–580, 1922
  The grading of carcinoma. Minnesota Med., 8: 726–
  730, Dec. 1925
  Carcinoma: grading and practical application. Arch.
  Path. and clin. Med., 2: 376–381, Sept. 1926
  The grading of cancer: its relationship to metastasis
  and prognosis. Texas State J. Med., 29: 520–525,
  Dec. 1933
  See also W. C. MacCarty
Brodie, Sir Benjamin Collins. English surgeon.
1783–1862
ABSCESS—chronic inflammation, sometimes tubercu-
  lous, of head of bone, especially of tibia.
  An account of some cases of chronic abscess of the

tibia. Med.-chir. Trans., London, 17: 239–249, 1832
Also: Med. Classics, 2: 900–906, May 1938
Lecture on abscess of the tibia. London Med. Gaz.,
36: 1399–1402, 1845
Also: Med. Classics, 2: 907–918, May 1938
DISEASE—1. chronic synovitis, especially of the knee
joint.
*Pathological researches respecting the diseases of the
joints.* Med.-chir. Trans., London, 4: 207–277, 1813
*Further observations on the diseases which affect the
synovial membranes of joints.* Ibid., 5: 239–254, 1814
Also: Med. Classics, 2: 919–928, May 1938
*Pathological and surgical observations on the diseases
of the joints.* London, Longman, 1818. 329 pp.
DISEASE—2. hysteric pseudo-fracture of the spine.
Lectures illustrative of certain local nervous affections.
London, Longman, 1837. 88 pp. pp. 46–49
JOINT—see disease 1.
KNEE—chronic synovitis; see disease 1.
OPERATION—for fissure or ulcer of anus, the muscle
fibers of the sphincter being divided at one side by a
history drawn from the anus laterally outward; see
pile.
PILE—sentinel p.; a mass of inflamed, traumatized
anal mucosa at lower end of fissure-in-ano.
*Lectures on diseases of the rectum. Lecture III. Pre-
ternatural contraction of the sphincter ani.* London
Med. Gaz., 16: 26–31, 1835
Also: Med. Classics, 2: 929–940, May 1938
*On preternatural contraction of the sphincter ani:
on ulcer on the inside of the rectum.* In: *Clinical lec-
tures on surgery,* London, 1846
Also: Phila., 1846. Ch. 36, p. 322
TUMOR—serocystic, of breast; cystadenoma or
chronic cystic mastitis.
Lectures on sero-cystic tumors of the breast. London
Med. Gaz., 25: 808–814, 1840
Also: Med. Classics, 2: 941–954, May 1938
Some diseases of the breast. Med. Times, 10: 163–
164, 1844
*Sero-cystic tumors of the breast. Clinical lectures on
surgery.* 1846. Lecture 24, p. 206
Studied influence of pneumogastric nerve on gastric
secretion.
*Experiments and observations on the influence of the
nerves of the eighth pair on the secretions of the stomach.*
Philos. Trans., 104: 102–106, 1814
Operated for varicose veins in 1814.
*Observations on the treatment of varicose veins of the
legs.* Med.-chir. Trans., 7: 195–210, 1816
Reported intermittent claudication in man.
*Lectures illustrative of various subjects in pathology
and surgery.* London, Longman, 1846. p. 361
Brodie, Bernard B. New York biochemist. 1909–
METHOD—
The determination of salicylic acid in plasma with S.
Udenfriend and A. F. Coburn, J. Pharmacol., 80:
114–117, Jan. 1944
Brodie, Charles Gordon. Scottish anatomist. 1786–
1818
LIGAMENT—transverse humeral 1.
Dissections illustrated. London, (1892–95). 142 pp.
Brodie, Maurice. American bacteriologist. 1903–
Introduced poliomyelitis vaccine.
Active immunization against poliomyelitis with W.
H. Park, J. A. M. A., 105: 1089–1093, Oct. 5, 1935

Brodie, Thomas Gregor. English physiologist. 1866–
1916
METHOD—
The determination of the coagulation time of blood
with A. E. Russell, J. Physiol., 21: 403–407, May
1897
Brodmann, Korbinian. Armenian anatomist. 1868–
1918
AREAS—fifty-two discrete areas in the human brain.
*Vergleichende Lokalisationslehre der Grosshirnrinde
in ihren Prinzipien dargestellt auf Grund des Zellen-
baues.* Leipzig, Barth, 1909. 324 pp.
Reprinted, 1925. 324 pp.
Brodny, Max Leopold. Boston urologist. 1905–
CLAMP—
A new instrument for urethrography in the male. J.
Urol., 46: 350–354, Aug. 1941
Brödel, Max. Baltimore physician. 1870–1941
LINE—a longitudinal white line on the anterior sur-
face of the kidney near the convex border; same as
Hyrtl's exsanguinated renal zone.
STITCH—for fraible organs, at right angles to the
framework.
*A more rational method of passing the suture in
fixation of the kidney.* Amer. Med., 4: 176–178, Aug.
2, 1902
Broesike, Gustav. German anatomist. 1853–
FOSSA—parajejunal.
*Ueber intraabdominale (retroperitoneale) Hernien
und Bauchfelltaschen, nebst einer Darstellund der
Entwiklung peritonealer Formationen.* Berlin, Fischer,
1891. 206 pp.
Brokaw, Augustus V. L. St. Louis surgeon. 1853–
1907
RING—of rubber tubing threaded with catgut strands
and employed in intestinal anastomosis.
*The use of segmented rubber rings in intestinal anasto-
motic and other operations.* Internat. J. Surg., 2: 251–
256, Nov. 1889
*Intestinal anastomotic operations with segmented
rubber rings; with some practical suggestions to their
use in other surgical procedures.* Med. News, Phila.,
55: 634–637, 1889
Bronfenbrenner, Jacques Jacob. American bac-
tericlogist. 1883–
SOLUTION—china blue rosolic acid whey; for cultivation of colon-typhoid group.
*On methods of isolation and identification of the mem-
bers of the colon-typhoid group of bacteria. The preparation of milk and milk-whey as culture medium* with
C. R. Davis and K. Morishima, J. med. Res., 39:
345–348, Jan. 1919
Bronstein, J. Moscow bacteriologist
TEST—for differentiating diphtheria from pseudo-
diphtheria.
*Zur Frage über Differenzierung der Diphtherie- und
Pseudodiphtheriebacillen* with G. N. Grünblatt, Zbl.
Bakt., Abt. 1, 32: 425–428, Sept. 25, 1902
Brooke, Henry Ambrose Grundy. English derma-
tologist. 1854–1919
DISEASE—keratosis follicularis contagiosa.
(no title) In: Internat. Atlas, No. 7, Plate 22, 1892
TUMOR—adenoid cystic epithelioma, a relatively
uncommon form of epidermoid carcinoma.
Epithelioma adenoides cysticum. Brit. J. Dermat., 4:
269–286, Sept. 1892

Brooke, Ralph. English surgeon. 1900–
OPERATION—
The treatment of fractured patella by excision; a study of morphology and function. Brit. J. Surg., 24: 733–747, Apr. 1937

Brookes, Theodore Prewitt. St. Louis surgeon. 1887–
TREATMENT—of fracture-dislocation of cervical vertebrae.
On reducing and treating cervical dislocations with F. H. Ewerhardt, Arch. Phys. Therap, X-ray, Radium, 13: 463–468, Aug. 1932
Dislocations of the cervical spine. Their complications and treatment. S. G. O., 57: 772–782, Dec. 1933

Brookover, Charles. Chicago
MODIFICATION—formaldehyde, of Golgi's bichromate and silver nitrate method.
The o'factory nerve, the nervus terminalis and the pre-optic sympathetic system in amia calva, L. J. com. Neurol., 20: 49–118, Apr. 1910

Brooks, Barney. American surgeon. 1884–
APPARATUS—for measuring temperatures in the extremities.
Intra-arterial injection of sodium iodid: preliminary report. J. A. M. A., 82: 1016–1019, Mar. 29, 1924
New methods for study of diseases of the circulation of the extremities. J. Bone and Joint Surg., 7: 316–318, Apr. 1925
See also N. Allison

Brophy, Truman William. American surgeon. 1848–1928
OPERATION—for cleft palate.
Premaxilla pushed back in the repair of hare-lip. In his: *Oral surgery; a treatise on disease, injuries and malformations of the mouth and associated parts.* Phila., Blakiston, 1915. 1090 pp. pp. 658–665
Cleft lip and cleft palate. Phila., Blakiston, 1923. p. 252

Brossa, G. A. Italian physician
REACTION—a flocculation test for cancer.
Una semplice prova sulla labilita colloidale del sangue nel carcinoma with G. Bozzolo, Gior. Accad. med. Torino, 4 s., 32: 95–101, 1926
Adsorbimento capillare e labilita di sieri patologici (carcinoma). Ibid., 93: 189–200, Sept. 1930

Brotman, I. See W. F. Hamilton

Broun, Goronwy Owen. St. Louis physician. 1895–
TEST—
A test for bile salts in urine. Proc. Soc. exp. Biol., N. Y., 23: 596–598, Apr. 1926
See also R. A. Kinsella

Broussais, Francois Joseph Victor. French physician. 1772–1838
Taught that irritability of the mucous membrane of the alimentary canal was a point of primary importance in the causation of disease; obsolete opinion.
De l'irritation et de la folie. Bruxelles, 1828

Browder, Eli Jefferson. Brooklyn surgeon. 1894–
OPERATION—
A surgical method for the prevention of thrombophlebitis of the cavernous sinus: report of a case with M. C. Myerson. Arch. Otolaryng., 21: 574–583, May 1935

Brown, Alice Lenore. American scientist. 1888–
APPARATUS—
A simple apparatus for delicate injections. Anat. Rec., 24: 295–297, Dec. 1922

Brown, C. L. M. English chemist
REACTION—
Differentiation of dextrose and levulose with E. A. Lum, Pharm. J., 131: 63 (only), July 15, 1933

Brown, Charles Leonard. Boston physician. 1899–
ENCEPHALOMYELITIS—
Acute serous encephalitis; a newly recognized disease of children with D. Symmers, Amer. J. Dis. Child., 29: 174–181, Feb. 1925
Also, abstr.: J. nerv. ment. Dis., 61: 181–186, Feb. 1925

Brown, Denis. London surgeon
SPLINT—
Talipes equino-varus. Lancet, 2: 969–974, Nov. 3, 1934

Brown, E. D. See T. H. Sollman

Brown, F. A. Jr. See R. Elman

Brown, Francis Robert. Dundee surgeon
OPERATION—for inguinal hernia.
The use of strips of hernial sac as fascial (living) sutures. Brit. med. J., 1: 858 (only), May 10, 1930

Brown, George Elgie. Rochester, Minn. physician. 1885–1935
Determined vasomotor index, which is the increase in surface temperature divided by the oral temperature under standard heat conditions.
The treatment of peripheral vascular disturbances of the extremities. J. A. M. A., 87: 379–383, Aug. 7, 1926
See also A. W. Adson, E. A. Hines, Jr., B. T. Horton

Brown, George Van Ingen. Milwaukee surgeon 1862–
OPERATION—for cleft palate.
The surgical treatment of cleft palate. A new method which is primarily a reconstructive application of parts of many old operative procedures revised to form what is in effect a new operation. J. A. M. A., 87: 1379–1384, Oct. 23, 1926

Brown, H. C. See P. H. Manson-Bahr

Brown, H. R. See T. Smith

Brown, Henry Paul, Jr. Philadelphia surgeon. 1888–
OPERATION—for intussusception: dorsal slit.
Acute intussusception in children: observations on thirty-one cases admitted to the Children's Hospital in Philadelphia. Ann. Surg., 81: 637–645, Mar. 1925

Brown, Herman. Philadelphia physician. 1900–
METHOD—
The determination of uric acid in blood. J. biol. Chem., 68: 123–133, Apr. 1926

Brown, J. B. See V. P. Blair

Brown, James Howard. American pathologist. 1884–
METHOD—
A method for the differential staining of Gram-positive and Gram-negative bacteria in tissue sections with Lena Brenn, Johns Hopk. Hosp. Bull., 48: 69–73, Feb. 1931
SOLUTION—milk; a culture medium.
Transparent milk as a bacteriological medium with P. E. Howe, J. Bact., 7: 511–514, Sept. 1922
See also A. R. Kimpton

Brown, John. English physician. 1735–1788
Father of the now obsolete doctrine that all disease is due either to excess or lack of stimulus.
Elementa medicinae. Edinburgi, Elliot, 1780. 421 pp.

Brown, Lawrason. American physician. 1871-1937
POINTS—five, of pulmonary tuberculosis.
A study of the occurrence of hemoptysis, pleurisy, rales, tubercle bacilli and x-ray findings in 1000 consecutive cases admitted to the Trudeau sanatorium. By F. H. Heise and L. Brown, Amer. Rev. Tuberc. 6: 1078-1083, Feb. 1923
The lungs and the early stages of tuberculosis. New York, Appleton, 1931

Brown, Philip King. American physician. 1869-1940
Described extreme leucopenia.
A fatal case of acute primary infectious pharyngitis with W. Ophüls, Trans. Med. Soc. California, pp. 91-101, 1901
See also W. B. Coffey

Brown, Philip Walling. Rochester, Minn. physician. 1896-
Suggested term "regional enteritis."
Chronic inflammatory lesions of the small intestine (regional enteritis) with J. A. Bargen and H. M. Weber, Trans. Amer. Gastro-enterol. Ass., pp. 2-7, 1934

Brown, Robert. English botanist. 1773-1858
MOVEMENT—dancing motion of minute particles suspended in a liquid.
A brief account of microscopical observations made in the months of June, July, and August, 1827, on the particles contained in the pollen of plants; and on the general existence of active molecules in organic and inorganic bodies. London, Taylor, 1828. 16 pp.; 7 pp.
Discovered the rôle of pollen in generation of plants. Ibid.
Discovered cell nucleus, 1831.
Observations on the organs and mode of fecundation in Orchideae and Asclepiadeae. Trans. Linn. Soc., London, 16: 685-746, 1829-32

Brown, T. M. See H. F. Swift

Brown, Thomas Kenneth. St. Louis gynecologist. 1898-
MEDIUM—for culture of gonococci.
Pyridium in the treatment of gonorrheal vaginitis in children with S. D. Soule and H. L. Kleine, J. Missouri Med. Ass., 31: 313-315, Aug. 1934

Brown, Thomas Richardson. American physician. 1872-
TEST—for estimating diastase in feces.
The normal amount of diastatic ferment in the feces and its variation in certain diseases of the pancreas and in achylia gastrica. Johns Hopk. Hosp. Bull., 35: 200-204, July 1914
Discovered eosinophilia in trichinosis.
Studies on trichinosis, with especial reference to the increase of the eosinophilic cells in the blood and muscle, the origin of these cells and their diagnostic importance. J. exp. Med., 3: 315-347, May 1898
See also W. S. Thayer

Brown, Sir Walter Langdon. English physiologist. 1870-1946
SCHEME—of the autonomic system as a whole.
The sympathetic nervous system in disease. London, Frowde et al., 1920. 161 pp.

Brown, William. Virginia physician. 1752-1792
Prepared the first pharmacopeia printed in America.
Pharmacopoeia simpliciorum et efficiarum in usum Nosocomi militaris ad Exercitum Federatum Americae Civitatum. Phila., Styner and Cyst, 1778. 2 ed., 1781

Browne, Denis John. London surgeon. 1892-
OPERATION—
The operation for cleft palate. Brit. J. Surg., 20: 7-25, July 1932

Browne, J. S. L. See J. B. Collip

Browne, John. English physician. 1642-1700?
Described cirrhosis of liver.
A remarkable account of a liver, appearing glandulous to the eye. Philos. Trans., London, 15: 1266-1268, 1685

Browning, Carl Hamilton. Glasgow scientist. 1881-
SOLUTION—brilliant green peptone, for enrichment of B. typhosus.
The isolation of typhoid bacilli from faeces by means of brilliant green in fluid medium with W. Gilmour and T. J. Mackie, J. Hyg., 13: 335-342, Oct. 1913

Brownlee, Inez E. See E. E. Osgood

Brownlee, John. English physician. 1868-1927
SIGN—edema of eyelids.
Public health administration in epidemics of measles. Brit. med. J., 1: 534-537 (536), Apr. 17, 1920
THEORY—
Investigations into the periodicity of infectious diseases by the application of a method hitherto only used in physics. Pub. Health, London, 28: 125-134, Mar. 1915

Brown-Séquard, Charles Edouard. French physiologist. 1817-1894
DISEASE or PARALYSIS or SIGN or SYNDROME—a lesion involving half of spinal cord gives paralysis on one side and loss of sensation on other.
De la transmission croisée des impressions sensitives par la moëlle épinière. C. R. Soc. Biol., 1850, 2: 33-34, 1851
Explication de l'hémiplégie croisée du sentiment. Ibid., 70-73
Recherches expérimentales sur la transmission croisée des impressions sensitives dans la moëlle épinière Gaz. hebd. de méd., Paris, 2, 1855
Also: Paris, Martinet, 1855. 19 pp.
EPILEPSY—epileptiform convulsions occurring after experimental injuries of the spinal cord in animals.
Recherches expérimentales sur la production d'une affection convulsive épileptiforme, à la suite de lésions de la moëlle épinière. Arch. gen. de méd., 5 s., 7: 143-149, Feb. 1856
Nouvelles recherches sur l'epilepsie due à certaines lésions de la moëlle épinière et des nerfs rachidiens. Arch. de Physiol. norm. et path., 2: 211-220; 422-441; 496-503, 1869
ELIXIR—sterilized testicular fluid for treatment of nervous and mental diseases.
Expérience démontrant la puissance dynamogénique chez l'homme d'une liquide extrait de testicules d'animaux. Arch. de Physiol. norm. et path., 5 s., 1: 651-658, 1889
Du rôle physiologique et thérapeutique d'un suc extrait de testicules d'animaux d'après nombre de faits observés chez l'homme. Ibid., 739-746
Nouveaux faits relatifs à l'injection sous-cutanée, chez l'homme, d'un liquide extrait des testicules de mammifères. Ibid., 2: 201-208, 1890
Exposé de faits nouveaux à l'égard de l'influence sur les centres nerveux d'un liquide extrait de testicules d'animaux. Ibid., 443-455
Nouveaux faits relatifs à l'influence sur les centre

nerveux de l'homme d'un liquide extrait de testicules d'animaux. Ibid., 641–648

TREATMENT—organotherapy; administration of animal organs or their extracts. See also ELIXIR.

Remarques sur les effets produits sur la femme par des injections sous cutanées d'un liquide retiré d'ovaires d'animaux. C. R. Soc. Biol., 5 s., 2: 456–457, 1890

Traitement de l'acromégalie par certains liquides organiques. Ibid., 45: 527 (only), May 20, 1893

Made important studies of sympathetic nerves. Garrison and Morton

Experimental researches applied to physiology and pathology. Med. Exam., Phila., 8: 481–504, 1852

Note sur la découverte de quelques-uns des effets de la galvanisation du nerf grand sympathique au cou. Gaz. méd. de Paris, 3 s., 9: 22–23, 1854

Sue les résultats de la section et de la galvanisation du nerf grand sympathique au cou. Ibid., 30–32

Excised adrenals, producing Addison's disease.

Recherches expérimentales sur la physiologie et la pathologie des capsules surrénales. Arch. gén. de méd., 5 s., 8: 385–401; 572–598, 1856

Also: C. R. Acad. Sci., Paris, 43: 422–425; 542–546, 1856

Also: Paris, Rignoux, 1856. 45 pp.

Found a dilatation of the vessels of the posterior limb in an animal in whom a lateral half of the spinal cord had been divided. Argyll Robertson

Summary of a paper (to be presented) on the resemblance between the effects of the section of the sympathetic nerve in the neck and of a transverse section of a lateral half of the spinal cord. By E. Brown-Séquard. Communicated by James Paget. Proc. roy. Soc., 8: 594–596, 1867

Studied pathways of conduction in spinal cord.

Recherches sur la transmission des impressions de tact, de chatouillement, de douleur, de température et de contraction (sens musculaire) dans la moëlle épinière. J. Physiol. Path. gen., 6: 124–145; 232–248; 581–646, 1863

Observed that "sleep resembles a slight attack of epilepsy."

Leçons sur les nerfs vasomoteurs.... Paris, 1872. p. 121

Bruce, Sir David. British Army surgeon. 1855–1931

SEPTICEMIA—Malta fever; demonstrated causative organism in 1886 and named it Microeoccus melitensis.

Note on the discovery of a microorganism in Malta Fever. The micrococcus of Malta Fever. Practitioner, London, 38: 161–170, Sept. 1887; 40: 241–249, Apr. 1888

Observations on Malta Fever. Brit. med. J., 1: 1101–1105, May 18, 1889

Found that nagana, the tsetse fly disease of Zuzuland, is due to a trypanosome (T. brucei).

Preliminary report on the tsetse fly disease or Nagana, in Zululand. Durban, Bennett and Davis, 1895

Discovered the trypanosome as the etiologic agent of African sleeping sickness, 1903. (See also A. Castellani)

Reports of the Sleeping Sickness Commission of the Royal Society. London, 1903–19. 17 parts.

The Croonian lectures on trypanosomes causing disease in man and the domestic animals in Central

Africa. Lancet, 1: 1323–1330, June 26; 2: 1–6 July 3; 55–63, July 10, 1915

See also J. E. Dutton

Bruce, W. J. New York scientist

DETERMINATION—of reaction.

A simple method for determining the reaction of feces. J. Lab. clin. Med., 5: 61–62, Oct. 1919

Bruch, A. See A. Conor

Bruck, Alfred. Berlin physician. 1865–

DISEASE—deformity of bones, multiple fractures, ankylosis of joints, and atrophy of muscles.

Ueber eine seltene Form von Erkrankung der Knochen und Gelenke. Dtsch. med. Wschr., 23: 152–155, Mar. 4, 1897

Bruck, Carl. German physician. 1879–

TEST—serochemical, for syphilis.

Die Serodiagnose der Syphilis. Berlin, 1909

Ueber Fällungserscheinungen beim Vermischen von Syphilisseren mit alkoholischen Luesleberextrakten with S. Hidaka, Z. Immun Forsch., 8: 476–482, Jan. 9, 1911

Beitrag zur Serodiagnose der Syphilis durch eine neue Methode. Abstr.: Münch. med. Wschr., 69: 569 (only), Apr. 14, 1922

Handbuch der Serodiagnose der Syphilis. Berlin, Springer, 1924

Demonstrated that persons infected with the gonococcus showed an allergic reaction to the cutaneous application of killed gonococci.

Ueber spezifische Behandlung gonorrhoischer Prozesse. Dtsch. med. Wschr., 35: 470–474, Mar. 18, 1909

See also A. von Wassermann

Brudzinski, Josef. Polish physician. 1874–1917

SIGN—contralateral reflex: in meningitis, when passive flexion of the lower limb on one side is made, a similar movement will be seen in the opposite leg.

Ueber die kontralateralen Reflexe an den unteren Extremitäten bei Kindern. Wien. klin. Wschr., 21: 255–261, Feb. 20, 1908

SIGN—neck s.: in meningitis, when the neck is bent, flexure movements of the ankle, knee and hip are produced.

Un signe nouveau sur les membres inférieurs dans les méningites chez les enfants: (signe de la nuque). Arch. de méd. d. enf., 12: 745–752, Oct. 1909

SIGN—cheek s.: in tuberculous meningitis, when pressure is made on both cheeks below the zygoma, both arms are jerked upward and the elbows are flexed.

Ueber neue Symptome von Gehirnhautentzündung und Reizung bei Kindern, insbesondere bei tuberkulösen. Berl. klin. Wschr., 53: 686–690, June 19, 1916

SIGN—symphysis s.: pressure over the symphysis pubis causes both lower extremities to flex. Ibid.

Brüche Ernst Wilhelm von Austrian physiologist 1819–1892

MUSCLE—longitudinal part of ciliary m.

TUNIC—tunica nervea; the retinal layers, exclusive of rod and cone layer, with its fibers and nuclei.

Anatomische Untersuchungen über die sogenannten leuchtenden Augen bei den Wirbelthieren. Arch. f. Anat., Physiol. u. wiss. Med., pp. 387–406, 1845

Anatomische Beschreibung des Augapfels. Berlin, 1847

REACTION—for urea.

Ueber die Nachweisung von Harnstoff mittelst Oxalsäure. S. B. Akad. Wiss. Wien, Math.-naturw. Cl., 3 Abth., 85: 280, 1882

TEST—emulsion t. for fatty acids.
Ueber die physiologische Bedeutung der theilweisen Zerlegung der Fette im Dünndarme. Ibid., 61, 1870
REAGENT—for protein substances. Ibid., p. 250
Wrote classical work on phonetics.
Grundzüge der Physiologie und Systematik der Sprachlaute für Linguisten und Taubstummenlehrer. Wien, Gerold's Sohn, 1856
Maintained that normal urine may contain sugar.
Ueber die reducirenden Eigenschaften des Harns gesunder Menschen. S. B. Akad. Wiss. Wien, Math.-naturw. Cl., 28, 1858

Brückner, Josef. Budapest physiologic chemist
REAGENT—for ergosterol.
Ueber eine empfindliche und spezifische Reaktion des Ergosterins. Biochem. Z., 270: 346–348, May 10, 1934

Brügger, H. See L. Ruzicka

Bruening, Friedrich. German surgeon. 1879–
Suggested, with O. Stahl, resection of splanchnic nerves in treatment of hypertension.
Die Chirurgie des vegetativen Nervensystems. Berlin, Springer, 1924

Bruenn, H. G. See R. L. Levy

Bruere, Paul. Maubeuge pharmacist
TEST—for boiled milk.
Comprimés enzymos opiques pour le contrôle rapide des laits pasteurisés. J. Pharm. Chim., Paris, 24: 488–493, Dec. 1906

Bruesch, S. R. See H. A. Davenport

Brugsch, Joachim Theodor. Münich physician. 1909–
TEST—for porphyrin in urine.
Zum qualitative Porphyrinnachweis im Harn (Porphyrinschnellprobe). Münch. med. Wschr., 81: 1546–1547, Oct. 5, 1934

Brugsch, Theodor. German physician. 1878–
TEST—for uric acid in blood.
Methode zum Harnsäurenachweis bei Verwendung geringer Blutmengen. Abstr.: Klin.-therap. Wschr., 21: 427 (only), 1914

Bruhl, I. See G. M. Débove

Brulé, Marcel. French physician. 1883–
TEST—hemokonia t.
Recherches récentes sur les ictères: les rétentions biliaires par l'insuffisance hépatique. Paris, Masson, 1919

Brun, Hippolyte de. French physician
SYMPTOM—
Le point épigastrique dans l'emphysème pulmonaire et dans les cardiopathies. Rev. de Méd., 25: 981–1012, Dec. 1905

Brunn, Albert von. German anatomist. 1849–1895
MEMBRANE—epithelium of olfactory region of nose.
Sinnesorgane. Jena, Fischer, 1897. 109 pp.
NESTS—cell-nests, in ureter.
Ueber drüsenähnliche Bildungen in der Schleimhaut des Nierenbeckens, des Ureters und der Harnblase beim Menschen. Arch. mikr. Anat., 41: 294–302, 1893

Brunn, Fritz. German physician
Treated angina pectoris by paravertebral injection of alcohol.
Die paravertebrale Injektion zur Bekämpfung visceraler Schmerzen with F. Mandl, Wien. klin. Wschr., 37: 511–514, 1924

Brunner, Heinrich. German chemist

REACTION—for atropine.
Beiträge zur Auffindung des Digitalins und Atropins. Ber. dtsch. chem. Ges., 6: 96–98, Feb. 10, 1873

Brunner, Johann Conrad. Swiss anatomist. 1653–1727
GLANDS—in submucous layer of duodenum; discovered by Brunner in 1672, published in 1687.
De glandulis in duodeno intestino detectis. Heidelberg, 1687
Made experimental excision of spleen and pancreas of dog in 1683. Garrison found one dog had extreme thirst and polyuria.
Experimenta nova circa pancreas accedit diatribe de lympha et genuino pancreatis usu. Amstelaedami, apud Wetstenium, 1683. 168 pp.

Bruns, Paul von. German surgeon. 1846–1916
Described plexiform neurofibroma (Rankenneuroma).
Das Rankenneurom, ein Beitrag zur Geschwulstlehre. Tübingen, Laupp, 1870. 68 pp.

Bruns, Victor von. German surgeon. 1812–1883
Pioneer in laryngoscopic surgery and removed a laryngeal polyp by the bloodless method, 1862.
Die erste Ausrortung eines Polypen in der Kehlkopfshöhle durch Zerschneiden ohne blutige Eröffnung der Luftwege, nebst einer kurzen Anleitung zur Laryngoskopie. Tübingen, Laupp u. Siebeck, 1862. 76 pp.
Die Laryngoskopie und die laryngoskopische Chirurgie. Tübingen, Laupp u. Siebeck, 1865

Brunschwig, Alexander. Chicago surgeon. 1901–
OPERATION—
Resection of head of pancreas and duodenum for carcinoma—pancreaticoduodenectomy. S. G. O., 65: 681–684, Nov. 1937
The surgery of pancreatic tumors. St. Louis, Mosby, 1942
One stage pancreaticoduodenectomy. S. G. O., 77: 581–584, Dec. 1943

Brunschwig, Hieronymus. German surgeon. 1450–1533
Wrote first important printed surgical treatise in German. Garrison
Dis ist das Buch der Chirurgia Hautwirckung der Wundartzny von Hyeronimo Brunschwig. Strassburg, (Grüninger), 1497

Brunton, Sir Thomas Lauder. Scottish physician. 1844–1916
Recommended amyl nitrite in treatment of angina pectoris.
On the use of nitrite of amyl in angina pectoris. Lancet, 2: 97–98, July 27, 1867
Also in: F. A. Willius and T. E. Keys, *Cardiac Classics,* pp. 561–564, 1941

Brushfield, T. London physician
DISEASE—
Epiloia with W. Wyatt, Brit. J. Child. Dis., 23: 178–185, July–Sept.; 254–265, Oct.–Dec. 1925

Bruskin, Ya M. Russian surgeon
METHOD—transfusion of placental blood.
(Use of umbilical and placental blood for massive transfusion in surgery.) with P. S. Farberova, Sovet. vrach. zhur., 20: 1546–1554, Oct. 30, 1936
Also, abstr.: J. A. M. A., 107: 2098, Dec. 19, 1936

Bryan, Joseph Hammond. American laryngologist. 1856–1935
Wrote on sinusitis.

Diagnosis and treatment of abscess of the antrum.
J. A. M. A., 13: 478–483, Oct. 5, 1889
A further contribution to the study of suppurative disease of the accessory sinuses, with report of cases.
New York Med. J., 62: 450–456, Oct. 12, 1895

Bryan, W(illiam) Ray. American physiologist. 1905–
Described—
The unusual occurrence of a high incidence of spontaneous mammary tumors in the Albany strain of rats with G. H. Klinck, Jr. and J. M. Wolfe, Amer. J. Cancer, 33: 370–388, July 1938

Bryant, Frank Augustus. New York physician. 1851–
TEST—
Acromium auscultation: a new and delicate test in the early diagnosis of incipient pulmonary tuberculosis.
J. A. M. A., 62: 1635–1636, May 23, 1914

Bryant, Thomas. London surgeon. 1828–1914
FORCEPS—torsion, for hemostasis.
Illustrated in his: *Practice of surgery.* London, Churchill, 1876. 2 ed., p. 406
LINE—vertical side of iliofemoral triangle; also test line for detecting shortening of femur.
Clinical lecture on the diagnostic value of the iliofemoral triangle in cases of injury of the hip-joint, more particularly of impacted fracture. Lancet, 1: 119–120, Jan. 22, 1876
OPERATION—lumbar colotomy.
The operation of colotomy. In his: *Practice of surgery.* London, Churchill, 1876. 2 ed., pp. 680–684
SPLINT—to keep legs and thighs parallel and to obviate necessity for perineal band in treatment of hip disease and hip injuries.
On the value of parallelism of the lower extremities in the treatment of hip disease and hip injuries, with the best means of maintaining it. Lancet, 1: 159–160, Jan. 31, 1880
TRIANGLE—the iliofemoral; see LINE

Bryce, James. Scottish physician
TEST—determination of a degree of immunity against small-pox conferred by vaccination by repeating the inoculation after a lapse of several days; if the first is successful, the second will rapidly overtake it. (Dorland)
Practical observations on the inoculation of cow-pox, pointing out a test of a constitutional affection in those cases in which no fever is perceptible. Edinburgh, Creech, 1802. 236 pp.

Bsteh, O. German surgeon
TECHNIC—of closure of duodenal stump.
Zur Feststellung der Resezierbarkeit eines tiefsitzenden Duodenalulcus. Chirurg., 7: 249–253, Apr. 15, 1935

Buard, Georges Gustav Paul. Bordeaux physician. 1872–
TEST—for indole in bacterial cultures.
Recherche de l'indol dans les cultures microbiennes.
C. R. Soc. Biol., 65: 158–160, July 7, 1908

Bubis, Jacob Louis. Cleveland gynecologist. 1885–
KNIFE—
The Bubis hysterectomy knife. West. J. Surg., 48: 243 (only), Apr. 1940

Buchanan, Andrew. Scottish physician. 1798–1882
Extracted the fibrin ferment of the blood.
On the coagulation of the blood and other fibriniferous liquids. London Med. Gaz., n.s., 1: 617–621, Aug. 1, 1845
Also: Proc. Glasgow Phil. Soc., 2, 1844–48

Buchanan, Robert Earle. Chicago bacteriologist. 1883–
SOLUTION—basal ammonium sulphate.
The gum produced by Bacillus radicicola. Zbl. Bakt., 2 Abt., 22: 371–396 (382; 391), 1909

Buchmann, P. St. Petersburg surgeon
OPERATION—for bony ankylosis of elbow.
Behandlung knöcherner Ellbogengelenksankylosen mittels Überpflanzung von ganzen Gelenken. Zbl. Chir., 19: 582–586, May 9, 1908

Buchner, Hans. German bacteriologist. 1850–1902
ALEXIN—an defensive protein; term is now synonymous with complement.
BODIES—defensive proteins.
THEORY—of immunity of cells of body which has recovered from an infection.
Die Naegei'sche Theorie der Infectionskrankheiten in ihren Beziehungen zur medizinischen Erfahrung. Leipzig, Engelmann, 1877. 112 pp.
Ueber die Disposition verschiedener Menschenrassen gegenüber den Infektionskrankheiten und über Akklimatisation. Hamburg, 1887. 34 pp.
METHOD—for anaerobic cultures.
Ueber die vermeintlichen Sporen der Typhusbacillen. Zbl. Bakt., 4: 353–358; 385–390, 1888
METHOD—of staining spores.
Ueber Cholerabacillen mit Demonstration. Aerztl. Int.-Bl., 31: 549–551, 1884
Discovered bactericidal effect of blood-serum.
Ueber die bakterientödtende Wirkung des zellenfreien Blutserums. Zbl. Bakt., 5: 817–823; 6: 1–11, 1889

Buchwald, Hermann Edmund. German physician. 1903–
ATROPHY—progressive atrophy of skin.
Ueber eigenartige, beim Baden entstehende Hautausschläge. Leipzig, 1929. 15 pp.

Buck, Gurdon. New York surgeon. 1807–1877
EXTENSION—
(Abstract and discussion of paper on new treatment of fractures of the femur.) Bull. New York Acad. Med., 1: 181–188, 1860
An improved method of treating fractures of the thigh. Trans. New York Acad. Med., 2: 232–250, 1861
Also: Med. Classics, 3: 764–782, Apr. 1939
FASCIA—
A new feature in the anatomical structure of the genitourinary organs not hitherto described. Trans. Amer. Med. Ass., 1: 367–371, 1848
Also: Med. Classics, 3: 784–789, Apr. 1939
METHOD—of treating edema of larynx.
On the surgical treatment of morbid growths within the larynx, illustrated by an original case and statistical observations, elucidating their nature and forms. Trans. Amer. Med. Ass., 6: 509–535, 1853
OPERATION—
The knee-joint anchylosed at a right angle—restored nearly to a straight position after the excision of a wedge-shaped portion of bone, consisting of the patella, condyles and articular surface of the tibia. Amer. J. Med. Sci., 10: 277–284, 1845
Also: Med. Classics, 3: 791–800, Apr. 1939
First to tie the primitive and internal carotids simultaneously, 1848. (Garrison)
A case of deep wound of the parotid region, in which a ligature was simultaneously applied to the common and internal carotid arteries. New York Med. Times, 5: 37–42, Nov. 1855

Buckell, G. T. See J. C. Torrey
Buckley, J. Philip. Manchester, England surgeon
OPERATION—for femoral hernia.
A method of treating the sac in the radical cure of femoral hernia. Lancet, 2: 1409–1410, Dec. 19, 1914
Bucknall, Rupert T. H. English surgeon
OPERATION—for hypospadias.
A new operation for penile hypospadias. Lancet, 2: 887–890, Sept. 28, 1907
Buckstein, Jacob. New York roentgenologist. 1890–
AIR INSUFFLATOR—for colonic aerograms.
Clinical roentgenology of the alimentary tract. Philadelphia, Saunders, 1940. 652 pp. p. 384
Bucky, Gustav. German-St. Louis radiologist. 1880–
DIAPHRAGM—used in x-ray work.
A grating-diaphragm to cut off secondary rays from the object. Arch. Roentgen Ray, Lond., 18: 6–9, June 1913
Budd, George. London physician. 1808–1882
DISEASE or CIRRHOSIS—chronic hepatic enlargement without jaundice caused by intestinal intoxication.
JAUNDICE—acute parenchymatous hepatitis; acute yellow atrophy of liver.
On diseases of the liver. London, Churchill, 1845. 401 pp. 2 ed., 1852
Also: in German, Berlin, 1846
Budd, J. W. See V. C. Hunt
Budd, William. English physician. 1811–1880
Established contagiousness of typhoid fever.
On intestinal fever: its mode of propagation. Lancet, 2: 694–695, Dec. 27, 1856
Typhoid fever. London, Longman, 1873
Budge, Albrecht. Greifswald physician. 1846–1885
Injected periosteal lymphatics.
Die Lymphwurzeln der Knochen. Arch. f. mikr. Anat., 13: 87–94, 1876
Budge, Julius Ludwig. German ophthalmologist. 1811–1884
With Waller observed that anterior roots of two lowest cervical and six upper dorsal nerves supplied filaments connected with the certival sympathetic passing to iris; applied term "cilio-spinal region."
Ueber den Einfluss des Nervensystems auf die Bewegung der Iris. Arch. f. physiol. Heilk., 11: 773–826, 1852
Erwiederung auf die Aeusserungen des Herrn Dr. A. Waller. Bonn. Georgi, 1852. 12 pp.
Ueber die Bewegung der Iris. Braunschweig, Vieweg u. Sohn, 1855
Büdinger, Konrad. Vienna surgeon. 1867–
DISEASE—of Büdinger, Ludloff and Laewen; torn cartilage of patella.
Ueber Ablösung von Gelenkteilen und verwandte Prozesse. Dtsch. Z. Chir., 84: 311–365, Oct. 1906
Ueber traumatische Knorpelrisse im Kniegelenk. Ibid., 92: 510–536, Mar. 1908
Bülow, Dr. German physician
TEST—for acetone in urine.
Eine Methode zur quantitativen Bestimmung des Acetons im Harn. Klin. Wschr., 4: 428 (only), 1925
Buerger, Leo. New York physician. 1879–1943
BOUILLON—basal ascitic fluid, for studying fermentation by bacteria.
The differentiation of streptococci by means of fermentative tests. J. exp. Med., 9: 428–435, July 17, 1907

DISEASE—thrombo-angiitis obliterans.
Thrombo-angiitis obliterans: a study of the vascular lesions leading to presenile spontaneous gangrene. Amer. J. Med. Sci., 136: 567–580, Oct. 1908
Is thrombo-angiitis obliterans related to Raynoud's disease and erythromelalgia? Ibid., 139: 105–107, Jan. 1910
Is thrombo-angiitis obliterans an infectious disease? S. G. O., 19: 582–588, Nov. 1914
Circulatory disturbances of the extremities, including gangrene, vasomotor and trophic disorders. Phila., Saunders, 1924. 628 pp. pp. 213–385
EXERCISES—for feet afflicted with Buerger's disease. See DISEASE, 1910
STAINING METHOD—for capsules.
A new method for staining the capsules of bacteria: preliminary communication. Med. News, 85: 1117–1118, Dec. 10, 1904
Observations on the staining of encapsulated bacteria with particular reference to pneumococci and streptococci. J. infect. Dis., 4: 426–433, June 15, 1907
Bürger, Max Theodor Ferdinand. German physician. 1885–
TEST—of circulatory efficiency.
Ueber die klinische Bedeutung des Valsalva'schen Versuches. Münch. med. Wschr., 2: 1066–1067, Aug. 19, 1921
Ueber die Bedeutung des intrapulmonalen Drucks für den Kreislauf und den Mechanismus des Kollapses bei akuten Anstrengungen. Klin. Wschr., 5: 777–780, Apr. 30, 1926
Bürgi, Emil. Swiss pharmacologist. 1872–
THEORY—two different substances causing identical therapeutic manifestations when combined are increased in their effects if they possess identical pharmacological points of attack.
Ueber das Kombinieren von Arzneien. Ann. a. Tomarkin-Found., 1: 67–83, 1931
Bürker, Karl. German physiologist. 1872–
COUNTING-CHAMBER—
Eine neue Form der Zählkammer. Arch. ges. Physiol., 107: 426–451, Apr. 10, 1905
Erfahrungen mid der neuen Zählkammer nebst einer weiteren Verbesserung der selben. Ibid., 118: 460–466, June 25, 1907
METHOD—for estimation of coagulation time of blood.
Ein Apparat zur Ermittelung der Blutgerinnungszeit. Ibid., 118: 452–459, June 25, 1907
Bugbee, E. P. See O. Kamm
Bugbee, Henry Greenwood. New York urologist. 1881–
Reported—
Retention of urine due to congenital hypertrophy of the verumontanum with Martha Wollstein, J. Urol., 10: 477–490, Dec. 1923
Bugie, Elizabeth. See S. A. Waksman
Buhl, Ludwig von. German pathologist. 1816–1880
DISEASE—chronic fatty degeneration of lungs, in consecutive desquamative pneumonia.
Die akute Fett degeneration der Neugeborenen. In: C. von Hecker and L. Buhl: *Klinik der Geburtskunde. Beobachtungen und Untersuchungen aus der Gebäranstalt zu München.* Leipzig, 1861. 2 vols. Vol. 1, p. 296
Lungenentzündung, Tuberculose und Schwindsucht

München, Oldenbourg, 1872. pp. 54
Also, in English: New York, Putnam, 1874. pp. 50
LAW—Buhl-Dittrich's l.; in every case of acute miliary tuberculosis there exists within the body at least one old focus of caseation. Ibid.
PNEUMONIA—desquamative p. Ibid.
Buhlert, Dr. Königsberg i. Pr. physician
SOLUTION—ammonium sulphate.
Zur Methodik der bakteriologischen Bodenuntersuchung with O. Fickendey, Zbl. Bakt., 2 Abt., 16: 399–405, 1906
Buie, Louis Arthur. Rochester, Minn. surgeon. 1890–
HEMORRHOIDECTOMY—
Proctoscopic examination and the treatment of hemorrhoids and anal pruritus. Phila., Saunders, 1931. 178 pp. pp. 96–117
See also F. W. Rankin
Bujwid, Odo. Warsaw bacteriologist
REACTION—for cholera.
Eine chemische Reaction für die Cholerabacterien. Z. Hyg. InfektKr. 2: 52–53, 1887
Bulbulian, A. H. See W. M. Boothby
Bulíř, Jaromír. Prague physician
BROTH—mannitol infusion, for detection of B. coli in water.
Bedeutung und Nachweis des Bacterium coli im Wasser und eine neue Modifikation der Eijkmanschen Methode. Arch. Hyg., Berl., 62: 1–14, 1907
Bulkley, K. See J. A. Blake
Bulkley, Lucius Duncan. Louisville dermatologist. 1845–1928
The first skin specialist in America.
Analysis of one thousand cases of skin-disease, with cases and remarks on treatment. Amer. Pract., Louisville, 1875
Also: Louisville, Morton, 1875. 29 pp.
Described—
On herpes gestationis: a rare affection of the skin, peculiar to pregnancy. Amer. J. Obstet. and Dis. Women and Child., 6: 580–612, Feb. 1874
Bull, Carroll Gideon. New York physician. 1883–1931
METHOD—of immunization of rabbits for production of monovalent immune sera.
The influence of typhoid bacilli on the antibodies of normal and immune rabbits. J. exp. Med., 23: 419–429, Mar. 1, 1916
Buller, Frank. Montreal ophthalmologist. 1844–1905
OPERATION—
Temporary ligation of the canaliculi as a means of preventing wound infections in operations on the eye. Trans. Amer. Ophth. Soc., 9: 633–638, 1902
SHIELD—
A protective bandage for the eye. Lancet, 1: 690 (only), May 16, 1874
Bullis
FEVER—described at Camp Bullis, Texas.
Bullis fever (Long Star fever—tick fever); an endemic disease observed at Brooke General Hospital, Fort Sam Houston, Texas. By J. C. Woodland, M. M. McDowell and J. T. Richards, J. A. M. A., 122: 1156–1160, Aug. 21, 1943
Bulloch, William. English physician. 1868–1941
Outlined relation of adrenal gland to virilism.
On the relation of the suprarenal capsules to the sexual

organs with J. H. Sequeira, Trans. Path. Soc. London, 56: 189–208, 1905
Established immunity of females to hemophilia.
Haemophilia with P. Fildes, London, Dulau & Co., 1911
Bullock, Frederich Dabney. New York physician. 1878–1937
Found sarcoma of liver in rats following ingestion of cysticerus fasciolaris (the larva of the cat tapeworm, Taenia crassicollis).
The experimental production of sarcoma of the liver of rats with M. R. Curtis, Proc. New York Path. Soc., 20: 149–175, Oct.–Dec. 1920
Bullowa, J. G. M. See D. Polowe
Bulmer, Ernest. Birmingham physician
Reported on use of histidine in treatment of peptic ulcer.
The histidine treatment of peptic ulcer with a note on fifty-two cases. Lancet, 2: 1276–1278, Dec. 8, 1934
Bulson, Albert Eugene, Jr. Fort Wayne, Ind. ophthalmologist. 1867–1932
OPERATION—
Correction of iridodialysis by operation. Amer. J. Ophth., 3: 357–358, May 1920
Bumke, Oswald Conrad Edward. German neurologist. 1877–
PUPIL—dilatation of pupil following psychic stimulus; not present in dementia precox.
Die Pupillenstörungen bei Geistes- und Nervenkrankheiten. Jena, Fischer, 1904. 262 pp.
See also J. Morgenroth
Bumm, Ernst von. German gynecologist. 1858–1925
Cultivated gonococcus in pure culture.
Der Mikroorganismus der gonorrhoischen Schleimhaut—Erkrankungen "Gonococcus-Neisser." Dtsch. med. Wschr., 11: 508–509, July 16, 1885
Also: Wiesbaden, Bergmann, 1885
Bumpus, Hermon Carey Jr. Rochester, Minn. urologist. 1888–
RESECTOSCOPE—the Braasch-Bumpus r.
Punch operation for prostatic obstruction. Surg. Clin. N. Amer., 7: 1473–1478, Dec. 1927
Hypertrophy of the prostate gland. In: *Minor surgery of the urinary tract.* Philadelphia, Saunders, 1932 Ch. 4, pp. 41–59
Bunge, Gustav von. German physiologist. 1844–1920
LAW—secreting cells of mammary gland take from the blood plasma mineral salts in exact proportion in which they are needed for developing and building up the offspring.
Der Kali-, Natron- und Chlorgehalt der Milch, verglichen mit dem anderer Nahrungsmittel und des Gesammtorganismus der Säugethiere. Dorpat, Mattiesen, 1874. 41 pp.
METHOD—for determination of hippuric acid.
Ueber die Bildung der Hippursäure with O. Schmiedeberg, Arch. exp. Path. Pharmak., 6: 233–255 (235), Nov. 17, 1876
THEORY—there is a causal relation between alcoholism in a father and inability to suckle a child in his daughter.
Die Alkoholfrage. Basel, Reinhardt, (1886). 44 pp.
Bunge, Rålf. Halle physician. 1906–
STAIN—for flagella.
Zur Kenntnis der geisseltragenden Bakterien. Fort. d. Med., 12: 653–670, Sept. 1, 1894

STAIN—to differentiate tubercle from smegma bacilli.
Smega- und Tuberkelbacil'en with A. Trantenroth,
Ibid., 14: 889–902, Dec. 1; 929–942, Dec. 15, 1896
Buniva, Michele Francesco. Italian physician. 1761–
1834
PHENOMENON—development on revaccination of
typical vaccina at point of reactionless previous in-
sertion of virus.
*Istruzione intorno alla vaccinazione, preceduta da un
discorso storico sulla sua utilita.* Torino, 1804. 160 pp.
Bunker, John Wymond Miller. Michigan scientist.
1886–
SOLUTION—veal infusion polypeptide, for production
of diphtheria toxin.
Studies of the diphtheria bacillus in culture. J. Bact.,
4: 379–407 (404–405), July 1919
Bunnell, Sterling. San Francisco surgeon. 1882–
ANESTHESIA METHOD—
*Positive pressure for thoracic surgery with nitrous
oxid—oxygen anesthesia.* Amer. J. Surg., Anesthesia
suppl., 37: 98–105, Oct. 1923
METHOD—of suture of tendons.
*Repair of tendons in the fingers and description of two
new instruments.* S. G. O., 26: 103–110, Jan. 1918
*Primary repair of severed tendons: the use of stainless
steel wire.* Amer. J. Surg., 47: 502–516, Feb. 1940
OPERATION—
Physiological reconstruction of a thumb after total loss.
S. G. O. 52: 245–248, Feb. 1931
Bunnell, W. W. See J. R. Paul
Bunyan, John. English surgeon
BAG or METHOD—
Envelope method of treating burns. Proc. Roy. Soc.
Med., London, 34: 65–70, 1940
*The treatment of burns and wounds by the envelope
method.* Brit. med. J., 2: 1–7, July 5, 1941
Burchardt, Dr. German physician
Described erythrasma.
Ueber eine bei Chloasma borkommende Pilzform.
Med. Zeitung, 2 F., 2: 141–142, July 20, 1859
Burdach, Karl Friedrich. German neurologist. 1776–
1847
COLUMN—the postero-external c. of spinal cord.
FIBER—nerve fibers connected with Burdach's nu-
cleus.
FISSURE—between lateral surface of insula and inner
surface of operculum.
NUCLEUS—the cuneate n.
OPERCULUM—o. insulae; part of cerebrum above
the insula, or island of Reil.
TRACT—the cuneate fasciculus; a continuation of
the oblongata into the posterior columns of the spinal
cord.
*Beitrag zur Nähernkenntniss des Gehirns in Hinsicht
auf Physiologie Medicin und Chirurgie.* Leipzig,
bei Breitkopf und Harten, 1806
*Anatomische Untersuchungen bezogen auf Natur-
wissenschaft und Heilkunst.* Leipzig, bei Hartmann,
1814
Von Baue und Leben des Gehirns. Leipzig. 3 vols.,
1819, 1822, 1826
Die Physiologie als Erfahrungswissenschaft. Leipzig,
Königsberg, 1826–40. 6 vols.
Burden, V. G. See J. B. Deaver
Burdon-Sanderson, Sir John Scott. English physician. 1828–1905

Made records of heart beat with capillary electrom-
eter.
*On the time-relations of the excitatory process in the
ventricle of the heart of the frog* with F. J. M. Page,
J. Physiol., 2: 384–435, 1879
*On the electrical phenomena of the excitatory process in
the heart of the frog and of the tortoise, as investigated
photographically* with F. J. M. Page, Ibid., 4: 327–
338, 1883
Burger, G. See R. S. Morris
Burget, G. E. See K. H. Martzloff
Burggraeve, Adolphe. French pharmacologist. 1806–
1902
Originator of dosimetric therapy. (Garrison)
Manuel pratique de médecine dosimétrique. Paris,
Chanteaud, 1873. 384 pp.
Burian, Richard. Leipzig physiologist. 1871–
REACTION—for xanthine bases.
*Diazoaminoverbindungen der Imidazole und der
Purinsubstanzen.* Ber. dtsch. chem. Ges., 37: 696–
707, 1904
*Weitere Beiträge zur Kenntnis der Diazoaminover-
bindungen der Purinbasen.* Z. physiol. Chem., 51:
425–437, 1907
See also R. Kolisch
Burke, G. T. See W. J. Stone
Burke, Victor. San Francisco bacteriologist. 1882–
METHOD—
*Notes on the Gram stain with description of a new
method.* J. Bact., 7: 159–182, Mar. 1922
Burkholder, Jacob F. Chicago ophthalmologist
1861–
FASICULUS—f. lateralis minor, from lateral part
of pons.
FASICULUS—f. fusiformis; on dorsal surface of
medulla oblongata.
The anatomy of the brain.... Chicago, Engelhard,
1905. 174 pp.
Burky, Earl LeRoy. Baltimore ophthalmologist
1898–
TOXIN—
*Staphylococcus toxin and antitoxin: experimental and
clinical studies with special reference to ophthalmology*
Internat. Clin., 3: 258–289, Sept. 1936
Burlingham, C. C. See W. D. Shipley
Burn, J. H. See H. H. Dale
Burnam, C. F. See H. A. Kelly
Burnet, Frank MacFarlane. Australian physician
Cultivated influenza virus.
*Propagation of the virus of epidemic influenza on the
developing egg.* Med. J. Australia, Sydney, 2: 687–
689, 1935
Burnett, Sir William. English surgeon. 1779–1861
FLUID—disinfecting; same as solution.
SOLUTION—
Reports on the solution of chloride of zinc.... London,
Clowes, 1857. 28 pp.
Burnham, Walter. American surgeon. 1808–1883
Performed abdominal hysterectomy.
*Extirpation of the uterus and ovaries for sarcomatous
disease.* Nelson's Amer. Lancet, Plattsburgh, N. Y.
7: 147, 1853
Burns, Allan. Scottish anatomist. 1781–1813
SPACE—between layers of deep cervical fascia.
*Observations on the surgical anatomy of the head and
neck.* Edinburgh, Bryce, 1811. 415 pp.

Wrote early work on endocarditis.
Observations on some of the most frequent and important diseases of the heart.... Edinburgh, Bryce, 1809. 322 pp.
Same: 2 ed., 1811
Same: Baltimore, Lucas, 1823. 512 pp.
Described chloroma. Ibid.
Burns, J(onathan) Edward. Kansas City, Mo. urologist. 1883–
OPERATION—
A new operation for exstrophy of the bladder. J. A. M. A., 82: 1587–1590, May 17, 1924
Introduced thorium nitrate.
Thorium—a new agent for pyelography: preliminary report. Ibid., 64: 2126–2127, June 26, 1915
Burow, Karl August von. Königsberg surgeon. 1809–1874
SOLUTION—mild aluminum acetate, for scalp wounds.
Alum, dr. V; lead acetate, oz. i; wasser, oz. viii. Dtsch. Klin., 9: 147–148, Apr. 18, 1857
Burq, V. French neurologist. 1823–1884
Established a system of metallotherapy called burquism.
Métallothérapie. Nouveau traitement par les applications métalliques. Paris, Germer-Baillière, 1853. 48 pp.
Burr, George Oswald. Minneapolis botanist. 1896–
Demonstrated need of body for certain unsaturated fatty acids (vitamin F).
On the nature and role of the fatty acids essential in nutrition with Mildred M. Burr, J. biol. Chem., 86: 587–621, Apr. 1930
Burri, Robert. Swiss bacteriologist. 1867–
STAINING METHOD—of organisms.
Das Tuscheverfahren als einfaches Mittel zur Lösung einiger schwierigen Aufgaben der Bakterioskopie. Jena, Fischer, 1909. 42 pp.
Burrows, M. T. See A. Carrel
Burrows, Waters Field. New York surgeon. 1879–
PACK—
Rectal packing with E. C. Burrows, J. A. M. A., 78: 1293–1294, Apr. 29, 1922
Burton, C. C. See R. L. Ramos
Burton, Henry. London physician. 1799–1849
LINE or SIGN—blue line on gums in lead poisoning.
On a remarkable effect upon the human gums produced by the absorption of lead. Med.-chir. Trans., London, 23: 63–79, 1840
Burton, John. London physician. 1697–1771
Suggested that puerperal fever is contagious.
An essay towards a complete new system of midwifery, theoretical and practical. London, Hodges, 1751
Bury, Judson Sykes. London dermatologist. 1852–
DISEASE—erythema elevatum diutinum.
A case of erythema with remarkable nodular thickening and induration of the skin, associated with intermittent albuminuria. Illust. Med. News, London, 3: 145–148, 1888
Busch, Ch. K. Strassburg physician
MIXTURE—osmic.
Ueber eine Färbungsmethode secundärer Degenerationen des Nervensystems mit Osmiumsäure. Neurol. Zbl., 17: 476 (only), May 15, 1898
Buschke, Abraham. Berlin dermatologist. 1868–
DISEASE—of Busse-Buschke; blastomycosis of skin.
Ueber eine durch Coccidien hervorgerufene Krankheit des Menschen. Dtschr. med. Wschr., Vereinsb., 21:

14 (only), Jan. 17, 1895
Described tonsils as portals of infection.
Die Tonsillen als Eingangspforte für eitererregende Mikroorganismen. Dtsch. Z. Chir., 38: 441–461, 1894
Bush, Francis. English physician
Introduced the stomach-pump.
On the common syringe with a flexible tube, as applicable to the removal of opium and other poisons from the stomach. London Med. and Phys. J., 48: 218–220, Sept. 1822
Busquet, P. French surgeon
DISEASE—exostoses on dorsum of foot due to osteoperiostitis of metatarsal bones.
De l'ostéo-périostite ossifiante des metatarsiens. Rev. d. chir., 17: 1065–1099, Dec. 1897
Busse, Otto. German physician. 1847–1922
DISEASE—of Busse-Buschke; blastomycosis of skin.
Ueber parasitäre Zelleinschlüsse und ihre Züchtung. Dtsch. med. Wschr., Vereinsb., 21: 14 (only), Jan. 17, 1895
Butcher, B. H. Iowa scientist
SOLUTION—basal chinate salt, for differentiating colon-aerogenes group.
Utilization of chinic acid in the differentiation of the colon-aerogenes group. Abst. Bact., 8: 295 (only), Aug. 1924
Butenandt, Adolf Friedrich Johann. Danzig physiologic chemist. 1903–
Prepared hormone progesterone in crystalline form.
Ueber die chemische Untersuchung der Sexualhormone. A. f. ang. Chem., 44: 905–908, Nov. 11, 1931
Neuere Ergebnisse auf dem Gebiet der Sexualhormone. Wien. klin. Wschr., 47: 897–901; 934–936, 1934
Ueber einen Abbanu des Stigmasterins zu corpusluteum-wirksamen Stoffen; ein Beitrag zur Konstitution des Corpus-luteum- Hormons. Ber. dtsch. chem. Ges., 67: 1611–1616, 1934
Ueber die Darstellung des Corpus-luteum Hormons aus Stigmasterin; die Konstitution des Corpus-luteum-Hormons with U. Westphal, Ibid., 2085–2091, Dec. 1934
Synthesized testosteron.
Uber Testosteron. Umwandlung des Dehydro-androsterons in Androstendiol und Testosteron; ein Weg zur Darstellung des Testosterons aus Cholesterin with G. Hanisch, Z. physiol. Chem., 237: 89–97, Nov. 9, 1935
Butler, Allan Macy. Boston pediatrician. 1894–
METHOD—for determination of ascorbic acid.
Distribution of ascorbic acid in the blood and its significance with Margaret Cushman, J. clin. Invest., 19: 459–467, May 1940
See also F. Albright
Butlin, Sir Henry Trentham. London surgeon. 1845–1912
OPERATION—excision of tongue.
A lecture on removal of the contents of the anterior triangle of the neck in cases of malignant diseases of the tongue. Brit. med. J., 1: 285–289, Feb. 11, 1905
Butt, E. M. See A. M. Hoffman
Butt, Hugh Roland. Rochester, Minn. physician. 1910–
Used vitamin K in treatment of hemorrhagic disease.
The use of vitamin K and bile in treatment of the hemorrhagic diathesis in cases of jaundice with A. M.

Snell, Proc. Staff Meet. Mayo. Clin., 13: 74-80, 1938
See also A. M. Snell
Butte, See G. Arthaud
Butzengeiger, Otto. German physician. 1885–
Introduced avertin.
Klinische Erfahrungen mit Avertin (E 107). Dtsch. med. Wschr., 1: 712-713. Apr. 22, 1927
Buxbaum, A. German physician
Demonstrated gall stones by x-ray.
Ueber die Photographie von Gallensteinen in vivo. Wien. med. Pr., 39: col. 534-538, 1898
Buxton, Bertram Henry. New York pathologist
Described two varieties, A and B, of Bacillus paratyphosus.
A comparative study of the bacilli intermediate between B. coli communis and B. typhosus. J. med. Res., 3: 201-230 (228), 1902
See also W. Coleman
Buzaglo, J. H. Amsterdam histologist
STAIN—for connective tissue.
Une coloration pouvant remplacer celle de Van Gieson. Bull. d'Hist. Appl., 11: 40-43, Jan. 1934
Buzby, B(enjamin) Franklin. Camden, N. J. surgeon. 1891–
OPERATION—for slipping patella; a wedge-shaped tibial graft (Albee) is combined with plication.
Recurring external dislocations of the patella. Ann. Surg., 97: 387-393, Mar. 1933
Buzzi, Fausto. Berlin dermatologist

METHOD—of staining eleidin. Mallory
Keratohyalin und Eleidin. Mschr. f. prakt. Dermat., 8: 149-163, 1889
Byford, William Heath. Chicago gynecologist. 1817–1890
TABLE—for gynecologic operations.
(*Dr. Byford's gynaecological table.*) Chicago Med. Rev., 2: 421-422, Sept. 20, 1880
Bylon, David. Dutch physician
Described dengue, 1779.
Korte aantekening wegens eene algemeene ziekte, doorgaans genaamd knokkel-koorts. Verh. v. h. Batav. Genootsch. v. Kunst. en Wetensch., Batavia, 2: 17-30, 1780
Knokkel-koorts. Ibid., 2: 331-340, 1823
Byrne, John. Brooklyn surgeon. 1825–1902
Introduced the cautery knife as a means of removing cancer of cervix.
Clinical notes on the electric cautery in uterine surgery. New York, Wood, 1873. 68 pp.
A digest of twenty year's experience in the treatment of cancer of the uterus by galvanocautery. Boston Med. and Surg. J., 121: 435-436, Oct. 31, 1889
Bywaters, Eric George Lapthorne. English physician
Described crush syndrome.
Crush injuries with impairment of renal function with D. Beall, Brit. med. J., 1: 427-432, Mar. 22, 1941
A case of crush injury with renal failure. By D. Beall, with E. G. L. Bywaters, R. H. R. Belsey and J. A. R. Miles, Ibid., 432-434

C

Cabot, Hugh. Rochester, Minn. urologist. 1872–1945
OPERATION—
Principles of treatment of hypospadias with W. Walters and V. S. Counseller, J. Urol., 33: 400-407, Apr. 1935
The treatment of hypospadias in theory and practice. New Engl. J. Med., 214: 871-876, Apr. 30, 1936
OPERATION—
The management of the incompletely descended testis. South. Surgeon, 4: 331-344, Oct. 1935
TECHNIC—of nephropexy.
In his: *Modern urology.* Philadelphia, Lea and Febiger, 1936. vol. 2, pp. 480-484
Cabot, Richard Clarke. Boston physician. 1868–1939
RING BODIES—in erythrocytes.
Ring bodies (nuclear remnants?) in anemic blood. J. med. Res., 9: 15-18, Feb. 1903
In Oct. 1905, at Massachusetts General Hospital, was first to employ a full-time, paid "social service" worker. (Cushing)
Social service and the art of healing. New York, Moffat et al., 1909. 192 pp.
Reported fatal case of jaundice attributed to cinchophen.
Case records of the Massachusetts General Hospital with H. Cabot, Boston M. & S. J., 192: 1122-1126, June 4, 1925
Cadet, F. fils. See Dupuytren
Cadogen, William. English physician. 1711–1797
Wrote work on pediatrics.
An essay upon nursing, and the management of children. London, Roberts, 1748
Wrote book on gout.
A dissertation on the gout, and all chronic diseases, jointly considered, as proceeding from the same causes;

what those causes are; and a rational and natural method of cure proposed. London, 1771. (8 ed. in 1 year)
Also: reprint of 10 ed., Ann. Med. Hist., 7: 67-90, Mar. 1925
Also: reprint of 10 ed. New York, Hueber, 1925. 114 pp.
Cadwalader, Thomas. American physician. 1708–1779
Described lead colic and lead palsy.
An essay on the West India dry-gripes. . . . to which is added an extraordinary case in physick. Philadelphia, B. Franklin, 1745
Cagniard-Latour, Baron Charles. French scientist. 1777–1859
In 1836 discovered the organic nature of yeast.
Mémoire sur la fermentation vineuse. Ann. Chim. (Phys.), Paris, 68: 206-222, 1838
Cahn, Arnold. German physician
Introduced acetanilide (antifebrine).
Das Antifebrin, ein neues Fiebermittel with P. Hepp, Zbl. klin. Med., 7: 561-564, 1886
Kalle's antifebrin, the new febrifuge with P. Hepp, New York, Merck, 1887. 16 pp.
Caius, John. English physician. 1510–1573
Published famous pamphlet on the sweating sickness.
A boke, or counseill against the disease commonly called the sweate, or sweatyng sicknesse . . . 1552
Also: in C. G. Gruner's *Scriptores de sudore anglico.* 1847. pp. 310-351
Also: fascimile, New York. 1937
Cajal. See Ramon y Cajal
Calandra, Eduardo. Palermo pathologist. 1880–

SOLUTION—picric acid litmus milk; for differentiating between typhoid and colon bacilli.
Differentialdiagnose des Typhusbacillus und des Bacterium coli durch besondere gefärbte Kulturböden. Zbl. Bakt., 54: 567–574, 1910

Calberla, Ernst. Freiburg i/Br physician
LIQUID—for preservation of histologic specimens.
Der Befruchtungsvorgang beim Ei von Petromyzon Planeri. Ein Beitrag zur Kenntniss des Baues und der ersten Entwicklung des befruchten Wirbelthiereies. Z. wiss. Zool., 30: 437–479 (442), Mar. 7, 1878

Caldani, Leopoldo Marco Antonio. Italian anatomist. 1725–1813
LIGAMENT—from coracoid process to clavicle and first rib.
Institutiones anatomicae. Venetiis, Pezzani, 1791. 2 vols.

Caldas, J. See R. dos Santos

Caldwell, Elbert Hayes. American surgeon. 1901–
NUT CRACKERS—
OPERATION—
Fractures of the condyles of the tibia. S. G. O., 63: 518–522, Oct. 1936

Caldwell, Eugene Wilson. American engineer. 1870–1918
APPARATUS—stereofluoroscopic.
A new method of obtaining stereoscopic effects in the fluoroscope. Electrical Rev., N. Y., 39: 601–603, Nov. 16, 1901

Caldwell, George W. New York otolaryngologist. 1866–
OPERATION—of Caldwell-Luc.
Diseases of the accessory sinuses of the nose, and an improved method of treatment of suppuration of the maxillary antrum. New York Med. J., 58: 526–528, Nov. 4, 1893

Caldwell, William Edgar. New York obstetrician. 1880–
CLASSIFICATION—of female pelves.
Anatomical variations in the female pelvis and their effect in labor with a suggested classification with H. C. Moloy, Amer. J. Obstet. Gynaec., 26: 479–505, Oct. 1933
PLATES—Caldwell-Moloy x-ray p.
The use of the Roentgen ray in obstetrics. Part I. Roentgen pelvimetry and cephalometry; technique of pelvioroentgenography with H. C. Moloy and P. C. Swenson. Amer. J. Roent. and Rad. Therap., 41: 305–316, Mar. 1939

Callander, C. Latimer. San Francisco surgeon. 1892–1947
AMPUTATION—
A new amputation in the lower third of the thigh. J. A. M. A., 105: 1746–1753, Nov. 30, 1935
Tendoplastic amputation through the femur at the knee; further studies. Ibid., 110: 113–118, Jan. 8, 1938
See also E. I. Bartlett

Callander, L. Dougal. English physician
TOURNIQUET—
Tourniquet for all purposes. Lancet, 1: 1166 (only), June 29, 1940

Callaway, Thomas. English physician. 1791–1848
TEST—for dislocation of humerus; circumference of shoulder through axilla and over acromium is greater on affected side.
A dissertation upon dislocations and fractures of the

clavicle and shoulder-joint. London, Highley, 1849; 178 pp.
(Jacksonian essay for 1846)

Callisen, Hendrik. Danish surgeon. 1740–1824
OPERATION—lumbar colotomy by a vertical incision
Grundsätze der heutigen Chirurgie. Wien, Hörling, 1786–92. 3 vols.

Calman, Arthur Samuel. New York surgeon. 1883–
METHOD—
Submucous hemorrhoidectomy. Amer. J. Surg., 44: 577–580, June 1939
The submucous method in the treatment of anorectal diseases. Ibid., 53: 428–433, Sept. 1941

Calmeil, Louis Florentin. French physician. 1798–1895
Described general paralysis of insane.
De la paralysie considérée chez les aliénes. Paris, Baillière, 1826

Calmette, Léon Charles Albert. Lille, France bacteriologist. 1863–1933
REACTION or TEST—ophthalmic r.
Sur un nouveau procédé de diagnostic de la tuberculose chez l'homme par l'ophthalmo-réaction a la tuberculine. C. R. Acad. Sci., Paris, 144: 1324–1326, June 17, 1907
Un nouveau procédé de diagnostic de la tuberculose chez l'homme. Pr. méd., 49: 388–389, June 19, 1907
SERUM—antivenomcus s.
Contribution à l'étude du venin des serpents; immunisation des animaux et traitement de l'envenimation. Ann. Inst. Pasteur, 8: 275–291, May 1894
Contribution a l'étude des venins, des toxines et des sérums antitoxiques. Ibid., 9: 225–251, Apr. 1895
Le vénin des serpents. Soc. d'éd. scient., Paris, 1896
Sur le mécanisme de l'immunisation contre les venins. Ann. Inst. Pasteur, 12: 343–347, May 1898
Les venins, les animaux venimeux et la sérothérapie antivenimeuse. Paris, Masson, 1907. 396 pp.
SOLUTION—basal peptone salt, for cultivation of tubercle bacilli.
Milieux de culture pour le bacille tuberculeux with L. Massol and M. Breton, C. R. Soc. Biol., 67: 580–583, Nov. 27, 1909
TUBERCULIN—see REACTION or TEST
L'infection bacillaire et la tuberculose chez l'homme et chez les animaux. Paris, Masson, 1920
Also, in English: Baltimore, Williams and Wilkins, 1923
Developed preventive treatment for children against tuberculosis, with non-virulent culture B C G (Bacillus Calmette-Guerin).
Sur la vaccination préventive des enfants nouveau-nés contre la tuberculose par le B C G. Ann. Inst. Pasteur, 41: 201–232, Mar. 1927

Calori, Luigi. Italian anatomist. 1807–1896
BURSA—between trachea and arch of aorta.
Sulle borse mucose sottocutanee del corpo umano; annotazioni anatomiche. Mem. Accad. d. sc. d. Ist. di Bologna, 8, 1857

Calot, Jean Francois. French surgeon. 1861–
OPERATION or TREATMENT—for scoliosis.
Note sur la correction opératoire des scolioses graves. Paris, Masson, 1897 (?). 5 pp.
Note sur quelques modifications apportées à la technique du redressement des maux de Pott. Paris, Masson, 1897 (?)

Die Behandlung der tuberkulosen Wirbelssaulenent-zuudung. Stuttgart, 1907

Calvé, Jacques. French surgeon. 1875–
DISEASE—Calvé-Perthe's d. or osteochondritis deformans juvenalis coxae.
Sur une forme particulière de pseudocoxalgie greffée sur des deformations caractéristiques de l'extremité superieure du fémur. Rev. Chir., 62: 54–84, July 1910
Described osteochondritis of vertebral body.
Sur une affection particulière de la colonne vertébrale chez l'enfant simulant le mal de Pott: ostéo-chondrite vertébrale infantile? J. radiol. et d'électro., 9: 22–27. Jan. 1925
A localized affection of the spine suggesting osteochondritis of the vertebral body, with the clinical aspect of Pott s disease. J. Bone & Joint Surg., 7: 41–46, Jan. 1925

Calvert, Edwin G. B. London physician
METHOD—for determination of blood sugar.
Diagnosis and treatment of diabetes mellitus in hospital and general practice. Lancet, 1: 1310–1314, June 28; 2: 14–18, July 5, 1924

Camara, Pedro de la. Madrid physician
MODIFICATION—of von Domarus' fluid for blood cell counting.
Investigaciones sobre la sangre "in vitro" . . . with J. G. Alvarez, Arch. cardiol. y hemat., 13: 315–334, Aug. 1932

Camerer, John Friedrich Wilhelm. German physician. 1842–1910
LAW—children of the same weight have same food requirements regardless of their ages.
Children's growth in weight and height. In: Pfaundler and Schlossmann's *Diseases of children.* English transl. by S. Amberg.
Phila. and London, 1: 409–424, 1908

Cameron, Donald F. American surgeon
Advocated use of sodium iodid for pyelogram.
Aqueous solutions of potassium and sodium iodids as opaque mediums in roentgenography: preliminary report. J. A. M. A., 70: 754–755, Mar. 16, 1918
Sodium and potassium iodids in roentgenography with C. C. Grandy, Ibid., 1516–1517, Mar. 25, 1918

Camitz, Helge Georg. Gothenburg surgeon. 1883–
OPERATION—for fracture of neck of femur.
Die Pseudoarthrosen (nebst wahrscheinlichen Vorstadien) nach medialen Frakturen des Collum femoris und deren Behandlung. Acta. chir. scand., 68, suppl. 19, 1931. 108 pp.

Cammidge, Percy John. English physician. 1872–
REACTION or TEST—pancreatic r., for ascertaining presence of pancreatitis or malignant disease of pancreas.
The chemistry of the urine in diseases of the pancreas. Lancet, 1: 782–787, Mar. 19, 1904
Also, abstr.: Brit. med. J., 1: 776–778, Apr. 2, 1904

Camp, J. D. See E. V. N. Allen

Campbell, A. W. See H. Head

Campbell, Henry Fraser. American physician. 1824–1891
THEORY—of secretion.
Essays on the secretory and the excito-secretory system of nerves. Philadelphia, Lippincott, 1857

Campbell, John Robert, Jr. Boston physician. 1898–
TREATMENT—
The treatment of diabetes insipidus with pituitary posterior lobe extract applied intranasally with H. L.

Blumgart, Amer. J. med. Sci., 176: 769–782, Dec 1928

Campbell, K. N. See F. A. Coller

Campbell, Walter Ruggles. Toronto physician. 1890–
METHOD—for determination of fractional plasma proteins.
Sulfites as protein precipitants with Marion I. Hanna J. biol. Chem., 119: 9–14, June 1937
See also G. W. Howland

Campbell, Willis Cohoon. Memphis, Tenn. orthopedist. 1880–1941
OPERATION—
An operation for the correction of "drop-foot." J Bone and Joint Surg., 5: 815–825, Oct. 1923
End-results of operation for correction of drop-foot J. A. M. A., 85: 1927–1931, Dec. 19, 1925
OPERATION—for fusion of ankle.
Reconstruction of ankylosed joints: with special reference to the after treatment. Med. J. and Rec., 122: 255–260, Sept. 2, 1925
OPERATION—
Malunited Colles' fractures. J. A. M. A., 109: 1105–1108, Oct. 2, 1937
OPERATION—
An operation for extra-articular fusion of the sacroiliac joint. S. G. O., 45: 218–219, Aug. 1927
Also: *Operative orthopedics.* St. Louis, Mosby, 1939

Camper, Petrus. Dutch physician. 1722–1789
ANGLE—facial a.; indicates slope of forehead and is a criterion of race.
ANGLE—maxillary a.
CHIASM—c. tendinum; passing of tendons of flexor digitorum profundus through tendons of flexor digitorum sublimis.
LIGAMENT—deep perineal fascia.
LINE—from external auditory meatus to point just below nasal spine.
Demonstrationum anatomico-pathologicarum libri ii. Amsteloedami, Schreuder et Mortier, 1760–62
Sämmtliche kleinere Schriften. Leipzig, Crusius, 1784–90. 3 vols. Same, in French, 1803
FASCIA—superficial layer of superficial fascia over lower portion of abdomen. Discovered processus vaginalis of peritoneum. (Garrison)
Icones herniarum. ed. a Sam. Thom. Soemmering Frankfort, Varrentrapp et Wenner, 1801. 16 pp.
Discovered fibrous structure of lens.
Dissertation de visu. Lugd. Bat., 1746

Campos, Moise. Paris ophthalmologist. 1872–
LIGAMENT OF—cordiform.
La portion réfléchie de la membrane hyaloïde. Arch. d'Ophthal., 18: 748–753, Dec. 1898

Campos, Oswaldo Pinherio. Rio de Janeiro surgeon. 1900–
OPERATION—
Acromioclavicular dislocation. Amer. J. Surg., 43: 287–291, Feb. 1939

Cannas. Italian ophthalmologist
OPERATION—for ptosis.
Una modificazione al processo operativo della ptosi. XVI. Cong. dell'assoc. oftalm. ital. Ann. di Ottalm e Lavori della clin. Oculistica di Napoli, 31: 772, 1902
Reference of four lines in Jahresb. f. Ophth., p. 357, 1902

Cannon, R. Keith. London physiologist

METHOD—
Estimation of alcohol in blood with R. Sulzer, Heart,
11: 148-150, Apr. 5, 1924
Cannon, Walter Bradford. Boston physiologist.
1871-1945
METHOD—for determination of coagulation time.
*Factors affecting the coagulation time of blood. I. The
graphic method of recording coagulation used in these
experiments* with W. L. Mendenhall, Amer. J.
Physiol., 34: 225-231, May 1, 1914
POINT or RING—tonic contraction ring often visible
in right half of transverse colon.
*The movements of the intestines studied by means of the
röntgen rays.* Ibid., 6: 251-277, Jan. 1, 1902
THEORY—of sympathin formation of sympathetic
stimulation.
Emotional stimulation of adrenal secretion with D.
de la Paz, Amer. J. Physiol., 28: 64-70, Apr. 1,
1911
*Studies on the conditions of activity in endocrine organs.
XXVI. A hormone produced by sympathetic action on
smooth muscle* with Z. M. Bacq, Ibid., 96: 392-412,
Feb. 1, 1931
*Studies on conditions of activity in endocrine organs.
XXIX. Sympathin E and sympathin I.* with A.
Rosenblueth, Ibid., 104: 557-574, June 1, 1933
Observed movements of stomach and intestines by
means of roentgen rays.
*The movements of the stomach studied by means of the
röntgen ray.* Amer. J. Physiol., 1: Proc. xiii-xiv, 1898
Also: Ibid., 1: 359-382, May 1, 1898
*The movements of the intestines studied by means of
the röntgen rays.* Ibid., 6: 251-277, Jan. 1, 1902
Produced exophthalmic goiter experimentally.
Experimental hyperthyroidism with C. A. L. Binger
and R. Fitz. Ibid., 36: 363-364, Mar. 1, 1915
Demonstrated that cats enraged by dogs respond
with an increased output of epinephrine, a rise in
blood sugar and an elevation in blood pressure.
Bodily changes in fear, hunger, pain and rage. New
York, Appleton, 1915. 2 ed., 1929
See also O. K. O. Folin
Canstatt, Carl Friedrich. German physician. 1807-
1850
Wrote on geriatrics.
Die Krankheiten des höheren Alters und ihre Heilung.
Erlangen, Enke, 1839. 2 vols.
Cantani, Arnoldo. Italian physician. 1837-1893
DIET—of meat for diabetes.
Diabete mellito. Tratt. ital. di patol. e terap. med.,
Milano, 4: 115-224, n.d.
Also, in French. Paris, Delahage, 1876
Also: *Der diabetes mellitus.* Trans. by S. Hahn,
Berlin, 1877
SERUM—for injection in infectious diseases.
Sulle infezioni miste. Napoli, Sangiovanni, 1903,
223 pp.
TREATMENT—of cholera by repeated injection into
bowel of large quantity of water containing tannic
acid and tincture of opium. (Dorland)
*L'enteroclisi tannica calda come cura abortiva del
cholera e l'ipodermoclisi al principio dello stadio
algido del cholera.* Napoli, Detken, 1884. 20 pp.
Cantani, Arnoldo, Jr. Naples physician
AGAR—sperm; culture medium.
Zur Verwendung des Sperma als Nährbodenzusatze.
Zbl. Bakt., 22: 601-604, Dec. 7, 1897

BOUILLON—basal ascitic fluid; culture medium.
*Ueber eine praktisch sehr gut verwendbare Methode,
albuminhaltige Nährböden für Bakterien zu bereiten.*
Ibid., 53: 471-473, 1910
Cantor, Meyer O. Detroit surgeon. 1907-
TUBE—
New simplified intestinal decompression tube. Amer.
J. Surg., 72: 137-142, July 1946
*Use and abuse of intestinal decompression tube: a
study based upon two hundred cases* with C. S. Ken-
nedy and R. P. Reynolds, Ibid., 73: 437-449, Apr.
1947
Cantwell, Frank V. Trenton surgeon. 1862-1910
OPERATION—for epispadias.
*Operative treatment of epispadias by transplantation of
the urethra.* Ann. Surg., 22: 689-694, Dec. 1895
Capaldi, Achille. Naples physician
BOUILLON—egg yolk, for cultivation of tubercle
bacilli.
Zur Verwendung des Eidotters als Nährbodenzusatz.
Zbl. Bakt., 20: 800-803, Nov. 28, 1896
MEDIUM—for colon-typhoid differentiation.
Ein weiterer Beitrag zur Typhusdiagnose. Z. Hyg.
InfektKr., 23: 475-476, 1896
SOLUTION—basal mannitol salt, for studying acid
production by B. coli.
*Beiträge zur Kenntniss der Säurebildung bei Typhus-
bacillen und Bakterium coli. Eine differential-diagnos-
tische Studie* with B. Proskauer, Ibid., 452-474 (456),
1896
Capek, A. German physician
Reported trichomonas urethritis.
*Die Flagellaten-Urethritis des Mannes; vorläufige
Mitteilung.* Med. Klin., 23: 1535-1539, Oct. 7, 1927
Cappelen, Axel. Norwegian surgeon. ?-1919
Sutured stab wound in heart in 1895. (D. H. Wil-
liams in 1893 sutured wound of pericardium; E. C.
Cutler)
Valvus cordis; sutur of hjertet. Norsk. mag. f. haege-
vidensk, 11: 285-288, Sept. 4, 1896
Capps, Joseph Almarin. Chicago physician. 1872-
Introduced blood volume studies (Blix, "haemato-
krit") to America.
*A study of volume index. Observations upon the volume
of erythrocytes in various disease conditions.* J. med.
Res., 10: 367-401, Dec. 1903
Studied peritoneal sensitivity.
*Experimental observations on the localization of the
pain sense in the parietal and diaphragmatic perito-
neum* with G. H. Coleman, Arch. intern. Med., 30:
778-789, Dec. 1922
REFLEX or SIGN—pain in shoulder with pleurisy.
*An experimental and clinical study of pain in the
pleura, pericardium and peritoneum.* New York,
Macmillan, 1932. 99 pp.
Capuron, Joseph. French physician. 1767-1850
POINTS—the iliopectineal eminences and the sacro-
iliac joints.
Cours théorique et pratique d'accouchemens. . . . Paris,
1811. 728 pp.
Carabba, Victor. New York surgeon. 1898-
METHOD—
Gastrostomy: a clamp method. Amer. J. Surg., 27:
484-486, Mar. 1935
SOLUTION—sclerosing.
Sclerosing injections in surgery. Ann. Surg., 99: 668-
675, Apr. 1934

Carabelli, George C. Vienna dentist. 1787–1842
TUBERCLE—on lingual surface of a molar tooth.
Systemetisches Handbuch der Zahnheilkunde. Wien,
Braumüller und Seidel, 1844

Carco, P. See S. Citelli

Cardan, Gerolamo. French physician. 1501–1576
Most celebrated physician of his time. (Garrison and
Morton)
*Metaposcopia, libris xiii et octingentis faciei humanae
eiconibus complexa.* Parisiis, apud T. Jolly, 1658
(Written in 1550)

Carden, Henry Douglas. English surgeon. ?–1872
AMPUTATION—through femoral condyles, with
single flap.
On amputation by single flap. Brit. med. J., 1: 416–421,
Apr. 16, 1864
Also: London, Richards, 1864. 25 pp.

Carey, Mathew. Philadelphia physician. 1760–1839
Described yellow fever.
*A short account of the malignant fever, lately prevalent
in Philadelphia.* Philadelphia, the author, 1793

Cargile, Charles Hastings. Bentonville, Ark. surgeon.
1853–
MEMBRANE—prepared ox peritoneum.
*A report on experiments made with Cargile membrane,
for the purpose of determining its value in preventing
the formation of peritoneal adhesions* with R. T.
Morris, Med. Rec., 61: 773–775, May 17, 1902;
note, Ibid., 717, May 3

Carle, Antonio. Italian physician. 1854–1927
Demonstrated transmissibility of tetanus.
Studio esperimentale sull'eziologia del tetano with G.
Rattone. Giorn. R. Accad. Med. di Torino, 3 s., 32:
174–180, 1884

Carleton, Harry Montgomerie. Oxford scientist
MODIFICATION—
*Note on Cajal's formalin-silver nitrate impregnation
method for the Golgi apparatus.* J. R. micr. Soc., 42:
321–328, Dec. 1919

Carlson, Anton Julius. American physiologist. 1875–
Recorded stomach movements by means of a balloon
inserted through a gastric fistula; studied physiology
of stomach.
Contributions to the physiology of the stomach. Amer.
J. Physiol., 31: 151–168, Dec. 2, 1912; 175–192,
Jan. 1; 212–222, Jan. 1; 318–327, Feb. 1; 32: 245–
263, Sept. 2, 1913

Carlson, W. E. See Chastek

Carman, Russell Daniel. American physician. 1875–
1926
SIGN—of carcinoma of stomach; loss of pliability of
stomach wall by fluoroscopy.
*The roentgen diagnosis of diseases of the alimentary
canal* with A. Miller, Philadelphia, Saunders, 1917.
558 pp. pp. 190–191

Carnochan, John Murray. American surgeon. 1817–
1887
OPERATION—ligation of carotids on both sides for
elephantiasis.
*Case of elephantiasis graecorum, treated by ligature of
the common carotid artery on both sides.* Amer. J.
med. Sci., 54: 109–115, July 1867
OPERATION—removal of Meckel's ganglion and
most of fifth nerve for neuralgia.
*Excision of the trunk of the second branch of the fifth
pair of nerves, beyond the ganglion of Meckel, for*

severe neuralgia of the face: with three cases. Ibid., 35:
134–143, Jan. 1858

Carnot, Nicolas Léonard Sadi. French scientist.
1796–1832
THEOREMS—thermodynamic.
*Réflexions sur la puissance motrice du feu et sur les
machines propres à développer cette puissance.* Paris,
Bachelier, 1824
Also, transl. by W. F. Magie In: *Harper's Scientific
memoirs.* New York, 1899. vol. 6
Also, transl. by W. Ostwald In: Ostwald's *Klassiker
der exakten Wissenschaften.* Leipzig, 1892. No. 37

Carnot, Paul. French physician. 1869–
TEST—for atonic dilatation of stomach.
Sur le passage pylorique des solutions de glucose with
A. Chassevant, C. R. Soc. Biol., 58: 1069–1072,
June 24, 1905
*Des modifications subies, dans l'estomac et le duo-
dénum, par les solutions acides ingérées* with
A. Chassevant, Ibid., 59: 106–109, July 8, 1905

Carnoy, Jean Baptiste. Louvain biologist. 1836–1899
FLUID or SOLUTION—a sclerosing f.; Carnoy-
Cutler s.; alcohol, 6 vols., acetic acid, 1 vol., chloro-
form 3 vols.
Les globules polaires de l'ascaris clavata. La Cellule,
3: 247–324, (276), 1887

Carpano, Matteo. Rome veterinarian
AGAR—hemolyzed blood; for cultivation of gonococci.
*Su un terreno molto adatto per l'isolamento e le ordinarie
culture del "Micrococcus gonorrhoeae" (Neisser).* Ann.
Igiene (sper.), Roma, 29: 599–603, Sept. 30, 1919

Carpenter, Charles Milton. American scientist.
1895–
Suggested and aided in developing the radiotherm.
The production of fever in man by short radio waves
with A. B. Page, Science, 71: 450–452, May 2, 1930
See also Alice D. Leahy

Carpenter, Thorne Martin. Boston scientist. 1878–
METHOD—for determination of respiratory quotient.
*A comparison of methods for determining the respir-
atory exchange of man.* Washington, Carnegie Inst.,
Publ. No. 216, 1915. 265 pp.
*The Carpenter form of the Haldane gas analysis ap-
paratus. Changes made in the apparatus and details
regarding its use.* J. biol. Chem., 83: 211–230, July
1929
Studied metabolism in women before and after
childbirth.
*The energy metabolism of mother and child just before
and just after birth* with J. R. Murlin, Arch. intern.
Med., 7: 184–222, Feb. 15, 1911

Carpue, Joseph Constantine. English surgeon.
1764–1846
OPERATION—the Indian method of rhinoplasty.
*An account of two successful operations for restoring a
lost nose from the integuments of the forehead, in the
cases of two officers of His Majesty's Army: to which
are prefixed historical and physiological remarks on the
nasal operation; including descriptions of the Indian
and Italian methods.* London, Longman, 1816
Wrote pioneer work on electrotherapy.
An instruction to electricity and galvanism. London,
Phillips, 1803
Wrote on lithotomy.
*A history of the high operation for the stone, by inci-
sion above the pubis: with observations on the advantages attending it, and an account of the various methods*

of lithotomy from the earliest periods to the present time. London, Longman, 1819

Carr, Francis Howard. London physician. 1874–

TEST—for vitamin A deficiency.

Colour reactions attributed to vitamin A with E. A. Price, Biochem. J., 20: 497–501, 1926

See also G. Barger

Carrasquilla, Juan De Dios. Bogotá physician

SERUM—an antileprous s. (of little therapeutic value).

Tercera comunicacion sobre un procedimento serotápico aplicado al tratamiento de la lepra griega. Bogotá, 1896. 19 pp.

Carrel, Alexis. French-American surgeon. 1873–1944

Awarded Nobel prize in 1912.

CURVE OF CICATRIZATION—calculated or ideal.

The treatment of wounds; a first article. J. A. M. A., 55: 2148–2150, Dec. 17, 1910

Cicatrization of wounds. I. The relation between the size of a wound and the rate of its cicatrization with Alice Hartman, J. exp. Med., 24: 429–450, Nov. 1, 1916

Cicatrization of wounds. XIII. Factors initiating regeneration. Ibid., 34: 425–432, Nov. 1, 1921

FLUID—Carrel-Dakin f. used in treatment of wounds. See METHOD (2).

METHOD—of end-to-end suture of blood vessels.

La technique opératoire des anastomoses vasculaires et la transplantation des viscères. Lyon méd., 98: 859–864, 1902

The surgery of blood vessels, etc. Johns Hopk. Hosp. Bull., 18: 18–28, Jan. 1907

Results of the transplantation of blood vessels, organs and limbs. J. A. M. A., 51: 1662–1667, Nov. 14, 1908

METHOD—Carrel-Dakin treatment of wounds.

Traitement abortif de l'infection des plaies with Dakin, Daufresne, Dehelly and Dumas, Bull. Acad. Méd. Paris, 74: 361–368, Oct. 5, 1915

Fermeture secondaire des plaies de guerre with Dehelly and Dumas, Ibid., 75: 32–40, Jan. 11, 1916

Le traitement des plaies infectées with G. Dehelly, Paris, Masson, 1917. 177 pp.

Also, English transl. by A. A. Bowlby, New York, Hoeber, 1917. 238 pp.

METHOD—of intradermal injection against small-pox.

La fabrication du vaccin in vitro with T. H. Rivers, C. R. Soc. Biol., 96: 848–850, 1927

PLASMA—for cultivation of tissue.

Cultures de sarcome en dehors de l'organisme with M. T. Burrows, C. R. Soc. Biol., Paris, 69: 332–334, Nov. 5, 1910

Cultivation of tissues in vitro and its technique with M. T. Burrows, J. exp. Med., 13: 387–396, Mar. 1, 1911

SOLUTION—Locke's s. with agar.

An addition to the technique of the cultivation of tissues in vitro with M. T. Burrows, Ibid., 14: 244–247, Sept. 1, 1911

See also C. Beck

Carrell, William Beall. Dallas, Texas surgeon. 1883–

OPERATION—

Habitual dislocation of the shoulder. J. A. M. A., 89: 948–952, Sept. 17, 1927

Carrez, Cyrille. French physician

REAGENT—for glucose.

Les réactifs cuivriques et le dosage des sucres; réactif

cupro-lactique. Repert. de Pharm., 21: 193–199, May 10, 1909

Carrington, G. L. See F. P. Underhill

Carrion, Daniel A. Peru student. 1850–1885

DISEASE—verrugo peruana, related to Oroya fever; named for a young student who lost his life after a voluntary inoculation.

Concurso sobre Veruga peruana. Monit. méd., Lima, 1: 161–163, Oct. 1, 1885

La verruga peruana y Daniel A. Carrion, estudiante de la Facultad de medicine, muerto el 5 de octubre de 1885. Lima, Estado, 1886. 109 pp.

La erupcion en la enfermedad de Carrion (verruga peruana). By E. Odriozola, Monit. méd., Lima, 10: 309–311, 1895

Also, in French, 1898

Carroll, J. See W. Reed

Carson, James. English physician. 1772–1843

Suggested artificial pneumothorax for pulmonary tuberculosis, in 1821.

Essays, physiological and practical. Liverpool, Wright, 1822

An inquiry into the causes of respiration; of the motion of the blood; animal heat; absorption; and muscular motion; with practical inferences. London, Longman et al., 1833. 2 ed.

Carson, Norman Bruce. St. Louis surgeon. 1844–1931

OPERATION—

Diaphragmatic hernia diagnosed before operation with L. Huelsmann, Interstate M. J., 19: 315–327, Apr. 1912

Carter, Burr Noland. Cincinnati surgeon. 1895–

METHOD—of dividing adhesions containing lung tissue.

Intrapleural pneumolysis. Amer. Rev. Tuber., 24: 199–212, Sept. 1931

OPERATION—

The use of muscle flaps in the closure of chronic empyema cavities. Surgery, 3: 506–517, Apr. 1938

TECHNIC—

Reaction of a portion of the thoracic esophagus for carcinoma: a report of two cases. S. G. O., 71: 624–632, Nov. 1940

Carter, Cyril William. English biochemist

Discovered vitamin B5.

Maintenance nutrition in the adult pigeon, and its relation to torulin (vitamin B1) with H. W. Kinnersley and R. A. Peters, Biochem. J., 24: 1832–1851, 1930

Carter, Henry Rose. American physician. 1852–1925

Determined incubation period of yellow fever and influenced Reed's later researches. (Garrison and Morton)

A note on the interval between infecting and secondary cases of yellow fever from the records of yellow fever at Orwood and Taylor, Miss. in 1898. New Orleans Med. and Surg. J., 52: 617–636, May 1900

Carter, Henry Vandyke.

SPIROCHAETA CARTERI—spirillum minus, a species from the relapsing fever of India.

Note on the occurrence of a minute blood-spirillum in an Indian rat. Sci. Mem. Med. Off. Army of India, 1887, Calcutta, 3: 45–48, 1888

Carter, J. B. See A. B. Luckhardt

Cartland, George F. Kalamazoo, Mich. scientist. 1902–

UNITS—of gonadotropic substance.
The preparation and purification of extracts containing the gonad-stimulating hormone of pregnant mare serum with J. W. Nelson, J. biol. Chem., 119: 59–67, June 1937

Carus, Carl Gustav. German obstetrician. 1789–1869
CURVE OF—the normal axis of the pelvic outlet.
Lehrbuch der Gynäkologie. . . . Leipzig, Fleischer, 1820. 2 vols.

Carwardine, Thomas. English surgeon
OPERATION—
Excision of the rectum for cancer by a new method, and its results. Brit. med. J., 2: 1190–1193, Oct. 28, 1899

Cary, Charles Aaron. American scientist. 1880–
TEST—for amino acids in blood.
Amino-acids of the blood as the precursors of milk proteins. J. biol. Chem., 43: 477–489, Sept. 1920

Cary, William Hollenback. Brooklyn gynecologist. 1883–
Used x-ray visualization of the uterine cavity.
Note on determination of patency of fallopian tubes by the use of collargol and x-ray shadow. Amer. J. Obstet., 64: 462-464, Mar. 1914

Casal, Gaspar. Spanish physician. 1679–1759
Wrote original description of pellagra in 1735; not published until 1762.
Historia natural, y medica de el Principado de Asturias. Madrid, Martin, 1762. pp. 327–360
Also, reprint pub. by Oviedo, 1900

Casares-Gil, M. See Gil
Casey, Albert Eugene. New York pathologist. 1903–
METHOD—of counting blood platelets.
An accurate and practical method for blood platelet counting with A. M. Helmer, Proc. Soc. exp Biol., N. Y., 27: 655–656, Apr. 1930
Further note on the enumeration of blood platelets and red blood cells. Ibid., 28: 523–524, Feb. 1931

Casoni, Tommaso. Italian physician
TEST—for hydatids.
La diagnosi biologica dell'echinoccosi umana mediante l'intradermcreazione. Folia clin., chim. et micro., 4: 5–16, 1912

Caspari, Wilhelm. Frankfurt a M. physician. 1872–
DIET—restricted, eliminating vitamin B, in treatment of malignancy.
Erwiderung auf die Ausführungen von Herrn de Raadt über die Ernährung der Krebskranken. Strahlentherapie, 42: 803–808, Nov. 14, 1931

Casper, Leopold. Berlin physician. 1859–
TEST—phlorrhizin, for permeability of kidney.
Ueber functionelle Nierendiagnostik with P. F. Richter, Berl. klin. Wschr., 37: 643-644, July 16, 1900

Cass, J. W. See J. V. Meigs
Cassel. See F. Wild
Casselberry, William Evans. Chicago laryngologist. 1859–1916
POSITION—
A new method of feeding in cases of intubation of the larynx by position, head downward, on an inclined plane. Chicago Med. J. and Exam., 57: 201–203, Oct. 1888

Casserius, Julius. Italian anatomist. 1556–1616
ARTERY—internal carotid and middle meningeal.
FONTANEL—at junction of temporal, parietal and occipital bones.

NERVE—perforating or musculo-cutaneous.
PERFORATED MUSCLE OF—coraco-brachialis.
Tabulae anatomicae LXXVIII. Venetiis, 1627
MUSCLE—laxator tympani minor; anterior ligament of malleus.
De vocis auditusque organis historia anatomica. Ferrariae, typ. Cameralis, 1600–01. 2 pts.

Castaigne, Joseph. French physician. 1871–
TEST—methylene blue t. of toxopexic function of liver.
Valeur séméiologique de l'épreuve par le bleu de méthylène chez les hépatiques. By H. Chauffard et J. Castaigne, Pr. méd., p. 170 (only), Apr. 24, 1898
See also E. C. Achard, N. A. Gilbert

Castaneda, M. R. See H. Zinsser
Castellani, Aldo. Anglo-Indian physician. 1878–
BRONCHITIS—bronchospirochetosis.
Observations on the fungi found in tropical bronchomycosis. Lancet, 1: 13–15, Jan. 6, 1912
MIXTURE—
Note on the internal treatment of yaws. J. Trop. Med. and Hyg., 18: 61–63, Mar. 15, 1915
TESTS—identification of sugars.
The mycological detection and determination of certain carbohydrates and other carbon compounds in pathological work with F. E. Taylor, Brit. med. J., 2: 855-857, Dec. 29, 1917
Also, in French: Ann. Inst. Pasteur, 36: 789–804, 1922
VACCINE—
Note on typhoid-paratyphoid vaccination with mixed vaccines. Zbl. Bakt., 72: 536–540, Jan. 24, 1914
Further researches on combined vaccines. Ibid., 77: 63–73, Sept. 8, 1915
Discovered T. gambiense in human cerebrospinal fluid.
On the discovery of a species of trypanosoma in the cerebrospinal fluid of cases of sleeping sickness. Proc. roy. Soc., 71: 501–508, Apr. 1903
Discovered Treponema pertenue as cause of yaws.
On the presence of spirochaetes in some cases of parangi (yaws, framboesia tropica); preliminary note. J. Ceylon Branch, Brit. Med. Ass., 2: pt. 1, 54 (only), Jan.-June 1905
On the presence of spirochaetes in two cases of ulcerated parangi (yaws). Brit. med. J., 2: 1280 (only), Nov. 11, 1905.
Further observations on parangi (yaws). Ibid., 1330–1331, Nov. 18, 1905
Spirochaetes in yaws. Ibid., 1430 (only), Nov. 25, 1905
Wrote standard text on tropical medicine in English.
Manual of tropical medicine with A. J. Chalmers, London, Ballière, Tindall and Cox, 1910

Castle, William Bosworth. Boston physician. 1897–
PRINCIPLE or FERMENT—
Proved that pernicious anemia is result of inability of stomach to secrete a definite anti-pernicious anemia factor.
Observations on the etiological relationship of achylia gastrica to pernicious anemia with E. A. Locke, J. clin. Invest., 6: 2–3, Aug. 20, 1928
Observations on the etiological relationship of achylia gastrica to pernicious anemia. I. The effect of the administration to patients with pernicious anemia of the contents of the normal human stomach recovered

after the ingestion of beef muscle. Amer. J. med. Sci., 178: 748–764, Dec. 1929

Castro, Rodericus a. German physician. 1546?–1637
Wrote important treatise of medical jurisprudence.
Medicus-politicus: sive de officiis medico-politicis tractatus, quatuor distinctus libris. . . . Hamburgi, ex bibliop. Frobeniano, 1614. 277 pp.

Castroviejo, Ramon. New York ophthalmologist. 1904–
OPERATION—
Keratoplasty. An historical and experimental study, including a new method. Amer. J. Ophth., 15: 825–838, Sept.; 905–916, Oct. 1932
Keratoplasty; report of cases with special reference to complicated ones. J. Med. Soc. New Jersey, 32: 80–88, Feb. 1935

Cathelin, Fernand. French surgeon. 1873–
METHOD—introduction of anesthetics into epidural space through the sacro-coccygeal ligament.
Une nouvelle voie d'injection rachidienne. Méthode des injections épidurales par le procédé du canal sacré. Applications à l'homme. C. R. Soc. Biol., 53: 452–453, Apr. 27, 1901

Cathelineau, H. French chemist. 1861–
SOLUTION—basal ammonium sulphate.
Contribution a l'étude biologique du Bacillus viridis de Lasage. Ann. Inst. Pasteur, 10: 228–237, Apr. 1896

Catlin, George. American physician. 1796–1872
Called attention to bad effects of mouth breathing.
The breath of life; or malrespiration and its effects upon the enjoyments and life of man. New York, Wiley, 1861

Caton, Richard. Liverpool surgeon. 1842–1926
OPERATION—hypophysectomy.
Notes on a case of acromegaly treated by operation with F. T. Paul, Brit. med. J., 2: 1421–1423, Dec. 30, 1893

Cattell, Raymond Bernard. English psychologist. 1905–
TEST—
Cattell group intelligence scale; specimen set. London, (1933–37). 2 ed., 9 pamphl.
A guide to mental testing, for psychological clinics, schools, and industrial psychologists. London, London Univ. Press, 1936. 312 pp.

Cattell, Richard Bartley. Boston surgeon. 1900–
TECHNIC—
Radical pancreatoduodenal resection for carcinoma of the ampulla of Vater. Surg. Clin. N. Amer., 24: 640–647, June 1944
See also F. H. Lahey

Caulfield, Alfred Hans Waring. Canadian physician. 1879–
TEST—inhibition t. for early diagnosis of tuberculosis.
Investigations on pulmonary tuberculosis. J. med. Res., 24: 101–213, Jan. 1911
Factors in the interpretation of the inhibitive and fixation serum reactions in pulmonary tuberculosis. Proc. roy. Soc. London, s. B., 84: 373–389, Dec. 28, 1911

Caulk, John Roberts. St. Louis urologist. 1881–1938
CAUTERY PUNCH—
Infiltration anesthesia of the internal vesical orifice for the removal of minor obstructions: presentation of a cautery punch. J. Urol., 4: 399–408, Oct. 1920
An analytical study of one hundred cases of selected vesical neck obstructions operated by the author's cautery punch. Ibid., 11: 45–62, Jan. 1924

Cave, Edwin French. Boston surgeon. 1896–
OPERATION—
Combined anterior-posterior approach to the knee joint. J. Bone and Joint Surg., 17: 427–430, Apr. 1935
See also M. N. Smith-Petersen

Cave, Henry Wisdom. New York surgeon. 1887–
METHOD—
A method of closure of temporary external fecal fistula. S. G. O., 61: 499–502, Oct. 1935

Cavendish, Henry. English scientist. 1731–1810
Discovered hydrogen in 1766, and demonstrated composition of air.
Experiments on air. Philos. Trans., 74: 119–153, 1784

Caventou, Joseph Bienaimé. French chemist. 1795–1877
Isolated strychnine.
Mémoire sur un nouvel alcali végétal (la strychnine) trouvé dans la noix vomique with P. J. Pelletier, J. Pharm. Chim., Paris, 5: 142–177, 1819
See also P. J. Pelletier

Cavina, Giovanni. Italian surgeon
OPERATION—for inguinal hernia.
Alcune reflessioni sul trattamento dell'ernia inguinale. "Scritti di chirurgia erniaria." Padova, Seminario, 1937. vol. 2, p. 133
Intorno al trattamento dell'ernia inguinale secondo il metodo Postempski. Policlinico, sez. prat., 45: 57–58, Jan. 10, 1938

Cavité
FEVER—a state in the Philippine Islands.

Cawley, Thomas. London physician
Wrote early work on diabetes.
A singular case of diabetes, consisting entirely in the quality of the urine; with an inquiry into the different theories of that disease. London med. J., 9: 286–308, 1788

Cayley, Dr. English physician
Induced pneumothorax to control hemoptysis.
. . . case of haemoptysis treated by the induction of pneumothorax so as to collapse the lung. Lancet, 1: 894–895, May 16, 1885

Cazenave, Pierre Louis Alphée. French dermatologist. 1795–1877
DISEASE—pemphigus foliaceus.
Pemphigus chronique génerale; forme rare du pemphigus foliacé. . . . Ann. d. mal. de la peau, 1: 208–210, 1844
LUPUS—
Lupus erythematodes. Des principales formes du lupus et de son traitement. Gaz. d. hôp., 3 s., 2: 393, 1850; 4: 113, 1852
See also L. T. Biett

Cecca, Raffaele. Bologne surgeon
OPERATION—for varicose veins.
Contributo clinico alla cura delle varici (con metodo proprio). La Clinica Chir., 16: 1427–1440, Sept. 30, 1908

Ceci, Antonio. Italian surgeon. 1852–1920
Performed amputations by "kinematization" as suggested by Vanghetti.
Tecnica generale della amputazioni mucosi. Amputazioni plastico-ortopediche con metodo proprio secundo la proposta del Vanghetti. Dimostrazioni pratiche. Arch. ed Atti Soc. Ital. di chir., Roma, 18, 1906

Cecil, Arthur Bond. Los Angeles surgeon. 1885–
OPERATION—for hypospadias.

Surgery of hypospadias and epispadias in the male.
Trans. Amer. Ass. Genito-Urin. Surg., 24: 253–302,
1931

Cecil, Russell LaFayette. New York physician. 1881–
STRAIN—of streptococcus used in preparing stock
vaccine for arthritis.
*The bacteriology of the blood and joints in chronic in-
fectious arthritis* with E. E. Nicholls and W. J.
Stainsby, Arch. intern. Med., 43: 571–605, May
1929
The etiology of rheumatoid arthritis. Amer. J. med.
Sci., 81: 12–25, Jan. 1931

Cegka, Josephus Joannes.
SIGN—in adherent pericarditis, the outline of cardiac
dulness remains unchanged during different phases
of respiration. Robertson
*Nouvellae observationes de valore diagnostico ausculta-
tionis ac percussionis.* Pragae, Spurny, (1837). 22 pp.

Celli, A. See E. Marchiafava

Celozzi, Domenico. Florence physician
SOLUTION—placenta digest blood; culture medium.
*Nuovo terreno di cultura d'uso generale in microparas-
sitologia umana.* Sperimentale, 72: 291–308, 1918

Celsus, Aulus Aurelius Cornelius. Roman gentle-
man. 53 B.C.–7 A.D.
AREA CELSI—alopecia areata.
KERION CELSI—trichophytosis.
PAPULES—lichen agrius.
VITILIGO CELSI—anesthetis leprosy.
De medicina. Florentiae, Nicolaus (Laurentius),
1478
De re medica libri octo. Haganoae, Secerium, 1528.
288 ff.
Same, ed. by E. Milligan. Edinburgi, 1831. 2 ed.
Same, in Latin with English transl. by W. G. Spencer,
London, Heinemann, 1935–38. 3 vols. Loeb Classical
Library.

Cenci, F. Italian physician
Used convalescent serum prophylactically against
measles.
*Alcune esperienze di sieroimmunizzazione e sierote-
rapia nel morbillo.* Riv. di clin. Pediat., Firenze, 5:
1017–1025, 1907

Cerenville, Édouard de. Swiss surgeon. 1843–1915
Performed thorocoplasty to collapse underlying tuberculous tissue.
*De l'intervention opératoire dans les maladies du
poumon.* Rev. med. de la Suisse Rom., Genève, 5:
441–467, 1885

Cervello, Vincenzo. Italian physician. 1854–1918
TREATMENT—for tuberculosis, by placing patient in
atmosphere filled with formalin vapor.
Sulla cura della tuberculosi polmonare. Palermo,
Reber, 1899. 37 pp.

Cesalpinus, Andreas. Italian physician. 1519–1603
Regarded by the Italians as a discoverer of the circulation (1571–93) before Harvey (1616), but not
supported by any convincing experiments. Garrison
Peripateticarum quaestionum, libri quinque. Venetiis,
apud Iuntas, 1571
Quaestiones medicae. Venetiis, apud Iuntas, 1593

Cesaris-Demel, Antonio. Turin pathologist. 1866–
BROTH—liver infusion, for cultivation of colon-
typhoid group.
*Ueber das verschiedene Verhalten einiger Mikroorga-
nismen in einem gefärbten Nährmittel.* Zbl. Bakt., 26:
529–540 (532), Nov. 16, 1899

Cestan, Étienne Jacques Marie Raymond. French
physician. 1872–1934
PARALYSIS or SYNDROME—
*Du myosis dans certaines lésions bulbaires en foyer
(hémiplégie du type Avellis associée ou syndrome ocu-
laire sympathique)* with L. Chenais, Gaz. d. hôp.,
Paris, 76: 1229–1233, Oct. 29, 1903
See also F. Raymond

Chabert, Philibert. French veterinarian. 1737–1814
DISEASE—symptomatic anthrax.
Description et traitement du charbon dans les animaux.
Paris, de l'imp. royale, 1780. 28 pp.

Chabrol, Étienne. French physician. 1883–
TEST—for bile salts.
*Une nouvelle technique de dosage des sels biliaires
(réaction phospho-vanillique)* with R. Charonnat,
Jean Cottet and P. Blonde, C. R. Soc. Biol., 115:
834–838, 1934

Chadwick, James Read. Boston gynecologist. 1844–
1905
SIGN—
*The value of the bluish coloration of the vaginal en-
trance as a sign of pregnancy.* Trans. Amer. Gynec.
Soc., 11: 399–418, 1887

Chaffin, Rafe Chester. Los Angeles surgeon. 1882–
FORCEPS—
Gastro-intestinal suturing forceps. S. G. O., 32: 465
(only), May 1921
OPERATION—vaginal subtotal hysterectomy.
*Cystocele, with or without descent of the uterus. With
especial reference to the technic of the interposition
operation.* Amer. J. Surg., 33: 183–187, Aug. 1919
*Procidentia: a new operation for cure of fourth degree
prolapse.* Ibid., 37: 239–243, Aug. 1937
*Procidentia: the Chaffin vaginal subtotal hysterectomy
for the cure of fourth degree prolapse—review of technic
and results.* Ibid., 66: 328–338, Dec. 1944
TREATMENT—
*Vesicovaginal fistula: a new method of postoperative
treatment and a simplified method of ureterocystostomy.*
Amer. J. Surg., 31: 484–488, Mar. 1936
*Vesicovaginal fistula: an improvement in the Chaffin
method of postoperative treatment, using Chaffin suction drainage.* Ibid., 71: 305–311, Mar. 1946

Chagas, Carlos. Brazil physician. 1879–1934
DISEASE—Brazilian trypanosomiasis. Discovered the
T. cruzi, the causal organism in American trypanoso-
miasis (Chagas' disease).
Neue Trypanosomen. Arch. f. Schiffs- u. Tropen-
Hyg., Leipzig, 13: 120–122, 1909
Nova entidato morbida do homen. Memor. do Inst.
Oswaldo Cruz, 2: 219, 1911
*American trypanosomiasis; study of the parasite and
of the transmitting insect.* Proc. Inst. Med., Chicago,
3: 220–242, 1921

Chagres
FEVER—a malignant type of malarial fever occurring
along the Chagres River in South America.

Chain, Ernst Boris. English scientist
Awarded Nobel prize in 1945, with Sir Alexander
Fleming and Sir Howard Walter Florey, for their
discovery of penicillin. Prepared a highly concen-
trated and active form of penicillin.
Penicillin as a chemotherapeutic agent with H. W.
Florey, A. D. Gardner, N. G. Heatley, M. A. Jen-

nings, J. Orr-Ewing and A. G. Sanders, Lancet, 2: 226–228, Aug. 24, 1940

See also A. Fleming

Chalatow, S. S. See N. N. Anichkov

Chalier, J. See E. Weill

Chalmers, A. J. See A. Castellani

Chamberlain, William Edward. American roentgenologist. 1892–

TECHNIC—for demonstrating slipping of sacroiliac joints by x-ray.

The symphysis pubis in the roentgen examination of the sacroiliac joint. Amer. J. Roentgenol., 24: 621–625, Dec. 1930

The x-ray examination of the sacroiliac joint. Delaware Med. J., 4: 195–201, Sept. 1932

Chamberland, C. See L. Pasteur

Chamberlen, Peter. English obstetrician. 1601–1683

FORCEPS—the original form of obstetric forceps, invented by Chamberlen about 1670.

In preface to: *Traité des maladies des femmes grosses, et de celles qui font accouchées.* By Mariceau, Paris, 1681. Transl. by Hugh Chamberlen, 1696

Chambers, Helen. London physician. 1880–1935

Prevented growth of tumors by radiation, which causes protective substances to be given off.

Experiments upon immunity to tumour growth with Gladwys M. Scott and S. Russ, Lancet, 1: 212–216, Feb. 4, 1922

Chambers, Robert. New York biologist. 1881–

APPARATUS—for micro-injection.

Micrurgical studies in cell physiology. I. The reaction of the chlorides of Na, K, Ca, and Mg on the protoplasm of Amoeba proteus with P. Reznikoff, J. gen. Physiol., 8: 369–401 (375), Apr. 20, 1926

Champetier de Ribes, Camille Louis Antoine. French obstetrician. 1848–1935

BAG—for dilating cervix uteri.

De l'accouchement provoqué: dilatation du canal génital (col de l'utérus, vagin et vulve) a l'aide de ballons introduits dans la cavité utérine pendant la grossesse. Ann. de Gynécol. et Obstet., Paris, 30: 401–438, Dec. 1888

Championnier, J. M. L. See Lucas-Championnier

Champy, Christian. French physician. 1885–

METHOD—iodide of osmium for Golgi bodies.

Granules et substances réduisant l'iodure d'osmium. J. Anat., Paris, 49: 323–343, July–Aug. 1913

Chandler, J. P. See A. Bodansky

Channing, Walter. American physician. 1786–1876

Wrote on anesthesia in obstetrics.

A treatise on etherization in childbirth. Boston, Ticknor, 1848

Chantemesse, André. French bacteriologist. 1851–1919

REACTION—ophthalmic r. for typhoid fever.

L'opthalmo-diagnostic, de la fièvre typhoïde. Bull. Acad. Méd. Paris, s. 3., 58: 138–139, July 23, 1907

SERUM or VACCINE—antityphoid s.

De l'immunité contre le virus de la fièvre typhoïde, conférée par des substances solubles with F. Widal, Ann. Inst. Pasteur, 2: 54–59, Feb. 1888

Chaoul, Henri. Berlin roentgenologist. 1887–

THERAPY—

Die Röntgen-Nahbestrahlung maligner Tumoren with A. Adam, Strahlentherapie, Berlin, 48: 31–50, Sept. 6, 1933

Chapin, C. W. See G. W. McCoy

Chapman, Nathaniel. American physician. 1780–1853

MIXTURE—for gonorrhea.

PILL—

Wrote first book on therapeutics and materia medica in United States.

Discourses on the elements of therapeutics and materia medica. Philadelphia, Webster, 1817. 2 vols.

Chapman, W. H. See S. B. Wolbach

Chappuis, J. French physician

Studied biliary concretions by x-ray.

Caculs du rein. Calculs de la vesicule biliaire with H. Chauvel, Bull. Acad. Méd. Paris, 35: 410–411, 1896

Chaput, Henri. French surgeon. 1857–1919

OPERATION—for artificial anus.

Thérapeutique chirurgicale des affections de l'intestin, du rectum et du péritoine. Paris, Doin, 1896. 244 pp.

Charcellay, J. L. Tours physician

HYPOTHESIS—the extra sound in gallop rhythm is assigned to the vigorous and audible contractions of auricles.

Mémoire sur plusiours cas remarquables de défaut de synchronisme des battements des bruits des ventricules du coeur. Arch. gen de Med., 3: 393–409, 1838

Charcot, Jean Martin. French neurologist. 1824–1893

ARTHROPATHY or JOINT DISEASE—occurring in diseases of spinal cord.

Sur quelques arthropathies qui paraissent dependre d'une lesion du cerveau ou de la moelle epiniere. Arch. Physiol. norm. path., 1: 161–178; 379–400, 1868

Ataxie locomotrice progressive; arthropathie de l'epaule gauche resultats necroscopiques. Ibid., 2: 121–125, 1869

Also: *Lecons sur les maladies du systeme nerveux faites a la Salpetriere.* Paris, s. 2, 65, 1873

Also, English transl.: *Lectures on the nervous system.* London, New Sydenham Soc., 1881. Ser. 2, p. 56

CIRRHOSIS—hypertrophic c. of liver.

Leçons sur les maladies du foie, des voies biliaires et des reins. Paris, Prog. méd., 1877

DISEASE—progressive neuropathic muscular atrophy.

Deux cas d'atrophie musculaire progressive avec lésions de la subsistance grise et des faisceaux antérolatéraux de la moelle épinière with A. Joffroy, Arch. Physiol. norm. path., 2: 744–760, 1869

DISEASE—of Erb-Charcot; spastic spinal paralysis.

Du tabès dorsal spasmodique. Prog. méd., Paris, 4: 737–738, Nov. 4; 773; 793, 1876

DISEASE—Charcot-Marie-Tooth type of peroneal form of muscular atrophy.

Sur une forme particulière d'atrophie musculaire progressive, souvent familiale, débutant par les pieds et les jambes, et atteignant plus tard les mains with P. Marie, Rev. de méd., Paris, 6: 97–138, Feb. 1886

EDEMA—

L'oedème bleu des hystériques. Prog. méd., 12: 259–264, Oct. 11; 275–278, Oct. 18, 1890

FEVER—hepatic f., resulting from impacted gallstones.

Note sur les altérations du foie consecutives a la ligature du canal cholédoque with Gombault, Arch. Physiol. norm. path., 8: 272–299, 1876

Leçons sur les maladies du foie, dés voies biliaires et des reins. Bureau de prog. méd., Paris, 1877

SCLEROSIS—amyotrophic laterals.
Des amyotrophies spinales chronique. Prog. med., 2: 573, 1874
Also: *Leçons sur les maladies du systeme nerveux.* ... 2 s., 147–272, 1874
SIGN—intermittent limping in arteriosclerosis of legs and feet.
Sur la claudication intermittente. C. R. Soc. Biol. (Mémoires), 1858, 5: 225–238, 1859
VERTIGO—laryngea.
Du vertige laryngé. Prog. méd., 7: 317–319, Apr. 26, 1879
Described lightning pains in locomotor ataxia.
Douleurs fulgurantes de l'ataxie sans incoordination des mouvements: sclérose commençante des cordons postérieurs de la moelle épinière with A. Bouchard, Gaz. méd. de Paris, 3 s., 21: 122–124, 1866
Demonstrated atrophy of anterior horns of spinal cord in infantile paralysis.
Une observation de paralysie infantile s'accompagnant d'une altération des cornes antérieures de la substance grise de la moelle with A. Joffroy, C. R. Soc. Biol., 1869, 5 s., 1: 312–315, 1870
See also P. Marie
Chargaff, S. See F. W. Bancroft
Chargin, Louis. New York physician. 1881–
TREATMENT—of syphilis.
Studies of velocity and the response to intravenous injections. V. The application of the intravenous drip method to chemotherapy as illustrated by massive doses of arsphenamine in the treatment of early syphilis with W. Leifer and H. T. Hyman, J. A. M. A., 104: 878–883, Mar. 16, 1935
Charleton, Walter. English physician. 1619–1707
Wrote first book in which a new physiology based on experimental grounds was propounded.
Natural history of nutrition, life, and voluntary motion. ... London, Herringman, 1659. 210 pp.
Charlouis, M. Dutch physician in Java
DISEASE—frambesia tropica.
Ueber Polypapilloma tropicum (Framboesia). Viertelj. f. Dermat. u. Syph., 8: 431–466, 1881
Also, trans. by A. E. Garrod: New Sydenham Soc., pp. 287–319, 1897
Charlton, Alice M. See W. D. Frost
Charlton, W. See W. Schultz
Charonnat, R. See E. Chabrol
Charrière, Joseph Francois Bernard. Paris surgeon. 1803–1876
ETHER INHALER—
Des inspirations de vapeur éthérée. Gaz. méd., Paris, 3 s., 2: 81–82, Jan. 30, 1847
Charrin, Albert. French bacteriologist. 1856–1907
DISEASE—
La maladie pyocyanique. Paris, 1889
SOLUTION—basal salt.
Les propriétés du bacille pyocyanogène en fonction des qualités nutritives du milieu with A. Dissard, C. R. Soc. Biol., Paris, 9 s., 5, pt. 2: 182–186, 1893
Charrin, Salomon. French physician
ICTERUS—neonatal, cyanotic.
Maladie bronzée hématique des enfants nouveau-nés (tubulhématie rénale de M. Parrot). Paris, Thesis, No. 442, 1873
Chasis, H. See H. W. Smith
Chassaignac, Charles Marie Edouard. French surgeon. 1804–1879

MUSCLE—axillary m., inconstant.
Note sur le système musculaire. Arch. gen. de méd.. 2 s., 4: 465–468, Mar. 1834
Chassevant, A. See P. Carnot
Chastaing, P. French chemist
REACTION—for morphine.
Action de l'acide sulfurique sur des mélanges de morphine et d'acides bibasiques with E. Barillot, C. R. Soc. Biol., 105: 941–943, 1887
Chastek
PARALYSIS—occurring in foxes on farm of Mr. Chastek.
A deficiency disease of foxes. By R. G. Green (Minnesota) and C. A. Evans, Science, 92: 154–155, Aug. 16, 1940
A deficiency disease of foxes produced by feeding fish: B1 avitaminoses analogous to Wernicke's disease of man. By R. G. Green, with W. E. Carlson and C. A. Evans, J. Nutrit., 21: 243–256, Mar. 10, 1941
Chatfield, Mabel. See F. L. Meleney
Chatin, Gaspard Adolph. French physician. 1813–1901
Presented evidence that iodine would prevent endemic goiter and cretinism.
Existence de l'iode dans les plantes d'eau douce. Conséquences de ce fait pour la géognosie, la physiologie végétale, la therapeutique et peut-être pour l'industrie. C. R. Acad. Sci., 30: 352–354, 1850
Chauchard, H. See A. Vernes
Chauffard, Anatole Marie Emile. French physician. 1855–1932
SYNDROME—when tumor of pancreas is in body or tail, jaundice is absent or long delayed, and severe pain is due to pressure on nerves behind pancreas.
Le cancer du corps du pancréas. Bull. Acad. Méd. Paris, 60: 242–255, Oct. 20, 1908
Described hereditary hemolytic jaundice.
Pathogénie de l'ictère hémolytique congénital. Ann. de méd., 1: 1–17, Jan. 1914
See also V. C. Hanot
Chauffard, H. See J. Castaigne
Chauliac, Guy de. See Guy de Chauliac
Chaussier, Francois. Paris physician. 1746–1828
LINE—median raphe of the callosum.
Exposition sommaire de la structure et des différentes parties de l'encéphale ou cerveau; suivant la méthode adoptée a l'École de médecine de Paris. Paris, Barrois, 1807. 200 pp.
SIGN—pain in epigastrium preceding eclampsia.
Considérations sur les convulsions qui attaquent les femmes enceintes. Paris, Compère jeune, 1824. 23 pp. 2 ed.
Repr. from: *Proc.-verb. de la distribution des prix aux élèves sages-femmes.*
Chauveau, Jean Baptiste Auguste. French physician. 1827–1917
HAEMOTACHROMETER—for measuring circulation rate.
Vitesse de la circulation dans les arteres du cheval d'apres les indications d'un nouvel hemodromometre with G. Bertolus and L. Laroyenne, J. Physiol. Path. gen., 3: 695–716, Oct. 1860
Made direct records of heart impulse.
Appareils et experiences cardiographiques with E. J. Marey, Mem. Acad. imp. de Med., Paris, 26: 268–319, 1863
Chauvel, H. See J. Chappuis

Chavaillon. See G. Faroy

Chavassieu, M. Lyon physician
TEST—for glucose.
Le métadinitrobenzène comme réactif des sucres with
M. Morel, C. R. Soc. Biol., 2: 582–583, 1906

Cheadle, Walter Butler. London pediatrician. 1836–
1910
DISEASE—infantile scurvy.
Scurvy and purpura. Brit. med. J., 2: 520–522, Nov.
9, 1872
*Clinical lecture on three cases of scurvy supervening on
rickets in young children.* Lancet, 2: 685–687, Nov.
16, 1878
Recommended general use of iodine for exophthalmic
goiter.
Exophthalmic goitre. St. George's Hosp. Rep., 4:
175–192, 1869

Cheatle, Sir George Lenthal. London surgeon. 1865–
DISEASE—
Cystiphorous desquamative epithelial hyperplasia.
In: *Tumors of the breast. Their pathology, symptoms,
diagnosis, and treatment* with M. Cutler, London,
Arnold, 1031
Also: Philadelphia, Lippincott, 1931 596 pp. pp.
91–134
OPERATION—
*An operation for the radical cure of inguinal and
femoral hernia.* Brit. med. J., 2: 68–69, July 17, 1920

Chediak, A. Argentina physician
METHOD—dry blood m. for diagnosis of syphilis.
*La microreacción Chediak para el diagnóstico de la
sífilis, efectuada con una gota de sangre seca.* Dia.
méd., 11: 294–297, Apr. 10, 1939

Chessman, John C. New York surgeon
Early contributor to American laryngology.
*Case of a remarkable disease of the larynx and trachea;
with a plate.* Trans. Physico-Med. Soc., 1: 413–414,
1817

Cheever, David. Boston surgeon, 1876–
METHOD—of dilating papilla of Vater.
*Instrumental dilatation of the papilla of Vater and the
dislodgment of calculi by retrograde irrigation. A
contribution to the surgery of the bile passages.* Arch.
Surg., 18: 1069–1077, Apr. 1929

Chen, Ko Kuei. Madison, Wis. chemist, 1898–
REACTION—for ephedrine.
Introduced ephedrine for therapeutic use.
*The action of ephedrine, the active principle of the
Chinese drug, Ma Huang* with C. F. Schmidt, J.
Pharmacol., 24: 339–357, Dec. 1924
*The action and clinical use of ephedrine, an alkaloid
isolated from the Chinese drug, Ma Huang* with C.
F. Schmidt, J. A. M. A., 87: 836–842, Sept. 11, 1926
*Ephedrine and pseudoephedrine, their isolation, con-
stitution, isomerism, properties, derivatives and syn-
thesis; (with a bibliography)* with C. H. Kao, J. Amer.
Pharmacol. Ass., 15: 625–639, 1926
*The CuSO₄-NaOH test of ephedrine isomers and re-
lated compounds.* Ibid., 18: 110–116, 1929
Ephedrine and related substances with C. F. Schmidt,
Baltimore, Williams & Wilkins, 1930

Chen, Mei-Yü. See C. D. Leake

Chenais, L. See E. J. M. R. Cestan

Cherney, Leonid Sergius. San Francisco surgeon.
1907–

INCISION—
*A modified transverse incision for low abdominal opera-
tions.* S. G. O., 72: 92–95, Jan. 1941
New transverse low abdominal incision. California
West Med., 59: 215–218, Oct. 1943

Chéron, H. See H. Dominici

Cherry, Ian S. Chicago physiologist
METHOD—for determination of lipolytic activity in
serum.
*The specificity of pancreatic lipase; its appearance in
the blood after pancreatic injury* with L. A. Crandall,
Jr., Amer. J. Physiol., 100: 266–273, Apr. 1932

Cheselden, William. London surgeon. 1688–1752
LITHOTOMY—lateral; see Alexander Reid
LITHOTOMY—suprapubic.
A treatise on the high operation for the stone. London,
Osborn, 1723
OPERATION—for artificial pupil.
*An account of some observations made by a young
gentleman who was born blind, or lost his sight so early
that he had no remembrance of ever having seen, and
was couch'd between 13 and 14 years of age.* Philos.
Trans., 35: 447–452, 1729

Chesny, Alan Mason. St. Louis physician. 1888–
AGAR—indicator lactose; for isolation of typhoid and
dysentery bacilli from stools.
*The use of phenol red and brom-cresol purple as indi-
cators in the bacteriological examination of stools.*
J. exp. Med., 35: 181–186, Feb. 1922
DOCTRINE—an immunity to syphilis persists even
if the original infection has been eliminated.
Immunity in syphilis. Baltimore, Williams & Wilkins,
1927. 85 pp.

Chevalier, Arthur. French physician
Developed compound objective of the compound
microscope, 1820. Garrison
*L'étudiant micrographe. Traité théorique et pratiqu du
microscope et des préparations.* Paris, Delahaye, 1865.
2 éd., augmentée.

Chevallier, André. French physician. 1905–
TEST—for vitamin A in blood.
Sur la détection de la vitamine A dans le sang with
Yvonne Choron, C. R. Soc. Biol., 118: 889–891,
Feb. 12, 1935

Chevassu, Maurice. French urologist. 1877–
SEMINOMA OF TESTIS—
Tumeurs du testicle. Thesis de Paris, 1906. 239 pp.

Chevreul, Michel Eugène. Paris physician. 1787–
1889
Investigated sugar in diabetic urine.
Note sur le sucre de diabétes. Ann. de Chimie, Paris,
95: 319–320, July 31, 1815
Made an important study of animal fats.
*Recherches chimiques sur les corps gras d'origine ani-
male.* Paris, Levrault, 1823. 484 pp.
Isolated creatine from muscle.
*Neues eigenthümliches stickstoffhaltiges Princip, in
Muskelfleisch gefunden.* J. f. Chem. u. Physik.,
Nürnberg, 65: 455–456, 1832

Cheyne, George. English physician. 1671–1743
DISEASE—hypochondria.
*The English malady; or, a treatise of nervous diseases
of all kinds as spleen, vapours, lowness of spirits,
hypochondrical and hysterical distempers, etc.* London,
Powell et al., 1733

Cheyne, John. Scottish physician. 1777–1836
ASTHMA—Cheyne-Stokes or cardiac a.

SIGN or RESPIRATION—Cheyne-Stokes r.
A case of apoplexy, in which the fleshy part of the heart was converted into fat. Dublin Hosp. Rep., 2: 216–223, 1818
Also: Med. Classics, 3: 705–709, Mar. 1939
Also in F. A. Willius and T. E. Key's Cardiac Classics. St. Louis, Mosby, 1941 pp. 317–320
Described cerebral dropsy or acute hydrocephalus.
An essay on hydrocephalus acutus, or dropsy in the brain.
Forms Essay III in Vol 2 of *Essays on the diseases of children, with cases and dissections.* Edinburgh, Mundell, 1801–08. 218 pp.

Cheyne, Sir William Watson. English surgeon. 1852–1932
OPERATION—
The radical cure of hernia, with a description of a method of operating for femoral hernia. Lancet, 2: 1039–1041, Nov. 5, 1892

Chiari, Hans. Prague physician. 1851–1916
DISEASE or SYNDROME—obstruction with thrombosis of hepatic veins.
Erfahrungen über Infarctbildungen in der Leber des Menschen. Z. Heilk., 19: 475–512, 1898
Ueber die selbständige Phlebitis obliterans der Hauptstämme der Venae hepaticae als Todesursache. Beitr. path. Anat., 26: 1–17, 1899
NETWORK—fibers which sometimes extend across right auricle of heart.
Ueber Netzbildungen im rechten Vorhofe des Herzens. Ibid., 22: 1–10, 1897

Chickering, H. T. See O. T. Avery

Chierici, E. Italian physician
TEST—for hexoses and pentoses in urine.
Sulla ricerca della formaldeide nell'urina. Ateneo parmense, 2: 8–12, Jan.–Feb. 1930

Chievitz, Mme Ingoborg. Copenhagen physician
METHOD—for early diagnosis of whooping cough.
Recherches sur la coqueluche with A. H. Meyer, Ann. Inst., Pasteur, 30: 503–524, Oct. 1916

Chievitz, Johan Henrik. Copenhagen anatomist. 1850–1901
ORGAN—mandibular branch of parotid duct.
Beiträge zur Entwicklungsgegeschichte der Speicheldrüsen. Arch. Anat. Physiol., Anat. Abt., pp. 400–436, 1885

Child, Charles Gardner, III. New York surgeon. 1908–
TECHNIC—
Carcinoma of duodenum; one-stage radical pancreaticoduodenectomy, preserving the external pancreatic secretion; case report. Ann. Surg., 118: 838–842, Nov. 1943
Pancreaticojejunostomy and other problems associated with the surgical management of carcinoma involving the head of the pancreas; report of five additional cases of radical pancreaticoduodenectomy. Ibid., 119: 845–855, June 1944

Chitral.
FEVER—an acute infectious fever occurring in the Chitral Valley in India.

Chittenden, Russell Henry. American physiochemist. 1856–1943
DIET—containing 47 to 55 gm. of protein.
Physiological economy in nutrition.... New York, Stokes, 1904. 478 pp.
Studied the minimum nutritive requirements of the

body in relation to its capacity for work and nitrogenous equilibrium. Ibid.

Chodat, Robert. Genf botanist. 1865–1934
REACTION—for polypeptides.
Ueber den Nachweis von Peptiden in Harn mittels der p-Kresol-Tyrosinase-Reaktion with R. H. Kummer, Biochem. Z., Berlin. 65: 392–399, July 18, 1914
See also A. Bach

Chomel, Auguste Francois. French pathologist. 1788–1858
Reported case of carcinoma of infrapapillary portion of duodenum.
Cancer du duodénum. Gaz. d. hôp., 25: 37 (only) Jan. 24, 1852

Chopart, Francois. French surgeon. 1743–1795
JOINT—the mediotarsal articulation.
OPERATION—amputation of foot at mediotarsal articulation.
Note by Lafiteau in A. F. Fourcroy's:
La médecine éclairée par les sciences physiques. Paris, Buisson, 1792. pp. 85–88
Traité des maladies chirurgicals, et des opérations qui leur conviennent with P. J. Desault, Paris, Villier, 1797. 2 vols.

Choron, Yvonne. See A. Chevallier

Christensen, E. Saarbrüchen physician
REACTION—for hormones and vitamins.
Eine chemische Reaktion auf Vitamine und Hormone. Münch. med. Wschr., 75: 1883 (only), Nov. 2, 1928

Christian, Henry Asbury. Boston physician. 1876–
DISEASE or SYNDROME—Hand-Schüller-Christian d.; craniohypophyseal xanthomatosis.
Defects in membranous bones, exophthalmos and diabetes insipidus. In: *Contributions to medical and biological research, dedicated to Sir William Osler.* New York, Hoeber, 1919. vol. 1, pp. 390–401
Also: Med. Clin. N. Amer., 3: 849–871, Jan. 1920
DISEASE—Weber-Christian d.
Relapsing febrile nodular nonsuppurative panniculitis. Arch. intern. Med., 42: 338–351, Sept. 1928

Christiansen, Johanne Ostenfeld. Copenhagen physician. 1882–
Curves—CO₂ dissociation c.
The absorption and dissociation of carbon dioxide by human blood with C. G. Douglas and J. S. Haldane, J. Physiol., 48: 244–271, July 14, 1914
METHOD—for preparation of Mett tubes.
Einige Bemerkungen über die Mettsche Methode nebst Versuchen über das Aciditätsoptimum das Pepsinwirkung. Biochem. Z., 46: 257–287, 1912

Christman, Adam, A. Ann Arbor, Mich. physiochemist. 1896–
METHOD—for detection of carbon monoxide in blood.
A convenient and accurate method for the determination and detection of carbon monoxide in blood with E. L. Randall, J. biol. Chem., 102: 595–609, Oct. 1933

Chrobak, Rudolf. German gynecologist. 1843–1910
OPERATION—abdominal hysterectomy.
Zur Exstirpatio uteri myomatosi abdominalis. Zbl. Gynäk., 15: 169–174, Feb. 28, 1891

Churchill, Edward Delos. Boston surgeon. 1895–
OPERATION—removal of lung for carcinoma.
The surgical treatment of carcinoma of the lung. J. Thorac. Surg., 2: 254–266, Feb. 1933

OPERATION—segmental pneumonectomy.
  Segmental pneumonectomy in bronchiectasis: the lingula segment of the left upper lobe with R. Belsey, Ann. Surg., 109: 481–499, Apr. 1939
OPERATION—for hyperparathyroidism.
  Parathyroid tumors associated with hyperparathyroidism: eleven cases treated by operation with O. Cope, S. G. O., 58: 255–271, Feb. 15, 1934
  The operative treatment of hyperparathyroidism. Ann. Surg., 100: 606–612, Oct. 1934
Churchman, John Woolman. American physician. 1877–1937
  Demonstrated germicidal action of gentian-violet against staphylococci.
  The selective bactericidal action of gentian violet. J. exp. Med., 16: 221–247, Aug. 1, 1912
  The selective bacteriostatic action of gentian violet and other dyes. J. Urology, 11: 1–18, Jan. 1924
Chvostek, Frantisek, Sr. Austrian surgeon, 1835–1884
SIGN or TREMOR—sudden spasm on tapping one side of face, seen in postoperative tetany.
  Beitrag zur Tetanie. Wien. med. Pr., 17: 1201–1203, Sept. 10; 1225–1227, Sept. 17; 1253–1258, Sept. 24; 1313–1316, Oct. 8, 1876
Chvostek, Franz. (Jr.) German surgeon. 1864–
PHENOMENON—increased sensitivity of nerves in tetanus.
  Ueber das Verhalten der sensiblen Nerven, des Hörnerven und des Hautleitungswiderstandes bei Tetanie. Z. klin. Med., 19: 489–538, 1891
  Also, abstr.: Wien. klin. Wschr., 3: 838–840, Oct. 23, 1890
  Beiträge zur Lehre von der Tetanie. I. Die mechanische Uebererregbarkeit der motorischen Nerven bei Tetanie und ihre Beziehung zu den Epithelkörpern. Wien. klin. Wschr., 20: 487–493, Apr. 25, 1907
  Beiträge zur Lehre von der Tetanie. II. Das kausale und die auslösenden Momente. Der akute Anfall von Tetanie nach Tuberkulininjektion. Ibid., 625–632, May 23, 1907
  Described bone lesions in parathyroid disease.
  Myasthenia gravis und Epithelkörper. Ibid., 21: 37–44, Jan. 9, 1908
Ciaccio. Carmelo. Palermo pathologist. 1877–
METHOD—for lipoids.
  Contributo alla conoscenza dei lipoidi cellulari. Anat. Anz., 35: 17–31, Aug. 10, 1909
  Contributo alla distribuzione ed alla fisio-pathologia cellulare dei lipoidi. Arch. Zellforsch., 5: 235–363, Aug. 2, 1910
Ciniselli, Luigi. Italian surgeon. 1803–1878
METHOD—galvanopuncture of aneurysm.
  Sulla risoluzione dei tumori per mezzo dell'azione eletro-chimica della corrente continua. Milano, Rechiedei, 1869. 8 pp.
Ciocaltau, Vintila. Bucharest physician
TEST—for blood.
  La diphénylamine, indicateur des hémorragies occultes. C. R. Soc. Biol., 90: 135–137, 1924
Cipollina, A. Genua physician
TEST—for levulose in urine.
  Ueber den Nachweis von Zucker im Harn. Dtsch. med. Wschr., 27: 334–336, May 23, 1901
Cirillo, Domenico. Italian physician. 1739–1799

OINTMENT—used for syphilis.
  Osservazioni pratiche intorno alla lue venerea Venezia, Pezzana, 1786. 288 pp.
Citelli, Salvatore. Italian scientist. 1875–
TEST—for cancer, hemoclastic.
  Un rilievo degno di nota sulla reazione emoclasica nei tumori maligni with P. Carcò, Boll. Soc. ital. biol. sper., 4: 783–785, 1929
Citois, Francois. Poitiers, 1572–1652
  In 1616 described "Poitou colic", which long afterward was found to be lead colic. Garrison
  De novo et populari apud Pictones dolore coico bilioso. Poitiers, 1616
Citron, Heinrich. Berlin physician. 1864–
TEST—for blood in feces.
  Technische und diagnostische Beiträge zur Blutanalyse der Faeces. Dtsch. med. Wschr., 34: 190–192, Jan. 30, 1908
  Ueber den Nachweis kleinster Blutwengen in der klinischen und forensischen Medizin. Berlin. klin. Wschr., 47: 1001–1004, May 30, 1910
Civiale, Jean. French physician. 1792–1867
OPERATION—lithotrity.
  Sur la lithotritie, ou broiement de la pierre dans la vessie. Paris, 1826. 29 pp.
Civinini, Filippo. Italian anatomist. 1805–1844
PROCESS or SPINE—small eminence of outer edge of external pterygoid plate.
  Line anatomiche. Fasc. 2. In osteologia: sulla scissura di glaser nel temporale. Pistoja, Bracali, 1830 31 pp.
Clado, Spirog. Paris surgeon
POINT—of tenderness in appendicitis; where external border of rectus muscle is crossed by interspinal line.
  Appendice caecal: anatomie - embryologie - anatomie comprxee bacteriologie normale et pathologique. C. R. Soc. Biol., 44: 133–172, 1892
Clairmont, Paul. Zurich surgeon. 1876–1942
OPERATION—for recurrent dislocation of shoulder.
  Ein neues Operationsverfahren zur Behandlung der habituellen Schulterluxation mittels Muskelplastik with H. Ehrlich, Arch. klin. Chir., 89: 798–822, 1909
  Ueber neue Operationsmethoden bei habitueller Schulterluxation. Abstr.: Wien. klin. Wschr., 30: 1507–1508, Nov. 22, 1917
  Showed that fluid in a closed segment of small bowel is poisonous when injected into the vein of another animal.
  Zur Frage der Autointoxication bei Ileus with E. Ranzi, Arch. klin. Chir., 73: 696–782, 1904
  See also R. Kraus
Clarens. See A. Job
Clark, Alonzo. New York physician. 1807–1887
DICTUM—do not measure the opium but measure the respiratory rate.
TREATMENT—of peritonitis with opium.
  On the treatment of puerperal peritonitis by large doses of opium. New York, 1855
Clark, Anson Luman. Oklahoma City urologist. 1893–
  Introduced, with H. F. Helmholz, ketogenic diet in therapeutics of bacteria.
  Escherichia coli bacilluria under ketogenic treatment. Proc. Staff Meet., Mayo Clinic, 6: 605–608, Oct. 14, 1931
  Bacilluria under ketogenic treatment. J. A. M. A., 98: 1710–1711, May 14, 1932
Clark, Byron Bryant. American scientist. 1908–

METHOD—
A bicolorimetric method for the determination of methemoglobin with R. B. Gibson, J. biol. Chem., 100: 205–208, Mar. 1933

Clark, C. P. See F. B. Kingsbury

Clark, Earl Perry. American biochemist. 1892–
METHOD—for estimation of serum calcium.
A study of the Tisdall method for the determination of blood serum calcium with a suggested modification with J. B. Collip, J. biol. Chem., 63: 461–464, Mar. 1925

Clark, Guy Wendell. Berkeley, Calif. biochemist. 1887–
METHOD—of determination of calcium content of blood plasma.
The micro determination of calcium in whole blood, plasma, and serum by direct precipitation. J. biol. Chem., 49: 487–517, Dec. 1921

Clark, John Goodrich. Baltimore gynecologist. 1867–1927
OPERATION—
A more radical method of performing hysterectomy for cancer of the uterus. Johns Hopk. Hosp. Bull., 6: 120–124, July–Aug. 1895
OPERATION—repair of posterior vaginal wall.
Prolapsus uteri; ultimate results in 100 cases. Surg. Clin. N. Amer., pp. 77–100, Feb. 1921

Clark, Mary E. See J. H. Kastle

Clark, W. G. See H. M. Tsuchiya

Clark, William Mansfield. American chemist. 1884–
METHOD—
The colorimetric determination of hydrogen ion concentration and its applications in bacteriology with H. A. Lubs, J. Bact., 2: 1–34, Jan.; 109–136, Mar.; 191–236, May 1917
SOLUTION—for differentiation of colon-aerogenes group.
The differentiation of bacteria of the colon-aerogenes family by the use of indicators with H. A. Lubs, J. infect. Dis., 17: 160–173, July 1915
VESSEL—hydrogen-electrode; for determination of hydrogen ions.
The determination of hydrogen ions. Baltimore, Williams & Wilkins, 1923. 2 ed., Chapt. 14
See also L. A. Rogers

Clarke, Sir Charles Mansfield. English physician. 1782–1857
ULCER—of neck of uterus.
Observations on those diseases of females which are attended by discharges. London, Longmans, 1814–21

Clarke. Jacob Augustus. English physician. 1817–1880
BUNDLE—of nerve fibers extending between Clark's and Burdach's columns.
On the anatomy of the spinal chord. Arch. Med., London, 1: 200–208, 1857–59

Clarke, John. English physician. 1761–1815
Wrote early account of laryngismus stridulus and tetany in children.
Commentaries on some of the most important diseases of children. London, Longman, 1815. 198 pp. pp. 86–97

Clarke, John James. 1827–1895
Described kala-azar.
Kala azar, the black disease. Ann. San. Rep. Prov. Assam., 1882 Appendix A.

Clarke, T(homas) Wood. Utica, N. Y. pediatrician. 1878–
Reported first case of sulph-hemoglobinemia in United States.
The rare forms of cyanosis: polycythemia, methemoglobinemia, and sulph-hemoglobinemia. Med. Rec., 76: 143–145, July 24, 1909
Sulph-hemoglobinemia, with a report of the first case in America. Ibid., 78: 987–991, Dec. 3, 1910

Clauberg, Carl. German physician
METHOD—for assaying of luteal principle.
Zur Physiologie und Pathologie des Sexualhormone, im besonderen des Hormons des Corpus luteum. I. Der biologische Test für das Luteohormon (das spezifische Hormon des Corpus luteum) am infantilen Kaninchen. Zbl. Gynaek., 54: 2757–2770, Nov. 1, 1930

Claude, Henri. French physician
TEST—for hyperthyreosis.
L'épreuve des extraits hypophysaires chez les basedowiens with A. Baudouin and R. Porak, Bull. Soc. méd. Hôp. Paris, 30: 1094–1112, June 19, 1914

Claudius, M. Copenhagen physician
METHOD—of staining bacteria in tissue.
Méthode de coloration a la fois simple et contrastante des microbes. Ann. Inst. Pasteur, 11: 332–335, Apr. 1897

Clausen, Samuel Wolcott. Rochester, N. Y. pediatrician. 1888–
METHOD—
A method for the estimation of potassium in blood. J. biol. Chem., 36: 479–484, Nov. 1918

Clay, Charles. English surgeon. 1801–1893
Performed supracervical hysterectomy.
Observations on ovariotomy, statistical and practical. Also, a successful case of entire removal of the uterus and its appendages. Trans. Obstet. Soc. Lond., (1863), 5: 58–74, 1864

Claybrook, Edwin B. Cumberland, Md. surgeon. 1871–
SIGN—of rupture of abdominal viscus: transmission of breath and heart sounds through abdominal wall.
A new diagnostic sign in injuries of the abdominal viscera. S. G. O., 18: 105–106, Jan. 1914

Clayfield, W. English physician
Constructed the first gasometer. Arnett. For description see T. Beddoes and J. Watt: *Considerations on the medicinal use and on the production of factitious airs.* London, 1796. 3 ed., Pt. III, p. 103
For diagram see frontispiece, H. Davy: *Researches chemical and physiological.* London, 1800

Cleland, Archibald. English physician
Performed catherization of Eustachian tube.
Instruments proposed to remedy some kinds of deafness proceeding from obstructions in the external and internal auditory passages. Philos. Trans., 1732–41, 9: 124, 1747

Cleland, John Burton. Australian microbiologist. 1878–
Proved that Aëdes aegypti (Stegomyia fasciata) is capable of transmitting dengue fever.
On the transmission of Australian dengue by the mosquito Stegomyia fasciata with B. Bradley and W. McDonald, Med. J. Australia, Sydney, 3: 179–184, Sept. 2; 200–205, Sept. 9, 1916

Clerc, C. See C. Jeannin

Cleret, M. See P. E. Launois

Clevand, D. See L. E. Davis

Cleveland, (N.) R. See J. M. Wolfe

Clifton, Charles Egolf. California bacteriologist. 1904–
TECHNIC—
Large-scale production of penicillin. Science, 98: 69–70, July 16, 1943

Climenko, D. R. See O. W. Barlow

Cline, J. K. See R. T. Major, R. R. Williams

Cloetta, Max. Swiss pharmacologist. 1868–1904
Introduced digalen.
Ueber Digalen (Digitoxin solubile). Münch. med. Wschr., 51: 1466–1468, 1904
Die Darstellung und shemische Zusammensetzung der aktiven Substanzen aus der Digitalisblättern, ihre pharmakologischen und therapeutischen Eigenschaften. Arch. exp. Path. Pharmak., 112: 261–342. 1926

Cloquet, Jules Germain. French surgeon. 1790–1883
FASCIA—areolar tissue closing femoral ring.
GLAND—in femoral canal.
HERNIA—pectineal crural h.
LIGAMENT—Haller's habenula; persistent relic of fetal canal connecting tunica vaginalis with peritoneal cavity.
SEPTUM—crurale internum.
Recherches anctomiques sur les hernies de l'abdomen. Paris, Thèse, 1817
Recherches sur les causes et l'anatomie des hernies abdominales. Paris, Méquignon-Marvis, 1819. 176 pp.
Observation sur une hernie vulvaire, suive de quelques réflexions sur la nature et le traitment de cette maladie. Paris, Migneret, 1821. 15 pp.

Cloquet, Jules Hippolyte. French surgeon. 1787–1840
GANGLION—a swelling of the naso-palatine nerve in the anterior palatine canal.
Mémoire sur les ganglions nerveux des fosses nasales; sur leurs communications et sur leurs usages. Paris, Migneret, 1818. 18 pp.

Closs, K. See J. M. Holst

Clough, Mildred Clark. Baltimore physician. 1888–
SYNDROME—of Clough and Richter: anemia in which red corpuscles exhibit a severe degree of autoagglutination.
A study of an autoagglutinin occurring in a human serum. Johns. Hopk. Hosp. Bull., 29: 86–93, Apr. 1918

Clover, Joseph Thomas. English physician. 1825–1882
APPARATUS—
On an apparatus for administering nitrous oxide gas and ether, singly or combined. Brit. med. J., 2: 74–75, July 15, 1876

Clowes, William. English physician. 1540–1604
Wrote on syphilis.
A short and profitable treatise, touching the cure of the morbus gallicus by inunctions. London, Daye, 1579

Clurman, A. W. See O. Teague

Clute, Howard Merrill. Boston surgeon. 1890–1946
CLAMP—
Duodenal stump closure in gastric resections with a modified Furniss clamp. New Engl. J. Med., 214: 724–725, Apr. 9, 1936
INCISION—
Cutting the costal arch for upper abdominal exposure with H. L. Albright, S. G. O. 67: 804–809, Dec. 1938

TECHNIC—of jejunostomy.
Jejunostomy for postoperative feeding with L. M. Bell, Ann. Surg., 114: 462–471, Sept. 1941

Clute, R. See F. Albright

Clutton, Henry Hugh. London surgeon. 1850–1909
JOINTS—
Symmetrical synovitis of the knee in hereditary syphilis. Lancet, 1: 391–393, Feb. 27, 1886

Coates, J. C. See J. W. McLeod

Coats, George. London ophthalmologist. 1876–1915
DISEASE—retinitis exudative.
Forms of retinal disease with massive exudation. Ophth. Hosp. Rep., 17: 440–525, Tab. 12 and 13, 1908

Cobbold, Thomas, Spencer. English physician. 1826–1886
Most distinguished helminthologist of his time. Garrison and Morton
Entozoa. London, Groombridge, 1864

Cober, Tobias. German physician. d. ca. 1625
Noted relation between typhus fever (morbus Hungaricus) and pediculosis.
Observationum medicarum castrensium hungaricarum. Helmstadii, Lüderwald, 1685. pp. 49–51

Coburn, Alvin Frederick. New York physician. 1899–
Described "phase reaction" of rheumatic fever.
A precipitinogen in the serum prior to the onset of acute rheumatism with Ruth H. Pauli, J. exp. Med., 59: 143–162, Jan. 1, 1939
See also B. B. Brodie

Coca, Arthur Fernandez. New York bacteriologist 1875–
METHOD—of slide titration.
A slide method for titrating blood-grouping sera. J. Lab. clin. Med., 16: 405–407, Dec. 1931
TEST—compatibility, for direct matching of blood samples.
The examination of the blood preliminary to the operation of blood transfusion. J. Immunol., 3: 93–100, Jan. 1918

Cock, Edward. English surgeon. 1805–1892
OPERATION—urethrotomy by an incision along median line of perineum and taping urethra at apex of prostate.
A few words on the means to be adopted for establishing a communication between the bladder and the exterior of the body, when the urethra has become impermeable. The last resource available in certain cases. Guy's Hosp. Rep., 12: 267–275, 1866

Cockayne, Edward Alfred. English physician. 1880–
DISEASE—localized epidermolysis bullosa.
Recurrent bullous eruption of the feet. Brit. J. Dermat., 50: 358–362, July 1938

Cockburn, William. English physician. 1669–1739
REMEDY—for dysentery; secret.
Nature and cure of distempers of seafaring people. London, Newman, 1696

Cockcroft, W. H. See C. E. Dolman

Code, Charles Frederick. Rochester, Minn. physiologist. 1910–
PREPARATION—histamine-in-beeswax.
Chronic histamine action with R. L. Varco, Proc. Soc. exp. Biol., N. Y., 44: 475–477, 1940
Prolonged action of histamine with R. L. Varco, Amer. J. Physiol., 37: 225–233, Aug. 1942

Codivilla, Alessandro. Bologna surgeon. 1851–1913
Advocated skeletal traction.
On the means of lengthening, in the lower limbs, the muscles and tissues which are shortened through deformity. Amer. J. Orthop. Surg., 2: 353–369, Apr. 1905

Codman, Ernest Amory. Boston surgeon. 1869–1940
REGISTRY—
The registry of cases of bone sarcoma. S. G. O., 34: 335–343, Mar. 1922
Bone sarcoma, an interpretation of the nomenclature used by the Committee on the Registry of Bone Sarcoma of the American College of Surgeons. New York, Hoeber, 1925
TREATMENT—
Depressed fracture of the malar bone. A simple method of reduction. Boston M. and S. J., 162: 532 (only), Apr. 21, 1910
TREATMENT—of subacromial bursitis.
On stiff and painful shoulders. The anatomy of the subdeltoid or subacromial bursa and its clinical importance. Ibid., 154: 613–620, May 31, 1906
Bursitis subacromialis, or periarthritis of the shoulder-joint. (Subdeltoid bursitis.) Ibid., 159: 533–537, Oct. 22; 576–582, Oct. 29; 615–616, Nov. 5; 644–648, Nov. 12; 677–681, Nov. 19; 723–726, Nov. 26; 756–759, Dec. 3, 1908
TUMOR—
Epiphyseal chondromatous giant cell tumors of the upper end of the humerus. S. G. O., 52: 543–548, Feb. 15, 1931

Codnere, J. T. See F. S. Patch

Codronchi, Giovanni Battista. 1547–1628
Wrote on forensic medicine.
Methodus testificandi, inquibusvis casibus medicis oblatis. In his: *De vitiis vocis, libri duo.* Francofurti, Wecheli, 1597. pp. 148–232

Coenen, Hermann. Breslau surgeon. 1875–
PHENOMENON—of Henle-Coenen; if an aneurysmal sac still pulsates after ligation of the artery proximal to it, collateral circulation is sufficient to prevent gangrene.
Zur Indikationsstellung bei der Operation der Aneurysmen und bei den Gefässverletzungen. Zbl. Chir., 40: 1913–1916, Dec. 13, 1913

Coffey, J. R. See A. W. Adson

Coffey, Robert Calvin. Portland Ore. surgeon. 1869–1933
OPERATION—for carcinoma of rectum.
The major procedure first in the two-stage operation for relief of cancer of the rectum. Ann. Surg., 61: 446–450, Apr. 1915
Cancer of the rectum and rectosigmoid. Amer. J. Surg., 14: 161–214, Oct. 1931
Demonstrated importance of mucous membrane valve in uretero-intestinal anastomosis.
Physiological implantation of the severed ureter or common bile duct into the intestine. J. A. M. A., 56: 397–403, Feb. 11, 1911
Transplantation of ureters into the large intestine in the absence of a functioning urinary bladder. S. G. O., 32: 383–391, May 1921
Transplantation of the ureters into the large intestine. Ibid., 47: 593–621, Nov. 1928
Production of aseptic uretero-enterostomy by a suture transfixing the ureteral wall and the intestinal mucosa. J. A. M. A., 94: 1748–1750, May 31, 1930

Coffey, Walter Bernard. San Francisco surgeon 1868–1944
OPERATION—for angina pectoris.
Surgical treatment of angina pectoris: report of additional cases and review of literature. By P. K Brown and W. B. Coffey, Arch. intern. Med., 34 417–445, Oct. 1924
TREATMENT—for cancer.
Extract of adrenal cortex substance. Report of it preparations and use—with some clinical notes with J. D. Humber, California and West. Med., 33 640–652, Sept. 1930
Cancer studies in relation to results of treatment with an aqueous extract made from the cortex of the suprarenal gland: a five-year review on treatment results in inoperable and hopeless malignancies: report on 7,51 cases with J. D. Humber, Ibid., 44: 160–178, Mar 1936

Cogswell, Mason Fitch. American surgeon. 1761–1830
Ligated common carotid on Nov. 4, 1803.
Account of an operation for the extirpation of a tumor in which a ligature was applied to the carotid artery New Engl. J. Med. and Surg., 13: 357–360, 1824

Cohen, Barnett. American scientist. 1891–
METHOD—for determination of hemoglobin; acid hematin method.
The colorimetric determination of hemoglobin: a practical procedure with A. H. Smith, J. biol. Chem. 39: 489–496, Oct. 1919

Cohen, H. H. See F. H. Falls

Cohen, Harriet R. See T. Kuttner

Cohen, Henry. Liverpool biochemist. 1900–
METHOD—for determination of magnesium.
The magnesium content of the cerebro-spinal and other body fluids. Quart. J. Med., 20: 173–186, Jan. 1927

Cohen, I. See H. Neuhof

Cohen, J. See A. E. Sobel

Cohen, J. I. See G. Macgill

Cohen, Milton Bronner, Cleveland physician. 1894–
TEST—
The intracutaneous salt solution test: preliminary report of a simple method for determining the efficiency of the circulation in the extremities. J. A. M. A., 84: 1561–1562, May 23, 1925
See also W. G. Stern

Cohen, W. See L. M. Gompertz

Cohn, Ferdinand Julius. Breslau botanist. 1828–1898
LAW—specific forms of bacteria have a fixed and unchanging basis.
MEDIUM or SOLUTION—for cultivating bacteria.
Introduced morphological classification of bacteria.
Untersuchungen über Bacterien. Beitr. z. Biol. d. Pflanzen, 1, Heft 2, 127–224; Heft 3, 141–208, 1872; 2, Heft 2, 249–276, 1876
Ueber Bacterien, die kleinsten lebenden Wessen. Samml. gemeinvers. wiss. Vortr., No. 165, 1872
Also: in English Rochester, N. Y., Phinney, 1881. 10 pp.
Also: Bull. Hist. Med., 7: 49–92, Jan. 1939
Declared that animal and vegetable protoplasm are analogous, if not identical, substances.
Zur Naturgeschichte des Protococcus pluvialis. Breslau, 1850
Untersuchungen über die Entwicklungsgeschichte der mikroskopischen Algen und Pilzen. Bonn, 1853

Cohn, Hermann Ludwig. German oculist. 1838–1906

TEST—for color perception by use of variously colored embroidery patterns.
Studien über angeborene Farbenblindheit. Breslau, Morgenstern, 1879. 288 pp.
Advocated examination of eyes of school children.
Die Hygiene des Auges in den Schulen. Wien, Leipzig, Urban and Schwarzenberg, 1883
Die ärztliche Überwachung der Schulen zur Verhütung der Verbreitung der Kurzsichtigkeit. Arb. d. VII internat. Cong. f. Hyg. u. Demog., Wien, 1, Heft 12, 9–28, 1887–88

Cohn, M. See A. Ellinger

Cohnheim, Julius Friedrich. Berlin pathologist. 1839–1884

AREA—dark areas outlined by bright matter, seen on cross section of a muscle fiber.
Ueber den feineren Bau der quergestreiften Muskelfaser. Arch. f. path. Anat., 34: 606–622, 1865
THEORY—emigration of leukocytes is the essential feature of inflammation.
Ueber Entzündung und Eiterung. Arch. f. path. Anat., 40: 1–79 (52–57), 1867
Neue Untersuchungen über die Entzündung. Berlin, Hirschwald, 1873. 85 pp.
Also, transl. by A. B. McKee: *Lectures on general pathology.* London, New Sydenham Soc., 1889
THEORY—of embryonal rests as origin of tumors in general.
Vorlesungen über allgemeine Pathologie. Berlin, Hirschwald, 1877. 2 vols. 1: 622–691
Also, transl. by A. B. McKee: *Lectures on general pathology.* London, New Sydenham Soc., 1889. 2: 746–820
Investigated sugar-forming ferments of salivary glands and pancreas.
Zur Kenntniss der zuckerbildenden Fermente. Arch. f. path. Anat., 28: 241–253, 1863
Described and named pseudoleukemia.
Ein Fall von Pseudoleukämie. Ibid., 33: 451–454, July 1865
Wrote on ʾinfarction.
Untersuchungen über die embolischen Processe. Berlin, Hirschwald, 1872
Proved infectiousness of tuberculosis by inoculating rabbits with tuberculous material.
Die Tuberkulose vom Standpunkte der Infectionslehre. Leipzig, Edelmann, 1880. 44 pp.
Also, English transl. by D. H. Cullimore London, Ballière, 1880

Coindet, Jean Francois. Swiss physician. 1774–1834
Showed value of iodine in thyroid disorders.
Découverte d'un nouveau remède contre le goitre. Ann. d. chim. et phys., Paris, 15: 49–59, 1820

Coiter, Volcher. Groningen anatomist. 1534–1600?
Investigated formation and growth of bones (1566), comparative osteology of animals (1575) and of children, described muscles of nose and eyelids, and experimented on decapitated animals with remarkable intelligence. Garrison
Tabulae externarum partium humani corporis. Bononiae, apud A. Benaccium, 1564
De ossibus et cartilaginibus corporis humani tabulae. Bononiae, apud J. Bossium, 1566
Externarum et internarum principalium humani

corporis partium tabulae. . . . Noribergae, T. Gerlatzeni, 1573. 133 pp.
Diversorum animalium sceletorum explicationes. Noribergae, Gerlachii, 1575

Coke, Frank. English physician
REACTION—cutaneous protein, for hay-fever and asthma.
Asthma and anaphylaxis. Brit. med. J., 1: 372–376, Mar. 12, 1921
Colds and hay fever. London, Baillière, 1933. 148 pp.

Coke, Harry. London scientist
INDEX—dispersion; of blood serum, an aid to diagnosis of malignancy.
A brief preliminary report on the lipoid-globulin cholesterol ratios in cancer. J. State Med., 41: 105–115, Feb. 1933

Cole, Harold Harrison. American physiologist. 1897–
METHOD—of extraction of gonadotrophic substance.
The potency of blood serum of mares in progressive stages of pregnancy in effecting the sexual maturity of the immature rat with G. H. Hart, Amer. J. Physiol., 93: 57–68, May 1930

Cole, Lewis Gregory. New York roentgenologist, 1874–
SIGN—deformity of duodenum indicates ulcers
Motor phenomena of the stomach, pylorus and cap observed Roentgenographically. Amer. J. Physiol. 42: 618–619, Mar. 1, 1917

Cole, Rufus Ivory. Baltimore physician. 1872–
Produced a serum specific to human platelets by injecting an animal with emulsion of human blood platelets.
Note on the production of an agglutinating serum for blood platelets. Johns Hopk. Hosp. Bull., 18: 261–262, June–July 1907
Differentiated various types of pneumococci.
Treatment of pneumonia by means of specific serums. J. A. M. A., 61: 663–666, Aug. 30, 1913
See also O. T. Avery

Cole, Sydney William. English physiologist. 1877–
SOLUTION—trypsinized casein; culture medium.
On a substitute for peptone and a standard nutrient medium for bacteriological purposes with H. Onslow, Lancet, 2: 9–11, July 1, 1916
TEST—for glucose.
The detection of small amounts of glucose in urine. Ibid., 2: 859–860, Sept. 20, 1913
TEST—for lactose.
The estimation of lactose and glucose by the copper-iodide method. Biochem. J., 8: 134–142, 1914
See also F. G. Hopkins

Cole, William Harder. American physiologist. 1892–
METHOD—for detection of chloroform in tissues.
The pyridine test as a quantitative method for the estimation of minute amounts of chloroform. J. biol. Chem., 71: 173–180, Dec. 1926
See also E. A. Graham

Cole, Wyman Charles Corydon. Detroit pediatrician. 1893–
METHOD—
Intraperitoneal blood transfusion: report of two hundred and thirty-seven transfusions on one hundred and seventeen patients in private practice with J. C. Montgomery, Amer. J. Dis. Child., 37: 497–510, Mar. 1929

Colebrook, Leonard. English physician

TREATMENT—
Treatment of human puerperal infections, and of experimental infections in mice, with prontosil with Méave Kenny, Lancet, 1: 1279–1286, June 6, 1936
See A. E. Wright

Coleman, Claude C. Richmond, Va. neurosurgeon. 1879–
SYNDROME—cervical spine trauma associated with injury of head and shoulder girdle.
Treatment of fracture-dislocation of the spine associated with cord injury with J. M. Meredith, J. A. M. A., 111: 2168–2172, Dec. 10, 1938

Coleman, G. H. See J. A. Capps

Colman, Katherine R. See A. R. Rose

Coleman, Marion B. See A. B. Wadsworth

Coleman, Warren, New York physician. 1869–
METHOD—of blood culture for typhoid bacilli.
The bacteriology of the blood in typhoid fever. An analysis of 1602 cases with B. H. Buxton, Amer. J. med. Sci., 133: 896–903, June 1907
See also P. A. Shaffer

Coley, B. L. See Helen Q. Woodard

Coley, William Bradley. New York surgeon. 1862–1936
FLUID or MIXTURE or SERUM or TOXIN or TREATMENT—for inoperable sarcoma.
Contribution to the knowledge of sarcoma. Ann. Surg., 14: 199–220, Sept. 1891
The treatment of malignant tumors by repeated inoculations of erysipelas: with a report of ten original cases. Amer. J. med. Sci., 105: 487–511, May 1893
OPERATION—
The radical cure of femoral hernia. Ann. Surg., 44: 519–528, Oct. 1906
Reported tuberculosis of clavicle.
Tubercular osteitis of the clavicle simulating malignant disease; operation; recovery. New York Med. J., 54: 230, Aug. 29, 1891

Collens, William S. Brooklyn physician. 1897–
TEST—venous filling time.
Two quantitative tests of peripheral vascular obstruction with N. D. Wilensky, Amer. J. Surg., 34: 71 (only), Oct. 1936
Peripheral vascular diseases with N. D. Wilensky, Springfield, Ill., Thomas, 1939. 243 pp. p. 27

Coller, Frederick Amasa. Ann Arbor, Mich. surgeon. 1887–
CLINICAL RULE—
The replacement of sodium chloride in surgical patients with R. M. Bartlett, D. L. C. Bingham, W. G. Maddock and S. Pedersen, Ann. Surg., 108: 769–782, Oct. 1938
Postoperative salt intolerance with K. N. Campbell, H. N. Vaughan and L. Vivian Iob, Ibid., 119: 533–542, Apr. 1944
METHOD—
The delayed closure of contaminated wounds. A preliminary report with W. L. Valk, Ibid., 112: 256–270, Aug. 1940
Did important work on water needs of patient.
Dehydration attendant on surgical operations with W. G. Maddock, J. A. M. A., 99: 875–880, Sept. 10, 1932
Water balance in surgery patients. Editorial, S. G. O., 59: 115–116, July 1934
See also W. G. Maddock

Colles, Abraham. Dublin surgeon. 1773–1843
FASCIA—deep layer of superficial perineal f.
LIGAMENT—reflected inguinal l.
SPACE—under perineal fascia.
Anatomy of the perineum. In: *A treatise on surgical anatomy.* Dublin, Gilbert and Hodges, 1811. pp. 174–180
Also: Med. Classics, 4: 1033–1037, June 1940
FRACTURE—
On a fracture of the carpal extremity of the radius Edinburgh Med. and Surg. J., 10: 182–186, 1814
Also: *The works of . . .* London, New Sydenham Soc. 1881. p. 411
Also: Med. Classics, 4: 1038–1042, June 1940
LAW or IMMUNITY—a child that is affected with congenital syphilis, its mother showing no signs of the disease, will not infect its mother. (Obsolete)
Syphilis in infants. Chapt. 14 of: *Practical observations on the venereal disease.* London, Sherwood et al. 1837. pp. 173–177
Also: Philadelphia, Waldie, 1837
Also, in German, Hamburg, 1839
Also: Med. Classics, 4: 1073–1080, June 1940
Tied the subclavan artery in 1811 and in 1813.
On the operation of tying the subclavian artery. Edinburgh, Med. and Surg. J., 11: 1–25, 1815
Also: *The works of . . .* London, New Sydenham Soc. 1881, pp. 337–366
Also: Med. Classics, 4: 1043–1072, June 1940

Collet, J. Thomas. French physician
SYNDROME—myosis, enophthalmos, sweating and combined paralyses.
De la myopie et de la presbyopie; des véritables modifications oculaires qui les déterminent. Paris, 1853 99 pp.

Collier, J. See J. S. R. Russell

Collip, James Bertram. Canadian biochemist. 1892–
EMMENIN—
The chemical nature of emmenin with J. S. L. Browne and D. L. Thomson, Endocrinology, 18: 71–74, Jan.–Feb. 1934
FACTOR—A. P. L.: anterior-pituitary-like.
The ovary-stimulating hormone of the placenta. Preliminary paper. Canad. med. Ass. J., 22: 215–219, Feb.; 761–774, June 1930
Improved insulin.
The original method as used for the isolation of insulin in semipure form for the treatment of the first clinical cases. J. biol. Chem., 55: XL–XLI, Feb. 1923
Treated tetany with parathyroid hormone.
A case of tetany treated with parathyrin with D. B. Leitch, Canad. med. Ass. J., 15: 59–60, Jan. 1925
Isolated parathyroid hormone.
The extraction of a parathyroid hormone which will prevent or control parathyroid tetany and which regulates the level of blood calcium. J. Biol. Chem., 63: 395–438, Mar. 1925
Further studies on the physiological action of a parathyroid hormone with E. P. Clark, Ibid., 64: 485–507, June 1925
See also E. P. Clark

Colman, W. S. See V. A. H. Horsley

Colombo
FEVER—resembling paratyphoid fever, occurring in Colombo, Ceylon.

Colonna, Paul Crenshaw. American surgeon. 1892–

OPERATION—
A new type of reconstruction operation for old un-
united fracture of the neck of the femur. J. Bone and
Joint. Surg., 17: 110–122, Jan. 1935

Colp, Ralph. New York surgeon. 1893–
Described a form of granulomatous, ulcerating and
stenosing terminal ileitis.
A case of nonspecific granuloma of the terminal ileum
and the cecum. Surg. Clin. N. Amer., 14: 443–449,
Apr. 1934

Colston, John Archibald Campbell. Baltimore
urologist, 1886–
OPERATION—excision of entire upper urinary tract
by electrocautery knife for carcinoma of kidney.
Complete nephroureterectomy; a new method employing the principle of electro-coagulation to the intramural
portion of the ureter. J. Urol., 33: 110–137, Feb. 1935
See also J. E. Dees

Combe, James Scarfe. Scottish physician. 1796–1833
Described condition now known as Addison's dis-
ease.
History of a case of anaemia. Trans. Med.-Chir. Soc.
Edinburgh, 1: 194-204, 1824

Côme, Frère. (Jean Baseilhac). 1703–1781
Devised several new instruments for use in suprapubic lithotomy. Garrison and Morton
Nouvelle méthode d'extraire la pierre de la vessie
urinaire. Paris, Houry, 1779

Comolli, Antonio. Modena, Italy pathologist. 1879–
SIGN—triangular swelling corresponding to outline of
scapula, in fractures of that bone.
Ueber ein deutliches Zeichen bei gewissen Schulter-
blattbrüchen. Zbl. Chir., 59: 937–940, Apr. 9, 1932

Concato, Luigi Maria. Italian physician. 1825–1882
DISEASE—tuberculous inflammation of serous mem-
branes.
Sulla poliorromennite scrofolosa o tisi delle sierose.
G. ingern. d. sci. med. Napoli, n.s., 3: 1037–1053,
1881

Condamin, René. Lyon surgeon. 1863–
OPERATION—for umbilical hernia.
De l'omphalectmie et de la suture à trois étages dans
la cure radicale de hernies ombilicales. Étude des
indications et de quelques procédés operatoires récents.
Arch. prov. de chir., 1: 193–221, Sept. 1892

Condy, Henry Bollman. English physician
FLUID—a disinfecting solution of sodium and potas-
sium permanganates.
On the purification of water and air, and the use of the
alkaline permanganates as purifying agents. London,
Davies, 1862. 16 pp.

Cone, W. See W. G. Penfield

Conn, Harold Joel. American scientist. 1886–
SOLUTION—glycerol ammonium chloride—for cul-
tivation of actinomycetes.
The use of various culture media in characterizing ac-
tinomycetes. New York Agri. Exp. Sta., Geneva,
N. Y. Tech. Bull., No. 83, 1921. pp. 26, p. 7

Conn, Harold Russell. Akron, Ohio surgeon. 1889–
OPERATION—
A new method of operative reduction for congenital
luxation of the patella. J. Bone and Joint Surg., 23:
370–383, Apr. 1925

Connell, F. Gregory. Oshkosh, Wis. surgeon. 1864–
OPERATION—
Fundusectomy: a new principle in the treatment of

gastric and duodenal ulcer. S. G. O., 49: 696–701,
Nov. 1929
SUTURE—
Intestinal suture, all knots inside. Medicine, 7: 277–
294, Apr. 1901

Connell, J. T. See C. C. Warden

Connell, Karl Albert. New York physician. 1878–
1941
REBREATHING TUBE—
An apparatus—anaesthetometer—for measuring and
mixing anaesthetic and other vapors and gases.
S. G. O., 17: 245–255, Aug. 1913

Connell, M. E. Milwaukee surgeon
METHOD or SUTURE—
An experimental contribution looking to an improved
technique in enterorrhaphy, whereby the number of
knots is reduced to two, or even one. This suture is
applicable in pylorectomy, gastroenterostomy, anastomosis, circular and oblique enterorrhaphy. Med. Rec.,
42: 335–337, Sept. 17, 1892

Conner, Lewis Atterbury. American physician. 1867–
METHOD—of aspiration of pericardium.
On the diagnosis of pericardial effusion with special
reference to physical signs on the posterior aspect of
the thorax. Amer. Heart J., 1: 421–433, Apr. 1926

Connor, Charles Lloyd. American pathologist. 1891–
METHOD—
Studies on lipochromes: III. The quantitative estimation of carotin in blood and tissues. J. biol. Chem., 77:
619–626, May 1928

Connors, John Fox. New York surgeon. 1873–1935
TREATMENT—
Treatment of lung abscess and emphyema by packing.
Ann. Surg., 94: 38–54, July 1931
TREATMENT—of penetrating wound of chest by
drawing lung into wound and suturing it there.
Penetrating stab wounds and bullet wounds of the
chest . . . with J. B. Stenbuck, Ibid., 97: 528–546,
Apr. 1933
TREATMENT—conservative, of fractures of skull.
Fractures of the skull with L. T. Wright, Ibid., 100:
996–1007, Nov. 1934

Conolly, John. English alienist, 1795–1866
SYSTEM—of non-restraint for treating insane.
Treatment of the insane without mechanical restraints.
London, Smith, Elder, 1856. 380 pp.

Conor, Alfred. French physician. 1870–
Described fièvre boutonneuse, a form of typhus in
Tunisia.
Un fievre éruptive observée en Tunisie with A. Bruch,
Bull. Soc. Path. Exot., Paris, 3: 492–496, 1910

Conradi, Heinrich. German bacteriologist, 1876–
MEDIUM—for typhoid bacilli: see also Drigalski-
Conradi m.
Ein Verfahren zum Nachweis der Typhus-erreger im
Blut. Dtsch. med. Wschr., 32: 58–61, Jan. 11, 1906
See also K. W. von Drigalski

Conseil, E. See C. J. H. Nicolle

Contamin, Antoine. French physician. 1883–
Radiated tumor cells as a means of stimulating im-
munity to tumor growth.
Rayons X et cancer expérimental de la souris. Bull.
Ass. franc. p. l'étude du cancer, 3: 160–168, Apr.18,
1910

Contargiris, Athanase. Athens, Greece surgeon.
1892–

OPERATION—
Correction of drop-foot by the posterior arthrodesis.
J. Bone and Joint Surg., 13: 54–57, Jan. 1931
Contino, A. Italian ophthalmologist
EPITHELIOMA—of conjunctiva.
Neue Beobachtungen und Untersuchungen über die Papillome des Limbus und der Hornhaut. Arch. f. Augenheilk., 68: 366–413, Apr. 1911
GLAUCOMA—
Del glaucoma anteriore emorragico. Ann. ottalm., 64: 433–436, July 1936
Conwell, H. Earle. Fairfield, Ala. surgeon. 1893–
TECHNIC—for strapping for fracture of clavicle.
Fractures of the clavicle: a simple fixation dressing, with a summary of the treatment and results attained in ninety-two cases. J. A. M. A., 90: 838–839, Mar. 17, 1928
Cook, A. See J. Barcroft
Cook, Henry Wireman. Baltimore physician. 1877–1940
MODIFICATION—of Riva-Rocci sphygmomanometer.
Blood pressure determinations in general practice, introducing a practical instrument for routine use. J. A. M. A., 40: 1199–1202, May 2, 1903
Cook, J. W. See G. Barry
Cook, James. English mariner. 1728–1779
Demonstrated that in long voyages scurvy could be prevented by employment of certain articles in diet, as suggested by Lind.
The method taken for preserving the health of the crew of H. M. S. The Resolution during her late voyage round the world. Philos. Trans., London, 66: 402–406, 1776
Cooke, C. See H. Southworth
Cooke, Jean Valjean. St. Louis pediatrician. 1883–
METHOD—
A simple clinical method for the assay of penicillin in body fluids and for the testing of penicillin sensitivity of bacteria. J. A. M. A., 127: 445–449, Feb. 24, 1945
Cooke, Wiliam Ernest. English physician
MODIFICATION—of the neutrophil nuclear count.
WEIGHTED MEAN OF—Cooke and Ponder.
The polynuclear count; the nucleus of the neutrophil polymorphonuclear leucocyte in health and disease, with some observations on the macropolycyte with E. Ponder, London, Griffin, 1927. 79 pp.
Cooley, Thomas Benton. Detroit pediatrician. 1871–1945
ANEMIA—"erythroblastic" or Mediterranean disease (thalassemia).
Anemia in children with splenomegaly and peculiar changes in the bones: report of cases with E. R. Witwer and Pearl Lee, Amer. J. Dis. Child., 34: 347–363 Sept. 1927
Erythroblastic anemia: additional comments with Pearl Lee, Ibid., 43: 705–708, Mar. 1932
Coolidge, William David. American scientist. 1873
TUBE—x-ray t.
A powerful roentgen ray tube with a pure electron discharge. Phys. Rev., 2: 409, 1913
Also: Amer. J. Roentgenol., n.s. 1: 115–124, Jan. 1914
See also A. Knudson
Cooper, Sir Astley Paston. English surgeon. 1768–1841
DISEASE—chronic cystic d. of breast.

IRRITABLE BREAST—neuralgia in breast. Described a relationship between conditions of pelvic organs and breast diseases.
Illustrations of the diseases of the breast. London, Longman, 1829
Also in: *Lectures . . .* 1831, vol. 2, lecture 20, p. 125
FASCIA—f. transversalis.
HERNIA—retroperitoneal h.
LIGAMENT—a fold of fascia transversalis attached to iliopectineal eminence and pubic spine.
TENDON—a semilunar extension of anterior aponeurosis of transversalis fascia.
The anatomy and surgical treatment of internal and congenital hernia. London, Longman, 1804
Same, 2 ed., London, Longman, 1827
Same, Amer. ed., Philadelphia, Lea and Blanchard, 1844
OPERATION—tying external iliac artery: performed in 1808.
Case of femoral aneurism, for which the external iliac artery was tied by Sir A. Cooper, Br., with an account of the preparation of the limb, dissected at the expiration of eighteen years. Taken from Sir Astley Cooper's notes. Guy's Hosp. Rep., 1: 43–52, 1836
TESTICLE—irritable t.; neuralgia.
Observations on the structure and diseases of the testis. London, Longman, 1830
Performed myringotomy.
Observations on the effects which take place from the destruction of the membrana tympani of the ear. Philos. Trans., 1800
Farther observations on the effects which take place from the destruction of the membrana tympani of the ear; with an account of an operation for the removal o. a particular species of deafness. Ibid., 91: 435–450 1801
Ligated abdominal aorta.
Case of ligature of the aorta (1817). Surgical essays London, 1818. Pt. 1, pp. 101–130
Published book on treatment of fractures and dislocations.
A treatise on dislocations and fractures of the joints London, 1823. 2 ed., 1824. 3 ed.
Ligated, successfully, the common carotid artery, in 1808.
A case of aneurism of the carotid artery. Med.-chir Trans., London, 1: 1–12; 222–233, 1809
An account of the first successful operation, performe on the common carotid artery, for aneurism, in th year 1808: with the post-mortem examination, in 1821 From the notes of Sir Astley Cooper, Bart. Guy' Hosp. Rep., 1: 53–58, 1836
Some experiments and observations on tying the ca rotid and vertebral arteries, and the pneumo-gastric phrenic and sympathetic nerves. Ibid., 457–475; 65
Cooper, C. See T. D. Spies
Cooper, G. A. See O. H. Foerster
Cooper, Georgia. See C. Krumwiede
Cooper, William Morris. New York surgeon. 1894
TECHNIC—
The treatment of varicose veins: a study based upon series of more than 35,000 injections of various scleros ing solutions given on 3,164 cases, and 293 cases o extensive and recurrent varisose veins treated by pre liminary ambulatory ligation and subsequent inje tions. Ann. Surg., 99: 799–805, May 1934

Coopernail, George Peter. Bedford, N. Y. surgeon. 1876–
OPERATION—
Femoral hernia. Amer. J. Surg., 22: 458–460, Dec. 1933
SIGN—ecchymosis in perineum, scrotum or labia.
A sign in fracture of the pelvis. Med. Rec., 89: 417 (only), Mar. 4, 1916
Cope, O. See E. D. Churchill
Cope, Vincent Zachary. English surgeon. 1881–
SIGN—of appendicitis: if appendix is in proximity to psoas muscle, pain will be caused by extending the thigh.
The early diagnosis of the acute abdomen. London, Oxford Press, 1928. 5 ed., p. 43
TEST—thigh rotation causes increased pain in acute appendicitis if inflamed appendix is adherent to fascia over obturator internus muscle.
The thigh-rotation or obturator test: a new sign in some inflammatory conditions. Brit. J. Surg., 7 : 537 (only), Apr. 1920
Copher, G. H. See E. A. Graham
Copland, James. English physician. 1791–1870
Discriminated between inflammation of cecum, appendix and pericecal tissue.
Cecum. In his: *A dictionary of practical medicine . . .* London, (1832)—58. 3 vols.
Corbus, Budd Clarke. Chicago urologist. 1876–
FILTRATE—gonococcus bouillon.
Intradermal injections of gonococcal bouillon filtrate with V. J. O'Connor, J. Urol., 24: 333–342, Sept. 1930
Intradermal immunization in gonorrhea: an experimental clinical report. J. A. M. A., 98: 532–537, Feb. 13, 1932
TEST—
A skin test for diagnosis of gonococcus infections. J. Urol., 35: 112–125, Jan. 1936
Corcoran, Arthur Curtis. Indianapolis physician. 1909–
METHOD—of Corcorand and Page, of determination of diodrast-iodine in plasma and urine.
Effects of hypotension due to hemorrhage and of blood transfusion on renal fuiction in dogs with I. H. Page, J. exp. Med., 78: 205–224, Sept. 1, 1943
METHOD—of Corcoran and Page, of determination of inulin.
Applications of diphenylamine in the determination of levulose in biological media. I. The determination of inulin. II. The determination of levulose in small amounts of blood with I. H. Page, J. biol. Chem., 127: 601–608, Mar. 1939
Cords, Richard. Cologne ophthalmologist. 1881–
ANGIOPATHIA RETINAE JUVENILIS—
Papillitis und Glaukom. Zugleich ein Beitrag zur juvenilen Phlebitis der Zentralvene. Arch. f. Ophthal., 105: 916–963, 1921
APPARATUS—for recording eye movements.
Über Hebelnystagmographie. Ibid., 118: 771–784, Aug. 20, 1927
Cordus, Valerius. 1515–1544
Published early pharmacopoeia.
Pharmacorum conficiendorum ratio, vulgo vocant dispensatorium. Norimbergae, Petreius, 1540? 535 pp.
Corelli, Humberto Horacio. Buenos Aires physician. 1882–
Introduced perirenal insufflation.

Un nuevo procedimiento para explorar el rinon with E. Sordelli, Rev. Asoc. méd. Argentina, 34: 424, June 1921
Sur le pneumopéritoine et sur une méthode personnelle pour voir le rein sans pneumopéritoine. Bull. Soc. méd. Hôp., Paris, 65: 1409–1412, Oct. 28, 1921
Coriat, Isador Henry. Boston neurologist. 1875–
METHOD—of testing for apraxia.
The clinical tests for apraxia and their value in the diagnosis of brain disease. Boston Med. and Surg. J., 165: 89–92, July 20, 1911
Cornaro, Luigi. Venetian gentleman. 1467–1566
Author of "the best treatise on personal hygiene and the simple life." Garrison
Trattato de la vita sobria. Padova, Perchacino, 1558
Also: *The art of living long.* Milwaukee, Butler, 1916. 214 pp.
Cornell, Virgil Heath. American pathologist. 1890–
TEST—
A simple field test to detect quinine in urine with S. Kaye, Military Surg., 93: 133–134, Aug. 1943
Corner, George Washington. American anatomist. 1889–
Produced crude extract containing hormone progesterone and established the quantitative test.
Physiology of the corpus luteum: II. Production of a special uterine reaction (progestational proliferation) by extracts of the corpus luteum. Amer. J. Physiol., 88: 326–339, Mar. 1929
See also W. M. Allen
Corning, James Leonard. New York neurologist. 1855–1923
ANESTHESIA or METHOD—local anesthesia followed by application of an Esmarch bandage.
On the prolongation of the anesthetic effects of the hydrochlorate of cocaine when subcutaneously injected; an experimental study. New York Med. J., 43: 317–319, Sept. 19, 1885
Local anesthesia in general medicine and surgery. New York, 1886
ANESTHESIA or METHOD—spinal anesthesia.
PUNCTURE—tapping of spinal membranes to obtain cerebospinal fluid.
Spinal anesthesia and local medication of the cord. New York Med. J., 42: 483–485, Oct. 31, 1885
A further contribution on local medication of the spinal cord with cases. Med. Rec., 33: 291–293, Mar. 17, 1888
Corper, Harry John. American pathologist. 1884–
AGAR—basal ammonium phosphate; for cultivation of tubercle bacilli.
The cultivation of recently isolated and laboratory strains of human tubercle bacilli on artificial media. Amer. Rev. Tuberc., 3: 461–472, Oct. 1919
MEDIUM—
The certified diagnosis of tuberculosis: practical evaluation of a new method for cultivating tubercle bacilli for diagnostic purposes. J. A. M. A., 91: 371–374, Aug. 11, 1928
Correll, John Trumbull. Kalamazoo biochemist. 1909–
Reported—
Certain properties of a new physiologically absorbable sponage with E. C. Wise, Proc. Soc. exp. Biol., N. Y., 58: 233–235, Mar. 1945
Correns, Carl Franz Joseph Erich. German physician. 1864–1934

Rediscovered, with Tschermak, Mendel's principle of heredity.

Bestimmung, Vererbung und Verteilung des Geschlechtes bei den höheren Pflanzen. Berlin, Bornträger, 1928. 138 pp.

Corrigan, Sir Dominic John. Dublin physician. 1802–1880

CIRRHOSIS—of lungs or fibroid phthisis.

On cirrhosis of the lungs. Dublin J. Med. Sci., 13: 266–286, 1838

DISEASE—aortic incompetency or regurgitation; called "maladie de Corrigan" by Trousseau.

PULSE or SIGN—water-hammer pulse, a jerky pulse with a full expansion, followed by a sudden collapse, occurring in aortic regurgitation.

On permanent patency of the mouth of the aorta or inadequacy of the aortic valve. Edinburgh M. and S. J., 37: 225–245, 1832

Also: Med. Classics, 1: 701–727, Feb. 1937

Also: F. A. Willius and T. E. Keys' *Cardiac Classics.* St. Louis, Mosby, 1941. pp. 422–440

LINE—a purple line at junction of teeth and gum in chronic copper-poisoning. (Dorland)

Cases of slow copper poisoning, with observations. Dublin Hosp. Gaz., 1: 229–232, 1854

SIGN—expanding pulsation indicative of aneurysm of abdominal aorta.

Aneurism of the aorta; singular pulsation of the arteries, necessity of the employment of the stethoscope. Lancet, 1: 586–590, 1829

Also: Med. Classics, 1: 689–699, Feb. 1937

Corson, W. C. See R. A. Phillips

Corti, (Alphonso) Marchese. Italian anatomist. 1822–1888

ARCHES—made up of rods of Corti.

CANAL—space between outer and inner rods.

CELLS—hair-cells on outer surface of organ of Corti.

GANGLION—spiral g.: sending filaments to organ of Corti.

MEMBRANE—over organ of Corti.

ORGAN—terminal acoustic apparatus within scala media, including rods of Corti and auditory cells.

RODS—forming the arches.

TUNNEL—same as canal.

Recherches sur l'organe de l'ouie des mammifères. Z. wiss. Zool., Leipzig, 3: 109–169, 1851

Corvisart des Marets, Baron Jean Nicholas de. French physician. 1755–1821

DISEASE—chronic hypertrophic myocarditis.

FACIES—characteristic of cardiac insufficiency.

Distinguished between functional and organic heart disease, and between hypertrophy and dilatation of the heart.

Essai sur les maladies et les lésions organiques du coeur et des gros vaisseaux; extrait des leçons cliniques. Paris, Migneret, 1806. 484 pp. p. 56

Also, transl. by J. Gates. Philadelphia, Finley, 1812. 344 pp.

Also, in German. Berlin, Rintel, 1814. p. 90

Also, abstr.: F. H. Willius and T. E. Keys' *Cardiac classics.* St. Louis, Mosby, 1841. pp. 281–290

Corvisart, Lucien R. F. E. (le baron). French physician. 1824–

Proposed name tetany.

De la contracture des extrémités ou tétanies. Paris, 1852. 108 pp.

Showed that proteids are converted by pancreatic juice into ordinary digestive products.

Collection de mémoires sur une fonction peu connue du pancréas, la digestion des aliments azotés. Paris, Masson, 1857–63. 10 pts.

Costa, S. French physician

AGAR—gum infusion, for isolation of gonococcus

Milieu non albumineux pour l'isolement, la culture et la conservation du gonocoque with L. Boyer, C. R. Soc. Biol., 87: 856–858, Sept. 15, 1922

Costello, William Birmingham. English surgeon. 1800–1867

Suggested possibility of etiologic relationship between chronic bone disease and formation of urinary calculi.

Lithotrity. Case of stone in the bladder, from injury to the loins.—Meningitis. Lancet, 2: 109–110, 1832

Cotard, Jules. French neurologist. 1840–1887

SYNDROME—paronia with delusions of negation, a suicidal tendency and sensory disturbances.

Du délire hypochondriaque dans une forme grave de la mélancolie auxieuse. Ann. méd.-psych., Paris, 6 s., 4: 168–174, 1880

Cotte, Gaston. Lyon surgeon. 1879–

OPERATION—presacral neurectomy.

La sympathectomie hypogastrique a-t-elle sa place dans la therapeutique gynécologique? Pr. méd., 33: 98–99, Jan. 24, 1925

Cottet, Jean. See E. Chabrol

Cottet, Jules. French physician

INDEX—of kidney function.

Contribution à l'étude clinique du rapport uréique hémato-urinaire. Pr. méd., 42: 762–765, May 12, 1934

Cotting, Benjamin Eddy. American surgeon. 1812–1898

OPERATION—for ingrowing toe-nail.

A few fragmentary remarks on the radical relief of infleshed toe-nail. Boston M. and S. J., 116: 324–325, Apr. 7, 1887

Cottle, E. Wyndham. London physician. ?–1919

Described angiokeratoma, "Mibelli's disease."

Warty growths. St. George Hosp. Rep., 9: 753–762, (758), 1877–78.

Cotton, Frederic Jay. Boston surgeon. 1869–1938

APPARATUS—

Nitrous oxide-oxygen-ether anesthesia: notes on administration; a perfected apparatus with W. M. Boothby; S. G. O., 15: 281–289, Sept. 1912

FRACTURE—

"Fender fracture" of the tibia at the knee with R. Berg, New Engl. J. Med., 201: 989–995, Nov. 14, 1929

METHOD—of impacting fracture of neck of femur.

Artificial impaction of hip fracture. Ann. Surg., 63: 366–371, Mar. 1916

OPERATION—for stabilization of knee joint.

Artificial ligaments at the knee. A technique with G. M. Morrison, New Engl. J. Med., 210: 1331–1332, June 21, 1934

POSITION—in treatment of Colles' fracture: hand flexed and adducted.

Adequate reduction and care in Colles's fracture. New Method. Boston M. and S. J., 181: 651–656, Dec. 4, 1919

TREATMENT—of fractured os calcis by impaction

Os calcis fracture. Ann. Surg., 64: 480–486, Oct. 191

Cotton, Richard Payne. English physician. 1820–1877

Described paroxysmal tachycardia.

Notes and observations upon a case of unusually rapid action of the heart (232 per minute). Brit. med. J., 1: 629–630, 1867

Cotton, T. See T. Lewis

Cutugno, Dominico. See Dominicus Cotunnius

Co-Tui, Frank Wang. New York surgeon. 1895–
SIGN—
Umbilical displacement and deviation of linea alba in acute abdominal conditions with J. Meyer, J. A. M. A., 90: 1779 (only), June 2, 1928
TREATMENT—
Kaolin in treatment of external gastrointestinal fistulas. Ann. Surg., 91: 123–125, Jan. 1930
The excoriations around external gastro-intestinal fistulae: experimental studies on their eticlogy and further experience with the kaolin powder treatment. Ibid., 98: 242–248, Aug. 1933

Cotunnius, Dominicus. Italian anatomist. 1736–1822
AQUEDUCT, CANAL or RECUSSUS—of the vestibule.
NERVE—nasopalatine n.
SPACE—within the membranous labyrinth.
De aqueductibus aurius humanae internae. Neapoli, 1760
Same. Viennae, Graeffer, 1774. 187 pp.
Also: *Opuscula medica.* Neapoli, ex off. Biblio. et Typo., 1826–27. 2 vols.
Also: *Opera posthuma.* ed. by P. Ruggiero Neapoli, typis Tramater, 1830–33. 4 vols.
DISEASE—sciatica.
Originated terms "ischias" and "sciatica." Described acute nephritis with anasarca and albumin in urine. W. Dock
De ischiade nervosa commentarius. Neopoli, apud Fratres Simonis, 1764
Also: Vienna, Graeffer, 1770
Also: *A treatise on the nervous sciatica, or, nervous hip gout.* London, printed for J. Wilkie, 1775
Also, in German, Leipzig, 1792

Coué, Emile. French physician. 1857–1926
Teacher of auto-suggestion.
Self mastery through conscious auto-suggestion. London, Allen and Unwin, 1922. 92 pp.

Coulon, A. de. See A. Borrel

Councilman, William Thomas. American physician. 1854–1933
Introduced term "amebic dysentery."
Amoebic dysentery with H. A. Lafleur, Johns Hopk. Hosp. Rep., 2: 395–548, Dec. 1891

Counseller, V. S. See H. Cabot, J. R. Learmonth

Couret, Maurice John. New Orleans pathologist. 1874–
AGAR—autolyzed tissue, for cultivation of amoebae.
The cultivation of amoebae in pure culture upon autolyzed tissues with J. Walker, J. exp. Med., 18: 252–258, Sept. 1913

Cournand, Andre. New York physician. 1895–
TECHNIQUE—
Catherization of the right auricle in man with H. A. Ranges, Proc. Soc. exp. Biol., N. Y., 46: 462–466, Apr. 1941

Courtois, Adolph. French neurologist. 1903–

SIGN—
Sur un syndrome comitio-parkinsonien: étude anatomo-clinique. Paris, 1928. 97 pp.

Courtois, Bernard. French physician. 1777–1838
Discovered and isolated iodine.
Découverte d'une substance nouvelle dans le vareck. Ann. Chim., Paris, 88: 304–310, 1813

Courtois, M. L. Heus. French surgeon
PUMP—
Mémoire sur les asphyxies (a), avec la description d'un nouvel instrument propre a rappeler le méchanisme de la respiration. J. de Méd., Chir., Pharm., 82: 361–377, Mar. 1790

Courvoisier, Ludwig J. Basel surgeon. 1843–1918
LAW or SIGN or SYNDROME—a much distended gall bladder from obstruction of common duct indicated tumor rather than calculus.
Casuistisch-Statistische Beitrdge zur Pathologie und Chirurgie der Gallenwege. Leipzig, Vogel, 1890. 387 pp. pp. 57–58
Devised posterior gastroenterostomy.
Gastro-Enterostomie nach Wolfler bei inoperablem Pyloruscarcinom. Tod. Zbl. Chir., 10: 794–797, 1883

Coutard, Henri. Paris roentgenologist. 1876–
METHOD—protracted fraction m. of short wave treatment of neoplasms.
Un cas d'epithélioma spino-cellulaire de la région latérale du pharynx, avec adénopathie angulo-maxillaire, quéri depuis six mois par la röntgenthérapie. Bull. de l'Assoc. franc. pour l'étude du cancer, Paris, 10: 160–168, 1921
Zusammenfassung der Grundlagen der röntgentherapeutischen Technik der tiefgelegenen Krebse. Strahlentherapie, 37: 50–58, 1930

Couto, Miguel. Brazil physician. 1864–1934
DISEASE—visceral lipomatosis.
Da polysteatose visceral curavel. Arch. brasil. med., 4: 475–483, 1914
La polystéatose viscérale chronique. Ann. méd., Par., 22: 449–459, 1927

Cowell, Ernest Marshall. Croydon surgeon. 1886–
OPERATION—
Femoral hernioplasty. Lancet, 1: 816–818, Apr. 8, 1939

Cowgill, George Raymond. American physician. 1893–
FORMULA—for vitamin B requirement of man;

$$\frac{\text{Vitamin B mg. equivalent}}{\text{Calories}} = 0.0000284 \text{ weight in grams}$$

PREDICTION CHART—of the adequacy or inadequacy of vitamin B content of diet of an individual of known weight.
The vitamin B requirement of man. New Haven, Yale Univ. Press, 1934. 261 pp.

Cownley, A. J. See B. H. Paul

Cowper, William. English surgeon. 1666–1709
GLANDS—near bulb of corpus spongiosum.
LIGAMENT—that part of fascia lata attached to crest of pubes.
An account of two new glands and their excretory ducts, lately discovered in human bodies. Philos. Trans. 21: 364–369, 1700
Described aortic insufficiency.
III. Of ossifications or petrifactions in the coats of the arteries, particularly in the valves of the great artery.

Ibid., 24: 1970–1977, 1706
Also: F. A. Willius and T. E. Keys' *Cardiac classics*,
St. Louis, Mosby, 1941. pp. 109–114
Operated on the maxillary antrum.
Of the nose. In: J. Drake's *Anthropologia Nova*.
London, 1707, pp. 526–549
Cox, G. L. See E. E. Glynn
Cox, Willem Hendrik. Dutch physician. 1861–1933
MODIFICATION—of Golgi's corrosive-sublimate
method of staining ganglion-cells.
*Imprägnation des centralen Nervensystems mit Queck-
silbersalzen.* Arch. mikr. Anat., 37: 16–21, 1891
Crabtree, Ernest Granville. Boston urologist. 1883–
THEORY—of infection of kidneys.
Some observations on the etiology of renal infections.
Lancet—Clinic, 115: 96–99, Jan. 29, 1916
Craig, Charles Franklin. U. S. Army surgeon. 1872–
CRAIGIA—a genus of flagellate protozoans; two
species cause dysentery-like symptoms. Named
Paramoeba by Craig.
A new intestinal parasite of man: Paramoeba hominis.
Amer. J. med. Sci., 132: 214–220, Aug. 1906
*Further observations on Paramoeba hominis, an in-
testinal parasite of man.* Arch. intern. Med., 6: 1–11,
July 1910
Reported on undulant fever.
*Malta fever: its occurrence in the United States Army,
with a review of the literature.* Amer. J. med. Sci.,
125: 105–115, Jan. 1903
*The symptomatology and diagnosis of Malta fever,
with the report of additional cases.* Int. Clin., 15 s., 4:
89–115, 1906
Demonstrated existence of malaria carriers.
*Intracorpuscular conjugation in the malarial plasmodia
and its significance.* Amer. Med., 10: 982–986, Dec.
9; 1029–1032, Dec. 16, 1905
See also P. M. Ashburn
Craig, Winchell McKendree. Rochester, Minn. sur-
geon. 1892–
OPERATION—for cardiospasm.
*Treatment of intractable cardiospasm by bilateral
cervicothoracic sympathetic ganglionectomy: report of
a case* with H. J. Moersch and P. P. Vinson, Proc.
Staff Meet. Mayo Clinic, 9: 749–753, Dec. 12, 1934
OPERATION—for hypertension.
*Hypertension and subdiaphragmatic sympathetic de-
nervation* with A. W. Adson, Surg. Clin. N. Amer.,
19: 969–980, Aug. 1939
See also B. T. Horton
Craigie, David. Scottish physician. 1793–1866
Described and named relapsing fever.
*Notice of a febrile disorder which has prevailed at
Edinburgh during the summar of 1843.* Edinburgh M.
and S. J., 60: 410–418, 1843
Described leukemia.
*Case of disease of the spleen, in which death took place
in consequence of the presence of purulent matter in
the blood.* Ibid., 64: 400–413, Oct. 1, 1845
Cramer, William. English scientist. 1878–
METHOD—of counting blood platelets.
The clinical significance of the blood-platelets with
R. G. Banperman, Lancet, 1: 992–994, May 11,
1929
TEST—for reducing sugars.
*On the cause and significance of an abnormal relation
obtained in testing urine for sugar with Fehling's
solution.* Biochem. J., 9: 71–77, 1915

A new test for reducing sugars in urine. Ibid., 156–
160
Noted increase in platelets of blood after ultraviolet
irradiation.
The effect of light on the organism with A. H. Drew,
Brit. J. exp. Path , 4: 271–282, Oct. 1923
Crampton, C(harles) Ward. New York physician.
1877–
INDEX or TEST—for measuring vasotone, by com-
paring blood pressure and pulse rate in standing and
lying positions.
A test of condition: preliminary report. Med. News, 87:
529–535, Sept. 16, 1905
Blood ptosis: a test of vasomotor efficiency. New York
Med. J., 98: 916–918, Nov. 8, 1913
Crandall, L. A. Jr. See I. S. Cherry
Crane, Augustus Warren. American physician. 1868–
1937
Introduced kymography.
Röntgenology of the heart. Amer. J. Röntgenol., 3:
513–524, 1916
Crane, Martin Powers. Philadelphia physician. 1903–
MODIFICATION—of the Jezler method of the
Takata-Ara test for liver function.
*A modified mercuric chloride reaction (Takata-Ara)
in cirrhosis and in neoplasms of the liver.* Amer. J.
med. Sci., 187: 705–711, May 1934
Cranwell, Daniel J. Buenos Aires surgeon. 1870–
OPERATION—for diaphragmatic hernia.
*Diagnostic et traitement de la hernie diaphragmatique
(forme chronique).* Rev. Chir., 37: 33–54, Jan. 1908
Crawford, Adair. English scientist. 1748–1795
Experimented on animal calorimetry.
Experiments and observations on animal heat. London,
Murray, 1779
Crecca, William Daniel. Newark, N. J., surgeon.
1893–
GUIDE—
*Improved technic for blind nailing of the neck of the
femur: the Crecca-Cetrulo guide.* Amer. J. Surg., 61:
93–98, July 1943
Credé, Carl Caecil Benno (-Hörder). German
surgeon. 1847–1929
ANTISEPTIC—silver citrate.
*Silber und Silbersalze als Antiseptica in chirurgischer
und bacteriologischer Beziehung.* Verh. dtsch. Ges.
Chir., 25, pt. 2, 1896
Same, in English, New York, 1896. 8 pp.
Introduced injections of colloidal metals (collargol,
etc.). Garrison
Silber als äusseres und inneres Antisepticum. Arch.
klin. Chir., 55: 861–871, 1897
Credé, Carl Siegmund Franz. Berlin gynecologist.
1819–1892
METHOD—of expressing the placenta.
First mentioned in: (*Handgriff zur Entfernung der
Placenta.*) Klin. Vortr. Geburtschülfe, Berlin,
Hirschwald, 1854. 927 pp. pp. 599–603
First exact description in: *Methode der Entfernung
des Fruchtkuchens bei natürlicher Geburt.* Mschr. f
Geburtsk., 16: 337–342, 1860
*De optima in partu naturali placentam amovendi
ratione.* Lipsiae, Edelmannum, (1860)
METHOD—use of a drop of 2% solution of silver
nitrate in each eye of a newborn child, to prevent
ophthalmia neonatorum.
Die Verhütung der Augenentzündung der Neuge-

borenen (Ophthalmoblennorrhoea neonatorum) der häufigsten und wichtigsten Ursache der Blindheit. Berlin, Hirschwald, 1884. 63 pp.

Crendiropoulo, Maud. Egyptian physician
AGAR—alkaline peptone, for diagnosis of cholera.
Sur un nouveau milieu pour le diagnostic du cholera with A. Panayotatou, Zbl. Bakt., 55: 248–250, July 9, 1910

Cretan
BUTTON—an endemic ulcer (oriental sore) of Canea in the Island of Crete.

Browne, Sir James Crichton. See J. C. Browne

Crile, George Washington. Cleveland surgeon. 1864–1943
CANULA—for direct transfusion of blood.
The technique of direct transfusion of blood. Ann. Surg., 46: 329–332, Sept. 1907
OPERATION—production of regional anesthesia by intraneural infiltration.
On the physiologic action of cocain and eucain when injected into tissues. In his: *Experimental and clinical research into certain problems relating to surgical operations.* Philadelphia, Lippincott, 1901. pp. 88–162
OPERATIONS—on thyroid gland.
The thyroid gland. Philadelphia, Saunders, 1922. 288 pp. pp. 223–252
OPERATION—for hypertension, by interruption of adrenal sympathetic nervous system.
The surgical treatment of essential hypertension. Report of progress in 106 cases. Cleveland Clin. Quart., 3: 201–204, July 1936
Blood pressure changes in essential hypertension after excision of the celiac ganglion and denervation of the aortic plexus with G. Crile, Jr., Ibid., 3: 268–277, Oct. 1936
OPERATION—
A radical operation for malignant tumors of the thyroid gland with G. Crile, Jr., S. G. O., 64: 927–934, May 1937
THEORY—of peptic ulcer formation by sympathico-adrenal hyperirritability.
Peptic ulcer. South. Surg., 2: 273–280, Dec. 1933
THEORY—exhaustion t. of shock.
On experimental research into surgical shock, Philadelphia, Lippincott, (1899). 160 pp.
Suggested denervation of the suprarenal glands.
Indications and contra-indications for denervation of the adrenal glands. Ann. Surg., 100: 667–669, Oct. 1934

Cripps, William Harrison. English surgeon. 1850–1923
OPERATION—a method of colotomy in iliac region.
Cancer of the rectum: its pathology, diagnosis, and treatment. London, Churchill, 1880. 191 pp. pp. 135–142

Crismer, Leon. Belgian chemist. 1858–
TEST—for glucose.
La safranine comme reactif de la glucose. Ann. Soc. med.-chir. Liege, 27: 630–633, Oct. 1888

Crissey, Roy Henry. Lansing, Mich. surgeon. 1885–
OPERATION—
A method of radical cure of femoral hernia. J. Mich. S. M. Soc., 25: 18–19, Jan. 1926

Crocker, H. R. See W. T. Fox

Crocq, Jean B. Belgian physician. 1868–1925
Described acrocyanosis.

De l'"acrocyanose." Abstr.: Semaine med., 16: 298 (only), 1896

Crohn, Burrill Bernard. New York physician. 1884–
Demonstrated advantages of aluminum hydroxide as an antacid in treatment of peptic ulcer.
The clinical use of a colloidal aluminum hydroxide as a gastric antacid. J. Lab. clin. Med., 14: 610–614, Apr. 1929
Described "regional ileitis."
Regional ileitis: a pathologic and clinical entity with L. Ginzburg and G. D. Oppenheimer, J. A M. A., 97: 1323–1328, Oct. 15, 1932

Cron, R. S. See C. H. Davis

Crone-Münzebrock, E. German surgeon
OPERATION—gastrostomy.
Zur Technik der Gastrostomie. Zbl. Chir., 53: 2075–2076, Aug. 14, 1926

Croner, Wilhelm. German chemist. 1867–
TEST—for lactic acid.
Ueber eine neue Milchsäureprobe with W. Cronheim, Berl. klin. Wschr., 42: 1080 (only), 1905

Cronheim, W. See W. Croner

Croone, William. London physician. 1633–1684
"Is memorable for two monographs on muscular physiology (1667) and embryology of the chick (1671–2), which were far in advance of their time." Garrison
His widow endowed the Croonian lectures.
De ratione motus musculorum. Londini, Thomson, 1664. 34 pp.

Cross, Charles Frederick. English scientist
TEST—for hydrochloric acid.
A new solvent for cellulose with E. J. Bevan, Chem. News, 63: 66 (only), Feb. 6, 1891

Cross, Howard Benjamin. Baltimore bacteriologist, 1873–1921
STAIN—for phagocytes and bacteria.
A contribution to the staining of phagocytes and exudates. Johns Hopk. Hosp. Bull., 32: 51–52, Feb. 1921

Crossman, Germain. Rochester, N. Y. scientist
MODIFICATION—
A modification of Mallory's connective tissue stain with a discussion of the principles involved. Anat. Rec., 69: 33–38, Aug. 1937

Crouzel, Edouard. Bordeaux pharmacologist
TEST—for santonin in urine.
Applications de la réaction colorée de la sántonine éliminée par les urines. Ann. chim. anal. chim. appli., 7: 219–220, 1902

Crouzon, Octave. French physician. 1874–1938
Described cranio-facial dysostosis.
Dysostose cranio-faciale héréditaire. Bull. Soc. méd. Hôp. Paris, 3 s., 33: 545–555, 1912

Crowe, Samuel James. Baltimore physician. 1883–
Showed relationship between pituitary and reproductive system.
Experimental hypophysectomy with H. W. Cushing and J. Homans, Johns Hopk. Hosp. Bull., 21: 127–169, May 1910

Cruchet, Jean René. French surgeon. 1875–
Described torticollis.
Traité des torticolis spasmodiques. Paris, 1907

Cruikshank, William Cumberland. English physician. 1745–1800
DISEASE—(Dr. Cruikshank was the patient).
On subjective abberations of the sense of smell. Arch. Surg., (Hutchinson), 2: 302–305 (303), 1891

Traced lymph vessels from periosteum into cortex.
*The anatomy of the absorbing vessels of the human
body.* London, Nicol, 1786. 192 pp.
Demonstrated that skin, like lungs, gives off CO_2.
*Experiments upon the insensible perspiration of the
human body.* London, 1795
Investigated passage of impregnated ovum through
Fallopian tube, 1778.
*Experiments in which, on the third day after impregna-
tion, the ova of rabbits were found in the Fallopian
tubes, and on the fourth day after impregnation in the
uterus itself.* Philos. Trans., 87: 197–214, 1797

Crussell, Gustav Samuel. Swedish physician. 1810–
1858
Showed effect of galvanic electrolysis in treatment
of urethral stricture.
*Ueber den Galvanismus als chemisches Heilmittel
gegen örtliche Krankheiten.* St. Petersburg, Kray,
1841–43. 158 pp.

Crutchfield, W(illiam) Gayle. Richmond, Va.
surgeon. 1900–
METHOD—
*Skeletal traction for dislocation of the cervical spine;
report of a case.* South. Surg., 2: 156–159, 1933
*Further observations on treatment of fracture-disloca-
tions of the cervical spine with skeletal traction.* S.
G. O., 67: 513–517, Oct. 1936

Cruveilhier, Jean. French pathologist. 1791–1873
ATROPHY—progressive muscular a.
Sur la paralysie musculaire, progressive, atrophique.
Bull. Acad. Méd. Paris, 18: 490–502, Mar. 8; 546–
584, Mar. 29, 1853
SYNDROME—of Cruveilbier-Baumgarten; dilated
veins in abdominal wall, patent umbilical vein,
caput Medusa and loud venous murmur at umbilicus.
E. L. Armstrong et al.
Maladies des veines. In: *Anatomie pathologique du
corps humain.* Paris, Baillière, 1829–35. Vol. 1,
XVI Livr., pl. VI
Traité d'anatomie pathologique générale. Paris, Bail-
lière, 1852. Vol. 2, Classe 8, ordre 3, p. 315
ULCER—simple gastric u.
Anatomie pathologique du corps humain. Paris,
Baillière, 1829–35. t. I, livr. X; 1835-42 t. II, livr.
XXX
Described and illustrated disseminated sclerosis.
Ibid., II, livr. XXXVIII, pl. 5
Described hypertrophy of pyloric muscle.
Rétrécissement du pylore. In: Ibid., Vol. 12, p. 1,
fig. VI
Described diverticula of colon.
Traité d'anatomie pathologique générale. Paris. Bail-
lière, 1849. Vol. 1, p. 590

Cuignet, Ferdinand Louis Joseph. French oph-
thalmologist. 1823–
Introduced a method of retinoscopy.
Kératoscopie. Rec. d'ophth., Paris, 1: 14–23, 1873–74

Culbertson, C. G. See E. Rupel

Cullen, Glenn Ernest. American biochemist. 1890–
METHOD—for determination of plasma pH.
*Studies of acidosis. XIX. The colorimetric determina-
tion of the hydrogen ion concentration of blood plasma.*
J. Biol. Chem., 52: 501–515 (507), June 1922
See also P. Drucker, D. D. Van Slyke

Cullen, Thomas Stephen. Baltimore gynecologist.
1868–

SIGN—
*Bluish discoloration of the umbilicus as a diagnostic
sign where ruptured extra-uterine pregnancy exists.*
In: *Contributions to medical and biological research,
dedicated to Sir William Osler, in honor of his seven-
tieth birthday, July 12, 1919, by his pupils and co-
workers.* New York, Hoeber, 1919. pp. 420–421
Described necrosis of abdominal wall.
*A progressively enlarging ulcer of the abdominal wall
involving the skin and fat, following drainage of an
abdominal abscess apparently of appendiceal origin.*
S. G. O., 38: 579–582, May 1924

Cullen, William. Scottish physician. 1712–1790
He was one of the first to give clinical or infirmary
lectures in Great Britain, and these lectures were the
first ever given in the vernacular instead of Latin,
1757. Garrison
Synopsis nosolgiae methodicae. Edinburgi, 1769
Lectures on the materia medica as delivered by . . .
London, Lowndas, 1773. 512 pp.
The works . . . Edinburgh, Blackwood, 1827. 2 vols.

Cuming, Ralph. English naval surgeon
Performed interscapular-thoracic amputation.
Removal of the arm, scapula and clavicle. Letter by
A. Copland Hutchinson, London M. Gaz., 5: 273,
1829–30

Cumming, William. English physician. 1812–1886
Studied retina.
*On a luminous appearance of the human eye, and its
application to the detection of disease of the retina and
posterior part of the eye.* Med.-chir. Trans., 29: 383–
396, 1846

Cummings, D. E. See L. U. Gardner

Cuneo, Bernard. Paris surgeon. 1873–
OPERATION—for exstrophy of bladder.
*Traitement de l'exstrophie de la vessie par la creation
d'une vessie nouvelle.* Pr. med., 20: 31 (only), Jan.
10, 1912

Cunningham, Andrew. Scottish scientist
SOLUTION—basal fuchsin peptone, for studying fermentation.
*Practical bacteriology; an introductory course for stu-
dents of agriculture.* Edinburgh, Oliver and Boyd,
1924. p. 18

Cunningham, David Douglas. Calcutta physician.
1843–1914
Described bodies, later known as Leishman-Donovan b.
*On the presence of peculiar parasitic organisms in the
tissue of a specimen of Delhi boils.* Sci. Mem. Med.
Off. Army of India, 1884, Calcutta, 1: 21–31, 1885

Cunningham, Mrs. Eileen Roach. Nashville medi-
cal librarian. 1894–
CLASSIFICATION—
A classification for medical literature. Nashville,
Tenn., Cullom and Ghertner Co., 1937. 2 ed., pp.
104. Also, 1929

Cunningham, John Henry. Boston urologist. 1877–
APPARATUS—for intrarectal administration of ether
vapor and oxygen.
*A method of producing ether narcosis by rectum, with
the report of forty-one cases* with F. H. Lahey, Boston
M. and S. J., 152: 450–457, Apr. 20, 1905
Rectal anesthesia. New York M. J., 91: 904–909, Apr.
30, 1910
MEDIUM—for pyelography; does not require steriliza-
tion.

An antiseptic pyelographic medium with R. C. Graves and T. L. Davis, J. Urol., 10: 255–260, Sept. 1923

Cunningham, R(obert) S(ydney). American anatomist. 1891–
Described—
The development of leucocytes, lymphocytes, and monocytes from a specific stem-cell in adult tissues with Florence R. Sabin and C. A. Doan, Carnegie Institution. Contrib. to Embryology, (No. 84), 16: 227–276, Jan. 1925
Described—
The supravital staining of normal human blood cells with Edna H. Thompkins, Folia Haematol., 42: 257–270, 1930
See also Florence R. Sabin

Cunningham, T(homas) Donald. Boston physician. 1889–
METHOD—vital staining.
A method for the permanent staining of reticulated red cells. Arch. intern. Med., 26: 405–409, Oct. 1920

Cunningham, William Francis. New York surgeon. 1889–
TREATMENT—
The prevention and treatment of abdominal wall excoriation in gastric and intestinal fistulas by copper bronzing powder. J. A. M. A., 98: 1643, May 7, 1932

Cuny, Louis. French scientist
TEST—for bismuth.
Sur le dosage colorimetrique de petites quantites de bismuth with G. Poirot, J. Pharm. Chim., Paris, s. 7, 28: 215–223, 1923

Curdy, Robert James. Kansas City ophthalmologist. 1868–
OPERATION—
The operative treatment of squint. J. Missouri M. Ass., 13: 16–19, Jan. 1916

Curie, Marie Sklodowska. Polish-French chemist. 1867–1934

Curie, Pierre. French scientist. 1859–1906
Discovered radium; isolated radium chloride in 1898.
Sur une substance nouvelle radio-active, contenue dans la pechblende. By P. Curie with M. S. Curie, C. R. Acad. Sci., 127: 175–178; 1215–1217, 1898
Radio-active substances. Chem. News, London, 88: 85 et seq., 1903
Loi de disparition de l'activité induite par le radium après chauffage des corps activés with J. Danne, C. R. Acad. Sci., 138: 748–751, 1904
Action physiologique de l'émanation du radium. By C. Bouchard, with P. Curie and V. Bolthazard, Ibid., 1384–1387, 1904
LAW—all substances may be made radio-active by influence of emanations of radium.
THERAPY—with radium.

Curie, P. See A. H. Becquerel

Curling, Thomas Blizard. London physician. 1811–1888
ULCER—of duodenum following burns of skin.
On acute ulceration of the duodenum, in cases of burn. Med.-chir. Trans., 25: 260–281, 1842
Acute perforating ulcer of the duodenum, after a severe burn. (*Under the care of Mr. Curling*). Lancet, 1: 484 (only), May 5, 1866
Wrote early description of myxedema; suggested that cretinism may be due to thyroid deficiency.
Two cases of absence of the thyroid body, and symmetrical swellings of fat tissue at the sides of the neck, connected with defective cerebral development. Med.-chir. Trans., 33: 303–306, 1850

Curran, Edward James. Kansas City ophthalmologist. 1878–
PERIPHERAL IRIDOTOMY—
A new operation for glaucoma involving a new principle in the aetiology and treatment of chronic primary glaucoma. Arch. of Ophthal., 49: 131–155, Mar. 1920

Currie, James. Scottish physician. 1756–1805
Introduced cold bathing in fevers, especially typhoid, and checked results with clinical thermometer.
Medical reports on the effects of water, cold and warm, as a remedy in fever and febrile diseases; whether applied to the surface of the body, or used as a drink; with observations on the nature of fever; and on the effects of opium, alcohol and inanition. Liver, Cadell and Davies, 1797. 252 pp.

Curschmann, Hans. German physician. 1875–
METHOD—of testing sensation of muscular contraction.
Zur Methodik der Muskel- und Gelenksensibilitätsbestimmung. Dtsch. med. Wschr., 31: 1222–1224, Aug. 3, 1905
Suggested term dystrophia myotonica.
Ueber familiäre atrophischen Myotonie. Dtsch. Z. Nervenheilk., 45: 161–202, 1912
Zur Nosologie und Symptomatologie der myotonischen Dystrophie. Dtsch. Arch. klin. Med., 149: 129–144, 1925
See Johann Hoffmann

Curschmann, Heinrich. Leipzig physician. 1846–1910
SPIRALS—coiled mucinous fibrils in sputum of bronchial asthma.
Ueber Bronchiolitis exsudativa und ihr Verhältniss zum Asthma nervosum. Dtsch. Arch. klin. Med., 32: 1–34, Nov. 8, 1882

Curtis, Arthur Hale. Chicago gynecologist. 1881–
APPARATUS—
Transfusion of blood by a new method, allowing accurate measurement with V. C. David, J. A. M. A., 56: 35–36, Jan. 7, 1911
The transfusion of blood. Further notes on a new method. Ibid., 57: 1453–1454, Oct. 28, 1911
TECHNIC—of amputation of cervix.
In his: *A textbook of gynecology.* Philadelphia, Saunders, 1942. 4 ed., pp. 585–586

Curtis, B. F. See J. A. Booth
Curtis, G. M. See C. B. Davis, F. J. Phillips
Curtis, L. See R. H. Ivy
Curtis, M. R. See F. D. Bullock
Curtman, L. J. See W. G. Lyle

Cushing, Harvey Williams. American surgeon. 1869–1939
HEMANGIOBLASTOMA—
Tumors arising from the blood-vessels of the brain. Angiomatous malformations and hemangioblastomas. with P. Bailey, Springfield, Ill., Thomas, 1928. 219 pp.
OPERATION—decompression, over cerebellum.
The establishment of cerebral hernia as a decompressive measure for inaccessible brain tumors; with the description of intermuscular methods of making the bone defect in temporal and occipital regions. S. G. O., 1: 297–314, Oct. 1905

OPERATION—exposure of gasserian ganglion and three divisions of fifth nerve by direct route.
A method of total expiration of the gasserian ganglion for trigeminal neuralgia by a route through the temporal fossa and beneath the middle meningeal artery. J. A. M. A., 34: 1035–1041, Apr. 28, 1900
The major trigeminal neuralgias and their surgical treatment based on experience with 332 gasserian operations. Amer. J. med. Sci., 160: 157–184, Aug. 1920
OPERATION—
Concerning surgical intervention for the intracranial hemorrhage of the new-born. Ibid., 130: 563–581, Oct. 1905
OPERATION—for hydrocephalus.
The special field of neurological surgery. Cleveland Med. J., 4: 1–25, Jan. 1905
OPERATION—on pituitary.
The pituitary body and its disorders. Philadelphia, Lippincott, 1912. 341 pp.
LAW—increase of intracranial tension causes increase of blood-pressure to a point slightly above pressure exerted against medulla. Dorland
Concerning a definite regulatory mechanism of the vasomotor center which controls blood pressure during cerebral compression. Johns Hopk. Hosp. Bull., 12: 290–292, Sept. 1901
Some experimental and clinical observations concerning states of increased intracranial tension. Amer. J. med. Sci., 124: 375–400, Sept. 1902
SYNDROME—angle tumor s.
Tumors of the nervus acusticus and the syndrome of the cerebellopontile angle. Philadelphia, Saunders, 1917. 296 pp.
SYNDROME—of pituitary basophilism.
The basophil adenoma of the pituitary body and their clinical manifestations (pituitary basophilism). Johns Hopk. Hosp. Bull., 50: 137–195, Mar. 1932
TECHNIC—
On the avoidance of shock in major amputations by cocainization of large nerve-trunks preliminary to their division: with observations on blood-pressure changes in surgical cases. Ann. Surg., 36: 321–345, Sept. 1902
Showed that intestinal tract can be sterilized by fasting.
Experimental and surgical notes upon the bacteriology of the upper portion of the alimentary canal, with observations on the establishment there of an amicrobic state as a preliminary to operative procedures on the stomach and small intestine with L. E. Livingood, Johns Hopk. Hosp. Rep., 9: 543–591, 1900
Also in: *Contributions to the science of medicine, dedicated by his pupils to William Henry Welch on twenty fifth anniversary of his doctorate.* Baltimore, Johns Hopkins Press, 1900. pp. 1059
Successfully treated facial paralysis in man by anastomosis of spinal accessory and facial nerves.
The surgical treatment of facial paralysis by nerve anastomosis. Ann. Surg., 37: 641–659, May 1903
Coined term "third circulation" for fluid bathing central nervous system.
Studies in intracranial physiology and surgery. The third circulation. The hypophysis. The gliomas. London, Oxford Univ. Press, 1926. 146 pp.
Gave early clinical report on coexistance of ulcers in gastro-intestinal tract with intracranial lesions.

Peptic ulcers and the interbrain. S. G. O., 55: 1–34, July 1932
See also P. Bailey, S. J. Crowe
Cushing, Hayward Warren. Boston surgeon. 1854–1934
OPERATION—
An improved method for the radical cure of femoral hernia. Boston M. and S. J., 119: 546–548, Dec. 6, 1888
SUTURE—
The "right-angle" continuous intestinal sutures. Ibid., 141: 57–59, July 20, 1899
Also: Med. and Surg. Reports of City Hospital. Boston, 1889. p. 83
Cushman, Margaret, See A. M. Butler
Cushny, Arthur Robertson. English physician. 1866–1926
THEORY—
The secretion of urine. London, Longmans, Green, 1917. 241 pp.
Described auricular fibrillation.
Paroxysmal irregularity of the heart and auricular fibrillation with C. W. Edmunds, In: *Studies in pathology written . . . to celebrate the quarter-centenary of Aberdeen University.* Ed. by W. Bulloch, Aberdeen, 1906. pp. 95–110
Custer, Richard Philip. Philadelphia physician. 1903–
METHOD—celloidin, for embedding tissues.
Adaptation of the Leitz ultropak for rapid tissue diagnosis. J. Lab. clin. Med., 18: 644–647, Mar. 1933
Cutler, D. Ward. Manchester zoologist
Cultivated Entamoeba histolytica.
A method for the cultivation of Entamoeba histolytica: (preliminary note.) J. Path. Bact., 22: 22–27, 1918
Cutler, Elliott Carr. Cleveland surgeon. 1888–
CARDIOVALVULOTOME.
The present status of the surgical procedures in chronic valvular disease of the heart with C. S. Beck, Arch. Surg., 18: 403–416, Jan. 1929
Did early work on relief of cardiac decompensation by total thyroidectomy.
Total thyroidectomy for angina pectoris with M. T. Schnitker, Trans. Amer. Surg. Ass., 52: 18–37; 45, 1934
See also A. Graham, J. L. Stoddard
Cutler, Jacob. Philadelphia physician. 1900–
METHOD—graphic, of sedimentation rate.
The graphic presentation of the blood sedimentation test. Amer. J. med. Sci., 171: 882–901, June 1926
The practical application of the blood sedimentation test in general medicine. Observations based upon approximately 5000 patients over a period of six years. Ibid., 183: 643–657, May 1932
Cutler, Max. New York surgeon. 1899–
Treated chronic mastitis with ovarian hormone.
The cause of "painful breasts" and treatment by means of ovarian residue. J. A. M. A., 96: 1201–1205, Apr. 11, 1931
See also G. L. Cheatle
Cutter, Ephraim. American surgeon. 1832–1917
Treated uterine tumors by galvanism.
New electrods and battery for electrolysis of uterine fibroids. Boston M. and S. J., 94: 177–182. Feb. 17, 1876
Cutting, W. C. See E. K. Marshall, Jr.

Cuvier, Georges Léopold Chrétien Frédéric Dagobert, le baron. French naturalist. 1769–1832
CANAL—ductus venosus, a fetal blood vessel.
DUCTS—venous trunks in fetus, opening into auricle of heart.
SINUSES—as ducts.
Leçons d'anatomie comparée . . . Paris, Baudouin, (1800)–05. 5 vols.
Cuvier
First stated theory of morphologic types (vertebrate, molluscan, articulate, radiote). Garrison
Le règne animal. Paris, Fortin, Masson & Cie, 1836–49. 20 vols.
The animal kingdom arranged in conformity with its organization. Transl. by H. McMurtie, New York, Carvill, 1831
Cuyler, William Kenneth. Durham, N. C. endocrinologist. 1900–
STAIN—
A spermatozoal stain for clinical studies with Margaret Baptist. J. clin. Endocrinol., 2: 571–572, Sept. 1942
Cybulski, Napoleon. St. Petersburg physiologist. 1854–1920
PHOTOHEMOTACHOMETER—for measuring circulation rate.
Die Bestimmung der Stromgeschwindigkeit des Blutes in den Gefässen mit dem neuen Apparat-Photohämotachometer. Arch. ges. Physiol., 37: 382–394, 1885
Cyon, Elie de. Russian physiologist. 1843–1912
Discovered vasomotor reflexes.
Die Reflexe eines der sensiblen Nerven des Herzens auf die motorischen der Blutfefässe with C. F. Ludwig, Arb. a. d. Physiol. Anst. zu Leipzig, 1866, 1: 128–149, 1867
Cyrillo. See D. Cirillo
Czaplewski, Eugen. Polish bacteriologist. 1865–
AGAR—alkaline serum glucose, for cultivation of diphtheria bacilli.
Ueber neue Serumnährböden. Dtsch. med. Wschr., 46: 828–829, July 22, 1920
STAIN and METHOD—for acid-fact organisms.
Die Untersuchung des Auswurfs auf Tuberkelbacillen. Jena, Fischer, 1891. 124 pp.
Czermak, Johann Nepomuk. Bohemian physician. 1828–1873
SPACES—in interglobular substance of dentin.
Beiträge zur mikroskopischen Anatomie der menschlichen Zähne. Z. wiss. Zool., Leipzig, 2, 1850
Also: *Observationes novae de structura dentium penitiori.* Wurtzburg, 1850
VAGUS PRESSURE—pressure on carotid triangle produces lowering of heart rate.

Ueber mechanische Vagus-Reizung beim Menschen. Jenaische Z. f. Med. u. Naturwiss. Leipzig, 2: 384–386, 1865–66
Devised method of exploring nose and nasopharynx by means of small mirrors.
Physiologische Untersuchungen mit Garcia's Kehlkopfspiegel. S. B. Akad. Wiss. Wien, 29: 557–584, 1858
Ueber den Kehlkopfspiegel. Wien. med. Wschr., 8: 196–198, Mar. 27, 1858
Beiträge zur Laryngoskopie. Ibid., 9: 145–148, Mar. 5; 165–168, Mar. 12; 180–183, Mar. 19, 1859
Ueber die Inspektion des Cavum pharyngo-nasale und der Nasenhöhle durch Choanen vermittelst kleiner Spiegel. Ibid., 9: 518–520, Aug. 6, 1859; 10: 257–264, Apr. 28, 1860
Also: Paris, Baillière, 1860
Also: London, New Sydenham Soc., 1861
Czerny, Vincenz. Heidelberg surgeon. 1842–1916
OPERATION—for inguinal hernia.
Studien zur Radikalbehandlung der Hernien. Wien. med. Wschr., 27: 495–500, May 26; 527–530, June 2; 553–556, June 9; 578–581, June 16, 1877
OPERATION—total hysterectomy by vaginal route.
Ueber die Ausrottung des Gebärmutterkrebses. Ibid., 29: 1171–1174, 1879
OPERATION—hysterectomy.
Zur Hysterotomie. Zbl. Gynäk., 3: 519–520, 1879
Zur Laparo-Hysterotomie. Wien. med. Presse, 20: 1265–1268, 1879
OPERATION—enucleation of subperitoneal uterine fibroids by vaginal route.
Ueber die Enukleation subperitonealer Fibrome der Gebärmutter durch das Scheidengewölbe; vaginale Myoniotomie. Wien. med. Wschr., 31: 501–505, Apr. 30; 525–529, May 7, 1881
SUTURE—for intestine.
Zur Darmresection. Berl. klin. Wschr., 637–642, Nov. 8, 1880
Nachtrag zur Darmresection. Ibid., 683–684, Nov. 29, 1880
Operated on a vesical diverticulum.
Resektion eines Blasendivertikels. Beitr. klin. Chir. 19: 247–252, 1897
Reported gastrojejunocolic fistula as complication of gastric surgery.
Zur Behandlung der Fissur und des Vorfalls des Mastdarms. Ibid., 37: 765–769, 1903
Czokor, Johann. Vienna physician
SOLUTION or STAIN—cochineal s.
Die Cochenille-Carminlösung. Arch. mikr. Anat., 18: 412–414, 1880

D

Dabney, William Cecil. Virginia physician. 1849–1894
Described epidemic pleurodynia.
Account of an epidemic resembling dengue, which occurred in and around Charlottesville and the University of Virginia, in June, 1888. Amer. J. med. Sci., 96: 488–494, Nov. 1888
Daça de Valdes, Benito. Spanish. 1591?–?
Wrote scientific work on spectacles.

Uso de los antojos para todo genero de vistas. Sevilla, Diego Perez, 1623
DaCosta, J. C. See W. W. Keen
DaCosta, Jacob Mendes. American physician. 1833–1900
Described irritable heart in soldiers.
On irritable heart: a clinical study of a form of functional cardiac disorder and its consequences. Amer. J. med. Sci., 61: 17–52, Jan. 1871

On strain and over action of the heart. Washington, 1874. 28 pp.

Described phantom tumors of abdomen.

Clinical lecture on spurious or "phantom" tumors of the abdomen. Philadelphia Med. Times, 1: 449–451, Sept. 15, 1871

Daddi, Lamberto. Turin physiologist

STAIN—for fat in tissues.

Nouvelle methode pour colorer la graisse dans les tissus. Arch. ital. Biol., 26: 143–146, Oct. 8, 1896

Da Fano, Corrado Donato. Italian-English scientist. 1879–1927

METHOD—cobalt nitrate.

Method for the demonstration of Golgi's internal apparatus. J. Physiol., 53: XCII–XCIV, 1920

Dagnini, Giuseppe. Italian physician. 1866–1928

REFLEX—pressure, of eyeball.

Il reflesso oculo-cardiaco di Dagnini nella pubertà femminile: studio su 230 giovani donne bolognesi, dagii 11 ai 17 anni di età. By Guido Dagnini, Cuore et circol., 21: 9–30, Jan. 1937

Dakin, Henry Drysdale. New York chemist. 1880–

FLUID, SOLUTION or TREATMENT—Carrel-Dakin s.

On the use of certain antiseptic substances in the treatment of infected wounds. Brit. med. J., 2: 318–320, Aug. 28, 1915

A handbook of antiseptics with E. K. Dunham, New York, 1918

A report of the use of dichloramin—T (tolueneparasulphonichloramin) in the treatment of infected wounds with W. E. Lee, J. E. Sweet, B. M. Hendrix and R. G. LeConte, J. A. M. A., 69: 27–30, July 7, 1919

METHOD—of producing a reticulocyte response in anemia.

Observations on the chemical nature of a hematopoietic substance occurring in liver with R. West, J. biol. Chem., 109: 489–517, May 1935

OXIDATION THEORY—

The oxidation of butyric acid by means of hydrogen peroxide with formation of acetone, aldehydes and other products. J. biol. Chem., 4: 77–89, Jan. 1908

Comparative studies of the mode of oxidation of phenyl derivatives of fatty acids by the animal organism and by hydrogen peroxide. Ibid., 4: 419–435, June; 5: 173–185, Oct.; 303–309, Dec. 1908; 6: 203–243, June 1909

Oxidations and reductions in the animal body. London, Longmans, 1912

See also A. Carrell

Daland, Ernest Merrill. Boston surgeon. 1891–

OPERATION—

Repair of large defects after removal of cancer of the lips. S. G. O., 69: 347–357, Sept. 1939

Dale, Sir Henry Hallett. London physiologist. 1875–

Awarded Nobel prize in 1936, with O. Loewi, for work on transmission of nerve impulse.

The vasodilator action of histamine and of some other substances with A. N. Richards, J. Physiol., 52: 110–165, July 10, 1918

On the pituitary active principles and histamine with H. W. Dudley, J. Pharmacol., 18: 27–42, Aug. 1921

The vaso-dilator action of histamine, and its physiological significance. By J. H. Burn and H. H. Dale, J. Physiol., 61: 185–214, Apr. 23, 1926

Chemical transmission of the effects of nerve impulses.

(Linacre lecture) Brit. med. J., 1: 835–841, May 12, 1934

Release of acetylcholine at voluntary motor nerve endings with W. Feldberg and M. Vogt, J. Physiol., 86: 353–380, May 4, 1936

Demonstrated that most important pharmacologic action of an extract of posterior lobe of pituitary gland is its oxytocic activity.

The action of extracts of the pituitary body. Biochem. J., 4: 427–447, Nov. 10, 1909

Showed that histamine produces arteriolar precapillary contraction with capillary dilatation, a condition known as secondary shock.

The physiological action of B-iminazolyl-ethylamine with P. P. Laidlaw, J. Physiol., 41: 318–344, 1910

Histamine shock with P. P. Laidlaw, Ibid., 52: 355–390, Mar. 25, 1919

Demonstrated inhibitory action of acetylcholine on heart.

The action of certain esters and ethers of choline, and their relation to muscarine. J. Pharmacol., 6: 147–190, Nov. 1914

Isolated acetylcholine from ox and horse spleen.

The presence of histamine and acetylcholine in the spleen of the ox and the horse with H. W. Dudley, J. Physiol., 68: 97–123, Oct. 23, 1929

See also G. Barger

Dalgarmo, George. Scottish educator. 1626?–1687

Invented alphabet for deaf-mutes.

Didascalocophus, or the deaf and dumb man's tutor. Oxford, Halton, 1680

Dalimier, Robert. French physician

BOUILLON—opsine, a culture medium.

Le milieu de culture d'acides-aminés complets pour les micro-organismes with E. Lancereau, Pr. méd., 21: 419 (only), May 21, 1913

Dallas, Alexander. American surgeon. 1850–

OPERATION—

The treatment of inguinal hernia. Med. News, 59: 622–623, Nov. 28, 1891

Also: Trans. Med. Soc. New York, pp. 387–402, 1893

Dalidorf, Gilbert. American pathologist. 1900–

APPARATUS—for estimating capillary resistance in purpura; number of petechiae produced under negative pressure in a small area may be counted.

A sensitive test for subclinical scurvy in man. Amer. J. Dis. Child., 46: 794–802, Oct. 1933

Dalrymple, John. English oculist. 1804–1852

DISEASE—cycloceratitis.

Pathology of the human eye. London, Churchill, 1852

Dalton, John. English chemist. 1766–1844

DALTONISM—color-blindness.

Extraordinary facts relating to the vision of colors: with observations. (Read Oct. 31, 1794), Mem. Lit. and Phil. Soc., Manchester, 5, pt. 1: 28–45, 1798

Dalton, John Call, Jr. American physiologist. 1825–1889

PARIETAL FISSURE—in brain; same as fissure of Pausch.

Topographical anatomy of the brain. Philadelphia, Lea, 1885. 3 vols.

Daly, Ivan de Burgh. English physiologist

MANOMETER—

A blood velocity recorder. J. Physiol., 61: xxi–xxii, Aug. 6, 1926

Dam, Henrik. Copenhagen and Rochester, N. Y. biochemist

Awarded Nobel prize in 1943, with E. A. Doisy, for their work on vitamin K.
UNIT—of activity of vitamin K.
Cholesterinstoffwechsel in Hühnereiern und Hühnchen. Biochem. Z., 215: 475–492, Nov. 21, 1929
The antihemorrhagic vitamin of the chick: occurrence and chemical nature. Nature, 135: 652–653, Apr. 27, 1935
Determination of vitamin K by the curative blood-clotting method with J. Glavind, Biochem. J., 32: 1018–1023, June 1938
Isolated vitamin K from alfalfa.
Isolierung des Vitamins K in hochgereinter Form. Helvet. Chim. Acta, Basel, 22: 310–313, 1939
Dambrin, C. See J. A. Sicard
Damiens, A. French scientist. 1866–
REAGENT—for absorption of carbon monoxide.
Sur un nouveau réactif de l'oxyde de carbone. C. R. Acad. Sci., Paris, 178: 849–854, 1924
Damoiseau, Louis Hyacinthe Céleste. French physician. 1815–1890
CURVE or SIGN—an S-shaped line on chest wall, showing upper border of pleural effusion.
Recherches cliniques sur plusieurs points du diagnostic des epanchements. Extrait des Arch. gén. de Méd., 1844
Du diagnostic et du traitement de la pleurésie. Paris, 1845. 64 pp.
Dana, Charles Loomis. New York neurologist. 1852–1935
OPERATION—resection of posterior roots of spinal nerves to relieve pain, athetosis, spastic paralysis, etc.; operation was first performed by R. Abbe on December 31, 1888.
A clinical study of neuralgias, and of the origin of reflex or transferred pains. New York M. J., 46: 87–91, July 23; 121–127, July 30, 1887
SYNDROME—of Putnam and Dana; a sclerosis of lateral and dorsal columns of spinal cord.
The degenerative diseases of the spinal cord, with a description of a new type. J. nerv. ment. Dis., 18: 205–216, Apr. 1891
Also, abstr.: New York M. J., 53: 279–281, Mar. 7, 1891
Dance, Jean Baptiste Hippolyte. French physician. 1797–1832
SIGN—depression in right iliac region due to displacement in intussusception at ileo-cecal junction.
Invaginations morbides des intestins. Répertoire gén. d'anat. et de physiol. path., 1826. tome 1.
Described tetany.
Observations sur une espèce de tétanos intermittent. Arch. gén. de méd., Paris, 26: 190–205, 1831
Dancel, Jean Francois. French physician. 1804–
TREATMENT—of obesity by a diet containing as little water as possible. (Dorland)
Préceptes fondés sur la chimie organique pour diminuer l'embonpoint sans altérer la santé. Paris, Leblanc, 1850. 2 ed. 213 pp.
Dandy, Walter Edward. Baltimore surgeon. 1886–1946
METHOD—
Section of the sensory root of the trigeminal nerve at the pons. Preliminary report of the operative procedure. Johns Hopk. Hosp. Bull., 36: 105–106, Feb. 1925
An operation for the cure of tic douloureux: partial

section of the sensory root at the pons. Arch. Surg., 18: 687–734, Feb. 1929
OPERATION—
An operation for the removal of pineal tumors. S. G. O., 33: 113–119, Aug. 1921
OPERATION—
The diagnosis and treatment of hydrocephalus resulting from strictures of the aqueduct of Sylvius. S. G. O., 31: 340–358, Oct. 1920
An operative procedure for hydrocephalus. Johns Hopk. Hosp. Bull., 33: 189–190, May 1922
OPERATION—
An operation for the total extirpation of tumors in the cerebello-pontine angle. A preliminary report. Ibid., 344–345, Sept. 1922
OPERATION—excision of ruptured intervertebral disk.
Loose cartilage from intervertebral disk simulating tumor of the spinal cord. Arch. Surg., 19: 660–672, Oct. 1929
OPERATION—for spasmodic torticollis, by section of first four cervical roots and spinal accessories.
An operation for the treatment of spasmodic torticollis. Ibid., 20: 1021–1032, June 1930
Demonstrated origin of cerebro-spinal fluid and established internal hydrocephalus as a clinical entity.
An experimental and clinical study of internal hydrocephalus with K. D. Blackfan, J. A. M. A., 61: 2216–2217, Dec. 20, 1913
Internal hydrocephalus; an experimental, clinical and pathological study with K. D. Blackfan, Amer. J. Dis. Child., 8: 406–482, Dec. 1914
Internal hydrocephalus; second paper with K. D. Blackfan, Ibid., 14: 424–443, Dec. 1917
Described ventriculography.
Ventriculography following the injection of air into the cerebral ventricles. Ann. Surg., 68: 5–11, July 1918
Introduced encephalography.
Röntgenography of the brain after the injection of air into the spinal canal. Ibid., 70: 397–403, Oct. 1919
Daniell, John Frederick. English physicist. 1790–1845
CELL—a form of two-fluid cell for galvanic battery, DANIELL—a unit of electricity equal to 1.124 volts.
An introduction to the study of chemical philosophy; ... London, Parker, 1843. 2 ed., 764 pp.
Daniell, William C. Savannah, Ga. surgeon
Published first paper in America on use of pulley and weight in treatment of fracture of leg.
Method of treating fracture of the thigh bone. Amer. J. med. Sci., 4: 330–333, 1829
Danielopolu, Daniel. Bucharest physician. 1884–
OPERATION—for hypertension, by resection of splanchnic nerves.
Recherches sur la sensibilité viscérale. Possibilité d'améliorer l'angine de poitrine par la résection des racines postérieures ou des nerfs spinaux correspondants. Bull. Soc. méd. Hôp. Paris, 47: 778–790, June 1, 1923
Daniels, L. E. See J. B. Doyle
Danielson, L. Medfield, Mass. physician
Described sleeping sickness in America.
The history of a singular and very mortal disease, which lately made its appearance in Medfield—symptoms of the disorder—its progress and termination—appearances on dissection—the different methods of treatment, and what eventually proved successful with

E. Mann, Med. and Agric. Register, Boston, 1: 65-69, May 1806

Danielssen, Daniel Cornelius. Norwegian physician. 1815-1894

DISEASE—of Danielssen-Boeck; leprosy.

Om spedalskheden with C. W. Boeck, Christiania, 1847

Also, in French, Paris, 1848. 2 vols.

Danilemsi, Aleksandr Iakovlyovich. 1838-?

Discovered trypsin.

Ueber specifisch wirkende Körper des natürlichen und künstlichen pancreatischen Saftes. Arch. f. path. Anat. u. Physiol., 25: 279-307, 1862

Danlos, Henri Alexandre. French physician. 1844-1912

SYNDROME—of Ehlers-Danlos; characterized by overextensibility of joints, hypertrophy of joints, hyperelasticity of skin, fragility of skin and pseudo-tumors following trauma.

Un cas de cutis laxa avec tumeurs par contusion chronique des coudes et des genoux. Bull. Soc. franc. de dermat. et Syph., Paris, 19: 70-72, 1908

Used radium for lupus.

Note sur le traitement du lupus érythémateux par des applications de radium with P. Bloch, Ibid., 12: 438-440, 1901

Danne, J. See M. S. Curie

Dantschakoff, Wera. Moscow histologist

METHOD—of serial sections by celloidin.

Zur Herstellung der Celloidinserien. Z. f. wiss. Mikr., 25: 32-37, June 23, 1908

Danysz, Jan. French physician. 1860-1928

PHENOMENON—decrease of neutralizing influence of an antitoxin when a toxin is added to it in divided portions instead of all at once. Dorland

Contribution à l'étude de la toxine tétanique sur la substance nerveuse. Ann. Inst. Pasteur, 13: 156-168, Feb. 1898

Contribution à l'étude de l'immunité. Propriétes des mélanges des toxines avec leurs antitoxines. Constitution des toxines. Ibid., 581-595, July 1899

Principes de l'évolution des maladies infectieuses. Paris, Baillière, 1918. 171 pp.

Also, transl. by F. M. Rackermann, Philadelphia, Lea and Febiger, 1921. 194 pp.

Dare, Arthur. Philadelphia physician. 1868-

HEMOGLOBINOMETER and METHOD—of determination of hemoglobin.

A new hemoglobinometer for the examination of undiluted blood. Philadelphia Med. J., 6: 557-561, Sept. 22, 1900

METHOD—for determination of alkalinity of blood.

A new method of hemo-alkalimetry and a new hemo-alkalimeter. Ibid., 11: 137-142, Jan. 17, 1903

A new hemo-alkalimeter. Proc. Path. Soc. of Philadelphia, 2 s., 6: 137-149, Apr. 1903

Darier, Ferdinand Jean. French physician. 1856-1938

DISEASE—psorospermosis; keratosis follicularis.

De la psorospermose folliculaire végétante. Étude anatomo-pathologique d'une affection cutanée non décrit ou comprise dans le groupe des acnés sébacées, conées, hypertrophiantes, des keratosis (ichthyoses) folliculaires, etc. Thesis de Paris, 1889

Also: Ann. de Dermat., 10: 597-642, July 25, 1889

DISEASE—pseudoxanthoma elasticum.

Pseudoxanthoma elasticum. Third Inter. Dermat. Cong., London, 1896

Also: Mschr. prakt. Dermat., 23: 609-617, Dec. 15, 1896

Sarcoid—

Un cas de tumeurs bénignes multiples (sarcoides sous-cutanées ou tuberculides nodulaires hypodermiques) with G. Roussy, Bull. Soc. franç. de Dermat., 15: 54-59, Feb. 4, 1904

Also: Ann. de Dermat., 5: 144-149, 1904

Des sarcoides sous-cutanées. Contribution à l'étude des tuberculides ou tuberculoses atténuées de l'hypoderme with G. Roussy, Arch. Méd. exp., 18: 1-50, Jan. 1906

Described acanthosis nigricans.

Dystrophie papillaire et pigmentaire. Ann. de Dermat., 3 s., 4: 865-875, July 1893

Darkshevitch, Liveri Osipovich. Russian neurologist. 1858-1925

FIBERS—of cerebrum running from optic tract to habenular ganglion.

NUCLEUS—of cells in upper part of aqueduct above third nucleus and extending into walls of third ventricle.

Kurs neronikh bolieznei. Kazan, Br. Bashmakovi, 1904-09. 3 vols.

Darling, Georgina. See W. J. Wilson

Darling, Samuel Taylor. Ancon, Panama physician. 1872-1925

DISEASE—histoplasmosis.

A protozoön general infection producing pseudotubercles in the lungs and focal necrosis in the liver, spleen and lymph nodes. J. A. M. A., 46: 1283-1285, Apr. 28, 1906

Notes on histoplasmosis—a fatal disorder met with in tropical America. Maryland med. J., 1: 125-129, Apr. 1907

Histoplasmosis: a fatal infectious disease resembling kala-azar found among the natives of tropical America. Arch. intern. Med., 2: 107-123, Aug. 1908

STAIN—for Entamaeba histolytica.

Romanowsky stain for entamebas. J. A. M. A., 59: 292 (only), July 27, 1912

Darmstädter, Ernst. German physician. 1877-1936

METHOD—for direct estimation of B-oxybutyric acid in urine.

Die quantitative Bestimmung der B-Oxybuttersäure im Harne. Z. phys. Chem., 37: 355-362, Feb. 21, 1903

Darnall, Carl Rogers. U. S. Army surgeon. 1867-1941

FILTER—for drinking water.

The purification of drinking water for troops in the field. Military Surg., 22: 253-285, Apr. 1908

Darrach, W. See R. L. Patterson, Jr.

Darrow, Daniel Cady. New Haven pediatrician. 1895-

FLUID and METHOD—for hypodermoclysis.

The changes in the distribution of body water accompanying increase and decrease in extracellular electrolyte with H. Yannet, J. clin. Invest., 14: 266-275, Mar. 1935

Dartigues, Louis. French surgeon. 1869-1940

OPERATION—for gynecomastia, with transplantation of nipple.

Mammectomie totale et autogreffe libre aréolomamelon-

naire: mammectomie bilatérale esthétique. Bull. Soc. Chir., Paris, 20: 739–744, 1928

Darwin, Charles Robert. English naturalist. 1809–1882

DARWINISM—theory of evolution: higher organisms have been developed from lower ones through influence of natural selection.
On the origin of species by means of natural selection. London, Murray, 1859. 502 pp.
The descent of man, and selection in relation to sex. London, Murray, 1871. 2 vols.
Described so-called Guilford's disease. In: *The variations of animals and plants under domestication.* New York, Appleton, 1868. 2 vols.

Dastre, Jules Albert Francois. French physician. 1844–1917

LAW—dilatation of splanchnic vessels is usually accompanied by constriction of surface vessels of body, and vice versa.
Recherches expérimentales sur le système nerveux vasomoteur. Paris, Masson, 1884. 344 pp.

Daufresne. See A. Carrel

Davaine, Casimir Joseph. French physician. 1812–1882
Gave an early confirmation of bacterial origin of disease.
Recherches sur les infusoires du sang dans la maladie connue sous le nom de sang de rate. C. R. Acad. Sci., Paris, 57: 220–223, July 27; 351–353, Aug. 10, 1863
Recherches sur la nature et la constitution anatomique-de la pustule maligne. Ibid., 60: 1296–1299, 1865
Discovered Bacillus anthracis in 1850.
Traité des entozaires et des maladies vermineuses de l'homme et des animaux domestiques. Paris, 1860

Davat. French surgeon

OPERATION—cure of varicocele by compressing veins by acufilopressure.
De l'obliteration des veines. Paris, 1833. 25 pp.
Same, 1836. 94 pp.

Davenport, Harold Alvin. Chicago anatomist. 1895–

METHOD—of staining nerve fibers.
Staining paraffin sections with protargol. 3. The optimum p H for reduction. 4. A two-hour staining method with Janet McArthur and S. R. Bruesch, Stain Techn., 14: 21–26, Jan. 1939
See also R. L. Swank

David, Jean Pierre. French surgeon. 1737–1784
DISEASE—same as Pott's d.: caries of vertebrae.
Dissertation sur les effets du mouvement et du repos dans les maladies chirurgicales. Paris, Vallat-La Chapelle, 1779. 164 pp.

David, K. Amsterdam pharmacologist
Isolated testosterone.
Über krystallinisches männliches Hormon aus Hoden (Testosteron), wirksamer als aus Harn oder aus Cholesterin bereitetes Androsteron with E. Dingemanse, J. Freud and E. Laquer, Z. physiol. Chem., 233: 281–282, June 7, 1935

David, N. A. See A. C. Reed

David, Vernon Cyrenius. Chicago surgeon. 1882–
MODIFICATION—of Rehn-Delorme operation for rectal prolapse.
Surgery of the rectum and anus. In: *Practice of surgery.* Dean Lewis, Hagerstown, Md., Prior, 1929. Vol. 7, Ch. 6
OPERATION—for posterior resection of colon and rectum.

Surgery of the rectum and anus. In: Nelson's *Loose-Leaf surgery.* Vol. 15, Ch. 3, pp. 160–242
See also A. H. Curtis

David, Walter. Berlin physician. 1890–
DISEASE—hemorrhagic disease with hormone deficiency.
Ueber "Purpura"—Erkrankungen bei Frauen. Med. Klinik, 22: 1755–1756, Nov. 12, 1926

Davidoff, Leo Max. New York neurologist. 1898–
OPERATION—
Treatment of hydrocephalus: historical review and description of a new method. Arch. Surg., 18: 1737–1762, Apr. 1929

Davidsohn, Heinrich. Berlin physician. 1884–
TEST—for differentiating human from cow's milk.
Neue Methode zur Unterscheidung von Frauenmilch und Kuhmilch, zugleich ein Beitrag zum Studium des lipolytischen Milchferments. Z. Kinderheilk., 8: 14–23, May 26, 1913

Davidsohn, Isreal. Chicago physician. 1895–
TEST—for infectious mononucleosis.
Infectious mononucleosis. Amer. J. Dis. Child., 49: 1222–1231, May 1935
The nature of the heterophilic antibodies in infectious mononucleosis with Phoebe H. Walker, Amer. J. Clin. Path., 5: 455–465, Nov. 1935
Serologic diagnosis of infectious mononucleosis. J. A. M. A., 108: 289–295, Jan. 23, 1937

Davidsohn, Isreal
TEST—
A method for recognition of blood subgroups A1 and A2 as a means of avoiding tranfusion reactions. Ibid., 112: 713–719, Feb. 25, 1939

Davidson, Edward Clark. Detroit surgeon. 1894–1933
TREATMENT—
Tannic acid in the treatment of burns. S. G. O., 41: 202–221, Aug. 1925
The prevention of toxemia of burns. Treatment by tannic acid solution. Amer. J. Surg., 40: 114–116, May 1926

Davie, T. B. See F. R. Edwards

Daviel, Jacques. French oculist. 1696-1762
OPERATION—extraction of cataract through corneal incision without incising iris.
SPOON—used in removing lens.
Sur une nouvelle methode guérir la cataracte par l'extraction du cristallin. Mém. Acad. roy. de chir., Paris, 2: 337–354, 1753

Davies, John Archibald V. Boston physician. 1896–
MICROMODIFICATION—of Hinton flocculation technic for syphilis.
A microflocculation test for syphilis. J. Lab. clin. Med., 22: 959–966, June 1937

Davis, Arthur George. Erie, Pa. surgeon. 1887–
EXERCISES—to strengthen anterior capsule of shoulder joint.
SIGN—in determination of function and stability of shoulder.
A conservation treatment for habitual dislocations of the shoulder. J. A. M. A., 107: 1012–1015, Sept. 26, 1936

Davis, B. J. See L. A. Rogers
Davis, C. R. See J. J. Bronfenbrenner
Davis, Carl Braden. Chicago surgeon. 1877–
METHOD—a micromethod for determination of iodine.

Blood iodine studies. I. The quantitative determination of the iodine content of blood with G. M. Curtis, J. Lab. clin. Med., 18: 24–29, Oct. 1932
OPERATION—for slipping patella; transplantation of patellar ligament with plication of medial capsule. *Recurrent dislocation of the patella.* Surg. Clin. M. Amer., 3: 291–293, Apr. 1919
Davis, Carl Henry. Milwaukee gynecologist. 1883–
OPERATION—
Congenital absence of the vagina: report of two cases treated by a vaginal plastic operation with R. S. Cron, Amer. J. Obstet. Gynaec., 15: 196–201, Feb. 1928
Davis, D. See S. Weiss
Davis, D. M. See E. K. Marshall, Jr.
Davis, George Gilbert. Chicago surgeon. 1879–
OPERATION—
Ruptured urethra operation. S. G. O., 50: 105 (only), Jan. 1930
Davis, Gwilym George. Philadelphia surgeon. 1857–1918
INCISION—
A transverse incision for the removal of the appendix. Ann. Surg., 43: 106–110, Jan. 1906
OPERATION—arthrodesis of subastragular joints.
The treatment of hollow foot (pes cavus). Amer. J. Orthop. Surg., 11: 231–242, Oct. 1913
Davis, John Staige. Baltimore surgeon, 1872–1946
GRAFT or METHOD—
A method of splinting skin grafts. Ann. Surg., 49: 416–418, Apr. 1909
The use of small deep skin grafts. J. A. M. A., 63: 985–989, Sept. 19, 1914
The use of free grafts of whole thickness skin for the relief of contractures. S. G. O., 25: 1–8, July 1917
Plastic surgery: its principles and practice. Philadelphia, Blakiston, 1919
The small deep graft: relationship to the true Reverdin graft. Ann. Surg., 89: 902–916, June 1929
The small deep graft. Ibid., 91: 633–635, Apr. 1930
Davis, Lewis. American chemist. 1889–
SOLUTION—basal cystine tryptophane, for cultivation of B. diphtheriae.
Studies on diphtheria toxin. II. The role of the amino acids in the metabolism of Bacterium diphtheriae with N. S. Ferry, J. Bact., 4: 217–241, May 1919
Davis, Lincoln. Boston physician. 1872–
MEDIUM—serum, for cultivation of Ducrey bacillus.
Observations on the distribution and culture of the chancroid bacillus. J. med. Res., 9: 401–415, June 1903
Davis, Loyal Edward. Chicago surgeon. 1896–
OPERATION—lumbar sympathectomy by transperitoneal approach.
Sympathectomy in Raynaud's disease, erythromelalgia and other vascular diseases of the extremities with A. B. Kanavel, S. G. O., 42: 729–742, June 1926
Demonstrated nerve pathways from hypothalmus to pituitary.
Carbohydrate metabolism. The effect of hypothalmic lesions and stimulation of the autonomic nervous system with D. Cleveland and W. R. Ingram. Arch. Neurol. Psychiat., Chicago, 33: 592–615, Mar. 1935
Davis, Marguerite. See E. V. McCollum
Davis, Morris Edward. Chicago gynecologist, 1899–
Isolated ergotocin.
A new active principle in ergot and its effects on uterine

motility with F. L. Adair, G. Rogers, M. S. Kharasch and R. R. Lagault, Amer. J. Obst. & Gynec., 29 155–167, Feb. 1935
A study of a new and potent ergot derivative, ergotocin Ibid., Ibid., 30: 466–480, Oct. 1935
Davis, T. L. See J. H. Cunningham
Davis, Theodore McCann. Greenville, S. C. urologist 1889–
OPERATION—use of coagulating current for hypertrophied prostate.
The present status of prostatic resection. J. A. M. A. 99: 1928–1932, Dec. 3, 1932
Davis, Warren Beagle. Philadelphia surgeon. 1881–
OPERATION—osteouranoplasty.
Harelip and cleft palate: a study of four hundred and twenty-five consecutive cases. Ann. Surg., 87: 536–554 Apr. 1928
Davy, Sir Humphrey. English scientist. 1788–1829
Discovered anesthetic properties of nitrous oxide 1799.
Researches, chemical and philosophical; chiefly concerning nitrous oxide, or dephlogisticated nitrous air and its respiration. London, Johnson, 1800. 580 pp
Also in: *The collected works of . . .* London, Smith, Elder and Co., 1839. vol. 3
Invented safety lamp for coal miners, 1815.
On the safety lamp for coal miners; with some researches on flame. London, Hunter, 1818. 148 pp.
Dawbarn, Robert Hugh Mackay. American surgeon. 1860–915
SIGN—in acute subacromial bursitis; when the arm hangs at the side palpation over bursa causes pain but when arm is abducted pain disappears. (Dorland)
Subdeltoid bursitis: a pathognomic sign for its recognition. Boston M. and S. J., 154: 691 (only), June 14, 1906
Diagnosis of subdeltoid bursitis. Ibid., 155: 25 (only) July 5, 1906
Dawson, Andrew Ignatius. New York bacteriologist
AGAR—butter soap peptone; culture medium.
AGAR—flour peptone, for cultivation of B. coli.
Bacterial variations induced by changes in the composition of culture media. J. Bact., 4: 133–148, Mar 1919
Day, A. A. See A. U. Kendall
Deaderick, William Harvey. Rogersville, Tenn. surgeon. 1773–1858
Removed mandible in 1810.
Case of removal of a portion of the lower maxillary bone. Amer. Med. Recorder, Philadelphia, 6 516–517, July 1823
Dean, A. L. See H. T. Hollmann
Deane, Edmond. English. 1572–
Made first study of mineral waters of England, 1626 (Garrison)
Spadaerme Anglica, the English spaw, or, the glory of Knaresborough. Their nature, physical use, situation, and many admirable cures being exactly expressed in the subsequent treatise of the learned Dr. Dean and the sedulous observations of the rigerious Michae Stanhope. . . . Pub. by J. Taylor, York, Broad 1649. 39 pp.
Deanesly, R. London scientist
Introduced subcutaneous implantation of pellets of estrogens.
Factors influencing the effectiveness of administered

hormones with A. S. Parkes, Proc. R. Soc., B, 124: 279–298, Dec. 7, 1937
Further experiments on the administration of hormones by the subcutaneous implantation of tablets with A. S. Parkes, Lancet, 2: 606–608, Sept. 10, 1938

Deaver, John Blair. Philadelphia surgeon. 1855–1931
INCISION—for appendectomy; through sheath of right rectus muscle with retraction medially of muscle.
Appendicitis. J. A. M. A., 25: 46–50, July 13, 1895
Appendicitis. Philadelphia, Blakiston, 1896. 168 pp. p. 132
OPERATION—
The surgery of pylorospasm with V. G. Burden, Ann. Surg., 90: 530–534. Oct. 1929

DeBains, E. See C. J. H. Nicolle

DeBakey, M. E. See E. W. A. Ochsner

Débove, Georges Maurice. Paris physician. 1845–1920
DISEASE—essential splenomegaly.
La splénomégalie primitive with I. Bruhl, Bull. Soc. méd. Hôp. Paris, 3 s., 9: 596–613, July 29, 1892
TREATMENT—of tuberculosis by a special form of forced feeding.
Leçons cliniques et thérapeutiques sur la tuberculose parasitaire. . . . Paris, Delahaye et Lecrosuier, 1884. 92 pp.
TUBE—for lavage of stomach.
Lavage de l'estomac with A. Rémond, Paris, Rueff, 1892. 208 pp.

Debrand, Louis. French physician. 1859–
BROTH—extract, a culture medium.
Sur un nouveau procede de culture du bacilli du tétanos. Ann. Inst. Pasteur, 14: 757–768, Nov. 1900

Decastello, Alfred Von. Vienna physician. 1872–
Discovered fourth blood group.
Ueber die Isoagglutinine in Serum gesunder und kranker Menschen with A. Sturli, Münch. med. Wschr., 49: 1090–1095, July 1, 1902

Deckers, Frederick. Leyden physician. 1648–1720
Detected albumin in urine (1694) by boiling in presence of acetic acid. (Garrison)
Exercitationes medicae practicae circa medendi methodum, observationibus illustratae. Lugd. Bat. et Amstelodami, Gaesback, 1673. 693 pp. Ch. 5
Exercitationes practicae circa medendi methodum. Leyden, 1694

Declat, Gilbert. French physician. 1827–1896
LIQUID—for use in cholera.
Du choléra . . . In his: De l'acide phénique. . . . Paris, Delahaye, 1874. pp. 603–637

DeEds, Floyd. American pharmacologist. 1894–
METHOD—
A simple micro vessel with electrode for estimating the hydrogen ion concentration of blood and other body fluids with P. J. Hanzlik, J. biol. Chem., 60: 355–360, June 1924

Dees, John Essary. Baltimore physician. 1910–
TREATMENT—
The use of sulfanilamide in gonococcic infections: preliminary report with J. A. C. Colston, J. A. M.A., 108: 1855–1858, May 29, 1937.

Deetjen, Hermann. German physician. 1867–1915
BODIES—blood-plates.
Zerfall und Leben der Blutplättchen. Z. phys. Chem., 63: 1–26, Nov. 5, 1909

Defries, R. D. See N. E. McKinnon

Degen, K. See E. Joest

DeGowin, Elmer Louis. Iowa City physician. 1901–
MODIFICATION—of Rous-Turner solution for preservation of blood for transfusion.
Studies on preserved human blood: I. Various factors influencing hemolysis with J. E. Harris and E. D. Plass, J. A. M. A., 114: 850–855, Mar. 9, 1940

Dehelly, G. See A. Carrel

Dehio, Karl Konstantinovich. Russian physician. 1851–1927
METHOD—of giving water in divided amounts before percussion of stomach.
Zur physikalischen Diagnostik der mechanischen Insufficienz des Magens. Verh. des VII Congr. f. inn. Med., pp. 410–419, 1888

Dehio, W. Wiesbaden chemist
TEST—for acetone in urine.
Beitrag zum Nachweis von Aceton im Harn mit Nitro-p-phelyl-hydrazin und zur annähernden Bestimmung des Acetons. Z. anal. Chem., 104: 417–422, 1936

Dehn, William Maurice. Seattle, Wash. chemist. 1872–
TEST—for hippuric acid in presence of urea.
Some characteristic color reactions produced by sodium hypobromite with S. F. Scott, J. Amer. Chem. Soc., 30: 1418–1423, 1908

Deibert, O. See O. Teague

Deiters, Otto Friedrich Carl. German anatomist. 1834–1863
CELLS—on basilar membrane of cochlea.
FRAMES—plates in lamina recitularis uniting Deiter's phalanges with cells of Hensen.
NUCLEUS—origin of median root of auditory nerve.
PHALANGES—plates at ends of cells of reticular membrane of organ of Corti.
PROCESS—axis-cylinder p.
TRACT—vestibulospinal t.
Untersuchungen über Gehirn und Rückenmark des Menschen und der Säugethiere. Brunschweig, Vieweg u. Sohn, 1865. 318 pp.

Déjérine, Joseph Jules. Paris neurologist. 1849–1917
ATROPHY or DISEASE—hypertrophic interstitial neuritis of infancy.
Sur une forme particulière de maladie de Friedreich avec atrophie musculaire et troubles de la sensibilité. C. R. Soc. Biol., Paris, 9 s. 2: 43–53, 1890
Sur la névrite interstitielle hypertrophique et progressive de l'enfance. . . . with J. Sottas, Ibid., 5: 63–96, 1893
NEURITIS—peripheral or SYNDROME—resembling tabes dorsalis, with deep sensibility depressed, but with tactile sense normal.
Sur un cas de paraplégie par névrites périphériques, chez un ataxique morphiomane (Contribution à l'étude de la névrite périphérique). Ibid., 8 s., 4: 137–143, 1887
SYNDROME—the thalamus opticus s.
Le syndrome thalamique with G. Roussy, Rev. neurol., 14: 521–532, 1906
See also L. T. J. Landouzy

Déjérine-Klumpke, Augusta. French neurologist. 1859–1927
PARALYSIS—of hand with lesion of brachial plexus, eighth cervical and first dorsal nerves.
Contribution à l'étude des paralysies radiculaires du

plexus brachial. Paralysies radiculaires totales. Paralysies radiculaires inférieures. De la participation des filets sympathiques oculo-pupillaires dans ces paralysies. Rev. de méd., Paris, 5: 591–616, July; 739–790, Sept. 1885

Described lead palsies.

Des polynévrites en général et des paralysies et atrophies saturnines en particulier. Paris, Alcan, 1889

Delafield, Francis. New York pathologist. 1841–1915

FLUID—fixing f.

Handbook of pathological anatomy and histology with T. M. Prudden, New York, Wood, 1889. 3 ed., pp. 45

STAIN—hematoxylin

(Formula given in note by J. M. Prudden, no title) in: Z. wiss. Mik., 2: 288 (only), 1885

Also in: *Handbook* (as above), pp. 47–48

Delagénière, Henry. French surgeon. 1858–1930

METHOD—of osteoperiosteal grafting.

Greffes Ostéo-périostiques; technique et applications. J. Chir., 17: 305–324, Apr. 1921

Delamare, V. See E. C. Achard

Delamarre, Georges. French physician

Described, with his teacher, P. Marie, gastric crises in locomotor ataxia.

Des troubles gastriques dans l'ataxie locomotrice progressive. Paris, Thèse, No. 250, 1866. 46 pp.

Delater. See E. Sacquépée

Delaye, J. B. French physician

PARALYSIS—

Considérations sur une espèce de paralysie qui affecte particulièrement les aliénés. Paris, Thèse, 1824

Delbet, Pierre Louis Ernst. French physician. 1861–1925

SIGN—in aneurysm, although pulsation may have disappeared, collateral circulation is sufficient if nutrition in distal part is maintained.

Du traitement des anéurysmes externes. Rev. Chir., 8: 869–913, Nov.; 998–1011, Dec. 1888; 9: 21–61, Jan. 1889

Also: Pa⁻is, Alcan, 1889. 274 pp.

Deléarde, Albert-Eugène. French physician. 1869–

TEST—for blood.

Sur un nouveau procédé chimique de recherche du sang with Benoit, C. R. Soc. Biol., 64: 990–992, June 6, 1908

DeLee, Joseph Bolivar. Chicago obstetrician. 1869–1942

OPERATION—"prophylactic operation"; when distension of perineum is evident, episiotomy is performed and patient delivered with forceps.

The prophylactic forceps operation. Trans. Amer. Gynec. Soc., 45: 66–83, 1920

Del Huerto, Garcia. 1490–1570

Wrote first book on Indian materia medica and first textbook on tropical medicine.

Coloquios dos simples e drogas he cousas mediçinais da India. Goa, Joannes, 1563

Delmas, J. See J. Fiolle

Delorme, Edmond. French surgeon. 1847–1929

OPERATION—decortication of lung in empyema; pleurectomy.

Nouveau traitement des empyèmes chroniques. Gaz. de hôp., 67: 94–96, 1894

Du traitement des empyèmes par la décortication du poumon. Ibid., 69: 1445–1447; 1453–1456, 1896

Du traitement des empyèmes chroniques par la dé-

cortication du poumon. Cong. franç. de chir. Proc. verb., Paris, 10: 379, 1896; 14: 433, 1901

Urged pericardial resection or decortication.

Sur un traitement chirurgical de la symphyse cardo-péricardique. Gaz. de hôp., 71: 1150–1151, 1898

Delpech, Jacques Mathieu. French surgeon. 1777–1832

Pointed out that spinal caries (Pott's disease) is of tuberculous nature.

Précis élémentaire des maladies réputées chirurgicales. Paris, 3: 629; 638 et seq., 1816

Performed subcutaneous section of tendon Achilles for club-foot.

Considérations sur la difformité appelée pieds-bots. (Section sous-cutanée du tendon d'Achille, le 9 mai 1816.) Clin. chir. de Montpellier, 1: 147–231, (184–192), 1823

Delprat, Guillaume Daniel. San Francisco surgeon 1896–

TEST—

The rose bengal test for liver function: an historical sketch and an improved technic with W. P. Stowe, J. Lab. clin. Med., 16: 923–925, June 1931

Deming, Clyde LeRoy. New Haven surgeon. 1885–

OPERATION—nephropexy.

Nephroptosis: causes, relation to other viscera, and correction by a new operation. J. A. M. A., 95: 251–257, July 26, 1930

Demoivre, Abraham. 1667–1754

FORMULA—expectation of life is equal to $\frac{2}{3}$ of difference between age of person and 80.

Annuities on lives with several tables, exhibiting at one view, the values of lives, for difcrent rates of interest; . . . London, Millar, 1752. 133 pp.

De Morgan, Campbell. English physician. 1811–1876

SPOTS—red spots, sometimes seen on skin of cancer patients.

The origin of cancer: considered with reference to the treatment of the disease. London, Churchill, 1872. 87 pp.

Denig, Rudolf Carl Robert. New York ophthalmologist. 1867–

OPERATION—

Circumcorneal transplantation of buccal mucous membrane as a curative measure in diseases of the eye. Arch. Ophthal., 1: 351–357, Mar. 1929

Denigès, Georges. French chemist. 1859–1935

REACTION—for butyric acid.

Caractérisation et dosage de l'acide butyrique. Repert. de pharm., 29: 262–264, 1917

REACTION—for morphine.

Nouvelle réaction de la morphine. C. R. Soc. Biol., 151: 1062–1063, 1910

REACTION—for strychnine.

Réaction microchimique de la strychnine. Repert. de pharm., 15: 249–250, 1903

TEST—for acetone.

Sur les fonctions organiques pouvant se combiner au sulfate mercurique. Cas des acétones. C. R. Soc. Biol. 126: 1868–1871, June 27, 1898

TEST—for cryogénine in urine.

Recherche de la cryogénine dans l'urine. Repert. de pharm., 22: 441–442, 1910

Denis, Jean Baptiste. French physician. ?–1704

Wrote account of tranfusion of blood from animal to man, performed June 15, 1667. Gertrude L. Annan

Lettre écrite a . . . (Habert) de Montmor . . . touchant

une nouvelle maniere de guerir plusieurs maladies par la tranfusion du sang. Paris, Cusson, 1667. pp. 12–13
An extract of a letter . . . touching a late cure of an inveterate phrensy by the transfusion of blood. Philos. Trans., 2: 617–624, Feb. 10, 1667

Denis, Prosper Sylvain. French chemist. 1799–1863
PLASMIN—a substance obtained by treating blood with sodium sulphate and then with sodium chloride. (Dorland)
Recherches expérimentales sur le sang humain. . . . Paris, Denis, 1830. 358 pp.

Denis, Willey Glover. American biochemist. 1879–
METHOD—
Determination of magnesium in blood. J. biol. Chem., 41: 363–365, Mar. 1920
METHOD—
A method for the quantitative determination of protein in cerebrospinal fluid with J. B. Ayer, Arch. intern. Med., 26: 436–442, Oct. 1920
See also O. K. O. Folin

Denk, Wolfgang. Vienna surgeon. 1882–
OPERATION—for carcinoma of esophagus.
Zur Radikaloperation des Oesophaguskarzinoms Zbl. Chir., 40: 1065–1068, July 5, 1913

Dennett, William Sawyer. American ophthalmologist. 1849–1924
Invented electric light ophthalmoscope.
The electric light ophthalmoscope. Trans. Amer. Ophth. Soc., 21: 156–157, 1885

Dennis, Clarence. Minneapolis surgeon. 1909–
TECHNIC—
A modified Whipple operation for carcinoma of the head of the pancreas. Surgery, 12: 201–206, Aug. 1942
Neoplastic biliary obstruction: an improved type of radical pancreaticoduodenectomy for ampullary and pancreatic cancers with R. L. Varco, Ibid., 20: 72–81, July 1946

Denonvilliers, Charles Pierre. Paris surgeon. 1808–1872
APONEUROSIS or FASCIA—portion of recto-vesical fascia between rectum and prostate.
LIGAMENT—puboprostatic 1.
Anatomie du perinee. Bull. et mém. Soc. anat. de Paris, 11: 105–107, 1836

Denslow, Frank McDonald. Kansas City, Mo. surgeon. 1877–1936
Described syphilis of bladder.
Report of a case of syphilis of the bladder. J. A. M. A., 70: 154 (only), Jan. 19, 1918

Denys, Joseph. Belgian physician. 1857–
TUBERCULIN—same a t. bouillon filtrate.
Le bouillon filtré du bacille de la tuberculose dans le traitement de la tuberculose humaine. Louvain, Uystpruyst, 1905. 322 pp.
Described almost complete absence of platelets in purpura.
Études sur la coagulation du sang dans un cas de purpura aver diminution considérable des plaquettes. La cellule, 3: 445–461, 1887

Denzer, Bernard Solomon. New York pediatrician. 1886–
TROCAR—
The diagnosis of peritonitis and peritoneal transudates in infants by means of abdominal puncture with the capillary tube. Amer. J. med. Sci., 163: 237–245, Feb. 1922

Depage, Antoine. Belgian surgeon. 1863–1925

OPERATION—gastrostomy.
Nouveau procédé pour la gastrostomie. J. chir. et ann. Soc. belge de chir., 1: 715–718, Dec. 1901
Résultats d'une nouvelle méthode de gastrostomie. 6 observations. Ass. franç. de chir., 16: 332–335, Oct 2, 1903

Depaul, Jean Anne Henri. French surgeon. 1811–1883
TUBE—for performing insufflation of lungs.
Mémoire sur l'insufflation de l'air dans les voies aériennes chez les enfants qui naissent dans un état de mort apparente. Paris, Dupont, 1845. 48 pp.

Depisch, Franz. Vienna physician
Described insulin atrophy.
Ueber lokale Lipodystrophie bei lange Zeit mit Insulin behandelten Fällen von Diabetes. Klin. Wschr., 5: 1965–1966, Oct. 15, 1926

Derby, George Strony. Boston ophthalmologist. 1874–1931
OPERATION—
The scleroconjunctival stitch in cataract extraction, Amer. J. Ophth., 8: 381–382, May 1925

Dercum, Francis Xavier. Philadelphia neurologist 1856–1931
DISEASE—adiposis dolorosa.
A subcutaneous connective tissue dystrophy of the arms and neck, associated with symptoms resembling myxedema. University Med. Mag., 1: 140–150, Dec. 1888
Three cases of a hitherto unclassified affection resembling in its grosser aspects obesity, but associated with special nervous symptoms: adiposis dolorosa. Amer. J. med. Sci., 104: 521–535, Nov. 1892

Derick, C. L. See H. F. Swift
de Rouville, W. H. See J. L. Donhauser
De Sanctis, Sante. Italian psychologist. 1862–1935
TEST—of intelligence.
La valutazione della intelligenza in psicologia applicata. Psiche, Fir., 2: 153–174, 1913

Desault, Pierre Joseph. French surgeon. 1744–1795
APPARATUS or BANDAGE—for fractured clavicle.
Oeuvres chirurgicales, ou exposé de la doctrine et de la practique de P. J. Desault. Paris, 1798. 528 pp.
Also: Nouv. ed., Paris, Méquignon, 1801
Also, in English: Philadelphia, Fry and Kammerer, 1805. 413 pp.
Also: 3 ed., Paris, Méquignon, 1813
LIGATURE—of femoral artery for popliteal aneurysm.
Remarques et observations sur l'opération de l'anévrisme. In his: *Oeuvres chirurgicales. . . .* Paris, 1801. pp. 553–580
See also F. Chopart

Descartes, Renatus. French scientist. 1596–1650
"His *De homine* (1662) is usually regarded as the first European text-book on physiology." Garrison
De homine figuris et latinitate donatus a Florentio Schuyl. Lugdini Batavorum, apud Moyardum et Leffen, 1662
Compared eye to a camera obscura, and showed its accommodation to be due to changes in form of lens. Garrison
Dioptrica. 1637

Deschamp, Joseph Francois Louis. French surgeon. 1740–1824
COMPRESSOR—for artery.
NEEDLE—with eye near point, used in ligation of deep-seated arteries.

Observations sur la ligature des principales artères des extrémités, a la suite de leurs blessures, et dans les anévrismes, particulierement dans celui de l'artère poplitée, dont deux ont été opérés suivant la méthode de Jean Hunter. Paris, Chaude, 1793. 48 pp.

Deschiens, Robert. French physician. 1893–
MODIFICATION—of Boeck-Drbohlav medium for culture of trichomanos.
Simplification du milieu de Boeck-Drbohlav pour la culture du Trichomonas. C. R. Soc. Biol., 96: 13–14, Jan. 8, 1927

Desesquelles, Édouard. French physician. 1863–
TEST—for phenols in urine.
Sur un mode de recherche des phénols dans les urines. C. R. Soc. Biol., n.s., 2: 101–104, 1890

Desjardin, Abel. French Physician.
POINT—six cm. above umbilicus on line toward right axilla; point of pancreatic tenderness.
Étude sur les pancréatites. Paris, 1905. 206 pp.

Desmarres, Louis Augusta. French oculist. 1810–1882
DACRYOLITE, DACRYOLITH—masses of Nocardia faersteri in lacrimal canal.
Traité théorique et pratique des maladies des yeux. Paris, Germer-Baillière, 1847. 904 pp.
Opérations qui se pratiquent sur les yeux. Paris, 1850

Desormeaux, Antonin Jean. French neurologist. ?–1894
ENDOSCOPE—
De l'endoscopie et de ses applications au diagnostic et au traitement des affections de l'urèthre et de la vessie. Leçons cliniques. Paris, Baillière, 1865. 186 pp.

D'Espine, Adolph. French physician. 1846–1930
SIGN—in pulmonary tuberculosis bronchophony over spinous processes is heard at a lower level than in health. (Dorland)
La cure marine de la scrofule à l'asile Dollfus de Cannes. Bull. Acad. Méd. Paris, 52: 400–420, Nov. 8, 1904
Le diagnostic précoce de la tuberculose des ganglions bronchiques chez les enfants. Ibid., 57: 167–174, Jan. 20, 1907

Dessauer, Friedrich. German physician. 1881–
CURVES—for deep x-ray therapy.
Zur Therapie des Karzinoms mit Röntgenstrahlen: Vorlesungen über die physikalischei Grundlagen der Tiefentherapie. Dresd., Steinkopff, 1922. 74 pp.

Destrée, Edmond. Brussels physician. 1858–1902
SIGN—unequal dilatation of pupils in tuberculosis.
Ein prämonitorisches Symptom der Lungentuberculose. Wien. med. Pr., 35: 539 (only), Apr. 1, 1894
Also: Congr. int. di Roma, 1894

de Takats, Geza. Chicago surgeon. 1892–
METHOD—
Revascularization of the ischemic kidney with G. W. Scupham, Arch. Surg., 41: 1394–1413, Dec. 1940
TECHNIC—
The injection treatment of varicose veins with H. Quint, S. G. O., 50: 545–561, Mar. 1930
TEST—
Heparin—tolerance: a test of the clotting mechanism. Ibid., 77: 31–39, July 1943

Determann, Hermann. German physician. 1865–
SYNDROME—
"Intermittierendes Hinken" eines Arms, der Zunge und der Beine (Dyskinesia intermittens angiosclero-

tica). Dtsch. Ztschr. f. Nervenh., 29: 152–162, July 13, 1905

Detmold, William. New York surgeon. 1808–1894
OPERATION—
Abscess of the substance of the brain: the lateral ventricles opened by an operation. Amer. J. med. Sci., n.s., 19: 86–95, Jan. 1850

Deuterman, J. L. See C. F. Dixon

Deutsch, Eugen. German obstetrician. 1866–
MANEUVER—of pushing up and rotating fetus when it has become wedged at internal strait.
Beiträge zur Hofmeierschen Methode der Expression des Kindskopfes bei engem Becken unter Berücksichtigung des normalen. Berlin, Schade, 1891. 43 pp.

Deutschlander, Carl Ernst Wilhelm. German orthopedist. 1872–
DISEASE—march foot.
Ueber entzündliche Mittelfussgeschwülste. Arch. klin. Chir., 118: 530–549, 1921
Ueber eine eigenartige Mittelfusserkrankung. Zbl. Chir., 48: 1422–1426, Oct. 1, 1921

Deutschmann, Richard. German physician. 1852–1935
THEORY—infective, of sympathetic ophthalmitis.
Ein experimenteller Beitrag zur Pathogenese der sympathischen Augen-Entzündung. Arch. Ophth., Berlin, 28, 1 Abt.: 291–300, 1882

Deventer, Hendrik von. Dutch obstetrician. 1651–1724
DIAMETER—oblique of pelvis.
METHOD—treatment of pelvic presentation in labor by developing shoulders without previously freeing arms.
PELVIS—one shortened antero-posteriorly. Called "the father of modern midwifery." "Gave first accurate description of the pelvis and its deformities, and the effect of the latter in complicating labor. At the same time it is a pioneer work in the delineation of deformities of the spine." Garrison
Operationes chirurgical, novum lumen exhibentes obstetricantibus, quo fideliter manisfestatur ars obstetricandi, et quidquid ad eam requiritur instructum. Lugd. Bat., Dyckwisen, 1701. 274 pp.

Devergie, Marie Guillaume Alphonse. French physician. 1798–1879
DISEASE—pityriasis rubra pilaris.
Pityriasis pilaris, maladie de peau non decrite par les dermatologistes. Gaz. hebd. de méd. Paris, 3: 197–201, 1856
Traite pratique des maladies de la peau. Paris, Masson, 1857. 2 ed., 852 pp. pp. 454–464

Devine, Sir Hugh Berchmans. Australia surgeon.
OPERATION—exclusion of pylorus.
Basic principles and supreme difficulties in gastric surgery. S. C. O., 40: 1–16, Jan. 1925
Gastric exclusion. Ibid., 47: 239–243, Aug. 1928
OPERATION—colectomy.
Carcinoma of the colon. Brit. med. J., 2: 1245–1249, Dec. 28, 1935
Excision of the rectum. Brit. J. Surg., 25: 351–381, Oct. 1937
Operation on a defunctioned distal colon. Surgery, 3: 165–194, Feb. 1938

Devonshire colic. See G. Baker

Dewees, William Potts. Philadelphia obstetrician. 1768–1841

SIGN—expulsion of whitish mucus by a pregnant woman.
"Gave first full length course of lectures on obstetrics in America." Ravdin
A compendious system of midwifery. Philadelphia, Carey and Lea, 1824. 602 pp.
Wrote early work on pediatrics.
Treatise on the physical and medical treatment of children. Philadelphia, Carey and Lea, 1825
de Weeselow, Owen Lambert Vaughan. English physician. 1883–
METHOD—determination of blood chlorides.
The excretion of chlorides by the healthy and diseased kidney. Quart. J. Med., 19: 53–73, 1925
METHOD—determination of phosphate content of blood serum.
The chemistry of the blood in clinical medicine. London, Benn, 1924
Deycke, Georg. Constantinople physician
AGAR—albuminate; culture medium.
Studien über kulturelle Nährböden with Voigtlander, Zbl. Bakt., 29: 617–627, May 4, 1901
AGAR—alkaline albumin gelatin; for diagnosis of cholera.
Die Benutzung von Alkalialbuminaten zur Herstellung von Nährböden. Ibid., 17: 241–245, Feb. 23, 1895
SOLUTION—albumin peptone, to enrich medium for cholera vibrio.
Ueber einen neuen elektiven Nährboden für Cholerabacillen. Dtschr. med. Wschr., 19: 888–889, Sept. 14, 1893
TREATMENT—
Die Bekämpfung der Tuberkulose mit Partialantigenen. Z. f. ärztl. Fortbild., Jena, 16: 569–576, 1919
Dhommée, René. French physician
REAGENT—for albumin.
Dosage de l'albumine dans l'urine. J. Pharm. Chim., Paris, 7 s., 13: 241–249, 1916
Diamond, Joseph Solomon. New York City physician. 1881–
METHOD—of aspiration separate contents of stomach and duodenum.
The clinical association of secretin in the study of pancreatic junction with S. A. Siegel, New York State J. Med., 41: 869–875, Apr. 15, 1941
See also G. B. Wallace
Diaz, Francisco. Spanish surgeon. circa 1588
Published the first treatise on diseases of the kidney, bladder, and urethra, and is, in effect, the founder of urology. Garrison
Tratado de todas las enfermedades de los rinones, veziga, y carnosidates de la vergz, y urina. Madrid, Sanchez, 1588
Diaz, de Isla (Ruy). 1476–1542
Wrote on American (Haiti) origin of syphilis.
Tractado cótra el mal serpentino. Sevilla, D. de Robertis, 1539
Dibdin, William Joseph. 1850–1925
Introduced bacterial system of sewage purification.
The purification of sewage and water. London, Sanitary Publ. Co., 1897
Dick, George Frederick. American physician. 1881–
IMMUNIZATION—
METHOD—for production of streptococcus antitoxic serum.

Scarlet fever toxin in preventive immunization with Gladys H. Dick, J. A. M. A., 82: 544–545, Feb. 16, 1924
A scarlet fever antitoxin with Gladys H. Dick, Ibid., 82: 1246–1247, Apr. 19, 1924
Therapeutic results with concentrated scarlet fever antitoxin: preliminary report; preparation, standardization, and dosage of the antitoxin with Gladys H. Dick, Ibid., 84: 803–805, Mar. 14, 1925
TEST—
A skin test for susceptibility to scarlet fever with Gladys H. Dick, Ibid., 82: 265–266, Jan. 26, 1924
Dickey, Clifford Allen. San Francisco ophthalmologist. 1901–
OPERATION—for ptosis.
Superior-rectus fascia-lata sling in the correction of ptosis. Amer. J. Ophth., 19: 660–664, Aug. 1936
Dickinson, R. E. See W. W. Tuttle
Dickinson, Robert Latou. Brooklyn surgeon. 1861–
TECHNIC—for vaginal hysterectomy.
Hysterectomy by two suture-ligatures. J. Obstet. Gynaec. Brit. Empire, 24: 176–181, Sept. 1913
Dickinson, William Howship. English physician. 1832–1913
Demonstrated that proximal end of a severed nerve eventually atrophies.
On the changes in the nervous system which follow the amputation of limbs. J. Anat. and Physiol., London, 3: 88–96, Nov. 1868
Dickson, Albert Robb. Battle Creek, Mich. surgeon. 1888–
OPERATION—
Femoral hernia. S. G. O., 63: 665–669, Nov. 1936
Dickson, James Archibald. Cleveland surgeon. 1889–
OPERATION—for slipping patella.
Recurrent dislocation of the patella. Surg. Clin. No. Amer., 16: 997–1000, Aug. 1936
Dickson, James Gillespie. U. S. Army surgeon. 1893–
METHOD—for preparation of a Dirofilaria immitis antigen.
Filariasis in defense force, Samoan group: preliminary report with R. W. Huntington, Jr. and S. Eichold, U. S. Nav. M. Bull., 41: 1240–1251, Sept. 1943
Diday, Charles Joseph Paul Edouard. 1812–1894
Wrote on hereditary syphilis.
Traité de la syphilis des nouveau-nés et des enfants à la mamelle. Paris, Masson, 1854
Also, in English. 1859
Didot, Alphonse. Liege surgeon
OPERATION—for syndactylism.
Note sur la séparation des doigts palmés, et sur un nouveau procédé anaplastique destiné à prévenir la reproduction de la difformité. Bull. Acad. Méd. Belg., 9: 351–356, Mar. 25, 1850
Dieffenbach, Johann Friedrich. Prussian surgeon. 1792–1847
OPERATION—amputation at the hip.
OPERATION—for cleft palate.
OPERATION—plastic closure of triangular defects by displacing a quadrangular flap toward one side of the triangle. (Dorland)
Chirurgische Erfahrungen, besonders über die Wiederherstellung zerstörter Theile des menschlichen Körpers nach neuen Methoden. Berlin, Enslin, 1929–34. 3 vols. (in 4) and atlas

Die operative Chirurgie. Leipzig, Brockhaus, 1845–48. 2 vols.

Experimented on transfusion of blood and fibrin.

Die Transfusion des Blutes und die Infusion der Arzeneien in die Blutgefässe. Berlin, Enslin, 1828. 234 pp.

Performed early operations for hypospadias.

Guerison des jentes congenitales de la verge. Gaz. med. de Par., 5: 156–157, 1837

Treated strabismus by severing tendons of eye muscles.

Ueber die Heilung des angebornen Schielens mittelst durchschneidung des innern geraden Augenmuskels. Med. Zeitg., Berl., 8: 227, 1839

Ueber das Schielen und die Heilung desselben durch die Operation. Berlin, Förstner, 1842. 220 pp.

Diemerbrock, Isbrand van. Dutch physician. 1609–1674

Wrote important work on plague.

De peste libre quatuor. Arenaci, Jacobi, 1646. 337 pl.

Dietl, Joseph. Polish physician. 1804–1878

CRISIS—sudden, severe attacks of pain, due to partial turning of kidney on its pedicle. Przegl. lek. Kraków, 3: 225; 233; 241, 1864

Wandernde Nieren und deren Einklemmung. Wien. med. Wschr., 14: 563–566; 579–581; 593–595, 1864

Dietrich, Albert. Charlottenburg physician. 1873–

STAIN—for lipoids.

Zur Differenzialdiagnose der Fettsubstanzen. Verh. dtsch. Path. Ges., 14: 263–268, 1910

Dietrich, Siegfried. Berlin physician

REACTION—for ascorbic acid in urine.

Ueber eine Farbreaktion der Ascorbinsäure with G. Hundhausen, Klin. Wschr., 16: 222–223, Feb. 13 1937

Dietrich, Walther. Berlin physician

SOLUTION—glycerol yeast infusion peptone, for cultivation of tubercle bacilli.

Vergleichende Prüfung von Tuberkulinen verschiedener Herkunft. Dtsch. med. Wschr., 47: 406–407, Apr. 14, 1921

Dieudonné, Adolph. Munich physician. 1864–

MEDIUM—culture.

Blutalkaliagar, ein Elektivnährboden für Choleravibrionen. Zbl. Bakt., 1: 107–108, 1909

Dieulafoy, Georges. Paris physician. 1839–1911

ASPIRATOR—

*De l'aspiration pneumatique sous-cutanée. Méthode de diagnosti*r *et de traitement.* Paris, Masson, 1870. 12 pp.

Same. A treatise on the pneumatic aspiration of morbid fluids. Philadelphia, Lippincott, 1873. Plate on p. 389

Diez, Julio. Buones Aires surgeon

OPERATION—lumbar sympathectomy.

El tratamiento de las afecciones troficas y gangrenosas de los miembros par la resección dc los cadenas cérvicotoracica y lumbosacra del simpático. Presna méd. argentina, 12: 377–403, Sept. 1925

Digby, Kenelm Henry. China surgeon

SPLINT—

A flexible-knee traction splint for the lower limb. S. G. O., 43: 207–214, Aug. 1926

Di Guglielmo, G. Italian physician

ERYTHROBLASTOSIS—acute.

Eritremie acute. Boll. Soc. med. chir., n. s., 1: 665–673, 1926

Analogie e differenze tra eritremia acute e leucemia acuta. Haematologica, Pavia, 19: 341–352, 1938

Dill, D. B. See L. J. Henderson

Dimitri, V. Argentine physician

DISEASE—Parkes Weber—Dimitri.

Tumor cerebral congénito. (Angioma cavernoso). Rev. Asoc. med. argent., 36: 1029–1037, Dec. 1923

Dimitry, Theodore J. New Orleans ophthalmologist. 1879–

OPERATION—

Evolution of a sucking disk for intracapsular extraction of cataract. Arch. Ophth., 21: 261–265, Feb. 1939

Dimler, M. C. See H. V. Arny

Dimmer, Friedrich. Graz ophthalmologist. 1855–1926

APPARATUS—for photographing fundus oculi.

Ein Apparat zur Photographie des Augenintergrundes. Internat. Cong. Ophthalmology, X, Lucerne, Switzerland, Sept. 13–18, 1904. 143–146

Dimsdale, Thomas (Baron). English physician. 1712–1800

Did important work on vaccination.

The present method of inoculating for the small-pox. London, Owen, 1767

Dingemanse, E. Amsterdam physician

Reported increase of estrin in blood of many types of malignant growth.

Ueber das Vorkommen von hohen Mengen weiblichen (Sexual-) Hormons Menformon im Blut von Krebskranken (Maennern) with J. Freud, S. E. de Jongh and E. Laqueur, Arch. f. Gynaek., 141: 225–227, May 12, 1930

See also K. David

Dingley, L. A. See T. R. Elliott

Di Palma, Joseph Rupert. Brooklyn physician. 1916–

TEST—

A reactive hyperemia ring test in the study, evaluation, and prognosis of pedal lesions caused by arteriosclerosis obliterans and arterial embolism with J. Muss and Frances I. Foster, Amer. Heart J., 24: 345–364, Sept. 1942

Dische, Zacharias. Vienna physiologic chemist

REACTION—aldehyde r., for estimating glycogen content of liver.

Ueber eine neue kolorimetrische Mikrobestimmungsmethode der Kohlehydrate in Organen und Körpersäften with H. Popper, Biochem. Z., 175: 371–411, Aug. 30, 1926

REACTION—for lactic acid.

Ueber charakteristische Farbreaktionen der Milchsäure, des Methylglyoxals und der Kohlehydrate mit Carbazol und Schwefelsäure. Ibid., 189: 77–80, Oct. 7, 1927

Dissard, A. See A. Charrin

Distaso, A. French physician

SOLUTION—trypsinized serum; culture medium.

Sur des milieux de culture liquides et solides préparés avec le serum digéré et dilué. C. R. Soc. Biol., 79: 599–601, July 1, 1916

Dithmarsch

DISEASE—a place in Holstein.

Der morbus Dithmarsicus. Kiel, 1878

Dittel, Leopold von. German surgeon. 1815–1898

OPERATION—for vesicovaginal fistula.

Abdominale Blasenscheidenfistel-Operation. Wien. klin. Wschr., 6: 449–452, June 22, 1893

Dittrich, Franz. German pathologist. 1815–1859

PLUGS—in sputum or bronchial tubes in septic bronchitis.
Beiträge zur pathologischen Anatomie der Lungen-Krankheiten. Erlangen, Blaesing, 1850. 28 pp.

Dix, John. Hull surgeon
OPERATION—for aneurysm.
Two cases of aneurism, one of the carotid and one of the femoral artery, successfully treated by the wire compress. Brit. med. J., 2: 551-554, Oct. 30, 1875

Dixon, Claude Frank. Rochester, Minn. surgeon. 1893-
TREATMENT—of intestinal fistula by 10% tannic acid on eroded skin.
The management of external intestinal fistulas with J. L. Deuterman, J. A. M. A., 111: 2095-2101, Dec. 3, 1938

Dixon, M. See F. G. Hopkins

Dixon, Walter Ernest. English pharmacologist. 1871-1931
Drew attention to similarity between effects of nerve stimulation and certain drugs, especially muscarine, on heart.
The mode of action of specific substances with special reference to secretin with P. Hamill, J. Physiol., 38: 314-336, Mar. 22, 1909

Dixon Mann—see Mann

Doan, C. A. See R. S. Cunningham, Florence R. Sabin and B. K. Wiseman

Dobie, William Murray. English physician. 1828-1915
GLOBULE—in middle of transparent disk of muscle fibril.
LAYER or LINE—separating disks of sarcous matter in striated muscles.
Observations on the minute structures and mode of contraction of voluntary muscular fibre. Ann. and Mag. Nat. Hist., London, 3, 1849

Dobson, Matthew. English physician. ?-1784
Proved that sweetness of urine and blood serum in diabetes is due to sugar.
Experiments and observations on the urine in a diabetes. Med. Obs. amd Inq., London, 5: 298-316, 1776

Dochez, Alphonse Raymond. New York physician. 1882-
BROTH—phosphate.
Studies on the biology of streptococcus. I. Antigenic relationships between strains of streptococcus haemolyticus with O. T. Avery and Rebecca C. Lancefield, J. exp. Med., 30: 179-213, Sept. 1919
METHOD—"agar culture", for immunization of horses for antistreptococcus serum.
The significance of streptococcus hemolyticus in scarlet fever and the preparation of a specific antiscarlatinal serum by immunization of the horse to streptococcus hemolyticus-scarlatinae with Lillian Sherman, J. A. M. A., 82: 542-544, Feb. 16, 1924
See also O. T. Avery

Dock, Gail M. See W. A. Starin

Dodd, Katharine. See Annie S. Minot

Dodek, Samuel Mayer. Cleveland obstetrician. 1902-
METHOD—of delivery in posterior position.
The vertex occipitoposterior position; the treatment of more than 500 consecutive cases. J. A. M. A., 96: 1660-1664, May 16, 1931

Döbereiner, Johann Wolfgang. German physician, 1780-1849

Treated subject of light therapy on scientific basis. Garrison and Morton
Anleitung zur Darstellung und Anwendung aller Arten der kräftigsten Bäder und Heilwässer welche von Gesunden und Krankhen gebraucht werden. Jena, 1816

Doebner, O. German chemist
Discovered cinchophen or phenyl-cinchoninic acid.
Ueber a-Phenylcinchoninsäure und ihre Homolgen: Benzaldehyd, Brenztraubensäure und Anilin. Ann. d. Chem., 242: 290-300, 1887

Döhle, Karl Gottfried Paul. German pathologist. 1855-1928
AORTITIS—syphilitic.
Ein Fall von eigentümlicher Aortenerkrankung bei einem Syfilitischen. Kiel, Lipsius u. Tischer, 1885, 19 pp.
INCLUSION BODIES—in polynuclear leukocytes of blood in several diseases, especially scarlet fever.
Leukocyteneinschlüsse bei Scharlach. Zbl. Bakt., 61: 63-68, Nov. 23, 1912

Döllinger, Ignatius. German physiologist. 1770-1841
RING—around circumference of cornea, formed by thickening of Descement's membrane. Dorland
Illustrationem ichnographicam fabricae oculi humani offert. Wirceburgi, Nitribitt, 1817. 19 pp.

Doerr, Robert. German bacteriologist. 1871-
SOLUTION—mannitol nutrose, for differentiation of colon, typhoid and dysentery group.
Beitrag zum Studium des Dysenteriebacillus. Zbl. Bakt., 34: 385-398, Aug. 22, 1903
Showed relation of pappataci fever to sandfly, Phlebotomus.
Ueber ein neues invisibles Virus. Berl. klin. Wschr., 45: 1847-1849, Oct. 12, 1908
Weitere Unterschungen über das Pappatacifieber with V. K. Russ, Arch. f. Schiffs- u. Trophen-Hyg., Leipzig, 13: 693-706, 1909

Does, O. W. Boston physician
APPARATUS—
Apparatus for resuscitating asphyxiated children. Boston Med. and Surg. J., 120: 9 (only), Jan. 3, 1889

Doganoff, A. See E. Moro

Dogiel, Jan von. German scientist. 1830-1905
Invented stromuhr for measurement of velocity of blood.
Die Ausmessung der strömenden Blutvolumina. Arb. a. d. Physiol. Anst. zu Leipzig, 1867, 2: 196-271, 1868
See also C. F. W. Ludwig

Dogliotti, Achille Mario. Turin surgeon
METHOD—of blood transfusion by use of "multiple paraffinated tubes."
Dimostrazione di uno strumentario completo per la transfusione di sangue puro. Gior. d. Acad. di Med di Torino, 90: 99-108, Feb. 1927
METHOD—subarachnoid injection of absolute alcohol for relief from pain.
Traitement des syndromes douloureux de la périphérie par l'alcoolisation sub-arachnoidienne des racines postérieures a leur émergence de la moelle épinière. Pr. méd., 39: 1249-1252, Aug. 22, 1931
OPERATION—
First surgical sections, in man, of the lemniscus lateralis (pain-temperature path) at the brain stem, for the treatment of diffused rebellious pain. Current Re-

searches in Anest. and Analg., 17: 143–145, May–June 1938
Introduced peridural anesthesia.
Eine neue Methode der regionären Anästhesie: Die peridurale segmentäre Anästhesie. Zbl. Chir., 58: 3141–3145, Dec. 12, 1931
A new method of block anesthesia: segmental peridural spinal anesthesia. Amer. J. Surg., 20: 107–118, Apr. 1933

Dohrn, M. See E. Steinach

Doisy, Edward Adelbert. St. Louis biochemist, 1893–
Awarded Nobel prize in 1943, with H. Dam, for their work on vitamin K.
Vitamin K with S. B. Binkley, S. A. Thayer and R. W. McKee, Science, 91: 58–62, Jan. 19, 1940
Vitamin K with S. B. Binkley and S. A. Thayer, Chem. Rev., 28: 477–517, June 1941
METHOD—
The determination of sodium in blood with R. D. Bell, J. biol. Chem., 45: 313–323, Jan. 1921
Isolated crystalline estrogenic compound.
Folliculin from urine of pregnant women with C. D. Veler and S. A. Thayer, Amer. J. Physiol., 90: 329–330, Oct. 1929
The preparation of the crystalline ovarian hormone from the urine of pregnant women with C. D. Veler and A. Thayer, J. biol. Chem., 86: 499–509, Apr. 1930
See also E. Allen, R. D. Bell, O. K. O. Folin, P. A. Katzman, D. W. MacCorquodale, R. W. McKee

Dold, Hermann. German physician. 1882–
TEST—for syphilis.
Eine vereinfachte, frühzeitig makroskopisch ablesbare Luesflockungsreaktion (Trübungsreaktion). Med. Klin., 17: 940–942, July 31, 1921

Dole, V. P. See R. A. Phillips

Doléris, Jacques Amádée. French gynecologist. 1852–1938
OPERATION—for retroversion of uterus.
Introduction à la pratique gynécologique with R. Pichevin, Paris, Rueff, 1896. 2 vols.

Dollinger, Julius. Budapest surgeon
TECHNIC—of decompression of orbit.
Die Druckenlastung der Augenhöhle durch Entfernung der äusseren Orbitalwand bei hochgradigem Exophthalmus (Morbus Basedowii) und konsekutiver Hornhauterkrankung. Dtsch. med. Wschr., 37: 1888–1890, Oct. 12, 1911

Dolman, C. E. Toronto scientist
TEST—for enterotoxin.
A new method of detecting staphylococcus enterotoxin with R. J. Wilson and W. H. Cockcroft, Canad. Pub. Health J., 27: 489–493, Oct. 1936

Dolt, Maurice Louis. American bacteriologist. 1883–
SOLUTIONS—ammonium asparagin, for cultivation of colon group.
Simple synthetic media for the growth of B. coli and for its isolation from water. J. infect. Dis., 5: 616–626, Dec. 18, 1908

Domagk, Gerhard. German physician. 1895–
Awarded Nobel prize in 1939. Introduced prontosil as a therapeutic agent against hemolytic streptococci.
Ein Beitrag zur Chemotherapie der bakteriellen Infektionen. Dtschr. med. Wschr., 61: 250–253, Feb. 15, 1935
Chemotherapie der bakteriellen Infektionen. Ang. Chem., 48: 657–661, Oct. 19, 1935

Synthesized uleron.
Weitere Untersuchungen über die chemotherapeutische Wirkung sulfonamidhaltiger Verbindungen bei bakteriellen Infektionen. Klin. Wschr., 16: 1412–1418, Oct. 9, 1937

Domarus, Alexander von. German physician. 1881–
FLUID—for blood cell counting.
Die Bedeutung der Kammerzählung der Eosinophilen für die Klinik. Dtsch. Arch. f. klin. Med., 171: 333–358, Sept. 4, 1931

Dominici, Henri. French physician. 1867–1919
TUBE—for applying radium emanations which permits passage of B and Y rays only.
De l'utilisation du rayonnement gamma du radium en thérapeutique. Cong. franç. d. méd., 9 ses., 429–431 1908
Traitement des cancers profonds par le radium with H. Chéron, J. Physiophérap., 8: 135–151, Mar. 15, 1910

Donaggio, Arturo. Italian neurologist
REACTION or TEST—obstruction of urine after surgery.
Ulteriori dati sulla determinazione dell'esistenza e del comportamento di un "fenomeno d'ostacolo" da parte dell'orina e del liquido cefalo-rachidiano umani in condizioni diverse. Riv. neur., 6: 34–44, Feb. 1933

Donald, Archibold. Manchester gynecologist. 1860–1937
OPERATION—the Manchester o.
Operation in cases of complete prolapse. J. Obstet. Gynaec. Brit. Empire, 13: 195–196, Mar. 1908
A short history of the operation of colporrhaphy, with remarks on the technique. Ibid., pp. 256–259, 1921

Donath, Julius. German physician
REACTION—for morphine.
Zwei Morphinreactionen. J. prakt. Chem., 33: 563–564, 1886

Donath, W. F. See B. C. P. Jansen

Donati, Mario. Italian surgeon. 1886–1946
INSTRUMENT—
Strumento per chiusura, sezione e sutura del duodeno (con dimostrazione sull'animale). Arch. ed atti d'Soc. ital de chir., 1930, 37: 719–724, 1931
Also, abstr.: Arch. ital. di chir., 27: 853–854, Dec. 1930
Modello semplificato del mio strumento per sezione e chiusura del moncone del duodeno nella resezione gastro-duodenale. Boll. e. mem. Soc. piemontese de chir., 2: 395–398, Apr. 2, 1932

Donders, Frans Cornelis. Dutch physician. 1818–1889
LAW—rotation of eye around line of sight is not voluntary.
Astigmatisme en cilindrische glazen. Utrecht, Post, 1862. 136 pp.
Also: Berlin, Peters, 1862
Also, transl. by W. D. Moore, London, New Sydenham Soc., 1864
Measured reaction time of a psychical process.
Die Schnelligkeit psychischer Processe. Arch. Anat., Physiol. u, wiss. Med., Berlin, pp. 657–681, 1868

Donhauser, J(oseph) Lewi. Albany, N. Y. surgeon. 1883–
Described—
The human spleen as an haematoplastic organ, as exemplified in a case of splenomegaly with sclerosis of

the bone-marrow. J. exp. Med., 10: 559–574, July 8, 1908
Described—
Multiple myeloma, with special reference to soft tissue metastasis with W. H. de Rouville, Arch. Surg., 43: 946–1020, Dec. 1941

Donné, Alfred. French physician. 1801–1878
Described parasite Trichomonas vaginalis.
Animalcules observés dans les matiéres purulentes et le produit des sécrétions des organes génitaux de l'homme et de la femme. C. R. Acad. Sci., 3: 385–386, 1836
Discovered blood-platelets.
De l'origine des globules du sang, de leur mode deformation et de leur fin. Ibid., 14: 366–368, 1842

Donogany, Zakariás. Budapest physician
TEST—for blood.
Die Darstellung des Hämochromogens als Blutreaction mit besonderer Berücksichtigung des Nachweises von Blut in Harn. Arch. path. Anat. u. Physiol., 148: 234–243, 1897

Donovan, C. Surgeon in Indian Medical Service
BODIES—Leishman-Donovan b.; parasite of kala azar.
On the possibility of the occurrence of trypanosomiasis in India. Brit. med. J., 2: 79 (only), July 11, 1903
Medical cases from Madras General Hospital. Indian med. Gaz., 40: 411–414, Nov. 1905

Donovan, Michael D. Dublin physician. ?–1876
SOLUTION—
On a new chemical combination of arsenic, mercury, and iodine; and on its employment as a therapeutic agent. Dublin J. med. Sci., 16: 277–282, Nov. 1, 1839

Donzelot, E. See L. H. Vaquez

Dopter, Charles Henri Alfred. French bacteriologist. 1873–
SERUM—effective against parameningonococcus.
Diagnostic et traitement de la méningite cérébro-spinale. Paris, Baillière, 1918. 96 pp.
TYPE—of meningococcus.
Etude de quelques germes isolés du rhino-pharynx, voisins du méningocoque (paraméningocoques). C. R. Soc. Biol., 67: 74–76, July 10, 1909

Dorée, Charles. London chemist
REACTION—for cholesterol.
The origin and destiny of cholesterol in the animal organism. Part III. The excretion of cholesterol by the dog with J. A. Gardner, Proc. roy. Soc., 80: 227–239, May 14, 1908
(Same) *Part III. The absorption of cholesterol from the food and its appearance in the blood* with J. A. Gardner, Ibid., 81: 109–128, Apr. 5, 1909

Dorendorf, Hans. Berlin surgeon. 1866–
SIGN—of aneurysm of aortic arch; prominence of supraclavicular groove.
Ueber ein bisher wenig beachtetes Aneurysmensymptom. Dtsch. med. Wschr., 28: 554–555, July 31, 1902

Dorrance, George Morris. Philadelphia surgeon. 1877–
METHOD—
A study of the normal coagulation of the blood, with a description of the instrument used. Amer. J. med. Sci., 146: 562–566, Oct. 1913
Demonstration of an instrument for determining the coagulation time of the blood. Med. Times, 58: 138–139, May 1930

OPERATION—
Operative treatment of pulsating exophthalmos. Amer. J. Ophth., 13: 675–676, Aug. 1930
OPERATION—
The repair of cleft palate: concerning the palatine insertion of the superior constrictor muscle of the pharynx and its significance in cleft palate; with remarks on the "push-back" operation. Ann. Surg., 95: 641–658, May 1932
The operative story of cleft palate with E. Shirozy, Philadelphia, Saunders, 1933

Dorset, Marion. American bacteriologist. 1872–
MEDIUM—egg.
The use of eggs as a medium for the cultivation of bacillus tuberculosis. Amer. Med., 3: 555–556, Apr. 5, 1902
SERUM—
Further experiments concerning the production of immunity from hog cholera with C. N. McBryde and W. B. Niles, U. S. Dept. Agric., Bureau Anim. Indust., Bull. No. 102, 1908. 96 pp.
STAIN—
A new stain for bacillus tuberculosis. Amer. Pub. Health Ass. Rep., 24: 157–160, 1898

Dorsey, John Syng. American surgeon. 1783–1818
Ligated external iliac artery successfully.
Inguinal aneurism cured by tying the external iliac artery in the pelvis. Elect. Repertory, Philadelphia, 2: 111–115, 1811
Wrote first surgical work in United States.
The elements of surgery. 1813. 2 vols.

Doryland, C. J. T. North Dakota scientist
SOLUTION—glucose ammonium sulphate; culture medium.
Preliminary report on synthetic media. J. Bact., 1: 135–152, Mar. 1916

Douglas, Beverly. Nashville surgeon. 1891–
METHOD OF—skin grafting: sieve graft.
The sieve graft—a stable transplant for covering large skin defects. S. G. O., 50: 1018–1023, June 1930

Douglas, Claude Gordon. English physiologist. 1882–
BAG—
A method for determining the total respiratory exchange in man. J. Physiol., 42: xvii–xviii, July 15, 1911
See also J. O. Christiansen

Douglas, James. Scottish anatomist. 1675–1742
CULDESAC or POUCH or SPACE—between anterior wall of rectum and bladder.
LIGAMENTS—peritoneal folds limiting culdesac.
LINE—curved lower edge of inner layer of aponeurosis of internal oblique muscle.
SEMILUNAR FOLD—lower part of posterior wall of sheath of abdominal rectus muscle.
A description of the peritoneum. London, Roberts, 1730

Douglas, John. English surgeon. ?–1759
OPERATION—
Lithotomia Douglassiana, or; an account of a new method of making the high operation, in order to extract the stone out of the bladder. London, Woodward, 1720

Douglas, Stewart Ranken. London scientist. 1871–1936
AGAR—tellurite trypsinized serum; for cultivation of B. diphtheriae.

A new medium for the isolation of B. diphtheriae.
Brit. J. exp. Path., 3: 263-267, Dec. 1922
See also A. E. Wright

Douglass, William. American physician. 1692-1752
Described scarlet fever in New England.
The practical history of a new epidemical eruptive fever with an angina ulculculosa. Boston, Fleet, 1736

Doumer. See E. M. Labbé

Dover, Thomas. English physician. 1660-1741
POWDER—pulvis opii et ipecacuanhae. Formula given in Dover's:
The ancient physician's legacy to his country. . . . London, Bettesworth and Hitch, 1733. 188 pp.

Dowd, Charles North. New York surgeon. 1858-1931
CLOSURE—of intestinal fistula by means of a double metallic button.
Enterostomy for ileus. Ann. Surg., 45: 95-104, Jan. 1917
See also C. McBurney

Dowden, John Wheeler. Edinburgh surgeon. 1866-1936
OPERATION—
A new operation for the cure of femoral hernia. S. G. O., 27: 348-349, Sept. 1918

Dowell, Greensville. American surgeon. 1822-1881
OPERATION—
A treatise on hernia; with a new process for its radical cure, and original contributions to operative surgery, and new surgical instruments. Philadelphia, Brinton, 1876. 205 pp.

Dowman, Charles Edward. Atlanta, Ga. surgeon. 1882-1931
OPERATION—
Relief of diaphragmatic tic, following encephalitis, by section of phrenic nerves. J. A. M. A., 88: 95-97, Jan. 8, 1927

Down, John Langdon Haydon. London physician. 1828-1896
Delineated a clinical picture of mongolism.
Marriages of consanguinity in relation to degeneration of race. London Hosp. Clinical Lectures and Reports, 3: 224-236, 1866
Observations on an ethnic classification of idiots. Ibid., 259-262, 1866

Downes, Sir Arthur Henry. English physician. 1851-1938
Described bactericidal action of sunlight.
Researches on the effect of light upon bacteria and other organisms with T. P. Blunt, Proc. roy. Soc., 26: 488-500, Dec. 6, 1877

Downes, William A. New York surgeon. 1872-
OPERATION—
Cases illustrating the use of the rectus muscle in direct inguinal hernia. Abstr.: Ann. Surg., 53: 568-570, Apr. 1911
TECHNIC—
Management of direct inguinal hernia. Arch. Surg., 1: 53-73, July 1920

Downey, Hal. Minneapolis scientist. 1877-
CELLS—leukocytoid, in blood in infectious mononucleosis.
Acute lymphadenosis compared with acute lymphatic leukemia with C. A. McKinlay, Arch. intern. Med., 32: 82-112, July 1923

Downs, T. McK. See W. E. Lee

Doyen, Eugène Louis. Paris surgeon. 1859-1916

OPERATION—excision of gasserian ganglion.
L'extirpation du ganglion de Gasser. Arch. Prov. de Chir., 4: 429-444, July 1895
Editorial in Ann. Surg., 23: 69, 1896
METHOD—of intestinal anastomosis.
Nouveau procede d'enterorrhaphie. 11 Congr. française, Paris, 1897

Doyle, John Benedict. Rochester, Minn. neurologist. 1894-
Reported use of ephedrine in treatment of narcolepsy.
Narcolepsy: results of treatment with ephedrine sulphate with L. E. Daniels, J. A. M. A., 98: 543-545, Feb. 13, 1932

Doyne, Robert Walter. English ophthalmologist. 1857-1916
Reported angioid streaks in fundus oculi.
Diseases of the optic nerve. 1. Recurrent transient blindness. Trans. Ophth. Soc. of United Kingdom, 9: 148-152, 1889

Doyon. See L. Hugounenq

Dragendorff, Georg Johann Noël. German physician. 1836-1898
TEST—for bile acids in urine.
Auffindung der Gallensäuren im Harn. Repert. f. Pharm., 17: 657, 1869
Wrote on forensic chemistry.
Die gerichtlichchemische Ermittelung von Giften in Nahrungsmitteln, Luftgemischen, Speiseresten, Körpertheilen. . . . St. Petersburg, Schmitzdorff, 1868

Dragstedt, Lester Reynold. Chicago surgeon. 1893-
METHOD—of skin grafting.
A modified sieve graft; a full thickness skin graft for covering large defects with H. Wilson, S. G. O., 65: 104-106, July 1937
OPERATION—
Implantation of the hepatic duct into the duodenum or stomach with O. C. Julian, J. G. Allen, and F. M. Owens, Jr. Ibid., 77: 126-129, Aug. 1943
POUCH—of isolated stomach.
The fatal effect of the total loss of gastric juice with J. C. Ellis, Amer. J. Physiol., 93: 407-416, June 1, 1930
OPERATION—
Supra-diaphragmatic section of the vagus nerves in treatment of duodenal ulcer with F. M. Owens, Jr. Proc. Soc. exp. Biol., N. Y., 53: 152-154, June 1943
Supra-diaphragmatic section of the vagus nerves in the treatment of duodenal and gastric ulcers with W. L. Palmer, P. W. Shafer and P. C. Hodges, Gastroenterology, 3: 450-462, Dec. 1944
Discovered lipocaic hormone.
Observations on a substance in pancreas (a fat metabolizing hormone) which permits survival and prevents liver changes in depancreatized dogs with J. van Prohaska and H. P. Harms. Amer. J. Physiol., 117: 175-181, Sept. 1, 1936
See also J. G. Allen

Drake, Daniel. American physician. 1785-1852
Wrote early work on relation of geography to medicine.
A systematic treatise, historical, etiological, and practical, on the principal diseases of the Interior Valley of North America as they appear in the Caucasian, African, Indian and Esquimaux varieties of its population. Cincinnati, Smith, 1850. 878 pp.
Same, 2 ser., Philadelphia, Lippincott. 985 pp.

Draper, John William. See John William Draper Maury

Dratz, H. M. See K. S. Grimson

Orbohlav, J. See W. C. Boeck

Drechsel, Edmund. German chemist. 1843–1897
Discovered that protein molecule contains both mono- and di-amino acids.
Der Abbau der Eiweisstoffe. Arch. Anat. Physiol., Lpz., pp. 248–278, 1891

Drennan, Jennie Gillespie. New York physician. 1870–
AGAR—crystal violet infusion; for isolation of B. pestis.
A selective medium for the isolation of B. pestis from contaminated plague lesions and observations on the growth of B. pestis on autoclaved nutrient agar with O. Teague, J. med. Res., 36: 519–532, July 1917

Dresbach, Melvin. American physiologist. 1874–1946
APPARATUS—
An improved form of apparatus for perfusion of the excised mammalian heart. Quart. J. exp. Physiol., 8: 73–77, Apr. 4, 1914
SYNDROME—anemia in which red corpuscles appear sickle shaped.
Elliptical human red corpuscles. Science, 19: 469–470, Mar. 18, 1904
Elliptical human erythrocytes (a supplementary statement). Ibid., 21: 473–475, Mar. 24, 1905
See also A. Knudson

Dresel, Kurt. Berlin physician. 1892–
". . . likens the diencephalon to a thermostat." Fetterman
Die Bedeutung der vegetativen Zentren für die innere Medizin. Med. Klin., 19: 1417–1419, Oct. 28, 1923

Dressler, Dr. Würzburg physician
Disease—recurrent hemoglobinuria.
Ein Fall von intermittirender Albuminurie und Chromaturie. Arch. path. Anat. u. Physiol., 6: 264–266, 1854

Drew, A. H. See W. Cramer

Drewsen, V. See A. Baeyer

Dreyer, Georges. Oxford pathologist. 1873–1934
ANTIGEN—produced by treating killed tubercle bacilli with a solution of formaldehyde and acetone.
Some new principles in bacterial immunity, their experimental foundation, and their application to the treatment of refractory infections. Brit. J. exp. Path., 4: 146–176 (149–150), June 1923
TEST—Sigma reaction, for diagnosis of syphilis.
A simple quantitative serum-reaction for the diagnosis of syphilis and the expression of results in standard units with H. K. Ward, Lancet, 1: 956–961, May 7, 1921
Popularized theory that magnitude of breathing capacity is an index of physical fitness.
Investigations on the normal vital capacity in man and its relation to the size of the body. The importance of this measurement as a guide to physical fitness under different conditions and in different classes of individuals. Lancet, 2: 227–234, Aug. 9, 1919
The assessment of physical fitness with G. F. Hanson, London, Cassell, 1920. 115 pp.

Drigalski, Karl Wilhelm von. German bacteriologist. 1871–

MEDIUM—for detecting typhoid bacilli in blood.
Ueber ein Verfahren zum Nachweis der Typhusbacillen with H. Conradi, Z. Hyg. InfektKr., 39: 283–300, 1902

Drinker, Philip. Boston scientist. 1893–
APPARATUS—respirator.
The use of a new apparatus for the prolonged administration of artificial respiration. I. A fatal case of poliomyelitis with C. F. McKhann, J. A. M. A., 92: 1658–1660, May 18, 1929
An apparatus for the prolonged administration of artificial respiration. A design for adults and children with L. A. Shaw, J. clin. Invest., 7: 229–247, June 20, 1929

Drucker, Paul. Copenhagen pediatrician. 1891–
METHOD—of obtaining blood specimen from heel of small children.
Investigations on the hemoglobin and cell volume in certain pathological conditions in the small child. Acta ped., a, 3: 40–56, Oct. 15, 1923
A simple method for obtaining cutaneous (capillary) blood from infants and adults for calorimetric pH determination with G. E. Cullen, J. biol. Chem., 64: 221–227, May 1925

Drummond, David. English physician
OPERATION—Talma-Drummond-Morison o.
A case of ascites due to cirrhosis of the liver cured by operation with J. R. Morison, Brit. med. J., 2: 728–729, 1896
See also J. R. Morison

Drummond, J. C. See O. Rosenheim

Drury, Phoebe E. See J. L. Stoddard

Drysdale, Thomas Murray. American gynecologist. 1831–1904
CORPUSCLES—transparent microscopic cells seen in fluid of ovarian cysts.
On the granular cell found in ovarian fluid. Trans. Amer. Med. Ass., 24: 179–184, 1873

Duane, Alexander. New York oculist. 1858–1926
TEST—employment of candle-blaze and prisms to measure degree of ocular heterophoria.
Some new tests for insufficiencies of the ocular muscles . . . New York Med. J., 50: 113–118, Aug. 3, 1889

Dubini, Angelo. Italian physician. 1813–1902
DISEASE—electric chorea, myoclonic form of epidemic encephalitis.
Primi cenni sulla corea elettrica. Ann. univ. di med., Milano, 117: 5–50, 1846
Discovered parasite of ancylostomiasis.
Nuovo verme intestinale umano (Agchylostoma duodenale), constituente un sesto genere dei nematoidei proprii dell'uomo. Ibid., 106: 5–51, 1843

Dublin
METHOD—of expression of placenta by external manual manipulation. See John Harvie

DuBois, Delafield. New York scientist. 1882–
FORMULA or METHOD—
Clinical calorimetry: fifth paper: the measurements of the surface of area of man with E. F. DuBois, Arch. intern. Med., 15: 868–881, May 1915
A formula to estimate the approximate surface area if height and weight be known with E. F. DuBois and E. Floyd, Ibid., 17: 863–871, June 15, 1916

DuBois, E. F. See R. R. Hannon

Dubois, Paul. French obstetrician. 1795–1871

ABSCESS or DISEASE—of thymus in congenital syphilis.
*Du diagnostic de la syphilis considérée comme une des
causes possibles de la mort du foetus.* Gaz. méd. de
Paris, 21: 392-395, May 25, 1850
Described hyperemesis gravidarum.
*Considérations sur l'avortement dans les cas de vomis-
sements.* Bull. Acad. Méd. Paris, 17: 557-583, 1852
Dubois-Reymond, Emil Heinrich. German physi-
ologist. 1818-1896
LAW—variation of current density, and not absolute
value of current density at any given moment, acts
as stimulus to muscle or motor nerve. (Dorland)
Described electrotonus.
Ueber den sogenannten Froschstrom. Ann. d. Physik.,
Berlin, 58: 1-30, 1843
Untersuchungen über thierische Electricität. Berlin,
Reimer, 1848-60. 2 vol. in 3
Dubos, René Jules. New York bacteriologist. 1901-
Introduced gramicidin.
*Studies on a bactericidal agent extracted from a soil
bacillus. I. Preparation of the agent; its activity in
vitro.* J. exp. Med., 70: 1-10, July 1, 1939
(Same) *II. Protective effect of the bactericidal agent
against experimental pneumococcus infections in mice.*
Ibid., 11-17
Du Bose, Francis Goodwin. Selma, Alabama surgeon.
1873-
OPERATION—
A new operation for umbilical hernia. S. G. O., 21:
771-773, Dec. 1915
Dubovsky, Bertha J. San Francisco scientist
SOLUTION—liver digest, for cultivation and toxin
production of B. botulinus.
*An experimental study of the methods available for
the enrichment, demonstration and isolation of B.
botulinus in specimens of soil and its products, in
suspected food, in clinical and necropsy material* with
K. F. Meyer, J. Infect. Dis., 31: 501-540 (505),
Dec. 1922
Dubreuil, Georges. Lyon physician. 1879-
STAIN—for connective tissue.
*Modifications structurales et disparition des fibres
élastiques au cours de l'inflammation expérimentale du
mésentère de la grenouille.* Bibliograph. Anatom., 13:
133-148, June 6, 1904
Reported hypertrophy and hyperplasia of islands of
Langerhans in fetus of a diabetic mother.
*Ilots de Langerhans géants chez un nouveau-né, issu
de mère glycosurique* with Anderodias, C. R. Soc.
Biol., 83: 1490-1493, Nov. 9, 1920
Duchàcek, F. Prossnitz physician
SOLUTION—nitrate glucose.
SOLUTION—nitrate tartaric acid: culture media.
*Neue biologisch-chemische Untersuchungen über den
Bacillen typhi abdominalis und Bacterium coli com-
mune.* Zbl. Bakt., 37: 161-168 (162), Oct. 17, 1904
Duchenne, Guillaume Benjamin Armand. French
neurologist. 1806-1875
DISEASE—myelopathic or progressive muscular
atrophy; Aran-Duchenne or Duchenne-Griesinger d.
*Recherches faites à l'aide du galvanisme sur l'etat de
la contractilité et de la sensibilité électro-musculaires
dans les paralysies des membres supérieurs.* C. R.
Acad. Sci., Paris, 29: 667-670, 1849
Recherches sur la paralysie musculaire pseudohyper-

trophique ou paralysie myo-sceérosique. Arch. gén.
de méd., 1: 5-25; 179-209; 305-321; 421-443; 552-
588, 1868
Also: London, New Sydenham Soc., 1883
DISEASE or PARALYSIS—bulbar p.
*Paralysie musculaire progressive de la langue, du voil.
du palais et des lèvres.* Arch. gén. de méd., 16: 283-
296; 431-445, 1860
DISEASE—locomotor ataxia.
*De l'ataxie locomotrice progressive, recherches sur un
maladie charactérisée spécialement par des trouble
généraux de la coordination des mouvements.* Ibid., 12
641-652, 1858; 13: 36-62; 158-181; 417-451, 1859
PARALYSIS or SYNDROME—involving fifth and
sixth cervical nerves; upper arm form; same as
Erb's s.
*De l'électrisation localisée et de son application à la
pathologie et à la thérapeutique.* Paris, Baillière, 1855
2 ed., 1861. 3 ed., 1872
Same, in English, London, Hardwicke, 1871. 322 pp.
SYNDROME—collective signs of labioglossopharyn-
geal paralysis; see bulbar paralysis.
Treated deafness by faradization of ossicles and
chorda tympani.
*Exposition d'une nouvelle méthode de galvanisation,
dite galvanisation localisée.* Arch. gén. de méd., 4 s.,
23, 1850
Also: Paris, Rignoux, 1850. 51 pp.
Founder of electrotherapy.
See Paralysis or Syndrome.
Ducrey, Augusto. Italian physician. 1860-1940
BACILLUS—of chancroid.
DISEASE—soft cnancre.
Il virus dell'ulcera venerea. Gazz. internaz. d. sci.
med., Napoli, 11: 44, 1889
*Experimentelle Untersuchungen über den Ansteckungs-
stoff des weichen Schankers und über die Bubonen.*
Mschr. prak. Derm., 9: 387-405, Nov. 1, 1889
Also: Congres internat. de dermatol. et syphiliogr.,
Paris, 1889. p. 229
Dudgeon, Leonard Stanley. English physician.
1876-1938
METHOD—
*On the demonstration of particles of malignant growth
in the sputum by means of the wet-film method* with
C. H. Wrigley, J. Laryng., 50: 752-763, Oct. 1935
STRAIN or TYPE—of dysenteriae.
*Studies of bacillary dysentery occurring in the British
forces in Macedonia.* M. Res. Com., Special Report
Series, London, No. 40, 1919. 35 pp.
Dudley, Benjamin Winslow. Kentucky surgeon.
1785-1870
Successfully trephined for relief of epilersy.
(No title)
Abstr.: Amer. J. med. Sci., 11: 542 (only), Feb.
1833
Dudley, Emilius Clark. Chicago gynecologist. 1850-
1928
OPERATION—
A new operation for procidentia uteri. Amer. Gynec.
and Obstet. J., 5: 1-11, July 1894
Dudley, Harold Ward. London chemist. 1887-1935
Isolated ergmetrine.
*The substance responsible for the traditional clinical
effect of ergot* with C. Moir, Brit. med. J., 1: 520-
523, Mar. 16, 1935
See also H. H. Dale

Dudley, William Lofland. Cincinnati physician. 1859–
REAGENT—for testing for glucose.
  On a modification of Böttger's test for sugar. Amer. Chem. J., 2: 47–48, Apr. 1880
Dührssen, Jacobus Alfred. German obstetrician. 1862–1933
INCISIONS—of cervix, or hysterostomatomy, for prompt termination of labor.
  Kaiserschnitt, tiefe Cervixincisionen und mechanische Dilatation des Muttermundes. Berl. klin. Wschr., 30: 643–646, July 3; 676–679, July 10, 1893
OPERATION—cesarean section by vaginal route; performed Apr. 1895.
  Ueber vaginalen Kaiserschnitt. Samml. klin. Vortr., Leipzig, No. 232, Gynäkol. No. 84, pp. 1355–1388, 1898
Dührssen, Jacobus Alfred.
OPERATION—vaginal fixation of uterus.
  Ueber die operative Heilung der Retroflexio uteri auf vaginalem Wege an der Hand von 182 eigenen Operationsfählen. Aerztl. Prakt., Hamb., 6: 1555–1567, 1893
  Ueber eine neue Methode der Laparotomie (vaginale Coeliotomie). Berl. klin. Wschr., 31: 673–675, July 6: 695–698, July 23, 1894
TAMPON—of vagina with iodoform gauze in uterine hemorrhage.
  Die Anwendung der Jodoformgaze in der Geburtshülfe. Berlin, Fischer, 1888. 34 pp.
Duel, A. B. See C. A. Ballance
Dufau, E. See L. L. Grimbert
Duff, G. L. See W. G. MacCallum
Duflos, Adolf. Halle pharmacologist
REACTION—for morphine.
  Beiträge zur chemischen Kenntniss des Morphins und Narkotins. J. Chem. u. Physik., 61: 105–120, 1831
Dugas, Louis Alexander. American physician. 1806–1884
SIGN or TEST—with dislocated shoulder it is impossible to place elbow against side with hand on uninjured shoulder.
  Report on a new principle of diagnosis in dislocations of the shoulder-joint. Trans. Amer. Med. Ass., 10: 175–179, 1857
Duhring, Louis Adolphus. Philadelphia dermatologist. 1845–1913
DISEASE—dermatitis multiformis or herpetiformis.
  Dermatitis herpetiformis. J. A. M. A., 2: 225–229, Aug. 30, 1884
PRURITUS—
  Pruritus hiemalis—an undescribed form of pruritus. Philadelphia M. Times, 4: 225–230, Jan. 10, 1874
Wrote first book on dermatology published in United States.
  Atlas of skin disease. 1876
  A practical treatise on diseases of the skin. 1877
Duisberg, W. See R. Willstätter
Dujarier, Charles. Paris surgeon. 1870–1931
OPERATION—for femoral hernia.
  Cure radicale de la hernie crurale par voie inguinale. J. de Chir., 8: 113–128, Feb. 1912
  See also T. Tuffier
Dujarric de la Rivière, Auguste René. French physician. 1885–

AGAR—orange juice peptic digest; culture medium.
  Sur un nouveau milieu de culture: la "gelose a l'orange." C. R. Soc. Biol., 79: 843–844, Oct. 21, 1916
Duke, William Waddell. Kansas City, Mo. pathologist. 1883–1945
METHOD—for estimation of bleeding time.
  The relation of blood platelets to hemorrhagic disease; description of a method for determining the bleeding time and coagulation time and report of three cases of hemorrhagic disease relieved by transfusion. J. A. M. A., 55: 1185–1192, Oct. 1, 1910
Duke-Elder, Sir William Stewart. English ophthalmologist. 1898–
PIPETTE MANOMETER—to measure pressure in extra-scleral veins.
  The venous pressure of the eye and its relation to the intra-ocular pressure. J. Physiol., 61: 409–418, June 22, 1926
  The arterial pressure in the eye. Ibid., 62: 1–12, Oct. 30, 1926
Dukes, Clement. English physician. 1845–1925
DISEASE—same as fourth disease.
  On the confusion of two different diseases under the name of rubeola (rose-rash). Lancet, 2: 89–94, July 14, 1900
Dukes, Cuthbert Esquire. London pathologist. 1890–
CLASSIFICATION—
  Classification of cancer of the rectum. J. Path. and Bact., 35: 323–332, May 1932
Du Laurens, Andre. See Laurens
Dumas. See A. Carrel
Dumas, J. B. A. See J. L. Prevost
Dumont, Fritz L. Lausanne surgeon
AMPUTATION—osteoplastic, of leg; Haffter a.
  Eine neue Methode der Amputatio cruris osteoplastica. Dtsch. Z. Chir., 92: 497–509, Mar. 1908 (from Haffter's clinic)
Dumont, J. See E. Mosny
Dunbar, William Phillips. American physician. 1863–1922
ANTITOXIN or SERUM—from pollen of rag-weed, golden-rod, rye, etc., used in treatment of hay-fever.
REACTIONS—cutaneous protein, for hay-fever and asthma.
  Zur Ursache und specifischen Heilung des Heufiebers. Munchen, Oldenbourg, 1903. 60 pp.
  Ursache und Behandlung des Heufiebers. Leipzig, Weber, 1905
Duncan, Andrew. Edinburgh physician. 1744–1828
THEORY—of exstrophy.
  An attempt towards a systematic account of the appearances connected with that malconformation of the urinary organs, in which the ureters, instead of terminating in a perfect bladder, open externally on the surface of the abdomen. Edinburgh Med. and Surg. J., 1: 43–60; 132–142, 1805
Duncan, Andrew, Jr. Edinburgh physician. 1773–1832
Wrote on purpura with its deficient clot retractility.
  Case of purpura hemorrhagica (haemorrhoea petechialis). Edinburgh Med. and Surg. J., 18: 405–410, 1822
Duncan, Charles H. New York physician. 1880–
METHOD—autotherapy.
  Autotherapy. New York, Duncan, 1918. 361 pp.
Duncan, George Walton. Baltimore surgeon. 1914–

CRUSHER—
The uniform production of experimental shock by crush injury: possible relationship to clinical crush syndrome with A. Blalock, Ann. Surg., 115: 684–697, Apr. 1942

Dundas, Sir David. English surgeon
Described rheumatic endocarditis.
An account of a peculiar disease of the heart. Med.-Chir. Trans., London, 1: 37–46, 1809

Dunfermline. a city in Scotland
SCALE—a scheme for classifying children according to their degree of nutrition.

Dungern, Emil Adolf Wilhelm Joseph von. Heidelberg physician. 1867–
TEST—complement-fixation t. for diagnosis of malignant disease.
Ueber Serodiagnostik der Geschwülste mittels Komplementbindungsreaktion. Münch. med. Wschr., 59: 65–67, Jan. 9, 1912
TEST—for syphilis.
Ueber Serodiagnostik der Syphilis mit chemischen Substanzen (Koagulationsreaktion). Ibid., 62: 1212–1213, Sept. 7, 1915
Proved that blood groups are inherited and that agglutino-gens A and B behave like mendelian dominants.
Ueber Verebung gruppen-spezifischer Strukturen des Blutes with L. Hirschfeld, Z. ImmunForsch., 6: 284–292, 1910

Dunham, Edward Kellogg. New York pathologist. 1860–1922
BOUILLON—glucose serum, for studying fermentation by diplococci.
Comparative studies of diplococci decolorized by Gram's method, obtained from the spinal fluid and from the nares of cases of epidemic cerebrospinal meningitis. Public Health, 31: 10–20, 1905
PEPTONE or SOLUTION—for detection of cholera vibrio.
REACTION—"cholera-red" r.
Zur chemischen Reaction der Cholerabacterien. Z. Hyg., 2: 337–341, 1887
The bacteriological examination of the recent cases of epidemic cholera in the city of New York. Amer. J. med. Sci., 105: 72–80, Jan. 1893
See also H. D. Dakin

Dunlap, Knox. American surgeon. 1903–
KNIFE—for removing meniscus of knee.
A method for complete removal of the semilunar cartilage. J. Bone and Joint Surg., 24: 929–931, Oct. 1942

Dunlop, John. Pasadena, Cal. orthopedist. 1876–
METHOD—
Correction of compressed fractures of the vertebrae with C. H. Parker, J. A. M. A., 94: 89–93, Jan. 11, 1930
OPERATION—
The use of the index finger for the thumb: some interesting points in hand surgery. J. Bone and Joint Surg., 5: 99–103, Jan. 1923
TREATMENT—
Transcondylar fractures of the humerus in childhood. Ibid., 21: 59–73, Jan. 1939

Dunschmann, H. French physician
AGAR—bile salt gelatin; enrichment medium for typhoid bacilli.
Études sur la fièvre typhoide. Ann. Inst. Pasteur, 23: 29–69 (64), Jan. 1909

Du Petit, Francois Pourfoir. French physician 1664–1741
THEORY—of contralateral innervation.
Lettres d'un médecin des hôpitaux: un nouveau système du cerveau. ... Namur, 1710
Discovered vasomotor nerves.
Mémoire dans lequel il est démontré que les nerfs intercostaux fournissent les rameaux que portent des esprits dans les yeux. Mém. Acad. roy. d. sci., Paris, 1: 1–18, 1727

Duplay, Simon Emmanuel. French surgeon. 1836–1924
BURSITIS or DISEASE—subacromial or subdeltoid b.
De la péri-arthrite scapulo-humérale et des raideurs de l'epaule qui en sont la conséquence. Arch. gén. de méd., 20: 513–542, 1872
FIBROMA—of breast.
Des tumeurs dites bénignes du sein. Gaz. des hôp., Paris, 51: 602–603, July 2, 1878
OPERATION—plastic, on congenitally deformed penis (epispadias and hypospadias).
De l'hypospadias périnéo-scrotal et de son traitement chirurgical. Arch. gén. de méd., 133: 513–530, 1874

Dupré, Ernest Pierre. French physician. 1862–1921
SYNDROME—meningismus.
Le méningisme. Congr. franç. de méd., 1894, Paris, 1: 411–423, 1895

Dupuy-Dutemps, Louis. Paris ophthalmologist. 1871–
OPERATION—
Autoplastie palpébro-palpébrale intégrale. Réflection d'une paupière détruite dans tout son épaisseur par greffe cutanée et tarso-conjonctivale prise a l'autre paupière. Ann. d'ocul., 164: 915–926, Dec. 1927
OPERATION—dacryostomy.
Statistique de 290 cas dacryocystorhinostomies plastiques. Rev. gén. ophth., Paris, 38: 194, 1924

Dupuytren, Guillaume, Baron. French surgeon. 1777–1835
ABSCESS—in right iliac fossa.
Abcès développé dans le petit bassin. Rev. méd. fr. et etr., Paris, 1: 367–368, 1829
CLASSIFICATION—of burns.
Leçons orales de clinique chirurgicale. 1: 424, 1832
CONTRACTURE or CONTRACTION—of fingers.
De la rétraction des doigts par suite d'une affection de l'aponévrose palmaire. Description de la maladie. Opération chirurgicale qui convient dans de cas. J. univ. et hebd. de méd. et de chir. prat., Paris, 2 s., 5: 352–365, 1831
Also, in English: Lancet, London, 2: 222–225, 1834
Also, trans. by L. Clark: London, New Sydenham Soc., 1854
Also, in French and English: Med. Classics, 4: 127–150, Oct. 1939
DISEASE—of Dupuytren-Nélaton; central tumor of bone.
Leçons orales. Paris, 2: 129, 1839
ENTEROTOME—a cutting forceps used in making an artificial anus.
Mémoire sur une méthode nouvelle pour traiter les anus accidentels. Mem. Acad. de méd., Paris, 1: 259–316, 1828
FRACTURE—of lower part of fibula, with rupture of internal lateral ligament and dislocation of ankle.
Mémoire sur la fracture de l'extrémité inférieure du

pérone, les luxations et les accidens qui en sont la suite. Ann. méd.-chir. d. hôp. de Paris, 1: 1–212, 1819

Also, trans. by A. S. Doane: Phila., De Silver, Jr. and Thomas, 1833. pp. 160–197

Also: Med. Classics, 4: 151–172, Oct. 1939

HYDROCELE—

Hydrocèle multiloculaire, opération. Clin. d. hôp., Paris, p. 76, Apr. 1, 1828

PHLEGMON—of neck.

Phlegmons larges du cou. Bull. d. Thérap., 5: 271, 1833

SIGN—a crackling sensation on pressure over a sarcomatous bone.

Leçons orales. Paris, 2: 129, 1839

Sign—up and down movement of head of femur in congenital dislocation of hip.

Mémoire sur un déplacement originel ou congénital de la tête des femurs. Repert. gén. d'anat. et de physiol. path., Paris, 2: 82–93, 1826

Sur un déplacement congénital de la tête des femurs. Arch. gen. de méd., 13: 83–89, Jan. 1827

Invented a stomach tube.

Secours à administer dans les empoisonnemens, d'après la methode de M. Dupuytren. Reported by F. Cadet, fils. Bull. de Pharm., p. 62, Feb. 1810

Treated aneurysm successfully by compression.

Anévrisme à l'artère poplitée guéri par la compression. Bull. Fac. de Méd. de Paris, 6: 242, 1818

Advocated treatment of wry-neck by subcutaneous section of sternomastoid muscle.

First reported by C. Averill in: *A short treatise on operative surgery.* London, pp. 61–64, 1823

De la section du sterno-cléido-mastoidien pour guérir le torticolis ancien. Leçons orales. Paris, 3: 454–461, 1839

Excised the lower jaw. 1812

Observation sur une résection de la mâchoire inferieure. J. univ. d. sci. méd., Paris, 19: 77–98, 1820

Carcinome de l'os maxillaire inférieur. Amputation de l'os pratiquée pour la première fois par M. Dupuytren. Guérison. Leçons orales. Paris, 2: 421–453, 1829

Advocated reduction by traction in flexion of fractures of neck of femur.

Leçons orales. Paris, 2 ed., 1: 258, 1839

Durand, L. G. See L. Gaston-Durand

Durand, J. Lyon physician

DISEASE—Durand-Nicolas-Favre's d.; lympho-granuloma inguinale.

Lymphogranulomatose inguinale subaigue d'origine génitale probable, peut-être vénérienne with J. Nicholas and M. Favre, Bull. Soc. méd. Hôp. Paris, 35: 274–288, Feb. 6, 1913

See also A. Mouchet

Durande, Jean Francois. French physician. ?–1794

REMEDY—for gall stones.

Beobachtungen über die Wirkung der Mischung von Schwefeläther und dem flüchtigen Terpentinöl bey Leberschwerzen die von Gallensteinen entstehen. Helmstadt, Fleckeisen, 1791. 128 pp.

Duran Reynals, Francesc. See F. D. Reynals

Duret, C. French surgeon

OPERATION—construction of artificial anus for congenital atresia.

Observation sur un enfant né sans anus, et auquel il a

été fait une ouverture pour y suppléer. Rec. périod. Soc. de Méd. de Paris, 4: 45, 1793

Duret, Henry. Paris physician. 1849–1921

HEMORRHOIDS—

Recherches sur la pathogenie des hémorrhoides. Arch. gén. de méd., 7 s., 4: 641–665, et sec., Dec. 1879

Durham, Herbert Alton. Shreveport, La. surgeon. 1883–

OPERATION—

A procedure for the correction of internal rotation of the thigh in spastic paralysis. J. Bone and Joint Surg. 20: 339–344, Apr. 1938

Durham, Herbert Edward. English scientist. 1866–1945

SOLUTION—litmus whey; for cultivation of colon-typhoid group.

Some theoretical considerations upon the nature of agglutinins, together with further observations upon Bacillus typhi abdominalis, Bacillus enteritidis, Bacillus coli communis, Bacillus aerogenes, and some other bacilli of allied character. J. exp. Med., 5: 353–388 (379), Jan. 15, 1901

See M. von Gruber

Duroziez, Paul Louis. French physician. 1826–1897

DISEASE—congenital mitral stenosis.

Du retrécissement mitral pur. Arch. gén. de méd., Paris, 6 s., 30: 32–54, July; 184–197, Aug. 1877

MURMUR or SIGN—a double intermittent crural murmur always accompanying aortic insufficiency.

Du double souffle intermittent crural, comme signe de l'insuffisance aortique. Ibid., 17: 417–443, Apr: 588–605, May 1861

Also, abstr. in English transl. by E. Hausner in: F. A. Willius and T. E. Keys' *Cardiac classics.* St. Louis, Mosby, 1941. pp. 494–496

Duryee, A(bram) Wilbur. New York City physician. 1899–

TECHNIC—of capillary study.

Studies of human capillaries. Present day technique for the study of human capillaries with I. S. Wright, Amer. J. med. Sci., 185: 664–673, May 1933

Dutertre, J. B.

In 1635 gave first account of yellow fever and dengue fever, at Guadeloupe and St. Kitts. (Garrison and Morton)

Histoire générale des Antilles habitées par les Francais. Paris, 1667. Tom. 1

Dutrochet, René Joachim Henri. French chemist. 1776–1847

Investigated endosmosis and exosmosis.

Nouvelles observations sur l'endosmose et l'exosmose, et sur la cause de ce double phenomene. Ann. Chim. (Phys.), Paris, 35. 393–400, 1827; 37:191; 49:411; 52:159; 60:337, 1827–1835

Also: Paris, Baillière, 1828. 106 pp.

Dutton, Joseph Everett. English physician. 1877–1905

DISEASE—trypanosomiasis.

Preliminary note upon a trypanosoma occurring in the blood of man with Sir D. Bruce, Thompson Yates Lab. Reports, Liverpool, 4: 455–468, 1901

SPIROCHETA DUTTONI—species found in cases of African tick fever.

The nature of tick fever in the eastern part of the Congo Free State, with notes on the distribution and bionomics of the tick with J. L. Todd, Brit. med. J., 2: 1259–1260, Nov. 11, 1905

Duval, Charles Warren. American pathologist. 1876–
AGAR—glucose blood.
  Studies on the pneumococcus with P. A. Lewis, J.
  exp. Med., 7: 473–496 (474), Aug. 25, 1905
AGAR—parasite; for cultivation of B. leprae.
  *The cultivation of the leprosy bacillus and the experi-
  mental production of leprosy in the Japanese dancing
  mouse.* Ibid., 12: 649–665 (653), Sept. 1, 1910
BOUILLON—inulin; for cultivation of pneumococci.
  See AGAR—glucose blood. p. 484
SOLUTION—tryptic digest for cultivation of leprosy
  bacilli.
  *Further studies upon the leprosy bacillus. Its cultiva-
  tion and differentiation from other acid-fast species*
  with W. H. Harris, J. med. Res., 28: 165–198 (168),
  May 1911
  Discovered strain of dysentery bacilli known as
  lactose fermenter.
  The etiology of summer diarrhea in infants with E.
  H. Schorrer, Studies from the Rockefeller Inst. M.
  Research, 2: 42, 1904
  Another member of the dysentery group. J. A. M. A.,
  43: 381–383, Aug. 6, 1904
Duval, Mathias Marie. French anatomist. 1844–1907
NUCLEUS—an assemblage of multipolar ganglion-
  cells situated ventrolateral from hypoglossal nucleus
  in oblongata.
  Leçons sur la physiologie du système nerveux. . . .
  Paris, Doin, 1883. 119 pp.
  Précis d'histologie. Paris, Masson, 1897. 956 pp.
Duval, Pierre. French surgeon. 1874–

INCISION—to expose heart.
  De la péricardotomie thoraco-abdominale médiane
  (chirurgie du coeur et des gros vaisseaux de la base)
  with P. Barasty, Pr. méd., 26: 437–439, Aug. 29
  1918
Duverney, Joseph Guichard. French anatomist
  1648–1730
  Made important investigation on inner structure of
  ear which led him to write first treatise on otology.
  (Garrison)
  *Traité de l'organe de l'ouie, contenant la structure, les
  usages, et les maladies de toutes les parties de l'oreille.*
  Paris, Michallet, 1683. 210 pp.
  Same, in English. London, Baker, 1737, 145 pp.
  First to notice simultaneous extra-uterine and intra-
  uterine pregnancy. (Garrison)
  Oeuvres. Paris, 2: 355, 1708
Duyk, M. Belgian chemist
REACTION—for glucose.
  Sels de nickel reactifs des sucres réducteurs. Ann.
  chim. anal. chim. appli., 6: 364, 1901
  Also: Assoc. belge des chim., July 1901
Dwight, R. W. See H. Rogers
Dyel, M. Bohemian physician
PHENOMENON—
  *Différenciation de la névrite optique brightique d'avec
  la névrite optique par tumeur cérébrale.* Report in:
  Sem. méd., 21: 247 (only), July 24, 1901
Dyer, Elizabeth. American chemist. 1906–
REACTION—for cysteine and cystine
  A new color test for cysteine with O. Baudisch, J.
  biol. Chem., 95: 483–489, Mar. 1932

E

Eagle, Harry. American physician. 1905–
TEST—for syphilis.
  *Studies in the serology of syphilis: VIII. A new floc-
  culation test for the serum diagnosis of syphilis.* J.
  Lab. clin. Med., 17: 787–791, May 1932
METHOD—for preparation of purified fibrinogen.
  *The coagulation of blood by snake venoms and its
  physiologic significance.* J. exp. Med., 65: 613–639,
  May 1, 1937
METHOD—of intensive treatment of early syphilis.
  *An experimental evaluation of intensive methods for
  for the treatment of early syphilis. I. Toxicity and ex-
  cretion* with R. B. Hogan. Ven. Dis. Inf., 24: 33–44,
  Feb. 1943
  Same. *II. Therapeutic efficacy and margin of safety*
  with R. B. Hogan, Ibid., 69–79, Mar. 1943
  Same. *III. Clinical implications* with R. B. Hogan,
  Ibid., 159–170, June 1943
TEST—microflocculation test for syphilis.
  *A micromodification of the Eagle flocculation tech-
  nique* with A. F. Brand, Amer. J. Syph., Gonor.
  and Ven. Dis., 22: 22–31, Jan. 1938
Eagleton, Wells Phillips. American neurologist.
  1865–1946
CRITERIA—of septic thrombophlebitis of cavernous
  sinus.
  *Cavernous sinus thrombophlebitis and allied septic and
  traumatic lesions of the basal venous sinuses; a clinical
  study of blood stream infection.* New York, Macmillan,
  1926. 196 pp.
Eakin, R. E. See E. E. Snell

Easton, Edward Raymond. New York surgeon
  1892–
OPERATION—
  *The incidence of femoral hernia following repair of
  inguinal hernia—ectopic recurrence: a proposed opera-
  tion of external and internal herniorrhaphy.* J. A.
  M. A., 100: 1741–1744, June 3, 1933
Ebbinghaus, Hermann. German alienist. 1850–1909
TEST—for mental disease; patient is asked to com-
  plete sentences from which several words have been
  omitted.
  Grundzüge der Psychologie. Peipzig, 1911–13. 2 vols.
Ebeling, A. H. See O. J. Mink
Eberson, Frederick. American chemist. 1892–
YEAST AGAR—for cultivating bacteria.
  *A yeast medium for prolonging the viability of the
  meningococcus.* J. A. M. A., 72: 852–853, Mar. 22,
  1919
Eberth, Karl Joseph. Halle pathologist. 1835–1926
BACILLUS—B. typhus abdominalis.
  *Die Organismen in den Organen bei Typhus abdo-
  minalis.* Arch. f. path. Anat., 81: 58–74, 1880
Ebner, Anton Gilbert Viktor von. Vienna histolo-
  gist. 1842–1925
FIBRILS—in dentin and cementum of tooth.
  Strittige Fragen über den Bau des Zahnschmelzes.
  S. B. Akad. Wiss. Wien, Math.-naturw. Cl., 99:
  57–104, 1890
GLANDS—mucous g. of tongue.
  Die acinösen Drüsen der Zunge und ihre Beziehungen

zu den Geschmacksorganen. Graz, Leuschner, 1873. 66 pp.
METHOD—decalcifying. Mallory
Über den feineren Bau der Knochensubstanz. S. B. Akad. Wiss. Wien, 72: Pt. 3, 49–138, 1875
Ebstein, Wilhelm. Göttingen physician. 1836–1912
DISEASE—hyaline degeneration and necrosis of epithelial cells of renal tubules; cylinduria; seen in diabetic coma. (Dorland)
Ueber Drüsenepithelnekrosen beim Diabetes mellitus; mit besonderer Berucksichtigung des diabetischen Coma. Dtsch. Arch. f. klin. Med., 28: 143–242, 1880–81
METHOD—of carmin-fibrin, for quantitative estimation of pepsin.
Ueber Pepsinbildung im Magen with P. Grützner Arch. Physiol., 8: 122–151, 1874
SYMPTOM or PYREXIA—Pel-Ebstein s.; chronic relapsing pyrexia of Hodgkin's disease.
Das chronische Ruckfallsfieber, eine neue Infectionskrankheit. Berl. klin. Wschr., 24: 565–568; 837–842, 1887
TEST—for pyrocatechol in urine.
Einige Bemerkungen über die Reactionen des Brenzkatechin mit Bezug auf das Vorkommen desselben im menschlichen Harn. with J. Müller, Arch. f. path. Anat., 65: 394–397, 1875
TREATMENT—of obesity by diet without carbohydrates but including protein and fat.
Die Fettleibigkeit (Corpulenz) und ihre Behandlung nach physiologischen Grundsätzen. Wiesbaden, Bergmann, 1883. 3 Aufl.
Same, in English, London, Grevel, 1884. 89 pp.
ck, Nicolai Vladimirovich. Russian physiologist 1849–
FISTULA—an artificial communication made between portal vein and vena cava.
Kvoprosu o perevyazkie vorotnoi vent. Predvaritelnoye soobshtshenize. Voyenno—Med. J., St. Petersburg, 130: 2 sect., 1, 1877
cker, Alexander. German anatomist. 1816–1887
CONVOLUTION—posterior occipital c.
FISSURE—on dorsal surface of occipital lobe; transverse occipital f.
GYRUS—aftermost of occipital convolutions of cerebrum.
Die Hirnwindungen des Menschen nach eigenen Untersuchungen, insbesondere über die Entwickelung derselben beim Fötus, und mit Rücksicht auf das Bedürfniss der Aerzte dargestellt. Braunschweig, Vieweg, 1869. 56 pp.
Same, in English. New York, Appleton, 1873. 84 pp.
cker, Arthur David. Syracuse, N. Y. surgeon. 1913–
VARNISH—
A new skin varnish for maintaining sterility of the operative field. Surgery, 12: 631–634, Oct. 1942
ckman, M. See A. L. Barach
conomo, Constantin von. Vienna psychiatrist. 1876–1931
DISEASE—
Encephalitis lethargica. Wien. klin. Wschr., 30: 581–585, May 10, 1917
Encephalitis lethargica. Berlin, Urban und Schwarzenberg, 1929. 251 pp.
Same, in English. London, Oxford, 1931. 200 pp.
ddowes, Alfred. London physician. 1850–

SYNDROME—
Dark sclerotics and fragilitas ossium. Brit. med. J., 2: 222 (only), July 28, 1900
Edebohls, George Michael. New York surgeon. 1853–1908
INCISION—for appendectomy, performed during operation on kidney.
Notes on movable kidney and nephrorrhaphy. Amer. J. Obst., 31: 161–169, Feb. 1895
The technics of nephropexy, as an operation per se, as modified by combination with lumbar appendicectomy and lumbar exploration of the bile passages. Ann Surg., 35: 137–188, Feb. 1902
OPERATION—decapsulation of kidney for Bright's disease and puerperal eclampsia.
Chronic nephritis effecting a movable kidney as an indication for nephropexy. Med. News, 74: 481–483, Apr. 22, 1899
The cure of chronic Bright's disease by operation. Med. Record, 60: 961–970, Dec. 21, 1901
The surgical treatment of Bright's disease. New York, Lisiecki, 1904. 327 pp.
OPERATION—
Movable kidney; with a report of twelve cases treated by nephrorrhaphy. Amer. J. med. Sci., 105: 247–259, Mar.; 417–432, Apr. 1893
OPERATION—for uterine displacements.
Panhysterokolpectomy; a new prolapsus operation. Med. Record, 60: 561–564, Oct. 12, 1901
Edeiken, Louis. Philadelphia roentgenologist. 1894–
One of the first to employ roentgen therapy in the United States.
Small doses of x-ray for amenorrhea and sterility. Amer. J. Obstet. Gynaec., 25: 511–521, Apr. 1933
Edelmann, Adolf. Polish physician. 1885–1939
ANEMIA or DISEASE—
Ueber Anaemia infectiosa chronica und ihre Aetiologie. Wien. klin. Wschr., 38: 268–269, Mar. 5, 1925
Ueber ein neues Krankheitsbild, die Anaemia infectiosa chronica. Abstr. in: Münch. med. Wschr., 72: 667–668, Apr. 17, 1925
TEST—for urobilin in urine.
Eine Urobilinprobe im Harn und Stuhl für klinische Zwecke. Wien. klin. Wschr., 28: 978–979, 1915
Eden, Rudolf. Jena surgeon
OPERATION—bone grafts for habitual dislocation of shoulder.
Zur Operation der habituellen Schulterluxation unter Mitteilung eines neuen Verfahrens bei Abriss am inneren Pfannenrande. Dtsch. Z. Chir., 144: 269–280, Mar. 1918
Edgeworth, Harriet (Isabel). Tuscon, Ariz. biochemist. 1892–
Discovered beneficial effect of ephedrine in myasthenia gravis.
A report of progress on the use of ephedrine in a case of myasthenia gravis. J. A. M. A., 94: 1136 (only), Apr. 12, 1930
Edinger, Ludwig. Giessen physician. 1855–1918
METHOD—of testing gastric secretion.
Zur Physiologie und Pathologie des Magens. Dtsch. Arch. f. klin. Med., 29:555–578, Sept. 28, 1881
Edkins, John Sydney. London physiologist. 1863–1940
THEORY—of a gastric hormone.
On the chemical mechanism of gastric secretion. Proc. roy. Soc., s. B, 76: 376 (only), May 1, 1905

The chemical mechanism of gastric secretion. J
Physiol., 34: 133–144, Mar. 13, 1906

Edling, Lars. Swedish physician. 1878–
Used x-rays for diagnosis of pregnancy.
*Ueber die Anwendung des Röntgenverfahrens bei
der Diagnose der Schwangerschaft.* Fort. a. d. Geb. d.
Röntgenstr., Hamburg, 17: 345–355, 1911

Edmund, Carsten. Copenhagen physician. 1897–
APPARATUS—for measuring a slightly lowered dark
adaptation (night blindness).
Vision in light of reduced intensity with H. U. Möller,
Arch. Ophth., 54: 531–544, Nov. 1925

Edmunds, Arthur. London surgeon. 1874–
OPERATION—for hypospadias.
*Hunterian lecture on pseudohermaphroditism and
hypospadias; their surgical treatment.* Lancet, 1:
323–327, Feb. 13, 1926
OPERATION—for femoral hernia.
*Nicoll's operation for femoral hernia: some suggested
modifications.* Ibid., 2: 1287–1289, Dec. 17, 1927

Edmunds, C. W. See A. R. Cushny

Edmunds, W. See C. A. Ballance

Edwards, F. Ronald. Liverpool surgeon
METHOD—of preparation of dried plasma by means
of vacuum drying.
*The preparation and use of dried plasma for trans-
fusion* with J. Kay and T. B. Davie, Brit. med.
J., 1: 377–381, Mar. 9, 1940

Edwards, H. T. See L. J. Henderson

Edwards, William Frédéric. French physician. 1777–
1849
Studied effect of light on body.
De l'influence des agens physiques sur la vie. Paris,
Crochard, 1824
Same, in English. London, Highley, 1832. 488 pp.

Eegriwe, Edwin. German chemist
TEST—for lactic acid.
*Reaktionen und Reagenzien zum Nachweis organischer
Verbindungen.* Z. anal. Chem., 89: 121–125, 1932;
95: 323–327, 1933; 100: 31–36, 1935

Egas Moniz, Antonio Caetano de Abreu Freire.
Spanish surgeon. 1874–
TECHNIC—of prefrontal lobotomy.
*Tentatives opératoires dans le traitement de certaines
psychoses.* Paris, Masson, 1936. 248 pp.
Introduced cerebral encephalography and arteriog-
raphy.
*L'encéphalographie artérielle, son importance dans la
localisation des tumeurs cérébrales.* Rev. neurol., 2:
72–90, July 7, 1927
*Nouvelle technique de l'encéphalographie artérielle;
quelques cas de localisation de tumeurs cérébrales.*
Pr. méd., 36: 689–693, June 2, 1928

Egeberg, Chas. A. Norwegian army surgeon
Suggested gastrostomy, in 1837.
*Om Behandlingen af impenetrable Stricturer i Madrøret
(Oesophagus).* Norsk mag. f. Laegevidensk., 2: 97,
1841

Egerer, Grete. See P. A. Kober

Eggers, Carl. New York surgeon. 1879–
MODIFICATION—of Torek operation.
*Resection of the thoracic portion of the oesophagus for
carcinoma* S. G. O., 52: 739–746, Mar. 1931
Upper esophagostomy: its indications and uses. J.
Thoracic Surg., 7: 633–648, June 1938

Eggleston, Cary. New York physician. 1884–

METHOD—of determining dosage of digitalis.
Digitalis dosage. Arch. intern. Med., 16: 1–32, July
15, 1915

Eguchi, Ch. See K. Shiga

Ehlers, Edvard. German dermatologist. 1863–1937
SYNDROME—of Ehlers-Danlos; abnormally elastic
skin, over-extensibility of joints and thin atrophic
scars.
*Cutis laxa, Neigung zu Haemorrhagien in der Haut
Lockerung mehrerer Artikulationen.* Dermat. Z.
Berlin, 8: 173–174, 1901

Ehret, Heinrich. German physician. 1870–
DISEASE—paralysis of peronei muscles with contraction of their antagonists.
*Ueber eine functionelle Lähmungsform der Peroneal
muskeln traumatischen Ursprunges.* Arch. f. Unfallh.
2: 32–56, 1898

Ehrlich, H. See P. Clairmont

Ehrlich, J. C. See L. H. Sloan

Ehrlich, Paul. German scientist. 1854–1915
Awarded Nobel prize in 1908, with E. Metchnikoff
"in recognition for their work on immunity."
ANEMIA—Addison-Biermer-Ehrlich or pernicious a
*Ueber einen Fall von Anämie mit Bemerkungen übe
regenerative Veranderungen des Knochenmarks.* Char
ité-Annalen, Berlin, 13: 300–309, 1886
Ueber schwere anämische Zustände. Verh. d. Congr. f
inn. Med., 11: 33–64, 1892
Die Anaemia with A. Lazarus, Wien, Holder, 1898
1 Abt., 142 pp. 1900. 2 Abt., 200 pp.
BODIES—hemoglobinemic b.; small round granule
staining with acid dyes, seen in bodies of erythro
cytes in severe hemocytolysis from septic blood
poisoning.
*Farbenanalytische Untersuchungen zur Histologi
und Klinik des Blutes.* Berlin, Hirschwald, 1891
REACTION—with diazo reagent.
Ueber eine neue Harnprobe. Z. klin. Med., 5: 285-
288, 1882
SALVERSAN—"606"—Ehrlich-Hata preparation o
treatment.
*Die experimentelle Chemotherapie der Spirillose
(Syphilis, Rückfallfieber, Hühnerspirillose, Fram
bösie).* with S. Hata, Berlin, Springer, 1910. 164 pp
*Abhandlungen über Salvarsan (Ehrlich-Hata-Prä
parat 606 gegen Syphilis)*[4] ... Münch., Lehmann
1911–14. 4 vols.
NEOSALVARSAN—
*Ueber Laboratoriumsversuche und klinische Erprobun
von Helistoffen.* Chem. Zeitung, Köthen, 36: 637-
638, 1912
STAIN—
(*Hämatoxylinlösung.*) Z. wiss. Mikr., 3: 150 (only)
1886
STAIN—neutral.
*Ueber das Methylenblau und seine Klinischbakterio
skopische Verwerthung.* Z. klin. Med., 2: 710–713
1881
*Ueber die Methylenblaureaction der lebenden Nerven
substanz.* Dtsch. med. Wschr., 12: 49–52, Jan. 2
1886
TEST—for bile pigments (bilirubin) in urine.
Sulfodiazobenzol, als Reagens auf Bilirubin. Zb
klin. Med., 4: 721–723, Nov. 10, 1883
TEST—for indican in urine.
Ueber die Dimethylamidobenzaldehydreaction. Me
Woche, pp. 151–153, Apr. 15, 1901

THEORY—side-chain.
Das Sauerstoff-Bedürfniss des Organismus. Eine farbenanalytische Studie. Berlin, Hirschwald, 1885
Die Wertbestimmung des Diphtherieheilserums und deren theoretische Grundlagen. Klin. Jahrb., Jena, 6: 299–326, 1897
Complementophilen Gruppen der Amboceptoren with H. T. Marshall, Berlin, 1902 et subs.
In: Stud. Rockefeller Inst. M. Research, N. Y., 2, No. 7, 1904
Collected studies on immunity, with new contributions. . . . New York, Wiley, 1906. 586 pp.
Developed staining methods.
Beiträge zur Kenntniss der Anilinfärbungen und ihrer Verwendung in der mikroskopischen Technik. Arch. mikr. Anat., Bonn, 13: 263–277, 1877
Demonstrated specific hemolysins in normal sera for corpuscles of other species.
Zur Theorie der Lysinwirkung with J. Morgenroth, Berl. klin. Wschr., 36: 6–9, 1899
Ueber Haemolysine. Ibid., 36: 481–486, 1899; 37: 452–458; 681–687, 1900

Ehrmann, Charles Henri. French surgeon. 1792–1878
Removed laryngeal polyp.
Sur une opération de laryngotomie pratiquée dans un cas de polype du larynx. Extract of letter. C. R. Acad. Sci., Paris, 18: 593 (only), Apr. 1, 1844
Nouvelle communication relative à une opération de laryngotomie pratiquée dans un cas de polype du larynx. Ibid., 709 (only), Apr. 15, 1844
Laryngotomie pratique dans un cas de polype du larynx Strasbourg, Berger-Levrault, 1844. 31 pp.

Ehrmann, Rudolf. German physician. 1879–
TEST—for iodine in urine.
Ueber den Nachweis von Jod im Urin. Berl. klin. Wschr., 50: 1400 (only), July 28, 1913
TEST—for mydriatic substances
Ueber eine physiologische Wertbestimmung des Adrenalins und seinen Nachweis im Blut. Arch. exp. Path. Pharmak., 53: 96–111, July 18, 1905

Eichelberger, Lillian. See A. B. Hastings
Eichenberger, E. See L. Ruzicka
Eichholtz, Fritz. German physician
Synthesized and studied Avertin.
Ueber rektale Narkose mit Avertin (E 107). Dtsch med. Wschr., 53: 710–712, Apr. 22, 1927

Eichhorst, Hermann Ludwig. Swiss physician. 1849–1921
CORPUSCLES—microcystes seen in blood of patients with pernicious anemia.
Die progressive perniziöse Anämie. Leipzig, Veit und Comp., 1878. 375 pp.
DISEASE or NEURITIS—neuritis fascians.
Ueber Nervendegeneration und Nervenregeneration. Königsberg, Longrien, 1873. 30 pp.
TYPE—femorotibial t. of progressive muscular atrophy.
Ueber Heredität der progressiven Muskelatrophie. Berl. klin. Wschr., 10: 497–499, Oct. 20; 511–514, Oct. 27, 1873

Eichold, S. See J. G. Dickson
Eichstedt, Karl Ferdinand. Griefswald physician. 1816–1892
DISEASE—tinea or pityriasis versicolor; a contagious skin disease caused by Microsporon furfur.
Ueber die Krätzmilben des Menschen, ihre Entwick-

lung und ihr Verhältniss zur Krätze (Microsporon furfur). Neue Notizen a. d. Geb. d. Nat. u. Heilk., 38: col. 105–110; 39: col. 265–270, 1846
Pilzbildung in der Pityriasis versicolor. Ibid., col. 270–271, 1846

Eijkman, Christiaan. Dutch physician. 1858–1930
Awarded Nobel prize in 1929. Discovered deficiency in vitamin B to be responsible for beri-beri.
Polyneuritis bij hoenders. Geneesk. Tijdschr. Nederland-Indie, Batavie, 30: 295, 1890; 32: 353, 1893; 36: 214, 1896; 41: 3, 1901
Eine Beri Beri-ähnliche Krankheit der Hühner. Arch. path. Anat., 148: 523–532, 1892
Ein Versuch zur Bekämpfung der Beri-Beri. Ibid., 149: 187–194, 1897
BROTH—culture medium.
Die Garungsprobe bei 46° als Hilfsmittel bei der Trinkwasseruntersuchung. Zbl. Bakt., 2 Abt., 39: 75–80, Sept. 27, 1913
MODIFICATION—of Hammerschlag's method for determination of specific gravity of blood.
Blutuntersuchungen in den Tropen. Arch. path. Anat., 143: 448–476 (457), Mar. 9, 1896
SOLUTION—glucose peptone, for detection of B. coli.
(Same title as under BROTH), Zbl. Bakt., 37: 742–752, Dec. 30, 1904

Eilbott, Wilhelm. Frankfurt a. M. physician. 1900–
TEST—bilirubin elimination.
Funktionsprüfung der Leber mittels Bilirubinbelastung. Z. klin. Med., 106: 529–560, Nov. 29, 1927

Eilmann, H. J. See T. L. Ramsey

Einhorn, Alfred. Munich physician
See H. Braun
Synthetized procaine.
Ueber die Chemie der localen Anaesthetica. Münch. med. Wschr., 46: 1218–1220, Sept. 12: 1254–1257, Sept. 19, 1899

Einhorn, Max. New York physician. 1862–
BUCKET—
A new method of obtaining small quantities of gastric contents for diagnostic purposes. Med. Rec., 38: 63–64, July 19, 1890
DISEASE—gastric ulcer.
Ein klinischer Beitrag zur Kenntniss und Behandlung der "Erosionen des Magens." Berl. klin. Wschr., 32: 435–437, May 20; 457–460, May 27, 1895
TEST—bead t. for digestive function.
Eine neue Methode, die Funktionen des Verdauungsapparates zu prüfen. Arch. VerdauKr., 12: 26–38, 1906
Weiteres zu meiner Perlenverdauungsprobe. Ibid., 13: 35–48, 1907
Historic sketch of the bead test for determining the functions of the digestive tract, with demonstration. Post-Graduate, 27: 359–367, May 1912
TUBE—duodenal tube.
Die Gastrodiathanie. New York med. Mschr., 1: 559–560, 1889
A practical method of obtaining the duodenal contents in man. Med. Rec., 77: 98–101, Jan. 15, 1910
An intestinal tube. New York Med. J., 110: 456–459, Sept. 13, 1919
Introduced concept of achylia gastrica.
On achylia gastrica. Med. Rec., 41: 650–654, June 11, 1892

Einhorn, Moses. New York physician. 1896–

TUBE—bilumen gastro-enterostomy.
Nasal simultaneous gastroduodenal aspirator: its use in postoperative gastro-intestinal and abdominal surgery. S. G. O., 72: 48–57, Jan. 1941
Einsel, Isaac Henry. Cleveland physician. 1896–
MODIFICATION—of Sippy treatment of gastric ulcer.
Aluminum hydroxide in the treatment of peptic ulcer with W. L. Adams and V. C. Meyers, Amer. J. Digest. Dis. and Nutrition, 1: 513–516, Sept. 1934
Einthoven, Willem. Leyden physiologist. 1860–1927
Awarded Nobel prize in 1924.
STRING GALVANOMETER—an apparatus for detecting minute electric currents.
Beitrag zur Theorie des Capillar-Elektrometers. Arch. ges. Physiol., 79: 1–25; 26–38, 1900
Ueber das normale menschliche Elektrokardiogram und über die capillar-elektrometrische Untersuchung einiger Herzkranken with K. de Lint, Ibid., 80: 139–160, 1900
Un nouveau galvanometre. Arch. d. sci. exactes et nat., Haarlem, 2 s., 6: 625–633, 1901
Die Galvanometrische Registrirung des menschlichen Elektrokardiogramms, zugleich eine Beurthrilung der Anwendung des Capillar-Elektrometers in der Physiologie. Arch. ges. Physiol., 99: 472–480, 1903
Also: K. Akad. v. Wetensch. te Amst., Proc. Sect. Sci., 6: 107–115, 1903–4
Also, English transl. by E. A. Willius in E. A. Willius and T. E. Keys' *Cardiac classics*, St. Louis, Mosby, 1941. pp. 722–728
Eiselsberg, Anton Freiheer von. Vienna surgeon. 1860–1939
OPERATION—hypophysectomy.
Ueber operative Behandlung der Tumoren der Hypophysisgegend with L. v. Frankl-Hochwart, Neurol. Zbl., 26: 994–1001, Nov. 1, 1907
Operations upon the hypophysis. Ann. Surg., 52: 1–14, July 1910
OPERATION—pyloric exclusion, followed by gastroenterostomy.
Ueber die Magenresectionen und Gastroenterostomieen in Prof. Billroth's Klinik von März 1885 bis October 1889 Arch. klin. Chir., 39: 785–844, 1889
Unsere Erfahrungen mit der Bahandlung des Magen-und Duodenal-Ulcus. Wien. klin. Wschr., 39: 709–713, June 17, 1926
Experimentally produced tetany by excision of thyroid of cat; transplanted parathyroids.
Ueber erfolgreiche Einheilung der Katzenschilddrüse in die Bauchdecke und Auftreten von Tetanie nach deren Exstirpation. Ibid., 5: 81–85, Feb. 4, 1892
Applied principles of Witzel gastrostomy to enterostomy.
Ueber Auschaltung inoperabler Pylorus-Stricturen nebst Bemerkungen über die Jejunostomie. Arch. klin. Chir., 50: 919–939, 1895
Eisenberg, H. See G. W. Thorn
Eisenhardt, Willy. Königsberg physician. 1885–
TEST—for glucose in blood.
Quantitative Blutzuckerbestimmung mit Hilfe des Methylenblaus. Münch. med. Wschr., 67: 1328–1383, Nov. 26, 1920
Eisenlohr, Carl. Hamburg physician. 1847–1896
SYNDROME—weakness and numbness of extremi-

ties, dysarthria and paralysis of lips, tongue and palate.
Ueber einen eigentümlichen Symptomenkomplex bei Abdominaltyphus. Dtsch. med. Wschr., 19: 122–123, Feb. 9, 1892
Eisenmenger, Victor. German physician
TETRALOGY—Fallot t; Eisenmenger complex.
Die angeborene Defecte der Kammerscheidewand des Herzens. Z. klin. Med., 32 (Suppl.): 1–28, 1897
Eitelberg, Abraham. German otologist. 1847–
TEST—of conducting apparatus.
Ueber die vom Gehörorgane ausgelösten allgemeinen und lokalen Reflexerscheinungen. Jena, Fischer, 1895. 72 pp.
Ekkert, Ladislaus. Budapest physician
REACTIONS—for adrenaline and ephedrine.
Beitrag zu den Reaktionen des Suprarenins und Ephedrins. Pharm. Zentralhalle, 75: 208–209, Mar. 29, 1934
Elder, O. F. See E. G. Ballenger
Elfinger, A. See F. von Hebra
Elkin, Daniel C. Atlanta, Ga. surgeon. 1893–
OPERATION—suturing wounds of the heart.
Suturing wounds of the heart. Ann. Surg., 95: 573–577, Apr. 1932
Elkington, Joseph Russell. Philadelphia surgeon. 1910–
FORMULA—for amount of plasma to be given to a burned patient.
Plasma transfusion in the treatment of the fluid shift in severe burns with W. A. Wolff and W. E. Lee, Ann. Surg., 112: 150–157, July 1940
Ellefson, Lillian J. See I. C. Hall
Ellenbog, Ulrich. Austrian physician. 1440–1499
Wrote first work on industrial hygiene and toxicology, in 1473.
Von den gifftigen besen Tempffen und Reuchen. Augsburg, Ramminger, 1524
Same: Münch. Beitr. a Gesch. u. Literatur d. Naturwiss. u. Med., 2, Sonderheit, 20: 12, 1927
Same: Lancet, 1: 270–271, Jan. 30, 1932
Ellermann, Vilhelm. Copenhagen physician. 1871–1924
MEDIUM—for Bacillus fusiformis.
Ueber die Kultur der fusiformen Bacillen. Zbl. Bakt., 37: 729–730, 1904
TEST—for spermatozoa.
Bidrag til den forensiske Methodik. Paavisning af Spermatozoer ued Hjaelp af Jern-Heamatoxylinfarvning. HospitalsTid., 4: 1353–1356, Nov. 22, 1911
Demonstrated neoplastic nature of transmissible forms of leukemias in mice and fowls.
Experimentelle Leukämie bei Hühnern. Verh. dtsch. path. Ges., 12: 224–225, 1908
Ellinger, Alexander. German physician. 1870–1923
Noted that secretion of pancreatic juice in humans is continuous.
Beiträge zur Kenntnis der Pankreassekretion beim Menschen with M. Cohn, Z. phys. Chem., 45: 28–37, 1905
Ellinger, Phillip. German scientist. 1887–
Established chemical formula of lactoflavin (vitamin B_2).
The lyochromes: a new group of animal pigments with W. Koschara, Nature, London, 133: 553–556, Apr. 14, 1934

Elliot, John Wheelock. Boston surgeon. 1852–1925
POSITION—a support placed under small of back to
elevate gall bladder region, in operations on gall
bladder.
*Immediate suture of the gall-ducts and the gall-bladder
after extraction of stones, with cases.* Ann. Surg., 22:
86–98 (97), July 1895

Elliot, Robert Henry. Madras ophthalmologist.
1864–1936
OPERATION—trephining sclerocornea for relief of
increased tension in glaucoma.
*A preliminary note on a new operative procedure for
the establishment of a filtering cicatrix in the treatment
of glaucoma.* Ophthalmoscope, London, 7: 804–806,
Dec. 1909
*Some cases demonstrating the existence of the filtering
cicatrix.* Ibid., 807–808
*Sclero-corneal trephining in operative treatment of
glaucoma.* London, Pulman, 1913. 117 pp.

Elliotson, John. English surgeon. 1786–1868
Proved that glanders in horse is communicable to
man.
On the glanders in the human subject. Med.-chir.
Trans., London, 16: 171–218, 1830
*Additional facts respecting glanders in the human
subject.* Ibid., 18: 201–207, 1833
Ascertained that pollen is cause of hay fever.
Hay fever. London Med. Gaz., 8: 411–416, June 25,
1831
Catarrhus aestivus, or hay fever. Ibid., 12: 164–171,
May 11, 1833
Used hypnotism in surgery.
*Numerous cases of surgical operations without pain
in the mesmeric state; with remarks upon the opposition
of many members of the Royal Medical and Chirurgical
Society and others to the reception of the inestimable
blessings of mesmerism.* London, Baillière, 1843.
93 pp.

Elliott, John. Salisbury, N. C. scientist
METHOD—of transfusion, utilizing a vacuum tube.
Blood plasma. South. Med. and Surg., 103: 252–255
May 1941
See also W. L. Tatum

Elliott, Thomas Renton. London physician. 1877–
BALLON APPLICATION—
On the innervation of the ileo-colic sphincter. J. Physiol., 31: 157–168, May 3, 1904
Suggested that adrenalin is liberated when sympathetic nerve impulse arrives at a smooth-muscle
cell.
On the action of adrenalin. Ibid., XX–XXI, May 21,
1904
The action of adrenalin. Ibid., 32: 401–467, July 13,
1905
Suggested possibility of inducing artificial pneumothorax on affected side in treating pulmonary collapse.
*Massive collapse of the lungs following abdominal
operations* with L. A. Dingley, Lancet, 1: 1305–1309,
May 9, 1914

Ellis, A. W. M. See H. F. Swift

Ellis, Calvin. Boston physician. 1826–1883
CURVE or LINE or SIGN—an S-shaped line on
chest, showing upper border of pleuritic effusion.
The line of dulness in pleuritic effusion. Boston M.
and S. J., 90: 13–14, Jan. 1, 1874

Ellis, Henry Havelock. English physician. 1859–
1939
Scientifically studied sex.
Studies in the psychology of sex. Philadelphia, Davis,
1900–1928. 7 vols.

Ellis, J. C. See L. R. Dragstedt

Ellram, W. German chemist
TEST—for acetone in urine.
Acetone im Harn. Abstr.: Pharm. Zentralhalle, 20:
461, 1899

Ellsworth, R. See W. G. MacCallum

Elman, Robert. American surgeon. 1897–
METHOD—for determination of plasma volume.
*Studies on hypoalbuminemia produced by protein-
deficient diets. II. Rapid correction of hypoalbuminemia
with an ad libitum meat diet* with F. A. Brown, Jr.
and Harriet Wolf, J. exp. Med., 75: 461–464, Apr.
1942
TEST—of blood amylase.
*The quantitative determination of blood amylase with
the viscosimeter* with J. M. McConghan, Arch. intern.
Med., 40: 58–64, July 1927
TEST—neutralization, of acid introduced into stom-
ach.
*The behavior of gastric acidity in duodenal ulcer and
pyloric obstruction before and after gastro-enterostomy.*
S. G. O., 49: 34–42, July 1929
TEST—for urobilin.
*Studies on urobilin physiology and pathology. I. The
quantitative determination of urobilin* with P. D.
McMaster. J. exp. Med., 41: 503–512, Apr. 1, 1925
Described—
*Acute interstitial pancreatitis: a clinical study of
thirty-seven cases showing oedema, swelling, and in-
duration of the pancreas but without necrosis, haemor-
rhage, or suppuration.* S. G. O., 57: 291–309, Sept.
1933
See also L. A. Sachar, D. O. Weiner

Eloesser, Leo. San Francisco surgeon. 1881–
OPERATION—flap, for drainage of empyema.
An operation for tuberculous empyema. S. G. O., 60:
1096–1097, June 1935
OPERATION—reconstruction of nose.
Some notes on plastic operations. Ibid., 34: 532–537,
Apr. 1922
Reported removal of both lower lobes of lung in case
of bilateral bronchiectasis.
Bilateral lobectomy. Ibid., 57: 247–249, Aug. 1933

Elsberg, Charles Albert. New York surgeon. 1871–
METHOD—
*Clinical experiences with intratracheal insufflation
(Meltzer), with remarks upon the method for thoracic
surgery.* Ann. Surg., 52: 23–29, July 1910
MODIFICATION—of Crile canula for direct trans-
fusion of blood.
A simple canula for the direct transfusion of blood.
J. A. M. A., 52: 887–888, Mar. 13, 1909
OPERATION—for relief of syringomyelia.
*Diseases and treatment of surgical diseases of the
spinal cord and its membranes.* Philadelphia, Saunders,
1916. 330 pp. p. 170
Described extradural lesions due to hypertrophy of
ligamentum flavum.
*Experiences in spinal surgery; observations upon 60
laminectomies for spinal disease.* S. G. O., 16: 117–
132, Feb. 1913

Elschnig, Anton. Prague ophthalmologist. 1863–1939
CONJUNCTIVITIS MEIBOMIANA OF—
*Beitrag zur Aetiologie und Therapie der chronischen
Conjunctivitis.* Dtsch. med. Wschr., 34: 1133–1135,
June 25, 1908
GLOBULAR or BLADDER CELLS OF—
*Klinisch-anatomischer Beitrag zur Kenntnis des
Nachstares.* Klin. Mbl. Augenheilk., 49: 444–451
Apr. 6, 1911
THEORY—sympathetic ophthalmia is due to allergy.
*Studien zur sympathischen Ophthalmie. I. Wirkung
von Antigenen vom Augen innern aus.* Arch. Ophth.,
75: 459–473; 76: 509–546, 1910; 78: 549–585; 79:
428, 1911
Developed method of corneal grafting.
Keratoplasty. Arch. Ophth., New York, n. s., 4:
165–173, Aug. 1930
Elsdon-Dew, Ronald. Johannesburg physician
THEOREM—
*The effects of mixture of races on serological constitu-
tion.* S. African J. M. Sci., 1: 184–190, June 1936
Elser, William James. New York bacteriologist.
1872–
SOLUTION—basal Nährstoff-Heyden, for studying
fermentation by meningococci.
Studies on meningitis with F. M. Huntoon, J. med.
Res., 20: 373–541 (404), June 1909
Elsholtz, Johann Sigmund. German physician.
1623–1688
Wrote on blood transfusion.
Clysmatica nova: oder newe Clystier-Kunst. Berlin,
Reiche, 1665
Elsner, Christoph Friedrich. Königsberg physician.
1749–1820
ASTHMA—angina pectoris.
Abhandlung über die Brustbräune. Königsberg, 1778
Elsner, Hugo Ottomar. Berlin histologist. 1869–
MEDIUM or SOLUTION—hydrochinone potato in-
fusion, for differentiation of coli and typhoid bac-
teria.
*Untersuchungen über electives Wachsthum der Bac-
terium coli-Arten und des Typhusbacillus und dessen
diagnostische Verwerthbarkeit.* Z. Hyg. InfektKr., 21:
25–31 (28), 1895
Elting, Arthur Wells. Albany, N. Y. surgeon. 1872–
CELLS—large circular c. found in fat embolism.
Fat embolism, with study of two fatal cases with C. E.
Martin, Ann. Surg., 82: 336–353, Sept. 1925
OPERATION—
*The treatment of fistula-in-ano, with especial reference
to the Whitehead operation.* Ibid., 56: 744–752, 1912
Produced malaria by inoculation.
Ueber Malaria nach experimentellen Impfungen. Z.
klin. Med., 36: 491–526, 1899
Described—
*Primary carcinoma of the vermiform appendix, with
a report of three cases.* Ann. Surg., 37: 548–574, Apr.
1903
Elvehjem, Conrad Arnold. Wisconsin chemist. 1901–
Isolated nicotinic acid.
*The isolation and identification of the anti-black tongue
factor* with R. J. Madden, F. N. Strong, and D. W.
Woolley, J. biol. Chem., 123: 137–149, Mar. 1938
Elvers, Charles F. Baltimore urologist
APPARATUS—
A new apparatus for heating bacterial and blood smears.
Johns Hopk. Hosp. Bull., 35: 94–95, Mar 1924

Ely, Edward Talbot. American otologist. 1850–1885
OPERATION—
Skin-grafting in chronic suppuration of the middle ear.
Arch. Otol., 9: 343–345, 1880
Ely, Leonard Wheeler. San Francisco physician.
1868–
SIGN—hyperextension of leg at thigh, when patient
is lying prone, will produce pain if there is a lesion in
lumbar spine or at lumbosacral joint.
*Backache; lumbago; pain in the lower part of the
back.* Arch. Surg., 27: 189–202, July 1933
Emanuel, Gustav. German physician. 1879–
REAGENT, TEST—for investigating cerebrospinal
fluid.
*Eine neue Reaktion zur Untersuchung des Liquor
cerebrospinalis.* Berl. klin. Wschr., 52: 792–794,
July 26, 1915
Emerson, Gladys A., Emerson, O. H. See H. McL.
Evans
Emerson, J. H., Co. Cambridge, Mass.
RESUSCITATOR—
(accepted by Council on Physical Therapy, J. A.
M. A., 119: 414 (only), May 30, 1942.)
Emerson, K. See E. K. Marshall, Jr., R. A. Phillips,
G. W. Thorn
Emery, H. French physician
SOLUTION—spleen digest, for differentiation of coli
and typhoid bacilli.
*Recherche du bacille typhique dans l'eau; note sur un
procédé permettant de différencier le bacilli d'Eberth
du colibacille.* C. R. Soc. Biol., 53: 979–980, Nov. 16,
1901
Emery, Walter D'Este. English physician. 1870–
1923
TEST—for diagnosis of syphilis.
*The technique of a simplified form of the Wassermann
reaction.* Lancet, 2: 732–734, Sept. 3, 1910
Emile, Prosper Weil. See P. E. Weil
Emmet, Frederick Victor. St. Louis surgeon. 1897–
MODIFICATION—of Dickinson technic of vaginal
hysterectomy.
*Gellhorn-Dickinson technic for vaginal hysterectomy
for prolapse of the uterus.* Surg. Clin. No. Amer., 18:
1315–1334, Oct. 1938
*The results of a modern technic in vaginal hysterec-
tomy.* South. Med. J., 32: 715–720, July 1939
*Vaginal hysterectomy. An evaluation of Gellhorn-
Emmert modification of the Dickinson technique in 600
cases.* S. G. O., 79: 276–285, Sept. 1944
Emmet, Thomas Addis. New York gynecologist.
1828–1919
OPERATION—artificially formed vesico-vaginal fis-
tula to secure drainage of bladder in cystitis.
Chronic cystitis in the female, and mode of treatment.
Amer. Pract., 5: 65–92, 1872
OPERATION—method of repair of lacerated perin-
eum.
*A study of the etiology of perineal laceration, with a
new method for its proper repair.* Trans. Amer. Gynec.
Soc., 1882, N. Y., 8: 198–216, 1884
OPERATION—trachelorrhaphy, suture of edges of
lacerated cervix uteri.
*Surgery of the cervix in connection with the treatment of
certain uterine diseases.* Amer. J. Obstet., 1: 339–
362, 1869
Emmons, Chester Wilson. New York botanist. 1900–

CLASSIFICATION—
Dermatophytes: natural grouping based on the form of the spores and accessory organs. Arch. Dermat. and Syph., 30: 337–362, Sept. 1934

Emmons, William Frank. Canadian physician. 1896–
METHOD—diffraction, of determining cell diameter.
The clinical eriometer. Quart. J. Med., 21: 83–90, Oct. 1927

Endemann, (Samuel Theodor) Hermann (Carl). American chemist. 1842–
REACTION—for phenol.
Formaldehyde as a reagent. Bull. Pharm., 11: 365 (only) 1897

Enderlen, Eugen. Würzburg surgeon. 1865–
OPERATION—transplanting fresh anterior tibial artery between ventricles and superficial temporal vein.
1. Zur Frage der Operation von Hypophysistumoren 2. Zur Behandlung des Hydrocephalus. 3. Demonstrationen. Beitr. klin. Chir., 76: 888–891, 1911

Endo, S. German physician
MEDIUM—culture, for typhoid bacilli.
Ueber ein Verfahren zum Nachweis der Typhusbacillen. Zbl. Bakt., 35: 109–110, 1904

Engel, Carl. German physician. 1901–
Demonstrated passive transfer or Prausnitz-Küstner reaction for gonorrhea.
Die Gonorrhoe als Testkrankheit bakteriell-allergischer Vorgänge. Wien. klin. Wschr., 48: 48–51, Jan. 11, 1935

Engel, Gerhard. German physician
DISEASE—Engel-Recklinghausen's d.; generalized osteitis fibrosa cystica.
Ueber einen Fall von cystoider Entartung des ganzen Skelettes. Giessen, I. D., Pietsch, 1864

Engel, Gilson Colby. Philadelphia surgeon. 1898–
DIRECTION-FINDER—
Two-plane direction finder for nailing fractures of neck of femur with H. May, S. G. O., 66: 495–499, Feb. 1938
Two-plane direction and range finder for nailing fractures of the neck of the femur with H. May, J. A. M. A., 110: 1828–1829, May 28, 1938

Engel, L. L. See G. W. Thorn
Engel, P. See F. Silberstein
Engelmann, Theodor Wilhelm. German physiologist. 1843–1909
DISK—same as Hensen's d.; pale, thin disk dividing muscle-case into two portions. Dorland
Nouvelles recherches sur les phénomènes microscopiques de la contraction musculaire. Arch. néerl. d. sci. exactes et natur., La Hague, 13: 437–465, 1878
Ueber den Ursprung der Muskelkraft. Leipzig, Engelmann, 1893

Engle, E. T. See P. E. Smith
Engman, Martin Feeney. St. Louis dermatologist. 1869–
DISEASE—infectious eczematoid dermatitis.
An infectious form of an eczematoid dermatitis. Amer. Med., 4: 769–773, Nov. 15, 1902
Introduced bacterial vaccines in treatment of skin diseases.
The treatment of certain diseases of the skin by the intravenous injection of a foreign protein with R. A. McGarry, J. A. M. A., 67: 1741–1745, Dec. 9, 1916

Enlows, Ella M. A. American bacteriologist. 1889–

MEDIUM—
A sugar free medium for fermentation studies. Pub. Health Rep., 38: 2129–2132, Sept. 14, 1923

Eppinger, Hans. Prague physician. 1846–1916
Gave complete anatomic description of tuberculous tracheal ulceration.
Handbuch der pathologischen Anatomie. (Klebs) II Band. *Pathologische Anatomie des Larynx und der Trachea.* Berlin, Hirschwald, 1880. 132 pp.

Eppinger, Hans. Vienna physician. 1879–1946
Studied electrocardiographic changes in bundle-branch block.
Ueber die Folgen der Durchschneidung der Tawaraschen Schenkel des Reizleitungssystems with J. Rothberger, Z. klin. Med., 70: 1–20, 1910
Zur Klinik des Elektrocardiograms with O. Stoerk, Ibid., 71: 157–164, 1910
Introduced phenylhydrazine hydrochloride in treatment of polycythemia.
Zur Therapie der Polyzythämie with K. Kloss, Therap. Monatsh., Berlin, 32: 322–326, 1918

Epstein, Albert Arthur. New York physician. 1880–
ALBUMINURIA—reduction in protein content of plasma, elevated cholesterol, and inversion of albumin-globulin ratio, associated with generalized edema.
SYNDROME—albuminuric nephrosis.
The nephroses. Bull. N. Y. Acad. Med., 13: 621–644, 1937
TEST—
A method for hemolysis and agglutination tests with R. Ottenberg, Arch. intern. Med., 3: 286–288, May 1909
Showed that iso-agglutinins are inherited.
A simple method of performing serum reactions with R. Ottenberg, Proc. Path. Soc. N. Y., 8: 117–123, Oct. and Nov. 1908

Epstein, Alois. Prague pediatrician. 1849–1918
PSEUDODIPHTHERIA—
Ueber septische Erkrankungen der Schleimhäute bei Kindern. Prager med. Wschr., 4: 329–333, Aug. 20; 341–344, Aug. 27, 1879

Erb, Wilhelm Heinrich. Heidelberg neurologist. 1840–1921
ATROPHY or DYSTROPHY or DISEASE—progressive muscular dystrophy.
Ein Fall von progressive Muskelatrophie. . . . with Fr. Schultze, Arch. Psychiat. Nervenkr., 9: 369–1879
Ueber die "juvenile Form" der progressiven Muskelatrophie und ihre Beziehungen zur sogenannten Pseudohypertrophie der Muskeln. Dtsch. Arch. f. klin. Med., 34: 467–519, 1884
DISEASE—Erb-Charcot d.; spastic spinal paralysis.
Ueber einen wenig bekannten spinalen Symptomencomplex. Berl. klin. Wschr., 12: 357–359, June 28, 1875
Ueber die spastische Spinalparalyse (Tabes dorsal spasmodique, Charcot). Arch. path. Anat., 70: 241–267, June 9: 293–328, July 5, 1877
Die Ätiologie der Tabes. Samml. klin. Vortr., n. F., No. 53, (Inn. Med., No. 18, pp. 515–542), 1892
Ueber syphilitische Spinalparalyse. Neurol. Zbl., 11: 161–168, Mar. 15, 1892
DISEASE or SYNDROME—of Erb-Goldflam: myasthenia gravis pseudoparalytica.
Zur Casuistik der bulbären Lähmungen: 3. Ueber einem neuen, wahrscheinlich bulbären Symptomen-

complex. Arch. Psychiat. Nervenkr., 9: 336–350, 1878

PARALYSIS or SYNDROME—Duchenne-Erb. p.; of brachial plexus.
Ueber eine eigenthümliche Localisation von Lähmungen im Plexus brachialis. Verh. d. naturh.-med. Ver. zu Heidelb., n. F., 2: 130–137, 1874–77

SIGN or PHENOMENON—increased electric irritability of motor nerves in tetany.
Zur Lehre von der Tetanie, nebst Bemerkungen über die Prüfung der electrischen Erregbarkeit motorischer Nerven. Arch. Psychiat. Nervenkr., 4: 271–316, 1873

SIGN—Erb-Westphal s.; absence of patella tendon reflex in locomotor ataxia.
Ueber Sehnenreflexe bei Gesunden und bei Rückenmarkskranken. Ibid., 5: 792–803, 1875
Introduced method of electrodiagnosis by galvanic and induction currents.
Ueber die Anwendung der Electricität in der inneren Medicin. Samml. klin. Vortr., No. 46, (Inn. Med., No. 17, pp. 351–388), 1872

Erben, Siegmund. Vienna physician. 1863–
PHENOMENON, REFLEX or SIGN—temporary slowness of pulse on stooping or sitting down, said to characterize certain cases of neurasthenia. Dorland
Diagnose der Simulation nervöser Symptome. Berlin, Urban und Schwarzenberg, 1912. 194 pp.

Erdélyi, J. See E. Rosenthal

Erdheim, Jakob. Vienna physician. 1874–1937
LAW—calcioprotective; disturbances in calcium metabolism do not affect various tissues of body to an equal extent; dentin and enamel are protected against loss.
Rachitis und Epithelkorperchen. Denkschr. d. k. Akad. Wiss. Wien, Math.-naturw. Cl., 90: 363–388, 1914
Described parathyroid adenoma and noted relation to osteomalacia.
Zur normalen und pathologischen Histologie der glandula Thyreoidea, Parathyreoidea und Hypophysis. Beitr. path. Anat., 33: 158–236, 1903
Ueber Epithelkörperbefunde bei Osteomalacie. S. B. Akad. Wiss. Wien, Math.-naturw. Cl., 116: 311–370, 1907
Ueber den Kalkgehalt des wachsenden Knochens und des Callus nach der Epithelkorporschenexstirpation. Z. Path., 7: 175–230, 1911
Described aortic medionecrosis.
Medionecrosis aortae idiopathica. Arch. path. Anat., 273: 454–479, Sept. 6, 1929
Medionecrosis aortae idiopathica cystica. Ibid., 276: 187–229, Feb. 17, 1930

Erf, Lowell Ashton. Philadelphia physician. 1908–
TEST—
The glycine tolerance test in sprue and pernicious anemia with C. P. Rhoads, J. clin. Invest., 19: 409–421, Mar. 1940
See also S. M. Peck

Erichsen, Sir John Eric. English surgeon. 1818–1896
DISEASE—railway spine.
On railway and other injuries of the nervous system. London, Walton and Maberly, 1866. 144 pp.
On concussion of the spine, nervous shock, and other obscure injuries of the nervous system, in their clinical and medico-legal aspects. New York, Wood, 1875, 340 pp.

Erickson, Mary Josephine. American physician. 1892–
MEDIUM—testicular-infusion agar.
Cultivation of the gonococcus with H. Albert, J. infect. Dis., 30: 268–278, Mar. 1922

Erlanger, Joseph. American physician. 1874–
SPHYGMOMANOMETER—
A study of the errors involved in the determination of the blood-pressure in man, together with a demonstration of the improvements in the sphygmomanometer suggested thereby. Amer. J. Physiol., 10: xiv–xv, 1903
A new instrument for determining the minimum and maximum blood-pressures in man. Johns Hopk. Hosp. Rep., 12: 53–110, 1904
Awarded Nobel prize in medicine in 1944, with H. S. Gasser, for measuring and photographing electric current of nerve impulse.
The compound nature of the action current of nerve as disclosed by the cathode ray oscillograph with H. S. Gasser, Amer. J. Physiol., 70: 624–666, Nov. 1, 1924
Analysis of the action potential in nerve. Harvey Lectures, series 22, pp. 90–113, 1926–27.
See also H. S. Gasser

Erlenmeyer, Ernest. German scientist
REACTION—for creatine.
Ueber Diacetylkreatin und Benzylidenacetylkreatinin. Ann. Chim., 284: 49–52, 1895

Ermengem, Émile Pierre Marie van. Belgian bacteriologist. 1851–1932
BACILLUS—botulinus.
BROTH—for isolation of botulinus bacilli.
Contribution à l'étude des intoxications alimentaires. Recherches sur des accidents à caractères botuliniques provoqués par du jambon. Arch. de Parmacodyn., Gand, 3: 213–376, 1897
Ueber einen neuen anaëroben Bacillus und seine Beziehungen zum Botulismus. Z. Hyg. InfektKr., 26: 1–56, 1897
METHOD—for staining flagella.
Nouvelle méthode de coloration des cils des bactéries. Ann. Soc. de Méd. de Gand, 72: 231–236, 1893

Erni, H. Swiss physician
SIGN—cavernous tympany over apical cavity.
Das Klopfphänomen bei der Phthise mit Kavernen. Z. Tuberk. u. Heilst., 7: 128–132, 1905

Ernst, Paul. German pathologist. 1859–1937
BODIES—Babes-Ernst b. or granules; stain deeply with anilin dyes; seen in protoplasm of bacteria.
Ueber den Bacillus xerosis und seine Sporenbildung. Z. Hyg. InfektKr., 4: 25–46, 1889

Ernstene, A. C. See M. Dorothy Rourke

Erskine, Arthur Wright. Cedar Rapids, Iowa roentgenologist. 1885–
SPECULUM—
Expanding speculum for transvaginal roentgen therapy. Amer. J. Roent. and Radium Therapy, 42: 423–427, Sept. 1939

Ervin, D. M. See W. B. Wherry

Esbach, Georges Hubert. Paris physician. 1843–1890
REAGENT—for albumin in urine.
Dosage pratique de l'albumine: trois méthodes. Gaz. Méd., Paris, r. s., 3: 61–62, 1874
Dosage clinique de l'albumine. Pam. Paris, 1880

Esch, Peter. German gynecologist. 1874–
AGAR—maltose ascitic fluid, for cultivation of meningococci.
Ein Beitrage zur Züchtung des Meningococcus. Zbl. Bakt., 52: 150–154, 1909

Eschacïh, A. French physician
TEST—for blood.
Procede de recherche du sang dans l'urine, les selles et les liquides pathologiques (Note, presented by L. Grimbert), C. R. Soc. Biol., 82: 741, 1919

Escherich, Theodor. German physician. 1857–1911
BACILLUS—B. coli.
Die Darmbakterien des Saüglings und ihre Beziehungen zur Physiologie der Verdauung. Stuttgart, Enke, 1886
SIGN—of tetany, muscular contraction of lips, resembling a goat's snout.
Die Tetanie der Kinder. Wien, Hölder, 1909. 268 pp.
TEST—modification of von Pirquet reaction.
Die Resultate der Koch'schen Injectionen bei Scrophulose und Tuberkulose des Kindesalters. Jb. Kinderheilk., n.F., 33: 369–426, 1892

Esmarch, Johannes Friedrich August von. German surgeon. 1823–1908
APPARATUS—for transfusion of defibrinated blood.
In: *Handbuch der kriegschirurgischen Technik.* Kiel, 1885. 3 Aufl.
BANDAGE or TOURNIQUET—of India-rubber, applied to limb from distal part upward so as to expel blood.
Der erste Verband auf dem Schlachtfelde. Kiel, Schwers'sche Buchhandlung, 1869
Ueber künstliche Blutleere bei Operationen. Samml. Klin. Vortr., No. 58 (Chir. No. 19), 373–384, 1873
MASK—a frame of metal covered with gauze, used for administering ether or chloroform by inhalation.
Regeln für die Chloroformnarkose. Mitt. a. d. chir. Klin. zu Kiel, 3, 1884
METHOD—for anerobic culture.
Ueber eine Modification des Koch'schen Plattenverfahrens zur Isolirung und zum quantitativen Nachweis von Mikroorganismen. Z. Hyg. InfektKr., 1: 293–301, 1886

Esquirol, Jean Étienne-Dominique. French alienist. 1772–1840
Noted for his studies on insanity.
Des maladies mentales considérées sous les rapports médical, hygiénique et médico-légal Paris, Baillière, 1838. 2 vols. and atlas
Same, in English: Philadelphia, Lea and Blanchard, 1845. 496 pp.

Esser, Johannes Fredericus Samuel. Holland surgeon. 1878–1946
INLAY GRAFT—
Neue Wege für chirurgische Plastiken durch Heranziehung du zahnärztlichen Technik. Beitr. klin. Chir., 103: 547–555, Nov. 1916
Studies in plastic surgery of the face. I. Use of skin from the neck to replace face defects. II. Plastic operations about the mouth. III. The epidermic inlay. Ann. Surg., 65: 297–315, Mar. 1917

Essex, H. E. See S. B. Harper

Estes, William Lawrence, Jr. Bethlehem, Pa. surgeon. 1885–

METHOD—of dismantling gastrojejunal retrocolci anastomosis in jejunal peptic ulcer.
Advanced gastrojejunal ulcer. Ann. Surg., 96: 250–257, Aug. 1932
OPERATION—
Ibid.
TECHNIC—
Partial cholecystectomy. Arch. Surg., 36: 849–857, May 1938

Estlander, Jakob August. French surgeon. 1831–1881
OPERATION—thoracoplasty; resection of one or more ribs for chronic empyema.
Résection des côtes dans l'empyéme chronique. Rev. mens. de Med. et de Chir., Paris, 3: 157–170, 1879
Encore quelques mots sur la résection des côtes dans l'empyème chronique. Ibid., 885–888

Estor, Eugène. French surgeon. 1861–
OPERATION—for slipping patella; a bone block taken from patella is placed into external condyle of femur.
La luxation recidivante de la rotule . . . with H. Estor, Rev. d'orthop., 20: 330–335, July–Aug. 1933

Eustachius, Bartholomaeus. Rome physician. 1524–1574
Discovered Eustachian tube, thoracic duct, abducens nerve, described origin of optic nerves, cochlea, pulmonary veins, muscles of throat and neck and gave first correct picture of uterus. Garrison
Described suprarenal glands.
De glandulis quae renibus incumbunt. In 6th Chapt. of *Opuscula anatomica.* Venetiis, Luchinus, 1564
Tractatio de renibus et primo de eorum structura. In 6th Chapt. of *Opuscula anatomica.* Lugd. Bat., 1707
Wrote best treatise of his time on structure of teeth. Garrison
Libellus de dentibus. Venice, 1563

Eustis, Allan. Louisiana physician. 1876–
Produced urticaria experimentally by means of histamine.
Urticaria—an experimental lesion produced by the local application of betaimidazolyethylamine: its relation to intestinal toxemia. New Orleans Med. and Surg. J.,66: 730–735, Apr. 1914
Suggested existence in body of an enzyme which inactivates histamine.
The detoxicating effect of the liver of Cathartes aura upon solutions of B-imidazolylethylamin. Biochem. Bull., 4: 97–99, 1915

Evans, Alice Catherine. Washington, D. C. scientist. 1881–
FORMULA—
A buffered physiologic salt solution. J. infect. Dis., 30: 95–98, Jan. 1922
MODIFICATION—(R. M. C.) of Huddleson's opsonocytophagic test for brucellosis.
Studies on chronic brucellosis. IV. An evaluation of the diagnostic laboratory tests with F. H. Robinson and Leona Baumgartner Publ. Health Rep., 53: 1507–1525, Aug. 26, 1938
Indicated in 1918 close relationship between organisms causing undulant fever in man and infectious abortion in animals.
Studies on Brucella (Alkaligenes melitensis). U. S.

Pub. Health Ser. Hyg. Lab. Bull. No. 143. Washington, Govt. Printing Office, 1925

Evans, C. A. See Chastek

Evans, F. A. See T. P. Sprunt

Evans, G. L. See T. Lewis

Evans, Henry D. Maine scientist
METHOD—of generating formaldehyde for disinfection.
Formaldehyde disinfection with J. P. Russell, Rep. State Bd. Health, Maine, 1902–03, pp. 234–255, 1904
Disinfection by the formalin-permanganate method. Ibid., pp. 227–243, 1905

Evans, Herbert McLean. California physician. 1882–
Studied growth principle of anterior lobe of pituitary gland.
The effect of the anterior lobe administered intraperitoneally upon growth, maturity, and oestrous cycles of the rat with J. A. Long, Anat. Rec., 21: 62–63, Apr. 1921
Discovered vitamin E in wheat germ.
On the existence of a hitherto unrecognized dietary factor essential for reproduction with K. S. Bishop, Science, 56: 650–651, Dec. 8, 1922
Produced adenomas and fibroadenomas by injection of anterior hypophyseal extracts, rich in growth hormone, into rats for long periods of time.
Hyperplasia of mammary apparatus in precocious maturity induced by anterior hypophyseal hormone with Mariam E. Simpson, Proc. Soc. exp. Biol., N. Y., 26: 597–598, 1929
Isolated vitamin F (linolenic acid).
Vital needs of the body for certain unsaturated fatty acids. IV. Reproduction and lactation upon fat-free diets with S. Lepkovsky and Elizabeth A. Murphy, J. biol. Chem., 106: 431–440, Sept. 1934
(Same) *V. Reproduction and lactation upon diets containing saturated fatty acids as their sole source of energy.* Ibid., 441–450.
Isolated vitamin E.
The isolation from wheat germ oil of an alcohol, a-tocopherol, having the properties of vitamin E with O. H. Emerson and Gladys A. Emerson, Ibid., 113: 319–332, Feb. 1936
See also J. A. Long

Evans, W. A. Jr. See J. G. Gibson, II

Eve, Frank C(ecil). Hull, England physician
METHOD—
Actuation of the inert diaphragm by a gravity method. Lancet, 2: 995–997, Nov. 5, 1932
Resuscitation of the drowned today. J. A. M. A., 124: 964–967, Apr. 1, 1944

Evelyn, Kenneth Austin. Canadian physician. 1911–
METHOD—photoelectrometric, for determination of hemoglobin concentration.
A stabilized photoelectric colorimeter with light filters. J. biol. Chem., 115: 63–75, Aug. 1936

Ewald, Carl Anton. Berlin physician. 1845–1915

TEST or TEST-MEAL—for motility of stomach.
Beiträge zur Physiologie und Pathologie der Verdauung with J. Boas, Arch. f. path. Anat., 101: 325–375, 1885

Ewart, William. English physician. 1848–1929
SIGN—of pericardial effusion.
Practical aids in the diagnosis of pericardial effusion, in connection with the question as to surgical treatment. Brit. med. J., 1: 717–721, Mar. 21, 1896

Ewell, Thomas. American physician. 1785–1826
Wrote thesis on digestion.
Notes on the stomach and secretion. Philadelphia, the author, 1805. 28 pp.

Ewerhardt, F. H. See T. P. Brookes

Ewing, James. New York pathologist. 1866–1943
POSTULATES—of malignancy due to trauma.
The relation of trauma to malignant tumors. Amer. J. Surg., 40: 30–36, Feb. 1926
Modern attitude toward traumatic cancer. Arch. Path., 19: 690–728, May 1935
TUMOR—endothelial myeloma, or diffuse endothelioma.
Diffuse endothelioma of bone. Proc. New York Path. Soc., 21: 17–24, 1921
Further report on endothelial myeloma of bone. Ibid., 24: 93–101, 1924

Ewins, Arthur James. London physician
REACTIONS—for epinephrine.
Some color reactions of adrenine and allied bases. J. Physiol., 40: 317–326, May 3, 1910
Isolated acetylcholine in ergot.
Acetylcholine, a new active principle of ergot. Biochem. J., Cambridge, 8: 44–49, 1914

Exalto, J. Utrecht surgeon
Produced peptic ulcer in dogs identical with those observed in man.
Ulcus jejuni nach Gastroenterostomie. Mitt. Grenzgeb. Med. Chir., 23: 13–41, 1911

Exner, Sigmund. Austria physiologist. 1846–1926
METHOD—of demonstrating myelin sheaths.
Zur Kenntniss vom feineren Baue der Grosshirnrinde. S. B. Akad. Wiss. Wien. 83, Abth. 3: 151–167, (Sitz.) Feb. 3, 1881
PLEXUS—layer of nerve fibers near surface of cerebral cortex.
Untersuchungen über die Localisation der Functionen in der Grosshirnrinde des Menschen. Wien, Braumüller, 1881. 180 pp.

Exton, William Gustav. Newark, N. J. physician. 1876–1943
REAGENTS—for albumin in urine.
A simple and rapid test for albumin and other urinary proteins. J. A. M. A., 80: 529–530, Feb. 24, 1923
A simple and rapid quantitative test for albumin in urine. J. Lab. clin. Med., 10: 722–734, June 1925
TEST—one hour, two dose test of dextrose tolerance.
Diabetes as a life insurance selection problem with A. R. Rose, Proc. A. Life Insur. M. Dir. Amer., 18: 252–286, 1931

Eysell, A. See H. H. R. Schwartze

F

Faber. See F. Penzoldt

Faber, Knud Helge. Copenhagen physician. 1862–

SYNDROME—hypochromic anemia in middle-aged women.

Achylia gastrica mit Anämie. Med. Klin., 5: 1310–1312, Aug. 29, 1909

Fabian, A. A. See A. Sachs

Fabricius, Hieronymus of Aquapendente, anatomist and surgeon. 1533–1619
Wrote on embryology.
De formato foetu. Venetiis, Bolzettam, 1600
De formatione ovi et pulli. Patavii, Bency, 1621
Described valves in veins.
De venarum ostiolis. Padua, Pasquatus, 1603
Same, facsimile ed., transl. by K. J. Franklin, Springfield, Ill., Thomas, 1933

Fabry, Wilhelm. Hilden surgeon. 1560–1624
"Father of German surgery." Recommended amputation above diseased part in gangrene.
De gangraeno et sphacelo. Cologne, Reschedt, 1593
Classified burns.
De combustionibus. Basileae, Regis, 1607
"His most important work is his Century of Surgical Cases (1606–1646), the best collection of case-records of the time." Garrison
Feldt Arztny Buch. Basel, König, 1615
Observationum et curationum chirurgicarum centuriae. Lugduni, Huguetan, 1641

Faget, Jean Charles. French physician. 1818–1884
LAW or SIGN—in yellow fever pulse is at first accelerated, but, as temperature rises, it shows marked tendency to fall.
Monographie sur le type et la specificite de la fièvre jaune. Paris and New Orleans, 1875

Fagge, Charles Hilton. London physician. 1838–1883
Wrote on cretinism.
On sporadic cretinism, occurring in England. Med.-chir. Trans., London, 36: 155–170, 1871
Described heart murmurs.
On the murmurs attendant on mitral contraction. Guy's Hosp. Rep., London, 3 s., 16: 247–342, 1871

Fahr, Th. See F. Volhard.

Fahraeus, Robin. Swedish pathologist. 1888–
METHOD—for determination of sedimentation rate.
Om hamagglutinationen. . . . Hygeia, 80: 369–382, 1918
The suspension-stability of the blood. Acta med. Scandinav., 55: 1–228, 1921
TEST—for pregnancy. (Not specific)
Über die Ursachen der verminderten Suspensionstabilität der Blutkörperchen während der Schwangerschaft. (Vorläufige Mitteilung). Biochem. Z., 89: 355–364, Aug. 16, 1918

Fairhall, L. T. See J. C. Aub

Faivre, J. French physician
Made first accurate estimation of blood pressure in man. Major
Études expérimentales sur les lésions organiques du coeur. Gaz. méd. de Paris, pp. 726–730, Nov. 22, 1856
Same: Ann. Soc. de Méd. de Lyon, 2 s., 4: 180–188, 1856

Fajersztajn, J. Lemberg neurologist
SIGN—crossed sciatic s.; flexing sound thigh with leg straight causes pain on affected side.
Ueber das gekreuzte Ischiaspänomen. Wien. klin. Wschr., 14: 41–47, Jan. 10, 1901

Fallopio, Gabriele. Modena anatomist. 1523–1563

AQUEDUCT, CANAL or ISTHMUS—canal for facial nerve in petrous bone; facial canal.
HIATUS—opening in petrous bone for petrosal branch of vidian nerve.
MUSCLE—pyramidalis nasi.
LIGAMENT—round 1. of uterus.
TUBE—oviduct.
Discovered and described chorda tympani, semicircular canals, sphenoid sinus, trigeminal, auditory and glossopharyngeal nerves, and named vagina and placenta. Garrison
Observationes anatomicae. Venetiis, apud Ulmus, 1561
De humani corporis anatome compendium. Venetiis, apud P. & A. Meilto fratres, 1571
Distinguished between syphilitic and non-syphilitic condylomata and opposed use of mercury in syphilis.
De morbo gallico. Patavii, Gryphium, 1563

Fallot, Étienne Louis Arthur. French physician. 1850–1911
DISEASE or TETRALOGY—congenital cyanosis due to: 1. stenosis or obliteration of pulmonary artery; 2. hypertrophy of right ventricle; 3. dilatation and deviation of aorta to right; 4. intervertricular communication.
Contribution à l'anatomie pathologique de la maladie blue (cyanose cardiaque). Marseille Med., 25: 77–93; 138–158; 207–223; 270–286; 341–354; 403–420, 1888
Also, conclusions trans. by P. D. White in: *Heart disease.* New York, Macmillan, 1931. p. 309
Also, abstr. trans. by L. Morissette, in: F. A. Willius and T. E. Keys' *Cardiac Classics,* St. Louis, Mosby, 1941. pp. 689–690

Falls, Frederick Howard. American obstetrician. 1885–
TEST—
A skin test for the diagnosis of pregnancy with V. C. Freda and H. H. Cohen, Amer. J. Obstet. Gynaec., 41: 431–438, Mar. 1941

Falret, Jean Pierre. French physician. 1794–1870
DISEASE—manic-depressive or circular insanity.
Mémoire sur la folie circulaire, forme de maladie mentale caractérisée par la reproduction successive et régulière de l'état maniaque, de l'état mélancoliquèe, et d'un intervalle lucide plus ou moins prolongé. Bull. Acad. Méd. Paris, 19: 382–400, Feb. 7, 1854

Falta, Wilhelm. Vienna physician. 1875–
COEFFICIENT—percentage of ingested sugar eliminated from the system.
Die Therapie des Diabetes mellitus. Ergebn. inn. Med. u. Kinderh., 2: 74–141, 1908
Attempted to systematize endocrine disorders.
Die Erkrankungen der Blutdrüsen. Berlin, Springer, 1913
Also, in English, 1915

Fanconi, Guido. Zurich physician
ANEMIA—constitutional, infantile, pernicious-like.
Familiäre infantile perniziosaartige Anämie (perniziöses Blutbild und Konstitution). Jb. Kinderh., 3 F., 67: 257–280, Oct. 1927
SYNDROME—of renal dysfunction.
Der nephrotisch-glykosurische Zwergwuchs mit hypophosphatämischer Rachitis. Dtsch. med. Wschr., 62: 1169–1171, July 17, 1936
Der frühinfantile nephrotisch-glykosurische Zwerg-

wuchs mit hypophosphatämischer Rachitis. Jb.
Kinderh., 147: 299–338, Oct. 1936
Fanner, C. J. See O. K. Folin
Fantus, Bernard. Chicago physician. 1874–1940
ETHER SOAP—for removing oil from skin.
The therapy of the Cook County Hospital, Therapy of burns. J. A. M. A., 103: 1446–1447, Nov. 10, 1934
TREATMENT—of mercuric chloride poisoning.
Antidotes in mercuric chloride poisoning. An experimental study. J. Lab. clin. Med., 1: 879–894, Sept. 1916
Antidotes in mercuric chloride poisoning. Second communication. The value of phosphite and hypophosphite combinations with E. G. Hyatt, Ibid., 2: 813–818, Aug. 1917
Described establishment of first blood bank.
The therapy of the Cook County Hospital. Blood preservation. J. A. M. A., 109: 128–131, July 10, 1937
Farabeuf, Louis Hubert. French surgeon. 1841–1910
OPERATION—ischiopubiotomy.
Dystocie du détroit supérieur: mécanisme—diagnostic—traitement symphyséotomie. Gaz. hebd. de méd., 31: 265–280, June 9, 1894
Farahaugh, Charles C. Minneapolis scientist
STANDARDS—
A new set of potassium dichromate standards for determination of the icterus index with Grace Medes, J. Lab. clin. Med., 14: 681–682, Apr. 1929
Farber, S. See C. Heymans
Farberova, P. S. See Y. A. Bruskin
Farina, Guido. Italian surgeon
Sutured right ventricle of heart, June 8, 1896.
Sutura del ventricolo destro. Bull. d. r. Accad. di med. di Roma, 23: 248, 1896–97
Farmer, Chester Jefferson. Chicago chemist. 1886–
METHOD—for determination of vitamin C.
Ascorbic acid content of blood with A. F. Abt, Proc. Soc. exp. Biol., N. Y., 32: 1625–1629, June 1935
Farmer, Vincent. Hackensack, N. J. surgeon. 1897–
OPERATION—
Ventral hernia: a new technique in its repair. Amer. J. Surg., 21: 116–119, July 1933
Faroy, Georges. French physician. 1881–
AGAR—egg albumin serum, for cultivation of meningococci.
Nouveau milieu pour la recherche et la culture du meningocoque with Chavaillon, C. R. Soc. Biol., 78: 455–456, July 24, 1915
Farr, Robert Emmett. American surgeon. 1875–1932
FORCEPS—
Bone-holding forceps. J. A. M. A., 71: 1554 (only), Nov. 9, 1918
MOTOR—
Description of an electric motor for use in bone work. S. G. O., 20: 360 (only), Mar. 1915
MOUTH-GAG—
Modification of the Brophy mouth-gag. J. A. M. A., 62: 1557 (only), May 16, 1914
Developed local anesthesia.
Abdominal surgery under local anesthesia. Ibid., 73: 391–395, Aug. 9, 1919
Practical local anesthesia and its surgical technic. Philadelphia, Lea and Febiger, 1923. 529 pp.
Farr, Samuel. English physician. 1741–1895
Wrote first English work on forensic medicine.

Elements of medical jurisprudence; or, a succinct and compendious description of such tokens in the human body as are requisite to determine the judgment of a coroner, and of courts of law, in cases of divorce, rape, murder, etc.; to which are added directions for preserving the public health. London, Becket, 1788. 144 pp.
Farr, William. English physician. 1807–1883
LAW—during an epidemic of disease, the number of cases at first rises rapidly, then slowly, to a maximum, and then descends more rapidly than it rose. Dorland
Vital statistics. London, Stanford, 1885
Farre, John Richard. English physician. 1775–1862
TUBERCLES—felt beneath capsule of liver in hepatic cancer.
The morbid anatomy of the liver. . . . London, Hurst, Rees et al., 1812–15. 2 vols.
Fasiani, Gian Maria. Italian surgeon. 1887–
AGAR—veal autolysate peptone, for cultivation of anaerobes.
Sulla technica dell'isolemento e della cultura degli anaerobi with A. Zironi, Sperimentale, 71: 439–449, 1917
Fasting, G. F. C. See J. A. Bargen
Fauchard, Pierre. French dentist. 1680–1761
DISEASE—alveolodental periostitis or pyorrhea alveolaris or Rigg's d.
Le chirurgien dentiste, ou traité des dents. . . . Paris, Mariette, 1746. 2 ed., pp. 275–277. (First ed. of 1728 does not describe disease.)
Faught, Francis Ashley. American chemist. 1881–
SPHYGMOMANOMETER—
Blood pressure primer: the sphygmomanometer and its practical application. Philadelphia, Pilling, 1914. 121 pp.
TEST—for acetone.
In his: *Essentials of laboratory diagnosis.* Philadelphia, Davis, 1911. 3 ed., p. 212
Faure, Jean Louis. French surgeon. 1863–1944
OPERATION—excision of uterus.
Sur un nouveau procédé d'hystérectomie abdominale totale; la section médiane de l'utérus. Pr. méd., 2: 237–238, Oct. 19, 1897
Faure, W. See E. Steinach
Fauvel, Sulpice Antoine. French physician. 1813–1884
GRANULES—peribronchial abscesses.
Recherches sur la bronchite capillaire, purulente et pseudo-membraneuse (catarrhe suffocant, croup bronchitique), chez les enfants. Th. d. Paris, 1840. 106 pp.
Described presystolic murmur in mitral stenosis.
Mémoire sur les signes stethoscopiques du rétrécissement de l'orifice auriculo-ventriculaire gauches du coeur. Arch. gén. de Méd., Paris, 4 s., 1: 1–16, 1843
Favre, M. See J. Durand
Faxon, Henry Hardwick. Boston surgeon. 1899–
INCISION—
Logical approach to subphrenic abscess. Amer. J. Surg., 54: 114–126, Oct. 1941
Fay, Temple Sedgwick. Philadelphia surgeon. 1895–
Popularized "artificial hibernation treatment" (cryomotherapy).
Correlation of body segmental temperature and its relation to the location of carcinomatous metastasis. Clinical observations and response to methods of refrigeration with G. C. Henny, S. G. O., 66: 512–524, Feb. 15, 1938

Temperature factors in cancer and embryonal cell growth by L. W. Smith and T. Fay, J. A. M. A., 113: 653–660, Aug. 19, 1939

Fearon, William Robert. Dublin physiologist. 1892–
REACTION—for vitamin A.
A study of some biochemical colour tests. III. Colour reactions associated with vitamin A. Biochem. J., 19: 888–895, 1925
TEST—for bile pigments in urine.
Simple clinical test for bile. Lancet, 1: 291, Feb. 6, 1926
TEST—for nitrite in urine.
(a) *A modified Kjeldahl method for estimation of nitrogen.* (b) *Carbazol test for nitrites.* (c) *Color test for tryptophane in the urine.* Dublin J. M. Sci., 1: 28–32, Mar. 1920
Also, abstr.: J. A. M. A., 74: 1128, Apr., 17, 1920

Fechner, Gustav Theodor. Prussian philosopher. 1801–1887
LAW—intensity of a sensation produced by a varying stimulus varies directly as the logarithum of that stimulus. Dorland
De variis intensitatem vis galvanicae metiendi methodis. Assumto socio Carol. Hermann. Brandes. Lipsiae, Breitkopfio-Haertelianis, (1835) 52 pp.
Ueber ein wichtiges psychophysisches Grundgesetz und dessen Beziehung zur Schätzung der Sterngrössen. Abh. sachs. Ges. (Akad.) Wiss., 4: 455–532, 1859

Fede, Francisco. Italian physician. 1832–1913
DISEASE—sublingual fibroma.
Della produzione sottolinguale, o malattia del Riga. Atti del I. Congr. pediatr. ital., 1890, Napoli, pp. 251–260, 1891

Feldi, Fortunato. Italian physician. 1550–1630
Wrote important early treatise on medical jurisprudence.
De relationibus medicorum. Palermo, 1602

Federspiel, Matthew Nicholas. Milwaukee surgeon. 1879–
METHOD—of wiring fractured maxilla.
Maxillo-facial injuries. Wisconsin M. J., 33: 561–568, Aug. 1934
OPERATION—for double harelip.
Harelip and cleft palate. St. Louis, Mosby, 1927

Feer, Emil. Zurich physician. 1864–
DISEASE or NEUROSIS—
Eine eigenartige Neurose des vegetativen Systems beim Kleinkinde. Ergebn. d. inn. Med. u. Kinderkeilk., 24: 100–122, 1923
PHENOMENON—
Nagelveränderungen nach Scharlach und Masern. Münch. med. Wschr., 51: 1782–1783, Oct. 4, 1904

Fehleisen, Frederich. German physician. 1854–1924
COCCUS or STREPTOCOCCUS—of erysipelas.
Ueber Erysipel. Dtsch. Z. Chir., 16: 391–397, 1882
Suggested use of inoculation erysipelas in treatment of malignant tumors.
Die Etiologie der Erysipels. Berlin, 1883

Fehling, Hermann Johannes Karl. German gynecologist. 1847–1925
OPERATION—for prolapse of uterus.
Lehrbuch der Frauenkrankheiten. Stuttgart, Enke, 1893. 540 pp.
Early writer on periodic intermenstrual pain.
Zur Casuistik des Intermenstrualschmerzes, zugleich als Beitrag zur Casuistik der Castration. Arch. Gynaek., 17: 338–350, 1881

Fehling, Hermann von. German chemist. 1812–1885
SOLUTION—used in testing for sugar.
Quantitative Bestimmung des Zuckers im Harn. Arch. f. d. physiol. Heilk., 7: 64–73, 1848

Fehr, Johannes Michael. Secretary of the Imperial Leopoldian Academy of Natural Sciences. 1610–1688
Published an eulogy of Dr. Johannes Laurentius Bausch who died in 1665, a victim of trigeminal neuralgia.
Naturae genius, medicorum Celsus, Jason Argonautarum, Bauschius occubuit with E. Schmidt, Misc. Cur. med.-phys. Acad. nat. cur., Jenae, 2, 1671. D3 et seq.

Feil, A. See M. Klippel

Feinblatt, Henry M. Brooklyn physician. 1891–
METHOD—of blood transfusion.
An instrument utilizable for various operations: blood transfusion, hypodermoclysis, intravenous infusion, phlebotomy and withdrawal of fluids from body cavities. Amer. J. med. Sci., 169: 870–872, June 1925
A simple apparatus for blood transfusions. Med. J. & Rec., 122: 143, Aug. 4, 1925
Transfusion of blood. New York, Macmillan, 1926. 137 pp.

Feinbloom, William. New York optometrist
Developed new type of telescopic lenses.
A plastic contact lens. Amer. J. Optometry, 14: 41–49, Feb. 1937

Feldberg, Wilhelm. English physiologist. 1900–
Produced evidence that a chemical agent (acetylcholine) appears in transfer of nerve impulses from neuron to neuron in sympathetic ganglia. Garrison and Morton
The chemical transmitter at synapses in a sympathetic ganglion with J. H. Gaddum, J. Physiol., 80: 12P–13P, Nov. 18, 1933
See also H. H. Dale

Feldman, Jacob B. Philadelphia physician. 1884–
APPARATUS—
An instrument for qualitative study of dark adaptation. Arch. Ophth., 18: 821–826, Nov. 1937

Feldman, Samuel. New York dermatologist. 1877–1947
VARIANT—planopilaris.
Lichen planus (with acuminate and atrophic lesions). Abstr.: Arch. Derm. Syph., Chic., 43: 425 (only), Feb. 1941

Feldmann, I. German physician
Reported chordoma arising from sacral region.
Chordoma ossis sacri. Beitr. path. Anat., 48: 630–634, July 27, 1910

Felix, Arthur. London scientist
Described Vi antigens.
A new antigen of B. typhosus: its relation to virulence and to active and passive immunisation with R. Margaret Pitt. Lancet, 2: 186–191, July 28, 1934
See also E. Weil

Fell, George Edward. Buffalo physician. 1850–1918
APPARATUS—an instrument for performing artificial respiration and for preventing collapse of lung in chest operations. Used forced respiration in poisoning, July 23, 1887
Forced respiration in opium poisoning—its possibilities, and the apparatus best adapted to produce it. Buffalo M. & S. J., 27: 145–157, Nov. 1887

Fallenberg, Th. von. Bern chemist
Determined iodine need of human adult and devised
an adequate method for the microdetermination of
iodine as it occurs in nature.
*Das Vorkommen, der Kreislauf und der Stoffwechsel
des Jods.* Ergebn. Physiol., 25: 176-363, 1926
Fellinger, K. See K. Franke
Fellner, Bruno, Jr. Franzensbad physician
Suggested use of stethoscope in measurement of sys-
tolic and diastolic pressure.
*Neuerung zur Messung des systolischen und diastolis-
chen Druckes.* Dtsch. Ges. inn. Med., 24: 404-407,
1907
Fellner, O. O. See F. Silberstein
Fels, Erich. Breslau gynecologist. 1897-
Prepared, from corpus luteum extract, crystalline
material possessing progestin activity.
*Das rein dargestellte Hormon des Corpus luteum und
seine biologischen Wirkungen.* Dtsch. Ges. Gynaek.,
May 26-30, 1931. Abstr. in: Klin. Woch., 10: 1639
(only), Aug. 29, 1931
Felton, Lloyd Derr. American pathologist. 1885-
SERUM—for pneumonia.
*A study of the isolation and concentration of the specific
antibodies of anti-pneumococcus sera.* Boston M. &
S. J., 190: 819-825, May 15, 1924
Felty, Augustus Roi. American physician. 1895-
DISEASE or SYNDROME—
*Chronic arthritis in the adult, associated with spleneme-
galy and leukopenia; a report of five cases of an unusual
clinical syndrome.* Johns Hopk. Hosp. Bull., 35:
16-20, Jan. 1924
Fenger, Carl Emil. Copenhagen surgeon. 1814-1884
OPERATION—
*Ueber Anlegung einer künstlichen Magenöffung an
Menschen durch Gastrotomie.* Arch. f. path. Anat., 6:
350-384, 1854
Fenger, Christian. Chicago surgeon. 1840-1902
OPERATION—
*Operation for the relief of valve formation and stricture
of the ureter in hydro- or pyo-nephrosis.* J. A. M. A.,
22: 335-343, May. 10, 1894
TECHNIC—of vaginal hysterectomy.
The total extirpation of the uterus through the vagina.
Amer. J. med. Sci., 83: 17-47, Jan. 1882
Fenger, Frederic. Chicago chemist
METHOD—of extraction of commercial pepsin in
which peptic hydrolysis of gastric mucosa is avoided.
On the isoelectric precipitation of pepsin with R. H.
Andrew, J. biol. Chem., 73: 371-377, June 1927
Fennel, E. A. See E. R. Whitmore
Fenton, Henry J. Horstman. English scientist
REACTIONS—for organic acids.
Some colour-reactions of organic acids with phenols.
Proc. Cambridge Phil. Soc., 14: 386-387 Mar. 10,
1908
REACTION—
Note on a reaction of tartaric acid. Chem. News, 43:
110-111, Mar. 11, 1881
REACTION—for urea.
*A reagent for the identification of urea and certain other
nitrogen compounds.* J. Chem. Soc., 83: 187-190, 1903
TEST—for hexoses in urine.
On a new test for sugar. Lancet, 1: 215 (only), Jan.
26, 1907
Fenton, W. J. See I. Owen

Fenwick, Samuel. English physician. 1821-1902
DISEASE—primary atrophy of stomach.
*On atrophy of the stomach and on the nervous affections
of the digestive organs.* London, Churchill, 1880. 187
pp.
Féréol. See F. Glenard
Ferguson, A. G. See R. A. Hibbs
Ferguson, Albert Barnett. New York roentgenolog-
gist. 1895-
OPERATION—
*Surgical stimulation of bone growth by a new proce-
dure: preliminary report.* J. A. M. A., 100: 26-27,
Jan. 7, 1933
Ferguson, Alexander Hugh. Chicago surgeon. 1853-
1912
OPERATION—for hernia.
*On the radical cure of inguinal and femoral hernia by
operation.* Ann. Surg., 21: 547-564, 1895
*Oblique inguinal hernia; typic operation for its radical
cure.* J. A. M. A., 33: 6-14, July 1, 1899
The technic of modern operations for hernia. Chicago,
Cleveland Press, 1907. 366 pp.
Ferguson, Charles. American urologist. 1894-
OPERATION—
*Experimental transplantation of the ureters in the
bowel by a two-stage operation: a preliminary report.*
Military Surg., 69: 181-187, Aug. 1931
Ferguson, Russell Sweetser. New York physician.
1894-
METHOD—quantitative Aschheim-Zondek test.
Quantitative behavior of prolan A in teratoma testis.
Amer. J. Cancer, 18: 269-295, June 1933
Fermi, Claudio. Italian physician
SOLUTION—basal ammonium phosphate.
*Weitere Untersuchungen über die tryptischen Enzyme
der Mikroorganismen.* Arch. Hyg., Berl., 14: 1-44
(26), 1892
SOLUTION—glycerol ammonium tartrate; culture
medium.
*Die von den Mikroben bedingte Inversion des Rohr-
zuckers* with G. Montesano, Zbl. Bakt., 2 Abr. 1:
542-556 (547), Aug. 10, 1895
Fernald, Grace Maxwell. American psychologist.
1879-
METHOD—of teaching reading.
*The effect of kinaesthetic factors in the development of
word recognition in the case of non-readers* with H.
Keller, J. Education. Res., 4: 355-377, Dec. 1921
On certain language disabilities. Mental Measurement
Monographs, Serial No. 11. Baltimore, Williams &
Wilkins, 1930
Fernel, Jean Francois. French surgeon. 1497-1558
Described lead poisoning.
De naturali parte medicinae, libri septem. Parisiis,
1542
Therapeutics universalis. Francfurti, apud A. Weche-
lum, 1681
Gave early description of appendicitis; called it coarc-
tion of intestine.
Medicina. Lutetiae Parisiorum, apud A. Wechelum,
1554. 3 pts. in 1
Fernet, Cu. French physician
SYMPTOMS—of pulmonary tuberculosis: 1. modified
respiration at apices; 2. tracheo-bronchial adenitis;
3. congestion at bases.
De quelques signes du début de la tuberculose pul-

monaire chronique. Bull. Acad. Méd. Paris, 3 s., 40: 253–263, Oct. 11, 1898

Fernholz, E. See S. Ansbacher

Ferrari, R. C. See O. Ivanissevich

Ferraton, Louis. French surgeon. 1860–
DISEASE—of Perrin and Ferraton; snapping hip.
Hanche à ressort: ressaut fessier-trochantérien. Rev. d'Orth., 2 s., 6: 45–51, Jan. 1, 1905

Ferrebee, Joseph Wiley. New York physician. 1908–
Introduced intramuscular injection of desoxycorticosterone acetate and propinate for Addison's disease.
Desoxycorticosterone esters: certain effects in the treatment of Addison's disease with C. Ragan, D. W. Atchley and R. F. Loeb, J. A. M. A., 113: 1725–1731, Nov. 4, 1939

Ferree, Clarence Errol. Baltimore scientist. 1877–
PERIMETER—
An illuminated perimeter with campimeter features with G. Rand, Amer. J. Ophth., 5: 455–465, June 1922
TEST—
A new type of instrument for testing the light and color sense with G. Rand, Ibid., 14: 325–333, Apr. 1931
TESTS—of visual acuity.
The testing of visual acuity. I. Factors in the sensitive use of the test for the detection of errors of refraction with G. Rand, Ibid., 17: 29–36, Jan. 1934
(Same) II. The comparative merits of test objects and a new type of broken circle as test object with G. Rand, Ibid., 610–618, July 1934

Ferrier, Sir David. English physician. 1843–1928
Laid foundations of our knowledge concerning localization of cerebral function. Garrison and Morton
The functions of the brain. London, Smith, Elder & Co., 1876 (contains earlier work published in the West Riding Lunatic Asylum Reports)

Ferry, E. L. See T. B. Osborne

Ferry, Erwin Sidney. American scientist. 1868–
LAW—of optics; the critical frequency is proportional to logarithm of illumination intensity; Ferry-Porter l.
Persistence of vision. Amer. J. Sci., 3 s., 44: 193–207, Sept. 1892

Ferry, Newell Simmons. Detroit physician. 1876–
ANTITOXIN—
Studies of the properties of bouillon filtrates of the meningococcus: production of a soluble toxin with J. F. Norton and A. H. Steele, I. Immunol., 21: 293–312, Oct. 1931
Meningococcus antitoxin. I. Prophylactic and therapeutic tests on guinea pigs. Ibid., 23: 315–324, Oct. 1932
(Same) Therapeutic tests on monkeys. Ibid., 325–347
PHENOMENOM—
Reappearance of reaction at site of previous Dick test coincident with appearance of measles rash in a case of measles. J. A. M. A., 87: 241–242, July 24, 1926
See also L. Davis

Feulgen, Robert. Giessen physiologist. 1884–
REACTION—nuclear (microscopic) for nucleic acid.
Mikrokopisch-chemischer Nachweis einer Nucleinsäure vom Typus der Thymonucleinsäure und die darauf beruhende elektive Färbung von Zellkernen in mikrospolischen Präparaten with H. Rossenbeck, Z. phys. Chem., 135: 203–248, Apr. 23, 1924

Fevold, H. L. See F. L. Hisaw

Fiamberti, A. Mario. Brescia physician
EXAMINATION or TEST—permanganate, of cerebrospinal fluid.
Proposta di una reazione sul liquor. (Nota preventiva). with E. Rizzatti, Riv. pat. nerv., 35: 228–231, Jan.–Feb. 1930

Fibiger, Johannes. Denmark physician. 1867–1928
Awarded Nobel prize in 1926. Discovered, in stomach of rat, a cancer which he attributed to a nematode carried by cockroach.
(Researches on a worm, nematode, and its power of provoking the formation of papillary and carcinomatous new-growths in the stomach of a rat.) Acad. Roy. d. Sci. et d. Let. d. Denmark, 1913
Also: J. Hosp. Tid., Kbenh., 6: 417; 449; 473, 1913
Untersuchungen über eine Nematode (Spiroptera sp. n.) und deren Fähigkeit, papillomatöse und carcinomatöse Geschwulstebildungen im Magen der Ratte hervorzurufen. Z. Krebsforsch., 13: 217–280, 1913; 14: 295–326, 1914
On spiroptera carcinomata and their relation to true malignant tumors; with some remarks on cancer age. J. Cancer Res., 4: 367–387, Oct. 1919

Fichera, Gaetano. Italian physician. 1880–1935
TREATMENT—of cancer by hypodermic injection of autolyzed human fetal tissue.
Tumori. Torino, 1911. 425 pp.
I fattori interni nella sviluppo dei tumori e gli odierni saggi di terapia biologica. Milano, Hoepli, 1933. 213 pp.

Fichtner, Dr. Leipzig physician
AGAR—sputum, for cultivation of influenza bacilli.
Beiträge zur Züchtung des Influenzabacillus. Zbl. Bakt., 35: 374–384 (376), Dec. 18, 1903

Fick, Adolph. German physician. 1829–1901
METHOD or PRINCIPLE—of measuring cardiac output.
Ueber die Messung der Blutquantums in den Herzventrikeln. Abst. Verh. phy.-med. Ges. Würzburg, 1870, 2 (neue Folge), 16, 1872
Introduced myotonograph, the cosine lever, and an improved thermopile.
Untersuchungen über elektrische Nervenreizung. Braunschweig, Vieweg, 1864

Fickendey, O. See Buhlert

Ficker, Philip Martin. German bacteriologist. 1868–
BOUILLON—caffein, for typhoid bacilli.
DIAGNOSTICUM—emulsion of killed typhoid bacilli for use in Widal reaction.
REACTION—clumping of dead typhoid bacilli by blood-serum of persons affected with typhoid fever.
Ueber neue Methoden des Nachweises von Typhusbazillen with W. Hoffman, Hyg. Rundschau, p. 1, 1904
Weiteres über den Nachweis von Typhusbazillen. with W. Hoffman, Arch. Hyg., Berl., 49: 229–273, 1904
SOLUTION—sputum serum; for cultivation of tubercle bacilli.
Wachstum der Tuberkelbacillen auf sauren Gehirnnährböden. Zbl. Bakt., 27: 504–511, Apr. 20; 591–597, May 4, 1900

Field, W. H. See E. K. Tanner

Fielding, George Hunsley. English anatomist. 1801–1871

MEMBRANE—the tapetum.
On a new membrane in the eye; . . . Hull, Wilson, 1832. 28 pp.
Fieser, Louis Frederick. American chemist. 1899–
Synthesized vitamin Ki.
Synthesis of vitamin Ki. J. Amer. Chem. Soc., 61: 3467–3475, 1939
Filatoff, Nils Feodrovich. Moscow pediatrician. 1847–1902
DISEASE—fourth d.; an alleged exanthematous contagious disease.
SIGN—circumoral pallor in scarlet fever.
Lektsii ob ostrikh infektsionnikh bolieznyakh u dietei. (Lectures on acute infectious diseases of children.) Moskva, Lang. 1887. vol. 2, p. 113
Vorlesungen über akute Infektionskrankheiten im Kindesalter. Übers. v. L. Polonsky, Wien, 1897. p. 383
Filatov, Vladimir Petrovich. Russian surgeon. 1875–
Did important work on corneal transplantation.
Transplantation of the cornea. Arch. Ophth., N. Y., n. s., 13: 321–347, 1935
(Earlier papers in Russian journals).
Fildes, Paul Gordon. English bacteriologist. 1882–
AGAR—blood peptone; culture medium.
AGAR—body fluid; for cultivation of cocci.
The technique of the preparation of culture media containing albuminous fluids, in particular for the growth of the meningococcus. Lancet, 1: 492–493, Mar. 31, 1917
BOUILLON—pepsinized blood, for cultivation of B. influenza.
A new medium for the growth of B. influenza. Brit. J. exp. Path., 1: 129–130, Apr. 1920
LAW—presence of complement-fixing antibodies in cord blood of infant is diagnostic not of syphilis in infant but rather of syphilis in mother.
The prevalence of congenital syphilis amongest the newly born of East End of London. J. Obstet. Gynaec. Brit. Emp., 27: 124, 1915
See also W. Bulloch, J. McIntosh
Filehne, Wilhelm. German physician. 1844–1927
Introduced antipyrin.
Ueber das Antipyrin, ein neues Antipyreticum. Z. klin. Med., 7: 641–642, 1884
Introduced pyramidon.
Ueber das Pyramidon, ein Antipyrinderivat. Berl. klin. Wschr., 33: 1061–1063, 1896
Fillinger, Franz, v. Budapest physician
REAGENT—for reducing sugar.
Neues Verfahren der Zuckerbestimmung. Z. Untersuch. Nahr.-u. Genussm., pp. 605–607, Nov. 15, 1911
Findlay, Francis McRae. California surgeon. 1898–
TECHNIC—of closure of gastrojejunocolic fistula.
Treatment of gastrojejunocolic fistula by multiple stage operations. Arch. Surg., 32: 896–906, May 1936
Fine, Jacob. Boston physician. 1900–
TREATMENT—
The treatment of gaseous distension of the intestine by the inhalation of ninety-five per cent oxygen: description of an apparatus for the clinical administration of high oxygen mixtures with B. M. Banks, J. B. Sears and L. Hermanson, Ann. Surg., 103: 375–387, Mar. 1936
Fine, Pierre. French surgeon. 1760–1814

Performed first recorded colostomy for intestinal obstruction, in 1797. Garrison and Morton
Mémoire et observation sur l'entérotomie. Ann. Soc. de Méd. prat. de Montpellier, 6: 34–54, 1805
Finger, Ernst Anton Franz. Vienna pathologist. 1856–1939
AGAR—urea; for cultivation of gonococci.
Beiträge zur Biologie des Gonococcus und zur pathologischen Anatomie des gonorrhoischen Processes with A. Ghon and F. Schlagenhaufer, Arch. f. Dermat. u. Syph., 28: 3–24, (14), 1894.
Finkler, Dittmar. Bonn bacteriologist. 1852–1912
BACILLUS—
Untersuchungen über Cholera nostras with J. Prior, Dtsch. med. Wschr., 10: 579–582, Sept. 4, 1884
DISEASE—
Influenzapneumonie. Ibid., 16: 84–86, Jan. 30, 1890
Finlay, Carlos Juan. Havana physician. 1833–1915
First to put forth theory that mosquito is transmitter of yellow fever.
El mosquito hipoteticamente considerado come agente de transmision de la fiebre amarilla. An. r. Acad., de cien. med. . . . de la Habana, 18: 147–160, 1881
Also, English trans. by Dr. Finlay in: *Selected works.* Habana, pp. 27–43, 1912
Yellow fever: its transmission by means of the culex mosquito. Amer. J. med. Sci., 92: 395–409, 1886
Above papers in: Med. Classics, 2: 569–639, Feb. 1938
Finney, John Miller Turpin. Baltimore surgeon. 1863–1942
INCISION—for radical mastectomy.
Surgery of the breast. In: Keen's *Surgery.* Philadelphia, Saunders, 1919. Vol. 3, pp. 563–613 (606)
OPERATION—gastroduodenostomy.
A new method of gastroduodenostomy, end-to-side; with illustrations. Trans. South. Surg. Ass., 36: 576–578; 586–587, 1924
OPERATION—gastroenterostomy.
Gastro-enterostomy for cicatrizing ulcer of the pylorus. Report in: Johns Hopk. Hosp. Bull., 4: 53–55, May 1893
OPERATION—
A new method of pyloroplasty. Trans. Amer. Surg. Ass., 20: 165–177, 1902
Also: Johns Hopk. Hosp. Bull., 13: 155–161, July 1902
Thirteen years' experience with pyloroplasty. S. G. O., 18: 273–284, Mar. 1914
OPERATION—
Spasmodic torticollis with W. Hughson. Ann. Surg., 81: 255–269, Jan. 1925
Finsen, Niels Ryberg. Danish physician. 1860–1904
Awarded Nobel prize in 1903.
APPARATUS—system of lenses for applying violet rays of light in light treatment of disease.
LIGHT—consisting principally of violet and ultraviolet rays.
TREATMENT—of lupus vulgaris by direct application of light rays.
Om anvendelse medicinen af koncentrerede kemiske lysstraaler. Kjøbenhavn, Hegel, 1896. 52 pp.
La photothérapie. I. Les rayons chimiques et la variole. II. La lumière comme agent d'excitabilité. III. Traite-

*ment du lupus vulgaire par des rayons chimiques con-
centrés.* Paris, Carré et Naud, 1899. 99 pp.
Also, in German, 1899; in English, 1901
Finsterer, Hans. Vienna surgeon. 1877–
OPERATION—partial resection of stomach with
gastroenterostomy.
*Ausgedehnte Magenresektion bei Ulcus duodeni statt
der enfachen Duodenalresektion bzw. Pylorusausschal-
tung.* Zbl. Chir., 45: 434–435, June 29, 1918
Surgical treatment of ulcer of stomach and duodenum.
S. G. O., 36: 454–457, Apr. 1923
*Ist die ausgedehnte Resektion des Magens beim Ulcus
duodeni erlaubt oder nicht?* Zbl. Chir., 50: 1566–1569,
Oct. 20, 1923
Duodenal ulcer and its surgical treatment. New Orleans
M. & S. J., 76: 459–461, Apr. 1924
OPERATION—for recurrent dislocation of shoulder.
*Zur Frage nach der zweckmässigsten Behandlung der
habituellen Schulterluxation.* Wien. med. Wschr., 74:
1232–1237, June 7, 1924
Fiocca, Rufino. Italian physician
STAINING METHOD—for spores.
Ueber eine neue Methode der Sporenfärbung. Zbl.
Bakt., 14: 8–9, July 1, 1893
Fiolle, Jean. French surgeon. 1884–
INCISION—
*Découverte des vaisseaux profonds par des voies d'accès
larges* with J. Delmas, Paris, Masson, 1917. 122 pp.
Also, transl. by C. G. Cumston: *The surgical exposure
of the deep-seated blood-vessels.* London, Heinemann,
1921. 87 pp.
Firor, W. M. See G. W. Thorn
Fischer, August Henrich Wilhelm. Frankfurt a.
Main physician. 1901–
TECHNIC—injection of air into rectum after evacua-
tion of barium; contrast technic for polyps.
*Früh diagnose des Dickdarmkrebses, insbesondere
seine Differentialdiagnose gegen Tuberkulose mit
Hilfe der kombinierten Luft- und Bariumfüllung des
Dickdarms.* Dtsch. Ges. inn. Med., 35: 86–87, 1923
Fischer, Emil. German chemist. 1852–1919
METHOD—analysis of proteins by acid hydrolysis
(esterification).
*Untersuchungen über Amniosäuren, Polypeptide und
Proteine.* Berlin, Springer, 1906
TEST—for glucose.
*Verbindungen des Phenylhydrazins mit den Zucker-
arten.* Ber. dtsch. chem. Ges., 17: 579–584, 1884
Introduced veronal.
Ueber Veronal with J. v. Mering, Therap. d. Gegen-
wart, 45: 145–146, Apr. 1904
See also F. Penzoldt
Fischer, Hans. Munich physician. 1881–1945
Awarded Nobel prize in chemistry in 1930 for dis-
covery and isolation of hematin.
TEST—for hemibilirubin in urine.
*Ueber einen einfachen (spektroskopischen) Nachweis
des Hemibilirubins in pathologischen Harn.* Münch.
med. Wschr., 59: 2555–2556, Nov. 19, 1912
Fischer, H. See O. Neubauer
Fischer, Hermann. Breslau surgeon. 1831–1919
THEORY—of shock, a vasomotor paralysis.
Ueber den Shok. Samml. klin. Vortr., No. 10 (Chir.
No. 5), pp. 69–82, 1870
Fischer, Hermann. New York surgeon. 1871–

OPERATION—for hernia.
Lotheisen's operation for femoral hernia. Ann. Surg.,
69: 432–434, Apr. 1919
Fischer, Martin Henry. American physician. 1879–
SOLUTION or TREATMENT—used by rectal or
intravenous injection in anuria of Bright's disease or
eclampsia.
Some practical points in the treatment of nephritis.
Ohio M. J., 7: 400–403, Aug. 1911
Made important studies of edema.
*Oedema; a study of the physiology and the pathology
of water absorption by the living organism.* New York,
Wiley, 1910. 209 pp.
*Das Oedem als Kolloidchemisches Problem nebst
Bemerkungen über die allgemeine Natur der Wasser-
bindung in Organismen.* Kolloidchem. Beihefte,
Dresden, 1: 93–118, 1910
Fischer, O. See C. W. Braun
Fischer, Roger. French physician
TEST—for cancer.
*II. Réaction du sérum sanguin permettant le diagnostic
précoce du cancer chez l'homme.* Bull. Acad. Méd.
Paris, 89: 71–73, Jan. 16, 1923
Fischler, Franz Joseph. Heidelberg physician. 1876–
STAIN—for fatty acids and soaps.
*Ueber die Unterscheidung von Neutralfetten, Fett-
säuren und Seifen im Gewebe.* Zbl. allg. Path. u. path.
Anat., 15: 913–917, Nov. 30, 1904
Coined term alkalosis.
*Ueber die Fleischintoxikation bei Tieren mit Eck'scher
Fistel. Der Krankheitsbegriff der Alkalosis.* Dtsch.
Arch. klin. Med., 104: 300–339, 1911
Fish, Hamilton. Ouray, Ohio physician
STERILIZER—
A new sterilizer for country and private practice.
J. A. M. A., 33: 1308 (only), Nov. 18, 1899
Fish, Mildred. See A. F. Hess
Fish, Pierre Augustine. Washington, D. C. scientist.
1865–
MODIFICATION—of Golgi's bichromate and silver
nitrate method.
The use of formalin in neurology. Trans. Amer. Micr.
Soc., 17: 319–328, 1895
Fishberg, Arthur Maurice. New York physician.
1898–
TEST—concentration t. of renal function.
Technique of the concentration and dilution tests. In:
Hypertension and nephritis. Philadelphia, Lea and
Febiger, 1930, 1 ed., pp. 45–47; 1939, 4 ed., pp.
77–79
Fisher, Alfred George Timbrell. English surgeon.
1887–
OPERATION—for removal of meniscus.
Internal derangements of the knee joint. New York,
Macmillan, 1924, p. 61
Same, London, Lewis, 1933, 2 ed., p. 75
Fisher, Fritz. Strassburg surgeon
OPERATION—gastrostomy.
Mittheilung über Magenfistelbildung. Verh. dtsch.
Ges. Chir., 24: 229–239, 1895
Fisher, Theodore. London physician
SIGN—presystolic murmur in certain cases of adherent
pericardium.
*A diastolic bruit at the apex in the heart disease of
children.* Brit. med. J., 1: 906–907, Apr. 28, 1894

Fisher, William Henry. Toledo, Ohio surgeon. 1870–1936
INCISION—Y-shaped for drainage of parotid abscess.
Post-operative infective parotiditis. Ann. Surg., 78: 568–571, Nov. 1923

Fiske, Cyrus Hartwell. Boston biochemist. 1890–
METHOD—for determination of inorganic phosphorus.
The colorimetric determination of phosphorus with Y. Subbarow. J. biol. Chem., 66: 375–400, Dec. 1925

Fittipaldi, Emil Hugo. Naples physician
TESTS—for albuminoses and peptones in urine.
Eine neue schnelle Methode zum Nachweis von Albumosen und Peptonen im Harn. Dtsch. med. Wschr., 47: 42–43, Jan. 13, 1921

Fitz, Fred. New York
METHOD—for determination of free and total cholesterol.
The application to the calorimeter of the Schoenheimer and Sperry method for the determination of total and free cholesterol. J. biol. Chem., 109: 523–527, May 1935

Fitz, Reginald. American physician. 1885–
METHOD—for determination of alkali reserve.
Studies of acidosis. IV. The relationship between alkaline reserve and acid excretion with D. D. Van Slyke, J. biol. Chem., 30: 389–400, June 1917
See also F. M. Allen, W. B. Cannon, D. D. Van Slyke

Fitz, Reginald Heber. Boston physician. 1843–1913
LAW or SYNDROME—of acute pancreatitis.
Acute pancreatitis. A consideration of pancreatic hemorrhage, hemorrhagic, suppurative, and gangrenous pancreatitis, and of disseminated fat-necrosis. Boston M. & S. J., 120: 181–187, Feb. 21; 205–207, Feb. 28; 229–235, Mar. 7, 1889
Recognized true nature of and coined term appendicitis.
Perforating inflammation of the vermiform appendix; with special reference to its early diagnosis and treatment. Trans. Ass. Amer. Phys., 1: 107–144, 1886
Also: Amer. J. med. Sci., 92: 321–346, 1886
Also: Med. Classics, 2: 459–491, Jan. 1938
The relation of perforating inflammation of the vermiform appendix to perityphilitis. New York med. J., 47: 505–508, May 12, 1888
Described intrapleural lipoma of mediastinum.
Intrapleural lipoma; acute pericarditis; pericardial exploration. Amer. J. med. Sci., 130: 785–793, Nov. 1905

Flack, Martin William. English physiologist. 1882–1931
TEST—patient blows against column of mercury of a sphygmomanometer with glottis open, indicating a deficient "potential" in the venous return to heart.
The Milroy lectures on respiratory efficiency in relation to health and disease. Lancet, 2: 637–641, Sept. 24; 693–696, Oct. 1, 1921
Some considerations in the estimation of physical efficiency. Abstr.: Brit. med. J., 2: 921–923, Nov. 17, 1923
See also A. Keith

Flagg, Paluel Joseph. New York physician. 1886–
METHOD—of resuscitation by direct exposure intu-

bation and intratracheal insufflation of 10% carbon dioxid and 90% oxygen under measured pressure.
Treatment of asphyxia in the new-born: preliminary report of the practical application of modern scientific methods. J. A. M. A., 91: 788–791, Sept. 15, 1928

Flajani, Giuseppe. Italian surgeon. 1741–1808
DISEASE—exophthalmic goiter.
Sopra un tumor freddo nell'anterior parte del collo detto broncocele. In his: *Collezione d'osservazioni e riflessioni di chirurgia.* Roma, 3: 270–273, 1802

Flanders, F. F. See O. K. O. Folin

Flatau, Eduard. German neurologist. 1869–1932
LAW—the greater the length of fibers of spinal cord, the closer they are situated to periphery. Dorland
Atlas des menschlichen Gehirns und des Faserverlaufes. Berlin, Karger, 1894. 27 pp.
Same, in English: Glasgow, Bauerweister, 1894. 25 pp.
MODIFICATION—of Golgi's bichromate and sublimate method.
Ueber die zweckmässige Anwendung der Golgi'schen Sublimatmethode für die Untersuchung des Gehirns des erwachsenen Menschen. Arch. mikr. Anat., 45: 158–162, 1895

Flechsig, Paul Emil. Leipzig neurologist. 1847–1929
AREAS—on each half of medulla oblongata, marked out by fibers of vagus and hypoglossal nerves.
CUTICULUM—layer of flat cells on external surface of neurolgia. Dorland
FASCICULUS—anterior ground-bundle and lateral ground-bundle.
TRACT or COLUMN—anterior ground-bundle or principal tract.
Named "the pyramidal tract."
Die Leitungsbahnen im Gehirn und Rückenmark des Menschen auf Grund entwickelungsgeschichtlicher Untersuchungen. Leipzig, Engelmann, 1876. 382 pp.

Fleig, Charles Auguste. Montpellier physiologist. 1883–1912
REACTION—precipitin, for diagnosis of hydatid disease.
Recherche sur un séro-diagnostic au kyste hydatique par la méthode des précipitines with M. Lisbonne, C. R. Soc. Biol., 62: 1198–1201, 1907
TEST—for blood in urine.
Nouvelle réaction, a la fluorescine, pour la recherche du sang, en particulier dans l'urine. Ibid., 2: 192–194, July 23, 1910

Fleischer, Richard. Erlangen physician. 1848–
Described "march haemoglobinuria."
Ueber eine neue Form von Haemoglobinurie beim Menschen. Berl. klin. Wschr., 18: 691–694, Nov. 21, 1881

Fleischl, von Marxow, Ernst von. Austrian pathologist. 1846–1891
HEMOMETER—
Regeln für den Gebrauch des Hämometers. Med. Jahrb., Wien, 1886
TEST—for bile pigments.
Modification der Gallenfarbstoffprobe. Zbl. med. Wiss., 13: 561–562, July 31, 1875

Fleming, Alexander. English physician. 1823–1875
SOLUTION or TINCTURE—of aconite.
An inquiry into the physiological and medicinal

*properties of the Aconitum Napellus, to which are
added observations on several other species of Aconitum.*
London, Churchill, 1845. 160 pp.

Fleming, Sir Alexander. London physician. 1881–
Awarded Nobel prize in 1945, with his associates,
Sir Howard Walter Florey and Dr. Ernest Boris
Chain, for their discovery of penicillin. Introduced
penicillin in 1929.
METHOD—for titration of penicillin.
*On the antibacterial action of cultures of a penicllium,
with special reference to their use in isolation of B.
influenzae.* Brit. J. exp. Path., 10: 226–236, June 1929
MODIFICATION—of Wright slide cell technic, to
determine level of penicillin.
*Streptococcal meningitis treated with penicillin; meas-
urement of bacteriostatic power of blood and cerebro-
spinal fluid.* Lancet, 2: 434–438, Oct. 9, 1943
TEST—
A simple method of serum diagnosis of syphilis. Ibid.,
1: 1512–1515, May 29, 1909
Discovered lysozyme.
*On a remarkable bacteriolytic element found in tissues
and secretions.* Proc. roy. Soc., в. B, 93: 306–317,
May 1922
*Arris and Gale Lecture on lysozyme. A bacteriolytic
ferment found normally in tissues and secretions.*
Lancet, 1: 217–220, Feb. 2, 1929

Fleming, David. English naval surgeon
Performed first successful ligation of common carotid artery. Garrison
*Case of rupture of the carotid artery, and wounds of
several of its branches, successfully treated by tying the
common trunk of the carotid itself.* Med.-Chir. Jour
and Rev., London, 3: 2–4, Jan. 1817

Fleming, Howard Webster. San Francisco surgeon.
1891–
TREATMENT—of subdural hematoma.
*Chronic subdural hematoma: simple drainage as a
method of treatment; report of eight cases* with O. W.
Jones, Jr. S. G. O., 54: 81–87, Jan. 1932

Fleming, Robert. Geneva physiologist
REACTION—for cysteine.
A sensitive reaction for cysteine. Biochem. J., 24:
965–966, 1930

Flemming, Walther. German anatomist. 1843–1905
ACID DIFFERENTIATION—of safranin staining.
Mittheilungen zur Färbetechnik. Z. wiss. Mik., 1:
349–361 (350), 1884
METHOD—of decalcifying bone for histologic study.
Surrogate für Knochenschliffe. Ibid., pp. 47–49, 1886
ORANGE METHOD—of plasma staining; triple
stain.
*Ueber Theilung und Kernformen bei Leukocyten, und
über deren Attractionssphären.* Arch. mikr. Anat.,
37: 249–298, 1891
Neue Beitrage zur Kenntniss der Zelle. Ibid., pp.
685–751
SOLUTION—for fixation.
See ACID DIFFERENTIATION.
Also in: *Zellsubstanz, Kern und Zelltheilung.* Leipzig,
Vogel, 1882. p. 382
SOLUTION—picro-osmic acid. Ibid., p. 381
Wrote classic account of cell division and karyo-
kinesis. Garrison
Ibid.

Discovered centrosome.
Beobachtungen über die Beschaffenheit des Zellkerns.
Arch. mikr. Anat., 13: 693–717, 1876

Fletcher, Sir Walter Morley. Liverpool physiologist.
1873–1933
TEST—for lactic acid.
Lactic acid in amphibian muscle with F. G. Hopkins,
J. Physiol., 35: 247–309, Mar. 27, 1907

Fleury, Maurice G. French physician. 1860–1931
TEST—
Reaction caracteristique de la morphine. Ann. chim.
anal., 6: 417–418, 1901

Flexner, Simon. New York physician. 1863–1946
BACILLUS—B. dysenteriae.
DYSENTERY—
STRAIN—Flexner-Harris s. of B. dysenteriae.
On the etiology of tropical dysentery. Johns Hopk.
Hosp. Bull., 11: 231–242, Oct. 1900
*Bacteriological and clinical studies of the diarrheal dis-
eases of infancy with reference to Bacillus dysenteriae
(Shiga)* with L. E. Holt, Studies, Rockefeller Inst.
Med. Res., New York, 1904. Vol. 2, pp. 202
BACILLUS—pathogenic agent of poliomyelitis.
Showed that monkeys can be infected by applying
virus of poliomyelitis to nasopharynx.
The transmission of acute poliomyelitis to monkeys
with P. A. Lewis, J. A. M. A., 53: 1639 (only), Nov.
13, 1909
(Same) *A further note* with P. A. Lewis, Ibid., 1913
(only), Dec. 4, 1909
The nature of the virus of epidemic poliomyelitis with
P. A. Lewis, Ibid., 2095 (only), Dec. 18, 1909
Epidemic poliomyelitis with P. A. Lewis, Ibid., 54:
45–46, Jan. 1, 1910
*Epidemic poliomyelitis in monkeys: a mode of spon-
taneous infection* with P. A. Lewis, Ibid., 535 (only),
Feb. 12, 1910
SERUM—
*Concerning a serum-therapy for experimental infec-
tion with Diplococcus intracellularis.* J. exp. Med., 9:
168–185, Mar. 14, 1907
Serum treatment of epidemic cerebro-spinal meningitis
with J. W. Jobling, Ibid., 10: 141–203, Jan. 1, 1908
See also W. H. Welch

Flinn, F. B. See E. H. Maechling

Flint, Austin. American physician. 1812–1886
LAW—an elevation of pitch always accompanies
diminution of resonance in consequence of pulmonary consolidation.
*The analytical study of auscultation and percussion,
with reference to the distinctive characters of pulmonary
signs.* Trans. Internat. Med. Cong., 7 Sess., London,
2: 130–141, 1881
Also: Med. Classics, 4: 901–920, Apr. 1940
MURMUR or SIGN—a loud presystolic m. at apex
in aortic regurgitation; mitral direct m.
On cardiac murmurs. Amer. J. med. Sci., 44: 29–54,
1862
Also: Med. Classics, 4: 864–900, Apr. 1940
Also in: F. A. Willius and T. E. Keys' *Cardiac
classics.* St. Louis, Mosby, 1941. pp. 502–528
Coined term bronchio-vesicular breathing.
*A practical treatise on the physical exploration of the
chest and the diagnosis of diseases affecting the respiratory organs.* Philadelphia, Blanchard and Lea,
1856, p. 197

Flint, Austin, Jr. American physician. 1836-1915
Claimed that cholesterin is removed from blood by
liver and discharged from body as stercorin. Garrison
*Experimental researches into a new excretory function
of the liver; consisting in the removal of cholesterine
from the blood, and its discharge from the body in the
form of stercorine (the seroline of Boudet).* (New York,
1862?). 61 pp.
Wrote on nitrogen excretion.
*On the physiological effects of severe and protracted
muscular exercise; with especial reference to the influence of exercise upon the excretion of nitrogen.* New
Med. J., 13: 609-697, June 1871

Flint, Joseph Marshall. New Haven surgeon 1872-
TREATMENT—
*Acute traumatic subdeltoid bursitis: a new and simple
treatment.* J. A. M. A., 60: 1224-1226, Apr. 19,
1913

Florence, Albert. French physician. 1851-1927
CRYSTALS—formed by action of iodin on any liquid
containing lecithin, as semen.
REACTION or TEST—for spermatic fluid.
Du sperme et des taches des sperme en médecine légale.
Arch. d'Anthrop. crimin., 10: 417-434; 520-543,
1895; 11: 37-46; 146-165; 249-265, 1896
TEST—for urobilin, urobilinogen and blood in urine.
*Réactif clinique de l'urobiline, de l'urobilinogène et du
sang.* J. Pharm. Chim., Paris, s 7, 2: 160 (only),
1910

Florey, Sir Howard Walter. Oxford pathologist.
1898-
Awarded Nobel prize in 1945, with Sir Alexander
Fleming and Ernest Boris Chain, for their discovery
of penicillin.
UNITS—of penicillin.
General and local administration of penicillin. Lancet,
244: 387-397, Mar. 27, 1943
See also E. B. Chain and A. Fleming

Flosdorf, Earl William. Philadelphia bacteriologist.
1904-
METHOD—
*Procedure and apparatus for preservation in "lyo-
phile" form of serum and other biological substances*
with S. Mudd, J. Immunol., 29: 389-425, Nov. 1935
PROCESS—
The desivac process for drying from the frozen state
with F. J. Stokes and S. Mudd, J. A. M. A., 115:
1095-1097, Sept. 28, 1940

Flothow, Paul George. Seattle, Wash. neurologist.
1897-
OPERATION—for lumbar sympathectomy by an
antero-lateral oblique incision for extraperitoneal
approach.
*Anterior extraperitoneal approach to the lumbar
sympathetic nerves.* Amer. J. Surg., 29: 23-25, July
1935

Flourens, Marie Jean Pierre. French physiologist.
1794-1867
DOCTRINE or THEORY—entire cerebrum takes
part in every mental process.
Nouvelles expériences sur le système nerveux. Arch.
gén. de méd., 8: 422-426, 1825
Demonstrated that brain is organ of thought and
will power, while cerebellum presides over coordination of bodily movements. Garrison
Recherches expérimentales sur les propriétés et les

*fonctions du système nerveux, dans les animaux
vertébrés.* Ibid., 2: 321-370, 1823
Also: Paris, Crevot, 1824. 331 pp.
Located existence of a true cerebellar and labyrin-
thine vertigo. Garrison
*Expériences sur les canaux semi-circulaires de l'oreille,
dans les oiseaux.* Mém. Acad. roy. d. sci., Paris, 9:
455-477, 1828
Discovered anesthetic properties of chloroform.
Note touchant l'action de l'éther sur les centres nerveux.
C. P. Acad. Sci., 24: 340-344, 1847
Discovered vital node, the bilateral center of res-
piration in medulla oblongata. Garrison
Recherches expérimentales. Paris, Baillière, 1842. 2 ed.,
p. 204
Nouveaux détails sur le noeud vital. C. R. Acad. Sci.,
47: 803-806, 1858
Nouveaux éclaircissements sur le noeud vital. Ibid.,
48: 1136-1138, 1859

Flournoy, T. See C. Norris

Floyd, E. See D. DuBois

Floyer, Sir John. English physician. 1649-1734
*Described use of watch in timing pulse. The physician's
pulse-watch; or, an essay to explain the old art of feeling the pulse, and to improve it by the help of a pulse-
watch.* London, Smith and Walford. Vol. 1, 1707;
Vol. 2, 1710
Wrote treatise on diseases of old age.
*Medicine gerocomica; or, the Galenic art of preserving
old men's healths, explan'd in twenty chapters. . . .*
London, Isted, 1724. 135 pp.
Gave first account, derived by dissection, of changes
in lungs now called emphysema and assigns as cause
of spasmodic asthma "a contracture of the musculature fibers of the bronchi." Garrison
A treatise of the asthma. . . . London, Wilkins, 1726.
p. 203; 239

Fluhmann, Charles Frederic. San Francisco obstetrician. 1898-
TEST—for serum prolan.
*The significance of anterior pituitary hormone in the
blood of gynecologic patients.* Amer. J. Obstet. Gynaec.,
20: 1-15, July 1930

Foa, Pio. Italian pathologist. 1848-1923
DIPLOCOCCUS—found in pneumonia.
*Weitere Untersuchungen über die Aetiologie der
Pneumonie.* Dtsch. med. Wschr., 15: 21-22, Jan.
10, 1889

Fodor, Josef von. Budapest physician. 1843-1901
TEST—for carbon monoxide in blood.
*Das Kohlenoxyd in seinen Beziehungen zur Gesund-
heit.* Dtsch. Vrtljschr. f. off. Gesundhtspfl., 12: 377-
399, 1880

Földes, Franz. Budapest physiologist
TEST—for histidine.
Das Vorkommen des Histidins im menschlichen Urin.
Biochem. Z., 283: 199-209, Jan. 1935

Förster, Otfried. German neurologist. 1873-1941
OPERATION—section intradurally of 7, 8 and 9
dorsal nerve-roots on both sides in locomotor ataxia.
Dorland
*Ueber operative Behandlung gastrischer Krisen durch
Resektion der 7.-10. hinteren Dorsalqurzel* with H.
Küttner, Beitr. klin. Chir., 63: 245-256, 1909
Presented exhaustive treatise on theoretical and
practical aspects of radicotomy.

Ueber eine neue operative Methode der Behandlung spastischer Lähmungen mittels Resektion hinterer Rückenmarkswurzeln. Z. orthop. Chir., 22: 203–223, 1908

Foerster, Otto Hottinger. Milwaukee physician. 1876–
Introduced mapharsen in treatment of syphilis.
Mapharsen in the treatment of syphilis: a preliminary report with R. L. McIntosh, L. M. Wieder, H. R. Foerster and G. A. Cooper, Arch. Derm. and Syph., N. Y., 32: 868–892, Dec. 1935

Fol, Hermann. German pathologist. 1845–1892
SOLUTION or STAIN—
Lehrbuch der vergleichenden mikroscopischen Anatomie mit Einschluss der vergleichenden Histologie und Histogenie. Leipzig, Engelmann, 1884–96. 451 pp. p. 100

Foley, Frederic Eugene Basil. St. Paul urologist, 1891–
OPERATION—lumbar ureterolithotomy.
Management of ureteral stone. Operation versus expectancy and manipulation. J. A. M. A., 104: 1314–1318, Apr. 13, 1935
OPERATION—for hydronephrosis.
A new plastic operation for stricture at the ureteropelvic junction; report of 20 operations. J. Urol., 38: 643–672, Dec. 1937

Folin, Otto Knut Olof. American chemist. 1867–1934
DIET—for studying metabolism.
Approximately complete analyses of thirty "normal" urines. Amer. J. Physiol., 13: 45–65 (64), Feb. 1, 1905
METHOD—for determination of amino-acids.
A new colorimetric method for the determination of the amino-acid nitrogen in blood. J. biol. Chem., 51: 377–391, Apr. 1922
METHOD—of purification of picric acid.
Impure picric acid as a source of error in creatine and creatinine determinations with E. A. Doisy, Ibid., 28: 349–356, Jan. 1917
METHOD—for determination of total and inorganic sulfates.
On sulphate and sulphur determinations. Ibid., 1: 131–159, Jan. 1906
METHOD—for determination of hippuric acid.
A new method for the determination of hippuric acid in urine with F. F. Flanders, Ibid., 11: 257–263, Apr. 1912
METHOD—for determination of phenols in urine.
A colorimetric method for the determination of phenols (and phenol derivatives) in urine with W. Denis, Ibid., 22: 305–308, Sept. 1915
METHOD—for determination of total nitrogen in urine.
A new method for the determination of total nitrogen in urine with C. J. Fanner, Ibid., 11: 493–501, June 1912
Nitrogen determinations by direct nesslerization. I. Total nitrogen in urine with W. Denis, Ibid., 26: 473–496, Sept. 1916
A simplified macro-Kjeldahl method for urine with L. E. Wright, Ibid., 38: 461–464, July 1919
METHOD—for estimation of creatin and creatinin in urine.
Beitrag zur Chemie des Kreatinins und Kreatins im

Harne. Z. physiol. Chemie., 41: 223–242, Mar. 5, 1904
On the determination of creatinine and creatine in urine. J. biol. Chem., 17: 469–473, May 1914
METHOD—for preparation of cystine.
On the preparation of cystin. Ibid., 8: 9–10, July 1910
METHOD—of quantitative determination of ammonia.
Note on the determination of ammonia in urine. Ibid., 8: 497–498, Dec. 1910
METHOD—micro-chemical, for determination of ammonia.
On the determination of ammonia in urine with A. B. Macallum, Ibid., 11: 523–525, June 1912
MODIFICATION—of Naegeli's method for determination of acidity of urine.
The acidity of urine. Amer. J. Physiol., 9: 265–278, July 1903
TEST—for epinephrine.
A new colorimetric method for the determination of epinephrine with W. B. Cannon and W. Denis, J. biol. Chem., 13: 477–483, Jan. 1913
TEST—for tyrosine.
Tyrosine in proteins as determined by a new colorimetric method with W. Denis, Ibid., 12: 245–251, Aug. 1912
TEST—for quantity of urea.
PREPARATION—of protein free blood filtrates.
DETERMINATION—of nonprotein nitrogen.
A system of blood analysis with H. Wu, Ibid., 38: 81–110 (91–98), May 1919
TEST—for sugar in urine.
A qualitative (reduction) test for sugar in normal human urine. Ibid., 22: 327–329, Sept. 1915
Copper-phosphate mixture as sugar reagents. A qualitative test and a quantitative titration method for sugar in urine with W. S. McEllroy, Ibid., 33: 513–519, Mar. 1918
A revision of the copper phosphate method for the titration of sugar with E. C. Peck, Ibid., 38: 287–291, June 1919
TEST—for blood sugar.
A system of blood analysis with H. Wu, Ibid., 38: 81–110 (106–110), May 1919
(Same) Supplement I. A simplified and improved method for determination of sugar with H. Wu, Ibid., 41: 367–374, Mar. 1920
The determination of sugar in blood and in normal urine. Ibid., 67: 357–370, Feb. 1926
A new blood sugar method. Ibid., 77: 421–430, May 1928
Two revised copper methods for blood sugar determination. Ibid., 82: 83–93, Apr. 1929
An improved form of Folin's micro method for blood sugar determinations with H. Malmros, Ibid., 83: 115–120, July 1929
The micro method for the determination of blood sugar. New Engl. J. Med., 206: 727–729, Apr. 7, 1932
TEST—for uric acid.
Ueber die quantitative Bestimmung der Harnsäure im Harn with P. A. Shaffer, Z. physiol. Chem., 32: 552–572, July 6, 1901
A new method for the (calorimetric) determination of uric acid in urine with A. B. Macallum, Jr., J. biol. Chem., 13: 363–369, Dec. 1912
A system of blood analysis: improvements in the qual-

ity and method of preparing the uric acid reagent
with H. Trimble, Ibid., 60: 473–479, June 1924
Folius, Caecilius. Vienna anatomist. 1615–1650
MUSCLE—laxator tympani.
PROCESS—p. gracilis, of malleus.
Nova auris internae delineatio. Venetiis, 1645. 4 pp.
Folli, Francesco. Italian physician. 1624–1685
Is claimed to be the first to have advocated trans-
fusion of blood.
*Stadera medica nelle quale altre la medicina infusoria
. . . e le contrario alla trasfusion der sangue. . . .*
Florence, 1680, p. 35
Foltz, Jean Charles Eugene. French ophthalmolog-
gist. 1822–1876
VALVE—fold of membrane at lacrimal canaliculus.
Anatomie et physiologie des conduits lacrymaux.
Lyon, Vingtrinier, 1860. 23 pp.
Fonio, Anton. Bern physician. 1889–
COAGULÈNE—of Kocher and Fonio.
*Ueber die neue Blutstillungsmethode und Wundbe-
handlung durch das Coagulin Kocher-Fonio.* Cor.-
Bl. f. schweiz. Aerzte, 385–398, Mar. 29; 422–431,
Apr. 5; 456–463, Apr. 12, 1913
TECHNIC—of platelet counting.
*Ueber vergleichende Blutplättchenuntersuchungen: ein
Beitrag zur Frage der Methodik der Gerinnungs
bestimmungen.* Ibid., 45: 1505–1524, Nov. 27, 1915
Fontaine, Bryce Washington. Memphis, Tenn.
physician. 1877–1926
CANNULA—
*An improved cannula and trocar for use in paracente-
sis abdominis.* J. A. M. A., 84: 1179 (only), Apr. 18,
1925
Fontaine, René. French surgeon
METHOD—of treatment of fracture of head of radius.
*Les résultats éloignés du traitement des fractures de
l'extrémité supérieure du radius* with R. Bauer, J.
de Chir., 45: 170–190, Feb. 1935
*Fracture de la tête radiale traitée par des infiltrations
locales répétées. Guérison aver récupération fonction-
nelle intégrale.* Rev. de Chir., 74: 761–764, Dec. 10,
1936
See also R. Leriche
Fontan, Jules Antoine Émile. Toulon surgeon.
1849–1931
OPERATION—gastrostomy by a conical and valvular method.
Sur une nouvelle opération de gastrostomie. Abstr.,
Seance Cong. franc. de chir. Semaine méd., 16: 423,
1896
*Une nouvelle operation de gastrostomie (procédé
valvulaire).* Assoc. franc. de chir. Proc. verb., 10:
411–415, 1896
Fontana, Arturo. Torino physician. 1873–
STAIN—for Treponemata.
*Sopra alcune modificazioni apportate al metodo di
colorazione del Treponema pallidum col nitrato d'ar-
gento ammoniacale.* Pathologica, 5: 205 (only), Apr.
1, 1913
*Ueber die Silberdarstellung des Treponema pallidum
und anderer Mikroorganismen in Ausstrichen.* Dermatol. Z., 46: 291–293, 1925–26
Fontana, Felice. Italian scientist. 1730–1805
CANAL—ciliary c.
SPACES—between processes of ligamentum pectina-
tum of iris. Dorland

Opuscoli scientifici. Napoli, 1787. 159 pp.
Author of a treatise on venom of viper. Garrison
Ricerche fisiche sopra il veleno della vipera. Lucca,
Giusti, 1767. 170 pp.
Foot, Nathan Chandler. American pathologist. 1881–
METHOD—
*Notes on the rapid impregnation of reticular tissue
with silver.* J. Tech. Meth., 12: 117–119, 1929
MODIFICATION—of Bielschowsky's method.
*A technic for demonstrating reticulum fibers in Zenker-
fixed paraffin sections.* J. Lab. clin. Med., 9: 777–781,
Aug. 1924
MODIFICATION—of Hortega's silver carbonate
method for reticulum.
*A rapid method for the silver impregnation of reticu-
lum* with M. C. Ménard, Arch. Path., 4: 211–214,
Aug. 1927
SILVER STAIN—to differentiate theca from granu-
losa cells.
*A technique of silver impregnation for general labora-
tory purposes* with Ellen B. Foot, Amer. J. Path., 8:
245–254, Mar. 1932
Forbes, Alexander. Boston physiologist. 1882–
TREATMENT—stretching nerves to relieve tension
on suture line.
*A note concerning the effect on their function of stretch-
ing nerve trunks.* New Engl. J. Med., 199: 555 (only),
Sept. 20, 1928
See also E. D. Adrian
Force, J. N. See F. P. Gay
Forchheimer, Frederick. Cincinnati physician. 1853–
1913
SIGN—reddish eruption on soft palate in measles.
Diseases of the mouth in children (non-surgical).
Phila., Lippincott, 1892. 199 pp.
German measles (rubella). Twentieth Cent. Pract.,
N. Y., 14: 175–188, 1898
Ford, F. R. See A. Blalock
Fordyce, John Addison. New York dermatologist.
1858–1925
DISEASE—
*A peculiar affection of the mucous membrane of the
lips and oral cavity.* J. Cutan. Dis., 14: 413–419,
Nov. 1896
DISEASE—see Fox-Fordyce d.
Forel, Auguste Henri. Swiss neurologist. 1848–1931
BUNDLE—fibers running from nucleus ruber to
thalamus.
COMMISSURE—fibers extending across posterior pre-
frontal space.
DECUSSATION—ventral parts of fountain d.
*Beiträge zur Kenntniss des Thalamus opticus und
der ihn umgebenden Gibilde bei den Säugethieren.* S.
B. Akad. Wiss. Wien. 3, 1872
Forrestier, Jacques. French neurologist
METHOD—
A simplified method of bronchography with L. Leroux,
Radiology, 24: 743–748, June 1935
See also J. A. Siccard
Forlanini, Carlo. Italian physician. 1847–1918
Discussed artificial pneumothorax as a form of
treatment for pulmonary tuberculosis in 1882 and
applied it clinically in 1888. Cutler
*A contribuzione della terapia chirurgica della tisi
ablazione del polmone? Pneumotorace artificale?* Gazz.
d. osp. Agosto, Sett.-Ott. Nov. 1882

Primi tentativi di pneumotorace artificiale della tisi polmonare. Gazz. med. di Torino, 45: 381–384; 401–403, 1894

Formad, Henry F. American physician. 1847–1892

KIDNEY—of chronic alcoholism.

The "pig-backed" or alcoholic kidney of drunkards; a contribution to the post-mortem diagnosis of alcoholism. Trans. Ass. Amer. Phys., Phila., 1: 225–236, 1886

Fornaca, Luigi. Torino physician

TEST—for blood serum.

Su di una cromo-reazione del siero di sangue. Rif. med., 24: 789–792, July 20, 1908

Forrest, William S. American physician

FEVER—

The great pestilence in Virginia; being an historical account of the origin, general character, and ravages of the yellow fever in Norfolk and Portsmouth in 1855. New York, Derby and Jackson, 1856. 326 pp.

Forrester, G. C. See W. W. E. Jetter

Forrester-Brown, Maude F. See H. J. Stiles

Forssell, Gösta. Stockholm surgeon. 1876–

TECHNIC—or Stockholm method, of radium treatment of cancer of uterus.

Oversikt över resultaten av Kräftbehandling vid Radiumhemmet; Stockholm 1910—15. Hospitalstid., København, 8 R., 10: 273–283, 1917

Operated on primary duodenal diverticulum.

Ein Divertikel an der Pars descendens duodeni mittels Röntgenuntersuchung diagnostiziert und operativ enfernt with E. Key, Röntgenstrahlen, 24: 48–57, 1916

Forssman, John. Swedish physician. 1868–

ANTIGEN—heterophile.

Om heterogenetiska antigen och antikroppar. Svenska läk. säll. handl., 55: 65–71, 1929

Forster, John Cooper. English surgeon. 1824–1896

Reported first English cases of gastrostomy.

Description of the operation of gastrotomy. Guy's Hosp. Rep., 3 s., 4: 13–18, 1858

Contraction of esophagus from corrosive poison. Gastrotomy. Ibid., 5: 1–8, 1859

Fosbinder, Russell John. American chemist. 1904–

Described sulfathiazole.

Sulfanilamido derivatives of heterocyclic amines with L. A. Walter, J. Amer. Chem. Soc., 61: 2032–2033, Aug. 1939

Foshay, Lee. Cincinnati physician. 1896–

SERUM—

Serum treatment of tularemia. J. A. M. A., 98: 552 (only), Feb. 13, 1932

An antiserum for the treatment of tularemia. Ibid., 101: 1447–1449, Nov. 4, 1933

SKIN TEST—for diagnosis of tularemia.

Tularemia: accurate and earlier diagnoses by means of the intradermal reaction. J. infect. Dis., 51: 286–291, Sept.-Oct., 1932

TEST—antiserum intracutaneous, for brucellosis.

The nature of the bacterial-specific intradermal antiserum reaction. Ibid., 59: 330–339, Nov.-Dec., 1936

Foster, Curtis Smiley. Pittsburgh physician. 1874–1929

METHOD—for estimation of hepatic function.

A study of the tests of liver function with M. Kahn J. Lab. clin. Med., 2: 25–36, Oct. 1916

Foster, D. P. San Francisco scientist

METHOD—for estimation of fibrinogen.

Blood fibrin studies. I. An accurate method for the

quantitative analysis of blood fibrin in small amounts of blood with G. H. Whipple, Amer. J. Physiol., 58: 365–378, Jan. 1922

Foster, Frances I. See J. R. Di Palma

Foster, G. S. See Z. A. Lavoie

Foster, M. Louise. See C. A. Herter

Foth, Hermann. German scientist. 1865–

STAIN—for spores.

Zur Frage der Sporenfärbung. Zbl. Bakt., 11: 272–278, Mar. 9, 1892

Fothergill, John. English physician. 1712–1780

DISEASE—trifacial neuralgia.

Of a painful affection of the face. Med. Obs. and Inq., 5: 129–142, 1773

Also: *Works,* London, 1783. vol. 2, pp. 179–189

Also: Med. Classics, 5: 100–106, Oct. 1940

DISEASE—scarlatina anginosa.

SORE-THROAT or ULCERATIVE ANGINA. Wrote early account of diphtheria.

An account of the sore throat attended with ulcers. A disease which hath of late years appeared in this city, and the parts adjacent. London, Davis, 1748

Also: *Works.* London, 1783. vol. 1, pp. 333–404

Also: Med. Classics, 5: 58–99, Oct. 1940

Described angina pectoris.

Case of an angina pectoris with remarks. Med. Obs. and Inq., 5: 233–252; 252–258, 1774

Also: *Works.* London, 1783. vol. 2, pp. 249–268

Wrote original description of sick headache.

Remarks on that complaint commonly known under the name of the sick headache. Med. Obs. and Inq., 6: 103–137, 1778

Also: *Works.* London, 1784. vol. 3, pp. 219–243

Fothergill, William Edward. Manchester gynecologist. 1865–1926

OPERATION—

On the operative treatment of displacements of the pelvic viscera. Trans. Edinburgh Obstet. Soc., 33: 129–145, 1908

Anterior colporrhaphy and its combination with amputation of the cervix as a single operation. J. Obstet. Gynaec. Brit. Emp., 27: 146–147, Mar.–May 1915

Fouchet, André. French chemist. 1894–

TEST—for bile pigments in blood, feces and urine.

Méthode nouvelle de recherche et de dosage des pigments biliaires dans le sérum sanguin. C. R. Soc. Biol., 80: 826–828, Nov. 10, 1917

Foucry, M. French chemist

REACTION—for amines.

La quinone: réactif des amines. J. Pharm. Chim., Paris, s 8, 20: 116–118, 1934

Fourneau, Ernest. French physician. 1872–

Introduced stovaine, 1903.

Stovaine, anesthesique locale. Bull. Soc. Pharmacol., Paris, 10: 141–148, 1904

Introduced moranyl ("Fourneau 309").

Chimothérapie des trypanosomiases. Paris Méd., 49: 501–508, 1923

Fournier, Jean Alfred. Paris syphilologist. 1832–1914

SIGN or TIBIA—anterior bowing and fusiform thickening in congenital syphilis.

La syphilis héréditaire tardive. Paris, Rueff & Cie., 1886

SIGN—sharp edge characteristic of syphilitic skin lesion.

TREATMENT—of syphilis with mrecury.
*Leçons cliniques dur la syphilis. Etudiée plus particu-
lièrement chez la femme.* Paris, Delahaye, 1873. 1108
pp. 2 ed., 1881
Foville, Achille Louis Francois. French neurologist.
1799-1878
DECUSSATION—in cerebellum.
FASCICULUS—oblique f.
TRACT—direct cerebellar t. of spinal cord.
*Traité complet de l'anatomie, de la physiologie et de
la pathologie du système nerveux cérébro-spinal.* Paris,
Fortin, Masson, 1844
SYNDROME—crossed paralysis or peduncular s.
*Note sur une paralysie peu connue des certains muscles
de l'oeil, et sa liaison avec quelques points de l'anatomie
et la physiologie de la protubérance annulaire.* Bull.
Soc. Anat. Paris, 3: 393-414, 1858
Fowler, Edson Brady. Evanston, Ill. surgeon. 1865-
1942
Reported use of cow horn as fixation material in
fractures.
*Cows horn for fixation of fractures: its stimulating
effect on callous formation and a simplified technic.*
Illinois Med. J., 66: 231-233, Sept. 1934
Fowler, George Ryerson. Brooklyn surgeon. 1848-
1906
INCISION—angular, for anterolateral abdominal
section.
A treatise on appendicitis. Philadelphia, Lippincott,
1894. 190 pp. pp. 156-158
INHALER—
A folding Allis ether-inhaler. Med. Rec., 32: 34
(only), July 2, 1887
METHOD—of ureterointestinal anastomosis.
*Implantation of the ureters into the rectum in exstrophy
of the bladder, with a description of a new method of
operation.* Amer. J. med. Sci., 115:270-276, Mar.
1898
OPERATION—
*A new method for the radical cure of inguinal hernia:
intraperitoneal transplacement of the spermatic cord
and typical obliteration of the internal ring and in-
guinal canal.* Ann. Surg., 26: 503-623, 1897
OPERATION—
The radical cure of femoral hernia. Brooklyn Med. J.,
11: 728-740, Nov. 1897
OPERATION—
Decortication of the lung for chronic empyema. Med.
News, 78: 933-938, June 15, 1901
POSITION and TREATMENT—
*Diffuse septic peritonitis, with special reference to a
new method of treatment, namely, the elevated head and
trunk posture, to facilitate drainage into the pelvis,
with a report of nine consecutive cases of recovery.*
Med. Rec., 57: 617-623, Apr. 14, 1900
Also: Med. Classics, 4: 551-580, Feb. 1940
Performed thoracoplasty.
*A case of thoracoplasty for the removal of a large
cicatricial fibrous growth from the interior of the chest,
the result of an old empyema.* Med. Rec., 44: 838-
839, Dec. 30, 1893
Fowler, Sir James Kingston. English physician.
1852-1934
Gave first description of infraclavicular primary
infiltration and way tuberculosis spreads along
bronchi.

Pulmonary tuberculosis. London, MacMillan, 1921.
284 pp. p. 120
Fowler, Thomas. English physician. 1736-1801
SOLUTION—liquor potassi arsenitis.
*Medical reports of the effects of arsenic, in the cure of
agues, remitting fevers, and periodic headaches. . . .*
London, Johnson, 1786. 128 pp. p. 79
Fox, Edward Long. English physician. 1832-1902
TREATMENT—of myxedema.
*A case of myxedema treated by taking extract of thy-
roid by the mouth.* Brit. med. J., 2: 941 (only), Oct.
29, 1892
Fox, George Henry. American dermatologist. 1846-
1937
DISEASE—
*Two cases of a rare papular disease affecting the axillary
region* with J. A. Fordyce, J. cutan. Dis., 20: 1-5,
Jan. 1902
Fox, Lawrence Webster. American ophthalmologist.
1853-
OPERATION—
*The present status of Mules' operation and of delayed
implantation of a gold ball.* Ophthalmoscope, 7: 6-12,
Jan. 1, 1909
Fox, William Tilbury. English dermatologist. 1836-
1879
Wrote original description of porrigo (the present
impetigo).
On impetigo contagiosa, or porrigo. Brit. med. J., 1:
467-469, Apr. 30; 495-496, May 7; 553-555, May 21;
607-609, June 4, 1864
Wrote original description of dysidrosis.
*Clinical lecture on dysidrosis (an undescribed erup-
tion).* Ibid., 2: 265-266, Sept. 27, 1873
The minute anatomy of dysidrosis with H. R. Crocker,
Trans. Path. Soc. London, 29: 264-268, 1878
Wrote original description of erysipeloid. In: *Diseases
of the skin.* London, 1873. 3 ed., p. 108
Described acnitis which he called disseminated
follicular lupus.
*Clinical lecture on disseminated follicular lupus (stimu-
lating acne).* Lancet, 2: 35-36, July 13; 75-76, July
20, 1878
Described lymphangioma.
*On a case of lymphangiectodes, with an account of the
histology of the growth* with T. C. Fox. Trans. Path.
Soc. London, 30: 470-476, 1879
Described epidermolysis bullosa.
*Notes on unusual or rare forms of skin disease. IV.
Congenital ulceration of skin (two cases) with pemphi-
gus eruption and arrest of development generally.*
Lancet, 1: 766-767, May 31, 1879
Wrote original description of hydroa.
A clinical study on hydroa. Arch. Dermat., 6: 16-52,
Jan. 1880
Fracastoro, Girolamo. Veronese physician. 1483-
1553
Published poem first using word syphilis, which was
the name of a shepherd infected with the disease.
Syphilis, sive morbus gallicus. Verona, 1530. 36 1.
Stated "the modern theory of infection by micro-
organisms." Garrison Early writer on infection and
contagion; distinguished between three categories
of infection: "by contact, by fomites, and at a dist-
ance." Gave first authentic account of typhus fever.
De sympathia et antipathia rerum liber unus. De

contagione et contagiosis morbis et curatione. Venetiis, apud heredes L. Iuntae, 1546

Fränkel, Albert. German physician. 1848-1916
DISEASE—indurative pneumonia.

Klinische und anatomische Mitteilungen über indurative Lungenentzündung. Dtsch. med. Wschr., 21: 153-156, Mar. 7; 177-180, Mar. 14; 190-195, Mar. 21, 1895

Reported discovery of pneumococcus as cause of pneumonia.

Ueber die genuine Pneumonie. Verh. Kongr. inn. Med., 3: 17-31, 1884

Bakteriologische Mittheilungen. Z. klin. Med., 10: 401-461 (426-457), 1885

Weitere Beiträge zur Lehre von den Mikrococcen der genuinen fibrinösen Pneumonie. Ibid., 11: 437-458, 1886

Fränkel, Bernhard. German physician. 1836-1911
METHOD—of staining tubercle bacilli.

Ueber die Färbung des Koch'schen Bacillus und seine semiotische Bedeutung für die Krankheiten der Respirationsorgane. Berl. klin. Wschr., 21: 214-217, Apr. 7, 1884

Reported mycosis pharyngis.

Fall von gutartiger Mycosis des Pharynx. Abstr.: Berl. klin. Wschr., 10: 94 (only), Feb. 24, 1873

Removed malignant growth intralaryngeally.

Erste Heilung eines Larynx-Cancroids vermittelst Ausrottung per vias naturales. Arch. klin. Chir., 34: 281-286, 1887

Fraenkel, Eugen. Hamburg physician. 1853-1925
Described phlebitis in syphilis of stomach.

Zur Lehre von der acquirierten Magen-Darmsyphilis. Arch. path. Anat., 155: 507-531, Mar. 22, 1899

Fraenkel, Ludwig. German physician. 1870-1930
TECHNIC—of posterior colpotomy.

Die vaginale Inzision von Entzündungsherden im weiblichen Becken. By Alfred Hermstein, Assistant in Fraenkel's clinic in Breslau, Dtsch. med. Wschr., 50: 1172-1174, Aug. 29, 1924

Demonstrated that removal of corpus luteum of rabbit in early pregnancy resulted in absorption or premature expulsion of fetus.

Die Funktion des Corpus luteum. Arch. Gynaek., 68: 438-545, 1902

Neue Experimente zur Function des Corpus luteum. Ibid., 91: 705-761, 1910

Fraentzel. See L. Traube

Francis, Edward. American physician. 1872-
AGAR—basal infusion.

Cultivation of Bacterium tularense on mediums new to this organism. Pub. Health Rep., 37: 102-115, Jan. 20, 1922

Cultivation of Bacterium tularense on three additional mediums new to this organism. Ibid., 987-989, Apr. 28, 1922

Described and gave name to tularemia in 1914, from Tulare County, California.

Deer-fly fever, or Pahvant Valley plague: a disease of man of hitherto unknown etiology. Ibid., 34: 2061-2062, Sept. 12, 1919

Tularaemia Francis 1921. The occurrence of tularemia in nature as a disease of man. Ibid., 36: 1731-1738, July 29, 1921

Tularaemia Francis 1921: a new disease of man. Bull. Hyg. Lab., No. 130, Mar. 1922. 87 pp.

Franco, Pierre. French surgeon. 1500-1561
He "did even more than Pare to put the operations for hernia, stone, and cataract upon a definite and dignified basis . . . and was the first to perform suprapubic cystotomy (1556)." Garrison

Petit traité contenant une des parties principalles de chirurgie, laquelle les chirurgiens hernières excercent. Lyon, Vincent, (1556). 144 pp.

Traité des hernies. Lyon, Payan, 1561

Frangenheim, Paul. German surgeon. 1876-1930
OPERATION—for slipping patella; fascial plus muscle graft over upper margin of patella.

Zur Behandlung der habituellen Patellarluxation. Arch. klin. Chir., 126: 426-435, 1923

Frank, Alfred Erich. Breslau physician. 1884-
Recognized connection between posterior lobe of pituitary and diabetes insipidus.

Ueber Beziehungen der Hypophyse zum Diabetes insipidus. Berl. klin. Wschr., 49: 393-397, 1912

Described thrombopenic purpura as a distinct entity.

Die essentielle Thrombopenie. Konstitutionelle Purpura—Pseudo-Hämophilie. Ibid., 52: 454-458, May 3; 490-494, May 10, 1915

Frank, Fritz. Cologne gynecologist. 1856-1923
OPERATION—suprasymphyseal transperitoneal cesarean section.

Die syprasymphysäre Entbindung und ihr Verhältniss zu den anderen Operationen bei engen Becken. Arch. Gynaek., 81: 46-94, 1907

Frank, I. L. See U. J. Salmon

Frank, Jacob. Chicago surgeon. 1856-1936
METHOD—of control of liver hemorrhage.

A new technique for operations upon the liver. S. G. O., 11: 418-423, Oct. 1910

Frank, Johann Peter. Palatinate physician. 1745-1821
First to signalize importance of diseases of spinal cord. Garrison

De vertebralis columnae in morbis dignitate. In his: *Delectus opusculorum medicorum.* Ticini, Galeatii, vol. 11, pp. 1-50, 1792

Differentiated between diabetes insipidus and diabetes mellitus. Garrison

De curandis hominum morbis epitome. Liber v. Mannheim, 1794

Frank, Robert Tilden. New York gynecologist. 1873-
METHOD—of obtaining estrin from urine, by chloroform extraction.

A new method for assaying the potency of the female sex hormone based upon its effect on the spontaneous contraction of the uterus of the white rat with C. D. Bonham and R. G. Gustavson, Amer. J. Physiol., 74: 395-399, Oct. 1. 1925

Clinical data obtained with the female sex hormone blood test with M. A. Goldberger, J. A. M. A., 90: 106-110, Jan. 14, 1928

The female sex hormone. Springfield, Ill., Thomas, 1929

METHOD—

The formation of an artificial vagina without operation. Amer. J. obstet. Gynaec., 35: 1053-1055, June 1938

OPERATION—

The formation of an artificial vagina by a new plastic technic with S. H. Geist, Ibid., 14: 712-718, Dec. 1927

Frank, Rudolf. Vienna surgeon. 1862-1913

OPERATION—
Ein neue Methode der Gastrostomie bei Carcinoma oesophagi. Wien. klin. Wschr., 6: 231–234, Mar. 30, 1893

Franke, Elizabeth. See S. R. Benedict

Franke, Kurt. Halle physician. 1909–
TEST—for bilirubin in urine.
Methylenblau, ein einfaches sehr empfindliches Reagens zum Nachweis von Bilirubin. Med. Klin., 27: 94–96, Jan. 16, 1931
Ueber quantitative Bilirubinbestimmung im Harn mit der Methylenblaumethode. By K. Fellinger and K. Menkes, Wien. klin. Wschr., 46: 133–134, Feb. 3, 1933

Frankel, Florence H. See Florence Hulton-Frankel

Frankel, Sigmund. Vienna chemist
REACTION—for epinephrine.
Ueber eine neue characteristische Adrenalinreaktion with R. Allers, Biochem. Z., 18:40–43, 1909

Frankenhäuser, Ferdinand. German gynecologist. ?–1894
GANGLION—cervico-uterine.
Die Nerven der Gebärmutter und ihre Endigung in den glatten Muskelfasern. Ein Beitrag zur Anatomie und Gynäkologie. Jena, Mauke, 1867. 82 pp.

Frankfeldt, Frank Meyer. New York proctologist. 1891–
DIATHERMY SNARE—
Diathermy dilators for rectal stricture. Trans. Amer. Proct. Soc., 38: 224–226, 1937

Frankl-Hochwart, L. v. See A. F. von Eiselsberg

Franklin, Philip. London laryngologist
TREATMENT—
Treatment of hay fever by intranasal zinc ionization. Brit. med. J., 1: 1115–1116, June 27, 1931

Franseen, Clifford Carlton. Boston physician. 1903–
METHOD—for determination of tissue phosphatase.
The phosphatase activity of tissues and plasma in tumors or bone with Regina McLean, Amer. J. Cancer, 24: 299–317, June 1935

Frantz, V. K. See A. O. Whipple

Franz, Carl August Otto. Berlin surgeon. 1870–
SYNDROME—cessation of thrill on ligation of vein proximal to arterio-venous aneurysm.
Klinische und experimentelle Beiträge betreffend das Aneurysma arteriovenosum. Arch. klin. Chir., 75: 572–623, 1905

Frapolli, Franciscus. Italian physician. ?–1773?
Published a careful account of pellagra in which he gave the malady its present name. Garrison
Animadversiones in morbum, vulgo pelagram. Milan, apud J. Galeautium, 1771. 37 pp.

Fraser, C. J. See P. J. Moloney

Fraser, Sir Thomas Richard. Scottish pharmacologist. 1841–1919
Did original work on physostigmine. Garrison
On the characters, actions and therapeutic uses of the ordeal bean of Calabar. . . . Edinburgh, Oliver and Boyd, 1863. 44 pp.
Did original work on strophanthus hispidus. Garrison
On the kombé arrow-poison (Strophanthus hispidus, D. C.) of Africa. J. Anat. and Physiol., London, 7: 139–155, Nov. 1872
Strophanthus hispidus: its natural history, chemistry, and pharmacology. Trans. Roy. Soc. Edinburgh, 35: 955–1027, 1890

Investigated immunization against cobra venom and obtained "antivenene," an anti-venom serum. Garrison and Morton
On the rendering of animals immune against the venom of the cobra and other serpents; and on the antidotal properties of the blood serum of the immunised animals. Brit. med. J., 1: 1309–1312, June 15, 1895

Frassineti, Pietro. Italian surgeon
OPERATION—
La chirurgia dell'ernia crurale. Modificazioni e dettagli di tecnica nel metodo crurale. Clin. Chir., 13: 517–554, Aug. 1937

Fray, Walter Wendell. Rochester, N. Y. physician. 1892–
METHOD—proportional m. of localizing pineal gland.
A roentgenological study of pineal orientation. I. A comparison of proportional and graphic methods in normal cases. Arch. Neurol. Psychiat., Chicago, 38: 1199–1207, Dec. 1937
(Same) *II. A comparison of the graphic and proportional methods in proven cases of brain tumor.* Radiology, 30: 579–587, May 1938

Frazier, Charles Harrison. Philadelphia surgeon. 1870–1936
OPERATION—
A further report upon the treatment of tic douloureux by the division of the sensory root of the gasserian ganglion with W. G. Spiller, Philadelphia Med. J., 10: 594–597, Oct. 25, 1902
Physiologic extirpation of the ganglion of Gasser. Further report on division of the sensory root for tic douloureux, based on the observations of four cases with W. G. Spiller, J. A. M. A., 43: 943–947, Oct. 1, 1904
Subtotal resection of sensory root for relief of major trigeminal neuralgia. Arch. Neurol. Psychiat., 13: 378–384, Mar. 1925
OPERATION—
Intracranial division of the auditory nerve for persistent aural vertigo. S. G. O., 15: 524–529, Nov. 1912
OPERATION—hypoglossolaryngeal anastomosis.
The treatment of paralysis of the recurrent laryngeal nerve by nerve anastomosis. Ann. Surg., 79: 161–171, Feb. 1924
OPERATION—hypophysectomy.
An approach to the hypophysis through the anterior cranial fossa. Ann. Surg., 57: 145–150, Feb. 1913
See also W. G. Spiller

Frazier, William Carroll. American bacteriologist. 1894–
MEDIUM—
A method for the detection of changes in gelatin due to bacteria. J. infect. Dis., 39: 302–309, Oct. 1926

Freda, V. C. See F. H. Falls

Frédet, Pierre. French surgeon. 1870–
OPERATION—pyloroplasty.
La sténose hypertrophique du pylore chez le nouveau-né. Arch. de mal. de l'appar. digest., 2: 393–417, 1908
La cure de la sténose hypertrophique du pylore chez les nourrissons par la pylorotomie extra-muqueuse. Jour. de Chir., 29: 385–408, Apr. 1927

Freedberg, A. S. See L. H. Sloan

Freeman, B. S. See R. B. Moreland

Freeman, Leonard. Denver surgeon. 1860–1935
OPERATION—
An operation for the relief of cardiospasm associated

with dilatation and tortuosity of the esophagus. Trans. Amer. Surg. Ass., 41: 19–24, 1923

Freeman, Walter Jackson. Washington, D. C. neurologist. 1895–
TECHNIQUE—
Psychosurgery; intelligence, emotion, and social behavior following prefrontal lobotomy for mental disorders with J. W. Watts, Springfield, Ill., Thomas, 1942 337 pp.

Freer, Otto Tiger. Chicago surgeon. 1857–1932
OPERATION—
The correction of deflections of the nasal septum with a minimum of traumatism. J. A. M. A., 38: 636–642, Mar. 8, 1902
The window resection operation for the correction of deflections of the nasal septum. Ibid., 41: 1391–1398, Dec. 5, 1903

Frehden, O. Vienna pharmacologist
TEST—for protein.
Die Anwendung der Tüpfelanalyse zur Untersuchung von Heilmitteln. II. Mitteilung. Ueber einige neue Nachweise von Aminen, unter besonderer Berücksichtigung von p-Phenylendiamin sowie eine neue Reaktion auf Eiweisskörper with L. Goldschmidt, Mikrochim. Acta, 1: 338–353, Aug. 30, 1937

Frei, Wilhelm Siegmund. Breslau physician. 1885–1943
TEST—intradermal, for lymphogranuloma inguinal.
Eine neue Hautreaktion bei "Lymphogranuloma inguinale." Klin. Wschr., 4: 2148–2149, Nov. 5, 1925
Ulcus vulvae chronicum elephantiasticum (Esthiomène) und sogenanntes Syphilöme anorectal als Folgeerscheinungen der Lymphogranulomatosis inguinalis with Alice Koppel, Ibid., 7: 2331–2336, Dec. 2, 1928

Freiberg, Albert Henry. Cincinnati surgeon. 1869–1940
DISEASE—enlargement of head of 2 and 3 metatarsal bones; called also Köhler II disease.
Infraction of the second metatarsal bone. S. G. O., 19: 191–193, Aug. 1914
OPERATION—piriformis myotomies.
SIGN—of contracture of piriformis.
Sciatic pain and its relief by operations on muscle and fascia. Arch. Surg., 34: 337–350, Feb. 1937

Freiburg (i. B., Germany)
METHOD—twilight sleep; called also scopolamin-morphin anesthesia, employed in conduct of labor.

Freireich, A. W. See A. O. Gettler

Freke, John. English physician. 1688–1756
Published original description of a case of myositis ossificans progressiva.
A case of extra-ordinary exostoses on the back of a boy. Philos. Trans., 41: 369–370, 1740

French, Thomas Rushmore. Brooklyn laryngologist. 1849–1929
Developed art of photographing larynx.
On photographing the larynx. Arch. Laryngol., 3: 221–222, July 1, 1882
(Same) Trans. Amer. Laryngol. Ass., pp. 59–68, 1883
(Same) Arch. Laryngol., 4: 235–243, Oct. 1883
On a perfected method of photographing the larynx. New York Med. J., 40: 653–656, Dec. 13, 1884

Frenkel, Heinrich. German physician. 1860–1931
MOVEMENT or TREATMENT—
Die Therapie atactischer Bewegungsstörungen. Münch. med. Wschr., 37: 917–920, Dec. 30, 1890

Frerichs, Friedrich Theodore von. Berlin physician 1819–1885
THEORY—that uremia is a poisoning by ammonium carbonate formed by action on urea of a ferment contained in blood.
Die Bright'sche Nierenkrankheit und deren Behandlung. Braunschweig, Vieweg, 1851. 286 pp.
Described disseminated sclerosis.
Ueber Hirnsklerose. Arch. ges. Med., Jena, 10: 334–350, 1849
Described appearance of tyrosin and leucin crystals in urine of patients with acute yellow atrophy of liver.
Offenes Schreiben an den Herrn Hofrath Dr. Oppolzer in Wien. Wien. med. Wschr., 4: 465–470, July 29, 1854
Ueber das Vorkommen von Leucin und Tyrosin im lebenden Organismus. Dtsch. Klinik, 7: 341–343, Aug. 4, 1855
Klinik der Leberkrankheiten. Braunschweig, 1858
Same: London, New Sydenham Soc., 1860. 2 vols.
Same: New York, Wood, 1879. 3 vols.
Described progressive lenticular degeneration (Kinnear Wilson's disease).
Klinik der Leberkrankheiten. Braunschweig, Vieweg u. Sohn, 1861. Bd. 2, pp. 62–64

Freud, J. See K. David, E. Dingemanse

Freud, Sigmund. Vienna neurologist. 1856–1939
THEORY—hysteria is due to a psychic trauma which was not adequately reacted to when it was received, and remains as an affect-memory. Dorland
Zur Psychopathologie des Alltagslebens. Berlin, Karger, 1904
Drei Abhandlungen zur Sexualtheorie. Leipzig, Deuticke, 1905
Selected papers on hysteria and other psychoneuroses. Transl. by A. A. Brill, Washington, Nerv. and Ment. Dis. Pub., 1909. 200 pp.
A general introduction to psycho-analysis. New York, Boni and Liveright, 1920
Made important investigation of position of auditory nuclei, of origin and central course of auditory nerve.
Ueber den Ursprung des N. acusticus. Mschr. Ohrenheilk., 20: 245–251, Aug.; 277–282, Sept. 1886

Freund, August von. German chemist
Described trimethylene, known as cyclopropane, used as an anesthetic.
Ueber Trimethylen. Mschr. Chem., 3: 625–635, July 13, 1882

Freund, Ernst. German physician. 1863–1946
REACTION—for cancer.
Ueber die Beziehungen zwischen Tumorzellen und Blutserum with G. Kaminer, Wien. klin. Wschr., 23: 1221–1223, Aug. 25, 1910
Zur Diagnose des Karzinoms with G. Kaminer, Ibid., 24: 1759–1764, Dec. 21, 1911
Die cytolytische Karzinomreaktion. Wien. med. Wschr., 72: 1329–1334, Aug. 5; 1390–1395, Aug. 12, 1922
Ueber die Quellen des Wachstum-Materiales der bösartigen Geschwülste with G. Kaminer, Wien. klin. Wschr., 36: 863–866, Dec. 6, 1923
Chemische Diagnose des Karzinoms. Ibid., 42: 257–260, Feb. 28, 1929

TEST—for peptone in urine.

Zur Methodik des Paptonnachweises im Urin. Wien. klin. Rundschau, Vienna, 12: 37–38, Jan. 16, 1898

Freund, Hermann Wolfgang. Strassburg physician. 1859–1925

Reported case of complete heart block associated with pregnancy.

Ein Fall von tödlichem Herzblock in der Geburt nebst Bemerkungen zur Frage "Herzkrankheiten und Schwangerschaft." Z. Geburtsch. u. Gynäk., 80: 175–212, 1917

Freund, Jules Thomas. New York pathologist. 1891–
EMULSIFIED VACCINES–

Sensitization to horse serum by means of adjuvants with Katherine McDermott, Proc. Soc. exp. Biol., N. Y., 49: 548–553, Apr. 1942

The effect of paraffin oil, lanolin-like substances and killed tubercle bacilli on immunization with diphtheric toxoid and bact. typhosum with Mary V. Bonanto, J. Immunol., 48: 325–334, May 1944

Freund, Leopold. Vienna physician. 1868–
Used x-rays for deep irradiation therapy.

Demonstration eines mit Röntgenstrahlen behandelten Falles von Naevus pigmentosus pilosus. Abstr.: Wien. klin. Wschr., 10: 73–74, Jan. 21, 1897

Freund, Wilhelm Alexander. German surgeon 1833–1918
ANOMALY—shortening of first rib.

Ueber primäre Thoraxanomalien; . . . Berlin, Karger, 1906. 28 pp.

OPERATION—

Eine neue Methode der Exstirpation des ganzen Uterus. Samml. klin. Vortr., No. 133 (Gynäk. No. 41), pp. 911–924, 1878

Zu meiner Methode der totalen Uterus-Exstirpation. Zbl. Gynäk., 2: 265–269, June 8, 1878

Frey, Emil Karl. Düsseldorf surgeon. 1888–
OPERATION—

Zur Technik der Ösophagogastrostomie. Zbl. Chir., 59: 845–847, Apr. 2, 1932

Die kardioplastische Ösophago-Gastrostomie. Ibid., 65: 2–5, Jan. 1, 1938

Frey, Margarete. See H. K. Barrenscheen

Frey, Max von. German physician. 1852–1932
HAIRS—mounted in a handle, used for testing sensitiveness of pressure points of the skin.
PRESSURE-POINTS—of sensation.

Untersuchungen über die Sinnesfunctionen der menschlichen Haut. I. Druckempfindung und Schmerz. Abh. sächs. Ges. (Akad.) Wiss., 1896, Leipzig, 23: 169–226, 1897

Frey, Walter. Kiel physician. 1884–
Showed that quinidine is effective in restoration of normal rhythm in auricular fibrillation.

Ueber Vorhofflimmern beim Menschen und seine Beseitigung durch Chinidin. Berl. klin. Wschr., 55: 450–452, May 13, 1918

Freyer, Sir Peter Johnson. Indian medican service. 1852–1921
OPERATION—

A new method of performing prostatectomy. Report in: Lancet, 1: 774–775, Mar. 17, 1900

A clinical lecture on total extirpation of the prostate for radical cure of enlargement of that organ: with four successful cases. Brit. med. J., 2: 125–129, July 20, 1901

Fricke, A. See H. R. A. Schridde

Friderichsen, Carl. Copenhagen physician. 1886–
SYNDROME—Waterhouse-Friderichsen.

Nebennierenapoplexie bei kleinen Kindern. Jb. Kinderb. u. phys. Erzieh., 87: 109–125, 1918

Fridericia, Louis Sigurd. Danish hygienist. 1881–
METHOD—for determination of alkali reserve of blood.

En klinisk Methode til Bestemmelse af Kulsyrespaendingen i Lungeluften. Hospitals-Tildende, Copenhagen, 5 Raekke, 7: 585–594, May 13, 1914

Frieben, Ernst August Franz Albert. German physician. 1875–
Described first case of cancer caused by Roentgen rays. Haagensen

Cancroid des rechten Handrückens. Abstr.: Dtsch. med. Wschr., 28: 335 (only), Nov. 13, 1902

Friedberger, Ernst. Greifswald physician. 1875–1932
AGAR—tellurite placenta infusion; for cultivation of Bacillus typhi exanthematici.

Ueber einen Nährboden zur Züchtung des Bacillus typhi exanthematici (Bacillus Proteus X Weil-Felix). with G. Joachimoglu, Münch. med. Wschr., 65: 805–807, July 23, 1918

Friedel, Gotthold. German surgeon. 1876–
OPERATION—for varicose veins.

Operative Behandlung der Varicen, Elephantiasis und Ulcus cruris. Arch. klin. Chir., 86: 143–159, 1908

Friedenwald, Jonas Stein. Baltimore ophthalmologist. 1897–
INSTRUMENT—

Freely movable instrument for ophthalmoscopy with yellow green light. Amer. J. Ophth., 7: 940–943, Dec. 1924

Ophthalmoscopy with yellow-green light. Visibility of the retinal capillaries. Ibid., 8: 177–179, Mar. 1925

Demonstration of a new ophthalmoscope. Trans. Sect. Ophth., A. M. A., pp. 359–363, 1932

Friediger, Adolf. Munich physician. 1879–
REAGENT—for fat in gastric and intestinal contents.

Dimethylamidoazobenzol als mikrochemisches Reagens auf Fett, insbesondere über seine Verwertbarkeit in kombinierten Färbungen in der Mikroskopie des Magen- und Darminhaltes. Münch. med. Wschr. 59: 2865–2866, Dec. 24, 1912

Friedlaender, Bernhard. Detroit physician. 1870–1939
MODIFICATION—of Linzenmeier test of sedimentation erythrocytes.

Blood sedimentation test as an aid in diagnosis in surgical infections. Amer. J. Obstet. Gynaec., 7: 125–144, Feb. 1924

Friedlaender, Ernst. Vienna physician. 1906–
REAGENT—for diagnosing urinary diseases.

Die Alizarinfärbung des Urinsediments als Diagnostikum in der internen Medizin (und Bemerkungen zur Kalktitration). Dtsch. med. Wschr., 48: 1035–1036, Aug. 4, 1922

Friedländer, Karl. German physician. 1847–1887
BACILLUS—of pneumonia.
VACCINE—prepared from bacillus.

Ueber die Schizomyceten bei der acuten fibrösen Pneumonie. Arch. path. Anat., 87: 319–324, Feb. 4, 1882

Die Mikrokokken der Pneumonie. Fort. d. Med., 1: 715–733, Nov. 15, 1883

DISEASE—
Ueber Arteriitis obliterans. Zbl. med. Wiss., 14: 65–70, Jan. 22, 1876
METHOD—of staining film on coverslips, for capsules.
Notiz, die Färbung der Kapselmicrococcen betreffend. Fort. d. Med., 3: 757–760, 1885
Friedlieb, Karl. German physician
APPARATUS—for gastric lavage.
Ein einfacher Saugapparat für Magenausspülungen. Dtsch. med. Wschr., 19: 1353–1354, Dec. 21, 1893
Friedman, Irving. New Haven physician. 1907–
OSCILLOMETER—
A new sensitive recording oscillometer with L. H. Ott and A. W. Oughterson. Amer. Heart J., 16: 575–581, Nov. 1938
Friedman, J. C. See S. Strouse
Friedman, Maurice Harold. Philadelphia physiologist. 1903–
MODIFICATION—of Aschheim-Zondek test for pregnancy.
Mechanism of ovulation in the rabbit: II. Ovulation produced by the injection of urine from pregnant women. Amer. J. Physiol., 90: 617–622, Nov. 1929
A simple, rapid procedure for the laboratory diagnosis of early pregnancies with M. E. Lapham, Amer. J. Obstet. Gynaec., 21: 405–410, Mar. 1931
Friedman, Townsend Baer. Chicago physician. 1905–
METHOD—of counting eosinophiles.
A rapid method for the determination of blood eosinophilia. J. A. M. A., 103: 1618 (only), Nov. 24, 1934
Friedmann, Friedrich Franz. Berlin physician
TREATMENT—of tuberculosis.
Erwiderung auf den Westenhöfer'schen Bericht über einen nach Friedmann behandelten Fall von Tuberkulose. Berl. klin. Wschr., 50: 1642 (only), Sept. 1, 1913
Ueber die wissenschaftlichen Vorstudien und Grundlagen zum Friedmann'schen Mittel. Ibid., 51: 1410–1419, July 27, 1914
Friedmann, Max. German physician. 1858–1925
DISEASE—relapsing infantile spastic spinal paralysis. Dorland
Ueber recidivierende (wahrscheinlich luetische) sogenannte spastische Spinalparalyse im Kindesalter. Dtsch. Z. Nervenheilk., 3: 182–206, Oct. 21, 1892
SYNDROME—due to progressive subacute encephalitis of traumatic origin.
Zur pathologischen Anatomie der multiplen chronischen Encephalitis. . . . Wien, Fromme, 1883. 50 pp.
Friedreich, Nicolaus Anton. German physician. 1761–1836
Described facial hemiplegia.
De paralysi muculorum faciei rheumatici. Wirceburgi, 1797.
Also: Med. Chir. Zeitg., Salzburg, 1: 415 (only), 1798
Friedreich, Nikolaus. German neurologist. 1825–1882
ATAXIA or DISEASE—hereditary or familial a.
FOOT—pes cavus, with hyperextension of toes, seen in hereditary ataxia.
Ueber degenerative Atrophie der spinalen Hinterstränge. Arch. path. Anat., 26: 391–419; 433–459; 27: 1–26, 1863

Ueber Ataxie mit besonderer Berücksichtigung der hereditären Formen. Ibid., 68: 145–245, 1876
DISEASE—
Paramyoklonus multiplex. Ibid., 86: 421–430, 1881
SIGN—diastolic collapse of cervical veins due to adherent pericardium.
Krankheiten des Herzens. Virchow's Handb. d. spez. Path. u. Ther., 5, pt. 2: 153–429 (308), 1855
Described hyperostosis of entire skeleton in 1868 and gave it name, Hagner's disease, after the two Hagner brothers affected. See Hagner
Frimadeau, Achille Henri Louis Anastase. French physician. 1885–
SIGN—if dilatation above an esophageal stricture is conical, stricture is fibrous; if cup shaped, stricture is malignant. Dorland
Diagnostic et étude des rétrécissements de l'oesophage par la radioscopie. Bordeaux, 1911. 77 pp.
Frisch, Anton. German physician. 1849–1917
BACILLUS—B. rhinoscleromatis.
Experimentelle Studien über die Verbreitung der Fäulnissorganismen in den Geweben und die durch Impfung der Cornea mit pilzhaltigen Flüssigkeiten hervorgerufenen Entzündungserscheinungen. Erlangen, Enke, 1874. 64 pp.
Frisch, Otto von. Vienna physician
SIGNS—of collateral circulation when artery is compressed: 1. living color; 2. arterial hemorrhage; 3. venous stasis distally.
Zur Indikationsstellung bei der Operation der Aneurysmen und bei den Gefässverletzungen. Zbl. Chir., 41: 89–91, Jan. 17, 1914
Fritsch, Ahasuerus. German physician. 1629–1701
Wrote early work on medical ethics. Garrison
Medicus peccans, sive tractatus de peccatis medicorum. Nuremberg, apud W. M. Endterum, 1684. 116 pp.
Fritsch, Gustav Theodor. German physician. 1838–1897
Established electric excitability of brain.
Ueber die elektrische Erregbarkeit des Grosshirns with E. Hitzig, Arch. Anat., Physiol. u. wiss. Med., Berlin, pp. 300–332, 1870
Fritsch, Rudolfo. Vienna chemist
TEST—for acetone.
Ueber den Nachweis von Gallensäuren. Z. anal. Chem., 49: 94–97, 1910
Fritzsche, E. German physician
Described acromegaly.
Ein Beitrag zur Pathologie des Riesenwuchses. Klinische und pathologisch-anatomische Untersuchungen. Leipzig, Vogel, 1884. 89 pp.
Fritzsche, H. See P. Karrer
Froehde, A. German chemist
REACTION—for albumin.
Notiz über eine neue Reaction der Eiweisskörper. Ann. Chem., 145: 376 (only), 1868
Frölich, Alfred. Austrian neurologist. 1871
SYNDROME—adiposity, genital atrophies, changes in secondary sexual characters, with lesions of pituitary. Dorland
Ein Fall von Tumor der Hypophysis cerebri ohne Acromegalie. Wien. klin. Rund., 15: 883–886, Nov. 23; 906–908, Nov. 30, 1901
Also, in German in: Res. Publ. Ass. nerv. ment. Dis., in: *The hypothalmus and central levels of autonomic function.* Baltimore, Williams & Wilkins, 1940

Also, abstr. in English transl. by Hilde Bruch in: *The Fröhlich syndrome; report of the original case.* Amer. J. Dis. Child., 58: 1282-1289, Dec. 1939

Frohner, A. German chemist

TEST—for acetone in urine.

Zur Stock'schen Acetonreaktion. Dtsch. med. Wschr., 27: 79 (only), Jan. 31, 1901

Froin, Georges. French physician. 1874-

SYNDROME—spinal fluid of transparent, clear, yellow color, large amounts of globulin, rapid coagulation and increased number of lymphocytes.

Inflammations méningées avec réactions chromatique, fibrineuse et cytologique du liquide céphalo-rachidien. Gaz. d. hôp., Paris, 76: 1005-1006, Sept. 3, 1903

Froment, Jules. Lyon physician. 1878-

SIGN—paper s. in ulnar paralysis.

La préhension dans les paralysies du nerf cubital et le signe du pouce. Pr. méd., 23: 409 (only), Oct. 21, 1915

Frommel, Richard Julius Ernst. German gynecologist. 1854-1912

DISEASE—

Ueber puerperale Atrophie des Uterus. Z. Geb. u. Gyn., 7: 305-313, 1882

OPERATION—

Über operative Behandlung des retroflektirten Uterus. Zbl. Gyn., 14: 94-95, Feb. 8, 1890

Frommer, Viktor. Berlin physician

TEST—for acetone in urine.

Neue Reaktion zum Nachweis von Aceton, samt Bemerkungen über Acetonurie. Berl. klin. Wschr., 42: 1008-1010, Aug. 7, 1905

Fronticelli, Enrico. Rome physician

TEST—for malaria and typhoid fever.

La reazione della uroeritrina per la diagnosi differenziale fra tifo e malaria. Policlinico, 31: 313-314, Mar. 10, 1924

Froriep, August. German anatomist. 1849-1917

GANGLION—of fourth occipital segment.

Ueber Anlagen von Sinnesorganen am Facialis, Glossopharyngeus und Vagus, über die genetische Stellung des Vagus zum Hypoglossus, und über die Herkunft der Zungenmusculatur. Beitrag zur Entwickelungsgeshichte des Saigethierkopfes. Arch. f. Anat. u. Entwick., Leipzig, pp. 1-55, 1885

Froriep, Robert. Berlin surgeon. 1804-1861

INDURATION or RHEUMATISM—myositis fibrosa.

Die rheumatische Schwiele. Weimar, 1843

Frost, William Dodge. Wisconsin scientist. 1867-

AGAR or BOUILLON—glucose; culture medium

A laboratory guide in elementary bacteriology. New York, MacMillan, 1902, 2 ed., p. 62

AGAR—milk serum; for isolation of B. diphtheriae.

A rapid cultural method of diagnosing diphtheria with Alice M. Charlton and Mary F. Little, J. A. M. A., 76: 30-31, Jan. 1, 1921

METHOD—

Rapid method of counting bacteria in milk. Science, 42: 255-256, Aug. 20, 1915

A rapid method of counting living bacteria in milk and other richly seeded materials. J. A. M. A., 66: 889-890, Mar. 18, 1916

See also Reba C. Haner

Frothingham, Langdon. American veterinarian. 1866-

AGAR—gelatin infusion; culture medium.

Laboratory guide for the bacteriologist. Philadelphia, Saunders, 1895. pp. 55

Described torulosis in horse.

A tumor-like lesion in the lung of a horse caused by a blastomyces (torula). J. med. Res., s 2., 3: 31-43, June 1902

Frouin, Albert. French scientist

SOLUTION—hydrolyzed serum, for cultivation of colon-typhoid group.

Production d'acides volatils par divers microbes cultivés sur des acides monoamines with Suzanne Ledebt, C. R. Soc. Biol., 70: 24-26, Jan. 7, 1911

Frugoni, Cesare. Italian physician. 1881-

SIGN or TEST—petechiae beneath a tourniquet in purpura.

Le "signe du lacet" dans les maladies à manifestations hémorrhagiques with F. Giugni, Semaine méd., 31: 25-28, Jan. 18, 1911

Fry, Hubert John Burgess. London physician. 1885-1930

TEST—precipitation, for cancer.

Remarks on a new flocculation reaction for the sero-diagnosis of malignant disease. Brit. med. J., 2: 4-9, July 4, 1925

Further observations on a flocculation reaction for the serum diagnosis of malignant disease. J. Path. Bact., 29: 353-364, Oct. 1926

Fuchs, Ernst. Vienna ophthalmologist. 1851-1930

ANTERIOR PIGMENT LAYER OF—of iris.

Beiträge zur normalen Anatomie der menschlichen Iris. Arch. f. Ophthal., 31 (3): 39-86, 1885

Über retinale Pigmentzellen im Irisstroma. Ibid., 103: 297-303, Dec. 23, 1920

ATROPHY—peripheral, of optic nerve.

Ueber die periphere Atrophie des Sehnerven. Ibid., 31 (1): 177-200, 1885

Fuchs, Hans J. German physician

TEST—for cancer; cytolytic t.

Ueber eine chemische Diagnose maligner Tumoren. Klin. Wschr., 4: 2350 (only), Dec. 3, 1925

Ueber eine Methode zur serochemischen Differentialdiagnostik von malignen Tumoren und Infektionskrankheiten. Med. Klinik, 24: 337-339, Mar. 2, 1928

Fuchs, Samuel. 1588-1630

Wrote an illustrated treatise on physiognomy and the estimation of character by the eyes. Garrison *Metoposcopia et ophthalmoscopia.* Argentinae, Glaserus, 1615. 140 pp.

Furstner, Carl. German psychiatrist. 1848-1906

DISEASE—

Ueber pseudospastische Parese mit Tremor. Neurol. Zbl., 15: 674-691, Aug. 1, 1896

Fütterer, G. See B. Anton

Fuhrmann, Franz. Graz physician. 1877-

SOLUTION—basal.

Zur Kenntnis der Bacterienflora des Flaschenbieres. I. Pseudomonas cerevisiae. Zbl. Bakt., 2 Abt., 16: 309-325 (319), 1906

Fuhs, Flora C. Brooklyn scientist

TEST—for albumin in urine.

A new test for albumin. Med. Rec., 61: 374 (only), Mar. 8, 1902

Fujita, Akiji. Japanese physician

TEST—for ascorbic acid (vitamin C).

Ueber die kolorimetrische Bestimmung von Vitamin

C. with D. Iwatake and T. Miyata, Biochem. Z., 277: 296–304, Apr. 17, 1935

Fuld, Ernst. German biologist. 1873–
METHOD—for estimation of enzyme content of gastric secretion.
Die Pepsinnestimmung mittels der Edestinprobe with L. A. Levison, Biochem. Z., 6: 473–501, 1907
TEST—for blood in feces.
Neue Briträge zur Methodik des okkulten Blutnachweises. Berl. klin. Wschr., 54: 186–187, Feb. 19, 1917

Fuld, Joseph Edward. New York surgeon. 1872–1937
FASCIA STRIPPER—
Difficult hernias: surgical treatment with special reference to a modified method of obtaining living fascial sutures. Amer. J. Surg., 18: 514–520, Dec. 1932
SUTURE—for tendon.
The restoration of hand injuries by plastic surgery. New York Med. J., 114: 692–699, Dec. 21, 1921

Fuller, A. T. London scientist
TEST—for sulfanilamide in urine and blood.
Is p-aminobenzenesulphonamide the active agent in prontosil therapy? Lancet, 1: 194–198, Jan. 23, 1937
Rapid clinical method for the estimation of sulphanilamide. Ibid., 1: 760–761, June 27, 1942
Discovered that b-hydroxybutyric acid excreted in urine by altered dietary intake inhibits growth of bacteria.
The ketogenic diet: nature of bactericidal agent. Ibid., 1: 855–856, Apr. 22, 1933

Fuller, Eugene. New York surgeon. 1858–1930
OPERATION—supra-pubic enucleation of prostate.
Six successful and successive cases of prostatestomy. J. Cutan. and Gen.-Urin. Dis., 13: 229–239, June 1895

Fulton, Charles Clarke. American chemist. 1900–
REACTION—for cocaine.
The identification of cocaine and novocaine. Amer. J. Pharm., 105: 326–339, July; 374–380, Aug. 1933
REACTION—for morphine.
Some new and improved tests for morphine and related alkaloids. J. Lab. clin. Med., 13: 750–762, May 1928
Some color reactions of morphine and its derivatives on heating in concentrated sulphuric acid solution. Ibid., 14: 13–29, Oct. 1928

Fulton, J. F. See J. W. Watts

Fumey, M. See A. C. Hollande

Funk, A. See W. Autenrieth

Funk, Casimir. German scientist. 1884–
METHOD—for isolation of dehydroandrosterone.
The male hormone with B. Harrow, Proc. Soc. exp. Biol. and Med., 26: 325–326, Jan. 1929
Did early work on vitamins.

On the chemical nature of the substance which cures polyneuritis in birds induced by a diet of polished rice. J. Physiol., 43: 395–400, 1911
Isolated nicotinic acid.
Studies on beri-beri. VII. Chemistry of the vitamin-fraction from yeast and rice-polishings. Ibid., 46: 173–179, June 19, 1913
Die Vitamine. . . . Wiesbaden, Bergmann, 1914. 193 pp.

Funke, Otto. German physician. 1828–1879
Discovered hemoglobin.
Ueber das Milzvenenblut. Z. rat. Med., Hedelb., n. F. 1: 172–218, 1851
Neue Beobachtungen über die Krystalle des Milzvenen- und Fisch-Blutes. Ibid., 2: 198–217, 1852

Furniss, Henry Dawson. New York surgeon. 1878–1942
METHOD—of intestinal anastomosis.
Instrument for intestinal anastomosis. Amer. J. Surg., 23: 379–380, Feb. 1934
MODIFICATION—
Uretero-intestinal anastomosis: a simplification of the Coffey technique. Ibid., 15: 12–14, Jan. 1932
SUCTION—
Modified Wangensteen suction drainage. S. G. O., 68: 118–119, Jan. 1939

Furstenberg, Albert Carl. Ann Arbor otolaryngologist. 1890–
PROCEDURE—cervical mediastinotomy.
Acute mediastinal suppuration. Trans. Amer. Laryng., Rhin. and Otol. Soc., 35: 210–227, 1929
TREATMENT—
Ménière's symptom complex; medical treatment with F. H. Lashmet and F. Lathrop, Ann. Otol., Rhin. and Laryng., 43: 1035–1046, Dec. 1934

Furth, Otto von. Vienna biochemist
REAGENT—
Ueber eine neue Modifikation des forensisch-chemischen Blutnachweises. Z. angew. Chem., 24: 1625–1628, Sept. 1, 1911

Furuhata, Tanemoto. Japanese physician
HYPOTHESIS—of inheritance of blood groups.
The isolation of immune hemagglutinin. Japan Med. World, 1: 1–10, Oct. 15, 1921
On the heredity of the blood groups. Ibid., 7: 197–208, July 15, 1927

Futaki, Kenzo. Tokyo physician. 1873–
Discovered parasite of rat-bite fever.
The cause of rat-bite fever with F. Takaki, T. Taniguchi and S. Osumi, J. exp. Med., 23: 249–250, Feb. 1, 1916
Spirochaeta morsus muris, N. S. P., the cause of rat-bite fever. Second paper with the same, Ibid., 25: 33–44, Jan. 1, 1917

Futcher, T. B. See W. G. MacCallum

G

Gabbe, Erich. German physician. 1891–
TEST—for lipoids in blood.
Ueber regelmässige Veränderungen der Lipoidmenge des Blutes nach Injektionen körperfremder Stoffe bei der sogenannten Reiztherapie. Münch. med. Wschr. 68: 1377–1380, Oct. 28, 1921

Gabbet, Henry Singer. English physician

STAINING METHOD—
Rapid staining of the tubercle bacillus. Lancet, 1: 757 (only), Apr. 9, 1887

Gabriel, William Bahall. English surgeon. 1893–
OPERATION—
Perineo-abdominal excision of the rectum in one stage. Lancet, 2: 69–74, July 14, 1934

SOLUTION—
The treatment of pruritus ani and anal fissure: the
use of anesthetic solutions in oil. Brit. med. J., 1:
1070–1072, June 15, 1929
Gad, Johannes. German physiologist. 1842–1926
Found contraction of muscle due to lactic acid
formation. Garrison
Zur Theorie der Erregungsvorgänge im Muskel. Abstr.:
Arch. Physiol., 164–175, 1893
Gaddum, John Henry. English biochemist. 1900–
TEST—for adrenaline.
A sensitive physical test for adrenaline with H. Schild,
J. Physiol., 80: 9P–10P, Nov. 18, 1933
See also W. Feldberg
Gaebler, O. H. See F. Breh
Gaehtgens, Walter. German bacteriologist. 1880–
AGAR—caffeine endo.
Ueber die Erhöhung der Leistungsfähigkeit des Endo-
schen Fuchsinagars durch den Zusatz von Koffein.
Zbl. Bakt., 39: 634–640, Oct. 10, 1905
AGAR—potato peptone; culture medium.
Ueber die Verwendung von Kartoffelwasser zur
Herstellung fester Bakteriennährböden. Ibid., 78:
45–48, May 9, 1916
TECHNIC—complement fixation, for syphilis.
Theoretisches und Praktisches über die Wirkung eines
karbolisierten wasserigen Pallidaantigens. Z. Immun-
Forsch., 63: 398–427, June 1929
Gaenslen, Frederick Julius. Milwaukee surgeon.
1877–1937
OPERATION—
The Schanz subtrochanteric osteotomy for irreducible
dislocation of the hip. J. Bone and Joint Surg., 17:
76–87, Jan. 1935
SIGN—pain on hyperextension of hip with pelvis
fixed by flexion of opposite hip.
Sacro-iliac arthrodesis: indications, author's technic
and end-results. J. A. M. A., 89: 2031–2035, Dec. 10,
1927
Low back pain: etiology, diagnosis and treatment.
Indust. Med., 4: 105–111, Mar. 1935
Gänsslen, Max. Tübingen physician. 1895–
"TOWER SKULL"—a defect sometimes found in
congenital hemolytic jaundice.
Die hämolytische Konstitution. Nach 105 Beobach-
tungen von hämolytischen Ikterus, 39 Beobachtungen
von leichten hämolytischen Konstitutionen und 19
Milzexstirpationen with E. Zipperlen and E. Schüz,
Dtsch. Arch. klin. Med., 146: 1–46, Jan. 1925
Gärtner, Gustav. Austrian physician. 1855–1921
BACILLUS—B. enteritidis, cause of food poisoning.
Ueber die Fleischvergiftung in Frankenhausen a. K.
und den Erreger derselben. Correspbl. ärztl. Ver.
Thüringen, 17: 573–600, 1888
METHOD—of fat reduction in obesity.
Diätetische Entfettungskuren. Leipzig, Vogel, 1913.
172 pp.
Same, in English, Philadelphia, Lippincott, 1914.
313 pp.
TONOMETER—for measuring blood pressure by
compressing ring applied to finger.
Ueber einen neuen Blutdruckmesser (Tonometer).
Wien. med. Wschr., 49: 1412–1418, July 22, 1899
Gaffky, Georg Theodor August. German bacteri-
ologist. 1850–1918
Grew pure cultures of B. typhosum.

Zur Aetiologie des Abdominaltyphus. Mitt. a. d. k.
Gesundheits., 2: 372–420, 1884
Gage, George Edward. American bacteriologist.
1883–
BOUILLON—lactose, used as presumptive test for B.
coli in water.
A comparative study of media for the detection of
Bacillus coli in drinking water. Zbl. Bakt., 47: 280–
287 (282), 1908
SOLUTION—basal salt.
Biological and chemical studies on nitroso bacteria.
Ibid., 2 Abt., 27: 7–48 (21), 1910
Gage, Simon Henry. Ithaca anatomist. 1851–1944
Described sphincter at entrance of bile duct into
duodenum.
The ampulla of Vater and the pancreatic duct in the
domestic cat (felis domestica). Amer. Quart. Micro.
J., 1: 128–169, 1879
Developed microscope.
The microscope. Ithaca, N. Y., Comstock, 1936. 16
ed. 617 pp.
Gagel, Otto. German neurologist, 1899–
Studied cells of origin of white rami.
Zur Histologie und Topographie der vegetativen Zentren
im Rückenmark. Z. Anat. u. Entw., München, 85:
213–250, Feb. 21, 1928
Gager, A. See A. Vernes
Gager, L. T. See C. A. Neymann
Gaine, Charles. English dentist
Described irregularities of teeth.
On certain irregularities of the teeth with cases illus-
trative of a novel method of successful treatment. Bath,
Oliver, 1858
Gaisböck, Felix. German physician
DISEASE—polycythemia hypertonica.
Die Bedeutung der Blutdruckmessung für die Praxis.
Dtsch. Arch. klin. Med., 83: 363–409, (396), 1905
Galbiati, Gennaro. Italian surgeon. 1776–1844
OPERATION—ischiopubiotomy.
Memoria sull'operazione del taglio della sinfisi del
pube; ... Napoli, Porcelli, 1819, 52 pp.
Gale, Joseph Wasson. Madison, Wis. surgeon. 1900–
OPERATION—division of scalene muscles with opera-
tions on phrenic nerve.
Scaleniotomy in the surgical treatment of pulmonary
tuberculosis with W. S. Middleton, Arch. Surg., 23:
38–46, July 1931
Galeazzi, Riccardo. Milan surgeon. 1866–
TREATMENT—
The treatment of scoliosis. J. Bone and Joint Surg., 11:
81–86, Jan. 1929
Galen, Claudius. Greek physician. 130–200?
AMPULLA—a dilatation of the vena magna galeni.
ANASTOMOSIS—between the superior and inferior
laryngeal nerves.
BANDAGE—for head.
FORAMEN—opening of anterior cardiac vein into
right auricle.
VEINS—deep cerebral or ventricular v.
VEIN—anterior cardiac v.
VENTRICLE—sacculus laryngis.
Opera omnia. Ediderunt Andreas Asulanus et J. B.
Opizo Greek text, 5 vols. Venetiis, Aldus et Andreas
Socer, 1525
Also, ed. by C. G. Kuhn. Leipzig, Cnoblock, 1821–33
20 vols.

Also, Daremberg transl. 1856
Also, Greek text with German transl. Leipzig, Hindrichs, 1906. 2 vols.
Also, in Greek Lipsiae, Teubner, 1914–22. 4 vols.
Also, *On the natural faculties*. Greek text with English transl. by A. J. Brock. London, Heinemann, 1923 Loeb Classical Library

Galilei, Galileo. Italian scientist. 1564–1642
Invented rude alcohol thermometer or thermoscope. Conceived the idea of using his own pulse to test the synchronous character of a pendulum's vibrations, which led him to the converse proposition of measuring the rate and variation of the pulse by a pendulum. Garrison
Le opere di. . . . Fierenze, 1718

Gall, Franz Joseph. German physician. 1758–1828
CENTER—posterior parietal region.
THEORY—function of brain can be localized in cerebral cortex.
Anatomie et physiologie du système nerveux en général et du cerveau en particulier with J. C. Spurzheim, Paris, Schoell, 1810–19. 4 vols.

Gallagher, T. F. See C. R. Moore

Gallais, Alfred. French physician
SYNDROME—
Le syndrome génito-surrénal; étude anatomo-clinique. Paris, 1912. 224 pp.

Galland, Walter Isaac. New York surgeon. 1889–
OPERATION—
An operative treatment for corns. J. A. M. A., 100: 880–881, Mar. 25, 1933

Galli, G. See G. Baccelli

Gallie, William Edward. Toronto surgeon. 1882–
OPERATION or TECHNIC—
The use of living sutures in operative surgery with A. B. Le Mesurier, Canad. med. Ass. J., 2: 504–513, July 1921
A clinical and experimental study of the free transplantation of fascia and tendon with A. B. Le Mesurier, J. Bone and Joint Surg., 4: 600–612, 1922
OPERATION—
Habitual dislocation of the patella with A. B. Le Mesurier, Ibid., 22: 575–582, July 1924
OPERATION—
An operation for the relief of recurring dislocation of the shoulder with A. B. Le Mesurier, Trans. Amer. Surg. Ass., 45: 392–398, 1927

Galli-Valerio, B. See M. Casares-Gil

Galton, Sir Francis. English scientist. 1822–1911
DELTA—a triangular arrangement of lines of a finger print near the base.
Finger prints. London, Macmillan, 1892. 216 pp.
LAW—of ancestral inheritance; in composition of an individual, two parents contribute one-half of total, four grandparents one-quarter, etc.
The average contribution of each several ancestor to the total heritage of the offspring. Proc. roy. Soc., 61: 401–413, 1897
LAW—of filial regression; offspring of parents unusual in heighth, talent, etc., regress to average of the stock.
Hereditary genius. London, Murray, 1869
Natural inheritance. London, Macmillan, 1889. 259 pp.

WHISTLE—
Whistles for determining the upper limits of audible sound in different persons. London, Tisley, n. d. 8 pp.
Coined term eugenics.
Inquiries into human faculty and its development. London, Macmillan, 1883

Galvani, Luigi. Bologna physiologist. 1737–1798
Discovered electric properties of excised tissues, the starting point of modern electrophysiology. Garrison
De viribus electricitatis in motu musculari commentarius. Comment. Bonon. Scient. et Art. Inst., Bologna, 7: 363–418, 1791

Gamaleya, Nikolai Fyodorovich. Russian bacteriologist. 1859–
SPIRILLUM—
Etiologiya choler'is. . . . St. Petersburg, Stasyulevich, 1893. 60 pp.

Gandy, Charles. French physician. 1872–
TYPE—of dwarfism; retrograde, endocrine.
Myxoedème acquis de l'adulte avec régression sexuelle à l'état prépubère; infantilisme réversif de l'adulte; dysthyroide et dysorchidie. Bull. Soc. méd. Hôp. Paris, 3 s., 23: 1226–1250, 1906

Gangee, Joseph Sampson. Birmingham surgeon. 1828–1886
TISSUE—absorbent dressing for wounds.
Absorbent and medicated surgical dressings. Lancet, 1: 417–418, May 1880

Ganser, Sigbert Joseph Maria. Dresden psychiatrist. 1853–1931
SYNDROME—acute hallucinatory mania.
Ueber einen eigenartigen hysterischen Dämmerzustand. Arch. Psychiat. Nervenkr., 30: 633–640, 1898

Gansser, E. See G. Hufner

Gant, Samuel Goodwin. New York surgeon. 1869–
CLAMP—used in operations on hemorrhoids.
Diseases of the rectum, anus, and colon. . . . Philadelphia, Saunders, 1923. Vol. 1, p. 504

Garcia, E. D. See V. Arreguine

Garcia, Manuel. Spanish singing teacher in London. 1805–1906
Invented modern laryngoscope.
"Observations on the human voice." Proc. roy. Soc., London, 7: 399–410, May 24, 1855
Observations physiologiques sur la voix humaine. Paris, Masson, 1855. 16 pp.

Garcia, O. See R. A. Kinsella

Gardiner, A. D. See E. Chain

Gardner, J. A. See C. Dorée

Gardner, Leroy Upson. Saranac Lake, N. Y. physician. 1883–1946
Performed animal experimentation with asbestosis.
Studies on experimental pneumonokoniosis; VI. Inhalation of asbestos dust: its effect upon primary tuberculous infection with D. E. Cummings, J. Indust. Hyg., 13: 65–81, Feb.; 97–114, Mar. 1931

Gardner, W. J. See W. A. Nosik

Garengeot, René Jacques Croissant de. French surgeon. 1688–1759
Described vaginal hernia.
Traité des operations de chirurgie. Paris, Huart, 1731. 2 ed., pp. 237; 369–371
Same, in English. London, Woodward, 1723. 581 pp.

Gargill, S. L. See B. E. Greenberg

Garland, George Minott. American physician. 1849–1926

CURVE or LINE—an S-shaped line on chest showing upper border of pleural effusion.

Some experiments upon the curved line of dulness with pleuritic effusion. Boston Med. and Surg. J., 91: 269–272, Sept. 17, 1874

Gariock, John Harry. New York surgeon. 1896–

METHOD—of closure of abdominal incision.

Appendectomy wound repair and hernia. Ann. Surg., 89: 282–286, Feb. 1929

Incisional hernia following operation for acute appendicitis. Surg. Clin. No. Amer., 19: 449–452, Apr. 1939

Garner, R. L. See W. S. Tillett

Garrè, Carl. German surgeon. 1858–1928

OSTEOMYELITIS—sclerosing non-suppurative.

Ueber besondere Formen und Folgezustände der akuten infektiösen Osteomyelitis. Beitr. klin. Chir., 10: 241–298, Apr. 1893

Garretson, James Edmund. American surgeon. 1828–1895

BANDAGE—for the lower jaw.

A treatise on the diseases and surgery of the mouth, jaws, and associate parts. Philadelphia, Lippincott 1869. 693 pp. p. 474

Garrod, Alfred Baring. London physician. 1819–1907

TEST—thread t. for uric acid in blood.

Observations on certain pathological conditions of the blood and urine in gout, rheumatism and Bright's disease. Med.-chir. Trans., 31: 83–97, 1848

Garrod, Archibald E. English physician. 1857–1936

Showed that constitutional variation in function can give rise to what he termed "chemical malformations", i.e., alcaptonuria, pentosuria, etc. Garrison and Morton

Inborn errors of metabolism. London, Frowde, 1909

TEST—for alkaptonuria.

Alkaptonuria: a simple method for the extraction of homogentisic acid from the urine. J. Physiol., 23: 512–514, Feb. 27, 1899

Garven, Hugh Shaw Dunn. Glasgow scientist

METHOD—gold chloride, for nerve endings in muscle.

The nerve-endings in the panniculus carnosus of the hedgehog, with special reference to the sympathetic innervation of striated muscle. Brain, 48: 380–441, Sept. 1925

Gasis, Demetrius. Athens physician

METHOD—of staining for tubercle bacilli.

Ueber eine neue Reaktion der Tuberkelbacillen und eine darauf begründete differenzialdiagnostische Färbungsmethode derselben. Zbl. Bakt., 1: 111–128, 1909

Gask, George Ernest. London surgeon. 1875–

OPERATION—anterior approach for cervicothoracic ganglionectomy.

TECHNIC—of periarterial sympathectomy.

The surgery of the sympathetic nervous system with J. P. Ross, Baltimore, Wood, 1934. 2 ed., 1937

Gaskell, Walter Holbrook. English physiologist. 1847–1914

Introduced term heart block.

On the action of the vagus nerve upon the frog's heart. Proc. Cambridge Philos. Soc., 4: 75–76, Mar. 7, 1881

Revived myogenic theory of heart impulses. Garrison

On the rhythm of the heart of the frog, and on the nature of the action of the vagus nerve. Philos. Trans., 173: 993–1033, 1882

On the innervation of the heart, with especial reference to the heart of the tortoise. J. Physiol., 4: 43–127, 1883

Established origin of preganglionic neurones (white rami). Garrison and Morton

On the structure, distribution and function of the nerves which innervate the visceral and vascular systems. Ibid., 7: 1–80, 1886

Gaspard, Marie Humbert Bernard. French physician. 1788–1871

Experimented with pyemia.

Memoire physiologique sur les maladies purulentes et putrides, sur la vaccine, etc. J. Physiol. exper., Paris, 2: 1–45, 1822; 4: 1–69, 1824

Gasperi, Frederico de. Paris physician

AGAR—glucose lactose, for cultivation of anaerobes.

Beitrag zur Züchtungs und Isolierungstechnik des Anaëroben Mikroorganismen with E. Savini, Zbl. Bakt., 58: 239–261 (248), Apr. 1, 1911

Gasperini, Gustavo. Italian physician

MIXTURE—nutrient medium for differentiating species of actinomyces.

Sul potere patogeno dell'actinomyces albus e sui rapporti fra attinomicosi e tubercolosi. Ricerche sperimentali. Proc. verb. d. Soc. Tosc. di Sc. nat., 1895

Also: Pisa, Nistri, 1895. 8 pp.

Gassendi, Pierre. French physician. 1592–1655

Demonstrated existence of vestigial foramen ovale in adult.

Elegans de septo cordis pervio observatia. In: L. Bonaciolus: *De foetus formatione. . . .* Lugduni Batavorum, Hegerum, 1640 pp. 270–272

Also, original with transl. by G. K. Tallmadge in Bull. Hist. Med., 7: 429–547 (438–442), May 1939

Also, English transl. by G. K. Tallmadge in: F. A. Willius and T. E. Keys' *Cardiac classics.* St Louis, Mosby, 1941. pp. 84–85

Gasser, Herbert Spencer. New York physician. 1888–

Awarded Nobel prize in 1944, with J. Erlanger, for study of functions of nerves.

Physiological action currents in the phrenic nerve An application of the thermionic vacuum tube to nerve physiology with H. S. Newcomer, Amer. J. Physiol. 57: 1–26, Aug. 1, 1921

A study of the action currents of nerve with the cathode ray oscillograph with J. Erlanger, Ibid., 62: 496–523 Nov. 1, 1922

See also J. Erlanger

Gasser, Johann Lorenz. Vienna anatomist. 1505–1577

GANGLION—on larger root of fifth cranial nerve.

Described and illustrated by a pupil of Lorenz Gasser, Antonius Balthasar Raymundus Hirsch, in a graduation thesis.

Paris quinti nervorum encephali disquisitio anatomica in quantum ad ganglion sibi proprium semilunare, ad originem nervi intercostalis pertinet. Vienna, July 31, 1765

Gassner, Georg. German bacteriologist

AGAR—metachrome yellow water blue infusion.

Ein neuer Dreifarbennährböden zur Typhus-Ruhr Diagnose. Zbl. Bakt., 80: 219–222, Nov. 15, 1917

AGAR—nutrose; for cultivation of colon-typhoi group.

Hefewassernährböden und ihre Bewertung. Ibid., 79:
308–317 (315), May 23, 1917
Solution- lactose yeast; culture medium. Ibid., p. 311
Gaston-Durand, Louis. Paris physician. 1879–
METHOD—of estimating diastase in feces.
*De dosage de l'amylase des féces dans le diagnostic
fonctionnel du pancréas.* Arch. des Mal. d. Appar.
Digest., 5: 76–96, 1911
Gatch, Willis Dew. American surgeon. 1878–
BED—
*The sitting posture: its postoperative and other uses.
With a description of a bed for holding a patient in this
position.* Ann. Surg., 49: 410–415, Mar. 1909
METHOD—
*Nitrous-oxide-oxygen anesthesia by the method of re-
breathing: with especial reference to the prevention of
surgical shock.* J. A. M. A., 54: 775–780, Mar. 5,
1910
METHOD—
Aseptic intestinal anastomosis: an experimental study.
Ibid., 59: 185–190, July 20, 1912
METHOD—acid-hematin m.
*Amount of blood loss during some of the more common
operations: preliminary report* with W. D. Little,
Ibid., 83: 1075–1076, Oct. 4, 1924
Gaté, Jean. French physician. 1883–
REACTION—formol-gel.
*Lymphogranulomatose inguinale subaiguë à foyers
purulents intra-ganglionnaires d'origine génitale pro-
bable, peut-être vénérienne.* Lyon, 1913. 159 pp.
*Une nouvelle reaction des serums syphilitiques; formol-
gelification* with G. Papacostas, C. R. Soc. Biol., 83:
1432–1434, Nov. 15, 1920
Gatellier, Jean. Paris surgeon. 1886–
OPERATION—
*The juxtaretroperoneal route in the operative treatment
of fracture of the malleolus with posterior marginal
fragment.* S. G. O., 52: 67–70, Jan. 1931
Gaucher, Philippe Charles Ernest. French derma-
tologist. 1854–1918
DISEASE or SPLENOMEGALIA—familial splenic
anemia.
*De l'epithélioma primitif de la rate: hypertrophie
idiopathique de la rate sans leucémie.* Thèse de doct.,
Paris, 1882. 31 pp.
Gauss, Carl Joseph. German physician. 1875–
TWILIGHT SLEEP—
Geburten in kunstlichen Dämmerschlaf. Arch. Gynaek.,
78: 579–631, 1906
Gavarret, Louis Denis Jules. French physician.
1809–1890
Wrote one of first treatises on statistics in study of
diseases. Garrison
*Principes généraux de statistique médicale, ou develop-
pement des règles qui doivent présider à son emploi.*
Paris, Bechet, 1840. 312 pp.
Gay, Frederick Parker. California pathologist. 1874–
1939
TEST—
*A skin reaction indicative of immunity against typhoid
fever. Studies in typhoid immunization, III* with J.
N. Force, Arch. intern. Med., 13: 471–479, Mar.
1914
Gayet, Charles Jules Alphonse. French physician.
1833–1904

Described acute superior haemorrhagic polioencephalitis; now called Wernicke's disease.
*Affection encephalique (encephalite diffuse probable)
localisee aux etages des pedoncles cerebraux et aux
couches optiques.* Arch. Physiol. norm. path., 2 s.,
2: 341–351, 1875
Gay-Prieto, José Antonio. Madrid dermatologist
TREATMENT—of lymphogranuloma inguinale.
*Contribución al estudio de la linfogranulomatosis in-
guinal subaguda o úlcera venérea adenógena de Nicolás
y Favre.* Actas dermo-sif., Madrid, 20: 122–175,
1927
*Zur Behandlung der Lymphogranulomatosis inguinalis
mit spezifischem Antigen.* Dermat. Wschr., 95: 1056–
1063, July 16, 1932
Gaza, Wilhelm von. Göttingen surgeon. 1883–
OPERATION—thoracic ramisectomy.
*Ueber paravertebrale Neurektomie am grenzstrange
und paravertebrale Injektionstherapie.* Klin. Wschr.,
3: 525–528, Mar. 25, 1924
Gee, Samuel Jones. London physician. 1839–1911
DISEASE—intestinal infantilism: Gee-Herter's or
Gee-Thaysen's d.
On the coeliac affection. St. Bartholomew's Hosp.
Rep., 24: 17–23, 1888
LINCTUS—
On osteal or periosteal cachexia. Ibid., 17: 9–12, 1881
Geiger, Philipp Lorenz. German chemist. 1785–1836
Isolated atropine.
Darstellung des Atropins with H. Hesse, Ann.
Pharm., 5: 43–81; 6: 44–65, 1833
Geiling, E. M. K. See J. J. Abel
Geist, S. H. See R. T. Frank, U. J. Salmon
Gelfan, Samuel. Edmenton, Canada physiologist.
1903–
First used divinyl ether (vinethene) on humans
(themselves).
The anesthetic action of divinyl oxide on humans with
I. R. Bell, J. Pharmacol., 47: 1–3, Jan. 1933
Gelineau, Jean Baptiste Edouard. French psychi-
atrist. 1859–
SYNDROME—
De la narcolepsie. Gaz. d. hop., 53: 626–628, July 8;
635–637, July 15, 1880
Gellé, Marie Ernst. French aurist. 1834–1923
TEST—of hearing.
*De l'exploration de la sensibilité acoustique au moyen
du tube interauriculaire.* Paris, Delahaye, 1876. 28 pp.
Gellhorn, George. St. Louis gynecologist. 1870–1936
MODIFICATION—of Dickinson technic for vaginal
hysterectomy.
Vaginal hysterectomy under local anesthesia. S. G. O.,
51: 484–490, Oct. 1930
Gelmo, P. Vienna chemist
Synthesized sulfanilamide.
Ueber Sulfanide der p-Amidobenzolsulfonsäure. J. f.
prakt. Chem., 77: 369–382, Apr. 3, 1908
Gély, Jules Aristide. French surgeon. 1806–1861
SUTURE—for intestine.
*Recherches sur l'emploi d'un nouveau procédé de suture
contre les divisions de l'intestin, et sur la possibilité
de l'adossement de cet organe avec lui-même dans cer-
taines blessures.* Paris, Germer-Baillière, 1844. 84 pp.
Generali, F. See G. Vassale
Genevrier, M. French Army surgeon

TREATMENT—
Du traitement des varices par les injections coagulantes, concentrées de sels de quinine. Bull. Soc. méd. mil. franc., Paris, 15: 169–171, May 19, 1921

Gengou, O. See J. J. B. V. Bordet

Gennari, Francesco. Italian anatomist. 1750–
BAND or LAYER—in cerebral cortex.
De peculiari structure cerebri nonnullisque ejus morbis. Parmae, 1782. 87 pp. pp. 72–75

Genth, Frederick Augustus, Jr. American chemist. 1855–
TEST—
A method for confirmation of the presence of saccharin in foods and beverages. Amer. J. Pharm., 81: 536–537, Nov. 1909

Georgi, F. See H. Sachs

Geraghty, John Timothy. Baltimore urologist. 1876–1924
OPERATION—
A new method of perineal prostatectomy which insures more perfect functional results. J. Urol., 7: 339–351, May 1922
See also N. M. Keith, L. G. Rowntree

Gerhard, William Wood. Philadelphia physician. 1809–1872
Made first accurate clinical study of tuberculous meningitis.
Cerebral affections of children. Amer. J. med. Sci., 13: 313–359, 1833; 14: 99–111, 1834
Differentiated typhoid from typhus fever.
On the typhus fever which occurred in Philadelphia in the spring and summer of 1836. Ibid., 20: 289–322, Aug. 1837

Gerhardt, Carl Adolph Christian Jacob. Berlin physician. 1833–1902
DISEASE—
Ueber Erythromelalgie. Berl. klin. Wschr., 29: 1125–1126, Nov. 7, 1892
LAW—in paralysis of recurrent laryngeal nerve vocal cords assume position between abduction and adduction.
Studien und Beobachtungen über Stimmbandlähmung. Arch. path. Anat., 27: 68–98; 296–321, 1863
Uber Diagnose und Behandlung der Stimmbandlähmung. Samml. klin. Vortr., No. 36, (Inn. Med., No. 13, pp. 271–282), 1872
TEST—for acetoacetic acid in urine.
Diabetes mellitus und Aceton. Wien. med. Pr., 6: 672, 1865
TEST—for bile pigments in urine and blood.
Ueber einige Gallenfarbstoffreactionen. Würz. phys.-med. Stzgsber., No. 2, p. 25, 1881

Gerlach, Joseph von. German anatomist. 1820–1896
METHOD—of staining nerve fibers.
Von dem Rückenmark. Stricker's Handb., 2: 665–693 (678), 1872
METHOD—methylen blue, for nerve endings.
Ueber die Einwirkung des Methylenblaus auf die Muskelnerven des lebenden Frosches. S. B. Bayer. Akad. Wiss., Math.-phys. Kl., München, 19: 125–135, (May 4, 1889), 1890
VALVE—at orifice of vermiform appendix.
Beobachtung einer tödlichen Peritonitis, als Folge einer Perforation des Wurmfortsatzes. Z. rat. Med., 6: 12–23, 1847
Described minute anatomy of kidney.

Beiträge zur Structurlehre der Niere. Arch. Anat. Physiol. u. wiss. Med., pp. 378–386, 1845

Gerlach, M. Posen physician
SOLUTION—basal.
Stickstoffsammelnde Bakterien with Vogel, Zbl. Bakt., 2 Abt., 8: 669–674, May 17, 1902

Gerlier, Félix. Swiss physician. 1840–1914
DISEASE or SYNDROME—pain along nerve trunks, paresis, vertigo, ptosis and muscular contractions.
Une épidémie de vertige paralysant. Rev. méd. de la Suisse Rom., Genève, 7: 5–29, 1887

Gernez, Léon. French surgeon. 1875–1937
MODIFICATION—of Witzel gastrostomy.
Sur la gastrostomie permanente. Bull. Soc. Nat. de Chir., 55: 1107–1110, Oct. 16, 1929
Nouvelle technique de gastrostomie with Ho-Dac-Di, Pr. méd., 38: 191–192, Feb. 5, 1930

Gerota, Dimitru. Berlin anatomist
CAPSULE or FASCIA—perirenal f.
Beiträge zur Kenntniss des Befestigungsapparates der Niere. Arch. f. Anat. u. Entwickl., pp. 265–285, 1895
NODES—subdiaphragmatic lymph n., sometimes involved in metastatic cancer of breast.
Zur Technik der Lymphgefässinjection. Eine neue Injections-masse für Lymphgefässe. Polychrome Injection. Anat. Anz., 12: 216–224, July 10, 1896

Gerrard, Alfred William. English scientist
IMPROVEMENT—of Hüfner's apparatus for estimating urea.
Some new forms of apparatus for estimating nitrogen in urine. Lancet, 2: 952 (only), Nov. 29, 1884

Gersdorff, Hans von (Schylhans). fl. 1500
Described amputations.
Feldtbuch der Wundtartznev. Strassburg, Schott, 1517

Gersh, Isidore. Chicago scientist. 1907–
TECHNIC—of freezing and drying specimens of tissue.
The Altmann technique for fixation by drying while freezing. Anat. Rec., 53: 309–337, Aug. 25, 1932

Gerson, Max Bernhard. Vienna-American physician. 1881–
CANCER TREATMENT—
Dietary considerations in malignant neoplastic diseases: a preliminary report. Rev. Gastroenterol., 12: 419–425, Nov.–Dec. 1945
See also Editorial, *Gerson's cancer treatment.* J. A.-M. A., 132: 645–646, Nov. 16, 1946
DIET—
Meine Diät; ein Ratgeber für Kranke und Gesunde Berlin, Ullstein, (1930). 168 pp.
Diatbehandlung bei Migräne und Lungentuberkulose. Wien. klin. Wschr., 45: 744–748, June 10, 1932
See also E. F. Sauerbruch

Gerster, Arpad Geyza Charles. American surgeon 1848–1923
OPERATION—use of gold plate to cover cranial defect.
Heteroplasty for defect of skull. Trans. Amer. Surg Ass., 13: 485–486, 1895

Geschickter, Charles Freeborn. Baltimore pathologist. 1901–
Demonstrated that gynecomastia or hypertrophy of breast of male monkey is induced by injection of estrin and anterior pituitary-like hormones.
Tumors of the breast related to the aestrin hormone

with D. Lewis and C. G. Hartman, Amer. J. Cancer, 21: 828–859, Aug. 1934

Gesellius, Franz. Russian physician

CANNULA—for blood transfusion.

Capillar-Blut (undefibrinirtes) zur Transfusion. Ein neuer Apparat zur Transfusion, sowohl zur einfachsen, als auch zur depletorischen. St. Petersburg, Münx, 1868. 49 pp.

Gessard, Carle. French physician. 1850–

Isolated Pseudomonas pyocyanea.

Sur les colorations bleue et verte des linges à pansements. C. R. Acad. Sci., 94: 536–538, Feb. 20, 1882

Gettler, Alexander Oscar. New York chemist. 1883–

METHOD—

Determination of alcoholic intoxication during life by spinal fluid analysis with A. W. Freireich, J. biol. Chem., 92: 199–209, July 1931

METHOD—for determination of chlorides.

A method for the determination of death by drowning. J. A. M. A., 77: 1650–1652, Nov. 19, 1921

METHOD—

Chloroform content of the brain following anesthesia with H. Blume, Arch. Path., 11: 841–846, June 1931

Ghedini, G. Genoa physician

REACTION—complement fixation for echinococcus disease.

Ricerche sul siero di sangue di individuo affetto da cisti da echinococce e sul liquido in essa contenuto. Gazz. d. osp., 27: 1616–1617, Dec. 23, 1906

Ghon, Anton. German bacteriologist. 1866–1936

Recognized importance of differentiating between lesions found in first infection tuberculosis and that resulting from reinfection.

Der primäre Lungenherd bei der Tuberkulose der Kinder. Berlin, Urban und Schwarzenberg, 1912. 143 pp.

Also, English transl. by King. London, Churchill, 1916. 172 pp.

See also E. A. F. Finger

Ghoreyeb, Albert A. W. Boston scientist

METHOD—

A new and quick method for staining spirochetes (treponemata) in smear preparations. J. A. M. A., 54: 1498–1499, May 7, 1910

Ghormley, Ralph Kalb. American surgeon. 1893–

OPERATION—

Use of the anterior superior spine and crest of the ilium in surgery of the hip joint. J. Bone and Joint Surg., 13: 784–798, Oct. 1931

See also B. T. Horton

Giacomini, Carlo. Italian anatomist. 1841–1898

BAND—anterior end of fascia dentata of hippocampus.

Guida allo studio delle circonvoluzioni cerebrali dell'uomo. Torino, Camilla & Bertolero, 1878. 96 pp.

Gianturco, Cesare. Rochester, Minn. radiologist. 1905–

Developed direct roentgen cinematography.

Roentgen ray motion pictures of the stomach. with W. C. Alvarez

Proc. Staff Meet. Mayo Clinic, 7: 669–671, Nov. 23, 1932

Giard, Alfred. Paris biologist. 1846–1908

GIARDIASIS—a protozoan of intestinal tract of man. Name applied by J. Künstler in: *Sur cinq Protozaires parasites nouveaux.* C. R. Acad. Sci., 45: 347–349, Aug. 14, 1882

Gibb. H. P. See F. E. Batten

Gibbon, John Heysham, Jr. Philadelphia physician. 1903–

TEST— (see also E. M. Landis)

Vasodilatation in the lower extremities in response to immersing the forearm in warm water with E. M. Landis, J. clin. Invest., 11: 1019–1036, Sept. 1932

Gibbons, Henry, III. San Francisco physician. 1906–

COUNT—of urine sediment.

A rapid quantitative method for examining the urine in renal disorders. Arch. intern. Med., 54: 758–763, Nov. 1934

Gibbons, Marjorie M. See F. W. Taylor

Gibbs, Owens Stanley. Edinburgh physician. 1898–

COAGULOMETER—

A clinical blood coagulometer. Quart. J. Med., 17: 321–318, Apr. 1924

Caused production of acetylcholine on stimulation of chorda tympani nerve.

Die humorale Übertragung der Chorda tympani-Reizung with J. Szelöczey, Arch. exp. Path. Pharmak., 168: 64–88, Oct. 4, 1932

Gibert, Camille Melchior. French dermatologist. 1797–1866

DISEASE—pityriasis rubra.

Traite pratique des maladies speciales de la peau. ... Paris, 1834. 2 ed., 1860 p. 402

Gibney, Virgil Pendleton. New York surgeon, 1847–1927

SPLINT or STRAPPING—

Sprained ankle. A treatment that involves no loss of time, requires no crutches, and is not attended with any ultimate impairment of function, New York Med. J., 61: 193–197, Feb. 16, 1895

Described hereditary deforming chondrodysplasis.

Multiple exostosis. (Case report). Med. Rec., 10: 300 (only), Apr. 24, 1875

Hereditary multiple exostosis; four cases, with remarks. Amer. J. med. Sci., 72: 73–80, July 1876

Gibson, Alexander George. English physician. 1875–

Described b-wave.

The significance of a hitherto undescribed wave in the jugular pulse. Lancet, 2: 1380–1382, Nov. 16, 1907

Gibson, Benjamin. Manchester surgeon. 1784–1812

Introduced couching cataract in new-born.

On the use of the couching-needle in infants of a few months old. Edinburgh Med. and Surg. J., 7: 394–400, Oct. 1811

Gibson, Charles Langdon. New York surgeon. 1864–1944

CHART—for recording repeated blood counts.

The value of the differential leucocyte in acute surgical diseases. Ann. Surg., 43: 485–499, Apr. 1906

OPERATION—for incisional hernia.

Post-operative intestinal obstruction. Ibid., 63: 442–451, Apr. 1916

Gibson, J. Lockhart. Brisbane ophthalmologist

GLIOMATA—

Intra-ocular glioma of optic nerve of each eye. Brit. J. Ophthal., 5: 67 (only), Feb. 1921

Gibson, John Graham, II. Boston physician. 1897–

METHOD—for determination of plasma volume.

Clinical studies of the blood volume. I. Clinical application of a method of employing the azo dye "Evans

blue" and the spectrophotometer with W. A. Evans, Jr., J. clin. Invest., 16: 301–316, May 1937
See also M. I. Gregersen

Gibson, R. B. See B. B. Clark

Gibson, S. See W. J. Potts

Gibson, Thomas Essington. San Francisco urologist. 1896–

OPERATION—
Hydronephrosis: standardization of surgical treatment. New Engl. J. Med., 222: 910–918, May 30, 1940

Gibson, William. American surgeon. 1788–1868

BANDAGE—for fracture of lower jaw.
Fracture of the lower jaw. In: *Institutes and Practice of Surgery.* Philadelphia, Parker, 1824. 2 vols. Vol. 1, pp. 381–385
Tied common iliac artery, 1812. Garrison
Case of a wound of the common iliac artery. Amer. Med. Recorder, Phila., 3: 185–193, 1820

Giemsa, Gustav. Hamburg chemist. 1867–

METHOD—of staining malarial parasites.
Färbemethoden für Malariaparasiten. Zbl. Bakt., 32: 307–313, Aug. 25, 1902
Zur Praxis der Giemsa-Färbung. Ibid., 1. Abt., 91: Orig., 343–346, Feb. 15, 1924

METHOD—of staining Spirochaeta pallida.
Bemerkungen zur Färbung der Spirochaete pallida (Schaudinn). Dtsch. med. Wschr., 31: 1026–1027, June 29, 1905
Same, abstr.: Zbl. Bakt., 37: 507 (only), Dec. 6, 1905
See also next reference.

METHOD—fixative, with corrosive sublimate-alcohol.
Ueber die Färbung von Feuchtpräparaten mit meiner Azur-Eosinmethode. Dtsch. med. Wschr., 35: 1751–1752, Oct. 7, 1909

Gierke, Edgar Otto Konrad von. German physician. 1877–

DISEASE—glycogen accumulation.
Ueber Speicherungen und Speicherungskrankheiten (Thesaurismosen). Med. Klin., 27: 576–579, Apr. 17: 611–614, Apr. 24, 1931

Gies, William John. American chemist. 1872–

REAGENT—
A reagent for the biuret test. J. biol. Chem., 7: LX, 1910

TEST—for albumin in urine.
A proteid reaction involving the use of chromate. Amer. J. Physiol., 8: XV–XVI, Feb. 2, 1903
See also J. L. Kantor

Giffin, Herbert Ziegler. Rochester, Minn. physician. 1878–

METHOD—
The estimation of urobilin and urobilinogen in the duodenal contents with A. H. Sanford and T. L. Szlapka, Amer. J. med. Sci., 155: 562–579, Apr. 1918

METHOD—
Clinical observations concerning the fragility of erythrocytes with A. H. Sanford, J. Lab. clin. Med., 4: 465–478, May 1919

Gifford, Harold. Omaha ophthalmologist. 1858–1929

OPERATION—
On strictly simple evisceration of the eye-ball. Arch. Ophth., 29: 422–425, 1900

OPERATION—
The treatment of recurrent pterygium. Ophth. Rev., 18: 1–8, Jan. 1909

OPERATION—
Delimiting keratotomy in the treatment of severe corneal ulcers. Trans. Amer. Acad. Ophth. and Otolaryngol., pp. 418–421, 1918

Gifford, Sanford Robinson. Chicago ophthalmologist. 1892–1944

OPERATION—
Iridencleisis with water tight closure of the conjunctiva. Trans. Amer. Acad. Ophth. and Otolaryngol., pp. 117–128, 1927

OPERATION—
The Machek operation for ptosis. Arch. Ophth., 8: 495–502, Oct. 1932
See also J. McD. Patton

Gigli, Leonardo. Florence gynecologist. 1863–1908

SAW—wire with saw teeth.

OPERATION—pubiotomy in obstructed delivery.
Ueber ein neues Instrument zum Durchtrennen der Knochen, die Drahtsäge. Zbl. Chir., 21: 409–412, May 5, 1894
Sinfisiotomia classica e taglio laterilizzato del pube. Clin. mod., Pisa, 8: 302–308, 1902

Gigli, T. Pavia chemist

REACTION—for uric acid.
Ueber eine Reaction der Harnsäure und eine volumetrische Bestimmungsmethode derselben. Chem. Zeitung, 22: 330–331, Apr. 27, 1898

Gil, Miguel Casares-. Swiss physician

STAIN—for flagella.
La méthode de Casares-Gil pour la coloration des cils des bactéries. By B. Galli-Valerio, Zbl. Bakt., 1 Abt., Orig., 76: 233–234, May 20, 1915

Gilbert, Judson Bennett. Schenectady urologist. 1898–

SYNDROME—choriogenic gynecomastia with testis tumors.
Studies in malignant testis tumors: 2. Syndrome of choriogenic gynecomastia: report of six cases and review of one hundred and twenty-nine. J. Urol., 44: 345–357, Sept. 1940

Gilbert, Nicholas Augustin. Paris physician. 1858–1927

DISEASE—
De l'ictère familial. Contribution a l'étude de la diathèse biliaire with J. Castaigne and P. Lereboullet, Bull. Soc. méd. Hôp. Paris, 17: 948–959, July 27, 1900
La cholémie simple familiale with P. Lereboullet, Sem. méd., 21: 241–243, 1901

Gilbert, Ruth. Albany, N. Y. physician. 1883–

AGAR—tellurite serum, for isolation of diphtheria bacilli.
The use of potassium tellurite in differential media with Eleanor M. Humphreys, J. Bact., 11: 141–151 Feb. 1926
See also H. Zinsser

Gilbert, W. Hamburg ophthalmologist

OPHTHALMIA LENTA—
Über chronische Verlaufsformen der metastatischer Ophthalmie ("Ophthalmia lenta"). Arch. f. Augen heilk., 96: 119–130, May 1925

Gilchrist, Thomas Casper. Baltimore dermatologist 1862–1927

DISEASE or MYCOSIS—blastomycosis. Discovered parasite of. . . .
A case of blastomycetic dermatitis in man. Johns Hopk. Hosp. Rep., 1: 269–290, 1896
See also E. Rixford
Gilford, Hastings. English physician. 1861–1941
DISEASE—senile dwarfism.
Progeria: a form of senilism. Practitioner, 73 : 188–217, 1904
Giliberti, V. See M. Osnato
Gill, Arthur Bruce. Philadelphia surgeon. 1876–
OPERATION—
Operation for correction of paralytic genu recurvatum. J. Bone and Joint Surg., 13 : 49–53, Jan. 1931
OPERATION—
A new operation for arthrodesis of the shoulder. Ibid., 287–295, Apr. 1931
OPERATION—
An operation to make a posterior bone block at the ankle to limit foot-drop. Ibid., 15: 166–170, Jan. 1933
OPERATION or PROCEDURE—
Arthrodesis for ununited fracture of the neck of the femur. Ibid., 21: 710–714, July 1939
Gill, William Davis. American surgeon. 1895–
TREATMENT or OPERATION—elevating fracture of malar bone.
Fractures about the orbit. South. Med. J., 21: 527–534, July 1928
Gilles de la Tourette, Georges. French neurologist. 1857–1904
DISEASE—motor incoordination with echolalia and coprolalia; convulsive tic.
Jumping, latah, myriachit. Arch. Neurol., Paris, 8: 68–74, July 1884
Étude sur une affection nerveuse caractérisée par de l'incoordination motrice accompagnée d'écholalie et de coprolalie (jumping, latah, myriachit). Ibid., 9: 19–42, Jan.; 158–200, Mar. 1885
Gillespie, James Donaldson. Scottish physician. 1823–1891
OPERATION—
On resection of the wrist-joint. Edinburgh Med. J., 16: 498–503, Dec. 1870
Gillette, William J. Toledo, Ohio surgeon. 1858–1925
METHOD—of control of liver hemorrhage.
Surgery of the liver, Report. S. G. O., 1: 361 (only), Oct. 1905
Gilliam, David Tod. American gynecologist. 1844–1923
OPERATION—
Round-ligament ventrosuspension of the uterus: a new method. Amer. J. Obstet., 41: 299–303, Mar. 1900
Gillies, Sir Harold Delf. English surgeon. 1882–
METHOD—
Reconstruction of the external ear with special reference to the use of maternal ear cartilage as the supporting structure. Rev. de chir. structive, 7: 169–179, Oct. 1937
OPERATION—
A new principle in the surgical treatment of "congenital cleft palate," and its mechanical counterpart with W. K. Fry, Brit. med. J., 1: 335–338, Mar. 5, 1921
OPERATION—
Fractures of the malar-zygomatic compound: with a description of a new x-ray position with T. P. Kilner and D. Stone, Brit. J. Surg., 41: 651–656, Apr. 1927

TUBED PEDICLE FLAPS—
The design of direct pedicle flaps. Brit. med. J., 2: 1008 (only), Dec. 3, 1932
Gilligan, D. Rourke. Boston scientist
METHOD—for determination of total blood and plasma volumes.
The effects on the cardiovascular system of fluids administered intravenously in man. I. Studies of the amount and duration of changes in blood volume with M. D. Altschule and Marie D. Volk, J. clin. Invest., 77 : 7–16, Jan. 1938
Gilmour, W. See C. H. Browning
Gimbernat, Antonio de. Spanish surgeon. 1734–1790
LIGAMENT—
Nuevo metoto de operar en la hernia crural. Madrid, 1793
Also, English transl. by T. Beddoes, London, Johnson, 1795. 70 pp.
Ginzburg, L. See B. B. Crohn
Giovannini, Sabastiano. Italian dermatologist. 1851–1920
DISEASE—nodular, of hair produced by a fungus.
Ueber die normale Entwicklung und über einige Veränderungen der menschlichen Haare. Vtljschr. f. Dermat. u. Syph., 19: 1049–1075 (1067), 1887
Recherches sur l'histologie pathologique de la pelade. Ann. de dermat. et de syph., 2: 921–957, Dec. 25, 1891
Girard, Alfred Conrad. American army surgeon. 1841–1914
TREATMENT—of seasickness.
In: *Letters from Europe . . . to Prof. Senn.* J. A. M. A., 22: 319 (only), Mar. 3, 1894
Atropin and strychnin combined: a specific for seasickness. Ibid., 46: 1925–1927, June 23, 1906
Girard, Charles. Berne surgeon. 1850–1916
AMPUTATION—interilio-abdominal.
Désarticulation de l'os iliaque pour sarcome. (Brief note) Rev. de Chir., 15 : 952, (only), 1895
Sur la désarticulation interilio-abdominale. Ibid., 18: 1141–1142, 1898
OPERATION—
Neue Methods der Gastrostomie mit Sphincterbildung. Correspond. f. schweizer Aerzte, 18: 345–346, June 1, 1888
OPERATION—
Du traitement des diverticules de l'oesophage. Cong. franç. de Chir., Proc. verb., 10 Session, Paris, 1896. pp. 392–407
OPERATION—for hypertrophy of breast.
Ueber Mastoptose und Mastopexie. Verh. dtsch. Ges. Chir., 39: 200–213, 1910
Girdner, John Harvey. New York physician. 1856–
PROBE—
On the detecting and locating of metallic masses in the human body by means of the induction balance and the telephonic probe. New York Med. J., 45: 393–396, Apr. 9, 1887
Giuffrida-Ruggieri, Vincenzo. Italian anthropologist. 1872–1922
STIGMA—abnormal shallowness of glenoid fossa.
Sulla dignita morfologica dei segui detti "degenerativi." Roma, Loescher, 1897. 117 pp.
Giugni, F. See C. Frugoni

Gius, John Armes. Portland, Ore. surgeon. 1908–
APPARATUS—
A new portable suction apparatus for use with the Miller-Abbott tube with C. A. Racely, Surgery, 15: 574–578, Apr. 1944

Givens, Maurice Hope. American biochemist. 1888–
MODIFICATION—
A modification of Rose's method for the estimation of pepsin. Hygienic Lab. Bull., 101: 71–78, Aug. 1915
See also A. Hunter

Gladstone, G. P. London bacteriologist
MEDIUM—basal synthetic.
Inter-relationship between amino-acids in the nutrition of B. anthracis. Brit. J. exp. Path., 20: 189–200, Apr. 1939

Glaessner, Karl. German surgeon. 1876–1944
Reported intubation of Wirsung's duct.
Ueber mensｇhliches Pankreassekret. Z. physiol. Chem. 40: 465–479, Jan. 26, 1904

Glaessner, Paul. Prague physician
AGAR—Nährstoff-Heyden, for cultivation of diphtheria bacilli.
Ueber die Verwertbarkeit einiger neuer Eiweisspräparate zur Kulturzwecken. I. Allgemeine Eignung mit besonderer Berücksichtigung der Diphtherie. Zbl. Bakt., 27: 724–732 (729), June 9, 1900

Glasgow, William Carr. St. Louis physician. 1845–1907
SIGN—systolic murmur in brachial artery in latent aneurysm of aorta.
A new and distinguishing sign of latent aneurysm of the aorta. New York Med. J., 60: 329–331, Sept. 15, 1894

Glauber, Johann Rudolf. German physician. 1604–1668
SALT—sodium sulphate; purgative.
Tractatus de natura salium.... Amsterodami, Janssonium, 1659

Glavind, J. See H. Dam

Glenard, Frantz. French physician. 1848–1920
DISEASE—splanchnoptosis.
TEST—girdle t. for disease.
THEORY—abdominal ptosis is a nutritional disease with atrophy and prolapse of intestine. Dorland
Application de la méthode naturelle à l'analyse de la dyspepsie nerveuse; détermination d'une espèce. Lyon Méd., 48: 449–464; 492–505; 532–543; 563–583, 1885
Enteroptose et neurasthenie. By Féréol and Glenard, Sem. méd., Paris, 6: 211–212, 1886
PROCEDURE—for examination of kidney.
Charactère, objectif et diagnostic du rein mobile (nephroptose); procédé néphroleptique. Paris, 1896

Glénard, Roger. French physician
Studied intestinal peristalsis.
Les mouvements de l'intestin en circulation artificielle. Paris thesis (Faculté des sciences), 1913
Also: Arch. d. mal. de l'appar. digest., 8: 61–95, 1915

Glenny, A. T. English physician
METHOD—intracutaneous, for "immunity index" of diphtheria toxin-antitoxin mixture.
Diphtheria toxoid as an immunising agent with Barbara E. Hopkins, Brit. J. exp. Path., 4: 283–288, Oct. 1923

Gley, Eugene. French physiologist. 1857–1903
GLANDS—parathyroids.

Demonstrated existence of iodine in thyroid gland and in blood.
Sur la fonction de la glande thyroide chez le lapin et chez le chien. C. R. Soc. Biol., 48: 841–847, 1891
Premiers resultats de recherches sur les modifications histologiques des glandules thyroidiennes apres la thyroidectomie with A. Nicolas, Ibid. 2: 216–218, Mar. 23, 1895

Gley, P. See L. H. Vaquez

Glisson, Francis. English physician. 1597–1677
CAPSULE—of liver.
CIRRHOSIS—of liver; chronic perihepatitis.
De hepate. London, 1664
Anatomia hepatis; cui praemittuntur quaedam ad rem anatomicam universe spectantia. Et ad calcem operi. subjiciuntur nonnulla de lymphae ductibus nuper repertis. Amsteloedami, Ravesteyn, 1659. 552 pp.
Wrote original and classic account of infantile rickets. Garrison
De rachitide, sive morbe puerili, qui vulgo the ricket dicitur, tratatus. London, typ. G. Du-Gardi, 1650, 416 pp.
Introduced concept of "irritability" as a specific property of all human tissues. His view was, however, "purely metaphysical." Garrison
Tractatus de ventriculo et intestinis. Cui praemittitus alius, de partibus continentibus in genere; et in specie de iis abdominis. Londini, H. Brome, 1677. 509 pp.

Glover, Donald Mitchell. Cleveland surgeon. 1895–
TECHNIC—
Fifteen years of the tannic acid method of burn treatment with A. F. Sydow, Amer. J. Surg., 51: 601–619, Mar. 1941

Gluck, Themistokles. German surgeon. 1853–
Improved technic of laryngectomy.
Kehlkopfchirurgie und Laryngoplastik. Therap. de Gegenwart., Berlin, 40: 169–179; 202–211, 1899
Resected lobe of lung.
Die Entwichelung der Lungenchirurgie. Verh. dtsch Ges. Chir., 36: pt. 2, 261–281, 1907

Gluzinski, Wladyslaw Antoni. Lemberg physician 1856–1935
TEST—for bile pigments.
Eine neue Reaction auf Gallenfarbstoffe. Wien. klir Wschr., 10: 1139–1140, Dec. 30, 1897

Glynn, Ernest Edward. English physician. 1873–1929
Used term "opsonocytophagie" to indicate phagocytic activity of blood in presence of serum opsonin and homologous leukocytes.
Variations in the inherent phagocytic power of leukocytes with G. L. Cox, J. Path. Bact., 14: 90–131, 1910

Glynn, John Hubert. American bacteriologist. 1902–
METHOD—
The application of the Gram stain to paraffin section. Arch. Path., 20: 896–899, Dec. 1935

Gmelin, Leopoldus. German physiologist. 1788–185
TEST— for bile pigments in urine.
Die Verdauung nach Versuchen with F. Tiedemann Heidelberg und Leipzig, 1826 (preface, p. 11)

Gobley, Théodore Nicolas. French chemist. 1811–1876
Introduced lecithin.
Recherches chimiques sur le jaune d'oeuf.... Paris De Fain et Thunot, 1846

Gocht, Hermann. Berlin surgeon. 1869–1938
OPERATION—for slipping patella, by reefing median capsule and fascia.
Die Ueberpflanzung der Kniebeugemuskeln auf den Kniestreckapparat. Arch. f. orthop. Chir., 16: 533–548, June 12, 1919

Godfrin, P. French scientist
TEST—for differentiating pathological albumin and egg albumin in urine.
Nouveau procédé permettant de reconnaitre facilement la presence de l'ovalbumine dans les urines. J. Pharm. Chim., Paris, 7 s., 14: 257–260, 1916
TEST—for albumin in urine.
Critique du procédé de recherche de l'albumine urinaire par la chaleur; nouveau procédé permettant de déceler les moindres troces d'albumine dans les urines. Ibid., pp. 294–303

Godlee, Sir Rickman John. London surgeon. 1849–1925
Reported successful operation for tumor of brain.
Excision of a tumor of the brain with A. H. Bennett, Lancet, 2: 1090–1091, Dec. 20, 1884
See also A. H. Bennett

Godman, John D. American surgeon. 1794–1830
FASCIA—at root of neck extending to pericardium.
Anatomical investigations, comprising descriptions of various fasciae of the human body; the discoveries of the manner in which the pericardium is formed from the superficial fascia, the capsular ligament of the shoulder joint from the brachial fascia; and the capsular ligament of the shoulder joint from the fascia lata. To which is added an account of some irregularities of structure and morbid anatomy; with a description of a new anatomical table. Philadelphia, Carey and Lea, 1824. 134 pp.

Gömöri, George. Hungarian-American physician. 1904–
METHOD—
Silver impregnation of reticulum in paraffin sections. Amer. J. Path., 13: 993–1001, Nov. 1937
STAIN—silver nitrate.
Microtechnical demonstration of insoluble lime salts in tissues. Ibid., 9: 253–260, Mar. 1933
STAIN—
A differential stain for cell types in the pancreatic islets. Ibid., 15: 497–500, July 1939

Goethe, Johann Wolfgang von. German scientist and poet. 1749–1832
One of the pioneers of evolution. Garrison
Ueber den Zwischenkiefer des Menschen und der Thiere. Jena, 1786. 48 pp.
Same, in German, 1790
Same, Nova Acta Acad. Leopold-Carol., Halle, 15: 1–48, 1831
Same, in English, 1863

Goetsch, Emil. New York physician. 1883–
SKIN REACTION—for hyperthyroidism.
Newer methods in the diagnosis of thyroid disorders: pathological and clinical. A. Functional activity of thyroid adenomata, as indicated by the cellular content of mitochondria. B. Adrenalin hypersensitiveness in clinical states of hyperthyroidism. New York State J. Med., 18: 259–267, July 1918

Goetsch, Johann Gotthilf Wilhelm August. German physician. 1879–

HYPOTHESIS—that carcinoma cells may become osteoblasts and form bone. (Obsolete)
Ueber den Einfluss von Karcinommetastasen auf das Knochengewebe. Beitr. path. Anat., 39: 218–251, 1906

Goettsch, E. See A. A. Weech

Goetze, Otto. German surgeon. 1890–
OPERATION—
Das Rektumkarzinom als Exstirpations-objekt; Vorschläge zur sakralen und abdominosakralen Operation. Zbl. Chir., 58: 1746–1766, July 11, 1931
OPERATION—phrenic resection.
Die radikale Phrenicotomie als selbständiger therapeutischer Eingriff bei einseitiger Lungen-Phthise. Klin. Wschr., 1: 1496–1502, July 22; 1544–1546, July 29, 1922

Gohrbandt, Erwin. German surgeon
TECHNIC—of closure of duodenal stump.
Zur Technik des Duodenalverschlusses. Zbl. Chir., 60: 1815–1817, Aug. 5, 1933

Goinard, Pierre. French surgeon
OPERATION—
Cure radicale de certaines hernies inguinales par fixation du tendon conjoint au ligament de Cooper. Pr. méd., 47: 872 (only), May 31, 1939

Goldberg, M. W.

Goldberg, S. W. St. Petersburg physician
Used radium in treatment of cancer.
Zur Frage der Beziehungen zwischen Becquerelstrahlen und Hautaffectionen with E. S. London, Dermat. Z., 10: 457–462, 1902

Goldberger, Esther W. See H. Vollmer

Goldberger, Joseph. American physician. 1874–1929
Produced pellagra experimentally by faulty diets and studied anti-pellagra vitamin.
The treatment and prevention of pellagra with C. H. Waring and D. G. Willets, U. S. Pub. Health Ser. Report, 29: 2821–2825, 1914
The experimental production of pellagra in human subjects by means of diets with G. A. Wheeler, Ibid., Hyg. Lab., No. 120, pp. 7–116, Feb. 1920
A further study of butter, fresh beef, and yeast as pellagra preventatives, with consideration of the relation of factor P-P of pellagra (and black tongue of dogs) to vitamin B with G. A. Wheeler, R. D. Lillie and L. M. Rogers, Ibid., 41: 297–318, 1926
See also J. F. Anderson

Goldberger, M. A. See R. T. Frank

Goldblatt, Harry. Cleveland physiologist. 1891–
Reported partial constriction of renal arteries of dogs is followed by a rise in blood pressure.
Studies on experimental hypertension: I. The production of persistent elevation of systolic blood pressure by means of renal ischemia with J. Lynch, R. F. Hanzal and W. W. Summerville, J. exp. Med., 59: 347–380. Mar. 1934

Goldflam, Samuel Vulfovich. Polish physician. 1852–
DISEASE—myasthenia gravis pseudoparalytica.
Ueber einen scheinbar heilbaren bulbärparalytischen Symptomencomplex mit Betheiligung der Extremitäten. Dtsch. Z. Nervenheilk., 4: 312–352, 1893

Goldhorn, L. B. New York pathologist
STAIN—
A rapid and certain method of staining Spirochaeta pallida. Abstr.: New York Path. Soc., s 2, 5: 169–173, May, 1905–Jan. 1906

Concerning the morphology and reproduction of Spirochaeta pallida and a rapid method for staining the organism. J. exp. Med., 8: 451–460, May 25, 1906

Goldman, A. See S. B. Grant

Goldmann, Edwin Ellen. Freiburg surgeon. 1862–1913

OPERATION—two-stage removal of pharyngeal diverticula.

Die zweizeitige Operation von Pulsionsdivertikeln der Speiseröhre, nebst Bemerkungen über den Oesophagusmund. Beitr. klin. Chir., 61: 741–749, 1909

Described eosinophils in lymph nodes in Hodgkin's disease.

Beitrag zu der Lehre von dem "Malignen Lymphom." Zbl. allg. Path. u. path. Anat., 3: 665–680, Sept. 10, 1892

Goldring, W. See H. W. Smith

Goldscheider, Johannes Karl August Eugen Alfred. Berlin physician. 1858–1935

DISEASE—epidermolysis bullosa.

Hereditäre Neigunz zur Blasenbildung. Mschr. prakt. Dermat., 1: 163–164, Aug. 1882

PERCUSSION—threshold.

Untersuchungen über Perkussion. Dtsch. Arch. klin. Med., 94: 480–528, Nov. 26, 1908

TEST—for cutaneous thermal sensibility.

Die spezifische Energie der Temperaturnerven. Mschr. prakt. Dermat., 3: 198–208; 225–241, 1884

Neue Thatsachen über die Hautsinnesnerven. Arch. Anat. Physiol., Physiol. Abt., Lpz., Suppl.-Bd., 1–110, 1885

Goldschmidt, L. See O. Frehden

Goldstein, Hyman Isaac. Camden, N. J. physician. 1887–

DISEASE—heredofamilial angiomatosis.

Hereditary hemorrhagia telangiectasia with recurring (familial) hereditary epistaxis. Arch. intern. Med., 27: 102–125, Jan. 15, 1921

Goldstein, Kurt. German neurologist. 1878–

SYNDROME—of cerebellar irritation.

Beiträge zur Kasuistik und Symptomatologie der Kleinhirnerkrankungen with F. Reichmann, Arch. Psychiat., Berlin, 56: 466–521, 1916

Goldstein, L. Würzburg physician

REACTION—for glycogen.

Beiträge zur Lehre von der Glycogenbildung in der Leber. Verh. physik.-med. Ges. in Würzburg, 7: 1–19, 1874

Goldthwait, Joel Ernest. Boston surgeon. 1866–

BRACE—back.

In his: *Diseases of the bones and joints; clinical studies* with C. F. Painter and R. B. Osgood, Boston, Heath, 1909. 685 pp. p. 543

OPERATION—

Permanent dislocation of the patella. The report of a case of twenty years' duration, successfully treated by transplantation of the patella tendons, with the tubercle of the tibia. Ann. Surg., 29: 62–68, Jan. 1899

Slipping or recurrent dislocation of the patella, with the report of eleven cases. Boston Med. and Surg. J., 150: 169–174, Feb. 13, 1904

Also: Amer. J. Orth. Surg., 1: 293–308, Feb. 1904

OPERATION—

An operation for the stiffening of the ankle-joint in infantile paralysis. Amer. J. Orthop. Surg., 5: 271–275, Jan. 1908

SIGN—flexion of straight leg at hip elicits pain in

sacro-iliac region in sprain of sacro-iliac ligaments.

In: *Diseases of the bones and joints* with C. F. Painter and R. B. Osgood, Boston, Leonard, 1910. pp. 539–540

The lumbo-sacral articulations. An explanation of many cases of "lumbago," "sciatica" and paraplegia. Boston Med. and Surg. J., 164: 365–372, Mar. 16, 1911

Suggested that many cases of lumbago and sciatica are due to injury of an intervertebral disk. Ibid.

Golgi, Camillo. Italian neurologist. 1844–1926

Awarded Nobel prize in 1906, with J. R. Ramon y Cajal.

APPARATUS—special part of protoplasm of tissue cells, demonstrated by staining by osmic acid or impregnation with silver.

Sulla fina anatomia degli organi centrali del sistema nervoso. Riv. sper. di freniat., Reggio-Emilia, 8: 165; 361, 1882; 9: 1; 161; 385, 1883; 11: 72; 193, 1885

CELLS—nerve c. with short processes in posterior horns of spinal cord.

Sulla struttura delle fibre nervosa midollate periferiche e centrali. Arch. per le sci. med., Torino, 4: 221–246, 1880

Studi istologici sul midollo spinale. Arch. ital. per le mal. nerv., Milano, 18: 155–165, 1881

Sull'origine centrale dei nervi. Gior. internaz. d. sci. med., Napoli, n.s. 3: 225–234, 1881

ERYTHROCYTE—

LAW—severity of a malarial attack depends on number of parasites in blood. Showed that malarial paroxysms are coincident with sporulation of parasites, and that parasite of quartan fever differs from that of tertian.

Sull'infezione malarica. Arch. per le sci. med., Torino, 10: 109–135, 1886

Sul ciclo evolutivo dei parassiti malarica nella febbre terzana. Ibid., 13: 173–196, 1889

METHOD—rapid, for impregnating neurons.

In his: *Untersuchungen über den feineren Bau des centralen und peripherischen Nervensystems.* Jena, Fischer, 1894

Goll, Friedrich. Swiss anatomist. 1829–1903

COLUMN—posteromedian, of spinal cord.

FIBERS—from Goll's nucleus to vermis of cerebellum.

NUCLEUS—in basal part of posterior pyramid of oblongata.

TRACT—fasciculus gracilis.

Ueber die feinere Anatomie des Rückenmarks. 1868

Golla, Frederick Lucien. English physician

TEST—for differentiating methylene blue from indigo blue in urine.

Green urine due to a proprietary pill with H. D. Rolleston, Brit. med. J., 1: 1064–1065, May 11, 1912

Golovine, Sergei Seliv. Moscow ophthalmologist

OPERATION—for frontal sinusitis.

Operative treatment of lesions of the frontal sinus. Transl. from French original MS by C. C. Whitman, Arch. Ophthal., 27: 294–314, 1898

Goltz, Friedrich Leopold. German physician. 1834–1902

EXPERIMENT—striking a frog on abdomen will stop heart's action.

Ueber Reflexionen von und zum Herzen (Klopfver-such). Königsb. med. Jahrb., 3: 271–274, 1862
Beiträge zur Lehre von den Functionen der Nerven-centren des Frosches. Berlin, Hirschwald, 1869. 130 pp.
THEORY—semicircular canals transmit sensations of position.
Ueber die physiologische Bedeutung der Bogengänge des Ohrlabyrinths. Arch. ges. Physiol., Bonn, 3: 172–192, 1870

Gombault, Francois Alexis Albert. Paris neurologist. 1844–1904
DEGENERATION or NEURITIS—
Contribution à l'étude anatomique de la névrite paren-chymateuse subaiguë ou chronique.—Névrite segmen-taire péri-axile. Arch. Neurol., Paris, 1: 11–38, July: 177–190, Oct. 1880
See also J. M. Charcot

Gomes, Bernardino Antonio Spanish scientist. 1768–1823
Obtained a substance which he named cinchonino, from cinchona bark.
Ensaio sobre o cinchonino, e sobre sua influencia em a virtude da quina, e de outras cascas. Mem. Acad. real. sci. de Lisboa, 3: 202–217, 1810

Gomez, D. M. See L. H. Vaquez
Gomori, George. See G. Gömöri
Gompertz, Louis Michael. New Haven physician. 1872–
TEST—
Studies on the action of histamin on human gastric se-cretion with M. G. Vorhaus, J. Lab. clin. Med., 11: 14–21, Oct. 1925
The effect of smaller doses of histamin in stimulating human gastric secretion with W. Cohen, Amer. J. med. Sci., 177: 59–64, Jan. 1929

Gongerot, Henri. French dermatologist. 1881–
DERMATITIS—
Nouveau cas de dermatite lichenoide purpurique et pigmentaire with P. Blum, Bull. Soc. fr. derm. syph., 41: 889–892, 1934

Gonin, Jules. Belgian ophthalmologist. 1870–1935
OPERATION—for retinal detachment.
Nouveaux cas de guérison opératoire de décollements rétiniens. Ann. d'ocul., Bruxelles, 164: 817–826, 1927
Le décollement de la rétine: pathogénie, traitement. Lausanne, Payot, 1934. 279 pp.

Gooch, Benjamin. English surgeon. c. 1700–1780?
SPLINT—of long, thin strips of wood attached to canvas or leather.
In his: *Cases and practical remarks in surgery.* 1758
Good, Clarence Allen. American physician. 1907–
METHOD—
The determination of glycogen with H. Kramer and M. Somogyi, J. biol. Chem., 100: 485–491, Apr. 1933
Goodale, Joseph Lincoln. Boston laryngologist. 1868–
Proved absorptive power of tonsil.
Ueber die Absorption von Fremdkörpern durch die Gaumentonsillen des Menschen mit Bezug auf die Entstehung von infectiösen Processen. Arch. Laryngol. u. Rhinol., 7: 90–95, 1898

Goodall, Alexander. English physician. 1876–
Showed that autolyzed yeast is moderately effective against pernicious anemia.
The treatment of pernicious anemia by marmite. Lancet, 2: 781–782, Oct. 8, 1932

Goodall, James Robert. Montreal surgeon. 1878–
Advocated use of placental blood for transfusion.
An inexhaustible source of blood for transfusion and its preservation. Preliminary report with F. O. Ander-son, G. T. Altimas and F. L. MacPhail, S. G. O., 66: 176–178, Feb. 1, 1938
Goodell, Helen. See Isolde T. Zeckwer
Goodell, M. See M. Sahyun
Goodenough, Florence Laura. American psychologist. 1886–
TEST—for intelligence, by drawings.
A new approach to the measurement of the intelligence of young children. Pedag. Semin., Worcester, 33: 185–211, 1926
An early intelligence test. Child. Develop., 5: 13–18, 1934
Goodlad, William. English surgeon
Ligated external iliac artery, July 29, 1811.
Case of inguinal aneurism cured by tying the external iliac artery. Edinburgh Med. and Surg., J., 8: 32–39, Jan. 1812
Goodman, Edward Harris. Philadelphia physician. 1880–1939
REAGENT—for albumin in urine.
A new method for the quantitative estimation of al-bumin in urine with Suzanne Stern, J. A. M. A., 51: 2055–2057, Dec. 12, 1908
Goodner, K. See F. L. Horsfall, Jr.
Goodpasture, Ernest William. American patholog-ist. 1886–
FIBRINOLYSIS TIME—
Fibrinolysis in chronic hepatic insufficiency. Johns Hopk. Hosp. Bull., 25: 330–336, Nov. 1914
STAIN—for bacteria.
An acid polychrome-methylene blue solution for rou-tine and special staining. J. A. M. A., 69: 998 (only), Sept. 22, 1917
STAIN—eosin-methylene blue, for pancreas. Ibid.
STAIN—carbol-anilin-fuchsin.
A study of rabies, with reference to a neural transmis-sion of the virus in rabbits, and the structure and sig-nificance of Negri bodies. Amer. J. Path., 1: 547–582, Nov. 1925
STAIN—peroxidase.
A peroxidase reaction with sodium nitroprusside and benzidine in blood smears and tissues. J. Lab. clin. Med., 4: 442–444, Apr. 1919
Goodsir, John. Scottish anatomist. 1814–1867
Discovered Sarcina ventriculi.
History of a case in which a fluid periodically ejected from the stomach contained vegetable organisms of an undescribed form. Edinburgh Med. and Surg. J., 57: 430–443, Apr. 1, 1842
Suggested cell theory (of Virchow). In: *Anatomical and pathological observations* with H. D. S. Goodsir, Edinburgh, Macphail, 1845. 127 pp.
Studied periosteum. Ibid., Ch. 20 and 21
Described minute anatomy of kidney.
Observations on the structure and some of the pathologi-cal changes of the kidney and liver.
In: *The anatomical memoirs of....* Edinburgh, Black, 1868. 2 vols.
Goormaghtigh, Norbert. Belgian physician. 1890–
CELLS—of kidney, possible producers of renin.
Les segments neuro-myo-artériels juxta-glomérulaires du rein. Arch. Biol., Paris, 43: 575–591, Nov. 15, 1932

L'appareil neuro-myo-artériel juxta-glomérulaire du rein: ses réactions en pathologie et ses rapports avec le tube urinifère. C. R. Soc. Biol., 124: 293–296, Dec. 19, 1937
Produced in mice by injection of follicular hormone a condition resembling Reclus' disease in morphology.
Realisation experimentale de la maladie de Reclus de la mamelle chez la souris with A. Amerlinck, Bull. de l'Ass. franc. p. l'etude du cancer, 19: 527–543, July 1930

Gordinier, Hermon Camp. Troy, N. Y. physician. 1864–1930
Wrote—
The gross and minute anatomy of the central nervous system. Philadelphia, Blakiston, 1899. 589 pp.

Gordon, Alexander. Aberdeen obstetrician. 1752–1799
Described contagious and infectious nature of puerperal infection.
A treatise on the epidemic puerperal fever of Aberdeen. London, Robinson, 1795. 124 pp.

Gordon, Alfred. Philadelphia neurologist. 1874–
REFLEX—extension of great toe when sudden pressure is made on deep flexor muscles of calf of leg.
A new reflex: paradoxic flexor reflex. Its diagnostic value. Amer. Med., 8: 971 (only), Dec. 3, 1904

Gordon, Ethel M. See F. D. White

Gordon, Harold. Louisville pathologist. 1894–
METHOD—
A precise silver impregnation method for blood cells. J. Lab. clin. Med., 22: 294–298, Dec. 1936

Gordon, Merwyn Henry. English physician. 1872–
TEST—biologic, for lymphadenoma.
In: T. Horder, *Rose research on lymphadenoma. Studies on the etiology of lymphadenoma.* Bristol, Wright, 1932
Also: Baltimore, Wood, 1932
Remarks on Hodgkin's disease. A pathogenic agent in the glands, and its application in diagnosis. Brit. med. J., 1: 641–644, Apr. 15, 1933
TRYPAGAR—
An experimental study of the cultural requirements of the meningococcus. Together with a description of an easily prepared medium for that micro-organism. Ibid., 2: 678–684, Nov. 18, 1916

Gore, S. N. Bombay scientist
TEST—for indican in urine.
A simple method for detecting and estimating indican in the urine by means of the cotton-wool plug test. Indian Med. Gaz., 59: 393–396, Aug. 1924

Gorgas, William Crawford. U. S. Army surgeon. 1854–1920
Organized sanitary conditions in Cuba and Panama Canal Zone.
A few general directions with regard to destroying mosquitoes, particularly the yellow fever mosquito. Washington, Gov. Print. Off., 1904
Sanitation of the tropics with special reference to malaria and yellow fever. J. A. M. A., 52: 1075–1077, Apr. 3, 1909
Sanitation in Panama. New York, Appleton, 1916. 298 pp.

Gorham, George Elmer. Albany, N. Y. physician. 1850–1925
BED—
The improved Gorham adjustable bed. Albany, Argus

Co., 1922. 19 pp. (First manufactured in 1892 and improved in 1922)

Gorham, L(emuel) Whittington. Albany, N. Y. physician. 1885–
SIGN—
The significance of transient localized pericardial friction in coronary thrombosis (pericarditis epistenocardica). Albany Med. Ann., 41: 109–130, Apr. 1920
THEORY—
Coronary occlusion with and without pain: analysis of one hundred cases in which autopsy was done with reference to the tension factor in cardiac pain with S. J. Martin, Arch. intern. Med., 62: 821–839, Nov 1938
Cardiac pain: an experimental study with reference to the tension factor with S. J. Martin, Ibid., 840–852
The tension theory of cardiac pain. Res. Publ. Ass nerv. ment. Dis., 23: 337–344, 1943

Gosio, Bartolomeo. Rome physician
SOLUTION—glycerol aspartic acid, for studying Vibrio cholera asiaticae.
Zersetzungen zuckerhaltigen Nährmateriales durch der Vibrio cholerae asiaticae Koch. Arch. Hyg., Bert. 22: 1–27 (25), 1894

Gosselin, Léon Athanese. French surgeon. 1815–1887
FRACTURE—V-shaped of distal end of tibia.
Des fractures en V et de leurs complications. Paris Claye, 1866. 15 pp.

Goth, A. Nashville pharmacologist
METHOD—
A simple clinical method for determining sulfonamide in blood. J. Lab. clin. Med., 27: 827–829, Mar. 1943

Gottheil, O. German physician
SOLUTION—carbohydrate glycerol; culture medium
Botanische Beschreibung einiger Bodenbakterien Beiträge zur Methode der Speciesbestimmung und Vorarbeit für die Entscheidung der Frage nach der Bedeutung der Bodenbakterien für die Landwirtschaft Zbl. Bakt., 2 Abt., 7: 430–435, et seq., (432), Ma 30, 1901

Gottlieb, Rudolf. Heidelberg pharmacologist. 1864–1924
Introduced dilaudid.
Vergleichende Messungen über die Gewöhnung de Atemzentrums am Morphin, Dicodid und Dilaudio Münch. med. Wschr., 73: 595–596, Apr. 9, 1926

Gottstein, Georg. Breslau surgeon. 1868–
OPERATION—for dilatation of esophagus.
Technick und Klinik der Oesophagoskopie. Mitt Grenzgeb. Med. Chir., 6: 560–604, 1900
Surgery of the esophagus. In: Keen's Surgery. Phila delphia, Saunders, 1908. 3: 780–824

Gottstein, Jacob. Breslau otologist. 1832–1895
FIBERS—part of expansion of auditory nerve in cochlea.
PROCESS—connecting basilar membrane of organ of Corti with an outer hair-cell.
Ueber den feinern Bau und die Entwicklung de Gehörschnecke beim Menschen und den Säugethierer Bonn, Cohen, 1871. 55 pp.

Gougerot, H. See C. L. de Beurmann

Gough, Alfred. Leeds surgeon
OPERATION—
A modification of the Fothergill operation for prolapse

J. Obstet. Gynaec., Brit. Empire, 38: 844-846, Winter, 1931

Goulard, Thomas. French surgeon. ?-1784

EXTRACT or SOLUTION—lead subacetate, for dressing infected parts (obsolete).

Traité sur les effets des préparations de plomb, et principalement de l'extrait de saturne, employé sous différentes formes, et pour différentes maladies chirurgicales. Montpellier, Gontier et Faure, 1760. 322 pp.

Gould, George Milbry. American ophthalmologist. 1847-1922

Showed that minute error of refraction may cause nervous irritation. Garrison

The psychological influence of errors of refraction and of their correction. Med. and Surg. Reporter, 59: 396-398, Sept. 29, 1888

Gould, Sylvester Emanuel. Detroit pathologist. 1900-

TEST—

The one-hour two-dose glucose tolerance test. Amer. J. Clin. Path., 7: 474-481, Nov. 1937

Gould, William Lawrence. Albany physician. 1897-

APPARATUS—

An adjustable extension for fractures of the upper third of the femur. Amer. J. Surg., 9: 527-529, Sept. 1930

HEMOGLOBINOMETER—

A new hemoglobinometer: a no-blood-drop method, using the principle of transillumination. New York State J. Med., 46: 1122-1124, May 15, 1946

Gouley, John William Severin. American surgeon. 1843-1920

CATHETER—a solid, curved instrument to be passed through a urethral stricture. Dorland

On external perineal urethrotomy, or an improved method of external division of the urethra in perinaeo, for the relief of obstinate stricture; with remarks on the preparatory and after-treatment. New York Med. J., 9: 449-478, Aug. 1869

Notes on urethral catheterism, catheters, and bougies. Ibid., 70: 660-666, Nov. 4: 701-706, Nov. 11, 1899

Gowers, Sir William Richard. English neurologist. 1845-1915

APPARATUS or HEMOMETER—

On the numeration of blood-corpuscles. Lancet, 2: 797-798, Dec. 1, 1877

The numeration of blood corpuscles, and the effect of iron and phosphorus on the blood. Practitioner, London, 21: 1-17, July 1878

(*Apparatus for the clinical estimation of the haemoglobin in the blood.*) Lancet, 2: 882 (only), Dec. 21, 1878

COLUMN OF—mass of fibers in front of direct cerebellar tract.

Diagnosis of diseases of the spinal cord. 1879

Also: *A manual of diseases of the nervous system.* Philadelphia, Blakiston, 1895. 2 ed. vol. 1, p. 183

CONTRACTION—of gastrocnemius on tapping muscles of leg. Ibid., p. 18

DISEASE—saltatory spasm. Ibid., London, Churchill, 1886-88. vol. 2, p. 79

MYOPATHY—distal form of.

A lecture on myopathy and a distal form. Brit. med. J., 2: 89-92, July 12, 1902

SOLUTION—

The numeration of blood-corpuscles. Lancet, 2: 901 (only), Dec. 21, 1878

SYNDROME—irregularity of pupillary light reflex sometimes seen in tabes dorsalis.

A manual of diseases of the nervous system. Philadelphia, Blakiston, 1895. 2 ed., vol. 1, p. 407

Described retinal vessels in hypertension.

The state of the arteries in Bright's disease. Brit. med. J., 2: 743-745, Dec. 9, 1876

Also, in: F. A. Willius and T. E. Keys' *Cardiac classics.* St. Louis, Mosby, 1941. pp. 605-611

Described epilepsy.

Epilepsy and other chronic convulsive diseases. London, Churchill, 1881

Successfully removed tumor of spinal cord.

A case of tumor of the spinal cord; removal; recovery. Med.-chir. Trans., London, 71: 377-430, 1888

Introduced aluminum chloride treatment of tabes. Garrison

A manual of diseases of the nervous system. Philadelphia, Blakiston, 1895. 2 ed., vol. 1, p. 437

Described ataxic paraplegia. Ibid., pp. 453-460

Described local panatrophy.

Local panatrophy. Rev. Neurol. and Psychiat., Edinburgh, 1: 3-4, 1903

Graaf, Regnier de. Dutch physician. 1641-1673

FOLLICLE or OVULE—(Name applied by Haller about 1730).

De mulierum organis generationi inservientibus tractatus novus; demonstrans tam homines et animalia caetera omnia, quae vivipara dicuntur, haud minus quam ovipara ab ovo originem ducere. Lugduni Batavorum, Hackiana, 1677. 334 pp.

Also: *Opera omnia.* Leyden, 1686

Also, Ch. XII, transl. by R. Knox, Edinburgh, 1848

Also, Ch. XII, transl. by G. W. Corner in: *Essays in biology, in honor of H. M. Evans.* Berkeley, Univ. Calif. Press, 1943

Described method of collecting pancreatic juice by means of temporary pancreatic fistula. Garrison

Disputatio medica de natura et usu succi pancreatici. Leyden, Hackiana, 1664

Published classic account of testicle.

De virorum organis generationi inservientibus, de clysteribus et de usu siphonis in anatomia. Leyden, Hackiana, 1668. 234 pp.

Grace, Roderick Vincent. New York surgeon. 1885-

FASCIA STRIPPER—

A subcutaneous fascial stripper. Ann. Surg., 90: 1109-1110, Dec. 1929

Grad, Hermann. New York gynecologist. 1872-

OPERATION—

The technique of formation of an artificial vagina. S. G. O., 54: 200-206, Feb. 1932

Gradenigo, Giuseppe. Italian physician. 1859-1926

SYNDROME—otitis, temporoparietal pain and abductor paralysis.

Sulla leptomeningite circonscritta e sulla paralis: dell'abducente di origine otitica. Gior. d. r. Accad. di med. di Torino, 4 s., 10: 59-64; 270; 361-367, 1904

Ueber circumscripte Leptomeningitis mit spinalen Symptomen und über Paralyse des N. abducens otitischen Ursprungs. Arch. f. Ohrenheilk., 62: 255-270, Aug. 26, 1904

Gradle, Harry Searls. Chicago ophthalmologist. 1883–
OPERATION—
A simple needle for diathermy treatment of retinal detachment. Amer. J. Ophthal., 18: 956–957, Oct. 1935
TONOMETER—
Tonometry; with description of a tonometer. Ophthal. Rev., 21: 468–471, Sept. 1912
Gradwohl, Rutherford Birchard Hayes. St. Louis physician. 1877–
TECHNIC—for cultivation of gonococci.
The diagnosis of gonorrhea by culture. J. A. M. A., 87: 242 (only), July 24, 1926
Cultural characteristics of the neisseria gonorrhoeae Urol. and Cur. Rev., 35: 434–442, July 1931
TEST—
The Hecht-Weinberg reaction as a control over the Wassermann reaction: a study based on one thousand parallel tests with both methods. J. A. M. A., 63: 240–242, July 18, 1914
The Hecht-Weinberg-Gradwohl test in the diagnosis of syphilis: its superiority over the Wassermann test in untreated and treated syphilitics. Ibid., 68: 514–521, Feb. 17, 1917
Graefe, Albrecht von. (Friederich Wilhelm Ernst Albrecht von Graefe). German ophthalmologist. 1828–1870
DISEASE—progressive ophthalmoplegia.
Demonstration in der Berliner medizinischen Gesellschaft vom 19. Februar 1868. Berl. klin. Wschr., 5: 127 (only), Mar. 16, 1868
KNIFE—used in extraction of cataract.
OPERATION—for cataract.
Ueber die Coremorphosis als Mittel gegen chronische Iritis und Iridochorioiditis. Arch. Ophthal., 2: 2 Abth., 202–257, 1856
Ueber die Iridectomie bei Glaucom und über den glaucomatösen Process. Ibid., 3: 2 Abth., 456–560, 1857
Also, transl. by T. Windsor, London, New Sydenham Soc., 1859
Ueber modificirte Linearextraction. Arch. Ophthal., 11: 3 Abth., 1–106, 1865
Nachiträgliche Bemerkungen über die modificirte Linearextraction. Ibid., 12: 1 Abth., 150–223, 1866
OPERATION—for strabismus.
Beiträge zur Lehre vom Schielen und von der Schiel-Operation. Ibid., 3: 1 Abth., 177–386, 1857
SIGN—lag of upper lid in looking downward, in exophthalmic goiter.
Ueber Basedow'sche Krankheit. Dtsch. Klinik., 16: 158–159, Apr. 16, 1864
Diagnosed embolism of retinal artery as a cause of sudden blindness.
Ueber Embolie der Arteria Centralis retinae als Ursache plötzlicher Erblindung. Arch. Ophthal., 5: 1 Abth., 136–157, 1859
Founder of modern knowledge of symptomatology of ocular paralyses. Garrison
Symptomenlehre der Augenmuskellähmungen. Berlin Peters, 1867. 175 pp.
Described conical cornea.
Angeborne, mit zahlreichen Haaren versehene Geschwulst auf der Hornhautgränze. Arch. Ophthal., 1: 1 Abth., 297–330, 1854
Ueber Ceratoconus. Berl. klin. Wschr., 60: 241–244, June 8: 249–254, June 15, 1868

Graefe, Alfred Carl. German ophthalmologist. 1830–1899
Made clinical analysis of disordered movements of eye.
Klinische Analyse der Motilitätsstörungen des Auges. Berlin, Peters, 1858
Graefe, Carl Ferdinand von. Warsaw surgeon. 1787–1840
OPERATION—for congenital cleft-palate.
Die Gaumennath, ein neuentdecktes Mittel gegen angeborene Fehler der Sprache. J. Chir. u. Augenheilk., Berlin, 1: 1–54, 1820
Introduced rhinoplasty.
Rhinoplastik, oder die Kunst den Verlust der Nase organisch zu ersetzen, in ihren früheren Verhältnissen erforscht und durch neue Verfahrungsweisen zur höheren Vollkommenheit gefördert. Berlin, (Reimer) 1818. 210 pp.
Same, in Latin Berolini, Reimerum, 1818. 168 pp.
First German surgeon to ligate innominate artery. 1822. Garrison
Account of Graefe's ligature of the Arteria Innominata. Communicated in a letter to Dr. Macleod, from Prof. Wagner of Berlin. London M. and Phys. J. 49: 475 (only), June 1823
Gräupner, Salo Ch. German physician
TESTS—for cardiac efficiency.
Die mechanische Prüfung und Beurtheilung der Herzleistung. Berl. Klinik, 174: 1–35, 1902
Die Messung der Herzkraft und deren Bedeutung für die Diagnose und Behandlung der chronischen Herzkrankheiten. München, Gmelin, 1905. 23 pp.
Funktionelle Bestimmung der Leistungsfähigkeit des Herzmuskels und deren Bedeutung für die Diagnostik der Herzkrankheiten. Dtsch. med. Wschr., 32: 1029–1032, June 28, 1906
Graham, A. S. See F. W. Rankin
Graham, Allen. Cleveland surgeon. 1886–
Demonstrated similarity of response to iodine in both adenomatous and non-adenomatous goiter.
Exophthalmic goiter and toxic adenoma: similarity of response to iodine with E. C. Cutler, Ann. Surg., 84: 497–508, Oct. 1926
Graham, Evarts Ambrose. St. Louis surgeon. 1883–
OPERATION—
Pneumectomy with the cautery: a safer substitute for the ordinary lobectomy in cases of chronic suppuration of the lung. J. A. M. A., 81: 1010–1012, Sept. 22, 1923
TEST—
Roentgenologic examination of the gallbladder: preliminary report of a new method utilizing the intravenous injection of tetrabromphenolphthalein with W. H. Cole, Ibid., 82: 613–614, Feb. 23, 1924
Visualization of the gallbladder by the sodium salt of tetrabromphenolphthalein with W. H. Cole and G. H Copher, Ibid., 1777–1778, May 31, 1924
Performed successful total pneumonectomy.
Successful removal of an entire lung for carcinoma of the bronchus with J. J. Singer, Ibid., 101: 1371–1374, Oct. 28, 1933
See also D. S. Allen
Graham, George Sellers. Albany pathologist. 1879–1942
STAIN—for oxydase granules.
TECHNIC—of oxydase test.
The oxidizing ferment of the myelocyte series of cell

and its demonstration by an alphanaphthol-pyronin method. J. med. Res., 35: 231–242, Nov. 1916
Benzidine as a peroxidase reagent for blood smears and tissues. Ibid., 39: 15–24, Sept. 1918

Graham, John Henry Porteus. English physician
Reported trench fever.
A note on a relapsing febrile illness of unknown origin Lancet, 2: 703–704, Sept. 25, 1915

Graham, Roscoe Reid. Toronto surgeon. 1889–
METHOD—of exteriorization of posterior wall duodenal ulcer.
Technical surgical procedures for gastric and duodenal ulcer. S. G. O., 66: 269–287, Feb. 15, 1938
OPERATION—"three interrupted sutures tied over a free omental graft."
The treatment of perforated duodenal ulcers. Ibid., 64: 235–238, Feb. 1, 1937
OPERATION—
A technique for total gastrectomy. Surgery, 8: 257–264, Aug. 1940

Graham, Thomas. Glasgow chemist. 1806–1869
LAW—regulating rate of diffusion of gas through membrane.
A short account of experimental researches on the diffusion of gases through each other, and their separation by mechanical means. Quart. J. Sci., 2 s., 6: 74–83, July–Sept. 1829
Investigated osmotic force.
On osmotic force. Philos. Trans., 144: 177–228, 1854
Introduced term colloid and made distinction between colloid and crystalloid substances.
Liquid diffusion applied to analysis. Ibid., 151: 183–224, 1861

Graham-Smith, George Stuart. English physician
INFUSION—heart; culture medium.
The behavior of bacteria in fluid cultures as indicated by daily estimates of the numbers of living organisms. J. Hyg., Camb., 19: 133–204 (136), Oct. 1920

Grainger, Richard Dugard. English neurologist 1801–1865
Discovered that gray matter in spinal cord and afferent roots is true medium of reflex action.
Observations on the structure and functions of the spinal cord. London, Highley, 1837. 159 pp.

Gram, Hans Christian Joachim. Copenhagen physician. 1853–1938
METHOD—
The results of a new method for determining the fibrin-percentage in blood and plasma. Acta med. scand., 56: 107–161, 1922
SOLUTION and STAIN—
Ueber die isolierte Färbung der Schizomyceten in Schnitt- und Trochenpräparaten. Fort. d. med., 2: 185–189, Mar. 15, 1884

Grancher, Jacques Joseph. French physician. 1843– physician. 1843–1907
DISEASE—
La spleno-pneumonie. Union med., Paris, 3 s., 36: 1078–1081, Dec. 23; 1108–1112, Dec. 27; 1117–1121, Dec. 29, 1883
SYSTEM—boarding out of children from tuberculous households in France.

Grandidier, Johann Ludwig. German physician. 1810–
Described hemophilia.

Die Haemophilie oder die Bluterkrankheit. Leipzig, Wigand, 1855

Grandy, C. C. See D. F. Cameron

Granger, Amedee. American roentgenologist. 1879–1939
SIGN—
A positive sign of extensive destruction of the mastoid of infants. Radiology, 14: 495–503, May 1930

Grant, Ronald Thomson. English scientist
Demonstrated function of glomus to regulate loss of heat and to maintain temperature of exposed parts.
Observations on arteriovenous anastomoses in human skin and in the bird's foot with special reference to the reaction to cold. Heart, 15: 385–407, July 1931

Grant, Samuel Becker. American physician. 1896–
Showed that alkalosis alone, without alteration of physiologically active fraction of blood calcium, may produce tetany.
A study of forced respiration: experimental production of tetany with A. Goldman, Amer. J. Physiol., 52: 209–232, June 1920

Granville, Joseph Mortimer. English physician. 1833–1900
HAMMER—for performing vibratory massage.
Percussion as a therapeutic agent in nervous diseases. Brit. med. J., 1: 339–340, Mar. 11, 1882
Nerve-vibration and excitation as agents in the treatment of functional disorder and organic disease. London, Churchill, 1833. 128 pp.

Graser, Ernst. German surgeon. 1860–1929
DIVERTICULUM—false, of sigmoid.
Ueber multiple falsche Darmdivertikel in der Flexura sigmoidea. Münch. med. Wschr., 16: 721–723, May 30, 1899
OPERATION—for dislocation of patella.
Behandlung der Luxatio patellae inverterata durch Osteotomie am Femur mit Drehung der Epiphyse. Zbl. Chir., 31: 169–170, 1904

Grassberger, Roland. Vienna physician. 1867–
AGAR—blood; for cultivation of influenza bacilli.
Beiträge zur Bakteriologie der Influenza. Z. Hyg. InfektKr., 25: 453–475, (462), 1897

Grassi, Battista. Italian pathologist. 1854–1925
Demonstrated presence of hookworm disease by fecal examination.
Intorno all'Anchilostoma duodenale (Dubini) with C. Parona and E. Parona, Gazz. med. lomb., Milano, 7 s., 5: 193–196, 1878
Showed, with A. Bignami, that parasites of malaria develop only in Anopheles mosquito.
Ciclo evolutive della semilune nell'Anopheles claviger. Ann. d'ig. sper., Roma, n. s. 9: 258–264, 1899

Graupner, Heinz. Leipzig scientist
METHOD—dioxane, of embedding tissue.
Über die Verwendung des Dioxans beim Einbetten mikroskopischer Objekte with A. Weissberger, Zool. Anz., 96: 204–206, Oct. 15, 1931

Graunt, John. English draper. 1620–1674
Wrote first book on vital statistics. Garrison
Natural and political observations mentioned in a following index, and made upon the bills of mortality. With reference to the government, religion, trade, growth, air, disease, and the several changes of the said city. London, Martyn, 1662

Graves, A. M. See E. W. A. Ochsner

Graves, R. C. See J. H. Cunningham, S. Warren

Graves, Robert James. Irish physician. 1796–1853
DISEASE—exophthalmic goiter.
Newly observed affection of the thyroid gland in females.
London Med. and Surg. J., 7, pt. 2: 516–517, 1835
Also: Med. Classics, 5: 25–43, Sept. 1940
Reported indirect fracture of rib as result of muscular violence associated with coughing in pulmonary tuberculosis.
Fracture of a rib produced by a violent fit of coughing.
Dublin J. Med. and Chem. Sci., 3: 353–355, 1833
Also: Amer. J. med. Sci., 13: 553–554, 1834

Graves, Sara Stowell. New York City scientist
TEST—
A precipitant for ammonia. (A substitute for Nessler's reagent.) J. Amer. Chem. Soc., 37: 1171–1181, May 1915

Graves, William Phillips. American gynecologist. 1370–1933
OPERATION—modification of Olshausen o. of ventral suspension for retroversion of uterus.
Operations for uterine malposition. In: *Gynecology.*
Philadelphia, Saunders, 1923. 1016 pp. pp. 726–728
OPERATION—
Method of constructing an artificial vagina. Surg. Clin. N. Amer., 1: 611–614, June 1921

Grawitz, Paul Albert. Greifswald pathologist. 1850–1932
CELLS—slumber c. in connective tissue.
Betheiligung der Leukocyten an der Gewebsneubildung.
Verh. d. X. internat. med. Cong., 1890, Berlin, 2, 3 Abth.: 9–11, 1891
TUMOR—of kidney.
Die sogenannten Lipome der Niere. Arch. f. path. Anat., 93: 39–63, July 2, 1883
Die Entstehung von Nierentumoren aus Nebennierengewebe. Arch. clin. Chir., 30: 824–834, 1884

Gray, Henry McIlree Williamson. English surgeon. 1870–1938
SIGN—of appendicitis.
Physical factors in the production of appendicitis. Points in diagnoses. Their influence on surgical treatment. Illinois Med. J., 48: 33–38 (36), July 1925
Revived debridement of wounds.
Treatment of gunshot wounds by excision and primary suture. Brit. med. J., 2: 317–320, Aug. 28, 1915

Gray, Seymour J. Chicago physician. 1911–
TEST—for liver function.
The colloidal gold reaction of blood serum in diseases of the liver. Arch. intern. Med., 65: 524–544, Mar. 1940

Greco, Aldo. Italian physician
TEST—for bilirubin in urine.
Un nuovo metodo per la ricerca qualitativa e quantitativa della bilirubina nelle urine col diazoreattivo di Daddi. Diag. e Tech. d. Lab., Naples, 2: 925–932, Nov. 25, 1931
Also, abstr.: J. A. M. A., 98: 1123 (only), Mar. 26, 1932

Greeff, Julius Hermann Adolf. Stuttgart physician. 1876–
TEST—for blood in urine.
Beitrag zum Nachweis geringer Blutmengen mit der Benzidinprobe. Med. Klin., No. 45: 1785–1786, Nov. 6, 1910

Green, Aaron Samuel. San Francisco ophthalmologist. 1878–1941

OPERATION—
An operation for keratoconus with report of two cases with L. D. Green, Amer. J. Ophthal., 3: 429–432, June 1920
OPERATION—
Vacuum method of intracapsular cataract extraction with L. D. Green, Ibid., 5: 92–96, Feb. 1922

Green, Horace. Vermont laryngologist. 1802–1866
Wrote on bronchitis.
A treatise on diseases of the air passages ... bronchitis, chronic laryngitis, clergyman's sore throat, etc. New York and London, Wiley and Putnam, 1846. 276 pp.
Described cystic and malignant laryngeal growths.
On the surgical treatment of polypi of the larynx, and edema of the glottis. New York. Putnam, 1852. 124 pp.

Green, Joseph Harry. English surgeon. 1791–1863
Performed thyroidectomy.
Removal of the right lobe of the thyroid gland. Lancet, 2: 351–352, June 13, 1829

Green, R. G. See Chastek

Green-Armytage, Vivian Bartley. English physician in India. 1882–
METHOD—of delivery in posterior position.
The occipito-posterior position; its complications and treatment; with observations on the insulin-glucose method in shock. Indian Med. Gaz., 62: 675–680, Dec. 1927

Greenberg, Boris Efim. Boston urologist. 1886–
METHOD—
A new method for staining spermatozoa with S. Berman, S. L. Gargill and R. C. Griffin. J. clin. Endocrinol., 3: 179–180, Mar. 1943

Greenberg, David Morris. California biochemist. 1895–
METHOD—
The calorimetric determination of the serum proteins. J. biol. Chem., 82: 545–550, May 1929

Greenberg, Geza. New York urologist. 1882–
URETHROSCOPE—
A new operating composite cysto-urethroscope. Ann. Surg., 37: 213–221, Aug. 1919

Greenblatt, R. B. See H. S. Kupperman

Greene, H. J. See L. Loewe

Greenfield, William Smith. London surgeon. 1846–1919
Described giant cells in tissues of Hodgkin's disease.
Specimens illustrative of the pathology of lymphadenoma and leucocythemia. Trans. Path. Soc. London, 29: 272–304, 1878
Described pathologic anatomy of thyroid in exophthalmic goiter.
Some diseases of the thyroid gland. Lancet 2: 1493–1497; 1553–1555, 1893

Greenhow, Edward Headlam. English physician. 1814–1888
DISEASE—
A case of vagabond's discoloration simulating the bronzed skin of Addison's disease. London Clin. Soc. Trans., 9: 44–47, 1876
Wrote on pneumoconiosis.
Specimen of diseased lung from a case of grinder's asthma. Specimen of coal-miner's black lung. Trans. Path. Soc., London, 16: 59–61, 1864
Added to knowledge of Addison's disease.
On Addison's disease; clinical lectures on Addison's

disease and a report on disease of the supra-renal capsules. London, Roche, 1866. 64 pp.
Addison's disease. Lancet, 1: 327 et seq., 1875
Also: London, Longmans, 1875. 212 pp.

Greenwald, Isidor. New York biochemist. 1887–
METHOD—for determination of phosphatides of blood.
The estimation of lipoid and acid-soluble phosphorus in small amounts of serum. J. biol. Chem., 21: 29–36, May 1915

Greenwood, Allen. American ophthalmologist. 1866–1942
OPERATION—
Combined iridencleisis and sclerectomy for chronic glaucoma. Amer. J. Ophth., 13: 301–303, Apr. 1930

Greenwood, Major. English physician. 1880–
RECONSTRUCTION—
On the determination of size of family and of the distribution of characters in order of birth from samples taken through members of the sibships with G. U. Yule, J. R. statist. Soc., 77: 179–199, Jan. 1914

Gregersen, J. P. Copenhagen physician
TEST—for blood.
Untersuchungen über okkulte Blutungen. Arch. verdauKr., 25: 169–195, 1919

Gregersen, Magnus I(ngstrup). American scientist. 1903–
METHOD—
Plasma volume determination with dyes; errors in colorimetry; use of the blue dye T-1824 with J. G. Gibson and E. A. Stead, Amer. J. Physiol., 113: 54–55, Sept. 1, 1935
An analysis of colorimetric methods in relation to plasma volume determinations. J. Lab. clin. Med., 23: 423–430, Jan. 1938
Simultaneous determinations of plasma volume with T-1824 and "available fluid" volume with sodium thiocyanate with J. D. Stewart, Amer. J. Physiol., 125: 142–152, Jan. 1939
MODIFICATION—
A practical method for the determination of blood volume with the dye T-1824; a survey of the present basis of the dye-method and its clinical applications. J. Lab. clin. Med., 29: 1266–1286, Dec. 1944

Gregory, Raymond Lestie. American biochemist. 1901–
TEST—for bile acids.
The quantitative determination of bile acids by means of a new color reaction and mono-chromatic light with T. A. Pascoe, J. biol. Chem., 83: 35–42, July 1929

Gréhant, Restor. French scientist. 1838–1910
METHOD—for determination of blood volume with carbon monoxide.
Mesure du volume de sang contenu dans l'organisme d'une mammifère vivant with C. E. Quinquaud, C. R. Acad. Sci., 94: 1450–1453, May 29, 1882

Greiffenhagen, Wilhelm. Esthonia surgeon
OPERATION—
Zur Technik der Splenopexis und Ätiologie der Wandermilz. Zbl. Chir., 24: 124–128, Feb. 6, 1897

Greig, David Middleton. Edinburgh scientist. ?–1936
Described hypertelorism.
Hypertelorism: a hitherto undifferentiated congenital cranio-facial deformity. Edinburgh med. J., 31: 560–593, Oct. 1924

Grenacher, Hans. Rostock scientist. 1884–
STAINS—alum carmine and alcoholic borax carmine.
Einige Notizen zur Tinctionstechnik, besonders zur Kernfärbung. Arch. f. mikr. Anat., 16: 463–471, 1879

Gretsel, Dr. Berlin physician
Described splenic anemia.
Ein Fall von Anaemia splenica bei einem Kinde. Berl. klin. Wschr., 3: 212–214, May 14, 1886

Grew, Nehemiah. English scientist. 1641–1712
Noticed "cells" in plants; "Was probably the first to note the existence of sex in plants." Garrison
The anatomy of plants.... (London), 1682. 304 pp.

Griesinger, Wilhelm. German neurologist. 1817–1868
DISEASE—anemia with dropsy, caused by ankylostomum duodenale.
Klinische und anatomische Beobachtungen über die Krankheiten von Egypten. Arch. f. physiol. Heilk., Stuttgart, 13: 528–575, et seq., 1854
DISEASE—pseudohypertrophic muscular dystrophy.
Ueber Muskelhypertrophie. Arch. d. Heilk., 6: 1–13, 1865
Described infantile splenic anemia.
Ein Fall von Anaemia splenica bei einem Kinde. Berl. klin. Wschr., 3: 212–214, May 14, 1866
From Policlinic of Dr. Griesinger, contributed by Dr. Gretsel, Assistant Physician

Gries, Peter. German scientist
TEST—for fecal material in water.
Notiz über die Anwendung von Diazoverbindungen zur Nachweisung von organischer Substanz im Wasser. Ber. dtsch. chem. Ges., 21: 1830–1832, 1888

Griffin, R. C. See B. E. Greenberg

Griffin, W. A. See W. Tileston

Griffith, Arthur Stanley. English physician
SOLUTION—citrated blood.
The cultivation of Spirochaeta icterohaemorrhagiae and the production of a therapeutic antispirochaetal serum. J. Hyg., Camb., 18: 59–68 (61), Apr. 1919

Griffith, Charles. Scottish surgeon
BONE SAW and NIPPERS—
Account of a circular saw, and of a new form of bone nippers. Edinburgh Med. and Surg. J., 2: 279–280, July 1815

Griffith, F. English medical officer
TECHNIC—for grouping and typing streptococci by micro-agglutination.
The serological classification of streptococcus pyogenes. J. Hyg., 34: 542–584, Dec. 1934

Grimaux, Louis Édouard. French chemist. 1835–1900
REACTION—for morphine.
Sur quelques réactions de la morphine et de ses congénères. C. R. Acad. Sci., 93: 217–219, 1881

Grimbert, Léon Louis. French chemist. 1860–1931
REACTION—for apomorphine.
Sur une réaction extrêmement sensible de l'apomorphine with A. Leclere, J. Pharm. Chim., Paris, 11: 23–24, 1915
REAGENT—for differentiating albumin and mucus in urine.
Sur le moyen de distinguer l'albumine vraie de la substance mucoinoide des urines with E. Dufau, Ibid., s 6. 24: 193–199, 1906
SOLUTION—basal peptone, for determining fermentation of Friedländer's pneumobacillus.

Recherches sur le pneumobacille de Friedländer.
Premier mémoire. Etude des fermentations provoquées
par cet organisme. Ann. Inst. Pasteur, 9: 840-853
(843), Nov. 1895
TEST—for bile pigments.
Recherche des pigments bilaires dans l'urine. J.
Pharm. Chim., Paris, s 6, 22: 487-492, 1905
TEST—for picric acid in urine.
Sur la recherches des dérivés picriques dans les urines.
Ibid., s 7, 13: 177-190, 1916
TEST—for cryogenine in urine.
Recherche de la cryogénine dans les urines. Ibid., 15:
305-306, 1917
See also W. Beckers

Grimm, Max. Helsingfors scientist
SOLUTION—basal ammonium sulphate.
Flüchtige organische Verbindungen als einzige Kohlen-
stoffquellen. Zbl. Bakt., 2 Abt., 41: 647-649, Aug. 29,
1914

Grimson, Keith Sanford. American surgeon. 1910-
OPERATION—
Total thoracic and partial to total lumbar sympathec-
tomy and celiac ganglionectomy in the treatment of
hypertension. Ann. Surg., 114: 753-775, Oct. 1941
OPERATION—
Surgery in obstinate megacolon: radical one-stage re-
section and ileosigmoidostomy with H. N. Vande-
grift and H. M. Dratz, S. G. O., 80: 164-173, Feb.
1945

Grindon, Joseph. St. Louis dermatologist. 1858-
DISEASE—ecbolic folliculitis.
A peculiar affection of the hair-follicle. J. Cutan. Dis.,
15: 256-259, June 1897
Reported cutaneous phenomena of typhoid fever.
The cutaneous phenomena of typhoid fever. Med.
Fortnightly, St. Louis, 3: 144-146, Mar. 1, 1893

Griswold, Rettig Arnold. Louisville, Ky. surgeon.
1898-
SPLINT—
Major fractures of the tibia and fibula; an apparatus
and a method of treatment. S. G. O., 58: 900-902,
May 1934

Gritti, Rocco. Milan surgeon. 1828-1920
AMPUTATION—patella is sectioned sagitally in
amputation of femur and is sutured to end of femur.
Dell'amputazione del femore al terzo inferiore e della
disarticolazione del ginocchio. Valore relativo di
cadauna, coll'indicazione di un nuovo metodo denomi-
nato amputazione del femore ai condili con lembo
patellare. Ann. univ. di med., Milano, 161: 5-32, 1857

Groat, William Avery. Syracuse, N. Y. physician.
1876-1945
TEST—
An improved clinical and a micro-chemical test for
blood. J. A. M. A., 61: 1897 (only), Nov. 22, 1913

Grocco, Pietro. Florence physician. 1857-1916
TRIANGLE or SIGN—dullness on back, on side
opposite to pleural effusion.
Triangolo paravertebrale opposto nella pleurite essu-
dativa. Lavori d. Cong. d. med. int., 1902, Roma, 12:
190, Oct. 1903

Gröer, Franz von. Vienna scientist. 1887-
SOLUTION—hydrolyzed placenta, for cultivation of
diphtheria bacillus.
Plazentabouillon als billiges und zuverlässiges Nähr-
medium zur Gewinnung von Diphtherietoxin. Zbl.
Bakt., 82: 333-336, Dec. 12, 1918

Grönblad, Ester Elizabeth. Stockholm ophthalmol-
ogist. 1898-
SYNDROME—
Angioid streaks—pseudoxanthoma elasticum. Acta
Ophthal., 7: 329 (only), 1929
Pseudoxanthoma elasticum and changes in the eye.
Acta derm. vener., Stockh., 13: 417-422, 1932-33
Angioid streaks.... Stockholm, Norstedt, 1932.
114 pp.

Groenouw, Arthur. Breslau ophthalmologist. 1862-
DISEASE or DYSTROPHY—bilateral nodular opaci-
ties of cornea.
Knötchenförmige Hornhauttrübung vererbt durch vier
Generationen. Klin. Mbl. Augenheilk., 90: 577-580,
May 1933

Groffith, Joseph. English surgeon
DEGENERATION—of undescended testicle.
The structural changes in the testicle of the dog when it
is replaced within the abdominal cavity. J. Anat. and
Physiol., 27: 483-500, July 1893

Grollman, Arthur. Baltimore physiologist. 1901-
DETERMINATION—
The determination of the cardiac output of man by the
use of acetylene. Amer. J. Physiol., 88: 432-445, Apr.
1, 1929
The cardiac output of man in health and disease,
Springfield, Ill., Thomas, 1932
See also J. R. Williams, Jr.

Gross, Morris. New York City physician
Invented a duodenal tube.
A duodenal tube; preliminary communication. New
York Med. J., 91: 77-78, Jan. 8, 1910

Gross, Oskar. German physician
METHOD—of estimation of enzyme content of gas-
tric secretion.
Die Wirksamkeit des Pepsins und eine einfache
Methode zu ihrer Bestimmung. Berl. klin. Wschr.,
45: 643-646, Mar. 30, 1908
TEST—for trypsin in feces.
Die Wirksamkeit des Trypsins und eine einfache
Methode zu ihrer Bestimmung. Arch. exp. Path.
Pharmak., 58: 157-166, Dec. 18, 1907
Zur Funktionsprüfung des Pankreas. Dtsch. med.
Wschr., 35: 706-708, Apr. 22, 1909

Gross, Robert Edward. Boston surgeon. 1905-
OPERATION—
Surgical ligation of a patent ductus arteriosus; report
of first successful case with J. P. Hubbard, J. A. M. A.,
112: 729-731, Feb. 25, 1939
Surgical management of the patent ductus arteriosus,
with summary of four surgically treated cases. Ann.
Surg., 110: 321-356, Sept. 1939

Gross, Samuel David. American surgeon. 1805-1884
DISEASE—encysted rectum.
In his: *System of surgery.* Philadelphia, Blanchard
and Lea, 3 ed., 1864. pp. 573-574
See also J. Pancoast

Grosz, Siegfried. German scientist
TEST—for methanamine in urine.
Eine Reaktion auf Hexamenthylentetramin. Wien.
klin. Wschr., 27: 755-756, May 28, 1914

Grote, L. W. See O. Kamm

Groves, Ernst W. Hey. Bristol surgeon. 1872-1944
OPERATION—
The crucial ligaments of the knee-joint: their function,
rupture, and the operative treatment of the same.
Brit. J. Surg., 7: 505-515, Apr. 1920

OPERATION—
A note on the operation for the radical cure of femoral hernia. Ibid., 10: 529–531, Apr. 1923

Groves, Thomas B. English scientist
REACTION—for morphine.
On some compounds of iodide and bromide of mercury with the alkaloids. Pharm. J., 18: 181–182, Sept. 1, 1858

Gruber, Joseph. Austrian aurist. 1827–1900
BOUGIE—for auditory meatus.
SPECULUM—for ear.
TEST—for hearing.
Lehrbuch der Ohrenheilkunde, mit besonderer Rücksicht auf Anatomie und Physiologie. Wien, Gerold's Sohn, 1870. 647 pp.

Gruber, Georg Benno Otto. Vienna pathologist. 1884–
TEST—for indican in serum.
Indikanbestimmung im Serum mit Ausschaltung der Eiweissstoffe als Azidverbindungen. Wien. med. Wschr. 82: 1253 (only), Oct. 1, 1932

Gruber, Max von. Munich bacteriologist. 1853–1927
REACTION—agglutination.
Theorie der activen und passiven Immunität gegen Cholera, Typhus und verwandte Krankheitsprocesse. Münch. med. Wschr., 43: 206–207, Mar. 3, 1896
Eine neue Methode zur raschen Erkennung des Cholera vibrio und des Typhusbacillus with H. E. Durham, Ibid., 285–286, Mar. 31, 1896

Gruber, Wenzel Leopold. St. Petersburg anatomist. 1814–1890
CLASSIFICATION—of cervical ribs.
Ueber die Halsrippen des Menschen mit vergleichend-anatomischen Bemerkungen. In: Mém. d. l'Acad. impér. d. sci. de St. Petersbourg, ser. 7, tome 13, No. 2, 1869
FOSSA—behind duodenojejunal angle.
HERNIA—mesogastrica interna.
Ueber einen Fall nicht incarcerirter, aber mit Incarceration des Ileum durch das Omentum complicirter Hernia interna mesogastrica. Oest. Z. prakt. Heilk., Wien, 9: 325–330, May 1; 341–345, May 8, 1863.

Gruby, David. Paris physician. 1810–1898
DISEASE—tinea tonsurans.
Recherches sur la nature, le siège et le développement du Porrigo decalvans ou phytoalopécie. C. R. Acad. Sci., 17: 301–303, 1843
Discovered achorion of favus.
Mémoire sur une végétation qui constitue le vraie teigne. Ibid., 13: 72–75, et seq., 1841
Found Oidium albicans in thrush.
Recherches anatomiques sur une plante cryptogame qui constitute le vrai muguet des enfants. Ibid., 14: 634–636, 1842
Described Trichophyton ectothrix, fungus responsible for sycosis barbae.
Sur une espèce de mentagre contagieuse résultant du développement d'un nouveau cryptogame dans la racine des poils de la barbe de l'homme. Ibid., 15: 512–515, 1842
Discovered and coined term trypanosome.
Recherches et observations sur une nouvelle espèce d'hématozoaire, Trypanosoma sanguinis. Ibid., 17: 1134–1136, 1843

Grün, E. See E. Meinicke
Grünbaum, Albert Sidney Frankau. English physician. 1869–

TEST—same as Widal t.
Blood and the identification of bacterial species. Sci. Prog., 5: 616–626, Oct. 1897

Gründblatt, G. N. See J. Bronstein
Grunewald, Richard. German chemist
TESTS—for levulose, pentose and glucuronic acid in urine.
Zum Nachweis von Kohlehydraten im Harn. Münch. med. Wschr., 54: 730–731, Apr. 9, 1907

Grünwald, Ludwig. German rhinologist. 1863–
OPERATIONS—for nasal suppuration and disease of ethmoid and sphenoid sinuses.
Die Lehre von den Nasenneiterungen.... München, Leipzig, Lehmann, 1893. 175 pp.
See also R. May

Grützner, P. See W. Ebstein
Gruner, Christianus Godofredus. German physician. 1744–1815
Showed possibility of venereal infection from a common drinking-cup. Garrison
Der gemeinschaftliche Kelch. Jena, 1785
Die venerische Ansteckung durch gemeinschaftliche Trinkgeschirre. Jena, 1787

Gruskin, Benjamin. Philadelphia pathologist. 1880–
TESTS—for malignancy, intradermal and serological.
Alergic phenomena in malignancy. Pennsylvania med. J., 36: 573–576, May 1933

Guarnieri, Giuseppi. Italian physician. 1856–1918
BODIES or CORPUSCLES—cytorrhyctes of variola and vaccina.
Sui parassiti del variolo e del vaccino. Atti. d. XI Cong. med. internaz., Roma, 1894, 2, patol. gen. ed. anat., patol., pp. 125–128

Gubler, Adolphe Marie. French physician. 1821–1879
HEMIPLEGIA or PARALYSIS—crossed h.
De l'hémiplégie alterne envisagée comme signe de lésion de la protubérance annulaire et comme preuve de la décussation des nerfs faciaux. Gaz. hebd. d. méd., 3: 749–754, Oct. 24; 789–792, Nov. 7; 811–816, Nov. 14, 1856
Mémoire sur les paralysies alternes en général, et particulièrement sur l'hémiplégie alterne, avec lésion de la protubérance annulaire. Ibid., 5: 721–723, Oct. 15; 765–769, Nov. 5; 801–804, Nov. 19; 835–838, Dec. 3; 883–886, Dec. 24, 1858
LINE—connecting apparent origins of roots of fifth nerve
Névralgie réflexe et plus tard anesthésie du tri jumaeu en rapport avec une névrite du tronc du facial, et une paralysie incomplète du côté correspondant de la face. Ibid., 3 s., 19: 743–745, Dec. 3, 1864
SIGN or TUMOR—swelling of wrist in lead poisoning.
De la tumeur dorsale des mains dans la paralysie saturnine des extenseurs des doigts. Union Méd., Paris, 3 s., 6: 2–8, July 2; 15–19, July 4; 26–30, July 7, 1868

Gudden, Bernard Aloys von. German neurologist. 1824–1886
ATROPHY—specific thalmic nuelei degenerate when certain areas of cerebral cortex are destroyed.
COMMISURE—inner and upper fibers of optic tract.
GANGLION—in cephalodorsal part of mammillary body.
LAW—degeneration of proximal end of a divided nerve is cellulipetal.
Experimentaluntersuchungen über das periphensche

und centrale Nervensystem. Arch. Psychiat. Nervenkr., 2: 693–723, 1870

Guedel, Arthur Ernest. American physician. 1883–
METHOD—
Nitrous oxide air anesthesia self administered in obstetrics; a preliminary report. Indianapolis Med. J., 14: 476–479, Oct. 15, 1911
STAGES and PLANES—of anesthesia.
Stages of anesthesia and a reclassification of the signs of anesthesia. Anesth. and Analg., 6: 157–162, Aug. 1927

Guelpa, Guillaume. French physician. 1850–1930
TREATMENT—
Starvation and purgation in the relief of disease. Brit. med. J., 2: 1050–1051, Oct. 8, 1910
Autointoxication et désintoxication. Paris, Doin, 1910. 318 pp.
Also, English transl. New York, Rebman Co.

Günsburg, Alfred. German physician
METHOD—of testing gastric secretion.
Ein Ersatz der diagnostischen Magenausheberung. Dtsch. med. Wschr., 15: 841–842, Oct. 10, 1889
REAGENT and TEST—for hydrochloric acid in gastric juice.
Eine neue Methode zum Nachweis freier Salzsäure im Mageninhalt. Zbl. klin. Med., 8: 737–740, Oct. 1, 1887

Günther, Hans. Bonn physician. 1884–
TEST—for bile pigments in urine or blood.
Bilirubinprobe. Med. Klin., 27: 1056–1057, July 3, 1910

Gürber, August. Würzburg physiologist. 1864–
TEST—for indican in urine.
Zur Methodik des Indikannachweises im Harn. Münch. med. Wschr., 52: 1578–1579, Aug. 15, 1905

Guérin, Alphonse Francois Marie. French surgeon. 1816–1895
FOLD or VALVE—in fossa navicularis of urethra.
GLANDS—within meatus of female urethra; same as Skene's glands.
SINUS—a diverticulum behind Guerin's fold.
Maladies des organs génitaux externes de la femme. Paris, Delahaye, 1864. 519 pp.
FRACTURE—of upper jaw.
Des fractures des maxillaires supérieurs. Nouveau moyen de les reconnaitre dans les cas fréquents ou elles ne s'accompagnent pas de déplacement. Arch. gen. de méd., 2: 5–13, July 1866

Guerin, Jules. French surgeon
OPERATION—advancement for strabismus.
Lettre sur le traitement du strabisme par la section des muscles de l'oeil. Gaz. méd. de Paris, 8: 424 (only), July 4, 1840

Guest, Arthur. English physician
CANNULA—for transfusion of blood.
A new type of cannula. Brit. med. J., 2: 878 (only), Dec. 20, 1941

Guiard, Firmin P. French physician. 1852–1920
Described pneumaturia in diabetes.
Du developpement spontane des gaz dans la vessie. Ann. d. mal. d. org. genito-urin., 1: 242 et seq., Mar.–May 1883

Guidi, Guido. See Vidius

Guilford, Simeon Hayden. American dentist. 1841–1919
DISEASE—certain familial "combined ectodermal defects."

A dental anomaly. Dental Cosmos, 25: 113–118, Mar. 1883

Guilhon, Jean. French scientist. 1906–
TEST—for iron pigments in liver.
Note au sujet d'une méthode pratique de recherche des pigments ferriques (hémosidérine) du foie. C. R. Soc. Biol., 115: 376–377, Jan. 27, 1934

Guillain, Georges. Paris physician. 1876–
REACTION—of cerebrospinal fluid.
Sur la réaction du benjoin colloidal with G. Laroche and P. Léchelle, C. R. Soc. Biol., 89: 30–32, 1923
SYNDROME—acute polyradiculoneuritis or virus encephalomyelitis.
Sur un syndrome de radiculo-nevrite avec hyperalbuminose du liquide cephalo-rachidien sans reaction cellulaire. Remarque sur les caracteres cliniques et graphiques des reflexes tendineux with J. A. Barré and A. Strohl, Bull. Soc. med. Hop. Paris, 40: 1462–1470, Oct. 13, 1916
Radiculoneuritis with acellular hyperalbuminosis of the cerebrospinal fluid. Arch. Neurol. Psychiat., Chicago, 36: 975–990, Nov. 1936

Guinon, Georges. French physician. 1859–1929
DISEASE—motor incoordination with echolalia and coprolalia.
Sur la maladie des tics convulsifs. Rev. de méd., 6: 50–80, Jan. 1886

Guist, Gustav. Vienna ophthalmologist
MICRO-ARC TRANSILLUMINATOR—
Die skelerale Durchleuchtung mit Bogenlicht. Z. Augenheilk., 48: 219–231, Aug. 1922
OPERATION—for retinal detachment.
Eine neue Ablatiooperation. Ibid., 74: 232–242, June 1931

Gull, Sir William Withey. English physician. 1816–1899
DISEASE—arteriosclerosis.
On the pathology of the morbid state commonly called chronic Bright's disease with contracted kidney. ("*Arterio-capillary fibrosis*") with H. G. Sutton Trans. Med.-Chir. Soc., 55: 273–326, 1872
DISEASE—myxedema of adults.
On a cretinoid state supervening in adult life in women. Trans. Clin. Soc. London, 7: 180–185, 1874 (Name suggested by Sir W. Osler in 1898)
RENAL EPISTAXIS—called also essential renal hematuria, angioneurotic hematuria or renal hemophilia.
A case of intermittent haematinuria, with remarks. Guy's Hosp. Rep., 3 s., 12: 381–392, 1866
A pioneer in use of static electricity in treatment of nervous diseases. Garrison
A further report on the value of electricity as a remedial agent. Ibid., 2 s., 8: 81–143, 1853
Described posterior spinal lesions in locomotor ataxia.
Cases of paraplegia. Ibid., 3 s., 2: 143–190, 1856
Cases of paraplegia. Second series. Ibid., 4: 169–208, 1858
Described and used term anorexia nervosa (apepsia hysterica).
(On anorexia hysterica ((Apepsia hysterica))). Med. Times and Gaz., 2: 534–535, Nov. 8, 1873
Anorexia nervosa (apepsia hysterica, anorexia hysterica.) Trans. Clin. Soc. London, 7: 22–28, 1874
See also T. Addison

Gulland, George Lovell. Edinburgh physician
REACTION—
The glycogen reaction in blood: its pathological and diagnostic import. Brit. med. J., 1: 880-882, Apr. 16, 1904

Gullstrand, Allvar. Swedish ophthalmologist. 1862-1934
Awarded Nobel prize in 1911, "for his work on the dioptrics of the eye."
LAW—when patient is made to turn his head while fixing on a distant object, if corneal reflex from either eye moves in direction in which head is turning, it moves toward weaker muscle.
Om Braünlinier vid Astigmatism. Nord. ophth. Tidsskr., Kjøbenh., 3: 1-18, 1890
Beitrage zur Theorie des Astigmatismus. Skandin. Arch. f. Physiol., 2: 269-359, 1890
Allgemeine Theorie der monochromatischen Abberationen und ihre nächsten Ergebnisse für die Ophthalmologie. Upsala, Berling, 1900. 204 pp.
Discovered intracapsular mechanism of accommodation.
Einführung in die Methoden der Dioptrik des Auges des Menschen. Leipzig, 1911

Gunn, Alexander. London pharmacologist. 1844-1914
REACTION—
A new characteristic reaction of adrenaline with E. F. Harrison. Pharm. J., 24: 718 (only), June 1, 1907

Gunn, Moses. American surgeon. 1822-1887
LIGAMENT—same as Bigelow, iliofemoral or Y 1.
Philosophy of certain dislocations of the hip and shoulder, and their reduction. Peninsular J. Med., 1: 97-100, Sept. 1853
Luxations of the hip and shoulder joints, and the agents which oppose their reduction. Detroit, Barnes et al., 1859. 2 ed., 20 pp.

Gunn, Robert Marcus. English ophthalmologist. 1850-1909
DOTS—on retina.
Peculiar appearance in the retina in the vicinity of the optic disc occurring in several members of the same family. Trans. Ophth., Soc., 3: 110-113, 1883
SYNDROME and PHENOMENON—
Congenital ptosis with peculiar associated movements of the affected lid. Ibid., 283-287

Gunning, Thomas Brian. American surgeon.
SPLINT—for fractured jaw.
The treatment of fracture of the lower jaw by interdental splints. New York Med. J., 3: 433-448, Sept.; 4: 11-29, Oct. 1866; 84: 274-277, Jan. 1867

Gurlt, Ernst Julius. Berlin surgeon. 1825-1899
Wrote excellent work on history of surgery. Garrison
Geschichte der Chirurgie und ihrer Ausübung.... Berlin, Hirschwald, 1898. 3 vols.

Gussenbauer, C. See T. Billroth

Gusserow, Adolf Ludwig Sigismund. German gynecologist. 1836-1906
Described pernicious anemia in pregancy.
Ueber hochgradigste Anämie Schwangerer. Arch. Gynaek., 2: 218-235, 1871

Gustavson, R. G. See R. T. Frank

Guth, I. Saarbrücken physician
BROTH—selenium extract, for enrichment of typhoid bacilli.
Selannährböden für die elektive Züchtung von Typhus-

bacillen. Zbl. Bakt., 77: 487-496 (490), Apr. 11, 1915

Guthrie, Charles Claude. Pittsburgh physiologist. 1880-
PIPETTE CONTROLLER—
An apparatus for quickly measuring the specific gravity of body fluids. J. Lab. clin. Med., 17: 1158-1162, Aug. 1932

Guthrie, George James. English surgeon. 1785-1856
MUSCLE—compressor urethrae m.
CATHETER—
Anatomy and diseases of the neck of the bladder and of the urethra. London, Burgess and Hill, 1834
On the anatomy and diseases of the urinary and sexual organs. London, Churchill, 1836. 284 pp.
Wrote on military surgery.
On gun-shot wounds of the extremities requiring the different operations of amputation, with their after treatment. London, Longman, 1815
Ligated peroneal artery.
Case of a wound of the peroneal artery, successfully treated by ligature. Med. chir. Trans., London, 7: 325-332, 1816
Amputated at hip joint.
Treatise on gunshot wounds. London, Longman, 1820. 2 ed., pp. 332-340

Guthrie, Samuel. Bloomfield, Mass. physician. 1782-1848
Discovered chloroform, independently of Liebig or Sauberian, and invented modern method of making it by distilling alcohol with chlorinated lime. Garrison
New mode of preparing a spirituous solution of chloric ether. Amer. J. Sci. and Arts (Silliman), 21: 64-65, 1831
On pure chloric ether. Ibid., 22: 105-106, 1832

Gutierrez, Robert. New York urologist. 1895-
PYELOGRAPHIC TRIANGLE, SYNDROME—
The clinical management of the horseshoe kidney. Part II. Amer. J. Surg., 15: 132-165, Jan. 1932
Horseshoe kidney. (In discussion). J. Urol., 27: 85-88, Jan. 1932; 32: 655-657, Dec. 1934
The clinical management of horseshoe kidney.... New York, Hoeber, 1934. 143 pp.

Gutman, Ethel Benedict. New York scientist
METHOD—
Estimation of "acid" phosphatase activity of blood serum with A. B. Gutman, J. biol. Chem., 136: 201-209, Oct. 1940

Gutman, S. Berlin chemist
REAGENT—for mercury in urine.
Ueber den Nachweis des Quecksilbers im Urin unter Zuhilfenahme eines neuen Lösungsmittels für Quecksilbersulfid. Biochem. Z., 89: 199-203, July 22, 1918

Guye, Ambroise Arnold Guillaume. Amsterdam laryngologist. 1839-1904
SIGN—aprosexia in children with adenoids.
Ueber Aprosexia ... die Unfähigheit.... Dtsch. med. Wschr., 13: 934-935, Oct. 27, 1887

Guyer, M. F. See F. E. Mohs

Guyon, Jean Casimir Felix. Paris surgeon. 1831-1920
PROCEDURE or SIGN—for examining kidney, one hand anterior and the other hand posterior for ballottment.
Lecons cliniques sur les maladies des voies urinaires. Paris, Baillière, 1881. 998 pp. p. 630

PROSTATIC-PELVIC   SYNDROME—malignant "freezing" of the male pelvis. Ibid.

Guyot, Edme Gilles. French postmaster. 1706–1786
First attempted catherization of Eustachian tube, 1724. Garrison
(*Instrument pour seringuer la trompe d'Eustache par la bouche.*) Hist. Acad. roy. d. sci., 1724, Paris, p. 37, 1726

Guyot, Francisque. French surgeon
OPERATION—
Sur la désarticulation tarso-métatarsienne; comparaison du procédé de Lefranc et du procédé de Marcellin Duval. Paris, 1874. 56 pp.

Gwathmey, James Tayloe. New York surgeon. 1865–1944
ANESTHESIA—oil-ether, by rectum.
Oil-ether anesthesia. New York Med. J., 98: 1101–1104, Dec. 6, 1913
Oil-ether anesthesia. An attempt to abolish inhalation anesthesia. Ibid., 99: 211–214, Jan. 31, 1914

Oil-ether colonic anesthesia: clinical experience with more than five thousand cases. J. A. M. A., 93: 447–452, Aug. 10, 1929
Ether-oil rectal analgesia in obstetrics: modified technic with C. O. McCormick, Ibid., 105: 2044–2047, Dec. 21, 1935

Gwyn, Norman Beechey. American physician. 1875–
Isolated paracolon bacillus (paratyphoid).
On infection with a para-colon bacillus in a case with all the clinical features of typhoid fever. Johns Hopk. Hosp. Bull., 9: 54–56, Mar. 1898

Gye, William Ewart. Scottish physician. 1884–
ORGANISM—of Gye and Barnard, of cancer.
THEORY—ultra-microscopic virus combined with an intrinsic chemical factor is concerned in production of Rous sarcoma.
The etiology of malignant new growths. Lancet, 2: 109–117, July 18, 1925

H

Haab, Otto. Zurich ophthalmologist. 1850–1931
REFLEX—cerebral cortex r.
Der Hirnrindenreflex der Pupille. Festschr. z. Feier d. . . . Karl Wilhelm v. Nägeli u. Albert v. Kölliker, Zurich, 1891

Haagensen, Cushman Davis. New York surgeon 1900–
CRITERIA—
Carcinoma of the breast. II. Criteria of operability with A. P. Stout, Ann. Surg., 118: 859–870, Nov.; 1032–1051, Dec. 1943

Haas, Sidney Valentine. New York pediatrician. 1870–
TREATMENT—of pylorospasm.
The hypertonic infant, the curative action of atropin on certain of its manifestations. Amer. J. Dis., Child., 15: 323–335, May 1918
The atropin treatment of pylorospasm and pyloric stenosis. Arch. Pediat., 36: 516–530, Oct. 1919
Also: New York State J. Med., 19: 365–371, Oct. 1919

Haasler, Fritz. Halle surgeon
OPERATION—retroduodenal choledochotomy, for stone.
Ueber Choledochotomie. Verh. dtsch. Ges. Chir., 27: 126–131, 1898

Habein, H. C. See M. H. Hoffman

Haberer, Hans von. German surgeon. 1875–
BONE CYST—of Haberer and Pommer.
Zur Frage der Knochenzystem. Arch. f. orth. Chir., 17: 1–16, 1920
OPERATION—partial gastrectomy.
Anwendungsbreite und Vorteil der Magenresektion Billroth I. Arch. klin. Chir., 114: 127–171, Aug. 3, 1920
Terminolaterale Gastroduodenostomie bei der Resektionsmethode nach Billroth I. Zbl. Chir., 492: 1321–1326, Sept. 9, 1922

Haberlandt, Ludwig. German physician. 1885–
HEART HORMONE—nodal; hormocardiol.
Ein Hormon der Herzbewegung. Umschau, 30: 735, 1926
Versuche mit alkoholischen Froschherzextrakten. Arch. ges. Physiol., 212: 587; 214: 471, 1926

Hachla, J. Vienna physician
AGAR—alkaline blood; enrichment medium for cholera vibrio.
Beitrag zur Frage elektiver Nährböden für Choleravibrionen with Th. Holobut, Zbl. Bakt., 52: 299–304, 1909

Hacker, Viktor von. Vienna surgeon. 1852–1933
METHOD—for dilatation of strictures of esophagus.
Ueber die nach Verätzungen enstehenden Speiseröhren-Verengerungen. Wien, Hölder, 1889. 147 pp.
OPERATION—exclusion for hypertrophic tuberculosis of cecum.
Ueber die Bedeutung der Anastomosenbildung am Darm für die operative Behandlung der Verengerungen desselben. Wien. klin. Wschr., 1: 359–362, July 16; 389–391, Aug. 2, 1888
OPERATION—gastrostomy.
Ueber die Verwendung des Musculus rectus abdominis zum Verschlusse der künstlichen Magenfistel. Wien. med. Wschr., 36: 1073–1078, July 31; 1110–1114, Aug. 7, 1886
See also T. Billroth

Haden, Russell Landram. Kansas City physician. 1888–
HEMATICRIT—
METHOD—for determination of hemoglobin.
The volume and hemoglobin content of the erythrocytes in health and disease. Folia Haematol., 31: 113–135, Jan. 1925
The technic of determination of the relative mass, the individual cell volume, and the volume index of the erythrocytes of man. J. Lab. clin. Med., 15: 736–746, May 1930
A new hemoglobinometer. Ibid., 16: 68–72, Oct. 1930
MODIFICATION—
A modification of the Folin-Wu method for making protein-free blood filtrates. J. biol. Chem., 56: 469–471, June 1923

Hadley, Philip Bardwell. Rhode Island biologist. 1881–
SOLUTION—glycerol glycocoll, for cultivation of B. diphtheria.
The growth and toxin production of Bacillus diphtheriae

upon proteid-free media. Amer. Pub. Health Ass.,
Public Health Papers, 32: 95–107, 1907
Hadra, Berthold Ernest. American surgeon. 1842–
1903
OPERATION—
*Wiring of the vertebrae as a means of immobilization
in fracture and Pott's disease.* Med. Times and Reg.,
22: 423–425, May 23, 1891
Also: Trans. Texas Med. Ass., 23: 187, 1891
Haeckel, Ernst Heinrich Philip August. Jena
naturalist. 1834–1919
LAW—an organism, in developing from ovum, goes
through same changes as did the species in developing from lower to higher forms of animal life; also
called gastrea theory.
*Die Gastraea-Theorie, die phylogenetische Classifica-
tion des Thierreichs und die Homologie der Keim-
blätter.* Jenaische Z. f. Naturw., 8: 1–55, 1874
*Ursprung und Entwickelung der thierischen Gewebe;
ein histogenetischer Beitrag zur Gastraea-Theorie.* Ibid.,
11: 206–275, 1885
Haenen, G. Brussels medical student.
TEST—for differentiation of typhoid from coli bacteria.
*De l'emploi de l'aldehyde paradimethylaminobenzoique
pour différencier le colibacille d'avec le bacille typhique.*
Arch. int. Pharmacodyn., 15: 255–261, 1905
Härtel, Friedrich Ferdinand. German surgeon.
1877–
METHOD—of injection for tic douloureux.
Intrakraniale Leitungsanästhesie des Ganglion Gasseri.
Zbl. Chir., 39: 705–708, May 25, 1912
*Die Behandlung der Trigeminusneuralgie mit intra-
kraniellen Alkoholeinspritzungen.* Leipzig, Vogel,
1912. 128 pp.
Härting, Friedrick Hugo. German physician
Described miners' cancer.
*Der Lungenkrebs, die Bergkrankheit in den Schnee-
bergen Gruben* with W. Hesse, Viertelj. f. gerichtl.
Med. u. öffen. Sanitäts., n. F., 30: 296–309; 31: 102–
132; 313–337, 1879
Haffkine, Waldemar Mordecai Wolff. Russian-
English bacteriologist. 1860–1930
SERUM—for prophylactic inoculation against plague.
*Experiment on the effect of protective inoculation in the
epidemic of plague at Undhera, Taluka Barada, Feb-
ruary and March,* 1898. (Bombay, 1898), 9 pp.
SERUM—an anticholera s.
Le choléra asiatique chez le cobaye. C. R. Soc. Biol., 44:
635–637, July 9, 1892
Inoculations de vaccins anticholéraiques a l'homme;
... Ibid., 740–741, July 30, 1892
Anti-cholera inoculation. Calcutta, Thacker, Spink,
1895. 66 pp.
Haffter, E. See F. L. Dumont
Hagedorn, Hans Christian. Copenhagen scientist.
1888–
METHOD—for determination of blood sugar.
*Zur Mikrobestimmung des Blutzuckers mittels Ferri-
cyanid* with B. N. Jensen, Biochem. Z., 135: 46–58,
Feb. 20, 1923
Die Ferricyanidmethode zur Blutzuckerbestimmung
with B. N. Jensen, Ibid., 137: 92–95, May 5, 1923
Introduced protamine insulin.
Protamine insulinate with B. N. Jensen, N. B. Krarup
and I. Wodstrup, J. A. M. A., 106: 177–180, Jan
18, 1936

Hagedorn, Werner. Madeburg surgeon. 1831–1894
TABLE—operating.
*Ein neuer Operationstisch mit Abflussvorrichtung in
der Mitte.* Zbl. Chir., 14: 513–516, July 9, 1887
Hagen, Fritz Bessel. German surgeon
METHOD—for evacuating pancreatic cyst.
Zur operativen Behandlung der Pankreascysten. Arch.
klin. Chir., 62: 157–169, 1900
Haggard, H. W. See Y. Henderson
Haggart, Gilbert Edmund. Boston surgeon. 1893–
METHOD—
*Sciatic pain of unknown origin: an effective method of
treatment.* J. Bone and Joint Surg., 20: 851–859,
Oct. 1938
Haglund, Patrick. Swedish surgeon. 1870–
DISEASE—bursitis in region of tendon Achilles.
*Ueber Fractur des Epiphysenkerns des Calcaneus,
nebst allgemeinen Bemerkungsn über einige ähnliche
juvenile Knochenkernverletzungen.* Arch. klin. Chir.,
82: 922–930, 1907
Hagner, Francis Randall. Washington, D. C. sur-
geon. 1873–
OPERATION—epididymo-vasostomy.
*The operative treatment of acute gonorrheal epididymi-
tis.* Med. Rec., 70: 565–568, Oct. 13, 1906
*A supplemental report on the operative treatment of
gonorrheal epididymitis.* Ibid., 76: 944–946, Dec. 4,
1909
OPERATION—for hypospadias.
Pseudohermaphrodism or complete hypospadias. Trans.
Amer. Ass. Genito-Urin. Surg., 15: 11–29, 1922
Hagner's disease.
In 1868 Nikolaus Friedrich of Heidelberg described
hyperostosis of entire skeleton and gave it name of
two Hagner brothers affected, Wilhelm and Karl.
Hyperostose des gesamten skeletts. Arch. path. Anat.
u. Physiol., 43: 83–87, Apr. 8, 1868
Haguenau. See R. Sicard
Hahn, Eugen. German surgeon. 1841–1902
OPERATION—gastrostomy.
Eine neue Methode der Gastrostomie. Zbl. Chir., 17:
193–195, Mar. 15, 1890
OPERATION—nephropexy.
*Die operative Behandlung der beweglichen Niere
durch Fixation.* Ibid., No. 29: 449–452, July 23, 1881
See O. Witzel
Hahn, Florian. Nürnberg surgeon
INSTRUMENT—
Nähapparat für Magen- und Darmresektionen.
Münch. med. Wschr., 58: 1919–1920, Sept. 5, 1911
Hahn, J. See D. Munro
Hahnemann, Christian Friedrich Samuel. German
physician. 1755–1843
Founded homeopathy.
Organon der rationellen Heilkunde. Dresden, Arnold,
1810. 222 pp.
Haight, Cameron. Michigan surgeon. 1901–
PROCEDURE—
*Certain technical considerations pertaining to lobec-
tomy; a preliminary report.* Univ. Hosp. Bull., Ann.
Arbor, Mich., 1: 25 (only), July; 29–30, Aug. 1935
TECHNIC—of anterior thoracoplasty.
*Complementary anterior thoracoplasty for pulmonary
tuberculosis: a technic employing parasternal division
of the costal cartilages.* J. Thoracic Surg., 5: 453–470,
June 1936

Haines, Walter Stanley. Chicago chemist. 1850–1923
REAGENT and TEST—for glucose.
On an improved test for detecting sugar in the urine.
Med. Examiner, 15: 569–572, Dec. 1, 1874
An improved test for the detection of glucose, especially in urine with G. P. Pond and R. W. Webster, J. A. M. A., 74: 301–302, Jan. 31, 1920
Halban, Josef von. Austrian gynecologist. 1870–1937
OPERATION—
Anatomie und Aetiologie der Genitalprolapse beim Weibe with J. Tandler, Wien, Braümuller, 1907. 273 pp.
THEORY—of lactation.
Die Entstehung der Geschlechtscharaktere. Eine Studie über den formativen Einfluss der Keimdrüse. Arch. Gynaek., 70: 205–308, 1903
Die innere Secretion von Ovarium und Placenta und ihre Bedeutung für die Function der Milchdrüse. Ibid., 75: 353–441, 1905
Halberstaedter, Ludwig. Breslau physician. 1876–
Announced specific sensitivity of ovaries to x-ray.
Die Einwirkung der Röntgenstrahlen auf Ovarien. Berl. klin. Wschr., 42: 64–66, Jan. 16, 1905
Halbertsma, Tjalling. Dutch gynecologist. 1841–1898
Introduced cesarean section in puerperal convulsions.
Eclampsia gravidarum: eene nieuwe indicatie voor sectio caesarea. Ned. Tijdschr. Geneesk., 2 R., 25, 2 D., 485–491, 1889
Haldane, John Scott. Scottish physiologist. 1860–1936
GAS ANALYSIS—for oxygen-carbon dioxide determinations.
A new form of apparatus for measuring the respiratory exchange of animals. J. Physiol., 13: 419–430, 1892
HAEMOGLOBINOMETER—
The colorimetric determination of haemoglobin. Ibid., 26: 497–504, June 14, 1901
MASK and THERAPY—
The therapeutic administration of oxygen. Brit. med. J., 1: 181–183, Feb. 10, 1917
METHOD—of collection of alveolar air.
The regulation of the lung-ventilation with J. G. Priestley, J. Physiol., 32: 225–266, May 9, 1905
METHOD—for determination of oxygen in oxyhaemoglobin.
A contribution to the chemistry of haemoglobin and its immediate derivatives. Ibid., 22: 298–306, 1898
Showed that respiration is regulated by carbon dioxide concentration in arterial blood.
See METHOD—of collection of alveolar air.
See also J. O. Christiansen, Stoke
Haldeman, K. O. See R. Soto-Hall
Halden, Wilhelm. Graz physician
REACTION—for vitamin D.
Ueber eine Farbreaktion zum Nachweis und zur Bestimmung von Vitamin D. Naturwissenschaften, 24: 296–297, May 8, 1936
A colour reaction for the detection and determination of vitamin D with H. Tzoni, Nature, 137: 909 (only), May 30, 1936
Hales, Stephen. English clergyman and physiologist. 1677–1761
PIEZOMETER—a glass tube inserted into an artery for purpose of ascertaining blood-pressure by height to which blood rises in tube.
First to devise a method of demonstrating force and movements of pulse. Garrison

Statical essays, containing haemostatics; or, an account of some hydraulic and hydrostatical experiments made on the blood and blood-vessels of animals. Vol. II. London, Innys, Manley et al., 1733
Also, 3 ed., 1769
Also: In F. A. Willius and T. E. Keyes' *Cardiac classics,* St. Louis, Mosby, 1941. pp. 131–155
Originator of artificial ventilation. Garrison
A description of ventilators. London, Innys, 1743
(Paper read before the Royal Society in May 1741.)
Hall, Edward Parks. Kansas City, Mo. rhinolaryngologist. 1876–1926
SPLINT—
A nasal splint. J. A. M. A., 62: 1636 (only), May 23, 1914
Hall, H. See M. Novak
Hall, Ivan Clifford. California bacteriologist. 1885–
AGAR—gentian violet glucose; culture medium.
The elimination of spurious presumptive tests for B. coli in water by the use of gentian violet with Lillian J. Ellefson, J. Bact., 3: 329–354, (336), July 1918
BROTH—gentian violet lactose. Ibid., p. 337
PROCEDURE—for culture tests for B. welchii.
Differentiation and identification of the sporulating anaerobes. J. infect. Dis., 30: 445–504, May 1922
SOLUTION—brain peptone, for enriching anaerobes.
Practical methods in the purification of obligate anaerobes. Ibid., 27: 576–590, (579), Dec. 1920
TESTICULAR INFUSION AGAR—
Testicular infusion agar—a sterilizable culture medium for the gonococcus. J. Bact., 1: 343–352, May 1916
Hall, John Basil. English surgeon. 1868–1926
OPERATION—
Splenopexy for wandering spleen. Ann. Surg., 37: 481–485, Apr. 1903
Hall, Josiah Newhall. Colorado physician. 1859–1939
SIGN—
Tracheal diastolic shock in the diagnosis of aortic aneurism. With a study of the value of the tracheal tug. Amer. J. med. Sci., 119: 10–14, Jan. 1900
Hall, M. G. See T. B. Bayles, H. Rogers
Hall, Marshall. English physiologist. 1790–1857
DISEASE—spurious hydrocephalus.
An easy on a hydrencephaloid affection in infants arising from exhaustion. London, Sherwood et al., 1836
METHOD—of artificial respiration.
On a new mode of effecting artificial respiration. Lancet, London, 1: 229 (only), 1856
Also: Lancet, New York, 1: 415 (only), May 1856
Prone and postural respiration in drowning, and other forms of apnoea or suspended respiration. London, Churchill, 1858. 216 pp.
Established difference between volitional action and unconscious reflexes.
On the reflex function of the medulla oblongata and medulla spinalis. Philos. Trans., 123: 635–665, 1833
Hall, Maurice Crowther. American zoölogist. 1881–1938
SWAB—NIH anal s.
Studies on oxyuriasis: I. Types of anal swabs and scrapers, with a description of an improved type of swab. Amer. J. trop. Med., 17: 445–453, May 1937
Found that carbon tetrachloride in small doses is specific for hookworm disease.

The use of carbon tetrachloride for the removal of hook-worms. J. A. M. A., 77: 1641–1643, Nov. 19, 1921

Hall, Richard John. New York surgeon
ANESTHESIA—cocaine for nerve blocking.
Hydrochlorate of cocaine. New York Med. J., 40: 643–644, Dec. 6, 1884

Halle, Max. German-American ophthalmologist. 1873–1939
OPERATION—dacryostomy.
Intranasale Tränensackoperation bei Säuglingen. Verh. Berl. med. Ges., (1928), 59: 2. Teil, 238–242, 1929

Haller, Albrecht von. Swiss physiologist. 1708–1777
ANSA or LOOP—formed by nerve which connects facial and glossopharyngeal nerves.
Disputationes anatomicae selectae. Gottingae, Vanderhoeck, 1746–52. 7 vols.
ARCHERS—external and internal arcuate ligaments of diaphragm.
De diaphragmatis musculis dissertatio anatomica. Bernae, 1733. 30 pp.
CIRCLE—1. of arteries in sclera, surrounding entrance of optic nerve.
CIRCLE—2. of veins beneath areola of nipple.
CIRCLE—3. of fibrocartilage to which mitral and tricuspid valves are attached.
CONES—coni vasculosi, making up globus major of epididymis.
CUL-DE-SAC—in pericardium, posterior to heart.
For foregoing, see *Disputationes* . . .
FRETUM or ISTHMUS—constriction between auricles and ventricles of fetal heart.
De aortae venaeque cavae gravioribus quibusdam morbis. Gottingae, 1749
Also: transl. by J. E. Erichsen, London, Sydenham Soc., 1844
HABENULA—remains of processus vaginalis of peritoneum.
LIGAMENT—a fold extending along ascending colon.
LINE—a fibrous band down anterior surface of pia mater of spinal cord.
OMENTUM—a process from greater omentum, which sometimes in fetal life becomes attached to testis, and may be included in an inguinal hernia. Dorland
PLEXUS—of nerves on outer surface of inferior constrictor of pharynx.
TRIPOD—celiac axis.
For foregoing, see *Disputationes.* . . .
First to have idea of muscular irritability and nerve sensibility. Garrison
De partibus corporis humani sensibilibus et irritabilibus. Comment. Soc. reg. scient., Gottingae, 1752, 2: 114–214, 1753
Also: *A dissertation on the sensible and irritable parts of animals.* . . . Transl. by M. Tissot, London, Nourse, 1755
Also: Baltimore, Johns Hopk. Press, 1936

Haller, H. L. See M. S. Schechter

Hallervorden, Julius. Landsberg neurologist. 1882–
SYNDROME—extrapyramidal.
Eigenartige Erkrankung im extrapyramidalen System mit besonderer Beteiligung des Globus pallidus und der Substantia nigra: ein Beitrag zu den Beziehungen zwischen diesen beiden Zentren with H. Spatz, Z. ges. Neurol. Psychiat., 79: 254–302, 1922

Halley, Edmund. English astronomer. 1656–1742
The virtual founder of vital statistics. Garrison

An estimate of the degrees of mortality of mankind, drawn from curious tables of the births and funerals at the city of Breslau, with an attempt to ascertain the price of annuities upon lives. Philos. Trans. 17: 596–610, 1693

Halliburton, W. D. See F. W. Mott

Hallion. See T. Tuffier

Hallman, Lois. See A. Bodansky

Hallopeau, Francois Henri. French dermatologist. 1842–1919
DISEASE—pustular dermatitis.
Sur une nouvelle forme de dermatite pustuleuse chronique en foyers à progression excentrique. Cong. internat. de Dermat. et de Syph., 1889, Paris, p. 344, 1890

Hallopeau, Paul. French surgeon. 1876–1924
OPERATION—pericardiectomy for constrictive pericarditis.
Un cas de cardiolyse. Bull. Soc. Chir. Paris, 47: 1120–1121, Oct. 26, 1921

Halstead, Albert Edward. Chicago surgeon. 1868–1926
OPERATION—hypophysectomy.
Remarks on the operative treatment of tumors of the hypophysis. S. G. O., 10: 494–502, May 1910

Halsted, William Stewart. Baltimore surgeon. 1852–1922
LAW—transplanted tissue will grow only if there is a lack of that tissue in the host. "Unless considerable deficiency in parathyroid tissue has been created, the autografts do not live."
Hypoparathyreosis, status parathyreoprivus, and transplantation of the parathyroid glands. Amer. J. med. Sci., 134: 1–12, July 1907
Auto- and isotransplantation, in dogs, of the parathyroid glandules. J. exp. Med., 11: 175–199, Jan. 9, 1909
LINE OF ANASTOMOSIS—between superior and inferior thyroid vessels from which parathyroid arteries may arise. See above, 1907
OPERATION—for aneurysm; gradual occlusion with metal bands.
The results of the complete and incomplete occlusion of the abdominal and thoracic aortas by metal bands. Trans. Sect. Surg. and Anat., Amer. Med. Ass., pp. 587–590, 1906
The effect of ligation of the common iliac artery on the circulation and function of the lower extremity. Report of a cure of iliofemoral aneurism by the application of an aluminum band to that vessel. Johns Hopk. Hosp. Bull., 23: 191–220, July 1912
OPERATION—for carcinoma of breast; first used by Halsted in 1882.
First described briefly in *The treatment of wounds with especial reference to the value of the blood clot in the management of dead spaces. IV. Operations for carcinoma of the breast.* Johns Hopk. Hosp. Rep., 2: 255–314, 1890
Also: Maryland Med. J., 24: 529–533, 1891
First described in detail in: *The results of operations for the cure of cancer of the breast performed at the Johns Hopkins Hospital from June, 1889 to January, 1894.* Johns Hopk. Hosp. Rep., 4: 297–350, 1894
Also: Ann. Surg., 20: 497–550, Dec. 1894
Also: Med. Classics, 3: 441–509, Dec. 1938
OPERATION—gastro- or entero-enterostomy.

Intestinal anastomosis. Johns Hopk. Hosp. Bull., 2: 1–4, Jan. 1891
OPERATION—for hernia.
The radical cure of hernia. (Report of case presentation.) Ibid., 1: 12–13, Dec. 1889; 111–112, Dec. 1890
The radical cure of inguinal hernia in the male. Ibid., 4: 17–24, Mar. 1893
Also: Ann. Surg., 17: 542–556, May 1893
Also: Med. Classics, 3: 412–440, Dec. 1938
SIGN—a "Swish" on firm pressure, in gelatinous carcinoma of breast.
A diagnostic sign of gelatinous carcinoma of the breast. J. A. M. A., 64: 1653 (only), May 15, 1915
SUTURE—mattress, of intestinal wall, to include serosa, muscularis and submucosa.
Circular suture of the intestine: an experimental study. Amer. J. med. Sci., 94: 436–461, Oct. 1887
Developed nerve block anesthesia with cocaine.
Practical comments on the use and abuse of cocaine; suggested by its invariably successful employment in more than a thousand minor surgical operations. New York M. J., 42: 294–295, Sept. 12, 1885
Successfully tied left subclavian artery within scaleni.
Ligation of the first portion of the left subclavian artery and excision of a subclavio-axillary aneurism. Johns Hopk. Hosp. Bull., 3: 93–94, July–Aug. 1892
Introduced rubber gloves in surgery. (No title.) Johns Hopk. Hosp. Rep., 4: No. 6, pl. XII, 1894
Ligature and suture material: the employment of fine silk in preference to catgut and the advantages of transfixion of tissues and vessels in control of hemorrhage; also an account of the introduction of gloves, guttapercha tissue and silver foil. J. A. M. A., 60: 1119–1126 (1123–1124), Apr. 12, 1913
Made classic contribution to swelling of arm following radical mastectomy.
The swelling of the arm after operations for cancer of the breast—Elephantiasis chirurgica—its cause and prevention. Johns Hopk. Hosp. Bull., 32: 309–313, Oct. 1921
Halverson, John Oliver. Philadelphia physiochemist. 1880–
METHOD—
The determination of small amounts of calcium, particularly in blood with O. Bergeim, J. biol. Chem. 32: 159–170, Nov. 1917
Hamann, E. E. See I. F. Huddleson
Hamberger, Georg Erhard. German surgeon. 1697–1755
Reported carcinoma of duodenum.
De ruptura intestini duodeni. Jena, Ritterianis, 1746
Also, in: A. Haller: *Disputationes ad morborum historiam et curationem facientes.* Lausanne, Bousquet et soc., vol. 3, p. 507, 1757
Hambrecht, Leonora. See L. W. Sauer
Hamburger, Franz. German physician. 1874–
TEST—subcutaneous, for tuberculosis.
Allgemeine Pathologie und Diagnostik der Kindertuberkulose. Leipzig, Deuticke, 1910. 147 pp.
Introduced so-called perkutan ointment, consisting of old tuberculin evaporated to a constant weight.
Eine Verbesserung der perkutanen Tuberkulinreaktion (Moro) with F. Stradner, Münch. med. Wschr., 66: 439 (only), Apr. 18, 1919
Hamburger, Hartog Jakob. German physician. 1859–1924
LAW—when blood is rendered acid, albumins and

phosphates pass from red corpuscles to serum, and chlorides pass from serum to cells; reverse occurs when blood is rendered alkaline.
Osmotischer Druck und Ionenlehre in den medicinischen Wissenschaften. Wiesbaden, Bergmann, 1902–04. 3 vols.
Hamel, Dr. Charlottenburg physician
Described basophilic granules in red blood cells in lead poisoning.
Ueber die Beziehungen der körnigen Degenerationen der rothen Blutkörperchen zu den sonstigen morphologischen Veränderungen des Blutes mit besonderer Berücksichtigung der Bleiintoxikation. Dtsch. Arch. f. klin. Med., 67: 357–376, May 23, 1900
Hamill, P. See W. E. Dixon
Hamilton, Bengt Leopold Knutsson. Swedish-American pediatrician. 1892–
TEST—
Effect of calcium administration to rachitic rabbits. with C. Schwartz. Proc. Soc. exp. Biol., N. Y., 29: 528–529, Feb. 1932
A method for the determination of small amounts of parathyroid hormone with C. Schwartz, J. Pharmacol., 6: 285–292, Nov. 1932
Presented evidence of increased function of parathyroid glands in children deficiently supplied with vitamin D.
Rickets and hyperparathyroidism with C. Schwartz, J. clin. Invest., 11: 817, July 1932
Hamilton, Frank Hastings. American surgeon. 1813–1886
BANDAGE—for lower jaw.
Illustrated in: *A practical treatise on fractures and dislocations.* Philadelphia, Lae, 1884. 17 Amer. ed., p. 158
TEST—when shoulder joint is dislocated, a straight rod applied along humerus can be made to touch outer condyle and acromium at same time. Ibid., p. 272
Hamilton, James Bruce. American anatomist. 1910–
Wrote on acne.
Male hormone substance: prime factor in acne. J. clin. Endocrinol., 1: 570–592, July 1941
Wrote on baldness.
Male hormone stimulation is prerequisite and an incitant in common baldness. Amer. J. Anat., 71: 451–480, Nov. 1942
Also, abstr.: J. Invest. Dermat., 5: 473–474, Dec. 1942
Hamilton, P. B. See R. A. Phillips
Hamilton, Robert. English surgeon. 1721–1793
Reported orchitis in mumps, 1773.
An account of a distemper, by the common people in England vulgarly called the mumps. Trans. Roy. Soc. Edinb., 1773, 2: pt. 2, 59–72, 1790
Hamilton, William Ferguson. American physiologist. 1893–
OPTICAL MANOMETER—
Pressure pulse contours in the intact animal. I. Analytical description of a high-frequency hypodermic manometer with illustrative curves of simultaneous arterial and intracardiac pressures with G. Brewer and I. Brotman, Amer. J. Physiol., 107: 427–435, Feb. 1, 1934
See also H. G. Barbour
Hamm, W. J. See V. P. Blair

Hamman, Louis. Baltimore physician. 1877–1946
SYNDROME—
Spontaneous interstitial emphysema of the lungs.
Trans. Ass. Amer. Phys., 52: 311–319, 1937
Spontaneous mediastinal emphysema. Johns Hopk.
Hosp. Bull., 44: 1–21, Jan. 1939
Hammarberg, Carl. Swedish anatomist. 1865–1893
Demonstrated clear distinction between cyto-archi-
tecture of sensory and motor regions.
*Studier öfver idiotiens klinik och patologi jamte under-
sökningar af hjärnbarkens normala anatomi.* Upsala,
Almqvist and Wiksells, 1893. 106 pp.
Hammarsten, Einar. Swedish pharmacologist. 1889–
Prepared crystalline secretin.
Versuche zur Reinigung von Sekretin with O. Wilander
and G. Ågren. Acta med. scand., 68: 239–247, 1928
See also G. Ågren
Hammarsten, Olof. Upsala physiologist. 1841–1932
TEST—for bile pigments in urine.
*Zum Nachweis der Gallenfarbstoffe, insbesondere im
Harn.* Z. anal. Chem., 39: 269–270, 1900
TEST—for globulin.
*Ueber die Anwendbarkeit des Magnesiumsulfates zur
Trennung und quantitativen Bestimmung von Serum-
albumin und Globulinen.* Ibid., 8: 467–502, 1883–84
THEORY—of coagulation of blood.
*Undersöknigar af de s. k. fibrinogeneratorerna fibrinet
samt fibrinogenets koagulation.* Upsala Läkaref. Förh.,
11: 538–579, 1875–6
Hammer, Adam. Vienna surgeon. 1818–1878
Described coronary thrombosis, with diagnosis be-
fore death.
*Ein Fall von thrombotischem Verschlusse einer der
Kranzarterien des Herzens.* Wien. med. Wschr., 28:
97–102, Feb. 2, 1878
Hammer, Bernard Wernick. Iowa bacteriologist.
1886–
TEST—
*The creatine test for acetylmethylcarbinol plus diacetyl
in butter cultures.* J. Dairy Sci., 18: 579–581, Sept.
1935
Hammerschlag, Albert. Vienna physician. 1863–
1935
METHOD or TEST—to determine specific gravity of
blood.
*Ueber das Verhalten des specifischen Gewichtes des
Blutes in Krankheiten.* Zbl. klin. Med., 12: 825–837,
Oct. 31, 1891
Hammett, Louis Plack. New York chemist. 1894–
TEST—
A new reagent for aluminum with C. T. Sottery,
J. Amer. Chem. Soc., 47: 142–143, Jan. 1925
Hammon, William McDowell. Boston physician.
1904–
TEST—for enterotoxin.
*Staphylococcus enterotoxin: an improved cat test,
chemical and immunological studies.* Amer. J. Pub.
Health, 31: 1191–1198, Nov. 1941
Hammond, William Alexander. American neurol-
ogist. 1828–1900
DISEASE—athetosis.
Athetosis. (Editorial) Med. Times and Gaz., 2:
747–748, Dec. 16, 1871
Also: *A treatise on the diseases of the nervous system.*
New York, Appleton, 1871. pp. 654–662
Athetosis. Med. Rec., 8: 309–311, June 16, 1873
Hampton, A. O. See F. Albright

Hamy, E. T. J. See J. L. A. de Quatrefages de Breau
Hanau, Arthur Nathan. Zurich pathologist. 1858–
1900
Successfully transplanted spontaneous carcinoma.
*Experimentelle Uebertragung von Carcinom von Ratte
auf Ratte.* Arch. klin. Chir., 39: 678–679, 1889
*Erfolgreiche experimentelle Uebertragung von Car-
cinom.* Fort. Med., 7: 321–339, May 1, 1889
Hancock, Henry. London surgeon. 1809–1880
AMPUTATION or OPERATION—at ankle.
On the operative surgery of the foot and ankle-joint.
London, Churchill, 1873. 476 pp.
Operated for appendicitis.
Disease of the appendix caeci cured by operation.
Lancet, 2: 380–381, Sept. 30, 1848
Also: London Med. Gaz., 7: 547–550, 1848
Also: *A short account of a case of disease of the ap-
pendix caeci cured by operation, with suggestions as to
the propriety of adopting a similar method of pro-
ceeding in certain cases of peritonitis.* London, Thomp-
son and Davidson, 1848. 12 pp.
Hancock, Virgil Kinney. Seattle, Wash. obstetrician.
1890–
TECHNIC—
Irradiated blood transfusion in treatment of infections
with E. K. Knott, Northwest. Med., 33: 200–204,
June 1934
Hand, Alfred, Jr. Philadelphia physician. 1868–
DISEASE—an early name for craniohypophyseal
xanthomatosis or Hand-Schiller-Christian's disease or
syndrome.
General tuberculosis. Trans. Path. Soc. Philadelphia,
16: 282–284, 1893
Polyuria and tuberculosis. Arch. Pediat., 10: 673–
675, Aug. 1893
Hand, L. V. See G. C. Moore
Handley, William Sampson. English surgeon. 1872–
INCISION—for radical mastectomy.
Cancer of the breast and its treatment. New York,
Hoeber, 1922. 2 ed., p. 241
OPERATION—for ascites.
The surgery of the lymphatic system. Brit. med. J.,
1: 922–928, Apr. 16, 1910
THEORY—of lymphatic permeation of metastases.
Cancer of the breast and its treatment. New York,
Hoeber, 1922. 2 ed., pp. 49–115
Attempted to re-establish lymph circulation in
lymphedema.
*Lymphangioplasty: a new method for the relief of the
brawny arm of breast-cancer and for similar conditions
of lymphatic oedema.* Lancet, 1: 783–785, Mar. 14,
1908
Handovsky, Hans. Prag pharmacologist. 1888–
METHOD—for determination of allantoin.
*Die Bestimmung des Allantoins im Harn durch
Titration.* Z. physiol. Chem., 90: 211–220, Apr. 11,
1914
Haner, Reba Cordellia. Wisconsin scientist
AGAR—for cultivation of pneumococci and streptococci.
*The characteristics of the microcolonies of some patho-
genic cocci* with W. D. Frost, J. infect. Dis., 28: 270–
274, Mar. 1921
Hanes, Granville Scott. Louisville, Ky. proctologist.
1865–1942

POSITION, TABLE—
In: L. A. Buie's *Practical proctology*. Philadelphia,
Saunders, 1938. pp. 29–31
Hanger, Franklin McCue. New York physician.
1894–
CEPHALIN TEST—
*The flocculation of cephalin-cholesterol emulsions by
pathological sera.* Trans. Ass. Amer. Phys., 53: 148–
151, 1938
*Serological differentiation of obstructive from hepatog-
enous jaundice by flocculation of cephalin-cholesterol
emulsions.* J. clin. Invest., 18: 261–269, May 1939
Hanisch, G. See A. F. J. Butenandt
Hanke, Martin Edward. Chicago physiochemist.
1898–
TUBE—
*A new type of centrifuge tube for preparation of blood
serum for accurate p H work.* Proc. Soc. exp. Biol.
N. Y., 30: 1129–1131, May 1933
Hanna, Marion I. See W. R. Campbell
Hannon, Robert Roger. American physician. 1890–
Clinically recognized hyperparathyroidism in 1906.
*A case of osteitis fibrosa cystica (osteomalacia?) with
evidence of hyperactivity of the parathyroid bodies.*
Metabolic study with E. Shorr, U. S. McClellan and
E. F. DuBois, J. clin. Invest., 8: 215–227, Feb. 20,
1930
Hannum, E. See F. McE. Huntoon
Hanot, Victor Charles. French physician. 1844–1896
CIRRHOSIS—biliary.
*Étude sur une forme de cirrhose hypertrophique du
foie (cirrhose hypertrophique avec ictère chronique)*
Thèse de Paris, No. 465, 1875. 155 pp.
SYNDROME—pigmentation of skin, hepatic cirrhosis
and diabetes.
*Cirrhose hypertrophique pigmentaire dans le diabète
sucré* with A. Chauffard, Rev. de méd., 2: 385–403,
1882
Sur la cirrhose pigmentaire dans le diabète sucré with
M. Schachmann, Arch. d. phys., 3 s., 7: 50–87, 1886
Hansemann, David Paul von. German pathologist.
1858–1920
Described asymmetrical mitotic figures as charac-
teristic of cancer cells.
*Ueber asymmetrische Zelltheilung in Epithelkrebsen
und deren biologische Bedeutung.* Arch. f. path. Anat.,
119: 299–326, Feb. 4, 1890
*Studies über die Specificität, den Altruismus und die
Anaplasie der Zellen, mit besonderer Berücksichtigung
der Geschwülste.* Berlin, Hirschwald, 1893. 96 pp.
Described interstitial cell sarcoma (of testicle).
*Ueber die sogenannten Zurischenzellen des Hodens
und deren Bedeutung bei pathologischen Veränderun-
gen.* Arch. f. path. Anat., 142: 538–546, 1895
Hansen, Frederick Carl Christian. Copenhagen
prosector. 1870–1934
SOLUTION—chrome haematoxylin.
*Ueber Eisenhämatein, Chromalaunhämatein, Toner-
dealaunhämatein, Hämateinlösungen und einige
Cochenillefarblösungen.* A. wiss. Mikr., 22: 45–90
(64), 1905
SOLUTION—picrofuchsin.
Eine zuverlässige Bindegewebsfärbung. Anat. Anz.,
15: 151–153, Nov. 10, 1898
Hansen, Gerhard Henrik Armauer. Norwegian
physician. 1841–1912
BACILLUS—B. leprae.

Forelöbige bidrag til spedalskhedens karakteristik.
Nordisk medicinskt Arvik., 1, 1869
Zur Pathologie der Aussatzes. Arch. f. Dermat., pp.
194–211, 1871
Hanson, Adolph Malanchton. Minnesota physician.
1883–
Isolated active principle of parathyroid glands.
*An elementary chemical study of the parathyroid
glands of cattle.* Military Surg., 52: 280–284, Mar.
1923
Hanson, G. F. See G. Dreyer
Hanus, Jos. Prag chemist
SOLUTION—for determination of iodine number.
*Die Anwendung von Jodmonobromid bei der Analyse
von Fetten und Oelen.* Z. Untersuch. Mahr.- u.
Genussm., 4: 913–920, Oct. 15, 1901
Hanzal, R. F. See H. Goldblatt
Hanzlik, P. J. See F. DeEds
Hapke, Franz. German physician
PHENOMENON—unusually prominent presenta-
tion of parietal bone of head of first one of twins.
*Ueber ein neues diagnostisches Phänomen der Zwill-
ingsschwangerschaft.* Emmendingen, Dölter, 1910.
73 pp.
Happold, F. C. See J. S. Anderson
Happold, H. C. See J. W. McLeod
Hardaway, William Augustus. American physician.
1850–1923
Described prurigo nodularis or Hyde's disease.
*A case of multiple tumors of the skin accompanied by
intense pruritus.* Report in: Arch. Dermatol., Phila.,
5: 385 (only), Oct. 1879
*Case of multiple tumor of the skin accompanied by in-
tense pruritus.* Ibid., 6: 129–132, Apr. 1880
Harde, E. French physician
MEDIUM—fish; culture m.
Milieux de cultures au poisson with A. Hauser, C. R.
Soc. Biol., 82: 1259–1260, Dec. 6, 1919
Harding, Harold E. London pathologist
MELANOMA—
A transplantable melanoma of the mouse with R. D.
Passey, J. Path. Bact., 33: 417–427, Apr. 1930
Harding, Victor John. Canadian biochemist. 1885–
METHOD—
*A colorimetric method for the estimation of amino-acid
α-nitrogen* with R. M. MacLean, J. biol. Chem., 20:
217–230, Mar. 1915
Hardisty, R. H. M. See R. F. Ruttan
Hardwick, Rose S. See R. M. Yerkes
Hardy, Arthur Cobb. Massachusetts physicist 1895–
RECORDING SPECTROPHOTOMETER—
A new recording spectrophotometer. J. Optical Soc.
of Amer., 25: 305–311, Sept. 1935
Harger, Rolla Neil. Indianapolis scientist. 1890–
METHOD—
*A simple micromethod for the determination of alcohol
in biologic material.* J. Lab. clin. Res., 20: 746–751,
Apr. 1935
TEST—
*A rapid chemical test for intoxication employing breath.
A new reagent for alcohol and a procedure for estimat-
ing the concentration of alcohol in the body from the
ratio of alcohol to carbon dioxide* with R. B. Lamb and
N. R. Hulpieu, J. A. M. A., 110: 779–785, Mar. 12,
1938

Harington, Charles Robert. London chemist. 1897–
Determined correct molecular structure of thyroxine
and synthesized thyroxine.
*Chemistry of thyroxine. Isolation of thyroxine from
the thyroid gland.* Biochem. J., 20: 293–299, 1926

Harkins, Henry Nelson. Detroit surgeon. 1905–
METHOD—for calculating plasma dosage in burns.
*The present status of intravenous fluid treatment of
traumatic and surgical shock* with R. D. McClure,
Ann. Surg., 114: 891–906, Nov. 1941
The treatment of burns. Springfield, Ill., Thomas, 1942.
457 pp. pp. 210–211
TECHNIC—
A Cooper's ligament herniotomy with S. A. Swensen,
Surg. Clin. N. Amer., 23: 1279–1297, Oct. 1943
TEST—for varicose veins.
*Pulmonary embolism following injection treatment of
varicose veins.* J. A. M. A., 115: 236 (only), July
20, 1940
TOXIC INDEX—
*The present status of blood examination in the diagno-
sis of surgical infections, with a study of twenty-seven
indices of infection reported in the literature.* S. G. O.,
59: 48–61, July 1934

Harley, George. English physician. 1829–1896
DISEASE—recurrent (paroxysmal) hemoglobinuria.
*On intermittent haematuria; with remarks upon its
pathology and treatment.* Med.-chir. Trans., 48: 161–
184, 1865

Harmer, Torr Wagner. Boston surgeon. 1881–
METHOD—of tendon suture.
Certain aspects of hand surgery. New Engl. J. Med.,
214: 613–617, Mar. 26, 1936
Injuries to the hand. Amer. J. Surg., 42: 639–658,
Dec. 1938

Harmer, William Douglas. English physician. 1873–
METHOD—fenestration, of x-ray treatment.
In his: *The relative value of radiotherapy in the treat-
ment of cancers of the upper air passages.* . . . London,
Murray, (1932). 85 pp.

Harmon, P. H. See E. O. Jordan

Harms, H. P. See L. R. Dragstedt

Harper, H. A. See Evelyn L. Blanchard

Harper, Samuel Bowman. Rochester, Minn. sur-
geon. 1912–
METHOD—drying red blood cells.
Preparation and experimental use of dried blood plasma
with H. E. Essex and A. E. Osterberg, Proc. Staff
Meet. Mayo Clin., 15: 689–694, Oct. 30, 1940

Harrass, Paul Georg Otto. German surgeon. 1879–
MEDIA—glucose liver; glucose brain.
*Zur Frage der aeroben Züchtung sogenannter obliga-
tanaerober Bakterien.* Münch. med. Wschr., 53:
2237–2240, Nov. 13, 1906

Harrington, Charles. Boston surgeon. 1856–1908
SOLUTION—for hand disinfection.
Some studies in asepsis. Ann. Surg., 40: 475–485,
Oct. 1904

Harris, A. See J. F. Mahoney

Harris, A. H. 2nd. See F. L. Horsfall, Jr.

Harris, Daniel Thomas. London scientist
TEST—to determine total volume of circulating blood.
*The value of the vital-red method as a clinical means for
the estimation of the volume of the blood.* Brit. J. exp.
Path., 1: 142–158, June 1920

Harris, Downey Lamar. St. Louis pathologist. 1875–
METHOD—
A method for the staining of Negri bodies. J. infect.
Dis., 5: 566–569, Dec 18, 1908

Harris, Franklin I. San Francisco surgeon. 1895–
TUBE—
*Intestinal intubation in bowel obstruction: technique
with a new single lumen mercury weighted tube.* S.
G. O., 81: 671–678, Dec. 1945

Harris, Henry Fauntleroy. American physician.
1867–1926
STAIN—alum hematoxylin.
*On the rapid conversion of haematoxylin into haematein
in staining reactions.* J. appl. Micr., 3: 777–780,
Mar. 1900

Harris, J(ames) Arthur. American scientist. 1880–
STANDARDS—
A biometric study of basal metabolism in man with
F. G. Benedict, Carnegie Inst. of Wash., Pub. 279,
1919. pp. 266

Harris, J. E. See E. L. DeGowin

Harris, L. J. See Y. L. Wang

Harris, Malcolm LaSalle. Chicago surgeon. 1862–
1936
OPERATION—
Hernia of the breast. Surg. Clin. Chicago, 1: 959–963,
Oct. 1917
SEGREGATOR—
*A new and simple method of obtaining the urine sepa-
rately from the two kidneys in either sex.* J. A. M. A.,
30: 236–238, Jan. 29, 1898
SUTURE—
Circular enterorrhaphy: a new method. Chicago Med.
Recorder, 3: 523–537, Sept. 1892

Harris, Norman MacLeod. Canadian physician.
1870–
Discovered and named Bacillus mortiferus.
Bacillus mortiferus (Nov. spec.). J. exp. Med., 6:
519–547, Feb. 4, 1905

Harris, P. N. See S. Warren

Harris, R. L. See T. C. Muer

Harris, Robert Inkerman. Toronto surgeon. 1889–
OPERATION—for lumbar sympathectomy by trans-
verse incision for extraperitoneal approach.
*The rôle of sympathectomy in the treatment of periph-
eral vascular disease.* Brit. J. Surg., 23: 414–424,
Oct. 1935

Harris, Seale. Birmingham, Ala. physician. 1870–
Suggested a syndrome due to excessive secretion or
action of insulin.
Hyperinsulinism and dysinsulinism. J. A. M. A.,
83: 729–733, Sept. 6, 1924

Harris, W. H. See C. W. Duval

Harris, Walter. English physician. 1647–1732
Wrote important treatise on acute diseases in infants (1689), remarkable for some prevision of doctrine of acidosis. Garrison
De morbis acutis infantum. Londini, Smith, 1689.
146 pp.

Harrison, E. F. See A. Gunn

Harrison, Francis Charles. Canadian bacteriologist
SOLUTION—
*Aesculin bile salt media for the isolation of B. coli and
B. typhosus* with J. Vanderleck, Zbl. Bakt., 51: 607–
623, 1909

Harrison, Geoffrey Arthur. English physician
METHOD—
A modification of Berberio's test for human seminal stains. Lancet, 2: 940–941, Oct. 29, 1932
Harrison, Ross Granville. American anatomist. 1870–
Cultivated and studied living explanted tissue in vitro.
The outgrowth of the nerve fiber as a mode of protoplasmic movement. J. exp. Zool., 9: 787–846, Dec. 1910
Harrison, T. R. See J. R. Williams, Jr.
Harrop, George Argale. Baltimore physician. 1890–
TEST—
The excretion of intravenously injected bilirubin as a test of liver function with E. S. Guzmán Barrón, J. clin. Invest., 9: 577–587, Feb. 20. 1931
Suggested that sodium chloride restriction precipitated crises in patients suffering from Addison's disease and could be used to establish a diagnosis in questionable cases.
The diagnosis and treatment of Addison's disease with A. Weinstein, L. J. Soffer and J. H. Trescher, J. A. M. A., 100: 1850–1855, June 10, 1933
Harrow, B. See C. Funk
Harsha, William McIntyre. Chicago surgeon. 1855–
OPERATION—
Bilateral resection of the jaw for prognathism. S. G. O., 15: 51–53, July 1912
Hart, G. H. See H. H. Cole
Hart, K. Berlin anatomist
MODIFICATION—of Weigert's elastic tissue stain.
Die Färbung der elastischen Fasern mit dem von Weigert angegebenen Farbstoff. Zbl. allg. Path. u. path. Anat., 19: 1–3, Jan. 15, 1908
Hart, Theodore Stuart. New York physician. 1869–
TEST—
The detection of B-oxybutyric acid in the urine. Amer. J. med. Sci., 137: 869–872, June 1909
Hartleb, R. See A. Stutzer
Hartley, Frank. New York surgeon. 1857–1913
OPERATION—for facial neuralgia.
Intracranial neurectomy of the second and third division of the fifth nerve; a new method. New York Med. J., 55: 317–319, Mar. 19, 1892
Hartman, Alice. See A. Carrel
Hartman, C. G. See C. F. Geschickter
Hartman, Frank Alexander. Buffalo physiochemist. 1883–
Elaborated extracts of adrenal cortex.
A substance which prolongs the life of adrenalectomized cats with C. G. MacArthur and W. E. Hartman, Proc. Soc. exp. Biol., N. Y., 25: 69–70, Oct. 1927
Hartman, Frank Wilbur. American physician. 1891–
APPARATUS—
Use of cellophane cylinders for desiccating blood plasma: a rapid, economical and bacteriologically safe method with F. W. Hartman, Jr., J. A. M. A., 115: 1989–1990, Dec. 7, 1940
TRANSFUSION APPARATUS—
New methods for blood transfusion and serum therapy. Ibid., 71: 1658–1659, Nov. 16, 1918
Transfusions reactions and citration within the needle. Ibid., 78: 15–18, Jan. 7, 1922
Hartman, H. R. See W. Walters
Hartmann, Alexis Frank. St. Louis pediatrician. 1898–

SOLUTION—6 molar concentration of sodium lactate in Ringer's solution.
Studies in the metabolism of sodium r-lactate: I. Response of normal human subjects to the intravenous injection of sodium r-lactate; II. Response of human subjects with acidosis to the intravenous injection of sodium r-lactate with M. J. E. Senn, J. clin. Invest. 11: 327–344, Mar. 1932
Theory and practice of parenteral fluid administration J. A. M. A., 103: 1349–1354, Nov. 3, 1934
See also P. A. Shaffer
Hartmann, Fritz. German neurologist. 1871–1937
APRAXIA—frontal.
Beiträge zur Apraxielehre. Mschr. Psychiat. Neurol. 21: 97–118; 248–270, 1907
Hartmann, Henri. French surgeon. 1860–
METHOD—of gastrostomy.
Note à propos d'un cas de gastrostomie. Gaz. hebd. méd. chir., 2: 325–326, Apr. 8, 1897
Hartmann, K. See K. Herxheimer
Hartmann, M. See P. Mühlens
Hartree, W. See A. V. Hill
Hartridge, Hamilton. English physiologist. 1886–
METHOD—
A spectroscopic method of estimating carbon monoxide. J. Physiol., 44: 1–21, Mar. 29, 1912
See also J. Barcroft
Hartwell, E. M. See H. N. Martin
Harvey, A. McG. See A. Blalock
Harvey, Gideon. London physician. 1640–1700
Wrote early work on scurvy.
The disease of London; or a new discovery of the scorvey ... London, James, 1675. 296 pp.
Harvey, Samuel Clark. American surgeon. 1886–
METHOD—
The quantitative determination of the chlorides in the urine. Arch. intern. Med., 6: 12–18, July 15, 1910
METHOD—of measuring wound healing by tensile strength of fibroblasts.
The velocity of the growth of fibroblasts in the healing wound. Arch. Surg., 18: 1227–1240, Apr. 1924
See also E. L. Howes
Harvey, William. English physician. 1578–1657
Discovered circulation.
Exercitation anatomica de motu cordis et sanguinis in animalibus. Frankfurti, G. Fitzeri, 1628
Also, transl. by R. Willis. London, Sydenham Soc., 1847. London, Bell, 1889. 72 pp.
Also in: Epoch-making contributions to medicine. ... By C. N. B. Camac, Phila., Saunders, 1909. pp. 27–111
Also in: Cardiac classics. By F. A. Willius and T. E Keyes, St. Louis, Mosby, 1941. pp. 18–79
Harvey, William Frederic. English-Indian scientist. 1873–
AGAR—alkaline egg; culture medium.
Bacteriology and laboratory technique. Section II. Ind. J. med. Res., 9: 66–131 (86), July 1921
AGAR—ascitic fluid blood; culture medium. Ibid., p. 84
AGAR—banana; culture medium. Ibid., p. 119
AGAR—basal infusion; culture medium. Ibid., p. 87; 92; 111
AGAR—brilliant green bile salt; for cultivation of colon-typhoid group. Ibid., p. 91

AGAR—glucose blood; for cultivation of gonococci. Ibid., p. 82

AGAR—lactose blood; for cultivation of colon-typhoid group. Ibid., p. 73

AGAR—litmus blood peptone; for cultivation of meningococci. Ibid., p. 76

AGAR—mannitol infusion; culture medium. Ibid., p. 111

AGAR—milk; culture medium. Ibid., p. 95

AGAR—oxalated blood; for cultivation of gonococci. Ibid., p. 77

AGAR—peptic blood digest; for cultivation of B. influenza. Ibid., p. 100

AGAR—phenol peptone; culture medium. Ibid., p. 90

AGAR—placenta blood serum; culture medium. Ibid., p. 78

AGAR—saponin blood; culture medium. Ibid., p. 76

AGAR—starch; culture medium. Ibid., p. 112

AGAR—trypsinized blood; for cultivation of B. influenza. Ibid., pp. 76–77

AGAR—whey infusion; for cultivation of gonococci. Ibid., p. 95

BROTH—ascitic fluid infusion; culture medium. Ibid., p. 83

BROTH—blood infusion; for cultivation of gonococci. Ibid., p. 82

BROTH—dehydrated; culture medium.
Desiccated nutrient media with K. R. K. Iyengar, Ibid., 9: 364–368 (366), Oct. 1921

BROTH—ferric tartrate infusion; culture medium.
Bacteriology and laboratory technique. Section II. Ind. J. med. Res., 9: 66–131 (107), July 1921

BROTH—lead acetate infusion; culture medium. Ibid.

INFUSION—starch beef; for cultivation of gonococci. Ibid., p. 112

MEDIUM—heart; for cultivation of anaerobes. Ibid., p. 94

SOLUTION—alkaline casein; for cultivation of anaerobic organisms. Ibid., p. 96

SOLUTION—basal neutral red peptone; for studying fermentation by bacteria. Ibid., p. 108

SOLUTION—blood clot digest; culture medium. Ibid., p. 100

SOLUTION—brown cresol purple milk; culture medium. Ibid., p. 88

SOLUTION—China blue rosolic acid milk; culture medium. Ibid., p. 95

SOLUTION—egg; culture medium. Ibid., p. 85

SOLUTION—egg peptone; for enrichment of V. cholera. Ibid., p. 86

SOLUTION—egg yolk; culture medium. Ibid., p. 121

SOLUTION—glycerol urea; culture medium. Ibid., p. 104

SOLUTION—hydrolyzed meat; culture medium. Ibid., p. 69

SOLUTION—trypsinized heart; culture medium Ibid., p. 114

SOLUTION—trypsinized meat and kidney; for cultivation of B. tetani. Ibid., p. 115

SOLUTION—wheat flour; culture medium. Ibid., p. 119

Harvie, John. London obstetrician
Described advantages of external manual expression of placenta over traction or internal manipulation (ninety years before Credé). Garrison
Practical directions showing a method of preserving the

perineum in birth, and delivering the placenta without violence; illustrated by cases. London, Wilson and Nicol, 1767. 48 pp.

Harz, Carl Otto. Munich botanist. 1842–1906
Identified micro-organism of actinomycosis and gave it its name.
Actinomyces bovis, ein neuer Schimmel in den Geweben des Rindes. Dtsch. Z. f. Thiermed., 5 (2 Suppl. Hft.), 125–140, 1879

Hashimoto, Hakaru. Japanese pathologist. 1881–
GOITER or STRUMA—
Zur Kenntniss der lymphomatösen Veränderung der Schilddrüse (Struma lymphomatosa). Arch. f. klin. Chir., 97: 219–248, Jan. 9, 1912

Haskell, Benjamin. Philadelphia surgeon. 1901–
METHOD—
The subcutaneous injection of alcohol for pruritus ani with C. D. Smith, J. A. M. A., 106: 1248–1249, Apr. 11, 1936
See also J. H. Allen

Haskins, Howard Davis. Portland, Ore. physician. 1871–1933
METHOD—
A rapid method for determination of the sedimentation rate of the red cells with results in health and disease with F. E. Trotman, E. E. Osgood and A. Mathieu, J. Lab. clin. Med., 16: 487–494, Feb. 1931
METHOD—
Methods of estimating hemoglobin with E. E. Osgood, Northwest Med., 25: 500–503, Sept. 1926
METHOD—
Modifications of Van Slyke's titration method for estimating the alkali reserve of blood with E. E. Osgood, J. Lab. clin. Med., 6: 37–41, Oct. 1920
MODIFICATION—of Shaffer-Hartman method for estimation of sugar in urine.
A uniform method for the estimation of glucose in blood and urine with W. P. Holbrook, Northwest Med., 23: 355–357, Aug. 1924
SOLUTION—for determination of hemoglobin.
A new permanent standard for Sahli's hemoglobinometer. J. biol. Chem., 57: 111–113, Aug. 1923
See also E. E. Osgood

Haslam, John. English physician. 1764–1844
Described pathology of dementia paralytica.
Observations on insanity; with practical remarks on the disease, and an account of the morbid appearances on dissection. London, Rivington, 1798. 147 pp.

Haslam, Thomas P. Iowa scientist
BROTH—brain liver infusion; culture medium.
Immunization with blackleg aggression. J. Immunol., 5: 539–546 (540), Nov. 1920

Haslewood, G. A. D. See G. Barry

Hasley, D. E. See I. F. Huddleson

Hasner, Joseph Ritter von. Prague ophthalmologist. 1819–1892
VALVE—at end of nasal duct.
Beiträge zur Physiologie und Pathologie des Thränenableitungsapparates. Prag, Calve, 1850. 104 pp.

Hass, Julius. Vienna surgeon. 1884–
OPERATION—subtrochanteric osteotomy in coxa vara.
Die Lorenzsche Gabelung und ihre Anwendungsgebiete. Ergebn. Chir. u. Orthop., 21: 457–488, 1928

Hasselbalch, K. A. Copenhagen scientist
FORMULA—for pH concentration of blood.

*Elektrometrische Reaktionsbestimmung des Blutes bei
Körpertemperatur* with C. Lundsgaard, Biochem.
Z., Berlin, 38: 77–91, Jan. 6, 1912

Hasson, James. London physician
REACTION—
Anaphylaxis following injection of pituitary extract.
Brit. med. J., 1: 242 (only), Feb. 8, 1930

Hastings, A(lbert) Baird. Chicago chemist. 1895–
FORMULA—
*The exchange of salt and water between muscle and
blood. I. The effect of an increase in total body water
produced by the intravenous injection of isotonic salt
solutions* with Lillian Eichelberger, J. biol. Chem.
117: 73–93, Jan. 1937
METHOD—
*Studies of acidosis. XX. The colorimetric determina-
tion of blood pH at body temperature without buffer
standards* with J. Sendroy, Jr. Ibid., 61: 695–710,
Oct. 1924

Hastings, Thomas Ward. New York physician.
1873–1942
STAIN—for malarial parasites.
*A method for preparing a permanent Nocht's stain
(Nocht-Jenner stain).* J. exp. Med., 7: 265–279,
June 10, 1905

Hata, Sahachiro. Japanese physician. 1876–1938
METHOD—
*A contribution to our knowledge of the cultivation of
Spirochaeta recurrens.* Zbl. Bakt., 72: 107–112, Nov.
26, 1914
PREPARATION or TREATMENT—
Salvarsantherapie der Rattenbisskrankheit in Japan.
Münch. med. Wschr., 59: 854–857, Apr. 16, 1912
See also P. Ehrlich

Hatcher, Robert Anthony. American pharmacolo-
gist. 1868–1944
METHOD—cat method of assaying digitalis.
Standardization of digitalis—a preliminary report.
J. Amer. Pharm. Ass., 8: 913–914, Nov. 1919

Hauck, Gustav. Berlin surgeon
OPERATION—gastrostomy.
*Zur künstlichen Epithelisierung der Witzelfistel nach
Narath.* Dtsch. Z. Chir., 171: 125–129, June 1922

Haudek, Martin. German physician. 1880–1931
NICHE, SIGN or SYNDROME—gastric ulcer cavity
filled with bismuth.
*Zur röntgenologischen Diagnose der Ulzerationen in
der Pars media des Magens.* Münch. med. Wschr.,
57: 1587–1591, July 26, 1910

Hauman, M. L. French botanist
SOLUTION—pectin peptone, for cultivation of B.
coli.
*Étude microbiologique et chimique du rouissage aérobie
du lin.* Ann. Inst. Pasteur, 16: 379–385, May 1902

Hauptmann, Alfred. German neurologist. 1881–
TREATMENT—
Luminal bei Epilepsie. München. med. Wschr., 59:
1907–1909, Aug. 27, 1912

Hauser, A. See E. Harde

Hauser, Gustav. German bacteriologist. 1856–1935
Isolated Proteus vulgaris.
METHOD—of anaerobic culture.
*Ueber Fäulnissbakterien und deren Beziehungen zur
Septicämie. Ein Beitrag zur Morphologie der Spalt-
pilze.* Leipzig, Vogel, 1885
METHOD—of staining spores.

*Entgegnung auf die Bemerkungen des Hrn. can
med. H. Schedtler über die Zooglöa-Bildung und da
Schwärmstadium der Proteusarten.* Münch. me
Wschr., 34: 492–494, June 28, 1887

Hausmann, Theodor. Rostock physician. 1868–
TEST—for urobilin.
Der Urobilinnachweis mittels Kupfersulfat. Dtsch
med. Wschr., 39: 360 (only), Feb. 20, 1913

Haüy, Valentin. French physician. 1745–1822
Originated methods of teaching blind to read b
means of raised letters.
Essai sur l'education des aveugles. . . . Paris, Imp. c
enf. aveugles, 1786. 126 pp.

Havens, Leon Clive. American physician. 1891–
BROTH—kidney and blood infusion, for cultivatio
of hemolytic streptococci.
*A toxic substance obtained by growing hemolyt
streptococci in a special medium* with Margaret
Taylor, Amer. J. Hyg., 1: 311–320, (313), Ma
1921

Haverhill
FEVER—occurred in Haverhill, Mass. in Jan. 1926
*Erythema arthriticum epidemicum; preliminary repor
By E. H. Place, L. E. Sutton and O. Willner, Bosto
M. and S. J., 194: 285–287, Feb. 18, 1926

Havers, Cloptan. English anatomist. 1650?–1702
CANALS, SPACES, LAMELIA—in bone.
*Osteologia nova or some new observations on the bone
and the parts belonging to them, with the manner
their accretion and nutrition, . . .* London, Smith
1691. 249 pp.

Hawk, Philip Bovier. Urbana, Ill. chemist. 1874–
MODIFICATION—
*A modification of Wohlgemuth's method for the quan
titative study of the activity of the pancreatic function
Arch. intern. Med., 8: 552–556, Oct. 15, 1911
See also H. A. Mattill

Hawkins, Caesar Henry. London surgeon. 1798–188
KELOID—
On warty tumors in cicatrices. London Med. Gaz., 13
481–482, Dec. 28, 1833

Hawley, George Waller. Bridgeport, Conn. surgeon
1875–1940
PIN AND STIRRUP DEVICE—
*A combination Finochietto and Steinmann pin tractio
stirrup.* J. A. M. A., 70: 22–23, Jan. 5, 1918
TABLE—orthopedic.
Fracture and orthopedic table. Ibid., 60: 1850–1851
June 14, 1913
*A new fracture, x-ray and orthopedic table: the author'
original orthopedic table redesigned.* Amer. J. Surg.
8: 19–25, Oct. 1932
Additional advantages of the Hawley table. S. G. O.
65: 228–231, Aug. 1937

Haxthausen, Holger. Copenhagen dermatologist
KERATOSIS—
Keratoderma climactericum. Brit. J. Derm. and
Syph., 46: 161–167, Apr. 1934
METHOD—culture.
*Les streptococcies épidermiques étudiées par une nou-
velle méthode de culture.* Ann. Dermat. et Syph.
Paris, 6 s., 8: 201–212, Apr. 1927

Hay, Matthew. Scottish physician. 1855–1932
TEST—
Test for the bile acids. In: L. Landois and W. Stirling

Text-book of human physiology. London, 1886. 2 ed., 1: 381

Hay, William Howard. American physician. 1866–
DIET—
Health via food. East Aurora, N. Y., Sun Diet Press, (1929). 299 pp.

Hayem, Georges. Paris physician. 1841–1933
APPARATUS—for counting blood corpuscles.
Hayem and Nachet's new apparatus for counting the blood-corpuscles. (Editorial) London Med. Rec., 3: 457–458, July 15, 1875
CORPUSCLES—blood-placques or haematoblasts.
Note sur les caractères et l'évolution des hématoblastes chez les ovipares. Mém. Soc. Biol., Paris, 1877, pp. 97–110, 1879
L'hématoblaste, troisième élément du sang. Paris, Presse univ. de Franc, 1923. 295 pp.
DISEASE—pseudoleukemia; Jaksch-Hayem d.
Du sang et de ses alterations pathologiques. Paris, 1889. p. 864
METHOD—for quantitative determination of hydrochloric acid in stomach contents.
Du chimisme stomachal with Winter, Paris, 1891. p. 72
SOLUTION—used in microscopic examination of blood.
Recherches sur l'anatomie normale et pathologiques du sang. Paris, Masson, 1878. 143 pp.
SYNDROME—of Hayem-Widal; jaundice with increased fragility of red corpuscles to hypotonic salt solution and moderate enlargement of spleen.
Sur une variété particuliére d'ictère chronique: ictère infectieux chronique splénomégalique. Pr. méd., 6: 121–125, Mar. 9, 1898
Nouvelle contribution à l'étude de l'ictère infectieux chronique splénomegalique. Bull. Soc. méd. Hôp. Paris, 25: 122–140, Jan. 24, 1908
Described chronic interstitial hepatitis.
Contribution à l'étude de l'hépatite interstitielle chronique aver hypertrophie (sclérose ou cirrhose hypertrophique du foie). Arch. de Physiol. norm. et path Paris, 2 s., 1: 126–157, Jan. 1874
Reported poor clot retractility in purpura.
Du caillot non rétractile; suppression de la formation du serum sanguin dans quelques états pathologiques. C. R. Acad. Sci., 123: 894–896, Nov. 25, 1896

Hayes, William Van Valzah. New York City physician. 1867–
MANEUVER—pushing intestines upward to left relieves pressure on mesenteric pedicle and duodenum and allows duodenal contents to pass to jejunum; visualized by x-ray.
Chronic intestinal stasis, medically considered. Abstr. in: Med. Rec., 85: 409–410, Feb. 28, 1914
Chronic intestinal stasis. New York, Elliott, 1914

Haygarth, John. English physician. 1740–1827
NODES—joint swellings in arthritis deformans.
A clinical history of the nodosity of the joints. In his: *A clinical history of diseases*. London, 1805. Vol. 2, p. 155

Hayner, John Clifford. New York surgeon. 1893–
OPERATION—
An analysis of the mechanism and surgical treatment of inguinal hernia: preliminary report of a new operation. J. Amer. Inst. Homeopathy, 25: 813–825, July 1932

Haynes, Herbert Hodge. Clarksburg, W. Va. surgeon. 1878–
SPLINT—
Skeletal fixation of fractures. Amer. J. Surg., 59: 25–36, Jan. 1943

Haynes, Irving Samuel. New York surgeon. 1861–
OPERATION—
Congenital internal hydrocephalus: its treatment by drainage of the cisterna magna into the cranial sinuses. Ann. Surg., 57: 449–484, Apr. 1913
Further experiences in the treatment of hydrocephalus by cisterna—sinus drainage (author's operation). New York State J. M., 16: 174–181, Apr. 1916

Hays, Harold Melvin. New York City rhinolaryngologist. 1880–1940
NASAL SYPHON APPARATUS—
Conservative treatment of the nasal sinuses. New York State J. M., 37: 137–144, Jan. 15, 1937

Hayward, George. Boston surgeon. 1791–1863
OPERATION—
Case of vesico-vaginal fistula, successfully treated by an operation. Amer. J. med. Sci., 24: 283–288, Aug. 1839

Hayward, Nancy J. London bacteriologist
METHOD—
The rapid identification of Cl. welchii by Nagler tests in plate cultures. J Path. Bact., 55: 285–293, July 1943

Head, Henry. English physician. 1861–1940
AREAS or ZONES—of hyperalgesia of skin, associated with diseases of viscera.
On disturbances of sensation with especial reference to the pain of visceral disease. Brain, 16: 1–133, 1893; 17: 339–480, 1894; 19: 153–276, 1896
Sensation and the cerebral cortex. Ibid., 41: 57–253, Sept. 1918
Demonstrated action of vagus in respiration.
On the regulation of respiration. Part I. Experimental. J. Physiol., 10: 1–70, 1889
Same. *Part II. Theoretical*. Ibid., 279–290
Showed that herpes zoster is a hemorrhagic inflammation of posterior nerve-roots.
The pathology of herpes zoster and its bearing on sensory localisation with A. W. Campbell, Brain, 23: 353–523, 1900
See also W. H. R. Rivers

Healy, William. Boston physician. 1869–
TEST—of intelligence.
A pictorial completion test. Psychol. Bull., 10: 80, 1913
Pictorial completion test. II. J. Appl. Psychol., 5: 225–239, 1921–22

Heath, Christopher. English surgeon. 1835–1905
OPERATION—division of ascending rami of lower jaw with a saw for ankylosis.
On the causes and treatment of closure and immobility of the jaws. Dublin Q. J. M. Sci., 35: 323–344, May 1, 1863

Heatley, N. G. See E. Chain

Heaton, George. Boston surgeon. 1808–1879
OPERATION—for inguinal hernia.
A review of a report of a committee of the American Medical Association on the permanent cure of reducible hernia or rupture. Boston, Chadwick, 1853. 31 pp.
The cure of rupture, reducible and irreducible, also of varicocele and hydrocele, by new methods. Boston, Houghton, 1877. 196 pp.

Hebb, Richard Graniger. London physician. 1848–1918

DISEASE—

A case of actinomycosis hominis. Westminster Hosp. Rep., London, 3: 150–154, 1888

Heberden, William. English physician. 1710–1801

ASTHMA—see syndrome of angina pectoris.

DISEASE or RHEUMATISM—of smaller joints, accompanied by nodosities.

NODES or SIGN—on sides of distal phalanges of fingers, commonly ascribed to gout.

Commentaries on the history and cure of diseases. London, Payne, 1802. Cap. 28

De nodis digitorum. In his: *Commentarii de morborum historia et curatione.* Londini, Payne, 1802

SYNDROME—of angina pectoris; substernal pain provoked by effort or excitement.

Some account of a disorder of the breast. Med. Trans. Col. Phys. Lond., 2: 59–67, 1768–70

On an angina pectoris. Ibid., 3: 1, 1785

Also: *Commentaries on the history and cure of diseases.* London, Payne, 1802. Cap. 28

Also: *Commentarii de morborum historia et curatione* London, Payne, 1802. Cap. 28

Also: *An introduction to the study of physic.* By William Heberden. With prefatory essay on LeRoy Crummer, New York, Hoeber, 1929. 159 pp.

Also: Chapter 70 in F. A. Willius and T. E. Keys' Cardiac classics. St. Louis, Mosby, 1941. pp. 222–224

Described night blindness.

On night blindness or nyctalopia. Med. Trans. Col. Phys. Lond., 1: 60–63, 1768

Described varicella.

On the chicken-pox. Ibid., 1: 427–436, 1768

Heberden, William, Jr. English physician. 1767–1845

Wrote a Latin epitome of pediatrics, "which is of such superlative excellence and brevity that it might well be attributed to the father." Garrison

Morborum puerilium epitome. Londini, Payne, 1804. 72 pp.

(Same) In English. 1807. 120 pp.

Hebra, Ferdinand von. Austrian dermatologist. 1816–1880

DISEASE—erythema exsudative multiforme. In: Hebra-Kaposi's: *Lehrbruch der Hautkrankheiten.* (Virchow's Handb. III) Erlangen, 1860. 1: 198

Ueber die Verwendung des Kautschuks bei der Behandlung von Hautkrankheiten. Arch. f. Dermat., 1: 1–7, 1869

PRURIGO—

Juckblattern. In: *Traité pratique des maladies de la peau.* Paris, 1854. p. 479

Wrote classic account of lichen ruber.

Lichen exsudativus ruber. Allg. Wien. med. Zeitg., 2: 75–76, May 12, 1857

Also in: *Atlas der Hautkrankheiten* with A. Elfinger, Wien, 1: 298, 1874

Made classification of skin diseases according to their pathologic anatomy.

Versuch einer auf pathologische Anatomie gegründeten Eintheilung der Hautkranken. Z. d. k. k. Gesellsch. d. Aerzte zu Wien, 1: 34–52; 142–155; 211–231, 1845

Gave classic account of eczema marginatum.

Acute Exantheme und Hautkrankheiten. Handb. d. spec. Path. u. Therap., 3, 1 Abth., 31: 316–363, 1860

Also: *Lehrbuch der Hautkrankheiten.* 1860

Also: London, New Sydenham Soc., 1866

Described impetigo herpetiformis.

Ueber einzelne während der Schwangerschaft, der Wochenbette und bei Uterinalkrankheiten der Fraue zu beobachtende Hautkrankheiten. Wien. med. Wschr 22: 1197–1201, 1872

Hebra, Hans von. Austrian dermatologist. 1847–190

Described rhinoscleroma. Garrison

Ueber ein eigenthümliches Neugebilde an der Nase Rhinosclerom. Wien. med. Wschr., 20: 1–5, Jan. 1870

Introduced thiosinamine. Garrison

Ueber die Wirkung des Allylsulfocarbamids (Thiosin amins) bei subcutaner Einverleibung. Abstr.: Wien med. Bl., 15: 605–606, Sept. 22, 1892

Described rhinophyma. Garrison

Das Rhinophyma. Vierteljschr. f. Dermat., 8: 603 619, 1881

Hecht, Adolf Franz. Vienna physician. 1876–

REAGENT and TEST—for mucus in feces.

Ein neuer mikrochemischer Schleimnachweis im Stuhl Wein. klin. Wschr., 21: 1554 (only), Nov. 5, 1908

Hecht, Hugo. Prague physician

TEST—for iodide in urine.

Eine einfache Jodprobe. Med. Klin., 12: 725 (only July 2, 1916

TEST—for syphilis.

Eine Vereinfachung der Komplementbindungs-rea tion bei Syphilis. Wien. klin. Wschr., 21: 1742–174 Dec. 10, 1903; 22: 338–340, Mar. 11, 1909

Wassermannsche Reaktion und Präzipitation. ImmunForsch., 24: 258–266, Nov. 23, 1915

Zur Methodik der Wassermannschen Reaktion. Dern Wschr., 68: 289–292, May 10, 1919

Die Grundlagen einer neuen Flockungsreaktion b Syphilis. Arch. Derm. u. Syph. Orig., 136: 296–30 Nov. 7, 1921

Hecht, Selig. American physiologist. 1892–

INSTRUMENT—

An adaptometer for measuring human dark adaptatie with S. Shlaer, J. Optic. Soc. Amer., 28: 269–27 July 1938

Hedin, R. I. See R. W. McNealy

Hedin, Sven Gustof. Swedish scientist. 1859–

HEMATOCRIT—for estimating relative volumes corpuscles and plasma.

Undersökningar med hematokriten. Nord. med. Ark Stockholm, 22: 1–12, 1890

Der Hämatokrit, ein neuer Apparat zur Untersuc ung des Blutes. Skand. Arch. f. Physiol., Leipzig, 134–140, 1891

Untersuchungen mit dem Hämatokrit. Ibid., 360–3 REACTION—for histidine.

Zur Kenntniss der Spaltungsproducte der Protei körper. Z. phys. Chem., 22: 191–196, 1896

Heerfordt, Christian Frederick. Copenhagen ph sician

SYNDROME—oveoparotid fever.

Ueber eine "Febris uveo-parotidea subchronica," der Glangula parotis und der Uvea des Auges lokalisi und häufig mit Paresen cerebrospinaler Nerven ko plizieret.* Arch. Ophthal., 70: 254–273, Apr. 13, 190

Heflebower, Roy Cleveland. U. S. Army physicis 1884–

DIAZO REACTION—of urine.

UROCHROMOGEN TEST—for urine.

The prognostic value of the urochromogen and diazo reactions in pulmonary tuberculosis. A preliminary report. Amer. J. med. Sci., 143: 221–229, Feb. 1912

Hegar, Alfred. Freiburg gynecologist. 1830–1914
OPERATION—perineorrhaphy.
Ueber die Exstirpation normaler und nicht zu umfänglichen Tumoren degenerirter Eierstöcke. Zbl. ges. Gynäk. Geburtsh., 1: 297–304, Nov. 10, 1877; 2: 25–39, Jan. 19, 1878
SIGN—softening of lower segment of uterus, indicative of pregnancy.
Ein neues sicheres diagnostisches Zeichen der Schwangerschaft in den ersten Monaten. described by C. Reinl of Hegar's clinic. Prager med. Wschr., 9: 253–254, June 25, 1884
Diagnose der frühesten Schwangerschafts-periode. Dtsch. med. Wschr., 21: 565–567, Aug. 29, 1895

Hegner, Robert William. Baltimore scientist. 1880–
METHOD—for preparation of washed cysts.
Excystation and infection in the rat with Giardia Lambia from man. Amer. J. Hyg., 7: 433–447, July 1927

Heiberg, Hjalmar. Christiania pathologist. 1837–1897
Suggested microbic nature of endocarditis.
Ein Fall von Endocarditis ulcerosa puerperalis mit Pilzbildungen im Herzen (Mycosis endocardii). Arch. f. path. Anat., 56: 407–414, Nov. 30, 1872

Heidelberger, Michael. New York scientist. 1888–
Made chemical study of antigenic constituents of pneumococcus.
The soluble specific substance of pneumococcus with O. T. Avery, J. exp. Med., 38: 73–79, July 1, 1923
(Same) *Second paper* with O. T. Avery, Ibid., 40: 301–316, Sept. 1, 1924
See also W. A. Jacobs

Heidenhain, Lothar. Worms a. Rh. surgeon. 1860–
Performed a successful lobectomy in man.
Ausgedehnte Lungenresection wegen zahlreicher eiternder Bronchectasieen in einem Unterlappen. Verh. dtsch. Ges. f. Chir., 30: 636–643, 1901

Heidenhain, Martin. Tübingen pathologist. 1864–
CHROME HAEMATOXYLIN—
Eine neue Verwendung des Hämatoxylin. Arch. mikr. Anat., 24: 468–470, 1885
Eine Abänderung der Farbung mit Hämatoxylin und chromsauren Salzen. Ibid., 27: 383–384, 1886
METHOD—of Mallory-Heidenhain; staining with azocarmine or aniline blue.
Ueber die Mallorysche Bindegewebsfärbung mit Karmin und Azokarmin als Vorfarben. Z. wiss. Mikr., Leipzig, 32: 361–372, 1915
STAIN—Biondi-Heidenhain s. Mallory
In: *Festschrift für Koelliker.* Leipzig, Engelmann, 1892. pp. 109–166
STAIN—iron hematoxylin.
Noch einmal über die Darstellung der Centralkörper durch Eisenhämatoxylin nebst einigen allgemeinen Bemerkungen über die Hämatoxylinfarben. Z. wiss. Mikr., 13: 186–199, 1896
TEST—for albumin.
Die Anilinfarben als Eiweissfällungsmittel. Münch. med. Wschr., 49: 437–440, Mar. 18, 1902
VANADIUM—HAEMATOXYLIN—
Hämatoxylinvanadium. Excyklop. mikr. Technik., 1: 518 (only), 1903

Heidenhain, Rudolph Peter Heinrich. German physician. 1834–1897
CELLS—of gastric glands.
Untersuchungen ü er den Bau der Labdrüsen. Arch. mikr. Anat., 6: 368–406, 1870
LAW—glandular secretion always involves change in structure of gland.
Ueber einige Verhältnisse des Baues und der Thätigkeit der Speicheldrüsen. Zbl. med. Wiss., 4: 130–133, Feb. 24, 1866
STAIN—triacid. Mallory
Beiträge zur Histologie und Physiologie der Dünndarmschleimhaut. Arch. f. ges. Physiol., 43, Suppl., 40, 1888
THEORY—of urinary secretion.
Versuche über den Vorgang der Harnabsonderung. Arch. ges. Physiol., 9: 1–27, 1874
Neue Versuche über die Aufsaugung im Dünndarm. Ibid., 56: 579–631, May 26, 1894
Studied effects of poisons on nerves of submaxillary gland.
Ueber die Wirkung einiger Gifte auf die Nerven der glandula submaxillaris. Ibid., 5: 309–318, 1872
Studied histologic changes in gastric glands during secretion.
Ueber die Absonderung der Fundusdrüsen des Magens. Ibid., 19: 148–166, 1879

Heile, Bernhard. Wiesbaden surgeon
OPERATION—
Zur Behandlung des Hydrocephalus. Dtsch. med. Wschr., 34: 1468–1470, Aug. 20, 1908

Heim, Ludwig Heinrich Wilhelm. German physician. 1857–
AGAR—meat extract salt; culture medium.
Zur Bereitungsweise von Nährmitteln. Zbl. Bakt., 17: 190–195 (193), Feb. 15, 1895
AGAR—hemoglobin.
Ueber Pneumoniecoccen. Dtsch. med. Wschr., 33: 1587–1588, Sept. 26, 1907

Heiman, Henry. New York physician. 1865–
AGAR—pleuritic serum, for cultivation of gonococci.
A further study of the biology of the gonococcus (Neisser), with contributions to the technique: a paper based on the morphological and biological examination of exudates in cases of chronic urethritis. Med. Rec., 50: 887–893, Dec. 19, 1896

Heine, Jacob von. German physician. 1800–1879
DISEASE—acute anterior or epidemic poliomyelitis; Heine-Medin d.
Beobachtungen über Lähmungszustände der untern Extremitäte und deren Behandlung. Stuttgart, Köhler, 1840. 78 pp.
(Same) II Aufl., Spinale Kinderlähmung. Stuttgart, Cotta, 1860. 204 pp.

Heine, Leopold. German oculist. 1870–
OPERATION—cyclodialysis in glaucoma.
Die Cyklodialyse, eine neue Glaukom-Operation. Dtsch. med. Wschr., 31: 824–826, May 25, 1905

Heineke, Walther Hermann. German surgeon. 1834–1901
OPERATION—pyloroplasty.
Reported by F. Fronmüller in: *Operation der Pylorusstenose.* Inaug. Dissert. (Erlangen), Fürth, p. 13, 1886

Heinemann, Paul Gustav. Chicago bacteriologist
AGAR—asparagin peptone; culture medium.

A substitute for potato as a culture medium. J. infect. Dis., 4: 282–284, Apr. 10, 1907
AGAR—litmus mannitol; culture medium
AGAR—meat extract; culture medium.
BOUILLON—culture medium.
SOLUTION—glucose yeast infusion.
A laboratory guide in bacteriology. Chicago, Univ. Chicago Press, 1905; 3 ed., 1915
Heinze, Berthold. Halle a. S. chemist
SOLUTION—basal.
Einige Berichtigungen und weitere Mitteilungen zu der Abhandlung: " Ueber die Bildung und Wiederverarbeitung von Glycogen durch niedere pflanzliche Organismen." Zbl. Bakt., 2 Abt., 14: 9–21 (18), Jan. 18, 1905
Einige Beiträge zur mikrobiologischen Bodenkunde. Ibid., 16: 640–653; 703–711, 1906
Heise, F. H. See L. Brown
Heiser, Victor George. New York physician. 1873–
TREATMENT—of leprosy by the injection of a mixture containing 60 c.c. of chaulmoogra oil, 60 c.c. of camphorated oil and 4 gr. of resorcin.
Leprosy—its treatment in the Philippine Islands by the hypodermic use of a Chaulmoogra oil mixture. Pub. Health Rep., Suppl. No. 20, Oct. 16, 1914. 25 pp.
Heister, Laurentius. German surgeon. 1683–1758
DIVERTICULUM—external jugular sinus.
FOLDS or VALVES—of mucosa in cystic duct and in neck of gall bladder.
Compedium anatomicum. Amsterdam, 1720
Introduced spinal braces, 1700.
Chirurgie. Nürnberg, Hoffman, 1719
Made first postmortem section of appendicitis, 1711. Garrison
Medicinische chirurgische und anatomische Wahrnehmungen. Rostock, Koppe, 1753. 1112 pp.
Also, in English. London, Reeves, 1755. 708 pp.
Hektoen, Ludvig. Chicago pathologist. 1863–
TEST—
Identification of human seminal stains; precipitin reaction of seminal fluid with G. J. Rukstinat, Arch. Path., 6: 96–99, July 1928
Produced experimental cirrhosis of liver.
Experimental bacillary cirrhosis of the liver. J. Path. and Bact., Edinburgh, 7: 214–220, 1901
Produced measles in man by injecting blood collected early in disease from measles patients.
Experimental measles. J. infect. Dis., 2: 238–255, Mar. 1, 1905
Pointed out possible danger from isoagglutination in transfusion of blood.
Isoagglutination of human corpuscles. Ibid., 4: 297–303, June 15, 1907
Held, Hans. German physician. 1866–
STAINING METHOD—for nerve tissue.
Beiträge zur Structur der Nervenzellen und ihrer Fortsätze. Zeweite Abhandlung. Arch. Anat. Phys., Anat. Abth., pp. 204–294 (227), 1897
Helferich, Friedrich. German surgeon. 1842–1927
OPERATION—
Die Gastrostomie als Hülfsoperation vor den Operationen am Pharynx und Oesophagus. Dtsch. Z. f. Chir., 55: 410–411, Apr. 1900
Heller, Arnold Ludwig Gotthelf. Kiel pathologist. 1840–1913
AORITIS—syphilitic, of Döhle-Heller.

Ein Fall von eigentümlicher Aortenerkrankung bei einem Syphilitischen I. D. Kiel, 1885
Die Aortensyphilis als Ursache von Aneurysmen. Münch. med. Wschr., 46: 1669–1671, Dec. 12, 1899
Heller, Ernst. Leipzig surgeon. 1877–
OPERATION—extramucous esophagocardioplasty.
Ausschaltung der Nervi vagi in ihrem intrathorakalen Verlauf für die Zwecke der Oesophaguschirurgie durch Novocain. Abstr.: Verh. dtsch. Ges. Chir., 42, Congr., 269–271, 1913
Extramuköse Cardiaplastik beim chronischen Cardiospasmus mit Dilatation des Oesophagus. Mitt. Grenzgeb. Med. Chir., 27: 141–149, 1913
Heller, Johann Florian. Vienna physician. 1813–1871
TEST—for albumin in urine.
Qualitative und quantitative Analyse albuminöser Flüssigkeiten. Arch. physiol. u. path. Chem. u Mikr., 1: 192–199, 1844
TEST—for glucose in urine.
Neue Diagnose des Zuckers. Ibid., 212–213
Höchst einfache und sichere Methode zur Diagnose des Zuckers in thierischen Flüssigkeiten; Unterscheidung des Harn-, Milch- und Rohrzuckers. Ibid. 292–298
Noticed retention of chlorides in pneumonic urine
Chemische Untersuchung des Harns, der Harnsedimente und Konkretionen am Krankenbette, nebst diagnostischen Beiträgen. Ibid., 4: 491–526 (522–525), 1847
Wrote famous classic on urinary concretions.
Die Harnconcretionen, ihre Entstehung, Erkennung und Analyse, mit besonderer Rücksicht auf Diagnose und Therapie der Nieren- und Blasenerkrankung. Wien Tendler, 1860. 197 pp.
TEST—for indican in urine. Ibid.
Heller, Julius. German physician. 1864–1931
SOLUTION—urine peptone; culture medium.
Der Harn als bakteriologischer Nährboden. Berl klin. Wschr., 27: 893–894, Sept. 29, 1890
Hellerström, Sven Curt Alfred. Stockholm physician. 1901–
Proved that etiologic agent of lymphogranuloma inguinale is a virus.
Meningo-enzephalitische Veränderungen bei Affe nach intracerebraler Impfung mit Lymphogranulom inguinale with E. Wassén, Verh. 8te. Internat Kong. Dermat. u. Syph., Kopenhagen p. 1147 1930
Hellfors, A. See M. Rosenberg
Hellin, Dyonizy. Polish pathologish. 1867–1935
LAW or RATIO—of multiple births.
Die Ursache der Multiparität der uniparen Tier überhaupt und der Zwillingsschwangerschaft bei Menschen. München, Seitz und Schaner, 1895. 70 pp
Helly, Konrad. Swiss pathologist. 1875–
FLUID—fixing.
Eine Modification der Zenker'schen Fixirungsflüssigkeit. Z. wiss. Mikr., 20: 413–415, June 9, 1904
Helmer, A. M. See A. E. Casey
Helmholtz, Hermann Ludwig Ferdinand von German physiologist. 1821–1894
LIGAMENT—anterior, of malleus.
Die Mechanik der Gehörknöchelchen und des Trom melfells. Bonn, Cohen, 1869. 60 pp.
THEORY—of sound perception.
Die Lehre von den Tonempfindungen als physiologisc

Grundlage für die Theorie der Musik. Braunschweig, Wieweg, 1863. 605 pp.
See also under Ligament.
THEORY—of color vision.
Ueber die Theorie der zusammengesetzten Farben. Arch. f. Anat., Physiol. u. wiss. Med., pp. 461–482, 1852
Handbuch der physiologischen Optik. Leipzig, Voss, 1867. 874 pp.
Demonstrated that muscles are main source of animal heat.
Ueber die Wärmeentwickelung bei der Muskelaction. Arch. f. Anat., Physiol. u. wiss. Med., pp. 144–164, 1848
Measured velocity of nervous impulse with pendulum-myograph of his invention.
Vorläufiger Bericht über die Fortpflanzungsgeschwindigkeit der Nervenreizung. Ibid., pp. 71–73; 276–364, 1850
Invented ophthalmometer, ophthalmoscope and phakoscope.
Beschreibung eines Augen-Spiegels zur Untersuchung der Netzhaut im lebenden Auge. Berlin, Förstner, 1851. 43 pp.
Ueber eine neue einfachste Form des Augenspiegels. Arch. f. physiol. Heilk., 11: 827–843, 1852
Helmholz, Henry Frederic. Rochester, Minn. pediatrician. 1892–
Introduced ketogenic diet in therapeutics of bacteriuria.
The ketogenic diet in the treatment of pyuria of children with anomalies of the urinary tract. Proc. Staff Meet., Mayo Clinic, 6: 609–613, Oct. 14, 1931
Helmont, Joannes Baptiste van. Belgian physician. 1577–1644
First to recognize physiologic importance of ferments and gases, particularly of carbonic acid, which he described as gas sylvestre. Introduced gravimetric idea in analysis of urine. Garrison
Opuscula medica inaudita. Coloniae Agrippinae, Kalcoven, 1844. 4 vols.
Ortus medicinae. Amsterodami, Elzevir, 1648
Helmstedter, Felix. French physician
Gave accurate description of aortic lesion associated with aneurysm.
Du mode de formation des anéurysmes spontanés. Inaug. Dissert., Strasbourg. Schultz & Cie, 1873. 31 pp.
Hemmeter, John Conrad. Baltimore physician. 1864–1931
APPARATUS—
An apparatus for washing out the stomach and sigmoid with a continuous current, with return stomach or rectal tube. New York Med. J., 61: 385–386, Mar. 30, 1895
METHOD—for studying gastric peristalsis.
An apparatus for obtaining records of the motor functions of the human and animal stomach on the kymographion. A preliminary report. Ibid., 769–772, June 22, 1895
Pioneer in radiography of stomach and in duodenal intubation.
Intubation of the duodenum. Abstr.: Johns Hopk. Hosp. Bull., 7: 79–80, Apr. 1896
Hemmings, A. W. See C. Rimington
Henderson, F. F. See F. B. Mallory

Henderson, Lawrence Joseph. Boston chemist. 1878–1942
ADAPTATION—of Sörensen's method for determination of hydrogen ion concentration.
On the intensity of urinary acidity in normal and pathological conditions with W. W. Palmer, J. biol. Chem., 13: 393–405, Jan. 1913
CHART—alignment; to determine CO_2 of blood.
Blood as a physiocochemical system. IX. The carbon dioxide dissociation curves of oxygenated human blood with A. V. Bock, D. B. Dill and H. T. Edwards. Ibid., 87: 181–196, June 1930
Henderson, Melvin Starkey. Rochester, Minn. surgeon. 1883–
INCISION—
Posterolateral incision for the removal of loose bodies from the posterior compartment of the knee-joint. S. G. O., 33: 698–699, Dec. 1921
OPERATION—
Recurrent or habitual dislocation of the shoulder. J. A. M. A., 70: 1–4, Jan. 5, 1918
(Same title) S. G. O., 33: 1–7, July 1921
"Tenosuspension" for habitual dislocation of the shoulder. Ibid., 43: 18–25, July 1926
Habitual dislocation of the shoulder: result of treatment especially by the tenosuspension operation. J. A. M. A., 95: 1653–1658, Nov. 29, 1930
Henderson, V. E. See G. H. W. Lucas
Henderson, Yandell. New Haven physiologist. 1873–1944
METHOD—of measuring circulation rate.
The circulation and its measurement with H. W. Haggard, Amer. J. Physiol., 73: 193–253, June 1, 1925
THEORY—of shock.
Acapnia and shock. I. Carbon-dioxide as a factor in the regulation of the heart-rate. Ibid., 21: 126–156, Feb. 1, 1908; 23: 345–373, Feb. 1, 1909; 24: 66–85, Apr. 1, 1909
Showed that poisonous effect of illuminating gas is due to its avidity for hemoglobin.
Carbon monoxid poisoning. J. A. M. A., 67: 580–583, Aug. 19, 1916
Hendon, George Albert. Louisville surgeon. 1871–1941
METHOD—
Simple enterostomy technic. Ann. Surg., 94: 156 (only), July 1931
Hendrix, B. M. See H. D. Dakin
Henke, Philipp Jakob Wilhelm. German anatomist. 1834–1896
TRIANGLE or TRIGONE—between descending portion of inguinal fold and lateral border of rectus muscle.
SPACE—between spinal column and pharynx and esophagus.
Topographische Anatomie des Menschen in Abbildung und Beschreibung. Atlas. Berlin, Hirschwald, 1878–9. 80 pl. fol.
Also: English trans. by Rothacker, 1884
Henle, Adolf Richard. German surgeon. 1864–
PHENOMENON—of Henle-Coenen; after ligation of artery proximal to aneurysmal sac, if sac still pulsates, collateral circulation is sufficient to prevent gangrene.
Zur Indikationsstellung bei der Operation der Aneurys-

men und bei den Gefässverletzungen. Zbl. Chir., 41:
91 (only), Jan. 17, 1914
Performed gastroduodenostomy.
Ein Fall von Gastroduodenostomie. Ibid., 25: 753–
756, July 23, 1898
Henle, Friedrich Gustav Jacob. German anatomist.
1809–1885
ANSA, CANALS, CELLS, LOOP, TUBES—of uriniferous tubules.
Zur Anatomie der Niere. Abh. d. J. Ges. d. Wissensch.
zu Göttingen, 10: 223, 1861–62
Same: Handb. d. syst. Anat. d. Mensch., 2: 300–305,
1862
First to describe epithelia of skin and intestines,
defined columnar and ciliated epithelium, and pointed
out that this tissue constitutes the true lining membrane of all free surfaces of the body and the inner
lining of its tubes and cavities. Garrison
*Symbolae ad anatomiam villorum intestinalium im-
primis eorum epithelii et vasorum lacteorum. Commentatio.* Berolini, Hirschwald, 1837. 37 pp.
Gave first clear statement of idea of a contagium
animatum. Garrison
Von den Miasmen und Contagien. In his: *Pathologische Untersuchungen.* Berlin, 1840. pp. 1–82
First to demonstrate smooth muscle in middle (endo-
thelial) coat of smaller arteries, a discovery which was
the starting point of present physiological theory of
vasomotor mechanism. Garrison
Gesässnerven. In his: *Allgemeine Anatomie.* Leipzig,
Voss, 1841. 1048 pp. pp. 510; 690
Henneberg, Richard. Berlin psychiatrist. 1868–
Used term cataplexy.
Ueber genuine Narkolepsie. Neurol. Zbl., 35: 282–
290, Apr. 1, 1916
Henneberg, Wilhelm. Berlin bacteriologist. 1871–
1936
SOLUTION—basal ammonium sulphate.
Weitere Untersuchungen über Essigbakterien. Zbl.
Bakt., 2 Abt., 4: 14–20 (18), Jan. 15, 1898
SOLUTION—basal nitrate, for determination of acetic
acid bacteria. Ibid., p. 19
Henneguy, Louis Felix. French physician. 1850–
1928
METHOD—of mounting with albumen and water.
Nouvelles recherches sur la division cellulaire indirecte.
J. Anat., Paris, 27: 397–423, 1891
METHOD—permanganate, of nuclear staining. Ibid.,
Henny, G. C. See T. S. Fay
Henoch, Eduard Heinrich. German pediatrician
1820–1910
CHOREA or DISEASE—spasmodic tic.
Beiträge zur Kinderheilkunde. N. F. Berlin, 1868. pp.
113
DISEASE or PURPURA—
*Vortrag über den Zusammenhang von Purpura und
Intestinalstörungen.* Berl. klin. Wschr., 5: 517–519,
Dec. 14, 1868
Ueber eine eigenthümliche Form von Purpura. Ibid.,
11: 622; 641–643, Dec. 21, 1874
Mondeville, Henri de. French surgeon. 1260–1320
"Made a valiant last stand for the principles of
avoiding suppuration by simple cleanliness as origi-
nally taught by Hippocrates, and which Mondeville
got from Theodoric." Garrison

Die Chirurgie . . . hrsg. von J. L. Pagel, Berlin,
1892
Published in French by Nicaise in 1893
Henriques, Valdemar. Copenhagen physiochemist.
1864–1936
METHOD—for determination of amino-acid nitrogen
in urine.
*Ueber die quantitative Bestimmung der Aminosäuren,
Polypeptide und der Hippursäure im Harne durch
Formoltitration* with S. P. L. Sörensen, Z. physiol.
Chem., 64: 120–143, Jan. 28, 1910
Henrotin, Fernand. American gynecologist. 1847–
1906
OPERATION—
*Vaginal hysterectomy in bilateral peri-uterine suppura-
tion.* Amer. J. Obstet., 26: 448–460, Oct. 1892
Henry, Adolf Felix Gerhard. Constantinople pathol-
ogist. 1894–
REACTION—melano flocculation, for malaria.
THEORY—of immunity in malaria.
*Contribution à l'étude sérologique de l'infection palus-
tre.* Gaz. hebd. Sci. méd., Bordeaux, 48: 311 (only),
May 15, 1927
Henry, Arnold Kirkpatrick. Irish surgeon in Cairo.
INCISION—
*A new method of resecting the left cervico-dorsal gan-
glion of the sympathetic in angina pectoris.* Irish J.
med. Sci., s. 5, No. 26: 157–167, Apr. 1924
OPERATION—
*Operation for femoral hernia by a midline extraperi-
toneal approach; with a preliminary note on the use of
this route for reducible inguinal hernia.* Lancet, 1:
531–533, Mar. 7, 1936
Henry, Joseph. Albany scientist. 1799–1878
Henry - unit of electric induction.
Scientific writings. Washington, Govt. Print. Off.,
1886, 2 vols.
Henschen, Karl. Zurich surgeon
OPERATION—for ascites.
*Dauerdrainage stagnierender ascitesergüsse in das
subkutane oder retroperitoneale Zellgewebe mit Hilfe
von Gummi- oder Fischblasenkondoms.* Zbl. Chir., 40:
41–43, Jan. 11, 1913
Henschen, Solomon Eberhard. Swedish physician.
1847–1930
Described word-hearing and visual centers. Garrison
Ueber die Hörsphäre. J. Psychol. Neurol., L z., 22:
319–474, 1918
*Ueber Sprach, Musik und Rechenmechanismen und
ihre Lokalisationen im Grosshirn.* Z. ges. Neurol.
Psychiat., 52: 273–298, 1919
Hensen, Viktor. German anatomist. 1835–1924
CANAL or DUCT—canalis reuniens.
CELLS—covering organ of Corti.
*Das Verhalten des Resonanz-Apparates im menschli-
chen Ohr.* S. B. preuss. Akad. Wiss., 2: 904–914,
July 24, 1902
Henshaw, Paul Stewart. American biophysicist.
1902–
HYPOTHESIS—carcinogenesis is result of gradualis-
tic tangential differentiation.
Implications from studies with physical carcinogens.
J. Nat. Cancer Inst., 5: 419–436, June 1945
Hensing, Frederick Wilhelm. German anatomist.
1719–1745
FOLD or LIGAMENT—left superior colic 1.

De peritonaeo. Giessae, 1742. 37 pp.
Observationes binas anatomiras de omento atque intestino colo exhibet. Giessae, Lammers, 1745. 11 pp.
Henssen, Otto. Freiburg i. Br. physician
AGAR—glycerol kidney; culture medium.
Ueber das Wachstum einiger Spaltpilzarten auf Nierenextrakt-Nährböden. Zbl. Bakt., 17: 401-411 (406), Apr. 1, 1895
Hepburn, Neil Jamieson. American physician. 1847-1918
Noticed constitutional effects of cocaine.
Some notes on hydrochlorate of cocaine. Med. Rec., 26: 534 (only), Nov. 15, 1884
Hepp, P. See A. Cahn
Herapath, William Bird. English scientist
TEST—for quinine in urine.
On the discovery of quinine and quinidine in the urine of patients under medical treatment with the salts of these mixed alkaloids. Phil. Mag., London, 4 s., 6: 171-175, Sept. 1853
Herbert, Herbert. English ophthalmologist
OPERATION—
On the "small flap" sclerotomy in glaucoma. Ophthalmoscope, 9: 762-768, Nov. 1, 1911
PITS—
Corneal pitting. Brit. J. Ophthal., 19: 261-264, May 1935
Herdman, W. A. See R. W. Boyce
d'Herelle, Felix. American bacteriologist. 1873-
Discovered bacteriophage phenomenon.
Technique de la recherche du microbe filtrant bacteriophage (Bacteriophagum intestinale). C. R. Soc. Biol., 81: 1160-1162, et seq., 1918
The bacteriophage and its behavior. Baltimore, Williams & Wilkins, 1926
An address on bacteriophagy and recovery from infectious diseases. Canad. med. Ass. J., 24: 619-628, May 1931
Héricourt, Jules. French physician. 1850-
SERUM—
De la vaccination contre la tuberculose par produits solubles des cultures tuberculeuses with C. Richet, Paris, Chamerot & Renouard, 1891
Hering, Carl Ewald Konstantin. Leipzig physiologist. 1834-1918
TEST—for binocular vision.
Die Lehre vom binocularen Sehen. Leipzig, Engelmann, 1868 146 pp.
THEORY—the psychophysical theory that facultative memory, the automatic power of protoplasm to do what it has done before, is the distinctive property of all living matter. Garrison
Ueber das Gädächtniss als eine allgemeine Funktion der organisierten Materie. Abh. d. k. Akad. d. Wissensch., Wien, 20: 253-278, 1870
THEORY—of color sense.
Zur Lehre vom Lichtsinne. S. B. Akad. Wiss. Wien., Math.-nat. Cl., 3 Abth., 66: 5-24, 1872; 68: 186-201, 229-244, 1873; 69: 85-104, 179-217; 70: 169-204, 1875
Hering, Heinrich Ewald. Austrian physician. 1866-
NERVE OF—"local reactions in the carotid sinus which, reflexly by way of the nerve of Hering and the medullary centers, will vary the heart rate, the respiration, and the like." Jackson
Der Karotisdruckversuch. Münch. med. Wschr., 70: 1287-1290, Oct. 19, 1923

Die Änderung der Herzschlazzahl durch Änderung des arteriellen Blutdruckes erfolgt auf reflektorischem Wege; Gleichzeitig eine Mitteilung über die Funktion des Sinus caroticus bzw. der Sinusnerven. Arch. ges Physiol., 206: 721-723, Dec. 22, 1924
Herisson, Jules. French physician
Invented a blood pressure apparatus.
Le Sphygmomètre; instrument qui traduit à l'oeil toute l'action des àrteres. Utilité de cet instrument dans l'étude de toutes les maladies; recherches sur les affections du coeur et le moyen de les distinguer entre elles. Paris, Crochard, 1834. 24 pp.
Same, in English. Philadelphia, Grigg and Elliott, 1835. 20 pp.
Herman, Martin. French bacteriologist
STAIN—
Sur la coloration du bacille tuberculeux. Ann. Inst. Pasteur, 22: 92-96, Jan. 1908
Herman. Friedrich. Erlangen anatomist. 1859-1920
SOLUTION or STAIN or FLUID—platino-aceto-osmic acid.
Beiträge zur Histologie des Hodens. Arch. mikr. Anat., 34: 58-106, 1889
Hermann, Ludimarus. German physician. 1838-1914
Showed increase elimination of CO_2 on contraction of muscle. Garrison
Untersuchungen über den Stoffwechsel der Muskeln, ausgehend vom Gaswechsel derselben. Berlin, Hirschwald, 1867. 128 pp.
Hermann, Otto. Vienna physician
REACTION—for serodiagnosis of syphilis.
Die Serodiagnose der Syphilis mittles Präzipitation von Natr. glycochol. unter Heranziehung des Cholesterins with A. Perutz, Med. Klin., 7: 60-63, Jan. 8, 1911
Hermannsdorfer, Adolf. Berlin surgeon
DIET—
Ueber Wund- und Tuberkulosediät. Jahrkurs. ärztl. Fortbild., 20: H. 8, 35-43, 1929
La influencia de una alimentación especial sobre la cicatrización de las heridas y sobre las afecciones tuberculosas graves. Rev. méd. germano-ibero-amer., 2: 677-684, Nov. 1929
Hermanson, L. See J. Fine
Hermestein, A. See L. Fraenkel
Herrick, Frederick Cowles. Cleveland surgeon. 1872-
METHOD—
A method of surgical approach to the lower ureter. Cleveland Med. J., 9: 963-966, Dec. 1910
Herrick, James Bryan. Chicago physician. 1861-
Described sickle-cell anemia.
Peculiar elongated and sickle-shaped red blood corpuscles in a case of severe anemia. Arch. intern. Med., 6: 517-521, Nov. 15, 1910
Same: Trans. Assoc. Amer. Phys., Phila., 25: 553-561, 1910
Described coronary thrombosis.
Clinical features of sudden obstruction of the coronary arteries. J. A. M. A., 59: 2015-2020, Dec. 7, 1912
Also in: F. A. Willus and T. E. Keys' Cardiac classics St. Louis, Mosby, 1941. pp. 817-829
Herrick, William Worthingtcn. American physician. 1879-1945
METHOD—
Demonstration of the Trichinella spiralis in the circu-

lating blood in man with T. C. Janeway, Arch. intern. Med., 3: 263–266, Apr. 1909

Herring, Percy Theodore. English physiologist. 1872–
BODIES—hyaline bodies of, in pituitary.
The histological appearances of the mammalian pituitary body. Quart. J. exp. Physiol., 1: 121–159, Apr. 1908

Herrmann, Elfriede. See F. E. Becher

Herrmann, Louis George. Cincinnati surgeon. 1900–
See M. R. Reid
Advocated—
Syphilitic peripheral vascular diseases: treatment by means of an intermittent negative pressure environment. Amer. J. Syph., 17: 305–320, July 1933
The Pavex (passive vascular exercise) treatment of obliterative arterial disease of the extremities with M. R. Reid, J. Med., 14: 524–529, Dec. 1933

Herrmannsdorfer, A. See E. F. Sauerbruch

Herschell, George Arich. English physician. 1856–
METHOD—of estimating absorptive power of stomach.
In his: *Indigestion.* . . . London, 1892. pp. 202. pp. 85–86

Hersman, C. F. St. Louis physician
DISEASE—
A case of progressive enlargement of the hands. Intern. Med. Mag., Phila., 3: 662–665, Oct. 1894

Herter, Christian Archibald. American physician. 1865–1910
DISEASE—intestinal infantilism; same as coeliac disease of Gee.
On infantilism from chronic intestinal infection: characterized by the overgrowth and persistence of flora of the nursling period. New York, Macmillan, 1908. 118 pp.
METHOD—
A method for the quantitative determination of indol with M. Louise Foster, J. biol. Chem., 1: 257–261, 1906
REACTION—for skatole.
In his: *Bacterial infections of the digestive tract.* New York, Macmillan, 1907. 360 pp. p. 141

Hertwig, Oscar. German scientist. 1849–1922
Demonstrated that spermatozoon enters ovum and that fertilization is accomplished by union of male and female pronuclei so formed.
Beiträge zur Kenntniss der Bildung, Befruchtung und Theilung des thierischen Eies. Morph. Jb., Leipz., 1: 347–434, 1875–6

Hertz, Arthur Frederick. English physician 1879–
Made important studies on alimentary tract.
The passage of food along the human alimentary canal with C. J. Morton et al, Guy s Hosp. Rep., 61: 389–427, 1907
Constipation and allied intestinal disorders. London, Frowde, 1909. 344 pp.

Hertzler, Arthur Emanuel. Kansas surgeon. 1870–1946
TRIANGLES—of topography of abdomen.
The regions of the abdomen from the surgeon's standpoint. St. Louis Cour. Med., 30: 1–8, Jan. 1904

Hervieux, Ch. See C. Porcher

Herxheimer, Karl. German dermatologist. 1861–
REACTION—inflammatory, in syphilitic tissues following salvarsan or other specific treatment. (Dorland)
Ueber eine bei Syphilitischen vorkommende Quecksil

berreaktion with Krause, Dtsch. med. Wschr., 28: 895–897, Dec. 11, 1902
Described chronic atrophic acrodermatitis.
Ueber Acrodermatitis chronica atrophicans with K. Hartmann, Arch. f. Dermat. u. Syph., 6: 57–76, 1902

Herz, Max. German physician. 1865–
TEST—for efficiency of myocardium.
Eine Funktionsprüfung des kranken Herzens. Dtsch. med. Wschr., 31: 215–218, Feb. 9, 1905

Herzfeld, Ernst. Zürich chemist. 1880–
TEST—for glucose in blood.
Ueber eine quantitative Zuckerbestimmungs-methode im Blute. Z. phys. Chem., 77: 420–424, Apr. 3, 1912

Herzog, Reginald O. Heidelberg physiologist
REACTION—for histidine.
Notiz über Histidin. Z. phys. Chem., 37: 248–249, 1902

Hess, Alfred Fabian. American physician. 1875–1933
TEST—of capillary resistance in purpura and scurvy.
Infantile scurvy: the blood, the blood-vessels and the diet with Mildred Fish, Amer. J. Dis. Child., 8: 385–405, Dec. 1914
Scurvy, past and present. Philadelphia, Lippincott 1920. 279 pp.
Advocated splenectomy for purpura.
A consideration of the reduction of blood platelets in purpura. Proc. Soc. exp. Biol., N. Y., 14: 96–97, 1917

Hess, Charles Leonard von. Chicago pharmacologist 1887–
MODIFICATION—of Abel's apparatus for vividiffusion.
The condition of the sugar in the blood with H. McGuigan, J. Pharmacol., 6: 45–55, Sept. 1914

Hess, W. C. See M. X. Sullivan

Hess, Walter. Swiss physiologist. 1881–
VISCOSIMETER—
Die Bestimmung der Viskosität des Blutes. Münch med. Wschr., 54: 2225–2229, Nov. 5, 1907

Hesse, H. See P. L. Geiger

Hesse, O. German physician
REACTION—for codeine.
Beitrag zur Kenntniss der Rinde von Aspidosperme Quebracho. Ber. dtsch. chem. Ges., 13: 2308–2309, 1880

Hesse, Walther. German bacteriologist. 1846–
AGAR—culture medium.
Die Methodik der bakteriologischen Wasseruntersuch ung with Niedner, Z. Hyg. InfektKr., 29: 454–462, 1898
Ein neues Verfahren zur Züchtung des Tuberkelbacil lus. Ibid., 31: 502–506, 1899
Methodik der Züchtung der Tuberkelbacillen au menschlichen Auswurf. Zbl. Bakt., 35: 386–387, Dec. 18, 1903
MEDIUM—for cholera vibrio.
Ueber den Einfluss der Alkalescenz des Nährbodens au das Wachsthum der Bakterien. Z. Hyg. InfektKr., 15 183–191, 1893
Ein neues Verfahren zur quantitativen Bestimmun der Darmbakterien, mit besonderer Berücksichtigun der Typhusbazillen. Ibid., 58: 441–448, 1908
See also F. H. Härting

Hesselbach, Franz Casper. German surgeon. 1759 1816
HERNIA—with a diverticulum through cribiforr fascia.

TRIANGLE—bounded by deep epigastric artery, Poupart's ligament and margin of rectus muscle.
Anatomisch-chirurgische Abhandlung über den Ursprung der Leistenbrüche. Würzburg, Baumgärtner, 1806. 32 pp.
Neues anatomisch-pathologische Untersuchungen über den Ursprung und das Fortschreiten der Leisten- und Schenkelbrüche. Würzburg, Stahel, 1814. 72 pp.

Hetsch, H. See R. E. W. Otto

Heublein, Arthur Carl. Hartford, Conn. physician. 1879–1932
METHOD—half of body treated daily with low intensity of roentgen output.
A preliminary report on continuous irradiation of the entire body. Radiology, 18: 1051–1062, June 1932

Heubner, Johann Otto Leonard. Berlin pediatrician 1843–1926
DISEASE—syphilitic endarteritis of cerebral vessels.
Die luetische Erkrankung der Hirnarterien, nebst allgemeinen Erörterungen zur normalen und pathologischen Histologie der Arterien sowie zur Hirncirculation. Leipzig, Vogel, 1874. 238 pp.
Originator of method of caloric feeding.
Säuglingsernährung und Sänglingsspitäler. Berlin, Hirschwald, 1897. 73 pp.

Heuer, George Julius. American surgeon. 1882–
OPERATION—
The surgery of mediastinal dermoids based upon an experience with four cases and a review of the literature. Ann. Surg., 90: 692–713, Oct. 1929

Heurteloup, Charles Louis Stanislas. French surgeon. 1793–1864
Designed best lithotrite of the time.
Lithotripsie. Paris, Béchet, 1833

Heuser, Carlos. Argentina surgeon. 1879–1934
Introduced iodized oil for x-ray visualization of uterine cavity.
La utero-salpingo-radiografía. Rev. Asoc. méd. argent., 41: 120–129, Jan.–Apr. 1928

Heusner, Ludwig. German surgeon
OPERATION—gastrostomy.
Ueber eine neue Methode zur Anlegung von Magenfisteln. Abstr.: Zbl. Chir., p. 986 (only), Oct. 17, 1896
First to successfully suture perforated gastric ulcer. Garrison and Morton
Ein Fall von einem frei in die Bauchhöhle perforirten Magengeschwür. Laparotomie. Naht der Perforationsstelle. Heilung. Reported by H. Kriegs, Berl. klin. Wschr., 29: 1244–1247, Dec. 5: 1280–1284 Dec. 12, 1892

Hewett, C. L. See G. Barry

Hewett, F(rederick) Charles Cresswell. English surgeon.
METHOD—
Thoracentesis: the plan of continuous aspiration. Brit. med. J., 1: 317 (only), Mar. 11, 1876

Hewlett, Albion Walter. Michigan physician. 1874–1925
METHOD—
The rate of blood flow in the arm with J. G. Van Zwaluwenburg Heart, 1: 87–97, 1909

Hewlett, Richard Tanner. English physician. 1865–1940
METHOD—of staining for capsules.
In his: *A manual of bacteriology.* Philadelphia, Blakiston, 1898. 439 pp. p. 86

Hewson, William. English physiologist. 1739–1774
Discovered lacteal and lymphatic vessels in birds, reptiles and fishes. Garrison
The state of the controversy concerning the discovery of the lacteals and lymphatics in birds, fish, and the animals called amphibious. London, 1769. 4 pp.
Account of the lymphatic system in birds, fish and turtles. Presented to the Royal Society, Mar. 8, 1770
A description of the lymphatic system in the human subject and in other animals illustrated with plates. Together with observations on the lymph, and the changes which it undergoes in some diseases. London, 1774. Also: Sydenham Soc., London, 1846. pt. 2, Ch. 4, 5, 6
Performed paracentesis.
The operation of paracentesis thoracis, proposed for air in the chest, with some remarks on the emphysema, and on wounds of the lungs in general. Med. Obs. and Inquiries, 2: 372–396, 1767
Established essential features of coagulation of blood. Isolated fibrinogen. Garrison
An experimental inquiry into the properties of the blood. Philos. Trans., 1770–71, 63: 323, 1773

Hey, William. Leeds surgeon. 1736–1819
AMPUTATION or OPERATION—of foot.
DERANGEMENT—internal of knee joint.
SAW—for enlarging orifices in bones.
Practical observations in surgery. London, Cadell, 1803. 537 pp.

Heyd, Charles Gordon. New York City surgeon. 1884–
SYNDROME—hepatorenal.
Called attention to "liver shock" following surgical procedures on gall bladder and biliary tract.
The liver and its relation to chronic abdominal infection. Ann. Surg., 79: 55–77, Jan. 1924
"Liver deaths" in surgery of the gall bladder. J. A. M. A., 97: 1847–1848, Dec. 19, 1931

Heyerdale, W. W. See J. J. McCallig

Heyfelder, Johann Ferdinand Martin. German physician. 1798–1869
Introduced ethyl chloride in anesthesia.
Die Versuche, mit dem Schwefeläther, Salzäther und Chloroform. Erlangen, Heyder, 1848

Heymann, Emil. German surgeon. 1878–
OPERATION—for recurrent dislocation of shoulder.
Zur Behandlung der habituellen Schulterluxation. Zbl. Chir., 54: 1411–1414, June 4, 1927

Heymans, Corneille. Belgian physician. 1892–
Awarded Nobel prize in 1938 "for his work on the sinus–aorta mechanism in breathing."
Le sinus carotidien et les autres zones vasosensibles réflexogènes. Paris, Presses Univ. de Franc, 1929. 122 pp.
Le sinus carotidien et la zone homologue cardio-aortique with J. J. Bouckaert and P. Regniers, Paris, Doin, 1933. 340 pp.
Spinal vasomotor reflexes associated with variations in blood pressure with J. J. Bouckaert, S. Farber and F. Y. Hsu, Amer. J. Physiol., 117: 619–625, Dec. 1936
The pressoreceptive mechanisms for the regulation of heart rate, vasomotor tone, blood pressure and blood supply. Experimental arterial hypertension. Role of the cardioaortic and carotid-sinus nerves in the reflex control of the respiratory center. New Engl. J. Med., 219: 147–159, Aug. 4, 1938

Heynsius, Adrian. Dutch physician. 1831–1885
TEST—for albumin in urine.
  Ueber die quantitative Bestimmung des Eiweisses in thierischen Flüssigkeiten. Chem. Zbl., 46: 795 (only), Dec. 15, 1875

Heyrovsky, Hans. Vienna surgeon. 1877–
OPERATION—esophagogastrostomy by the abdominal route.
  Casuistik und Therapie der idiopathischen Dilatation der Speiseröhre. Oesophagogastroanastomose. Arch. f. klin. Chir., 100: 703–715, Jan. 30, 1913

Hibbs, Russell Aubra. New York City surgeon. 1869–1932
OPERATION—
  An operation for progressive spinal deformities. New York Med. J., 93: 1013–1016, May 27, 1911
  A further consideration of an operation for Pott's disease of the spine, with report of cases from the service of the N. Y. Orthopaedic Hospital. Ann. Surg., 55: 682–688, May 1912
  An operation for Pott's disease of the spine. J. A. M. A., 59: 433–436, Aug. 10, 1912
  Treatment of vertebral tuberculosis by fusion operation: two hundred and ten cases. Ibid., 71: 1372–1376, Oct. 26, 1918
OPERATION—
  An operation for stiffening the knee-joint. Ann. Surg. 53: 404–407, Mar. 1911
  End-results in treatment of knee joint tuberculosis with H. L. von Lackum, J. A. M. A., 85: 1289–1292, Oct. 24, 1925
OPERATION—
  An operation for "claw foot." Ibid., 73: 1583–1585, Nov. 22, 1919
OPERATION—
  Scoliosis treated by the fusion operation: an end-result study of three hundred and sixty cases with J. C. Risser and A. G. Ferguson, J. Bone and Joint Surg., 13: 91–104, Jan. 1931

Hibler, Emanuel von. German bacteriologist. ?–1913
MEDIUM—brain, for cultivation of anaerobes.
  Beiträge zur Kenntnis der durch anaërobe Spaltpilze erzeugten Infektionserkrankungen der Tiere und des Menschen, sowie zur Begründung einergenauen bakteriologischen und pathologisch-anatomischen Differentialdiagnose dieser Prozesse. Zbl. Bakt., 25: 593–613 (604), May 5, 1899

Hibma, A. M. Utrecht medical student
TEST—for albumin in urine.
  Eine neue Eiweissreaktion. Dtsch. med. Wschr., 47: 272 (only), Mar. 10, 1921

Hickey, J. C. See W. C. Billings

Hickey, N. G. See A. M. Hoffman

Hickling, R. A. English scientist
METHOD—
  Vital staining of malignant cells in a peritoneal effusion. J. Path. Bact., 34: 789–791, Nov. 1931

Hickman, Henry Hill. English physician. 1800–1830
Did early work on anesthesia.
  A letter on suspended animation, containing experiments showing that it may be safely employed during operations on animals, with a view of ascertaining its probable utility in surgical operations on the human subject. Ironbridge, Smith, 1824

Hicks, John Braxton. English gynecologist. 1825–1897
SIGN—
  On the contractions of the uterus throughout pregnancy: their physiological effects and their value in the diagnosis of pregnancy. Trans. Obstet. Soc. London, 1871, 13: 216–231, 1872
VERSION—
  On a new method of version in abnormal labour. Lancet, 2: 28–30, July 14: 55 (only), July 21, 1860
  On combined external and internal version. Trans. Obstet. Soc. London, 1863, 5: 219–267, 1864
Studied condition of uterus in obstructed labor. Garrison
  On the condition of the uterus in obstructed labor; and an inquiry as to what is intended by the terms "cessation of labour pains," "powerless labour," and "exhaustion." Ibid., 1867, 9: 207–239, 1868
Treated blood with phosphate of soda to retard coagulation during transfusion.
  On transfusion, and new mode of management. Brit. med. J., 2: 151 (only), Aug. 8, 1868
  Cases of transfusion, with some remarks on a new method of performing the operation. Guy's Hosp. Rep., 3 s., 14: 1–14, 1869
Wrote important work on accidental concealed hemorrhage.
  On a form of concealed hemorrhage before the expulsion of the placenta, rarely noticed. Brit. med. J., 1: 207–208, Feb. 24, 1872

Hida, O. Tokio physician
BROTH—horse meat infusion, for cultivation of diphtheria bacilli.
  Ein für Diphtherietoxinbildung geeigneter Nährboden. Zbl. Bakt., 53: 412 (only), 1910
  See also Y. Teruuchi

Hidaka, S. See C. Bruck

Hieger, I. See G. Barry, E. L. Kennaway

Higgins, Charles Clair. Cleveland urologist. 1897–
DIET—an experimental diet for rats.
  The experimental production of urinary calculi. J. Urol., 29: 157–170, Feb. 1933
TECHNIC—
  Aseptic uretero-intestinal anastomosis. S. G. O., 57: 359–361, Sept. 1933
  (Same title) J. Urol., 31: 791–802, June 1934

Higgins, Charles H. Montreal pathologist
SOLUTION—glycerol ammonium chloride, for cultivation of cholera organisms.
  Notes upon an epidemic of fowl cholera and upon the comparative production of acid by allied bacteria. J. exp. Med., 3: 651–668, Nov. 1898

Higgins, George Marsh. American physician. 1890–
Showed that deprivation of ultraviolet rays in chickens deprived of other sources of vitamin D leads to hypertrophy and hyperplasia of parathyroid glands.
  The effects of selective solar irradiation on the parathyroid glands of chicks with C. Sheard, Amer. J. Physiol., 85: 299–310, May 1928
  The effects of ultraviolet irradiation on rachitic chickens with C. Sheard and R. M. Wilder, Anat. Rec., 58: 205–216, Jan. 25, 1934

Higgins, Harold Leonard. American scientist. 1887–
MODIFICATION—of Plesch's method of collection of alveolar air.

A study of prolonged fasting. Alveolar air. Publ. Carneg. Instn., 203: 168-181, 1915

Higgs, Sidney Limbrey. London surgeon
OPERATION—
"*Hammer-toe.*" Med. Press and Circular, 131: 473-475, June 10, 1931

Highmore, Nathaniel. English physician. 1613-1684
ANTRUM—maxillary.
BODY or CORPUS—mediastinum of testis.
Corporis humani disquisitio anatomica; in qua sanguinis circulatione in quavis corporis particula plurimis typis novis, ac aenygmatum medicorum succincta dilucidatione ornatem prosequutus est. Hague—Comitis, Broun, 1651. 262 pp.
Also: *Opera omnia.* Amstelaedami, 1682

Higinbotham, N. L. See Helen Q. Woodard

Hildebrand, Otto. German surgeon. 1858-1927
OPERATION—to prevent recurrent dislocation of shoulder by deepening glenoid fossa.
Beiträge zur operativen Chirurgie. Arch. f. klin. Chir., 66: 347-376, (360-364), 1902
OPERATION—
Eine neue Operationsmethode zur Behandlung des Hydrocephalus (int. chron.) der Kinder. Ibid., 127: 178-194, 1923

Hildenbrand, Johann Valentin von. Austrian physician. 1763-1818
DISEASE—typhus fever.
Ueber den ansteckenden Typhus. Wien, 1. A., 1810. 2 A., 1814
Also, in French, 1811. Also, in Italian, 1822. Also, in English transl. by S. D. Gross, 1829

Hilger, Albert. Swiss pharmacologist. 1839-1905
TEST—for bile pigments.
Zum Nachweis der Gallensäuren und Gallenfarbstoffe im Urin. Z. anal. Chem., 15: 105-106, 1876

Hill, Archibald Vivian. English physiologist. 1886-
Awarded Nobel Prize in 1922 for work on physiology of muscle.
The four phases of heat-production of muscle with W. Hartree, J. Physiol., 54: 84-128, Aug. 19, 1920
The mechanism of muscular contraction. Physiol. Rev., 2: 310-341, Apr. 1922

Hill, D. K. English physician
METHOD—
Determination of blood-volume in shocked patients. Lancet, 1: 177-178, Feb. 8, 1941

Hill, Hibbert Winslow. American bacteriologist. 1871-
MEDIUM—
Artificial milk: a substitute for ordinary milk as a laboratory medium. Public Health, 35: 379 (only), Oct. 1909
METHOD—for study of bacteria.
"*Hanging block*" *preparations for the microscopic observation of developing bacteria.* J. med. Res., 7 202-212, Mar. 1902

Hill, Sir Leonard Erskine. English physician. 1866-
SPHYGMOMETER—
A simple and accurate form of sphygmometer or arterial pressure gauge contrived for clinical use with H. Barnard, Brit. med. J., 2: 904 (only), Oct. 2, 1897
TEST—
A simple oxygen bed tent and its use in a case of edema

and chronic ulcer of the leg. J. Physiol., 55: xx-xxi, Nov. 18, 1921
Described pathology of cerebral circulation.
The physiology and pathology of the cerebral circulation. An experimental research. London, Churchill, 1896. 208 pp.

Hill, Richard Charles Jocelyn. English surgeon
PROBE—
Electric probe for location of metallic foreign bodies in the tissues. Brit. med. J., 2: 616 (only), Nov. 1, 1941

Hill, William. English laryngologist. 1858-1928
OPERATION—
Pharyngeal pouch treated by diverticulo-pexy. Proc. Roy. Soc. Med. (Sect. Laryng.), 11: 60-63, June 1, 1917

Hillary, William. English physician. ?1700-1763
Wrote on lead poisoning and sprue.
Observations on the changes of the air and the concomitant epidemical diseases in the island of Barbadoes.... London, Hitch and Hawes, 1759. 360 pp. 2 ed., 1766

Hilliard
LUPUS—marginatus, named after a patient affected.
A rare form of lupus (marginatus) by J. Hutchinson, Arch. Surg., 1: Plate 13 and 14, 1890

Hilsmann, Friedrich Alexander. German surgeon. 1849-
Performed pericardiocentesis for suppurative pericarditis.
Ueber die Paracentese der Perikardiums. Schriften der Univ. zu Kiel, 1875, Diss. Nr. 2, 1876

Hilton, John. English surgeon. 1804-1878
LAW—"The same trunks of nerves, whose branches supply the groups of muscles moving a joint, furnish also a distribution of nerves to the skin over the insertions of the same muscles . . . and the interior of the joint. . . ."
In: *Rest and pain.* London, Bell, 1863; also 5 ed., 1920. p. 168
LINE, WHITE—one and a half centimeters above anocutaneous junction. Ibid., 2 ed., New York, Wood, 1879, p. 166
METHOD—of draining abscess, by forceps and director, to avoid injury to important vessels and nerves. Ibid., p. 74

Hindenlang, Karl. Freiburg physician. 1854-1884
TEST—for albumin.
Die Metaphosphorsäure und ihre Verwerthbarkeit als Eiweissreagens des Harns. Berl. klin. Wschr., 18: 205-207, Apr. 11, 1881

Hindle, Edward. English physician.
Prepared prophylactic vaccine for immunization against yellow fever.
A yellow fever vaccine. Brit. med. J., 1: 976-977, June 9, 1928

Hines, Edgar Alphonso, Jr. Rochester, Minn. physician. 1906-
TEST—cold pressor t. for measuring variability of blood pressure.
A standard stimulus for measuring vasomotor reactions: its application in the study of hypertension with G. E. Brown, Proc. Staff Meet. Mayo Clinic, 7: 332-335, June 8, 1932
A standard test for measuring the variability of blood pressure; its significance as an index of the prehyper-

tensive state with G. E. Brown, Ann. intern. Med., 7: 209–217, Aug. 1933
The cold pressor test for measuring the reactibility of the blood pressure: data concerning 571 normal and hypertensive subjects. Amer. Heart J., 11: 1–9, Jan. 1936

Hinman, Frank. San Francisco urologist. 1880–
REFLUX—
Pyelovenous back flow: its relation to pelvic reabsorption, to hydronephrosis, and to accidents of pyelography with R. K. Lee-Brown, J. A. M. A., 82: 607–613, Feb. 23, 1924
Pyelovenous back flow with F. H. Redewill, Ibid., 87: 1287–1293, Oct. 16, 1926

Hinojoso, Alphonso Lopez de.
His *Summa y recopilacion de chirurgia*, (1578; 2 ed., 1595) was the first surgical book published in the New World, in Mexico City. Garrison

Hinterstoisser, Hermann. Vienna surgeon. 1861–
OPERATION—
Ueber einen durch Trepanation geheilten Fall von traumatischer Epilepsie (Jackson) nebst Bemerkungen zur Heteroplastik mittelst Celluloid. Wien. klin. Wschr., 4: 302–305, Apr. 16, 1891

Hinton, James. English surgeon. 1822–1875
Performed mastoidectomy.
Perforation of the mastoid process. Report in: Med. Times & Gaz., 2: 378 (only), Sept. 26, 1868

Hinton, William Augustus. Boston pathologist. 1883–
TEST—for syphilis.
A glycerol-cholesterol precipitation reaction in syphilis. Boston Med. and Surg. J., 196: 993–996, June 16, 1927
Hinton test for syphilis; third modification. J. Lab. clin. Med., 18: 198–205, Nov. 1932

Hippel, Arthur von. German ophthalmologist. 1841–1917
OPERATION—keratoplasty.
Eine neue Methode der Hornhauttransplantation. Arch. f. Ophth., Berlin, 34: 1 Abt., 108–130, 1888

Hippocrates. Greek physician. "Father of Medicine." 460?–359? B. C.
FACIES—indicative of approaching death.
Prognostics. Adams. Transl., par. 2. line 4
FINGERS—nails curve over ends, seen in diseases of lungs and heart. Ibid., par. 17, line 5
SUCCUSSION—sign in hydrothorax.
Diseases. Book 2
Described Cheyne-Stokes breathing, "as if the patient recollected something."
Epidemics. Book 1, 13, case 1

Hirsch, Edwin Frederick. Chicago pathologist. 1886–
AGAR—chocolate, for isolation of influenza bacilli.
An epidemic of pneumococcus bronchopneumonia with Marion McKinney, J. infect. Dis., 24: 594–617, (605), June 1919
METHOD—
A method for graphic demonstration of foreign inorganic matter and carbon in the lungs. J. A. M. A., 66: 950–951, Mar. 25, 1916

Hirsch, Oskar. German surgeon. 1877–
METHOD—endonasal.
Ueber endonasale Operationsmethoden bei Hypophysis-Tumoren mit Bericht über 12 operierte Fälle. Berl. klin. Wschr., 48: 1933–1935, Oct. 23, 1911

Hirschberg, Fritz. Berlin physician. 1888–
TEST—for blood.
Ueber die Pyramidonprobe zum Nachweis von okkultem Blut. Dtsch. med. Wschr., 49: 414–416, Mar. 30, 1923

Hirschberg, Julius. Potsdam ophthalmologist. 1843–1925
Introduced electromagnet into ophthalmology.
Der Electromagnet in der Augenheilkunde. Leipzig, Veit, 1885. 157 pp.

Hirschberg, Leonard Keene. Baltimore physician. 1877–
REACTION—for differentiating sucrose from other sugars.
Eine neue Methode, um Saccharose von Dextrose, Pentose, Lävulose, Laktose, Maltose und Invertzucker in Urin, Speichel oder andereer Sekreten zu trennen. Berl. klin. Wschr., 49: 409 (only), Feb. 26, 1912

Hirschbruck. German physician
AGAR—crystal violet litmus lactose; for diagnosis of cholera.
Die Choleradiagnose mit Hilfe eines Spezialagars with Schwer, Zbl. Bakt., 34: 585–591, (587), Sept. 12, 1903

Hirschfeld, Felix Victor Birch. German physician. 1842–
DISEASE—acute diabetes mellitus.
Vorläufige Mitteilung über eine besondere klinische Form des Diabetes. Zbl. med. Wiss., 18: 164–166, Mar. 8; 193–195, Mar. 15, 1890
Ueber eine neue klinische Form des Diabetes. Z. klin. Med., 19: 294–304, 1891

Hirschfeld, Hans. Berlin physician. 1873–1929
TEST—for pus.
Die makroskopische Oxydasereaktion als Mittel zum Eiternachweis in pathologischen Körperflüssigkeiten. Dtsch. med. Wschr., 43: 1620 (only), Dec. 27, 1917

Hirschfeld, Ludwik. Zurich physician. 1884–
BACILLUS—
A new germ of paratyphoid. Lancet, 1: 296–297, 1919
BIOCHEMICAL INDEX OF—
Serological differences between the blood of different races. The result of researches on the Macedonian front. Ibid., 2: 675–679, Oct. 18, 1919
TEST—coagulation, for syphilis.
Une nouvelle réaction du sérum syphilitique: la coagulo-réaction. Sem. med., 34: 361–363, Aug. 5, 1914
Ueber eine Gerinnungsreaktion bei Lues with R. Klinger, Dtsch. med. Wschr., 40: 1607–1610, Aug. 6, 1914

Hirschfeld, Ludwig Mauryey. Austrian anatomist. 1816–1876
GANGLION—hippocampal gyrus.
NERVE—of motion, arising from facial and distributed to palatoglossus and styloglossus.
Anatomia opisowa ciala ludzkiego. Warszawa, 1861–1870. 4 vols.
Recorded intracranial tumor of chondroma group.
Sur une tumeur cartilagineuse de la base du crane (enchondrome). C. R. Soc. Biol., 3: 94–96, 1851
See also E. A. W. J. von Dungern

Hirschfelder, Joseph Oakland. American physician. 1854–1920
TUBERCULIN—
The cure of tuberculosis by oxytuberculine, with ex-

periments on patients, animals, and cultures. Trans. Med. Soc. California, San Francisco, 27: 251–274, 1897

Hirschsohn, Ed. Dorpat.
REACTION—for cholesterol.
Ueber eine neue Reaction des Cholesterins. Pharm. Zentralhalle, 23: 357–358, July 10, 1902

Hirschsprung, Harald. Copenhagen physician. 1830–1916
DISEASE—congenital hypertrophic dilatation of colon
Stuhlträgheit Neugeborener in Folge von Dilatation und Hypertrophie des Colons. Jb. Kinderh., 27: 1–7, 1888
Die angeborene Erweiterung und Hypertrophie des Dickdarms. Paediatr. Arbeiten, Berlin, 1890. pp. 78–86

Hirsch, Maximilian. Vienna surgeon
METHOD—of gastroscomy.
Plastischer Ersatz des Ösophagus aus dem Magen. Zbl. Chir., 38: 1561–1564, Dec. 2, 1911

Hirst, Barton Cooke. American gynecologist. 1862–1935
TECHNIC—of cesarean section.
In his: Atlas of operative gynecology. Philadelphia, Lippincott, 1919. 292 pp. pp. 235–246

Hirst, George Keble. New York physician. 1909–
TECHNIC—
The quantitative determination of influenza virus and antibodies by means of red cell agglutination. J. exp. Med., 75: 49–64, Jan. 1942

Hirtz, E. J. French army surgeon
COMPASS—used in removal and localization of foreign bodies.
L'examen radiologique des blessés et la recherche des projectiles. Arch. de méd. et pharm. mil., 65: 499–521, 1916

His, Wilhelm, (Sr.). German anatomist. 1831–1904
BURSA—a dilatation at end of archenteron.
Beobachtungen über den Bau der Säugethier—Eierstockes. Arch. mikr. Anat., 1: 151–202, 1865
Die Häute und Höhlen des Körpers. Basel, Schweighauser, 1865
Unsere Körperform und das physiologische Problem ihrer Entstehung. Leipzig, Vogel, 1874
Anatomie menschlicher Embryonen. I. Embryonen des ersten Monats. Leipzig, Vogel, 1880. 3 pts., Leipzig, 1880–1885
CANAL—thyroglossal duct.
Beobachtungen zur Geschichte der Nasen- und Gaumenbildung beim menschlichen Embryo. Abh. sachs. Ges. (Akad.) Wiss., 27: 353–389, 1901
FLOOR-PLATE—
Zur Geschichte des Gehirns, sowie der centralen und peripherischen Nervenbahnen beim menschlichen Embryo. Ibid., 14: 341–392, 1888
RULE—reckon duration of pregnancy from first day of missed menstruation. See BURSA
ZONE—four thickenings which run entire length of medullary cord in fetus. See BURSA

His, Wilhelm, (Jr.) German physician. 1863–1934
BAND or BUNDLE—auriculoventricular b.
Die Thätigkeit des embryonalen Herzens und deren Bedeutung für die Lehre von der Herzbewegung beim Erwachsenen. Leipzig, Vogel, 1893. pp. 14–50
Also, abstr. in English transl. in F. A. Willus and

T. E. Key's *Cardiac classics.* St. Louis, Mosby, 1941 p. 695 (only).
DISEASE—of Werner-His; trench fever.
Ueber eine neue periodische Fiebererkrankung (Febris Wolhynica). Berl. klin. Wschr., 53: 322–323, Mar. 20, 1916

Hisaw, Frederick Lee. Wisconsin zoologist. 1891–
Produced crude extracts containing hormone progesterone.
Inhibition of ovulation and associated histological changes with R. K. Meyer and C. K. Weichert, Proc. Soc. exp. Biol., N. Y., 25: 754–756, June 1928
Demonstrated ability of progestin to nullify effect of posterior pituitary extract.
The corpus luteum hormone: II. Methods of extraction with H. L. Fevold and R. K. Meyer, Physiol. Zoöl., 3: 135–144, Jan. 1930

Hiss, Philip Hanson. Jr. New York bacteriologist. 1869–1913
Bacillus—of dysentery.
A study of a bacillus resembling the bacillus of Shiga, from a case of fatal diarrhea in a child; with remarks on the recognition of dysentery, typhoid, and allied bacilli with F. F. Russell, Med. News, 82: 289–295, Feb. 14, 1903
BOUILLON—
A contribution to the physiological differentiation of pneumococcus and streptococcus, and to methods of staining capsules. J. exp. Med., 6: 317–345 (323), Feb. 4, 1905
CULTURE MEDIUM—for typhoid-paratyphoid group.
On a method of isolating and identifying Bacillus typhosus, based on a study of Bacillus typhosus and members of the colon group in semi-solid culture media. Ibid., 2: 677–700, Nov. 1897
METHOD—for capsules; see STAIN
STAIN—copper sulphate, for capsules, to differentiate pneumococcus from streptococcus.
Beitrag zur physiologischen Differenzierung des Pneumococcus und des Streptococcus und zu den Methoden der Kapselfärbung. Zbl. Bakt., 31: 302–303, Mar. 24, 1902. See also, BOUILLON

Hitchcock, C. H. See H. F. Swift
Hitchcock, F. C. See J. Rosin
Hitchens, Arthur Parker. Washington, D. C. physician. 1877–
MEDIUM—
Advantages of culture mediums containing small percentages of agar. J. infect. Dis., 29: 390–407, Oct. 1921
SOLUTION—yeast autolysate blood; culture medium.
The production of yeast "vitamine" in the laboratory for the cultivation of bacteria. Abst. Bact., 6: 35, 1922

Hitschman, Fritz. Vienna obstetrician. 1870–1926
Described cyclic changes of endometrium.
Der Bau der Uterusschleimhaut des geschlechtsreifen Weibes mit besonderer Berücksichtigung der Menstruation with L. Adler, Mschr. Geburtsch. u. Gynäk., 27: 1–82, Jan. 1908

Hitzig, Eduard. German physician. 1838–1907
Defined limits of motor area in cerebral cortex of dog and monkey.
Untersuchungen über das Gehirn. Berlin, Hirschwald, 1874
See also G. T. Fritsch

Hitzig, William Maxwell. New York physician. 1904–
METHOD—of determining arm to lung time.
Measurement of circulation time for antecubital veins to pulmonary capillaries. Proc. Soc. exp. Biol., N. Y., 31: 935–938, May 1934

Hobart, Marcus Hatfield. Evanston, Ill. surgeon. 1888–
OPERATION—
Recurrent dislocation of the shoulder. Nicola operation. With report of cases. J. Bone and Joint Surg., 15: 733–736, July 1933
The Hobart operation; a new combination operation for recurrent dislocation of the shoulder. Ibid., 17: 1001–1004, Oct. 1935

Hochenegg, Julius. Vienna surgeon. 1859–
OPERATION—for rectal cancer.
Zur Therapie des Rectumcarcinoms. Wien. klin. Wschr., 10: 729–736, Aug. 12, 1897
Bestrebungen zur Kontinenzerzielung bei wegen Masdarmkrebs Operierten. Wien. med. Wschr., 79: 594–595. Apr. 27, 1929
OPERATION—hypophysectomy.
Operativ geheilte Akromegalie bei Hypophysentumor. Zbl. Chir., 35: 72–79, 1908
ULCER—non-specific of rectum.
Ueber Ulcus callosum recti und dessen Behandlung. Wien. klin. Wschr., 39: 522–524, May 6, 1926

Hochstetter, Ferdinand. German physician. 1872–
Described postcaval ureter in man.
Beiträge zur Entwicklungsgeschichte des Venensystems der Amnioten. Morphol. Jahrb., 4: 543–648, Dec. 8, 1893

Hodara, Menahem. Turkish physician. ?–1926
DISEASE—a kind of trichorrhexis nodosa seen in women in Constantinople.
Ueber die Trichorrhexis des Kopfhaares der Konstantinopeler Frauen. Mschr. prakt. Dermat., 19: 173–188, Aug. 15, 1894

Hodge, Hugh Lenox. Philadelphia gynecologist. 1796–1873
FORCEPS—obstetrical.
PLANE—through second sacral vertebra and upper border of os pubis, parallel to plane of pelvic inlet.
The principles and practice of obstetrics. Philadelphia, Blanchard and Lea, 1864. 550 pp.
PESSARY—
The "open-lever" or "horse-shoe" pessary. Med. & Surg. Reporter, Philadelphia, 15: 343–344, Oct. 20, 1866

Hodges, P. C. See L. R. Dragstedt

Hodgkin, Thomas. English physician. 1798–1866
DISEASE—granuloma leukemia; characterized by enlargement of lymph nodes, progressive anemia and death.
On some morbid appearances of the absorbent glands and spleen. Med.-chir. Trans., London, 17: 68–114, 1832
Also: *Selected essays.* London, New Sydenham Soc., 1901. pp. 159–183
Also: *Medical classics,* 1: 741–770, Mar. 1937
Described insufficiency of aortic valves.
On the retroversion of the valves of the aorta. Lond. Med. Gaz., 3: 433–443, 1829

Hodgson, Joseph. English physician. 1788–1869
DISEASE—aneurysmal dilatation of proximal part of aorta.
*A treatise on the diseases of the arteries and veins, con-*taining the pathology and treatment of aneurisms an wounded arteries. London, Underwood, 1815. 603 pp

Hoefer, Wolfgang. Austrian physician. 1614–1681
Wrote early account of cretinism.
Hercules medicus, sive locorum communium medcorum tomus unicus.... Viennae, 1657. p. 43

Hoefftcke, Carel A. English surgeon
SPLINT—of femur for non-union.
In his: *The ambulatory treatment of fractures an diseased joints.* London, Heinemann, 1923. 276 pp pp. 18–25

Högler, Franz. German physician
METHOD—of sciatic nerve injection with antipyrin solution.
Ueber perineurale Antipyrininjektionen bei Ischia. Wien. klin. Wschr., 34: 617–618, Dec. 22, 1921
Zur Technik der perineuralen Injektionen bei Ischia. Bemerkungen zur gleichnamigen Mitteilung von D Grünbaum in dieser Wochenschrift 1922 Nr. 4. Ibid 35: 343 (only), Apr. 13, 1922

Högyes, Andreas. Budapest physician. 1847–1906
METHOD—dilution m., of preventive inoculatio against rabies.
Lyssa. Nothnagel's Specielle Path. u. Ther., Wien 1897. vol. 5, p. 240

Hoehne, Ottomar. German obstetrician. 1871–1932
SIGN—
Zur Ätiologie und Diagnostik der Spontanruptur d hochgraviden Uterus. Zbl. Gynäk., 49: 66–70, Ja 10, 1925

Hölzel, Eduard. Munich anatomist
BOUILLON—glycogen, for cultivation of anthra bacilli.
Beiträge zur Züchtung, Isolierung und Desinfektio des Rauschbrandbacillus. Zbl. Bakt., 71: 147–16 (149), Oct. 4, 1913

Hoepfner. See M. Nonne

Hoernigk, Ludwig von. German physician. 1600–16 Wrote important book on forensic medicine an medical ethics. Garrison
Politia medica.... Frankfurt, 1638. 222 pp.

Hoff, Jacobus Hendricus Van't. Dutch chemist Berlin. 1852–1911
LAW—velocity of chemic reactions is increased tw fold or more for each rise of 10 degrees in temper ture.
Die Rolle des osmotischen Druckes in der Analog zwischen Lösungen und Gasen. Z. phys. Chem., 481–508, 1887

Hoffa, Albert. German surgeon. 1859–1908
DISEASE—inflammatory hyperplasia of fatty tissue of knee joint.
Beiträge zur Pathologie und Therapie der Kniegelen serkrankungen. Berl. klin. Wschr., 41: 13–16, Ja 4; 43–46, Jan. 11, 1904
The influence of the adipose tissue with regard to th pathology of the knee joint. J. A. M. A., 43: 795–79 Sept. 17, 1904
OPERATION—for brachial palsy.
Ueber die Endresultate der Sehnenplastiken. Arc klin. Chir., 81: 455–503 (473), 1906
OPERATION—for slipping patella, by reefing medi capsule and fascia.
Zur Behandlung der habituellen Patellarluxatio Ibid., 59: 543–549, 1899
OPERATION—Hoffa-Lorenz, for congenital disloc tion of hip.

Ueber die operative Behandlung der angeborenen Hüftgelenksverrenkungen. S. B. d. phys.-med. Ges. zu Würzb., 1890

Hoffheinz, Fritz. German physician. 1874–
Noted decalcifying disease of skeleton in instances of enlarged parathyroid glands.
Ueber Vergrösserungen der Epithelkörperchen bei Osteitis fibrosa und verwandten Krankheitsbildern. Arch. f. path. Anat., 256: 705–735, June 30, 1925

Hoffman, Arthur Max. Los Angeles physician. 1898–
Reported granulopenia following oral administration of alpha-dinitrophenol in treatment of obesity.
Neutropenia following amidopyrine with E. M. Butt and N. G. Hickey, J. A. M. A., 102: 1213–1214, Apr. 14, 1934

Hoffman, Frederick Ludwig. American physician. 1865–
Called attention to possible harmfulness of asbestos dust.
Mortality from respiratory diseases in dusty trades (inorganic dusts). U. S. Dept. Labor, Statistics, Bull. No. 231 458 pp. June 1918

Hoffman, G. R. See H. P. Smith, S. E. Ziffren

Hoffman, Max Harold. St. Paul, Minn. physician. 1896–
METHOD—of transfusion.
Transfusion of citrated blood with H. C. Habein, J. A. M. A., 76: 358–360, Feb. 5, 1921

Hoffman, W. See P. M. Ficker

Hoffman, William Joseph. New York surgeon. 1894–
UNCH—
New technique and instrument for obtaining biopsy specimens. Amer. J. Cancer, 15: 212–220, Jan. 1931
Punch biopsy in tumor diagnosis. S. G. O., 56: 829–833, Apr. 1933

Hoffmann, E. See F. R. Schaudinn

Hoffmann, Friedrich. German physician. 1660–1742
NODYNE or DROPS—compound spirit of ether.
Medicinae rationalis systematicae. Halae Magdeburgicae, 1729–39 4 v. in 8. Frankfurt, 1738. vo. 3, sect. 2, q. 533
Gave original description of chlorosis. Garrison
De genuina chlorosis indole, origine et curatione. Halis, 1730
Gave original description of rubella. Garrison
Opera omnia. Geneva, 2: 63, 1748

Hoffmann, Johann. German physician. 1857–191
TROPHY—a variety of progressive muscular a.
Weitere Britrage zur Lehre von der progressiven neurotischen Muskelatrophie. Dtsch. Z. Nervenheilk., 1: 95–120, Apr. 30, 1891
Weitere Beitrag zur Lehre von der hereditären progressiven spinalen Muskelatrophie im Kindesalter nebst Bemerkungen über den fortschreitenden Muskelschwund im Allgemeinen. Ibid., 10: 292–320, Apr. 30, 1897
IGN—digital reflex.
Ueber die diagnostische Bedeutung des Babinskischen Phaenomens im praeuraemischen Zustand. By Hoffmann's assistant, Hans Curschmann, who coined term Hoffmann's sign. Münch. med. Wschr., 39: 2054–2057, Sept. 20, 1911
IGN—increased irritability of sensory nerves in tetany.
Zur Lehre von der Tetanie. Dtsch. Arch. klin. Med., 43: 53–119, June 22, 1888

SYNDROME—
Ueber chronische spinale Muskelatrophie im Kindesalter, auf familiärer Basis. Dtsch. Z. Nervenheilk., 3: 427–470, May 4, 1893

Hoffmann, Michael. Munich surgeon. 1881–
INSTRUMENT—flexible gastroscope.
Optische Instrumente mit beweglicher Asche und ihre Verwendung für die Gastroskopie. Münch. med. Wschr., 58: 2446–2448, Nov. 14, 1911

Hoffmann-Wellenhof, Georg von. Austrian bacteriologist
BACILLUS—pseudodiphtheria b.
Untersuchungen über den Klebs-Löffler'schen Bacillus der Diphtherie und seine pathogene Bedeutung. Wien. med. Wschr., 3: 65–68, Jan. 21, 1888

Hofmann, Karl Andreas. Berlin chemist. 1870–
TEST—for lactic acid.
Trennung und Nachweis der Milchsäure als komplexes Eisen (3)—Natriumlactat. Ber. dtsch. chem. Ges., 53: 2224–2226, Dec. 30, 1920

Hofmeister, Franz. German physician. 1850–1922
Coined term "hunger diabetes"; fasting animals show glycosuria.
Ueber Resorption und Assimilation der Nährstoffe.
Ueber den Hungerdiabetes. Arch. exp. Path. Pharmak., 26: 355–370, Jan. 17, 1890

Hofmeister, Max Friedrich. German surgeon. 1854–
OPERATION—modification of Billroth II gastroenterostomy.
Beitrag zur Magenchirurgie. By R. Stumpf (Assistenzarzt), Beitr. klin. Chir., 59: 551–641, 1908

Hogan, James Joseph. Vallejo, Calif. physician. 1872–
TREATMENT—
The intravenous use of colloidal (gelatin) solutions in shock. J. A. M. A., 64: 721–726, Feb. 27, 1915
TREATMENT—
Treatment of acute alcoholic delirium. Ibid., 67: 1826 (only), Dec. 16, 1916

Hogan, R. B. See H. Eagle

Hogue, Mary Jane. Baltimore scientist. 1883–
MEDIUM—egg, for protozoa.
The cultivation of Trichomanos hominis. Amer. J. trop. Med., 1: 211–214, July 1921
METHOD—
Spirochaeta Eurygyrata. A note on its life history and cultivation. J. exp. Med., 36: 617–626, Dec. 1, 1922

Hoguet, Joseph Pierre. New York surgeon. 1882–1946
OPERATION or MANEUVER—conversion of direct and indirect sac into one.
Direct inguinal hernia. Ann. Surg., 72: 671–674, Dec. 1920

Hohlweg. W. See E. Steinach

Hohmann, Georg. German surgeon. 1880–
OPERATION—
Ueber Hallux valgus und Spreizfuss; ihre Entstehung und physiologische Behandlung. Arch. f. Orthop., 21: 525–550, 1923

Hoke, Michael. Atlanta, Ga. surgeon. 1872–1944
OPERATION—astragalectomy, stabilizing.
An operation for stabilizing paralytic feet. J. Orthop. Surg., 3: 494–507, Oct. 1921

Hoke, R. See R. Inada

Holbrook, William Paul. Portland, Ore. scientist. 1898–

TEST—
Blood uric acid; comparative results by three methods,
and technic necessary for accurate estimation with
H. D. Haskins, J. Lab. clin. Med., 11: 377–381,
Jan. 1926
See also H. D. Haskins
Holländer, Eugene. German physician. 1867–1932
DISEASE—of Simons and Holländer; progressive
lipodystrophie.
Ueber einen Fall von fortschreitendem Schwund des
Fettgewebes und seinen kosmetischen Ersatz durch
Menschenfett. Münch. med. Wschr., 57: 1794–1795,
Aug. 23, 1910
Holland, James William. Philadelphia physician.
1849–1922
TESTS—
Improved methods for the guaiac test for blood and the
oxidation test for indican. J. A. M. A., 48: 1942–1943,
June 8, 1907
Hollande, A. Charles. French physician. 1881–
SOLUTION—basal albumin, to study fermentation by
dysentery bacillus.
Emploi de l'ovalbuminate de soude et des papiers
réactifs tournesolés sucrés dans la différenciation des
bacilles dysenteriques; gélification de l'alcali-albumine
with M. Fumey, C. R. Soc. Biol., 80: 835–839 (836),
Nov. 10, 1917
Hollmann, Harry Triebner. Honolulu physician.
1878–
INTRODUCED—
Chaulmoogra oil in the treatment of leprosy with A. L.
Dean, J. Cutan. Dis., 37: 367–386, June 1919
The fatty acids of chaulmoogra oil in the treatment of
leprosy and other diseases. Arch. Dermat. and Syph.,
5: 94–101, Jan. 1922
Hollo, Julius. German physician
DRUG TESTS OF—
Experimentelle Analyse der subfebrilen Temperaturen
und ihre Ergebnisse. Berl. klin. Wschr., 55: 640–
643, July 8, 1918
Holly, L. E. See T. O. Menees, C. C. Warden
Holman, Emile Frederic. San Francisco surgeon.
1890–
OPERATION—
Partial resection of the lower scapula as an aid in
compressing apical tuberculosis abscesses and in con-
serving vital capacity. J. Thorac. Surg., 6: 496–501,
June 1937
Holman, William Ludlow. Canadian bacteriologist.
1879–
BOUILLON—basal serum, for studying fermentation
by bacteria.
The classification of streptococci. J. med. Res., 34:
377–444 (385), July 1916
SERUM BROTH—for cultivation of bacteria.
A method for making carbohydrate serum broth of
constant composition for use in the study of streptococci.
J. infect. Dis., 15: 209–214, July 1914
Holmes, Gordon Morgan. English physician
Recorded removal, by P. Sargent, of adrenal corti-
cal tumor.
A case of virilism associated with a suprarenal tumour:
recovery after its removal. Quart. J. Med., 18: 143–152,
Jan. 1925
Holmes, Oliver Wendell. Boston physician. 1809–
1894
Demonstrated that puerperal fever is contagious.

The contagiousness of puerperal fever. New Engl.
Quart. J. Med., 1: 503–530, Apr. 1843
Puerperal fever as a private pestilence. Boston, Tick-
nor and Fields, 1855. 60 pp.
Also: Medical essays. 1892, pp. 103–172
Also: Amer. Gynec. and Pediat., 6: 513–534, 1893
Also in: Epoch making contributions to medicine . . .
by C. N. B. Camac, Philadelphia, Saunders, 1909.
pp. 399–435
Also: Harvard classics, 38: 233–268, 1920
Also: Medical classics, 1: 245–268, Nov. 1936
Proposed terms "anesthesia" and "anesthetic" in
a letter to W. T. G. Morton, Nov. 21, 1846
Holmgren, Alarik Frithiof. Swedish physiologist.
1831–1897
TEST—for perception of colors.
YARNS—used in testing color sense.
Om den medfödda färgblindhetens diagnostik och teori.
Nord. med. Ark., Stockholm, 6: No. 24, 1–21; No.
28, 1–35, 1874
Also: Stockholm, Norstedt, 1874. 35 pp.
Demonstrated retinal action currents.
Om retinaströmmen. Upsala Läkarefor. Förh., 6:
419–455, 1870
Holmgren, J. Stockholm physician
TEST—for iodine in urine.
Nachweis von Jodverbindungen im Harn. Abstr.:
Dtsch. med. Ztg., 32: 572–573, July 15, 1911
Holobut, T. See J. Hachla
Holst, Axel. German physician. 1861–1931
Introduced study of food deficiencies in guinea-pigs.
Ueber experimentellen Scorbut. Ein Beitrag zur
Lehre von dem Einfluss einer einseitigen Nahrung.
Z. Hyg. InfektKr., 72: 1–120, 1912
Holst, F. See E. Schlesinger
Holst, Johan Martin. Oslo surgeon. 1892–
Declared that blood in thyrotoxicosis is rich in io-
dine.
Ueber den inneren Jodstoffwechsel bei primären Thyre-
otoxikosen (primär-Basedow) with G. Lunde, K.
Closs and O. C. Pedersen, Klin. Wschr., 7: 2287–
2290, Nov. 25, 1928
Holsti, Hugo Oesten Leonard. Finnish physician,
1850–1918
MEALS—"pure diets" used for study of pancreatic
secretion.
Om pankreas-sekretionen hos människan vid ett fall
av traumatisk fistel. Helsingfors, 1912. 93 pp.
Holt, L. E. See S. Flexner, W. H. Howell
Holth, Sören. Christiania ophthalmologist. 1863–1937
OPERATION—for glaucoma.
Iridencleisis antiglaucomatosa. Ann. d'ocul., 137:
345–375, May 1907
Sclérectomie avec la pince emporte-pièce dans le glau-
come, de préférence après incision à la pique. Ibid.,
142: 1–15, July 1909
On the technique in extralimbal tangential punch for-
ceps sclerectomy for chronic glaucoma. Acta ophth.,
Kbh., 3: 62–68, 1925
Holt-Harris, John Evan. Albany, N. Y. physician.
1876–
AGAR—
A new culture medium for the isolation of Bacillus
typhosus from stools with O. Teague, J. infect. Dis.,
18: 596–600, June 1916

Holtz, Friedrich. German surgeon.
Introduced A. T. 10 (dihydrotachysterol) in treatment of tetany.
Die Behandlung der postoperativen Tetanie. Abstr.: Arch. klin. Chir., 177: 32–34, 1933
Holzknecht, Guido. Vienna roentgenologist. 1872–1931
CHROMORADIOMETER—an apparatus for measuring x-ray dosage.
Das Chromoradiometer. Cong. intern. d'Electrol et de Radiol. Méd., 2: 377–379, 1902
Eine neue, einfache Dosirungsmethode in der Radiotherapie. (Das Chromoradiometer.) Wien. klin. Rundschau., 16: 685–687, Aug. 31, 1902
MOVEMENT—"en masse" of colon.
Die normale Peristaltik des Kolon. Münch. med. Wschr., 56: 2401–2403, Nov. 24, 1909
SPACE—middle lung field or retrocardiac or prevertebral.
Die röntgenologische Diagnostik der Erkrankungen der Brusteingeweide. Hamburg, Gräfe & Sillen, 1901. 229 pp.
UNITS—of roentgen-ray dosage equal to one-fifth the erythema dose. See chromoradiometer.
Holzmann, W. See H. C. R. Much
Homans, John. Boston surgeon. 1877–
OPERATION—excision of ulcers, varicose and postphlebitic.
Thrombophlebitis of the lower extremities. Ann. Surg., 87: 641–651, May 1928
SIGN—pain in calf on forcible dorsiflexion of ankle in thrombophlebitis.
Exploration and division of the femoral and iliac veins in the treatment of thrombophlebitis of the leg. New Engl. J. Med., 224: 179–186, Jan. 30, 1941
See also S. J. Crowe
Homburger, E. See O. W. Barlow
Home, Sir Everard. English surgeon. 1763–1832
LOBE—third lobe of prostate.
Practical observations on the treatment of the diseases of the prostate gland. London, Nicol. 1811. 280 pp.
Described hyperkeratosis (cutaneous horns). Garrison
Observations on certain horny excrescences of the human body. Philos. Trans., 81: 95–105, 1791
Published drawings of microscopic sections of cancer but mistook cells for lymph globules.
A short tract on the formation of tumours, and the peculiarities that are met with in the structure of those that have become cancerous, with their mode of treatment. London, Longman, 1830. 98 pp.
See also J. Hunter
Home, Francis. Scottish physician. 1719–1813
Described diphtheria.
An enquiry into the nature, cause, and cure of the croup. Edinburgh, Kincaid and Bell, 1765
Homén, Ernst Alexander. Finnish physician. 1851–1926
SYNDROME—due to lesion of lenticular nucleus.
Eine eigenthümliche Familienkrankheit, unter der Form einer progressiven Dementia, mit besonderem anatomischen Befund. Neurol. Zbl., 9: 514–518, Sept. 1, 1890
Homer, A. A. See F. B. Mallory
Homolle, Augustin Eugène. French physician 1808–1875

Isolated active principle in digitalis, amorphous digitalin.
Mémoire dur la digitale pourprée. J. Pharm.Chim., Paris, 3 s., 7: 57–83, 1845
Honigmann, Georg. German physician. 1863–1930
METHOD—of determination of hydrochloric acid deficit in stomach content.
Ueber das Verhalten der Salzsäure im carcinomatösen Magen with C. von Noorden, Z. klin. Med., 13: 87–99, 1887
Hooke, Robert. London scientist. 1635–1703
Invented compound microscope (1665) and first noticed cells in plants. Garrison
Micrographia or some physiological descriptions of minute bodies made by magnifying glasses; with observations and inquiries thereupon. London, Martyn and Allestry, 1665
Also: London, Allestry, 1667. 246 pp.
"Showed, in 1667, by attaching a bellows in the arteria aspera (trachea) of a dog with opened thorax, that artificial respiration can keep the animal alive without any movement of either chest or lungs. This experiment, which had also been performed by Vesalius, proved that the essential feature of respiration is not in its intrinsic movements. but in certain blood changes in the lungs." Garrison
An account of an experiment made by M. Hook, of preserving animals alive by blowing through their lungs with bellows. Philos. Trans., 2: 539–540, Oct. 21, 1667
A supply of fresh air necessary for life. Ibid., 1667, 3: 66, 1700
Hooper, C. W. See G. H. Whipple
Hoover, Charles Frank. Cleveland physician. 1865–1927
SIGN—in pericardial effusion of any magnitude, diminished expansion of chest is apt to occur because of interference of movements of diaphragm.
Definitive percussion and inspection in estimating size and contour of heart. J. A. M. A., 75: 1626–1630, Dec. 11, 1920
Hoover, Charles Ruglas. American chemist. 1885–
REACTION—
The detection of carbon monoxide. J. Ind. and Eng. Chem., 13: 770–772, Sept. 1921
Hope, James. London physician. 1801–1841
SIGN—double heart beat in aortic aneurysm.
A treatise on the diseases of the heart and great vessels. ... London, Kidd, 1832. 612 pp.
Also: 2 ed., 1835. Also: 1st Amer. ed., Philadelphia, Haswell and Johnson, 1842
Also, from above, Part III, Chapt. IX, Section 5 in: F. A. Willius ahd T. E. Keys' *Cardiac classics.* St. Louis, Mosby, 1941. pp. 405–415
Hopf, Gustav. Hamburg dermatologist
KERATOSIS—
Über eine bisher nicht beschriebene disseminierte Keratose (Akrokeratosis verruci formis). Derm. Z., 60: 227–250, Feb. 1931
See also E. Keining
Hopkins, Barbara E. See A. T. Glenny
Hopkins, Sir Frederick Gowland. English biologist. 1861–1947
Awarded Nobel prize in 1929, for discovery of vitamins in 1912. With C. Eijkman.
METHOD—
On the estimation of uric acid in urine: a new process

by means of saturation with ammonium chloride.
Proc. roy. Soc., 52: 93–99, June 16, 1892
On the estimation of uric acid in the urine. J. Path.
Bact., 1: 451–459, 1893
REACTION—glyoxylic r.
On the proteid reaction of Adamkiewicz, with contributions to the chemistry of glyoxylic acid with S. W.
Cole, Proc. roy. Soc., 68: 21–33, Jan. 17, 1901
*A contribution to the chemistry of proteids, Part I.
A preliminary study of a hitherto undescribed product
of tryptic digestion* with S. W. Cole, J. Physiol., 27:
418–428, Dec. 23, 1901
REAGENT—for tryptophane. Ibid.
Discovered vitamins.
*Feeding experiments illustrating the importance of
accessory factors in normal dietaries.* J. Physiol., 44:
425–460, July 15, 1912
*Report on the present state of knowledge concerning food
factors (vitamins).* London, H. M. Stat. Off., 1919.
107 pp.
Isolated pure glutathione, the nucleus of auto-oxidation in the cell.
On an autoxidisable constituent of the cell. Biochem.
J., 15: 286–305, 1921
*On glutathione. II. A thermostable oxidation-reduction
system* with M. Dixon, J. biol. Chem., 54: 527–563,
Nov. 1922
On glutathione, a reinvestigation. Ibid., 84: 269–320,
Oct. 1929
See also W. M. Fletcher, Edith G. Willcock

Hopkins, Heywood Hill. Rochester, N. Y. surgeon.
1896–
Used vitallium cup on Feb. 11, 1938
Arthroplasty on hip, with use of vitallium cup with
F. N. Zuck. Med. Bull. Veterans' Adminis., 15: 1–2,
July 1938

Hopkins, J(oseph) Gardner. New York physician.
1882–
BROTH—basal veal infusion, for studying fermentation.
*Classification of pathogenic streptococci by fermentation
reactions* with A. Lang, J. infect. Dis., 15: 63–84
(72), July 1914
METHOD—
A method for standardizing bacterial vaccines.
J. A. M. A., 60: 1615–1617, May 24, 1913
See also H. Zinsser

Hopmann, Carl Melchior. Cologne physician. 1844–
1925
PAPILLOMATA—of nose.
Die papillären Geschwülste der Nasenschleimhaut.
Arch. path. Anat., Physiol. u. Med., 93: 213–258,
Aug. 1, 1883

Hoppe, Hermann Henry. Cincinnati neurologist.
1867–
DISEASE—myasthenia gravis paralytica.
Ein Beitrag zur Kenntniss der Bulbar-Paralyse.
Berl. klin. Wschr., 29: 332–336, Apr. 4, 1892

Hoppe-Seyler, Ernst Felix Immanuel. German
chemist. 1825–1895
REACTION—for glucose.
*Ueber eine Reaction zum Nachweis von Zucker im
Urin, auf Indigobildung beruhend.* Z. physiol. Chem.,
17: 83–86, 1893
TEST—for bile pigments.
*Weitere Mittheilungen über die Eigenschaften des
Blutfarbstoffs.* Ibid., 2: 149–155, 1878

TEST—for carbon monoxid in blood.
*Ueber die Einwirkung des Kohlenoxydgases auf das
Hämatoglobulin.* Arch. path. Anat., 11: 288–289,
Mar. 1857
*Ueber die Einwirkung des Kohlenoxydgases auf das
Blut.* Ibid., 13: 104–105, 1858
Suggested term hemoglobin for red coloring matter
of blood.
*Ueber die chemischen und optischen Eigenschaften des
Blutfarbstoffs.* Ibid., 29: 597–600, 1864

Horbaczwski, Johann. Vienna physician
Synthesized uric acid in vitro in 1882 and proved that
it is derived from nuclein in 1889. Garrison
*Beiträge zur Kenntniss der Bildung der Harnsäure
und der Xanthinbasen,* . . . S. B. Akad. Wiss. Wien.
Math.-naturw. Cl., 100: 78–132, 1891

Horder, Lord (Thomas Jeeves). English physician.
1871–
Gave classical description of subacute bacterial endocarditis.
*Infective endocarditis, with an analysis of 150 cases
and with special reference to the chronic form of the
disease.* Quart. J. Med., 2: 289–324, Apr. 1909

Horner, Johann Friedrich. Swiss ophthalmologist.
1831–1886
PTOSIS, SYNDROME or TRIAD—mitosis, ptosis
and enophthalmos, caused by paralysis of cervical
sympathetic.
Über eine Form von Ptosis. Klin. Mbl. Augenheilk.,
7: 193–198, 1869

Horner, William Edmonds. Philadelphia surgeon.
1793–1853
Described tensor tarsi Hornerian, muscle supplying
lacrymal apparatus.
Description of a small muscle at the internal commissure of the eyelids. Philadelphia J. Med., and Phys.
Sci., 8: 70–80, 1824
Wrote first American text-book of pathology. Garrison and Morton
A treatise on pathological anatomy. Philadelphia,
Carey, 1829. 460 pp.
Discovered that cholera stools contain intestinal
epithelia.
Note on the anatomic characters of cholera. Amer. J.
med. Sci., 15: 545 (only), 1834; 16: 58–81; 277–
295, 1835

Horoszkiewicz, Stefan von. Krakow physician
TEST—for carbon monoxide in blood.
*Ueber die Wirkung des Chinins auf den Blutfarbstoff nebst Mitteilung einer einfachen Methode zum
Nachweis von Kohlenoxyd im Blut* with H. Marx,
Berl. klin. Wschr., pp. 1156–1157, Aug. 27, 1906

Horrax, Gilbert. Boston neurosurgeon. 1887–
TREATMENT—
*The recognition and treatment of chronic subdural
hematoma: a favorable intracranial condition frequently overlooked* with J. L. Popper, Surg. Clin. N.
Amer., 1489–1499, Dec. 1935

Horsfall, Frank Lappin, Jr. New York physician.
1906–
Introduced—
*Antipneumococcus rabbit serum as a therapeutic agent
in lobar pneumonia* with K. Goodner, C. M. MacLeod
and A. H. Harris, 2nd. J. A. M. A., 108: 1483–1490,
May 1, 1937

Horsley, John Shelton. American surgeon. 1870–
1945

OPERATION—modification of Billroth I gastro-duodenostomy.
Partial gastrectomy. S. G. O., 44: 214–220, Feb. 1927

Horsley, Sir Victor Alexander Hayden. English neurologist. 1857–1916

OPERATION—excision of area of motor cortex for relief of athetoid and convulsive movements of upper extremity.
Remarks on ten consecutive cases of operations upon the brain and cranial cavity to illustrate the details and safety of the method employed. Brit. med. J., 1: 863–865, Apr. 23, 1887
The function of the so-called motor area of the brain. Ibid., 2: 125–132, July 17, 1909

OPERATION—
Remarks on the various surgical procedures devised for the relief or cure of trigeminal neuralgia (tic douloureaux) with J. Taylor and W[t] S. Colman, Ibid., 2: 1139–1143, Nov. 28; 1191–1193, Dec. 5; 1249–1253, Dec. 12, 1891
Produced artificial myxedema in monkey by thyroidectomy.
(A recent specimen of artificial myxoedema in a monkey.) Abstr.: Lancet, 2: 827 (only), Nov. 8, 1884
"On the function of the thyroid gland." Proc. roy. Soc., 38: 5–7, Dec. 11, 1884
The Brown lectures on pathology. Brit. med. J., 1: 111–115, Jan. 17, 1885
Made early attempts to transplant thyroid gland.
Remarks on the function of the thyroid gland: a critical and historical review. Ibid., 1: 215–219, Jan. 30; 265–268, Feb. 6, 1892

Horton, Bayard Taylor. Rochester, Minn. physician. 1895–

SYNDROME—
A new syndrome of vascular headache: results of treatment with histamine: preliminary report with A. R. MacLean and W. McK. Craig, Proc. Staff Meet., Mayo Clin., 14: 257–260, Apr. 26, 1939

TEST—oxygen saturation, for arterio-venous fistula.
Arteriovenous fistula involving the common femoral artery identified by arteriography. Ibid., 8: 189–191, Mar. 29, 1933
Same: Amer. J. med. Sci., 187: 649–652, May 1934
Congenital arteriovenous fistulae of the extremities visualized by arteriography with R. K. Ghormley, S. G. O., 60: 978–983, May 1935
Described—
An undescribed form of arteritis of the temporal vessels with T. B. Magath and G. E. Brown, Proc. Staff Meet., Mayo Clin., 7: 700–701, Dec. 7, 1932

Horvath, A. A. See W. P. Yant
Horvitz, A. See L. A. Sachar
Hosoi, K. See V. C. Jacobsen
Hottinger, Robert. San Paulo, Brazil physician
BROTH—for culture media.
Nachprüfung und Kritik der üblichen Bouillonbereitung. Einfache Herstellung einer billigen guten Nährlösung. Zbl. Bakt., 63: 178–206, Dec. 4, 1912

Hotz, Ferdinand Carl. Chicago ophthalmologist. 1843–1909
OPERATION—blepharoplasty.
A method of utilizing cicatricial skin flaps in the operation for ectropium of the upper lid. Arch. Ophthal., N. Y, 25: 293–296, 1896

Hou, H. C. Chinese physician
DIET—high salt.
Influence of diet on the formation of urinary calculi. Chinese med. J., 50: 787–796, June 1936

Houssay, Bernardo A. Buenos Aires physiologist. 1887–
PHENOMENON—hypersensitivity of hypophysectomized animals to insulin and virtual disappearance after hypophysectomy of diabetes induced by de-pancreatization.
La diabetes pancreática de los perros hipofisoprivos with A. Biasotti, Rev. Soc. Argent. de Biol., Buenos Aires, 6: 251–296, 1930
The hypophysis and metabolism. New Engl. J. Med., 214: 961–971, May 14, 1936
Relations between the parathyroids, the hypophysis, and the pancreas. Harvey Lectures. Baltimore, Williams & Wilkins, 1936. Vol. 31, pp. 116–134

Houston, John. Dublin surgeon. 1802–1845
MUSCLE—compressor venae dorsalis penis.
An account of two newly discovered muscles for compressing the dorsal vein of the penis, in man and other animals; and also of a similar provision for compressing the veins of the chameleon's tongue. Dublin, Hodges and Smith, 1830
VALVES—folds of mucous membrane in rectum
WHITE LINE—in rectum.
Observations on the mucous membrane of the rectum. Dublin Hosp. Rep., 5: 158–165, 1830

Houstoun, (Houston) Robert. English surgeon ?–1734
Treated ovarian dropsy by tapping cyst.
An account of a dropsy of the left ovary of a woman, aged fifty-eight, cured by a large incision made in the side of the abdomen. Philos. Trans., (1724–24), 33: 8–15, 1726

Hovius, Jacobus. Dutch anatomist
CANAL—ciliary.
MEMBRANE—inner layer of choroid.
PLEXUS—in ciliary region.
De circulari humorum ocularium motu. Traj. ad Rhenum, van de Water, 1702. 44 pp.

Howard, Benjamin Douglas. New York physician. 1840–1900
METHOD—of artificial respiration.
Plain rules for the restoration of persons apparently dead from drowning. New York, Treat, 1869
The direct method of artificial respiration for the treatment of persons apparently dead from suffocation by drowning, or from other causes. With cases. Trans. Amer. Med. Ass., 22: 311–347, 1871

Howard, N. W. See M. X. Sullivan
Howard, R. P. See G. W. Thorn
Howe, Paul Edward. American pathologist. 1885–
METHOD—of determination of proteins in blood and of separation of serum albumin and globulin.
The use of sodium sulfate as the globulin precipitant in the determination of proteins in blood. J. biol. Chem., 49: 93–107, Nov. 1921
The determination of proteins in blood—a micro method. Ibid., 109–113
See also J. H. Brown

Howell, William Henry. American physiologist. 1860–1945
BODIES—in erythrocytes.
The life-history of the formed elements of the blood,

especially the red blood corpuscles. J. Morph., 4: 57–116, July 1890

DETERMINATION—of coagulation time of blood.
The condition of the blood in hemophilia, thrombosis and purpura. Arch. intern. Med., 13: 76–95 (80), Jan. 1914

METHOD—
The preparation and properties of thrombin, together with observations on antithrombin and prothrombin. Amer. J. Physiol., 26: 453–473, Oct. 1, 1910
Rapid method of preparing thrombin. Ibid., 32: 264–265, Sept. 2, 1913
Studied physiology of hypophysis.
The physiological effects of extracts of the hypophysis cerebri and infundibular body. J. exp. Med., 3: 245–258, Mar. 1898
Discovered anticoagulant, heparin. 1916
Two new factors in blood coagulation—heparin and pro-antithrombin with L. E. Holt, Amer. J. Physiol., 47: 328–341, Dec. 1918

Howes, Edward Lee. American surgeon. 1903–
Studied healing of wounds.
The strength of the healing wound in relation to the holding strength of the catgut suture. New Engl. J. Med., 200: 1285–1291, June 20, 1929
The clinical significance of experimental studies in wound healing with S. C. Harvey, Ann. Surg., 102: 941–946, Nov. 1935

Howland, Goldwin William. Toronto physician. 1875–
Described dysinsulinism with islet cell tumor of pancreas.
Dysinsulinism: convulsions and coma due to islet cell tumor of the pancreas, with operation and cure with W. R. Campbell, E. J. Maltby and W. L. Robinson, J. A. M. A., 93: 674–679, Aug. 31, 1929

Howland, John. American pediatrician. 1873–1926
MASK—for collection of alveolar air from infants.
Acidosis occurring with diarrhea with W. McK. Marriott, Amer. J. Dis. Child., 11: 309–325, May 1916
SCHEME OF DIET—for celiac disease.
Prolonged intolerance to carbohydrates. Trans. Amer. Pediat. Soc., 33: 11–19, 1921
See also B. Kramer, W. McK. Marriott

Hoyer, Heinrich Friedrich. Warsaw surgeon. 1834–1907
Described glomus tumors, or angioneuroma.
Ueber unmittelbare Einmündung kleinster Arterien in Gefässäste venösen Charakters. Arch. mikr. Anat., 13: 603–644, 1877

Hsu, F. Y. See C. Heymans

Hubata, Robert. U. S. Army physician
TEST—
A simple rapid test for detection of sulfonamide compounds in urine: a preliminary report. War Med., 5: 56–57, Jan. 1944

Hubbard, J. P. See R. E. Gross

Huber, Armin. Zürich physician
METHOD—of testing motor function of stomach.
Die Methoden zur Bestimmung der motorischen Thätigkeit des Magens. Correspond. f. schweiz. Aerzte, 20: 65–74, Feb. 1, 1890
See also N. M. Arthus

Huber, Carl. Heidelberg chemist
Prepared nicotinic acid by oxidation of nicotine.

Vorläufige Notiz über einige Derivate des Nicotins. Ann. Chem. u. Pharm., 141: 271, 1867

Huc. See E. Apert

Huchard, Henri. Paris physician. 1844–1910
ATAXIA—of hysteria.
Caractère, moeurs, état mental des hystériques. Arch. neurol., Paris, 3: 187–211, Mar. 1882
DISEASE—continued arterial hypertension, thought to be a cause of arteriosclerosis.
Principales causes de l'artério-sclérose. Rev. gen. de clin. et de therap., 23: 322–325, 1909

Huddleson, I. F(orest). American bacteriologist. 1893–
DIAGNOSTIC CRITERIA—of brucellosis; a positive cutaneous reaction (Brucellergin) with low or absent opsonins indicates active disease.
METHOD—for determination of opsonocytophagic power of blood.
A study of the opsono-cytophagic power of the blood and allergic skin reaction in Brucella infection and immunity in man with H. W. Johnson and E. E. Hamann, Amer. J. Pub. Health, 23: 917–929, Sept. 1933
METHOD—
Further studies on the isolation and cultivation of bacterium abortus (Bang) with D. E. Hasley and J. P. Torrey, J. infect. Dis., 40: 352–368, Feb. 1927

Hudgins, Archibald Perrin. Charleston, W. Va. gynecologist. 1902–
CANNULA—
X-ray studies in hysterosalpingography, using a new cannula. Amer. J. Obstet. Gynaec., 49: 431–435, Mar. 1945

Hudson, N. P. See A. Stokes

Hudson, William H. American surgeon. 1862–1915
OPERATION—
Subtemporal muscle drainage by the aid of silver wire drainage mats in cases of congenital hydrocephalus. Ann. Surg., 57: 338–340, Mar. 1913

Hübener, E. A. See P. T. Uhlenhuth

Huebscher, C. Basel surgeon
OPERATION—for slipping patella.
Ueber Operationen bei habitueller Luxation der Kniescheibe. Z. orthop. Chir., 24: 1–22, 1909

Hueck, Alexander Friedrich. German anatomist. 1802–1842
LIGAMENT—pectinate.
De mutationibus oculi internis respectu distantiae rerum. (Dorpat), Schünmanni, 1826. 74 pp.

Hueck, Hermann Richard. German surgeon. 1891–
OPERATION—for formation of thumb.
Ein Fall von Daumenersatz durch einen unbrauchbaren Finger. Dtsch. Z. Chir., 153: 321–330, Mar. 1920

Hüfner, Carl Gustav von. German physician. 1840–1908
Showed that 1 gm. of hemoglobin combines with 1.34 c.c. of oxygen.
Neue Versuche zur Bestimmung der Sauerstoffcapacität des Blutfarbstoffs. Arch. Anat. Physiol., Physiol. Abt., Lpz., pp. 130–176, 1894
Ueber das Molekulargewicht des Oxyhämoglobins with E. Gansser, Ibid., pp. 209–216, 1907

Huelsmann, L. See N. B. Carson

Hueper, Wilhelm C. American physician. 1894–

HYPOTHESIS—of cancer formation by allergic mutation.
In his: *Occupational tumors and allied diseases.*
Springfield, Ill., Thomas, 1942. pp. 896

Hueppe, Ferdinand Adolf Theophil. Wiesbaden physician. 1852–1938
MEDIUM—egg, culture.
Ueber die Verwendung von Eiern zu Kulturzwecken.
Zbl. Bakt., 4: 80–81, 1888

Hürthle, Karl. German surgeon. 1860–
CELL and CELL TUMOR—of thyroid gland.
Beiträge zur Kenntniss des Secretinsvorgangs in der Schilddrüse. Arch. ges. Physiol., 56: 1–44, Feb. 24, 1894
MODIFICATION—of syphygmomagraph.
Ueber eine Methode zur Registrirung des arteriellen Blutdrucks beim Menschen. Dtsch. med. Wschr., 22: 574–577, Sept. 3, 1896

Hüet, G. J. Dutch physician
ANOMALLY—of neutrophil.
(Familial anomaly of leukocytes.) Ned. tschr. geneesk., 75: pt. 4, 5956–5959, 1931
Also: Mschr. kindergeneesk., 1: 173–181, 1931–32
Über eine bisher unbekannte familiäre Anomalie der Leukocyten. Klin. Wschr., 11: 1264–1266, July 23, 1932

Hueter, Carl. German surgeon. 1838–1882
SIGN—in rupture of long head of biceps, flexion of elbow with forearm pronated is stronger than when supinated.
Zur Diagnose der Verletzungen des M. Biceps brachii.
Arch. klin. Chir., 5: 321–323, 1864

Hughes, Charles Hamilton. American neurologist. 1839–1916
REFLEX—
Note on the viril reflex. Alienist and Neurol., 12: 44–46, Jan. 1891

Hughes, T. P. See W. F. Petersen

Hughes, Wendell Lochead. Hempstead, N. Y. Ophthalmologist. 1900–
OPERATION—
A new method for rebuilding a lower lid: report of a case. Arch. Ophthal., 17: 1008–1017, June 1937

Hughson, W. See J. M. T. Finney

Hugounenq, Louis. French physician
SOLUTION—sucrose urea; culture medium.
A propos de la culture du bacille de Loeffler en milieu chimique défini with Doyon, C. R. Soc. Biol., 48: 401–403, Apr. 18, 1896

Huguenin, Gustav. Zurich physician. 1841–1920
EDEMA—acute, of brain.
Ueber Hirnoedem. Corresp. f. Schweizer Aerzte, 19: 321–330, June 1, 1889

Huguier, Pierre Charles. French surgeon. 1804–1873
OPERATION—reconstruction of thumb.
Considérations anatomiques et physiologiques pour servir a la chirurgie du pouce. Arch. gén. de méd., 1: 54–82, Jan. 1874
THEORY—uterine prolapse is usually due to lengthening of supravaginal part of cervix.
Mémoire sur les allongements hypertrophiques du col de l'utérus, dans les affections désignées sous les noms de descente, de précipitation de cet organe, et sur leur traitement par la résection ou l'amputation de la totalité du col, suivant la variété de la maladie. Paris, Baillière, 1860. 231 pp.

Described esthiomène.
Mémoire sur l'esthiomène ou dartre rongeante de la région vulvo-anal. Mém. Acad. nat. de Méd., Paris, 14: 501–596, 1848

Huhner, Max. New York surgeon. 1873–
TEST—
Sterility in the male and female and its treatment. New York, Rebman Co., 1913
The value of the spermatozoa test in sterility. Urol. and Cutan. Rev., 18: 587–595, Nov. 1914

Huldschinsky, Kurt. German physician. 1883–
Introduced light treatment for rickets.
Heilung von Rachitis durch künstliche Höhensonne.
Dtsch. med. Wschr., 65: 712–713, June 26, 1919

Hulen, Vard Houghton. American ophthalmologist. 1865–1939
OPERATION—
Vacuum fixation of the lens, and flap suture in the extraction of a cataract in its capsule. J. A. M. A., 57: 188–189, July 15, 1911

Hull, Alfred John. London surgeon. 1875–
OPERATION—for inguinal hernia.
Recurrence of inguinal hernia. Ann. Surg., 58: 479–482, Oct. 1913

Hull, Albert Wallace. Schenectady scientist. 1880–
FORMULA—to determine amount of roentgen absorptive power of any substance.
Absorption and scattering of x-rays. J. Radiol., 1: 27–39, Jan. 1920

Hulpieu, N. R. See R. N. Harger

Hulton-Frankel, Florence. New York physician.
AGAR—
Differentiation of typhoid, paratyphoid A and B by means of a dextrin-inosite medium with Katherine MacDonald, Proc. Soc. exp. Biol., N. Y., 15: 31–33, Dec. 19, 1917
Differentiation of typhoid and paratyphoid A and B bacilli by a dextrine-inosite medium. J. infect. Dis., 23: 380–381, Oct. 1918
SOLUTION—acetic acid and ammonia; culture medium.
*Studies on synthetic mediums. I. Study of the characteristics of some bacteria on a simple synthetic medium.
II. Sugar fermentations in synthetic mediums* with Helene Barber and Eleanor Pyle, Ibid., 24: 9–21 (17), Jan. 1919

Human, J. U. London physician
SIGN—
Chin retraction: a new sign in anesthesia. Brit. J. Anaesth., 15: 66–68, Jan. 1938

Humber, J. D. See W. B. Coffey

Humboldt, F. H. See C. Matteucci

Hummelsheim, Eduard Karl Marie Joseph. German ophthalmologist. 1868–
OPERATION—for paralysis of external rectus.
Ueber Sehnentransplantation am Auge. Ber. ophth. Ges., Heidelberg, pp. 248–253, 1907
Weitere Erfahrungen mit partieller Sehnenüberpflanzung an den Augenmuskeln. Arch. f. Augenh., 62: 71–74, 1908

Humphrey, Sir George Murray. English surgeon. 1820–1896
LIGAMENT—of knee.
On excision of the knee. Med.-chir. Trans., London, 41: 193–218, 1858

The results of thirty-nine cases of excision of the knee. Ibid., 52: 13-25, 1869

OPERATION—
Excision of the condyle of the lower jaw. Ass. Med. J., 160: 61-62, Jan. 26, 1856
Removed tumor from bladder.
Tumour in the bladder removed by perineal incision. Complete recovery. Med.-chir. Trans., 62: 421-427, 1879

Humphreys, Eleanor M. See Ruth Gilbert, Mary W. Wheeler

Humphreys, Frederick Brown. New York bacteriologist. 1878-
METHOD—acrolein, of identification of B. welchii in cultures.
Formation of acrolein from glycerol by B. welchii. J. infect. Dis., 35: 282-290, Sept. 1924

Hun, Henry. Albany, N. Y. neurologist. 1854-1924
Wrote—
An atlas of the differential diagnosis of the diseases of the nervous system; analytical and semeilogical neurological charts. Troy, N. Y., Southworth, 1913. 290 pp.

Hundhausen, G. See S. Dietrich

Hunner, Guy LeRoy. American urologist. 1868-
ULCER—of bladder.
Consideration of a new viewpoint on the etiology of renal tuberculosis in women. Amer. J. Obstet. Gynaec., 24: 706-728, Nov. 1932

Hunt, George Herbert. English physician. 1884-1926
Described trench fever.
Intermittent fever of obscure origin, occurring among British soldiers in France. The so-called "trench fever." Lancet, 2: 1133-1136, Nov. 20, 1915
See also Stoke

Hunt, James Ramsay. New York neurologist. 1872-1937
SYNDROME—geniculate.
On herpetic inflammations of the geniculate ganglion. A new syndrome and its complications. J. nerv. ment. Dis., 34: 73-96, Feb. 1907
SYNDROME—of paralysis agitans; lesion is in pallidal region of lenticular nucleus.
Progressive atrophy of the globus pallidus (primary atrophy of the pallidal system). Brain, 40: 58-148, May 1917
Primary atrophy of the pallidal system of the corpus striatum. A contribution to the nature and pathology of paralysis agitans. Arch. intern. Med., 22: 647-691, Nov. 1918

Hunt, Reid. American pharmacologist. 1870-
REACTION—pathogenesis of exophthalmic goiter.
Studies on thyroid with A. Seidell, Treas. Dept. U. S. Mar.-Hosp. Serv., Hyg. Lab. Bull., No. 47, 1909. 115 pp.
TEST—
The influence of thyroid feeding upon poisoning by acetonitrile. J. biol. Chem., 1: 33-44, Oct. 1905
On the influence of thyroid feeding and of various foods and of small amounts of food upon poisoning by acetonitril. Abstr.: Proc. Soc. exp. Biol., N. Y., pp. 15-16, Oct. 18, 1905
The acetonitril test for thyroid and of some alterations of metabolism. Amer. J. Physiol., 63: 257-299, 1923
Discovered hypotensive effect of acetylcholine.
On the physiological action of certain cholin derivatives and new methods for detecting cholin with R.

deM. Taveau, Brit. med. J., 2: 1788-1791, Dec. 22 1906
Showed that tissues are more sensitive to acetylcholine after treatment with eserine (physostigmine)
Vasodilator reactions. I and II. Amer. J. Physiol. 45: 197-267, Feb. 1, 1918

Hunt, Verne Carlton. Los Angeles surgeon. 1888-
TECHNIC—
Transduodenal resection of the ampulla of Vater for carcinoma of the distal end of the common duct, with restoration of the continuity of the common and pancreatic ducts with the duodenum with J. W. Budd Trans. West. Surg. Ass., pp. 419-449, 1934
Surgical management of carcinoma of the ampulla o Vater and of the periampullary portion of the duodenum. Ann. Surg., 114: 570-602, Oct. 1941

Hunter, Andrew. Ithaca, N. Y. biochemist. 1876-
MODIFICATION—of Krüger-Schmidt method for determination of uric acid.
The metabolism of endogenous and exogenous purines in the monkey with M. H. Givens, J. biol. Chem. 17: 37-53, Feb. 1914

Hunter, Donald. London physician. 1898-
Described hyperparathyroidism and generalized osteitis fibrosa.
Hyperparathyroidism: generalized osteitis fibrosa, with observations upon the bones, the parathyroid tumours, and normal parathyroid glands with H. M Turnbull, Brit. J. Surg., 19: 203-284, Oct. 1931

Hunter, George. Canadian biochemist. 1894-
REAGENT—for ergothioneine.
A new test for ergothioneine upon which is based a method for its estimation in simple solution and in blood-filtrates. Biochem. J., 22: 4-10, 1928
TEST—
A diazo-method for detecting bilirubin in urine Canad. Med. Ass. J., 23: 823-824, Dec. 1930

Hunter, John. Scottish surgeon. 1728-1793
CANAL—c. adductorius.
An account of Mr. Hunter's method of performing the operation for the popliteal aneurism. Communicated in a letter to Dr. Simmons by Mr. Everard Home, Surgeon. London Med., J., 7: 391-406, 1786
Also: Medical classics, 4: 449-457, Jan. 1940
CHANCRE—
A treatise on the venereal disease. London, 1786. 398 pp. p. 218
Also: *Works.* London, Longman, 1837
Also: Medical classics, 4: 458-527, Jan. 1940
GUBERNACULUM—testis.
A description of the situation of the testis in the foetus with its descent into the scrotum. First published in *Medical commentaries,* by William Hunter, 1762 part 1, p. 75
Also in: *Animal economy,* by John Hunter, 1786
Also: *Works.* London, Longman, 1837. Vol. 4, pp 1-19
Also: Medical classics, 4: 421-441, Jan. 1940
OPERATION—
An account of Mr. Hunter's method of performing the operation for the cure of the popliteal aneurism. By Everard Home, Trans. Soc. Improvement Med. and Chir. Knowledge, London, 1: 138-181, 1793
Additional cases to illustrate Mr. Hunter's method of performing the operation for the cure of the popliteal aneurism. By Everard Home, Ibid., 2: 235-256 1800

First to study teeth in a scientific manner. Garrison
Treatise on the natural history of the human teeth, explaining their structure, use, formation, growth and diseases. Part I, 1771. Parts I and II, called 2 ed., London, Johnson, 1778
Introduced artificial feeding by means of a flexible tube passed into the stomach, 1790. Garrison
A case of paralysis of the muscles of deglutition, cured by an artificial mode of conveying food and medicines into the stomach. Trans. Soc. Improvement Med. and Chir. Knowledge, London, 1: 182–188, 1793

Hunter, William. Scottish surgeon. 1718–1883
First to describe arterio-venous aneurysms. Garrison
The history of an aneurysm of the aorta, with some remarks on aneurysms in general. Med. Obs. and Inq., London, 1: 323–357, 1757
Observations upon a particular species of aneurism (arteriovenous aneurysm). Ibid., 1: 340, 1753–57; 2: 390, 1762
Discoverer of decidua reflexa and separate maternal and fetal circulation. Garrison
Anatomie uteri humani gravidi tabulis illustrata, Anatomy of the human gravid uterus exhibited in figures. Birminghamae, Baskerville, 1774
Also, reprint: London, Sydenham Soc., 1851
First to describe retroversion of uterus. Garrison
On retroversion of the uterus. Med. Obs. and Inq., 4: 409, 1771; 5: 388, 1776

Hunter, William. London pathologist. 1861–1937
SYNDROME—glossitis in pernicious anemia.
Further observations on pernicious anemia (severe cases): a chronic infective disease: its relation to infection from the mouth and stomach; suggested serum treatment. Lancet, 1: 221–224, Jan. 27; 296–299, Feb. 3; 371–377, Feb. 10, 1900

Huntington, George. American physician. 1850–1916
CHOREA or DISEASE—
On chorea. Med. and Surg. Reporter, Phila., 26: 317–321, Apr. 13, 1872
Recollections of Huntington's chorea as I saw it at East Hampton, Long Island, during my boyhood. J. nerv. ment. Dis., 37: 255–257, Apr. 1910

Huntington, R. W. Jr. See J. G. Dickson

Huntington, Thomas Waterman. San Francisco surgeon. 1849–1929
OPERATION—for ununited fracture.
Case of bone transference; use of a segment of fibula to supply a defect in the tibia. Ann. Surg., 41: 249–251, Feb. 1905

Huntoon, Frank McElroy. American bacteriologist. 1881–
AGAR—"hormone", for cultivation of gonococcus.
"Hormone" medium: a simple medium employable as substitute for serum medium. J. infect. Dis., 23: 169–172, Aug. 1918
BROTH—hormone heart infusion; culture medium. Ibid.
METHOD—
A simple method for staining the capsules of bacteria. J. Bact., 2: 241–243, May 1917
SERUM or SOLUTION—polyvalent antibody, used in pneumonia.
Antibody studies; III. Chemical nature of antibody with P. Masucci and E. Hannum, J. Immunol., 6: 185–200, Mar. 1921

STAIN—
A simple and reliable method of staining spores. J. A. M. A., 62: 1397 (only), May 2, 1914
See also W. J. Elser

Huot, E. French physician
Discovered an animal with an aglomerular kidney.
Sur les capsules surrenales, les reins, le tissu lymphoide des poissons lophobranches. C. R. Acad. Sci., 124: 1462–1467, June 21, 1897

Huppert, Hugo. Leipzig biochemist. 1832–1904
DISEASE—multiple myeloma.
Ein Fall von Albumosurie. Prager med. Wschr., 14: 35–36, Jan. 23, 1889
TEST—for bile pigments.
Ueber eine Fehlerquelle beim Nachweise von Gallenfarbstoff. Arch. d. Heilkunde, 4: 479–480, 1863
TEST—for homogentisic acid in urine.
Ueber die Homogentisinsäure. Dtsch. Arch. klin. Med., 64: 129–139, 1899

Hurler, Gertrud. Munich pediatrician
SYNDROME—congenital, multiple symmetrical skeletal deformities with disturbance of lipoid metabolism.
Ueber einen Typ multipler Abartungen, vorwiegend am Skelettsystem. Z. Kinderheilk., 24: 220–234, Jan. 20, 1920

Hurler, Konrad. Munich physician
SOLUTION—succinate meat extract; for cultivation of typhoid bacilli.
Vergleichende Untersuchungen über den Bacillus paratyphosus B, den Bacillus enteritidis Gärtner und die Rattenbacillen: Ratinbacillus, Bacillus ratti Danysz, Bac.llus ratti Dunbar und Bacillus ratti Issatschenko. Zbl. Bakt., 63: 341–372, May 25, 1912

Hurtley, William Holdsworth. London scientist. 1865–1936
TEST—
The tests for acetoacetic acid including a simple new test. Lancet, 1: 1160–1161, Apr. 26, 1913

Hu w tz, S. H. See L. G. Rowntree, G. H. Whipple

Husemann, August. German chemist
REACTION—for morphine.
Zur Erkennung des Morphins und Narcotins. Ann. Chem. u. Pharm., 128: 305–310, 1863

Hussey, Hugh Hudson, Jr. American physician. 1910–
METHOD—of measuring venous pressure.
Clinical application of venous pressure measurement. M. Ann. Dist. of Columbia, 5: 232–237, Aug. 1936

Husson, Camille Louis. French chemist
TEST—for hemoglobin.
Sur quelques reactions de l'hemoglobine et de ses derives. (Extrait), C. R. Acad. Sci., 81: 477–480, 1875

Hustin, Albert. Belgium physician. 1882–
Advocated use of sodium citrate as anticoagulant of blood.
Note sur une nouvelle méthode de transfusion. Bull. Soc. roy. d. sci. méd. de Bruxelles, 72: 104–111, 1914

Hutchins, Elliott Holdsworth. Baltimore surgeon. 1880–
OPERATION—
Operation for direct inguinal hernia. S. G. O., 54: 964–968, June 1932

Hutchinson, A. C. See R. Cuming

Hutchinson, Sir Jonathan. English physician. 1828–1913
DISEASE—degeneration of choroid; choroiditis guttata senilis.

In his: *Illustrations of clinical surgery*. London, Churchill, 1875. Vol. 1, pp. 49–52

DISEASE—
Infective angioma or naevus-lupus. Arch. Surg., 3: 166–168, 1892

DISEASE—recurrent summer eruption.
A care of summer eruption recurring with great severity for many years, but finally getting well (a form of Kaposi's disease). Clin. Soc. Trans., 22: 80–83, 1888

MELANOTIC WHITLOW—subungual melanoma.
Melanotic disease of the great toe, following a whitlow of the nail. Trans. Path. Soc., 8: 404–405, Mar. 3, 1857
Melanosis often not black; melanotic whitlow. Brit. med. J., 1: 491 (only), Mar. 13, 1886

PRURIGO—of dentition.
Summer prurigo, prurigo aestivalis, seu prurigo adolescentium, seu acne-prurigo. Med. Times and Gaz., 1: 161–163, 1878

SIGN or KERATITIS or TEETH or TRIAD—
Report on the effects of infantile syphilis in marring the development of the teeth. Trans. Path. Soc., 9: 449–456, July 14, 1858
Also: Medical classics, 5: 138–146, Nov. 1940
On the different forms of inflammation of the eye consequent on inherited syphilis. Ophth. Hosp. Rep., 1: 191–203; 226–244, 1858; 2: 54–105, 1859; 258–283, 1860
Also: Medical classics, 5: 147–245, Nov. 1940
Heredosyphilitic struma and on teeth as a means of diagnosis. Brit. med. J., 1: 515–517, 1861
Reported primary carcinoma of male urethra.
Epithelial cancer of the mucous membrane of the urethra. Trans. Path. Soc. London, 13: 167–169, Feb. 18, 1862
First to successfully operate in a case of intussusception in an infant. Garrison and Morton
A successful case of abdominal section for intussesception; with remarks on this and other methods of treatment. Med.-chir. Trans., 57: 31–75, 1874
Described hidradenitis destruens suppurativa.
In his: *Lectures on clinical surgery*. London, Churchill, 1879. Part 2, p. 298
Described varicella gangrenosa or dermatitis gangrenosa infantum.
On gangrenous eruptions in connection with vaccination and chicken-pox. Med.-chir. Trans., 65: 1–11, 1882
Asserted that long continued absorption of small quantities of arsenic may be followed by formation of epithelial new growths.
Arsenic cancer. Brit. med. J., 2: 1280–1281, Dec. 10, 1887
Described Hilliard's lupus. See Hilliard
See also Mortimer

Hutchinson, John. Newcastle-on-Tyne physician. 1811–1861
Invented spirometer and investigated vital capacity of man.
On the capacity of the lungs and on the respiratory functions, with a view of establishing a precise and easy method of detecting disease by the spirometer. Med.-chir. Trans., 29: 137–252, 1846

Hutchinson, Sir Robert. English physician. 1871–
SYNDROME—
On suprarenal sarcoma in children with metastases in the skull. Quart. J. Med., 1: 33–38, Oct. 1907

Hutinel, Victor Henri. Paris physician. 1849–1933
DISEASE—infectious erythema seen in typhoid, pneumonia, etc.
Notes sur quelques érythèmes infectieux. Arch. gén. d. méd., Paris, 2: 263–291, Sept.; 385–403, Oct. 1892

Huxham, John. English physician. 1694–1768
Described Devonshire colic (from cider-drinking) without ascertaining its true cause. Garrison
Opusculum de morbo colico Damnoniensi. Londini, 1739
First to observe paralysis of soft palate which attends diphtheria (and which he confused with scarlatina). Garrison
An essay on fevers and their various kinds . . . to which is now added, a dissertation on the malignant, ulcerous sore-throat. London, Hinton, 1757. 336, pp.
Advised vegetable diet for sailors to guard against scurvy. Homans
De scorbuto. Venice, 1766

Huxley, Thomas Henry. English physiologist. 1825–1895
LAYER—of root sheaths of hair follicle.
MEMBRANE—cellular m. of root sheath.
On a hitherto undescribed structure in the human hair sheath. London Med. Gaz., 36: 1340–1341, 1845

Hyatt, E. G. See B. Fantus

Hyde, James Nevins. Chicago dermatologist. 1840–1910
DISEASE—prurigo nodularis.
In his: *A practical treatise on diseases of the skin, for the use of students and practitioners*. Philadelphia, Lea's, 1883. Same, 1909, p. 174
Called attention to—
On the influence of light in the production of cancer of the skin. Amer. J. Med. Sci., 131: 1–22, Jan. 1906

Hyman, Albert Solomon. New York physician. 1893–
"ARTIFICIAL PACE-MAKER" for heart.
Resuscitation of the stopped heart by intracardiac therapy. Arch. intern. Med., 46: 553–568 (563), Oct. 1930

Hyman, Harold Thomas. New York pharmacologist. 1894–
TREATMENT—
Massive arsenotherapy in early syphilis by continuous intravenous drip method; clinical considerations. Arch. Dermat. and Syph., 42: 253–261, Aug. 1940
See also L. Chargin

Hyrtl, Joseph. Vienna anatomist. 1810–1894
RECESS—lodging head of malleus and greater part of incus.
Zur vergleichenden Anatomie der Trommelhöhle. Denkschr. d. math.-naturw. Cl. d. k. Akad. d. Wissensch., Wien, 1849
Discovered origin of coronary arteries.
Beweis, dass die Ursprüng der Coronar-Arterien während der Systole der Kammer von den Semilunarklappen nicht bedeckt werden und dass der Eintritt des Blutes in diesselben nicht während der Diastole stattfindet. S. B. Akad. Wiss. Math.-naturw. Cl., Wien, 14, 1854

I

Iason, Alfred Herbert. New York surgeon. 1891–
OPERATION—for hernia.
In his: *Hernia*. Phila., Blakiston, 1941. 1325 pp. p.
529; 593–597

Icaacson, V. I. See N. W. Janney

Icard, Séverin. Marseille physician. 1860–
REAGENTS—for determining death.
Le signe de la mort réelee en l'absence du médecin.
Paris, Maloine, 1907
Also, abstr.: Dtsch. med. Wschr., 33: 1752, Oct. 17,
1907

Icart, M. French surgeon
Reported use of wire for suturing a fracture.
*Lettre en réponse au mémoire de M. Pujol, sur une
amputation naturelle de la jambe: avec des réflexions
sur quelques autres cas relatif à cette operation.* J. de
méd., Paris, 44: 164–169, Aug. 1775

Ichikawa, K. See K. Yamagiwa

Ide, Sobei. Japanese physician
TEST—
Ide test—the new color test for syphilis with T. Ide,
Jap. J. Dermat. and Urol. (Abst. Sect.), 39: 22, Feb.
1936
Also: J. Lab. clin. Med., 21: 1190–1194, Aug. 1936

Ido, Yutaka. Tokio physician
Discovered Leptospira hebdomadis to be cause of
"seven day fever" of Japan.
*Spirochaeta hebdomadis, the causative agent of seven
day fever (Nanukayami)* with H. Ito and H. Wani,
J. exp. Med., 28: 435–448, Oct. 1918
See also R. Inada

Iglauer, Samuel. Cincinnati otolaryngologist. 1871–
PROCEDURE—for dilating stricture of esophagus.
*Impermeable stricture of the esophagus relieved by
retrograde bouginage with the aid of a cystoscope in-
serted through a gastrostomy.* Ann. Otol., Rhi. and
Laryng., 41: 1191–1202, Dec. 1932

Ihl, Anton. German chemist
REACTIONS—for carbohydrates.
The phenols as reagents for carbohydrates. Chem.
News, 51: 114–115, Mar. 6, 1885

Illyés, Géza von. Budapest surgeon. 1870–
Demonstrated ureteral calculi with x-ray and in-
dwelling opaque catheter.
Uretercatheterazés és radiographia. Orvosi hetilap,
Budapest, 45: 659–662, 1901
Same: *Ureterkatheterismus und Radiographie.* Dtsch.
Z. Chir., 62: 132–140, Dec. 1901

Imai, N. See K. Shiga

Inada, Ryukichi. Japanese physician. 1874–
Developed successful serum-therapy against infectious jaundice (Weil's disease) and discovered
that a spirochete is etiologic agent.
*The etiology, mode of infection, and specific therapy
of Weil's disease (spirochaetosis icterohaemorrhagiae).*
with Y. Ido, R. Hoke, R. Kaneko and H. Ito, J.
exp. Med., 23: 377–403, Mar. 1916

Ingals, Ephraim Fletcher. Chicago surgeon. 1848–
1918
OPERATION—
(Deflection of the nasal septum), Trans. Amer. Laryngol. Ass., 4: 61–69, 1882

Inghilleri, G. Italian physician
REAGENT—for reducing sugar.
*Ricerche dei componenti anormali delle orine. Ricerca
del glucosio.* Boll. chim. farm., 62: 225–227, 1923

Ingraham, Franc Douglas. Boston surgeon. 1898–
Developed fibrin foam.
*The use of products prepared from human fibrinogen
and human thrombin in neurosurgery: fibrin foam as
hemostatic agents; fibrin films in repair of dural defects and in prevention of meningocerebral adhesions*
with O. T. Bailey, J. Neurosurg., 1: 23–39, Jan. 1944

Ingram, W. R. See L. E. Davis

Ingrassia, Giovanni Filippo. Italian anatomist.
1510–1580
APOPHYSIS—lesser wing of sphenoid bone.
PROCESS OF—see apophysis.
Discovered stapes.
In Galeni librum de ossibus. Panorni, ex typog. J. B.
Maringhi, 1603
Differentiated varicella from scarlet fever. Garrison
and Morton
De tumoribus praeter naturam. Neapoli, 1553. pp.
194–195

Inouye, Katsuji. Japanese physiologist. 1876–
TEST—for bile acids.
*Ueber eine Farben- und spektralreaktion der Gallen-
säuren mit Vanillin und Schwefelsäure* with H. Ito,
Z. phys. Chem., 57: 313–314, 1908

Inouye, Zenjiro. Japanese physician
TEST—for blood.
Ein neues Verfahren zum Nachweise von Blut with
T. Yastomi, Arch. VerdauKr., 18: 223–239, Apr. 20,
1912

Iob, L. Vivian. See F. A. Coller

Ipsen, Karl. Innsbruck physician. 1866–1927
TEST—for carbon monoxide in blood.
*Ueber eine Methode zum chemischen Nachweis von
Kohlenoxydblut.* Vierteljahrschrift f. gerichtl, Med.,
3 F., 18: 46–65, 1899

Irving, Frederick Carpenter. Boston obstetrician.
1883–
METHOD—of tubal sterilization.
*A new method of insuring sterility following cesarean
section.* Amer. J. Obstet. Gynaec., 8: 335–337, Sept.
1924
MODIFICATION—
*A simple method of performing extra-peritoneal cesar-
ean section in potentially infected cases.* Med. Rec.
and Ann., 31: 300–302, Aug. 1937

Irwin, G. F. See R. A. Phillips

Irwin, W. F. American physician
Reported carcinoma of infrapapillary portion of
duodenum.
*Case of cancerous duodenum and scirrhus of the pan-
creas.* Philadelphia J. Med. and Phys. Sci., 8: 406–
413, 1823

Isaacs, Charles Edward. New York physiologist.
1811–1860
Wrote important work on kidney function.
*Researches into the structure and physiology of the
kidney.* Trans. New York Acad. Med., 1: 377–435,
1857

On the functions of the Malpighian bodies of the kidney.
Ibid., 437–456

Isaacs, K. See C. C. Sturgis

Isaacs, Raphael. Ann Arbor, Mich. physician. 1891–
Noted apparently constant haploid state of chromosomes in mitosis.
Development of the myeloblast in chronic myelogenous leukemia. Arch. Path., 9: 1298–1299, June 1930
See also G. R. Minot

Isambert, Emile. French physician. 1828–1876
DISEASE—acute miliary tuberculosis of larynx and pharynx.
De la tuberculose miliaire aigue pharyngo-laryngée.
Paris, 1871

Isayeff, V. I. See R. F. J. Pfeiffer

Iselin, Marc Henri. French surgeon. 1898–
OPERATION—arthroplasty on fingers.
Chirurgie de la main. Paris, Masson, 1933

Ishihara, Junko. 1864–
TEST—
Tests for colour-blindness. New York, Myrowitz, n. d., 6 pp.

Israel, James. German surgeon. 1848–1926
METHOD—of palpating kidney, bimanual, with patient in lateral position.
Chirurgische Klinik der Nierenkrankenheiten. Berlin, Hirschwald, 1901
First proved presence of actinomycosis in a human.
Homans
Neue Beobachtungen auf dem Gebiete der Mykosen des Menschen. Arch. path. Anat. u. Physiol., 74: 15–53, 1878
Described carbuncle of kidney.
Erfahrungen über Nierenchirurgie. Arch. klin. Chir., 47: 302–463, 1894

Israel, Oscar. Berlin physician. 1855–1907
STAIN—for actinomyces.
Ueber Doppelfärbung mit Orcëin. Arch. path. Anat. u. Physiol., 105: 169–172, 1886

Itard, Jean Marie Gaspard. French otologist. 1774–1838
CATHETER—for eustachian tube.
SIGN—anesthesia of tympanic membrane in otosclerosis.
Traité des maladies de l'oreille et de l'audition. Paris, Méquignon-Marvis, 1821. 2 vols.

Ito, H. See Y. Ido, R. Inada, K. Inouye

Ito, Tetsuta. Japanese physician
MEDIUM—culture.
The pure cultivation of spirochaeta icterohaemonhagiae (Inada) with H. Matsuzaki, J. exp. Med., 23: 557–562, Apr. 1, 1916
REACTION—specific intradermal, for lymphogranuloma inguinale.
VACCINE—prepared from Ducrey bacillus cultures.
Klinische und bakteriologisch-serologische Studien über Ulcus molle und Ducreysche Streptobazillen.
Arch. Derm. u. Syph., 116: 341–374, Apr. 1913

Ivanissevich. Oscar. Argentina surgeon. 1895–
METHOD—
El método argentino para la rinoplastia. Presna méd. argentina, July 30, 1921
Rhinoplasty: Argentine method with R. C. Ferrari, S. G. O., 71: 187–190, Aug. 1940

Ivy, Andrew Conway. Chicago physiologist. 1893–
METHOD—for determination of bleeding time.
The bleeding tendency in jaundice with P. F. Shapiro and P. Melnick, S. G. O., 60: 781–784, Apr. 1935
Demonstrated existence of duodenal hormone that specifically activates gall-bladder musculature.
The physiology of the gall-bladder. Physiol. Rev., 14: 1–102, Jan. 1934

Ivy, Robert Henry. American surgeon. 1881–
OPERATION—
Fractures of the upper jaw and matar bone with L. Curtis, Ann. Surg., 94: 337–346, Sept. 1931

Iwatake, D. See A. Fujita

Iyengar, K. R. K. See W. F. Harvey

J

Jaboulay, Mathieu. French surgeon. 1860–1913
AMPUTATION or OPERATION—
La désarticulation interilio-abdominale. Lyon Méd., 75: 507–510, Apr. 15, 1894
OPERATION—cervical sympathectomy for exophthalmic goiter.
Performed periarterial sympathectomy.
Chirurgie du grand sympathétique et du corps thyroide.
. . . Paris, Doin, 1900. 358 pp.
OPERATION—gastroduodenostomy.
La gastro-entérostomie. La jéjuno-duodénostomie. La résection du pylore. Arch. prov. de chir., 1: 1–22, July 1892
De la gastro-duodénostomie. Ibid., 551–554
OPERATION—gastrostomy.
Procédé pour pratiquer la gastrostomie et la cystostomie.
Abstr.: Gaz. hebd. méd. chir., 31: 89–90, Feb. 24, 1894
Attempted to control or end pelvic pain by sympathetic surgery, by cutting rami communicantes.
Le traitement de la névralgie pelvienne par la paralysie du sympathique sacré. Lyon Méd., 90: 102–104, Jan. 15, 1899
Extirpated celiac plexus.

La chirurgie du sympathique abdominal et sacré.
Trav. neul. chir., No. 1, 1900
Abstr.: Zbl. Chir., 28: 227–228, 1901
Chirurgie des centres nerveux, des viscères et des membres. Paris, Doin, 1902. 2 vols.

Jackson, Charles Thomas. Boston scientist. 1805–1880
Wrote book on anesthesia.
A manual of etherization: concerning directions for the employment of ether, chloroform, and other anesthetic agents by inhalation in surgical operations. Comprising also a brief history of the discovery of anesthesia. Boston, Mansfield, 1861. 134 pp.

Jackson, Chevalier. Philadelphia laryngologist. 1865–
SIGN—"asthmatoid wheeze" in foreign body in trachea or bronchus.
The mechanism of the physical signs, with especial reference to foreign bodies in the bronchi. Amer. J. med. Sci., 165: 313–320, Mar. 1923
Introduced modification of gastroscope.
Gastroscopy. Med. Rec., 71: 549–555, Apr. 6, 1907
Tracheo-bronchoscopy, esophagoscopy, and gastroscopy. St. Louis, 1907. 191 pp.
Described contact ulcer of larynx.

Contract ulcer of the larynx. Ann. Otol., Rhin. and Laryng., 37: 227–230, Mar. 1928
Introduced improved technics for—
Bronchoscopy, esophagoscopy and gastroscopy with C. L. Jackson, Phila., Saunders, 1934
See also W. W. Babcock

Jackson, Daniel Dana. Brooklyn chemist. 1870–1941
AGAR—
Liver broth: a medium for the determination of gas-forming bacteria in water with T. C. Muer, J. infect. Dis., 8: 289–294, Apr. 12, 1911
MEDIUM—
The use of lactose-bile medium in water analysis. Pub. Health, 32: 30–32, Dec. 5, 1906
A new solution for the presumptive test for bacillus coli. Biol. studies of pupils of W. T. Sedgwick. Univ. Chicago Press, 1906. pp. 292–299

Jackson, Dennis Emerson. American pharmacologist. 1878–
METHOD—of anesthesia.
A new method for the production of general analgesia and anesthesia with a description of the apparatus used. J. Lab. clin. Med., 1: 1–12, Oct. 1915

Jackson, Edward. American ophthalmologist. 1856–1942
OPERATION—
Operation on the tendon of the superior rectus muscle for paresis of the superior oblique. Ophth. Rev., 22: 61–70, Mar. 1903
TECHNIC—of retinoscopy.
The measurement of refraction by the shadow-test, or retinoscopy. Amer. J. Med. Sci., 89: 404–412, Apr. 1885

Jackson, Jabez North. Kansas City surgeon. 1868–1935
INCISION—
A new technic for breast amputation. J. A. M. A., 46: 627–633, Mar. 3, 1906
Radical operation in mammary cancer. Ibid., 54: 178–185, Jan. 15, 1910
MEMBRANE or VEIL—about cecum.
Membranous pericolitis. S. G. O., 9: 278–287, Sept. 1909
Membranous pericolitis and allied considerations of the ileocecal region. Ann. Surg., 57: 374–401, Mar. 1913

Jackson, James, (Sr). Boston physician. 1777–1868
Gave early account of alcoholic neuritis.
On a peculiar disease resulting from the use of ardent spirits. New Engl. J. Med. and Surg., 2: 351–353, Oct. 1822

Jackson, John Hughlings. English neurologist. 1834–1911
EPILEPSY—
Unilateral epileptiform seizures, attended by temporary defect of sight. Short report: Med. Times and Gaz., 1: 588 (only), June 6, 1863
A study of convulsions. St. Andrews Med. Grad. Ass. Trans., (1869), 3: 162–204, 1870
LAW—nerve functions that are latest developed are earliest to be destroyed.
RULE—after epileptic attacks, simple nervous processes are more quickly recovered from than complex ones.
The Hughlings Jackson lecture on the relations of different divisions of the central nervous system to one

another and to parts of the body. Lancet, 1: 79–87, Jan. 8, 1898
Also: Brit. med. J., 1: 65–69, Jan. 8, 1898
Also: Medical classics, 3: 936–971, June 1939
SYNDROME—unilateral palsy of motor tenth, eleventh and twelfth nerves.
On a case of paralysis of the tongue from hemorrhage in the medulla oblongata. Lancet, 2: 770–773,Nov. 30, 1872
Made important study of aphasia.
Loss of speech: its association with valvular disease of the heart, and with hemiplegia on the right side. Defects of smell. Defects of speech in chorea. Arterial regions in epilepsy. Clin. Lects. and Rep. Lond. Hosp., 1: 388–471, 1864

Jackson, Seguin Henry. English physician. 1750–1816
Classified skin diseases on basis of pathology.
Dermato-pathologia: or practical observations from some new thoughts on the pathology and proximate cause of diseases of the true skin. London, Reynell, 1792

Jacob, A. Hamburg neurologist
DISEASE—spastic, pseudosclerosis degeneration of brain.
Über eigenartige Erkrankungen des Zentralnervensystems mit bemerkenswertem anatomischem Befunde (spastische Pseudosklerose-Encephalomyelopathie mit disseminierten Degenerationsherden). Dtsch. Z. Nervensheilk., 70: 132–146, Mar. 11, 1921

Jacob, Arthur. Irish ophthalmologist. 1790–1874
ULCER—rodent, of eyelid.
Observations respecting an ulcer of peculiar character, which attacks the eyelids and other parts of the face. Dublin Hosp. Rep., 4: 231–239, 1827

Jacobaeus, Hans Christian. Swedish surgeon. 1879–1937
OPERATION—cauterizing pleural adhesions as auxiliary to artificial pneumothorax in pulmonary tuberculosis.
Endopleural Operationen unter der Leitung des Thorakoskops. Beitr. klin. Tuber., 35: 1–35, Dec. 23, 1915
Invented thorascoscope.
Ueber die Möglichkeit die Zystoscopie bei Untersuchung seröser Höhlungen anzuwenden. Münch. med. Wschr., 57: 2090–2092, Oct. 4, 1910

Jacobi, Eduard. Breslau physician. 1862–1915
AGAR—peptone; culture medium.
AGAR—meat infusion salt: culture medium.
Kleine Beiträge zur bakterioskopischen Methodik Härtung und Färbung von Plattenkulturen. Zbl. Bakt., 3: 536–540 (548), 1888
First described—Garrison and Morton
Fall zur Diagnose (Poikilodermia vascularis atrophicans). Verh. dtsch. Dermat. Ges., 1906, Berlin, 9: 321–323, 1907

Jacobs, Walter Abraham. New York chemist. 1883–
Prepared tryparsamide, a modification of arsphenamine.
Aromatic arsenic compounds. I. A plan of procedure for the synthesis of arsenicals for chemotherapeutic research with M. Heidelberger, J. Amer. Chem. Soc., 41: 1581–1587, Oct. 1919
Chemotherapy of trypanosome and spirochete infections. Chemical series. I. N-phenylglycineamide-p-arsonic acid with M. Heidelberger, J. exp. Med., 30: 411–415, Nov. 1, 1919

Jacobsen, Christian. Lübeck physician
HYPOTHESIS—reticulo-endothelial system, when sufficiently active (as when stimulated by one or a number of acute infectious processes), may attain in a measure ability to cope with neoplastic disease.
Der chronische Reiz des reticulo-endothelialen Systems —eine Krebshemmung. Arch. Dermat. u. Syph., 169: 562–576, Feb. 1934

Jacobsen, Victor Clarence. Troy, N. Y. physician. 1891–
METHOD—of lifting longitudinal wedge from "roof" of an artery to disclose a clot in situ.
In: *The pathology of cardiac infarction; based upon a study of sixty-four cases.* By L. W. Gorham, T. Ordway, V. C. Jacobsen and K. Hosoi, Trans. Amer. Climat. and Clin. Ass., 48: 105–113, 1932

Jacobson, Harry Pincus. Los Angeles physician. 1888–
CLASSIFICATION—of fungous diseases.
Fungous diseases. Springfield, Ill., Thomas, 1932. 317 pp.

Jacobson, Jacob. French physician
AGAR—for differentiation of dysentery bacilli.
Éther-éthylcinnamique comme milieu différentiel entre le Bacille dysentérique du type Flexner et le Bacillus dysenterique du type Hiss. C. R. Soc. Biol., 82: 726, July 21, 1919

Jacobson, Julius. German ophthalmologist. 1828–1889
OPERATION—for cataract.
Ein neues und gafahrloses Operations-Verfahren zur Heilung des grauen Staares. Berlin, Peters, 1863. 65 pp.

Jacobson, Ludwig Levin. Danish anatomist. 1783–1843
ANASTOMOSIS—part of tympanic plexus.
CANAL—tympanic c.
NERVE—tympanic portion of glossopharyngeal.
PLEXUS—tympanic p.
Supplementa ad otojatriam. Supplementum primum de anastomosi nervorum nova in aure detecta. Acta Reg. Soc. Med. Havniensis, 5: 293–303, 1818

Jacobsthal, Erwin. Hamburg physician
TEST—for serodiagnosis of syphilis.
Versuche zu einer optischen Serodiagnose der Syphilis. Z. ImmunForsch., Orig., 8: 107–128, Nov. 7, 1910

Jacoby, Martin Johann. German biochemist. 1872–
METHOD—for estimation of pepsin.
Ueber die Beziehungen der Verdauungswirkung und der Labwirkung. Biochem. Z., 1: 53–74, 1906

Jacquart, Henri. French physician
ANGLE—at anterior nasal spine between lines from auricular point and glabella.
Mensuration de l'angle facial. Gaz. méd. de Par., 3 s., 11: 753–754, Nov. 29, 1856

Jacquemier, Jean Marie. French obstetrician. 1806–1879
SIGN or SPOT—of violet on mucous membrane of vagina just below urethral orifice, seen after fourth week of pregnancy.
Recherches d'anatomie et de physiologie sur le système vasculaire sanguin de l'utérus humain pendant la gestation, et plus spécialement sur les vaisseaux utéro-placentaires. Arch. gén. de méd., 3 s., 3: 165–194, 1838

Jacquet, Leonard Marie Lucien. French dermatologist. 1860–1914
DISEASE or SYNDROME—reflex alopecia, connected with anomalies of teeth.
Des érythèmes papuleux fessiers post-érosifs. Rev. d. mal. de l'enf., 4: 208–218, 1886

Jadassohn, Josef. Breslau dermatologist. 1863–1936
DISEASE—maculopapular erythrodermia; macular atrophy.
Ueber eine eigenartige Form von "Atrophia maculosa cutis." Verh. dtsch. Derm. ges. Wien., pp. 342–358, 1892
Introduced patch test.
Zur Kenntnis der medicamentösen Dermatosen. Verh. dtsch. Derm. Kongr., Wien, pp. 103–129, 1896
Described granulosis rubra nasi.
Ueber eine eigenartige Erkrankung der Nasenhaut bei Kindern ("Granulosis rubra nasi"). Arch. Dermat., 58: 145–158, 1901

Jaeger, Michael. German surgeon. 1795–1838
OPERATION—
De extirpatione linguae. Erlangen, 1832

Jaeger, Dr., Jn. German surgeon
CHAIR—operating.
Ueber einen neuen Operationsstuhl. Oesterr. Z. f. prakt. Heilk., 4: 877–880, Dec. 3, 1858

Jaeger, Eduard, Ritter von. Jaxtthal Austrian oculist. 1818–1884
TYPES—test.
Schriftskalen. Wien, Seidel, 1860, 3te. Aufl.

Jaffe, H. L. See A. Bodansky
Jaffé, Karl. German surgeon. 1854–
OPERATION—for dilatation of esophagus.
Ueber idiopathische Oesophaguserweiterungen. Münch. med. Wschr., 44: 386–387, Apr. 13, 1897

Jaffé, Max. Königsberg physician. 1841–1911
REACTION—for creatinine.
Ueber den Niederschlag, welchen Pikrinsäure in normalen Harn erzeugt und über eine neue Reaction des Kreatinins. Z. physiol. Chem., 10: 391–400, 1886
TEST—for indican in urine.
Ueber den Ursprung des Indicans im Harns. Zbl. med. Wiss., 10: 2 (only), Jan. 6, 1872
Discovered urobilin in urine.
Beitrag zur Kenntniss der Gallen- und Harnpigmente. Ibid., 6: 241–245, Apr. 11, 1868
Also: J. prakt. Chem., 104: 401–406, 1868
Discovered urobilin in intestinal contents.
Ueber das Vorkommen von Urobilin im Darminhalt. Zbl. med. Wiss., 9: 465–466, July 29, 1871

Jager, L. de. Dutch chemist
REACTION—for normal urine.
Ein roter Farbstoff im Harn. Z. phys. Chem., 64: 110–119, 1910
TESTS—for albumin in urine.
Beiträge zur Harnchemie. Ibid., 62: 333–346, 1909
TEST—for blood in urine.
Een wijziging van de benzidineproef. Ned. Tydschr. v. Geneesk., 46: 2330–2331, Dec. 31, 1910
TEST—for glucose in urine.
Eine neue Zuckerprobe. Zbl. ges Physiol. u. Path. d. Stoffw., 12: 630–633, Aug. 1, 1911
Eine Modifikation der von mir beschriebenen Zuckerprobe. Z. inn. Med., 33: 625–626, June 22, 1912

akob, Alfons. Hamburg psychiatrist
PASTIC PSEUDOSCLEROSIS—
Ueber eigenartige Erkrankungen des Zentralnerven-
systems mit bemerkenswertem anatomischem Befunde.
Z. ges. Neurol. Psychiat., 64: 147–228, Feb. 15, 1921
akobsohn, Paul. Berlin physician
IGN—
Ueber den Fingerbeugereflex. Dtsch. med. Wschr.,
34: 1971–1973, Nov. 12, 1908
aksch, Rudolf von. Prague physician. 1855–
DISEASE or ANEMIA—pseudoleukemic anemia of
infants.
Ueber Leukämie und Leukocytose im Kindesalter.
Wien. klin. Wschr., 2: 435–437, May 30; 456–458,
June 6, 1889
TEST—for bile pigments in blood.
Nachweis von Gallenbestandtheilen in thierischen
Flüssigkeiten. Z. anal. Chem., 31: 725–726, 1892
Also: Verh. d. X Cong. f. inn. Med., p. 353, 1892
TEST—for melanin and melanogen in urine.
Beitrag zur Kenntniss des Verhaltens des Harnes bei
der Melanurie. Z. physiol. Chem., 13: 385–394, 1889
Described acetonuria and diaceturia.
Ueber Acetonurie und Diaceturie. Berlin, Hirschwald,
1885. 156 pp.
Jalaguier, Adolphe. French surgeon. 1853–1924
INCISION—Battle—Jalaguier—Kammerer i., for ab-
dominal section, with retraction of rectus inward.
Traitement de l'appendicite: procédé opératoire destiné
à assurer la reconstitution solide de la paroi abdomin-
ale après l'excision à froid de l'appendicite. Pr. méd.,
5: 53 (only), Feb. 2, 1897
METHOD—lateral cheek flap method for correcting
partial atresia of anterior nares.
Autoplasties. 1. Brûlures graves de la face et de la
main. 2. Obliteration des narines par cicatrice vicieuse
consécutive à une ulcération survenue après la rougeole.
Bull. Soc. Chir., 28: 890–893, July 30, 1902
Jalsma, F. See R. G. Spurling
Jameson, Horatio Gates. Baltimore surgeon. 1778–
1855
Performed total excision of upper jaw.
Case of tumor of the superior jaw. Amer. Med. Re-
corder, 4: 222–230, Apr. 1821
Jameson, Patrick Chalmers. Brooklyn ophthalmol-
ogist. 1867–1939
OPERATION—
Re-attachment of iridodialysis: a method which does
not incarcerate the iris. Arch. Ophthal., 38: 391–396,
July 1909
OPERATION—
External ocular muscles. I. The principles of muscle
recession with scleral suturing as applied to the cor-
rection of squint. Trans. Ophthal. Soc. U. Kingdom,
45: 405–419, 1925
OPERATION—
Subconjuncival section of the ductules of the lacrimal
gland as a cure for epiphora. Arch. Ophthal., 17:
207–212, Feb. 1937
Janes, Robert Meredith. Toronto surgeon. 1894–
OPERATION—
Primary tumors of ribs: report of eight cases and a
method of repair of the defect in the chest wall that
follows their removal. J. Thoracic Surg., 9: 145–163,
Dec. 1939

Janet, Pierre Marie Félix. French physician. 1859–
1947
DISEASE—psychasthenia.
Les obsessions et la psychasthénie. Paris, Alcan, 1903.
764 pp.
METHOD—of treatment of hysteria.
L'hystérie et l'hypnotisme, d'après la théorie de la
double personnalité. Rev. scient., Paris, 41: 616–623,
1888
Janeway, Henry Harrington. New York surgeon.
1873–1921
GASTROSTOMY—by means of a flap from anterior
stomach wall, converted into a tube.
The relation of gastrostomy to inoperable carcinoma of
the esophagus with a description of a new method of
performing gastrostomy. J. A. M. A., 61: 93–95,
July 12, 1913
Eine neue Gastrostomiemethode. Münch. med. Wschr.,
60: 1705–1707, Aug. 5, 1913
Janeway, Theodore Caldwell. American physician.
1872–1917
SPHYGMOMANOMETER—
In his: The clinical study of blood-pressure. . . . New
York, Appleton, 1904. 300 pp. pp. 89–93
See also W. W. Herrick
Janicke, O. German physician
Reported generalized myositis fibrosa.
Einen Fall von Myositis Interstitialis. Abstr.: Dtsch.
med. Wschr., 21: 117 (only), July 4, 1895
Janney, J. H. See A. T. Shohl
Janney, Nelson Wilson. New York physician. 1881–
TEST—of dextrose tolerance.
A blood sugar tolerance test with V. I. Isaacson,
Proc. Soc. exp. Biol., N. Y., 15: 15–16, Nov. 21,
1917
Also: J. A. M. A., 70: 1131–1134, Apr. 20, 1918
Janowsky, V. See S. Pollitzer
Jansen, Albert. German otologist. 1859–1933
OPERATION—for disease of frontal sinus.
Zur Eröffnung der Nebenhöhlen der Nase bei chron-
ischer Eiterung. Arch. f. Laryngol., 1: 135–157, 1894
Jansen, Barend Coenraad Petrus. Dutch physio-
chemist. 1884–
Isolated vitamin B from natural sources and gave
name aneurin to vitamin B_1.
Isolation of anti-beriberi vitamin with W. F. Donath,
Mededeel. Dienst. Volksgezondheid Nederland.
Indie., part 1, pp. 186–199, 1927
TEST—for vitamin B_1.
Wertbestimmung des Völkerbund-Standart-Präparats
für Vitamin B_1. Z. Vitaminforsch., 5: 254–256,
Oct. 1936
A chemical determination of aneurin (=vitamin B_1)
by the thiochrome reaction. Rec. trav. chim., 55: 1046–
1052, Nov. 15, 1936
Jansen, J. See G. M. Taylor
Jansen, Murk. Leiden surgeon. 1863–1935
THEORY—of dissociation of bone growth.
Dissociation of bone growth. (Exostoses and enchon-
dromata, or Ollier's dyschondroplasia and associated
phenomena). In: The Robert Jones Birthday Vol-
ume, Oxford, Univ. Press, 1928. pp. 43–72
Janský, Jan. Prague physician
Classified human blood into four groups.
Etudes hématologiques, dans les malades mentales.

Haematologické studie u psychotiků. Sborník klinický, Praze, 8: 85–139, 1907

Jarjavay, Jean Francois. French surgeon. 1815–1868

MUSCLE—depressor urethral m.
Recherches anatomiques sur l'urètre de l'homme. Paris, Labé, 1856. 230 pp.

Jarvis, William Chapman. New York laryngologist. 1855–1895

OPERATION and SNARE—
Surgical treatment of hypertrophic nasal catarrh. Trans. Amer. Laryngol. Ass., 1880, 2: 130–141, 1881
Removal of hypertrophied turbinated tissues by écrasement with the cold wire. Arch. Laryngol., 3: 105–111, Apr. 1, 1882

Javal, Louis Émile. Paris oculist. 1839–1907

OPHTHALMOMETER—
Un ophthalmomètre pratique with H. Schiötz, Ann. d'ocul., 86: 5–21, 1881
Contribution a l'ophthalmométrie. Ibid., 87: 213–221, 1882
Invented astigmometer.
Sur un nouvel instrument pour la détermination de l'astigmatisme. Ibid., 57: 39–43, 1867

Jaworski, Walery. Polish physician. 1849–1924

BODIES or CORPUSCLES—spiral mucous b. seen in secretion of stomach in hyperchlorhydria.
Methoden zur Bestimmung der Intensität der Pepsinausscheidung aus dem menschlichen Magen und Gewinnung des natürlichen Magensaftes zu physiologish-chemischen Versuchszwecken. Münch. med. Wschr., 34: 634–637, Aug. 16, 1887

TEST—in hour-glass stomach, a splashing sound will be heard on succussion of pyloric portion after siphonage.
Ueber Anwendung der Gase für therapeutische und diagnostische Zwecke bei Magenkrankheiten. Dtsch. Arch. f. klin. Med., 35: 79–92, July 2, 1884

Jean, G. French physician
Suggested section of splanchnic nerves for relief of pyloric spasm, hyperacidity and hypersecretion.
Les nerfs splanchniques au point de vue chirurgical. Arch. Méd. et Pharm. nav., 111: 292–302, 1921

Jeandelize, Pierre Marie Paul. French physician. 1872–
Suggested that epilepsy, tetany and convulsions of childhood may be due to parathyroid deficiency.
Insuffisance thyroidienne et parathyroidienne (à début dans le jeune âge); étude expérimentale et clinique. Nancy, 1902. 733 pp.

Jeannin, Cyrille. French obstetrician. 1874–
Reported case of complete heart block in which successful gestation occurred.
Dissociation auriculo-ventriculaire et grossesse with C. Clerc, Bull. Soc. méd. Hop. Paris, 51: 122–127, Feb. 10, 1927

Jeans, Philip Charles. Iowa City pediatrician. 1883–
TEST—photometric, for detecting vitamin A deficiency by determining ability to adapt to darkness.
A clinical method for determining moderate degrees of vitamin A deficiency with Zelma Zentmire, J. A. M. A., 102: 892–895, Mar. 24, 1934
The prevalence of vitamine A deficiency among Iowa children with Zelma Zentmire, Ibid., 106: 996–997, Mar. 21, 1936

Jefferson, Geoffrey. English surgeon
Reported—
Report of a successful case of embolectomy, with a review of the literature. Brit. med. J., 2: 985–987, Nov. 28, 1925

Jeffrey, Isabelle A. See J. A. Kasper

Jeffries, John Amory. American physician. 1859–1892

BACILLUS—
The bacteria of the alimentary canal, especially in the diarrhoeas of infancy. Boston Med. and Surg. J., 119: 217–223, Aug. 30, 1888

Jelinek, Bohdan. French chemist
TEST—for mustard gas.
Sur une réaction caractéristique de l'ypérite. Bull. Soc. Chim., 4: 1813–1815, Oct. 1937

Jelinek, Edmund. Vienna surgeon. 1852–1928
Introduced local anesthesia in operations on nose.
Das Cocain als Anästheticum und Analgeticum für den Pharynx und Larynx. Wien. med. Wschr., 34: 1364–1367, Nov. 15, 1884

Jelks, John Lemuel. Memphis surgeon. 1870–
OPERATION—
The treatment of peri-rectal abscesses. Trans. Mississippi Valley Med. Ass., 2: 222–225, 1900
OPERATION—
A new operation for rectal stricture. Trans. Amer. Proct. Soc., 32: 19 (only), 1931

Jenckel, Adolf. Göttingen surgeon
Reported indirect hepaticoduodenotomy.
Beitrag zur Chirurgie der Leber und der Gallenwege. Dtsch. Z. Chir., 104: 1–121, Feb. 1910

Jendrassik, Aladar. Baltimore chemist
REAGENT—for vitamin B₁.
A color test for water-soluble B. J. biol. Chem., 57: 129–138, Aug. 1923

Jendrässik, Ernst. Budapest physician. 1824–1891
Recognized diuretic action of mild mercurous chloride.
Das Calomel als Diureticum. Dtsch. Arch. klin. Med., 38: 499–524, Apr. 1886

Jenkins, H(ilger) Perry. Chicago physician. 1902–
MONOGRAM—
Guide to replacement therapy for loss of blood or plasma with P. W. Schafer and F. M. Owens, Jr., Arch. Surg., 47: 1–3, July 1943

Jenner, Edward. English physician. 1749–1823
Introduced preventive inoculation (vaccination) of cow-pox against small-pox.
An inquiry into the causes and effects of the variolae vaccinae, a disease discovered in some of the western counties of England, particularly in Gloucestershire, and known by the name of the cow-pox. London, Low, 1798. 75 pp.
Further observations on the variolae vaccinae or cow-pox. London, Low, 1799. 64 pp.
A continuation of the facts and observations relative to the variolae vaccinae, or cow-pox. London, Low, 1800. 42 pp.
Also in: *Epoch-making contributions to medicine . . .,* by N. C. S. Camac, Philadelphia, Saunders, 1909. pp. 213–296
Gave early reference to anaphylaxis or allergy. Garrison
See first reference, 1798, footnote to p. 13

Jenner, Harley Deming. Canadian physician. 1907–
METHOD—
  Plasma phosphatase. III. A clinical method for the determination of plasma phosphatase with H. D. Kay, Brit. J. exp. Path., 13: 22–27, Feb. 1932
Jenner, Louis Leopold. English physician. 1866–1904
STAIN—
  A new preparation for rapidly fixing and staining blood. Lancet, 1: 370–371, Feb. 11, 1899
Jenner, Sir William. English physician. 1815–1898
Instrumental in differentiating typhus from typhoid fever. Garrison
  On typhoid and typhus, an attempt to determine the question of their identity or non-identity, by an analysis of the symptoms, and of the appearances found after death in sixty-six fatal cases of continued fever, observed at the London Fever Hospital from January 1847 to February 1849. Month. J. Med. Sci., Edinburgh, 9: 663–680, Apr. 1849
  On the identity or non-identity of the specific cause of typhoid, typhus, and relapsing fever. Med.-cnir. trans.. 33: 23–42, 1850
Described emphysema of lungs.
  On the determining causes of vesicular emphysema of the lung. Ibid., 40: 25–37, 1857
Jennings, John Edward. Brooklyn surgeon. 1875–
INCISION—for radical mastectomy.
  Dissection of the axilla in radical operations for cancer of the breast. Ann. Surg., 83: 770–773, June 1926
Jennings, M. A. See E. Chain
Jennings, William Oscar. English physician. 1851–1914
TREATMENT—of drug addiction.
  Sur un nouveau mode de traitement de la morphinomanie. Paris, Baillière, 1887. 30 pp.
  The morphine habit and its voluntary renunciation. A personal revelation of a suppression after twenty-five years' addiction. New York, Wood, 1909. 492 pp.
Jensen, B. N. See H. C. Hagedorn
Jensen, Carl Oluf. Copenhagen physician. 1864–1934
Showed that carcinoma and sarcoma could be transplanted and retransplanted in mice and rats and that cancerous growth came wholly from the transplanted cells.
  Nogle Forsøg med Kraeftsvulster. Hosp. Tid., København., 10: 489–502, May 7, 1902
  Experimentelle Untersuchungen über Krebs bei Mäusen. Zbl. Bakt., 34: 28–34; 122–143, 1903
Jensen, Lloyd B. Illinois chemist. 1896–
TEST—
  A delicate test for blood pigments. Food Research, 1: 275–276, May–June, 1936
Jensen, Nathan Kenneth. Minneapolis surgeon. 1910–
Reported—
  The local implantation of sulfanilamide in compound fractures: a preliminary report with L. W. Johnsrud and M. C. Nelson, Surgery, 6: 1–12, July 1939
Jensen, Orla. Danish physiochemist
SOLUTION—milk digest, for cultivation of lactic acid bacteria.
  Der beste Nährboden für die Milchsäurefermente. Zbl. Bakt., 2 Abt., 4: 196–199, Mar. 5, 1898
Jepson, Paul Newton. Rochester, Minn. surgeon. 1893–

OPERATION—
  Transformation of the middle finger into a thumb. Minnesota Med., 8: 552 (only), Aug. 1925
Jersild, Olaf. Copenhagen physician
SYNDROME—rectal stenosis of lymphogranulomatosis.
  Les intradermo-réactions dans le chancre mou et dans la lymphogranulomatose inguinale considérées spécialement dans leurs rapports avec l'étiologie du syphilome ano-rectal. Ann. Dermat. et Syph., 1: 577–608, June 1930
  Elephantiasis genito-anorectalis. Derm. Wschr., 96: 433–438, Mar. 31, 1933
Jesty, Benjamin. Dorset, England farmer. 1737–1816
Performed successful cow-pox vaccination in 1774–1789. Garrison
His tombstone inscription says "having been the first person known that introduced the cow-pox by inoculation, and who from his great strength of mind made the experiment from the cow on his wife and two sons in the year 1774".
Jetter, Walter William Edward. Boston physician. 1905–
METHOD—
  The perchlorate method for determining concentration of alcohol in expired air as a medicolegal test with G. C. Forrester, Arch. Path., 32: 828–842, Nov. 1941
Jewett, Eugene Lyon. Orlando, Fla. surgeon. 1900–
NAIL—
  One-piece angle nail for trochanteric fractures. J. Bone and Joint Surg., 23: 803–810, Oct. 1941
Jewett, Hugh Judge. Baltimore urologist. 1903–
METHOD—
  A new method of ureteral transplantation for cancer of the bladder. A report of 15 clinical cases. J. Urol., 48: 489–513, Nov. 1942
  Uretero-intestinal anastomosis in two stages for cancer of the bladder: modification of original technique and report of 33 cases. Ibid., 52: 536–562, Dec. 1944
Jez, Valentin. German physician
EXTRACTS—antityphoid.
  Ueber Typhusbehandlung (Abdominaltyphus) mit einem Antityphusextract. Wien. med. Wschr., 49: 346–351, Feb. 18, 1899
Jezler, Adolf. Basel physician
METHOD—of Takata-Ara test for liver function.
  Beitrag zur funktionellen Leberdiagnostik. Z. klin. Med., 111: 48–70, July 18, 1929
  Die Takatasche Kolloidreaktion in Serum und Körperflüssigkeiten und ihre Beziehungen zu Störungen des Eiweissstoffwechsels der Leber. Ibid., 114:739–756, Dec. 1, 1930
Jianu, Amza. Bucharest surgeon
OPERATION—for facial paralysis by muscle transplantation.
  Die chirurgische Behandlung der Facialislähmung. Dtsch. Z. f. Chir., 102: 377–386, Nov. 1909
OPERATION—
  Gastrostomie und Osophagoplastik. Ibid., 118: 383–391, Aug. 1912
Joachimoglu, G. See E. Friedberger
Joanny. See A. Leri
Job, André. French chemist. 1871–1928
REAGENT—for urea.
  Type simplifié d'uréomètre à volume constant with Dr. Clarens, J. Pharm. Chim., Paris, 6 s., 30: 97–100, 1909

Jobert de Lamballe, Antoine Joseph. French surgeon. 1799–1867
OPERATION—autoplastic closure of vesicovaginal fistula.
Traité des fistules vésico-utérines, vésico-utéro-vaginales, entéro-vaginales et recto-vaginales. Paris, Baillière, 1852. 420 pp.
SUTURE—for divided intestine, upper end being invaginated into lower.
Traité théorique et pratique des maladies chirurgicales du canal intestinal. Paris, 1829. 2 vols.
Jobling, J. W. See S. Flexner
Jochmann, Georg. German physician. 1874–1915
AGAR—potato bouillon; for diagnosis of typhoid fever.
Zur Schnelldiagnose der Typhus bacillen. Eine Nachprüfung des von Weil angegebenen Nährbodens. Zbl. Bakt., 32: 460–467, Sept. 25, 1902
Introduced specific antiserum against infections with the meningococcus.
Versuch zur Serodiagnostik und Serotherapie der epidemischen Genickstarre. Dtsch. med. Wschr., 32: 788–793, May 17, 1906
See also E. Müller
Joerg, Eduard. German, Cuban and Pennsylvanian physician. 1808–1878
Described pulmonary atelectasis and its significance in determining whether or not air has entered lungs of a dead infant.
De morbo pulmonum organico, ex respiratione neonatorum imperfecta orto. Leipzig, Niesii, 1832. 59 pp.
Joest, Ernst. Dresden pathologist. 1873–1926
BODIES—
Über eigentümliche Kerneinschlüsse der Ganglienzellen bei der enzootischen Gehirn-Rückenmarksentzündung der Pferde with K. Degen, Z. Infektkr. Haustiere, 6: 348–356, 1909
Joffe, J. S. See S. A. Waksman
Joffroy, Alexis. Paris physician. 1844–1909
SIGN—absence of facial contraction in exophthalmic goiter when patient suddenly turns his eyes upward.
Nature et traitement du goitre exophthalmique. Prog. med., 18: 477–480, Dec. 23, 1893
See also J. M. Charcot
Johannsen, Wilhelm Ludwig. Danish botanist. 1857–1927
Divined mechanism of transmission of heredity.
Ueber Erblichkeit in Populationen und in reinen Linien. Jena, Fischer, 1903. 68 pp.
Johansson, Sven. Swedish surgeon. 1880–
DISEASE—epiphysitis of accessory center of ossification at apex of patella.
En förut icke beskriven sjukdom i patella. Hygiea, 84: 161–166, Mar. 16, 1922
Eine bisher anscheinend unbekannte Erkrankung der Patella. Z. orthop. Chir., 43: 82–87, 1924
OPERATION—for transfixion of fracture of neck of femur.
Zur Technik der Osteosynthese der Fract. colli femoris. Zbl. Chir., 59: 2019–2023, Aug. 20, 1932
On the operative treatment of medial fractures of the neck of the femur. Acta orthop. Scandinav., 3: 362–392, 1932
A case of pseudarthrosis of the neck of the femur, treated by a method of extra-articular osteosynthesis. Ibid., 4: 214–227, 1933
Johns, Albert. Dresden bacteriologist. 1839–1910

METHOD—for staining bacterial capsules.
Zur Färbung der Milzbrandbazillen. Dtsch. tierärztl. Wschr., 2: 289–292, Sept. 1, 1894
Johns, F. M. See C. C. Bass
Johnson, Clayton Richardson. Los Angeles roentgenologist. 1896–
STEREOROENTGENOMETER—for pelvimetry.
Mensuration and localization by means of the roentgen ray. Radiology, 8: 518–521, June 1927
Pelvimetry by stereoroentgenometry. Amer. J. Roentgenol. and Rad. Therapy, 38: 607–619, Oct. 1937
Johnson, F. C. See A. M. Stevens
Johnson, Sir George. English physician. 1818–1896
HYPOTHESIS—extra sound in gallop rhythm is assigned to vigorous and audible contractions of auricles.
Triple pericardial friction-sound, and on reduplication of the first sound of the heart. Lancet, 1: 337–343, Aug. 1876
TEST—
On picric acid as a test for albumen and sugar in the urine. Brit. med. J., 1: 504–507, Mar. 17, 1883
THEORY—of arteriosclerosis.
On certain points in the anatomy and pathology of Bright's disease of the kidney. II. On the influence on the minute blood-vessels upon the circulation. Med. chir. Trans., 51: 57–77, 1868
Johnson, George Arthur. New York scientist
BROTH—
Isolation of Bacillus coli communis from the alimentary tract of fish and the significance thereof. J. Infect. Dis. 1: 348–354, Mar. 19, 1904
Johnson, H. W. See I. F. Huddleson
Johnson, Herbert Lester Charles. American surgeon. 1890–
TREATMENT—prophylaxis against peritonitis.
An exposition of the preparation and administration of amniotic fluid concentrate. New Engl. J. Med. 212: 557–559, Mar. 28, 1935
Johnson, J. H. See C. McCrearry
Johnsrud, L. W. See N. K. Jensen
Johnston, C. G. See W. O. Abbott
Johnston, Christopher. Baltimore surgeon. 1822–1891
CHAIR—
Operating chair, for surgical and obstetrical operations and vaginal examinations. Maryland and Virginia Med. J., 15: plate following p. 92; 140 (only), Aug. 1860
Johnston, Herbert Allan. Anaheim, Calif. surgeon. 1873–
KEYED SCREW—
Combination of nail and screw for the fixation of fractures of the neck of the femur. Amer. J. Surg., 63: 329–336, Mar. 1944
Johnston, Thomas Baillie. Edinburgh anatomist. 1883–
THEORY—of exstrophy.
Extroversion of the bladder, complicated by the presence of intestinal openings on the surface of the extroverted area. J. Anat. and Physiol., 48: 89–106, Oct. 1913
Jolles, Adolf. Austrian chemist. 1862–
TEST—for albumin in urine.
Eine neue Eiweissprobe. Z. anal. Chem., 29: 406–407, 1890
Eine empfindliche Probe zum Nachweis von Albumin

im Harne. Z. physiol. Chem., 81: 205–206, Oct. 10, 1912
TEST—for bile.
Ueber den Nachweis von Gallenfarbstoffen im Harne. Ibid., 18: 545–557, 1894
Eine sehr empfindliche Probe zum Nachweis von Gallenfarbstoff im Harn. Arch. klin. Med., 78: 137–140, Oct. 15, 1903
TEST—for bromine in urine.
Eine einfache, sehr empfindliche Probe zum Nachweis von Brom im Harn. Z. anal. Chem., 37: 439–440, 1898
TEST—for glucuronic acid in urine.
Ueber den Nachweis von Glukuronsäure in diabetischen Harnen. Z. physiol. Chem., 81: 203–204, Oct. 10, 1912
TEST—for histonen in urine.
Ueber das Auftreten und den Nachweis von Histonen im Harne. Ibid., 25: 236–241, July 9, 1898
TEST—for indican in urine.
Ueber eine neue Indikan-Reaktion. Ibid., 87: 310–312, Sept. 17, 1913
Ueber eine neue Methode zur quantitativen Bestimmung des Indikans im Harne. Ibid., 94: 79–103, June 12, 1915
TEST—for iron in blood.
Ferrometer, Apparat zur quantitativen Bestimmung des Bluteisens für klinische Zwecke. Dtsch. med. Wschr., 23: 148–150, Mar. 4, 1897
TEST—for iron in urine.
Beiträge zur quantitativen Bestimmung des Eisens im Harne. Z. anal. Chem., pp. 149–158, 1897
TEST—for nitrite in urine.
Ueber den Nachweis von Nitriten im Harn. Z. anal. Chem., 32: 762–766, 1893
TEST—for pentoses.
Ueber den Nachweis der Pentosen in diabetischen Harnen. Z. inn. Med., 33: 693–696, July 13, 1912
TEST—for sucrose.
Ueber eine quantitative Methode zur Bestimmung der Saccharose im Harne neben allen anderen Zuckerarten. Biochem. Z., 43: 56–64, July 29, 1912
Jolly, Friedrich. German neurologist. 1844–1904
REACTION—myasthenic.
Pseudoparalysis myasthenica. Neurol. Zbl., 14: 34–36, Jan. 1, 1895
I. Ueber Myasthenia gravis pseudoparalytica. Berl. klin. Wschr., 32: 1–7, Jan. 7, 1895
Jolly, Justin Marie Jules. French physician. 1870–
BODIES—Howell-Jolly b. in blood.
Sur la formation des globules rouges des mammifères. C. R. Soc. Biol., 18: 528–531, Mar. 25, 1905
Sur l'évolution des globules rouges dans le sang des embryon de mammifères. Ibid., pp. 593–595, Apr. 1
Recherches sur la formation des globules rouges des mammifères. Arch. Anat. micros., 9: 133–314, June 10, 1907
Joltrain, E. See G. F. I. Widal
Jonas, August Frederick. Omaha surgeon. 1858–1934
OPERATION—
A modification in the operative method for inveterate and relapsed cases of talipes-equino-varus. Ann. Surg., 449–454, Apr. 1899
Jones, C. A. See F. Boerner
Jones, Chester Morse. Boston physician. 1891–
Described localization of pain from digestive tract.
Reference of pain produced at different points in the

esophagus, duodenum and proximal jejunum with P. H. Means and R. W. Vance, Communicated to Amer. Soc. Clin. Investigation, 1924
Abstr.: J. A. M. A., 82: 2078, June 21, 1924
Jones, Daniel Fiske. Boston surgeon. 1868–1937
OPERATION—
A two-stage combined abdominal-sacral operation for carcinoma of the rectum. J. A. M. A., 65: 757–764, Aug. 28, 1915
Jones, E. See G. W. Ross
Jones, Ernest Lloyd. English physician. 1862–1942
Made important contributions to study of specific gravity of blood.
On the variations in the specific gravity of the blood in health. J. Physiol., 8: 1–14, 1887
Further observations on the specific gravity of the blood in health and disease. Ibid., 12: 299–346, 1891
Jones, G. W. See R. R. Sayers
Jones, Henry Bence. English physician. 1814–1873
ALBUMIN—in urine of pseudoalbuminuria; when precipitated, it can be redissolved by boiling.
ALBUMINOSURIA—
BODIES—albumose b. found in urine in diseases of bone-marrow.
CYLINDERS—forming contents of seminiferous tubules, sometimes seen in urine.
REACTION—see ALBUMIN.
On a new substance occurring in the urine of a patient with mollities ossium. Philos. Trans., 138: 55–62, 1848
Jones, Harold Wellington. Philadelphia physician. 1877–
DIET—
The treatment of purpura hemorrhagica with L. Tocantins. J. A. M. A., 100: 83–88, Jan. 14, 1933
See also L. M. Tocantins
Jones, Helen. See G. W. Rake
Jones, Horry M. Chicago scientist. 1885–
APPARATUS—for determination of respiratory exchange.
A simple device for measuring basal metabolism: preliminary report. J. A. M. A., 75: 538–539, Aug. 21, 1920
Jones, L. E. See E. T. C. Milligan
Jones, O. W., Jr. See H. W. Fleming, H. C. Naffziger
Jones, Reginald Watson. Liverpool surgeon. 1902–
TECHNIC—
Fractures of the neck of the femur. Brit. J. Surg., 23: 787–808, Apr. 1936
Arthrodesis of the osteoarthritic hip. J. A. M. A., 110: 278–280, Jan. 22, 1938
Jones, Sir Robert. British surgeon. 1855–1933
APPARATUS or TREATMENT—for stretching shortened muscles.
On a simple method of dealing with Volkmann's ischemic paralysis. Amer. J. Orthop. Surg., 5: 377–383, Apr. 1908
OPERATION—on semilunar cartilage of knee.
Notes on derangements of the knee. Based upon a personal experience of over five hundred operations. Ann. Surg., 50: 969–1001, Dec. 1909
POSITION—acute flexion for fractures of distal end of humerus.
In his: *Orthopedic surgery* with R. W. Lovett, New York, 1929. 2 ed., p. 399
TREATMENT—of tuberculosis of spine with anterior and posterior molds. Ibid., pp. 219–231

Jones, Stephen George. Boston urologist. 1893–
METHOD—
A method of demonstrating tubercle bacilli in the urine.
J. A. M. A., 83 : 1917–1918, Dec. 13, 1924
Jones, Thomas Wharton. English physician. 1808–
1891
Discovered amoeboid power of leucocytes. Osler
Observations on the state of the blood and the blood-
vessels in inflammation. Trans. Roy. Med.-Chir
Soc., Lond., 36 : 391–402, 1853
Jones, William David. Rising City, Neb. surgeon
OPERATION—cholecystostomy.
An improved technique for the avoidance of fistula after
cholecystostomy. Ann. Surg., 27 : 53–58, 1898
Jones, William Howard. London physician. 1880–
1935
TECHNIC—of nupercaine anesthesia.
Spinal analgesia—a new method and a new drug—
percaine. Brit. J. Anest., 7 : 99–113, Apr. ; 146–156,
July 1930
Jongh, S. E. de
Jonnesco, Thomas. Bucharest surgeon. 1860–1926
FOLD—parietoperitoneal.
Anatomie des ligaments de l'appendice vermiculaire
et de la fossette iléo-appendiculaire with Juvara,
Prog. med., 19 : 273–276, Apr. 21 ; 303–306, Apr. 28 ;
321–325, May 5 ; 353–355, May 19, 1894
FOSSA—duodenojejunal f.
Anatomie topographique du duodénum et hernies
duodénales. Paris, Lecrosnier et Babé, 1889. 107 pp.
OPERATION—sympathectomy.
La résection totale et bilatérale du sympathique cervi-
cal. Arch. prov. de chir., 6 : 88–99, Feb. 1897
Angine de poitrine guerie par la résection du sympathi-
que cervico-thoracique. Bull. Acad. med., Paris, 84 :
93–102, Oct. 5, 1920
Jordan, Edwin Oakes. Chicago scientist. 1866–1936
AGAR—basal peptone bile.
The inhibitive action of bile upon B. coli. J. infect.
Dis., 12 : 326–334, May 1912
AGAR—lead acetate infusion.
Differentiation of the paratyphoid-enteritidis group.
II. Lead acetate agar with Ruth Victorson, Ibid., 21 :
554–555, Dec. 1917
BROTH—phenol infusion ; enrichment medium.
The relative abundance of Bacillus coli communis in
river water as an index of the self-purification of streams.
J. Hyg., 1 : 295–320, July 1901
MEDIUM—peptone tartrate, for salmonella group.
A new differential medium for the paratyphoid group
with P. H. Harmon, J. infect. Dis., 42 : 238–241,
Mar. 1928
Jordan, Ronald Charles. Cardiff physiologist
TEST—
Note on a quantitative skatole colour reaction for
fructose with J. Pryde, Biochem. J., 32 : 279–281,
Feb. 1938
Jores, Leonhard. Bonn physician. 1866–1935
Described suburethral glands.
Ueber die Hypertrophie des sogenannten mittleren
Lappens der Prostata. Arch. f. path. Anat., 135 :
224–247, 1894
Described hyperplastic type of intimal thickening.
Ueber die Arteriosklerose der kleinen Organarterien
und ihre Beziehungen zur Nephritis. Ibid., 178 :
367–406, 1904

Jorissenne, Gustav. Belgian physician
SIGN—non-acceleration of pulse on changing from
horizontal to erect position ; sign of pregnancy.
Nouveau signe de la grossesse. Ann. Soc. méd.-chi
de Liege, 21, 1882
Josafson, Arnold. Swedish physician
TEST—for cancer cells by centrifuging aspirated flu
and sectioning sedimented cells.
Primär lungkancer med svulstceller i pleuraexsud
och sputum. Hygiea, 63 : 435–445, Nov. 1901
Joseph. See A. Kamnitzer
Joseph, Eugen. German surgeon. 1879–
OPERATION—for recurrent dislocation of shoulde
Eine neue Operation zur Verhütung der habituelle
Schulterverrenkung. Berl. klin. Wschr., 1 : 525 (only
May 28, 1917
Joseph, Jacques. Berlin surgeon. 1865–1934
OPERATION—mammaplasty.
Zur Operation der hypertrophischen Hängebru
Dtsch. med. Wschr., 51 : 1103–1105, July 3, 1925
Josias, Albert Henri Louis. French physician. 185?
1906
Transmitted measles to animals.
Recherches expérimentales sur la transmissibilité
la rougeole aux animaux. Méd. Mod., Paris, 9 : 15
154, Mar. 9, 1898
Joslin, Elliott Proctor. Boston physician. 1869–
DIETS—diabetic diets.
The treatment of diabetes mellitus. Philadelphia, L
and Febiger, 1916. 440 pp.
The routine treatment of diabetes with insulin. J.
M. A., 80 : 1581–1583, June 2, 1923
Josué, Otto. French physician. 1869–1923
Produced arteriosclerosis experimentally.
Athérôme aortique expérimental par injections ré
tées d'adrénaline dans les veines. C. R. Soc. Biol., 5
1374–1376, Nov. 14, 1903
Jouan, C. French physician
SOLUTION—litmus whey ; for cultivation of colc
typhoid group.
Petit-lait tournesolé et succédanés. C. R. Soc. Bi
79 : 520–522, June 3, 1916
Joubert. See L. Pasteur
Jourdain, Anselme Louis Bernard Berchllle
Paris surgeon. 1734–1816
DISEASE—pyorrhea alveolaris. Fischer
Traité des maladies et des operations réelement chiru
cales de la bouche et des parties qui y corresponde
. . . Paris, 1778, 2 : 396
METHOD—of washing out antrum of Highm
through natural opening.
Recherches sur les differens moyens de traiter
maladies des sinus maxillaire. J. de méd., chir. phar
Paris, 27 : 52–71 ; 157–174, 1767
Joyce, James Leonard. English surgeon. 1882–1?
OPERATION—
A new operation for the substitution of a thumb. B
J. Surg., 5 : 499–504, Jan. 1918
The results of a new operation for the substitution c
thumb. Ibid., 16 : 362–369, Jan. 1929
Joyce, Thomas Martin. Portland, Ore. surge
1885–1947
TECHNIC—
Fascial repair of inguinal hernias : report of 760 ope
tions from January 1934 to January 1939. J. A. M.
115 : 971–977, Sept. 21, 1940

udd, Edward Starr. Rochester, Minn. surgeon. 1878–
PERATION—dilatation of bile ducts after cholecys-
tectomy.
The effect of removal of the gall-bladder with F. C.
Mann, S. G. O., 24: 437–442, Apr. 1917
PERATION—
Oesophageal diverticula. Ibid., 27: 135–141, Aug.
1918
Also in: Collected papers of Mayo Clinic. Phila.,
Saunders, 1918. 10: 15–25
Esophageal diverticula. Arch. Surg., 1: 38–52, July
1920
irgens, R. See E. A. Von Willebrand
ilian, O. C. See J. G. Allen, L. R. Dragstedt
illiard, Prof. Genf surgeon
ABLE—operating.
Operationstisch. Illustirte Monatsschrift der ärztli-
chen Polytechnik, Bern, 5: 267–268, Dec. 11, 1883
ing, Carl Gustav. German psychiatrist. 1875–
Made important contributions to psychiatry.
*Zur Psychologie und Pathologie sogenannter occulter
Phänomene.* Leipzig, Mutze, 1902. 121 pp.
Collected papers on analytical psychology. London,
Baillière et al., 1916. 392 pp.
inghaus, P. See W. Wolff
inker, F. E. English physician
PPARATUS or INHALER—
Description of a new apparatus for administering

narcotic vapours. Med. Times and Gaz., 2: 590 (only),
Nov. 30, 1867
*On a new apparatus for the administration of narcotic
vapours; and some observations on the variations of
pulse and respiration during the anaesthesia from
chloromethyl.* Ibid., 1: 171–173, Feb. 15, 1868
Junod, Victor Theodor. French physician. 1809–
1881
BOOT—with air-pump, to cause vacuum about a
member. Garrison
*Recherches physiologiques et thérapeutiques sur les
effets de la compression et de la raréfaction de l'air,
tant sur le corps que sur les membres isolés.* Paris,
Deville Cavellin, 1834. 25 pp.
Traité theorique et pratique de l'hémospasie. Paris,
Masson, 1875. 380 pp.
Jupille, F. See A. Besredka
Jurewitsch, W. St. Petersburg physician
BROTH—potato infusion, for cultivation of tubercle
bacilli.
*Kartoffelnährbouillon zur Züchtung der Tuberkel-
bacillen.* Zbl. Bakt., 47: 664–666, 1908
Jurin, James. English scientist. 1684–1750
Determined specific gravity of blood as 1.053 and
of blood serum as 1.030.
*Experiments relating to the specific gravity of human
blood.* Philos. Trans., 5: 320–326, 1719
Juvara. See T. Jonnesco

K

abat, H. See S. W. Ranson
ader, Bronislaw. Polish surgeon
PERATION—
Zur Technik der Gastrostomie. Zbl. Chir., 23: 665–670,
July 11, 1896
igi, H. See L. Ruzicka
aes, Theodor. German neurologist. 1852–1913
NE—of white matter forming anterior margin of
layer III of cortex.
*Die Anwendung der Wolters'schen Methode auf die
feinen Fasern der Hirnrinde.* Neurol. Zbl., 10: 456–
459, 1891
*Beiträge zur Kenntniss des Reichtums der Grosshirn-
rinde des Menschen an markhaltigen Nervenfasern.*
Arch. Psychiat. Nervenkr., 25: 695–758, 1893
afka, Victor. Hamburg physician
ROTEIN RELATION—of cerebrospinal fluid.
Der Eiweissquotient des Liquor cerebrospinalis. Klin.
Wschr., 5: 2068–2069, Oct. 29, 1926
EACTION—colloidal, of cerebrospinal fluid.
*Die kolloidchemische Untersuchung der Rückenmarks-
flüssigkeit mit Paraffinsolen.* Ibid., 2: 1890 (only),
Oct. 8, 1923
agan, Benjamin Milton. Baltimore physician.
1913–
ETHOD—
*A simple method for the estimation of total protein
content of plasma and serum: II. The estimation of
total protein content of human plasma and serum by
the use of the falling drop method.* J. clin. Invest., 17:
373–376, July 1938
ihlbaum, Karl Ludwig. German psychiatrist.
1828–1899
Described hebephrenia, 1863. Garrison

Described katatonia, 1874. Garrison
Die Katatonie. Berlin, Hirschwald, 1874. 104 pp.
Kahlden, Clemens von. Freiburg pathologist. 1809–
1903
Described granulosa cell tumor.
Ueber eine eigenthümliche Form des Ovarialcarcinoms.
Zbl. f. allg. Path., Jena, 6: 257–264, Apr. 20, 1895
Kahlenberg, Louis. American chemist. 1870–
REACTION—
On some new color reactions of cholesterol. J. biol.
Chem., 52: 217–225, May 1922
See also J. V. Steinle
Kahler, Otto. Austrian physician. 1849–1893
DISEASE—multiple myeloma.
*Zur Symptomatologie des multiplen Myeloms. Beo-
bachtung von Albumosurie.* Prag. med. Wschr., 14:
33–35, Jan. 23; 44–49, Jan 30, 1889
Kahn, B. S. See J. H. Roe
Kahn, Ed. Karlsruhe physician
TEST—for arsphenamine injuries.
*Urobilinogenreaktion als Signal bei Salvarsanschädi-
gungen.* Münch. med. Wschr., 70: 431 (only), Apr.
6, 1923
Kahn, Herbert. Karlsruhe physician
REACTION—a flocculation test for cancer.
*Die chemischen Veränderungen bei Krebskranken und
ihre Bedeutung für die Serodiagnostik der malignen
Geschwülste.* Klin. Wschr., 4: 178–179, Jan. 22;
222–224, Jan. 29, 1925
Kahn, Morton Charles. American scientist. 1895–
MILK—brown cresol purple.
A cultural study of anaerobic spore-bearing bacteria

with strains isolated by the Barber single cell technic.
J. med. Res., 43: 155–206, Jan. 1922
See also C. S. Foster

Kahn, Reuben Leon. American bacteriologist. 1887–
TEST—
A simple quantitative precipitation reaction for syphi-
lis. Arch. Derm. and Syph., 5: 570–578, May 1922
*Effect of dilution on the precipitation reaction for
syphilis proposed by author.* Proc. Soc. exp. Biol.,
N. Y., 19: 294–295, 1922
*Relation between serum and antigen in precipitation
reaction for syphilis proposed by author.* Ibid., 295–
296
*Kahn precipitation test for syphilis—improved pro-
cedure.* Ibid., 20: 325–332, 1923

Kaiser, Eduard. German scientist
GLYCERIN JELLY—for mounting. Mallory
*Instrumente, Präparirungs- und Conservirungsmetho-
den etc. Verfahren zur Herstellung einer tadellosen
Glycerin-Gelatine.* Bot. Zbl., 1: 25–26, 1880

Kaiserling, Carl. Berlin pathologist. 1869–
SOLUTION—
*Weitere Mittheilungen über die Herstellung möglichst
naturgetreuer Sammlungspräparate.* Arch. f. path.
Anat., 147: 389–417, Mar. 1, 1897

Kalal, Evelyn. See Ida Kraus
Kaliski, D. J. See R. Ottenberg
Kaminer, G. See E. Freund
Kamm, Oliver. American chemist. 1888–
Separated vasopressor and oxytocic factors of pos-
terior lobe of pituitary gland.
*The active principle of the posterior lobe of the pituitary
gland* with T. B. Aldrich, L. W. Grote, L. W. Rowe
and E. P. Bugbee, J. Amer. Chem. Soc., 50: 573–
601, Feb. 1928

Kammerer, Frederic. American surgeon. 1856–1928
INCISION—Battle-Jalaguier-Kammerer i.
*A modified incision at the outer border of the rectus
muscle for appendicitis.* Med. Rec., 52: 837–839, Dec. 11,
1897

Kamnitzer, Adolf. German physician. 1879–
TEST—for pregnancy.
*Ein neues Verfahren zur Feststellung der intra- und
extrauterinen Frühgravidität* with Joseph. Med.
Klinik, 18: 396–398, Mar. 26, 1922

Kanavel, Allen Buckner. Chicago surgeon. 1874–
1938
APPARATUS—Y tube inserted into Murphy drip.
*Pre-operative preparation and postoperative care of
surgical patients* with S. L. Koch, Bull. Amer. Coll.
Surg., 11: 14–28, July 1927
OPERATION—
*The removal of tumors of the pituitary body by an
infranasal route; a proposed operation with a descrip-
tion of the technic.* J. A. M. A., 53: 1704–1707, Nov.
20, 1909
SIGN—tenderness proximal to distal flexion crease in
tendon sheath infection.
Infections of the hand. Philadelphia, Lea & Febiger,
1925. 5 ed., p. 63
See also L. E. Davis

Kanenko, Renjiro. Japanese physician. 1886–
Distinguished Japanese encephalitis from encepha-
litis lethargica.
Über die Encephalitis epidemica in Japan with Y.
Aoki, Ergebn. d. inn. Med., 34: 342–456, 1928

Kant, Immanuel. German philosopher. 1724–1804
Attempted classification of mental diseases. Garri-
son and Morton
Anthropologie in pragmatischer Hinsicht abgefasst.
Königsberg, Nicolovius, 1798

Kanter, Aaron Elias. Chicago physician. 1893–
TEST—
A new biologic test for hormones in pregnancy urin.
with C. P. Bauer and A. H. Klawans, J. A. M. A.,
103: 2026–2027, Dec. 29, 1934

Kanthack, Alfredo Antunes. London pathologist.
1863–1898
AGAR—serous exudate; for diagnosis of diphtheria.
*Ein neues und bequemes Verfahren zur Bereitung vo
Serum-Agar-Agar als Hilfsmittel zur Erkennung de
Diphtherie* with J. W. W. Stephens, Zbl. Bakt., 19
609–610, May 8, 1896

Kantor, John Leonard. New York physician. 1890–
BIURET PAPER—
Additional experiments with the biuret reagent wit.
W. J. Gies, Proc. Soc. Biol. Chem., 1910, abstr. in
J. biol. Chem., 9: xvii-xviii, Apr. 1911
SIGN—string s. of regional ileitis.
Regional (terminal) ileitis; its roentgen diagnosis
J. A. M. A., 103: 2016–2021, Dec. 29, 1934

Kao, C. H. See K. K. Chen
Kapeller-Adler, Regina. German scientist
TEST—for histidine; for pregnancy.
*Über eine neue Methode zur quantitativen Histidin
bestimmung und über deren Andendbarkeit zur Unte
suchung von biologischen Flüssigkeiten, insbesonde
von Gravidenhamen.* Biochem. Z., 264: 131–14
Aug. 17, 1933

Kaposi, Moritz Kohn. Austrian dermatologist. 1837
1902
DISEASE—
Xeroderma pigmentosum. Med. Jahr. Wien., 12
619–633, 1882
Described pigmented sarcoma of skin. Garrison
Idiopathisches multiples Pigmentsarkom der Hau
Arch. Dermat. u. Syph., 4: 265–273, 1872
Described lymphoderma perniciosa. Garrison
*Ueber eine neue Form von Hautkrankheit, "Lymphe
dermia perniciosa," zugleich ein Beitrag zur Patho
ogie der Leukämie.* Med. Jahr. Wien., 15: 129–14
1885
Described—
*Lichen ruber monileformis— Korallenschnurartig
Lichen ruber.* Vrtlschr. f. Dermat., 2 s., 18: 572–58
1886

Kappis, Max. German surgeon. 1881–
METHOD—for closure of intestinal fistula by mea
of a T tube.
*Einige praktische Winke zur Behandlung des per
tonitischen Ileus.* Münch. med. Wschr., 58: 15–1
Jan. 3, 1911
METHOD—of blocking splanchnic nerves.
Zur Technik der Splanchnicusanästhesie. Zbl. Chi
47: 98 (only), Jan. 31, 1920
Splanchnikusanästhesie. Abstr.: Dtsch. med. Wsch
46: 535 (only), May 6, 1920
Advocated paravertebral anesthesia in urology.
*Über Leitungsanästhesie bei Nierenoperationen u
Thorakoplastiken, überhaupt bei Operationen a
Rumpf.* Zbl. Chir., 39: 249–252, Feb. 24, 1912

Kapsinow, R. See F. P. Underhill

Kardon, Eugen. Berlin physician
MODIFICATION—of Giemsa's stain.
Zur Kenntnis der neutrophilen und azurophilen Kör-nung, nebst einer neuen Färbemodifikation. Folio haematol., Archiv., 12: 39–49, July 4, 1911

Karell, Philippe. German physician. 1806–1886
DIET—for treatment of heart or kidney disease, starting with 800 c.c. of milk daily.
On the milk cure! Transl. from the author's manu-script by E. L. Carrick, Philadelphia, 1870. 24 pp.

Kark, Robert. Boston scientist
MODIFICATION—of Quick test for prothrombin.
Nutritional deficiency of vitamin K in man: a study of four non-jaundiced patients with dietary deficiency with E. L. Lozner, Lancet, 2: 1162–1164, Dec. 2, 1939

Károly, Csépai. Budapest physician
TEST—for blood.
Ueber eine neue spektroskopische hämochromogene Blutprobe der Faeces. Dtsch. med. Wschr., 35: 1191 (only), July 8, 1909

Karplus, Johann Paul. Vienna physiologist. 1866–1936
Performed experimental work on hypothalamus.
Gehirn und Sympathicus with A. Kreidl, Arch. ges. Physiol., 129: 138–144, Aug. 19, 1909; 135: 401–416, Dec. 5, 1910

Karr, Walter Gerald. Philadelphia biochemist. 1892–
METHOD—
A method for the determination of blood urea nitrogen. J. Lab. clin. Med., 9: 324–333, Feb. 1924

Karrer, Paul. Swiss chemist. 1889–
Synthesized vitamin E.
a-Tocopherol with H. Fritzsche, B. H. Ringier and H. Salomon, Helv. Chim. Acta, 21: 520–525, Apr. 1938

Kartulis, Stephanos. Greek physician. 1852–1920
AMOEBA—found in liver abscess in cases of dysentery.
Zur Aetiologie der Dysenterie in Aegypten. Arch. f. path. Anat., 105: 521–531, Sept. 1, 1886
See also Schiess Bey

Kasper, Joseph Arthur. Detroit pathologist. 1896–
TEST—
A simplified Benedict test for glycosuria with Isabelle A. Jeffrey, Amer. J. clin. Path., Tech. Sect., 8: 117–121, Nov. 1944

Kasper, W. See J. E. v. Purkinje

Kassowitz, Karl Erhard. Vienna pediatrician. 1886–
SCRATCH TEST—for determination of susceptibility to diphtheria.
Über cutane Hautreaktionen mittels Diphtherie-Toxin zum Nachweis der Diphtherie-Immunität. Klin. Wschr., Berlin, 3: 1317–1318, July 15, 1924

Kassowitz, Max. Vienna physician. 1842–1913
LAW—virulence of syphilis for child decreases with duration of infection in mother.
Die Vererbung der Syphilis. Med. Jb., Wien, pp. 359–495, 1875

Kast, Alfred. German physician. 1856–1903
Introduced sulphonal.
Sulfonal, ein neues Schlafmittel. Berl. klin. Wschr., 25: 309–314, Apr. 16, 1888
See also E. Baumann

Kastle, Joseph Hoeing. American chemist. 1864–
REAGENT—
A new reagent for the recognition and estimation of free hydrochloric acid in gastric contents with H. L. Amoss, J. biol. Chem., 3: xi–xii, 1907
REAGENT and TEST—for free acids.
Cyanogen iodide as an indicator for acids with Mary E. Clark, Amer. Chem. J., 30: 87–96, Aug. 1903
TEST—for blood.
Variations in the peroxidase activity of the blood in health and disease with H. L. Amoss, Hyg. Lab. U. S. P. H. & M. H. S., Bull. 31, 1906. 26 pp.
Demonstrated reversible action of lipase.
Concerning lipase, the fat-sp'itting enzyme, and the reversibility of its action with A. S. Loevenhart, Amer. Chem. J., 24: 491–525, 1900

Katayama disease
A town in Japan where the disease is common. It is marked by painful enlargement of liver and spleen, dropsy, anemia, and dysenteric symptoms, with or without fever and is caused by infestation with Schistosoma japonicum. Stedman

Katayama, Kuniyosi. Japanese physician
TEST—for carbon monoxide in blood.
Ueber eine neue Blutprobe bei der Kohlenoxydvergif-tung. Arch. path. Anat., 114: 53–64, Oct. 2, 1888

Kato, Kan. Japanese scientist. 1879–
TEST—for glycogen in tissues.
Beitrag zur Frage des mikrochemischen Nachweises des Glykogens. Arch. ges. Physiol., 27: 125–142, Mar. 5, 1909

Kato, Katsuji. Chicago pediatrician. 1885–
TEST—
Micro-prothrombin test with capillary whole blood: a modification of Quick's quantitative method. Amer. J. clin. Path., 10: 147–153, Feb. 1940

Katz, Georg. Berlin physician. 1894–
METHOD—of estimating sedimentation rate of erythrocytes.
Die Senkung der roten Blutkörperchen im Zitratblut bei Lungentuberkulose. Z. Tuberk., 35: 401–424, Mar. 1922
Zur Differentialdiagnose der Lungentuberkulose ver-mittels der Bestimmung der Sedimentierzeit der Erythrocyten. Klin. Wschr., 1: 1368 (only), July 1, 1922

Katzenstein, Moritz. German surgeon
OPERATION—transplantation of muscle in serratus paralysis.
Ueber funktionelle Heilung der Serratuslähmung durch Operation. Berl. klin. Wschr., 45: 2297–2300, Dec. 28, 1908
TEST—for efficiency of myocardium.
Ueber eine neue Funktionsprüfung des Herzens. Dtsch. med. Wschr., 30: 807–809, May 26, 1904

Katzman, Philip Aaron. St. Louis biochemist. 1906–
METHOD—of demonstrating prolan in urine.
Preparation of extracts of the anterior pituitary-like substances of urine of pregnancy with E. A. Doisy, J. biol. Chem., 98: 739–754, Nov. 1932
A quantitative procedure for determining normal ex-cretion of prolan with E. A. Doisy, Proc. Soc. exp. Biol., N. Y., 30: 1188–1191, May 1933

Kaufmann, Carl. Berlin physician. 1900–
TREATMENT—of amenorrhea.
Umwandlung der Uterusschleimhaut einer kastrierten Frau aus dem atropischen Stadium in das der sekre-torischen Funktion durch Ovarialhormone. Zbl. Gynäk., 56: 2058–2061, Aug. 20, 1932

Die Behandlung der Amenorrhöe mit hohen Dosen der Ovarialhormone. Klin. Wschr., 12: 1557–1562, Oct. 7, 1933

Kaufmann, M. French scientist
METHOD—of determination of blood amylase.
Sur le pouvoir saccharifiant du sang et des tissus chez les chiens diabétiques. C. R. Acad. Biol., 46: 130–132, Feb. 10, 1894

Kaufmann, Paul. Naples physician
SOLUTION—jequirity seed infusion peptone; culture medium.
Ueber einen neuen Nährboden für Bakterien. Zbl. Bakt., 10: 65–69, July 28, 1891

Kaufmann, Rudolf. Berlin physician. 1871–1927
METHOD—of staining for capsules.
Eine neue Methode zur Färbung von Bakterienkapseln. Hyg. Rundschau., 8: 873–875, Sept. 15, 1898

Kausch, Walther. Schöneberg surgeon. 1867–1928
OPERATION—choledochoenterostomy.
Ueber Gallenwag-Darmverbindungen. Arch. klin. Chir., 47: 574–626, Mar. 14, 1912

Kawahara, Mizuchi. Tokio physician
TEST—for pepsin.
Über eine neue Methode der quantitativen Pepsinbestimmung (Kongorotmethode). Arch. ges. Physiol., 206: 360–368, Nov, 22, 1924

Kawai, Ginnosuke. Japanese physician
TEST—for blood.
Ueber eine neue Farbenreaktion des Blutes und die Extrahierbarkeit des Blutfarbstoffes mittels Alkali. Beitr. Physiol., 3: 241–286, 1926

Kawlet, Jonas. Brooklyn scientist
METHOD—
A simplified micro determination of cholesterol in whole blood, serum, and plasma. J. Lab. clin. Med., 19: 883–884, May 1934

Kay, Herbert Davenport. Canadian biochemist. 1893–
METHOD—
Plasma phosphatase. I. Method of determination. Some properties of the enzyme. J. biol. Chem., 89: 235–241, Nov. 1930
See also R. T. Brain, H. D. Jenner

Kay, J. See F. R. Edwards
Kaye, John. See John Caius
Kaye, S. See V. H. Cornell
Kayser, Bernhard. German ophthalmologist. 1869–
RING—Kayser-Fleischer's r. (cornea).
Ueber einen Fall von angeborener grünlicher Verfärbung der Cornea. Klin. Wschr. f. Augenh., 40: 22–25, 1902

Kayser, Heinrich. German physician. 1853–1940
SOLUTION—blood bile; culture medium.
Zur Frühdiagnose und Bakteriologie des Typhus sowie Paratyphus. Zbl. Bakt., 42: 185–192, 1906
STAIN—modification of Proca's to distinguish living from dead bacteria.
Die Unterscheidung von lebenden und toten Bakterien durch die Färbung. Ibid., 62: 174–176, Jan. 30, 1912
See also A. Brion

Kazanjian, Varaztad Hovhannes. Boston otolaryngologist. 1879–
METHOD—of treating fractures of nose.
Injuries to the face and jaws resulting from automobile accidents. Trans. Amer. Acad. Ophth. and Otolaryngol., pp. 275–308, 1933

Kaznelson, Paul. Prague physician
Advocated splenectomy in treatment of purpura.
Verschwinden der hämorrhagischen Diathese bei einem Falle von "essentieller Thrombopenie" (Frank) nach Milzexstirpation. Splenogene thrombolytische Purpura. Wien. klin. Wschr., 24: 1451–1454, Nov. 16, 1916

Keating-Hart, Walter Valentin. French physician. 1870–1922
TREATMENT—of cancer by electric spark.
La fulguration et ses resultats dans le traitement du cancer d'après une statisque personnelle de 247 cas. Paris, Maloine, 1909. 98 pp.

Keegan, Denis Francis. English surgeon. 1840–1920
OPERATION—
Rhinoplastic operations, with a description of recent improvements in the Indian method. London, Baillière, 1900. 72 pp.

Keeley, Leslie G. Dwight, Ill. physician. 1832–1900
CURE—a proprietary treatment of alcohol and opium habits by means of gold chlorid.
The morphine eater; or, from bondage to freedom; the opium, morphine, and kindred habits, etc. Dwight, Ill., Palmer, 1881. 200 pp.

Keen, William Williams. Philadelphia surgeon. 1837–1932
OPERATION—
A case of interilio-abdominal amputation for sarcome of the ilium, and a synopsis of previously recorded cases with J. C. DaCosta, Internat. Clin., 13 s., 4: 127–147, 1904
First to tap the ventricles. Garrison
Exploratory trephining . . . Med. News, 53: 603–609, Dec. 1, 1888
See also S. W. Mitchell

Keetley, Charles Robert Bell. London surgeon. 1848–1909
OPERATION—
Temporary fixation of testis to thigh. A series of 2 cases operated on for undescended testis. Lancet, 2: 279–281, July 29, 1905

Kehr, Hans. German surgeon. 1862–1916
OPERATION—
Die Hepato-Cholangio-Enterostomie. Zbl. Chir., 31: 185–189, Feb. 20, 1904
OPERATION—cholecystectomy.
Die chirurgische Behandlung der Gallensteinkrankhei Berlin, Kornfeld, 1896. 239 pp.

Kehrer, Ferdinand Adolph. Heidelberg gynecologist. 1837–1914
OPERATION—improvement in cesarean section.
Ueber ein modificirtes Verfahren beim Kaiserschnitt. Arch. Gynäk., 19: 177–209, 1882

Keibel, Franz Karl Julius. German physician. 1861–1929
THEORY—of exstrophy.
Zur Entwickelungsgeschichte der Harnblase. Anat. Anz., 6: 186–192, Apr. 15, 1891

Keining, Egon. Hamburg physician. 1892–
DIET—equilibrated salt.
Ueber das Wesen der vegetativen Störungen, d Bedeutung der sogenannten salzfreien Diät und de Kationenrelation sowie über Gesichtspunkte für eir rationelle Ernährungsmethode with G. Hopf, Dtsch med. Wschr., 57: 181–185, Jan. 30, 1931

Keith, Sir Arthur. London physician. 1866–
BUNDLE—sino-atrial b.
NODE—sino-auricular n.
  The form and nature of the muscular connections be-
  tween the primary divisions of the vertebrate heart
  with M. W. Flack, J. Anat., Lond., 41: 172–189,
  Apr. 1907
  Also in F. A. Willius and T. E. Key's *Cardiac classics,*
  St. Louis, Mosby. 1941. pp. 747–762
THEORY—control stations for intestinal movements.
  The Cavendish lecture on a new theory of the causation
  of enterostasis. Lancet, 2: 371–375, Aug. 21, 1915
Keith, Norman Macdonnell. American physician.
1885–
CLASSIFICATION—of hypertension by changes in
ocular fundus.
  Some different types of essential hypertension: their
  course and prognosis with H. P. Wagener and N. W.
  Barker, Amer. J. med. Sci., 197: 332–343, Mar. 1929
DETERMINATION—of blood volume.
  A method for the determination of plasma and blood
  volume with L. G. Rowntree and J. T. Geraghty,
  Arch. intern. Med., 16: 547–576, Oct. 1915
  See also H. P. Wagener
Keith, Thomas. Edinburgh surgeon. 1827–1895
OPERATION—intraperitoneal ligation of ovarian
pedicle.
  On ovarian dropsy, with cases of ovariotomy. Edin-
  burgh med. J., 9: 299–311, Oct. 1863
Kekulé, Friedrich August von. German chemist.
1829–1896
Stated theory of open carbon chain and closed ben-
zene ring. Garrison
  Lehrbuch der organischen Chemie. 1860
Kekwick, A. See H. L. Marriott
Keller, Alexander G., Jr. Philadelphia scientist. 1895–
METHOD—
  A micro method for blood urea nitrogen. J. Lab. clin.
  Med., 17: 1146–1147, Aug. 1932
Keller, H. See Grace M. Fernald
Keller, William Lordan. U. S. Army surgeon. 1874–
GRAFT—
  Ten years of the tunnel skin graft. Ann. Surg., 91:
  924–936, June 1930
OPERATION—for hallux valgus.
  The surgical treatment of bunions and hallux valgus.
  New York med. J., 80: 741–742, Oct. 15, 1904
OPERATION—pleurectomy.
  The treatment of chronic empyema where the recog-
  nized surgical procedures have failed to produce ob-
  literation. Ann. Surg., 76: 549–580, Nov. 1922
OPERATION—for recurrent dislocation of shoulder.
  The treatment of chronic recurrent dislocation of the
  shoulder by crucial capsular plication. Ann. Surg., 81:
  143–148, Jan. 1925
OPERATION—for varicose veins.
  A new method of extirpating the internal saphenous
  and similar veins in varicose conditions; a preliminary
  report. New York med. J., 82: 385–386, Aug. 19, 1905
OPERATION—
  Annual stricture of the rectum and anus: treatment by
  tunnel skin graft; preliminary report. Amer. J. Surg.,
  20: 28–32, Apr. 1933
Kellie, George. English physician
HYPOTHESIS—skull and spinal column form rigid
container for central nervous system.

  On death from cold, and on congestions of the brain.
  An account of the appearances observed in the dissec-
  tion of two of three individuals presumed to have
  perished in the storm of 3rd November, 1821; with
  some reflexions on the pathology of the brain. Trans.
  Med.-Chir. Soc. Edinburgh, 1: 84, 1824
Kelling, Georg. Dresden surgeon
METHOD—of closure of pylorus.
  Ueber Prothesen bei Magen- und Darm- Vereinigun-
  gen. Arch. klin. Chir., 62: 739–737, 1900
TEST—for lactic acid in stomach.
  Ueber Rhodan im Mageninhalt, zugleich ein Beitrag
  zum Uffelmann'schen Milchsäure-Reagens und zur
  Prüfung auf Fettsäuren. Z. physiol. Chem., 18: 397–
  408, 1893
Kellogg, John Harvey. Battle Creek, Mich. surgeon.
1852–1943
OPERATION—
  Plication of the hernial sac in operating for femoral
  hernia. Amer. J. Surg., 4: 597–598, June 1928
Kelly, Adam Brown. Scottish laryngologist. 1865–
1941
SYNDROME—of Patterson and Kelly; hypochromic
anemia, achlorhydria and atrophic gastritis.
  Spasm at the entrance of the esophagus. Brit. J.
  Laryng., Rhin. and Otol., 34: 285–289, Aug. 1919
Kelly, Howard Atwood. Baltimore gynecologist.
1858–1943
CYSTOSCOPE—
  The examination of the female bladder and the catheteri-
  zation of the ureters under direct inspection. Johns
  Hopk. Hosp. Bull., 4: 101–102, Nov. 1893
  Cystoscopy and catheterization of the ureters in the
  male. Ann. Surg., 27: 475–486, 1898
PAD—
  Perineal and ovariotomy cushions. Amer. J. Obstet.,
  20: 1029–1031, 1887
METHOD—
  Uretero-ureteral anastomosis — uretero-ureterostomy.
  Ann. Surg., 19: 70–77, Jan. 1894
METHOD—
  Ureteral calculus; its diagnosis by means of the wax-
  tipped bougie. Escape of the calculus per vias naturales
  after forcible dilatation of the ureteral orifice. J. A.
  M. A., 34: 515–517, Mar. 3, 1900
METHOD—of nephropexy.
  Diseases of the kidneys, ureters and bladder with
  special reference to the diseases in women with C. F.
  Burnam, New York, Appleton, 1922. Vol. 1, Ch. 16,
  pp. 459–519
METHOD—of Kelly and Burnam; pelvic plication for
hydronephrosis. Ibid., Ch. 17
OPERATION—
  Supra-vaginal hysterectomy. Hysteromyomectomy with
  suspension of the stump in the lower angle of the ab-
  dominal incision. Med. News, 56: 695–698, June 28,
  1890
  Abdominal hysterectomy for fibroma uteri. Abstr.:
  South. Practitioner, 19: 1–21, Jan. 1897
OPERATION—
  The treatment of incontinence of urine in women.
  Therap. Gaz., 3 s., 28: 685–687, Oct. 15, 1912
OPERATION—modification of Mayo o.
  An operation for umbilical hernia. Ann. Surg., 51:
  694–696, May 1910

OPERATION—for uterine displacements.
Hysterorrhaphy. Amer. J. Obstet., 20: 33–46, Jan. 1887

TUBES—proctoscope and sigmoidoscope.
A new method of examination and treatment of diseases of the rectum and sigmoid flexure. Ann. Surg., 21: 468–478, 1895

Pioneer in use of cocaine anesthesia.
On the anesthetic use of the hydrochlorate of cocaine upon parts of the body other than the eye. Med. News, 45: 713–714, Dec. 27, 1884

Kelly, Joseph Dominic. New York otolaryngologist. 1888–

OPERATION—for restoration of laryngeal function following bilateral paralysis of vocal cords.
Surgical treatment of bilateral paralysis of the abductor muscles. Arch. Otolaryng., 33: 293–304, Feb. 1941

Kelman, Sarah R. See H. Albert

Kelser, Raymond Alexander. American pathologist. 1892–

SOLUTION—blood infusion peptone; culture medium.
The preparation of culture media from whole blood. J. Bact., 1: 615–617, Nov. 1916

Kendall, Arthur Isaac. American bacteriologist. 1877–

AGAR—sucrose mannitol; culture medium.
A double sugar medium for the cultural diagnosis of intestinal and other bacteria with Majorie Ryan, J. infect. Dis., 24: 400–404, Apr. 1919

MODIFICATION—of Endo's medium.
The isolation of Bacillus dysenteriae from stools with A. W. Walker, J. med. Res., 23: 481–485, Nov. 1910

SOLUTION—ammonium asparagin, for studying tubercle bacilli.
A comparison of the curves of lipolytic activity and proteolysis of certain rapidly growing human tubercle bacilli in media of varied composition. Studies in acid-fast bacteria. I X with A. W. Walker and A. A. Day, J. infect. Dis., 15: 460–466, Nov. 1914

SOLUTION—basal ammonium chloride.
Observations on the specificity and thermostability of the lipase developed during the growth of a rapidly growing tubercle bacillus in media of varied composition. Studies in acid fast bacteria. VIII with A. W. Walker and A. A. Day, Ibid., 455–459

SOLUTION—basal ammonium phosphate.
The metabolism of certain rapidly growing tubercle bacilli in media with inorganic salts as sources of nitrogen. Studies in acid fast bacteria. IV with A. A. Day and A. W. Walker, Ibid., 433–438

SOLUTION—fat free peptone.
The metabolism of certain rapidly growing human tubercle bacilli in broth free from lipoids and fatty substances. Studies in acid fast bacteria. II with A. A. Day and A. W. Walker, Ibid., 423–427

Kendall, E. K., Jr. See E. K. Marshall, Jr.

Kendall, Edward Calvin. American physiochemist. 1886–

TEST—for iodine in blood.
Determination of iodine in blood and in animal tissues with F. S. Richardson, J. biol. Chem., 43: 161–170, Aug. 1920

TEST—for reducing sugars.
The detection and identification of certain reducing sugars by condensation with p-brom-benzylhydrazide

with H. C. Sherman, J. Amer. Chem. Soc., 30: 1451 1455, 1908

Isolated thyroxine.
A method for the decomposition of the proteins of tl thyroid, with a description of certain constituents. biol. Chem., 20: 501–509, Apr. 1915
The isolation in crystalline form of the compound co taining iodine, which occurs in the thyroid, its chem cal nature and physiological activity. J. A. M. A., 64 2042–2043, June 19, 1915
Isolation of the iodine compound which occurs in tl thyroid. J. biol. Chem., 39: 125–147, Aug. 1919

Reported—
Isolation in crystalline form of the hormone essenti to life from the suprarenal cortex: its chemical natu and physiologic properties with H. L. Mason, B. F McKenzie, C. S. Myers and G. A. Moelsch, Pro Staff Meet. Mayo Clin., 9: 245–250, Apr. 25, 193
See also H. L. Mason, R. M. Wilder

Kennaway, Ernest Laurence. London physicia 1881–
Produced cancer by means of a pure hydrocarbo
Carcinogenic substances and their fluorescence spect with I. Hieger, Brit. med. J., 1: 1044–1046, June 1930
See also G. Barry, A. Leitch

Kennedy, C. S. See M. O. Cantor

Kennedy, F. See A. Wolf

Kennedy, Robert. Glasgow surgeon. ?–1924
OPERATION—
Suture of the brachial plexus in birth paralysis of t upper extremity. Brit. med. J., 1: 298–301, Feb. 1903

Kennedy, Robert Phelps. Rochester, N. Y. patho ogist. 1890–
METHOD—
The use of light filters in colorimetry with a method f the estimation of hemoglobin. Amer. J. Physiol., 7 56–63, Sept. 1926

Kennedy, William Thomson. New York surgeo 1884–
OPERATION—
Incontinence of urine in female: some functional o servations of urethra illustrated by roentgenogram Amer. J. Obstet. Gynaec., 33: 19–29, Jan. 1937
Incontinence of urine in female, urethral sphinct mechanism, damage of function, and restoration control. Ibid., 34: 576–589, Oct. 1937

Kenny, Sister Elizabeth. Australian nurse. 1884–
TREATMENT—
Infantile paralysis and cerebral diplegia: metho used for the restoration of function. Sydney, Ang and Robertson, 1937
Treatment of infantile paralysis in the acute sta St. Paul, Minn., Bruce Pub. Co., 1941

Kenny, Méave. See L. Colebrook

Kent, Albert Frank Stanley. English scientist. 186 BUNDLE—same as His b.
Researches on the structure and function of the ma malian heart. J. Physiol., 14: 233–254, 1893

SOLUTION—glycerol albumin; for cultivation virus vaccinia.
The virus of vaccinia and its cultivation. Lancet, 1391–1393, May 21, 1898

Kent, E. M., Jr. See B. B. Blades, D. B. Pfeiffer

Kent, Grace Helen. American psychologist. 187

TESTS—of intelligence.
  A graded series of geometrical puzzles. J. exp. Psychol.,
  1: 40–50, 1916
Kentish, Edward. English physician
  Used breathing capacity for diagnostic purposes.
  *A \ account of baths, and of a Madeira-House, at
  Br:stol; with a drawing and description of a pulmome-
  ter, and cases, shewing its utility in ascertaining the
  state of the lungs in diseases of the chest.* London, Long-
  man, 1813. 117 pp.
Kepler, E. J. See W. Walters, R. M. Wilder
Kerckring, Thomas Theodor. Dutch anatomist.
  1640–1693
OSSICLE—small bone of early life which becomes
  basilar process of occipital bone.
  Osteogenia foetum . . . Ludg. Bat., Boutesteyn, 1717
VALVES—He demonstrated intestinal valvulae con-
  niventes. Garrison
  Spicilegium anatomicum . . . Amstelodami, Frissi,
  1670. 280 pp.
Kermorgant. See E. Apert
Kerner, Christian Andreas Justinus. German
  physician. 1786–1862
  Described botulism.
  *Neue Beobachtungen über die in Würtemberg so
  häufig vorfallen tödtlichen Vergiftung durch den Genuss
  geräuchter Würste.* Tübingen, Osiander, 1820
Kernig, Vladimir Michailovich. St. Petersburg phy-
  sician. 1840–1917
SIGN—of meningitis.
  Über ein Krankeitssymptom der acuten Meningitis.
  Abstr.: St. Petersburg med. Wschr., 7: 398 (only),
  Nov. 13 (25), 1882
  *Om odnom malo izviestnom priznakie vospalenija
  mjagkoi mosgovoi obo!ochke.* Vrach, St. Petersburg.,
  5: 427–428; 446–447, 1884
  Ueber ein wenig bemerktes Meningitis-Symptom.
  Berlin. klin. Wschr., 21: 829–832, Dec. 29, 1884
Kerr, Harry Hyland. Washington, D. C. surgeon.
  1881–
OPERATION—
  *Intrathoracic dermoids with the report of a case of total
  extirpation at one sitting by a new method of thoracot-
  omy* with J. O. Warfield, Jr., Ann. Surg., 88: 607–
  629, Sept. 1928
  See also E. M. Parker
Kerr, Josephine E. See W. J. MacNeal
Kerr, W. J. See T. Lewis
Kerry, R. See F. Obermayer
Kessiakow, Chr. Duschkow. Sofia physician
TEST—for pus in urine.
  Eine chemische Reaktion für Eiter im Harne. Münch.
  med. Wschr., 75: 1341-1342, Aug. 3, 1928
Key, Ben Witt. New York ophthalmologist. 1883–
  1940
OPERATION—
  *Transplantation of the temporal half of the vertical
  recti tendons in a case of complete paralysis of the
  external rectus.* Arch. Ophthal., 2: 39–47, July 1929
OPERATION—
  *Extensive iridodialysis; operation, reattachment. A
  report of two cases.* Ibid., 7: 748–756, May 1932
  Transplanted cornea.
  Report of a case of transplantation of the human cornea.
  Trans. Amer. Ophthal. Soc., 28: 29–41, 1930
Key, Charles Aston. English surgeon. 1793–1849

OPERATION—lateral o. for lithotomy done with a
  straight staff.
  *A short treatise on the section of the prostate gland in
  lithotomy; with an explanation of a safe and easy
  method of conducting the operation on the principles of
  Cheselden.* London, Longman, 1824. 30 pp.
  Introduced principle of dividing stricture outside sac
  in strangulated hernia. Garrison
  *A memoir on the advantages and practicability of
  dividing the stricture in strangulated hernia on the
  outside of the sac.* London, Longman, 1833. 161 pp.
Key, Einar Samuel Henrik. Stockholm surgeon.
  1872–
OPERATION—embolectomy.
  Vorgestellt in der Gesellschaft der Aerzte in Stock-
  holm am 28. Januar 1913.
  Also: *Ein Fall operierter Embolie der Arteria femoralis.*
  Wien. klin. Wschr., 26: 936–939, June 5, 1913
  *Über Embolectomi als Behandlingsmethode bei em-
  bolischen Zirculationsstörungen der Extremitäten.*
  Acta chir Scand., 54: 339–416, 1922
  See also G. Forssell
Key, J(ohn) Albert. American surgeon. 1890–
OPERATION—synovectomy.
  *The reformation of synovial membrane in the knees of
  rabbits after synovectomy.* J. Bone and Joint Surg.,
  23: 793–813, Oct. 1925
Keyes, E. L. See W. H. van Buren
Keynes, Geoffrey Langdon. English surgeon. 1887–
OPERATION—
  The modern treatment of hernia. Brit. med. J., 1:
  173–179, Jan. 29; 595–596, Mar. 26, 1927
Kharasch, M. S. See M. E. Davis
Kielland, Christian. Munich gynecologist. 1871–
FORCEPS—
  *Eine neue Form und Einführungsweise der Geburts-
  zange, stets biparietal an den kindlichen Schädel gelegt.*
  Münch. med. Wschr., 62: 923 (only), July 6, 1915
Kienböck, Robert. Austrian physician. 1871–
ATROPHY—
  *Ueber acute Knochenatrophie bei Entzündungspro-
  zessen an den Extremitäten (fälschlich sogenannte
  Inaktivatätsatrophie des Knochen) und ihre Diagnose
  nach dem Röntgen-Bilde.* Wien. med. Wschr., 51:
  1346–1348, July 13; 1389–1392, July 20; 1427–1430,
  July 27; 1462–1466, Aug. 3; 1508–1511, Aug. 8;
  1591–1596, Aug. 24, 1901
DISEASE—osteochondrosis of carpal semilunar.
  *Über traumatische Malazie des Mondbeins und ihre
  Folgezustände: Entartungsformen und Kompresfrak-
  turen.* Fort. a. d. Geb. d. Röntgenstr., 16: 77–103,
  1910–11
LUXATION—of hand.
  Über Luxationen im Bereiche der Handwurzel. Ibid.,
  16: 103–115, 1910–11
SYRINGOMYELIA—
  *Kritik der sogenannten "traumatischen Syringo-
  myelie"* . . . Jb. Psychiat., 21: 50–210, 1902
TECHNIC—epilating doses of low voltage roentgen
  irradiation.
  Über Radiotherapie der Haarerkrankungen. Arch. f.
  Dermat. u. Syph., 83: 77–112, 1907
UNIT—of roentgen-ray dosage, equal to one tenth of
  erythema dose.
  Ueber Dosimeter und das quantimetrische Verfahren.
  Fort. a. d. Geb. d. Röntgenstr., 9: 276–295, 1906

Radiotherapie, ihre biologischen Grundlagen, Anwendungsmethoden und Indikationen. Stuttgart, Enke, 1907. 190 pp.

Kiernan, Francis. English physician. 1800–1874
SPACE—interlobar space of liver.
The anatomy and physiology of the liver. Philos. Trans., London, 710–770, 1833

Kikuth, Walther. German chemist. 1896–
Introduced atebrin.
Zur Weiterentwicklung synthetisch dargestellter Malariamittel. I. Über die chemotherapeutische Wirkung des Atebrin. Dtsch. med. Wschr., 58: 530–531, Apr. 1, 1932

Kilborne, F. L. See T. Smith

Kilian, Hermann Friedrich. German gynecologist. 1800–1863
LINE and PELVIS SPINOSA—
Schilderungen neuer Beckenformen und ihres Verhaltens im Leben. Mannheim, Bassermann und Mathey, 1854
PELVIS—an osteomalacic pelvis, "pelvis obtecta." Garrison
De spondylolisthesi gravissimae pelvangustiae caussa nuper detecta commentatio anatomico-obstetricia. Bonnae, Georgii, (1854). 34 pp.

Kiliani, Otto G. T. New York surgeon. 1863–1920
OPERATION—hypophysectomy.
Some remarks on tumors of the chiasm, with a proposal how to reach the same by operation. Ann. Surg., 40: 35–43, July 1904

Killian, Gustav. Mainz laryngologist. 1860–1921
OPERATION—for frontal sinusitis.
Die Killian'sche Radicaloperation chronischer Stirnhöhleneiterungen. Arch. Laryn. u. Rhin., 13: 59–88 1903
TUBES—used in removing foreign bodies from trachea and esophagus.
Introduced direct bronchoscopy. Garrison
Ueber directe Bronchoskopie. Münch. med. Wschr., 45: 844–847, July 5, 1898
Introduced suspension laryngoscopy.
Die Schwebelaryngoscopie. Arch. Laryn. u. Rhin., 27: 277–317, 1912

Killian, John Allen. New York biochemist. 1891–
TEST—for carbohydrate tolerance.
Studies in the diastatic activity of the blood and blood sugar curves indicating a decreased carbohydrate tolerance in hyperthyroidism. Proc. Soc. exp. Biol., N. Y., 17: 91–93, 1920
See also V. C. Myers

Kilner, T. P. See H. D. Gillies

Kilpatrick, James. American physician. ?–1770
Advocated inoculation.
An essay on inoculation, occasioned by the small-pox being brought into South Carolina in the year 1738. London, Huggonson, 1743

Kimball, Gilman. Lowell, Mass. surgeon. 1804–1892
Performed hysteromyomectomy.
Successful case of extirpation of the uterus. Boston M. and S. J., 52: 249–255, May 3, 1855

Kimball, O. P. See D. Marine

Kimble, Marion Stark. Madison, Wis. scientist
METHOD—
The photocolorimetric determination of vitamin A and carotene in human plasma. J. Lab. clin. Med., 24: 1055–1065, July 1939

Kimmelstiel, Paul. Boston pathologist. 1900–
DISEASE or SYNDROME—
Benign and malignant hypertension and nephrosclerosis; a clinical and pathological study with C. Wilson, Amer. J. Path., 12: 45–82, Jan. 1936

Kimpton, Arthur Ronald. Boston surgeon. 1881–
TUBE—
A new and simple method of transfusion with J. H. Brown, J. A. M. A., 61: 117–118, July 12, 1913

Kindborg, Erich. German physician
AGAR—fuchsin malachito green; for typhoid and dysentery organisms.
Verbesserter Säurefuchsinagar zur Typhus- und Ruhrdiagnose. Zbl. Bakt., 77: 442–446, Mar. 22, 1916

King, Albert Freeman Africanus. American physician. 1841–1914
Set forth mosquito theory of malaria transmission.
Insects and disease—mosquitoes and malaria. Pop. Sci. Month, N. Y., 23: 644–658, Sept. 1883

King, B. G. See A. H. Blakemore

King, Brien Thaxton. Seattle, Ore. surgeon. 1886–
OPERATION—
New and function-restoring operation for bilateral abductor cord paralysis: preliminary report. J. A. M. A., 112: 814–823, Mar. 4, 1939

King, Sir E. See R. Lower

King, Earl J. Toronto biochemist. 1901–
METHOD—
A convenient method for determining serum and bile phosphatase activity with A. R. Armstrong, Canad. med. Ass. J., 31: 376–381, Oct. 1934

King, J. H. See A. T. Shohl

King, John. South Carolina surgeon
Described operation for abdominal pregnancy.
Case of an extra-uterine foetus, produced alive, through an incision made into the vagina of the mother, who recovered after delivery, without any alarming symptoms. Med. Reposit., N. Y., n. s. 3: 388–394, 1817
An analysis of the subject of extrauterine foetation and of the retroversion of the gravid uterus. Norwich, Vt., Wright, 1818

King, Joseph Eggleston Johnson. New York surgeon. 1886–
OPERATION—
The treatment of brain abscess by unroofing and temporary herniation of abscess cavity with the avoidance of usual drainage methods. S. G. O., 39: 554–568, Nov. 1924

King, Thomas Wilkinson. English physician. 1809–1847
"The father of endocrinology." Seems to have anticipated endocrine action of thyroid.
Observations on the thyroid gland. . . . Guy's Hosp. Rep., 1: 429–447, 1836

Kingsbury, Francis Bullard. New York biochemist. 1886–
METHOD—
The rapid determination of albumin in urine with C. P. Clark, Gertrude Williams and Anna L. Post, J. Lab. clin. Med., 11: 981–989, July 1926
TEST—
The synthesis and elimination of hippuric acid in nephritis: a new renal function test with W. W. Swanson, Arch. intern. Med., 28: 220–236, Aug. 1921

Kingsley, George R. Philadelphia biochemist
METHOD—
   A rapid method for the separation of serum albumin and globulin. J. biol. Chem., 133: 731–735, May 1940
METHOD—
   The direct Biuret method for the determination of serum proteins as applied to photoelectric and visual colorimetry. J. Lab. clin. Med., 27: 840–845, Mar. 1942
Kinnersley, Henry Wulff. English biochemist
METHOD—of preparation of vitamin B₁.
   Crystalline preparations of vitamin B₁ from baker's yeast with J. R. O'Brien and R. A. Peters, Biochem. J., 27: 232–239, 1933
TEST—
   The formaldehyde-azo-test for vitamin B₁ with R. A. Peters, Ibid., 28: 667–670, 1934
   See also C. W. Carter
Kinney, Ethel M. Chicago scientist
METHOD—
   A simple method for staining reticulum. Arch. Path., 5: 283–284, Feb. 1928
Kinney, K. K. See J. H. Vastine
Kinnicutt, R. See J. H. Wright
Kinnier
SYNDROME—see Samuel Alexander Kinnier Wilson.
Kinsella, Ralph A. St. Louis physician. 1886–
AGAR—nutrose gelatian; culture medium.
   Cultivation and isolation of gonococci with G. O. Broun and O. Garcia, J. infect. Dis., 32: 1–7 (4), Jan. 1923
Kirchensten, A. See C. Spengler
Kircher, Anthanasius. Jesuit philosopher. 1602–1680
   "He was undoubtedly the first to state in explicit terms the doctrine of a contagium animatum as the cause of infectious disease." Garrison
   One of first users of microscope; described maggots in putrefying flesh and small "worms" in blood of plague patients.
   Scrutinium physico-medicum contagiosae luis, quae pestis dicitur. Romae, Mascordi, 1658. 252 pp.
Kirchhoff, Const. St. Petersburg
   Discovered that starch can be converted into glucose by dilute sulphuric acid, without the acid itself being changed. Garrison
   Ueber die Reinigung der Getreide-Stärke. J. f. Chem. u. Physick, Nuremb., 14: 389–398, 1815
Kirk, Esben. New York physician. 1905–
ROCEDURE—of lipoid determination.
   Gasometric microdetermination of lipids in plasma, blood cells, and tissues with I. H. Page and D. D. Van Slyke, J. biol. Chem., 106: 203–234, Aug. 1934
Kirk, Norman Thomas. U. S. Army surgeon. 1888–
ECHNIC—of supracondylar tendoplastic amputation.
   Amputations in war. J. A. M. A., 120: 13–16, Sept. 5, 1942
Kirk, Robert. Scottish physician
EST—
   On albumen tests. Glasgow med. J., pp. 314–324, Apr. 1884
Kirkes, William Senhouse. English physician. 1823–1864
   Described embolism from intracardiac coagula.

On some of the principal effects resulting from the detachment of fibrinous deposits from the interior of the heart, and their mixture with the circulating blood. Trans. Roy. Med.-Chir. Soc. London, 35: 281–324, 1852
   Also in F. A. Willus and T. E. Key's Cardiac classics. St. Louis, Mosby, 1941. pp. 474–482
Kirkpatrick, James. See Kilpatrick
Kirmisson, Edouard. French surgeon. 1848–1927
OPERATION—subtrochanteric osteotomy, for fracture of neck of femur.
   De l'ostéotomie sous-trochantérienne appliquée à certains cas de luxation congénitale de la hanche (flexion de la cuisse avec adduction considérable). Rev. d'Orthop., 5: 137–146, Mar. 1894
Kirschner, Martin. Greifswald surgeon. 1879–1942
OPERATION—for hernia.
   Die praktischen Ergebnisse der freien Fascien-Transplantation. Arch. klin. Chir., 92: 889–912, 1910
OPERATION—for spilling patella.
   Ein neues Operationsverfahren zur schonenden Eröffnung des Kniegelenkes. Beitr. klin. Chir., 71: 703–713, 1911
WIRE—for skeletal traction in fracture treatment.
   Ueber Nagelextension. Ibid., 64: 266–279, 1909
   Performed successful pulmonary embolectomy.
   Ein durch die Trendelenburgsche Operation geheilter Fall von Embolie der Art. pulmonalis. Arch. klin. Chir., 133: 312–359, 1924
Kirstein, Alfred. Berlin physician. 1863–1922
METHOD—direct-vision laryngoscopy.
   Autoskopie der Luftwege. Dtsch. med. Wschr., 21: 634–636, Sept. 19, 1895
   Autoskopie des Larynx und der Trachea; (Laryngoscopia directa, Euthyskopie, Besichtigung ohne Spiegel). Arch. f. Laryngol. u. Rhinol., 3: 156–164, 1895
Kissingen
SALTS—from water of a spring at Kissingen, Bavaria.
Kita, G. Tokio physician
SOLUTION—basal ammonium sulphate.
SOLUTION—basal nitrate, for cultivation of molds.
   Einige japanische Schimmelpilze. Zbl. Bakt., 2 Abt., 37: 433–452, May 22, 1913
Kitasato, Shiramiro. Japanese bacteriologist. 1852–1931
BACILLUS—pestis, of bubonic plague.
   Pest-byo-no genin shibare sa dai hito hokoku. Tokio 1894. 14 pp.
   The bacillus of bubonic plague with A. Yersin, Lancet, 2: 428–430, Aug. 25, 1894
   Cultivated bacillus tetani in pure culture.
   Ueber den Tetanusbacillus. Z. Hyg. Infekt Kr., 7: 225–234, 1889
   See also E. A. von Behring
Kitchen, S. F. See W. A. Sawyer
Kittelson, John Asdal. Sioux Falls, S. D. surgeon. 1887–
TREATMENT—
   The treatment of duodenal fistula: including a report of two new cases and a report of a new buffer solution. S. G. O., 56: 1056–1065, June 1933
Kitutsi, M. Japanese physician
REACTION—for pregnancy.
   Milk-diagnosis of pregnance (!) and diseases. Sapporo, Bungeido, 1915. 10 pp.

Kjeldahl, Johann. Danish chemist. 1849-1900
METHOD—for determination of amount of nitrogen in an organic compound.
En ny methode til kvaelstofbestemmelse i organiske stoffer. Medd. f. Carlsberg Lab., Kjøbenhavn, 2: 1-27, 1883
Neue Methode zur Bestimmung des Stickstoffs in organischen Körpern. Z. anal. Chem., 22: 366-382, 1883

Klapp, Rudolf. Marburg surgeon. 1873-
OPERATION—osteotomy.
Demonstrationen aus der praktischen chirurgie . . . 3. Anspitzende Osteotomie . . . Arch. klin. Chir., 177: 688-694 (692-694), 1933
OPERATION—for slipping patella.
Die Operationen an der unteren Extremität von Rudolf Klapp in Berlin. In: *Chirurgische Operationslehre.* By A. Bier, H. Braun and H. Kuemmell, Leipzig, 1920. 5: 330-668
TREATMENT—of scoliosis.
Funktionelle Bedeutung der Skoliose. Jena, Fischer, 1907. 95 pp.

Klauder, Joseph Victor. Philadelphia dermatologist. 1888-
ERYSIPELOID—fish hand.
Erysipeloid and swine erysipelas in man: a clinical and bacteriological review; swine erysipelas in the United States. J. A. M. A., 86: 536-541, Feb. 20, 1926

Klausen, S. W. See Clausen

Klausner, E. Prague dermatologist
SEROREACTION or TEST—for syphilis.
Ueber eine klinisch verwendbare Kutanreaktion auf tertiäre Syphilis. Wien. klin. Wschr., 26: 973-974, June 12, 1913
Die Kutireaktionen bei Syphilis mit besonderer Berücksichtigung der Pallidinreaktion. Arch. Dermat. u. Syph., 120: Orig., 444-522, June 1914

Klawans, A. H. See A. E. Kanter

Klebs, Theodor Albrecht Edwin. Berlin bacteriologist. 1834-1913
BACILLUS—Klebs-Löffler, of diphtheria.
Ueber Diphtherie; ihre parasitäre Natur, Verhältniss des localen Prozesses zur allgemeinen Infection, Contagiosität, Therapie (Chirurgie) und Prophylaxe. Verh. d. Cong. f. Inn. Med., 2 Cong., 2: 125-154 (138-154), 1883
TUBERCULIN—
Die Behandlung der Tuberculose mit Tuberculocidin. Hamburg, 1892
Transmitted syphilis to apes.
Ueber Syphilis-Impfung bei Thieren und über die Natur des syphilitischen Contagiums. Prag. med. Wschr., 3: 409-411, Oct. 9, 1878
Das Contagium der Syphilis. Eine experimentelle Studie. Arch. exp. Path. Pharmak., 10: 161-221, Feb. 25, 1879

Klecki, Valerian v. Krakau physician
BASAL BOUILLON—for studying fermentation.
Ein neuer Buttersäuregarungserreger (Bacillus saccharobutyricus) und dessen Beziehungen zur Reifung und Lochung des Quargelkases. Zbl. Bakt., 2 Abt., 2: 249-258 (254), May 9, 1896

Kleeberg, K. See J. Rudisch

Klein, Alexander. Amsterdam bacteriologist. 1865-

METHOD—of staining spores.
Eine einfache Methode zur Sporenfärbung. Zbl. Bakt., 25: 376-379, 1899

Klein, B. Kiew bacteriologist
TEST—for glucose and lactose in urine.
Zum bakteriologischen Nachweise von Zuckerarten im Harne with P. Soliterman, Dtsch. med. Wschr., 52: 959-960, June 4, 1926

Klein, Carl Christian von. Stuttgart surgeon. 1771-1825-
OPERATION—for trigeminal neuralgia.
Ueber die Möglichkeit der Zerstörung des Gesichtsnerven bei seinem Austritt aus dem Schädel. J. d. Chir. u. Augenh., 3: 46-61, 1822

Klein, Karl. Cologne physician
AGAR—alkaline serum.
Ein neuer Diphtheriennährboden. Dtsch. med. Wschr., 46: 297 (only), Mar. 11, 1920

Kleinberg, Samuel. New York surgeon. 1885-
BRACE—modification of Abbott b. for scoliosis.
Scoliosis. . . . New York, Hoeber, 1926. 311 pp., pp. 233-245

Kleine, Dr. German scientist
Worked out life cycle of trypanosome.
Positive Infektionsversuche mit Trypanosoma Brucei durch Glossina palpalis. Dtsch. med. Wschr., 35: 469-470, Mar. 18, 1909
Weitere wissenschaftliche Beobachtungen über die Entwicklung von Trypanosomen in Glossinen. Ibid., 924-925, May 27, 1909

Kleine, H. L. See T. K. Brown

Klemm, Paul. Dorpat surgeon. 1861-1921
TETANUS—cephalic.
Ueber den Tetanus hydrophobicus. Dtsch. Z. Chir., 29: 168-192, 1889

Klemperer, Georg. German physician. 1865-
TEST—for motor power of stomach.
Ueber die motorische Thätigkeit des menschlichen Magens. Dtsch. med. Wschr., 14: 962-966, Nov. 22, 1888
Used rabbit immune serum in treatment of pneumonia.
Versuche über Immunisirung und Heilung bei der Pneumokokkeninfection with F. Klemperer. Berl. klin. Wschr., 28: 869-875, Aug. 31, 1891

Klencke, Philipp Friedrich Hermann. German physician. 1813-1881
Showed that tuberculosis may be transmitted by cow's milk. Garrison
Uber die Ansteckung und Verbreitung der Scrophelkrankheit bei Menschen durch den Genuss der Kuhmilch. Leipzig, Kollmann, 1846. 90 pp.

Klett, A. Basel chemist
TEST—for indican in urine.
Nachweis von Indican im pathologischen Harn. Chem. Ztg., 24: 690 (only), Aug. 15, 1900

Kligler, Israel J. New York bacteriologist. 1889-1943
AGAR—yeast autolysate; culture medium.
Yeast autolysate as a culture media for bacteria. J. Bact., 4: 183-188, Mar. 1919
LEAD ACETATE AGAR—
A simple medium for the rapid differentiation of typhoid and paratyphoid bacilli. Amer. J. Pub. Health, 7: 805 (only), Oct. 1917

METHOD—
The cultivation and biological characteristics of Spiro-chaeta obermeieri (recurrentis) with O. H. Robertson, J. exp. Med., 35: 303–316, Mar. 1, 1922
SOLUTION—glucose peptone, for studying metabolism of colon-typhoid group.
Some regulating factors in bacterial metabolism. J. Bact., 1: 663–671, Jan. 1916
See also P. K. Olitsky
Klikowitsch, Stanislaus. St. Petersburg physician
Used nitrous oxide in obstetrics.
Ueber das Stickstoffoxydul als Anaestheticum bei Geburten. Arch. f. Gynek., 18: 81–108, 1881
Klimenko, W. N. St. Petersburg physician
BOUILLON—basal glycerol, for cultivation of whooping cough bacillus.
Morphologie und Biologie des Keuchhustenbacillus. Zbl. Bakt., 50: 305–315, 1909
Klimmer, Martin. German physician. 1873–
SOLUTION—nitrate peptone, to enrich cholera vibrio.
Technik und Methodik der Bakteriologie und Serologie. Berlin, Springer, 1923. p. 221
Klinck, G. H. Jr. See W. R. Bryan
Kline, Benjamin Schoenbrun. American physician. 1886–
TEST—
A microscopic slide precipitation test for syphilis with A. M. Young, J. A. M. A., 86: 928–931, Mar. 27, 1926
(Same) Second communication with A. M. Young, J. Lab. clin. Med., 12: 477–481, Feb. 1927
Klinefelter, Harry Fitch. Boston physician. 1912–
SYNDROME—
Syndrome characterized by gynecomastia, aspermatogenesis without A-Leydigism, and increased excretion of follicle-stimulating hormone with E. C. Reifenstein and F. Albright, J. clin. Endocrinol., 2: 615–627, Nov. 1942
Klinger, R. See L. Hirschfeld
Klippel, Maurice. French neurologist. 1858–
DISEASE—arthritic general pseudoparalysis.
De la pseudo-paralysie générale arthritique. Rev. d. méd., Paris, 12: 280–285, Apr. 1892
SYNDROME—short neck.
Anomalie de la colonne vertébrale par absence des vertèbres cervicales.—Cage thoracique remontant jusqu'à la base du crâne with A. Feil, Bull. Soc. anat. Paris, 87: 185–188, May 3, 1912
Un cas d'absence des vertebrés cervicales, avec cage thoracique remontant jusqu'à la base du crâne (cage thoracique cervicale) with A. Feil, Nouv. Iconogr. de la Salpetrière, 25: 223–250, 1912
Kloss, K. See H. Eppinger
Klotz, Oskar. Pittsburgh physician. 1878–1936
METHOD—gravimetric estimation of carbon in sputum.
Pulmonary anthracosis—a community disease. Amer. J. Pub. Health, 4: 887–916, Oct. 1914
METHOD—
A modified Jores' method for the preservation of colors in gross specimens with W. W. G. Maclachlan, Internat. Ass. Med. Museums Bull., 5: 59–60, June 1, 1915
Klumpke, A. Dejerine. See Dejerine-Klumpke
Knack, Andreas V. Hamburg physician. 1886–

TEST—for blood in urine.
Modifizierte Blutprobe im Urin. Dtsch. med. Wschr., 40: 1595, July 30, 1914
Ueber eine Blutprobe im Urin mit Trockenreagentien. Münch. med. Wschr., 63: 708, May 16, 1916
Knapp, Arnold Herman. New York ophthalmologist. 1869–
OPERATION—
Report of a series of extractions of cataract in the capsule after subluxation with the capsule forceps. Trans. Amer. Ophth. Soc., 13: 666–677, 1914
Report of one hundred successive extractions of cataract in the capsule after subluxation with the capsule forceps. Arch. Ophth., 44: 1–9, Jan. 1915
Knapp, Herman Jakob. New York ophthalmologist. 1832–1911
FORCEPS—
Demonstration of a roller-forceps constructed according to the mangle principle for pressing out trachoma granulations, with remarks. Trans. Amer. Ophthal. Soc., 6: 148–155, 1891
OPERATION—
On cataract extraction without iridectomy. Arch. Ophthal., 16: 54–71, 1887
STREAKS or STRIA—
On the formation of dark angioid streaks as an unusual metamorphosis of retinal hemorrhage. Ibid., 21: 289–292, Apr. 1892
Advanced inferior rectus for paralysis of superior oblique.
Three cases of tenotomy of the superior and inferior recti, with comments. Arch. Ophthal. and Otol., 4: 20–32, 1874
Used retrobulbar anesthesia.
On cocaine and its use in ophthalmic and general surgery. Arch. Ophthal., 13: 402–448, 1884
Knapp, Karl. German chemist
TEST—for sugar in urine.
Ueber eine neue Methode zur Bestimmung des Traubenzuckers. Ann. d. Chem. u. Pharm., 154: 252–254, 1870
Knapp, R. E. See F. C. Novy
Knaus, Hermann. Graz gynecologist. 1892–
METHOD—of testing reactivity of uterus to pituitrin.
Zur Ursache des Geburtseintrittes. Münch. med. Wschr., 75: 553–556, Mar. 30, 1928
THEORY—of "safe period" for intercourse.
Ueber den Zeitpunkt der Konzeptionsfähigkeit des Weibes im Intermenstruum. Ibid., 76: 1157–1161, July 12, 1929
Knies, Max. German ophthalmologist
Discovered fundamental cause of glaucoma, closing of Schlemm's canal.
Ueber das Glaucom. Arch. f. Ophthal., 22: 163–201, 1876
Knight, James. Maryland physician. 1810–
BRACE—back.
In his: Orthopaedia, or a practical treatise on the aberrations of the human form. New York, Putnam, 1874. 364 pp. p. 181; 184
Knight, Jonathan. New Haven physician. 1789–1864
TREATMENT—of aneurysm by digital compression.
Popliteal aneurism successfully treated by compression

with D. A. Tyler, Boston M. and S. J., 38: 293–296, May 10, 1848

Knisely, Melvin Henry. Chicago anatomist. 1904–
METHOD—
A method of illuminating living structures for microscopic study. Anat. Rec., 64: 499–524, Mar. 25, 1936

Knoop, Franz. Freiburg physiologist. 1875–
REACTION—for histidine.
Eine Farbenreaktion des Histidins. Beitr. chem. Physiol. Path., 11: 356 (only), 1908

Knop, Wilhelm. German chemist
REAGENT—for urea.
Stickstoffbestimmungsapparat (Azotometer). Chem. Zbl., 31: 244–254, 1860
Methode zur Bestimmung des Stickstoffs in Ammoniak- und Harnstoffverbindungen. Z. anal. Chem., 9: 226, 1870

Knott, E. K. See V. K. Hancock

Knudson, Arthur. Albany, N. Y. biochemist. 1889–
METHOD—
A chemical method of assaying the active principles of digitalis with M. Dresbach, J. Pharmacol., 20: 205–220, Oct. 1922
METHOD—
A chemical method of assaying strophanthin preparations with M. Dresbach, J. Amer. Pharm. Ass., 12: 390–396, May 1913
Studied—
Effect of high voltage cathode rays on rickets and on the activation of cholesterol with W. D. Coolidge, Proc. Soc. exp. Biol., N. Y., 24: 366–369, Jan. 1927
See also W. R. Bloor

Kobelt, Georg Ludwig. German physician. 1804–1857
TUBES—remains of tubules of wolffian body.
Die mannlichen und weiblichen Wollust-Organe des Menschen. . . . Freiburg, Emmerling, (1844). 61 pp.

Kober, Philip Adolph. American chemist. 1884–
COLORIMETER—
ESTIMATION—nephelometric, of protein in antitoxin.
Persaporation, perstillation and percrystallization. J. Amer. Chem. Soc., 39: 944–948, May 1917
METHOD—of determination of phosphatides of blood.
Nephelometric estimation of phosphorus with Grete Egerer, Ibid., 37: 2373–2381, Oct. 1915
NEPHELOMETER—
Nephelometry in the study of proteases and nucleases. J. biol. Chem., 13: 485–497, Jan. 1913
TEST—for proteins. Ibid.
Nephelometric determination of proteins; casein, globulin and albumin in milk. J. Amer. Chem. Soc., 35: 1585–1593, Oct. 1913

Koby, Frédéric Edouard. French ophthalmologist
ASTIGMATIC BEAM OF—
Une modification de la lampe à fente; utilisation d'un faisceau lumineux astigmatique. Rev. gen. d'Ophthal., Ges., 39: 53–59, 1925

Koch, E. German surgeon
METHOD—of closure of duodenal stump.
Zur Technik des Duodenalverschlusses nach Magenresektion. Zbl. Chir., 62: 2951–2955, Dec. 14, 1935

Koch, Frederick Conrad. American biochemist. 1876–

METHOD—
The estimation of urea in blood by the calorimetric urease method. In his: *Practical methods in biochemistry.* Baltimore, Williams & Wilkins, 1941. 3 ed., pp. 121–122
See also W. R. Tweedy

Koch, Robert. German physician. 1843–1910
Awarded Nobel prize in 1905.
BACILLUS—B. tuberculosis.
Die Aetiologie der Tuberculose. Berl. klin. Wschr., 19: 221–230, 1882
Also, in Italian: Gior. internaz. d. sc. med., Napoli, n. s. 4: 702–716, 1882
Also, in English: Canad. M. and S. J., 10: 649–655, 1882; Cincinnati Lancet and Clinic, n. s. 10: 428–439, 1883
Also: Klassiker der Med., No. 19, Leipzig, Barth, 1912
Also, in English: Amer. Rev. Tuberc., 25: 298–323, 1932
Also, in German and English: Medical classics, 2: 821–880, Apr. 1938
CULTURE MEDIUM—
Zur Untersuchung von pathogenen Organismen. Mitt. a. d. k. Gesundheits., 1: 1–48, 1881
LAW or POSTULATES—
Die Aetiologie der Tuberculose. Berl. klin. Wschr., 19: 221–230 (224), 1882
TUBERCULIN—old.
Weitere Mittheilungen über ein Heilmittel gegen Tuberculose. Zbl. Bakt., 8: 673–685, Nov. 18, 1890
Weitere Mittheilung über das Tuberkulin. Dtsch. med. Wschr., 17: 1189–1192, Oct. 22, 1891
TUBERCULIN—new.
Über neue Tuberkulinpräparate. Dtsch. med. Wschr., 23: 209–213, Apr. 1, 1897
Obtained pure cultures of B. anthracis.
Die Aetiologie der Milzbrandkrankheit, begründet auf die Entwicklungsgeschichte des Bacillus anthracis. Beitr. z. Biol. u. Pflanzen, Breslau, 2, Heft 2: 277–310 1877–
Also, with English transl.: Medical classics, 2: 745–820, Apr. 1938
Discovered cholera bacillus.
Bericht der nach Egypten entsendenten deutschen Cholera-Commission. Mitt. d. Ver. d. Aerzte in Nied.-Oest., 9: 258–264, 1883
Bericht über die Thätigkeit der deutschen Cholerakommission in Aegypten und Ostindien. Wien. med Wschr., 33: 1548–1550, 1883
Discussion on Conferenz zur Erorterung der Cholerafrage. Berl. klin. Wschr., 21: 478–483, Aug. 4, 188
Ueber die Cholerabakterien. Dtsch. med. Wschr., 10 725–728, Nov. 6, 1884

Koch, Sumner Leibnitz. Chicago surgeon. 1888–
METHOD—of tendon suture.
Division of the nerves and tendons of the hand with discussion of the surgical treatment and its results with M. L. Mason, S. G. O., 56: 1–39, Jan. 1933
Introduced aseptic pressure dressings in local burn therapy. See H. S. Allen
Surgical cleanliness, compression and rest as primary surgical principles in the treatment of burns. J. A M. A., 125: 612–616, July 1, 1944
See also H. S. Allen, A. B. Kanavel

KOCHER, THEODOR   233   KÖLLIKER, RUDOLPH ALBERT VON

Kocher, Theodor. Swiss surgeon. 1841–1917
Awarded Nobel prize in 1909.
OPERATION—excision of ankle joint.
Resection of the foot. In his: *Operative surgery.* New
York, Wood, 1894. pp. 206–209
OPERATION—excision of thyroid for goiter.
Zur Pathologie und Therapie des Kropfes. Dtsch. Z.
f. Chir., 4: 417–440, 1874
Exstirpation einer Struma retroesophagea. Corre-
spond. f. schweiz. Aerzte, 8: 702–705, 1878
Bericht über weitere 250 Kropfexstirpationen. Ibid.,
19, 1889
OPERATION—excision of tongue.
Ueber Radicalheilung des Krebses. Dtsch. Z. f.
Chir., 13: 134–166, 1880
OPERATION—for hernia.
Zur Radicalcur der Hernien. Correspond. f. schweiz.
Aerzte, 22: 561–576, Sept. 15, 1892
OPERATION—hypophysectomy.
*Ein Fall von Hypophysis-Tumor mit operativer Heil-
ung.* Dtsch. Z. f. Chir., 100: 13–37, 1909
OPERATION—modification of Billroth I gastro-
duodenostomy.
Zur Technik und zu den Erfolgen der Magenresection.
Correspond. f. schweiz. Aerzte, 23: 682–694, Oct.
15; 713–724, Nov. 1, 1893
*Zur Magenschirurgie bei Carcinom und bei Ulcus
simplex.* Ibid., 28: 610–623, Oct. 15, 1898
OPERATION—method of reducing dislocation of
shoulder.
Eine neue Reductionsmethode für Schulterverrenkung.
Berl. klin. Wschr., 7: 101–105, Feb. 28, 1870
REFLEX—contraction of abdominal muscles on com-
pression of testicle.
*Verletzungen und Krankheiten des Hodens und seiner
Hüllen, des Nebenhodens, Samenstrangs und der
Samenblasen.* Handb. d. allg. u. spec. Chir., 8, 2
Abth, 1–469, 1874
Performed successful drainage of gallbladder, in
June 1878.
Mannskopfgrosses Empyem der Gallenblase. Corre-
spond. f. schweiz. Aerzte, 8: 577–583, Oct. 1, 1878
Demonstrated myxedema after thyroidectomy;
called it "cachexia strumipriva".
Ueber Kropfexstirpation und ihre Folgen. Arch.
klin. Chir., 29: 254–337, 1883
Reported injury to intervertebral disk.
*Die Verletzungen der Wirbelsäule zugleich als Beitrag
zur Physiologie des menschlichen Rückenmarks.* Mitt.
Grenzgeb. Med. Chir., 1: 415–480, 1896

Kock, Joseph. German surgeon. 1846–1916
OPERATION—shortening of base of broad ligament
by vaginal route for uterine retroversion or prolapse.
Dorland
*Die normale und pathologische Lage und Gestalt des
Uterus. . . .* Bonn, Cohen, 1880. 84 pp.

Kodama, H. Japanese bacteriologist
AGAR—fuchsin sulphite serum: medium for cholera
vibrio.
Ein neuer elektiver Nährboden für Choleravibrionen.
Zbl. Bakt., 88: 433–435, Aug. 8, 1922

Koeberlé, Eugène. French surgeon. 1828–1915
FORCEPS—hemostatic.
*Opérations chirurgicales. L'hémostasie définitive rapide
par les pinces hémostatiques et la suppression de la*

*ligature out été inventées à Strasbourg en 1867 par.
. . .* Strasbourg, Schultz, 1893. 114 pp.
OPERATION—excision of uterine tumor.
Extirpation de l'utérus et des ovaires. Gaz. méd. de
Strasbourg, 23: 101, 1863
*Documents pour servir à l'histoire de l'extirpation des
tumeurs fibreuses de la matrice par la méthode sus-
pubienne.* Ibid., 24: 17, 1864

Köber, Heinrich. Breslau dermatologist. 1838–1904
DISEASE—epidermolysis bullosa hereditaria.
*Hereditäre Anlage zur Blasenbildung (Epidermolysis
bullosa hereditaria).* Dtsch. med. Wschr., 12: 21–22,
Jan. 14, 1886

Köhler, Alban. Wiesbaden roentgenologist. 1874–
DISEASE—of Pellegrini—Stieda—Köhler; calcifica-
tion of tibial collateral ligament following injury.
*Die normale und pathologische Anatomie des Hüftge-
lenkes und Oberschenkels in röntgenographischer Dar-
stellung.* Hamburg, 1905. Plate 7, Fig. 12, p. 140
DISEASE—tarsal scaphoiditis.
*Ueber eine häufige, bisher anascheinend unbekannte
Erkrankung einzelner kindlicher Knochen.* Verh.
dtsch. Röntg. Ges., 4: 110–112, 1908
Also: Münch. med. Wschr., 55: 1923–1925, Sept.
15, 1908
DISEASE—juvenile deforming metatarsophalangeal
osteochrondritis.
*Eine typische Erkrankung des 2. Metatarsophalangeal-
gelenks.* Ibid., 67: 1289–1290, Nov. 5, 1920
Introduced tele-radiography of heart.
*Technik der Herzstellung fast orthodiagraphischer
Herzphotogramme vermittels Röntgeninstrumentarien
mit kleiner Elektrizitätsquelle.* Wien. klin. Rundschau.,
19: 279–282, Apr. 23, 1905

Köhler, H. See W. Olszewski

Koehler, R. See E. Bataillon

Kölliker, Rudolph Albert von. German anatomist.
1817–1905
First demonstrated true development of spermatozoa,
showed that they originate in testicular cells and
fertilized ovum.
*Beiträge zur Kenntniss der Geschlechtsverhältnisse und
der Samenflüssigkeit wirbelloser Thiere.* Berlin, Logier,
1841
Über das Wesen der sogenannten Saamenthiere. N.
Notiz. a. d. Geb. d. Natur.—und Heilk., 19: 4–8, 1841
First to isolate smooth muscle. Garrison
Beiträge zur Kenntniss der glatten Muskeln. Z. wiss.
Zool., Leipz., 1: 48–87, 1848
Wrote first formal textbook on histology. Garrison
*Mikroskopische Anatomie, oder Geweblehre des
Menschen.* Leipzig, Engelmann, 1850–1854
Handbuch der Gewebelehre des Menschen. Leipzig,
Engelmann, 1852. 637 pp.
Showed that contraction of muscle produces an
electric current.
*Nachweis der negativen Schwankung des Muske-
stroms am natürlich sich contrahirenden Muskel* with
H. Müller, Verh. d. d. phys. med. Ges. i. Würzburg,
6: 528–533, 1856
First to investigate effect of veratrine upon muscular
contraction ("veratrinized muscle"). Garrison
*Physiologische Untersuchungen über die Wirkung
einiger Gifte.* Arch. f. path. Anat., 10: 3–7; 235–296,
(257–272, 1856)

Author of first work on comparative embryology. Garrison

Entwicklungsgeschichte des Menschen und der höheren Thiere. Leipzig, Engelmann, 1861. 468 pp.

Stated that hereditary characters are transmitted by cell nucleus. Garrison and Morton

Die Bedeutung der Zellenkerne für die Vorgänge der Vererbung. Z. wiss. Zool., Würzburg, 62: 1–46, 1885

Koelsch, G. A. See E. C. Kendall

König, Franz. German surgeon. 1832–1910

OPERATION—hypophysectomy.

In discussion of Friedmann und Maass:

Zur Totalexstirpation der Hypophysis cerebri. Berl. klin. Wschr., 37: 1040 (only), Nov. 12, 1900

OPERATION—twin flap technic for repair of cranial defect.

Der knöcherne Ersatz grosser Schädeldefekte. Zbl. Chir., 17: 497–501, July 5, 1890

Used cartilage transplants in man.

Zur Deckung von Defecten in der vorderen Trachealwand. Berl. klin. Wschr., 33: 1129–1131, Dec. 21, 1896

König, P. Göttingen physician

Coined term "chronic cystic mastitis" and introduced inflammatory theory.

Mastitic chronica cystica (interstitielle Mastitis, Cystadenoma mammae, Maladie de Reclus, etc.) Zbl. Chir., 20: 49–53, Jan. 21, 1893

Koepp, Leonhard. Halle a. S. ophthalmologist. 1884–

METHOD—of examination for detachment of vitreous body.

Die Mikroskopie des lebenden Augenhintergrundes mit starken Vergrösserungen im fokalen Lichte der Gullstrandschen Nernstspaltlampe. I. Die Theorie, Apparatur und Anwendungstechnik der Spaltlampenuntersuchung des Augenhintergrudes im fokalen Licht. Arch. f. Ophthal., 95: 282–306, Apr. 9, 1918

Kofoid, Charles Atwood. American zoologist. 1865–

METHOD—

Rapid method for detection of ova of intestinal parasites in human stools with M. A. Barber, J. A. M. A., 71: 1157–1561, Nov. 9, 1918

METHOD—of culturing amoeba and flagellates.

The advantages of Locke's blood medium in the culture of parasitic protozoa of the digestive tract with Ethel McNeil, Amer. J. Hyg., 15: 315–317, Jan. 1932

Koga, Kensai. Kioto physician

TREATMENT—of thrombo-angiitis obliterans by diluting blood by hypodermoclysis with normal salt solution.

Zur Therapie der Spontangangrän an den Extremitäten. Dtsch. Z. f. Chir., 121: 371–382, Feb. 1913

Kohman, Edward Frederick. American scientist. 1885–

MEDIUM—brain infusion.

The so-called reduced oxygen tension for growing the meningococcus. J. Bact., 4: 571–584 (577), Nov. 1919

Kohn, L. A. See C. Krumwiede

Kohs, Samuel Calmin. American psychologist. 1890–

TEST—of intelligence; block t.

Precentile norms for scaling data. J. Educ. Psychol., 9: 101, 1918

Kolaczek, Johannes. Breslau physician. 1842–1906

Described glomus tumor or angioneuroma.

Ueber das Angio-Sarkom. Dtsch. Z. f. Chir., 9: 1–48; 165–227, 1878

Kolisch, Rudolf. Vienna physician. 1867–1922

METHOD—of identification of nucleohiston in urine in cases of leukemia.

Ueber die Eiweisskörper des leukämischen Harnes mit besonderer Berücksichtigung des Histons with R. Burian, Z. klin. Med., 20: 374–380, 1896

REAGENT—for creatinine.

Eine neue Methode der Kreatininbestimmung im Harne. Zbl. inn. Med., 16: 265–269, 1895

Kolisko, A. See C. Breus

Koljubakin, S. L. Saratow surgeon

OPERATION—plastic tube from dura to drain hydrocephalus.

Die operative Therapie der Hirnwassersucht. Arch. klin. Chir., 128: 151–161, 1924

Kolle, Wilhelm. German bacteriologist. 1868–1935

VACCINE—killed cholera v.

Zur aktiven Immunisierung des Menschen gegen Cholera. Zbl. Bakt., 1 Abt., 19: 97–104, Feb. 5, 1896

See also R. F. J. Pfeiffer

Koller, Carl. Vienna and New York ophthalmologist. 1857–

Introduced cocaine as local anesthetic in operations on eye. Garrison

Ueber die Verwendung des Cocain zur Anaesthesirung am Auge. Wien. med. Bl., 7: 1352–1355, Oct. 23, 1884

Vorläufige Mittheilung über locale Anästhesirung am Auge. Klin. Mbl. Augenheilk., 22: Beilageheft, 60–63, 1884

Historical notes on the beginning of local anesthesia. J. A. M. A., 90: 1742–1743, May 26, 1928

Kolmer, John Albert. Philadelphia physician. 1886–

TEST—

Studies in the standardization of the Wassermann reaction. XXX. A new complement-fixation test for syphilis based upon the results of studies in the standardization of technic. Amer. J. Syph., 6: 82–110, Jan. 1922

Quantitative complement-fixation test in syphilis. Ibid., 496–498, July 1922

Changes in the technic of the Kolmer-Wassermann test. Amer. J. Syph. and Neurol., 19: 481–488, Oct. 1935

Introduced a poliomyelitis vaccine.

Concerning vaccination of monkeys against acute anterior poliomyelitis with special reference to oral immunization with Anna M. Rule, J. Immunol., 26: 505–515, June 1934

A successful method for vaccination against acute anterior poliomyelitis with Anna M. Rule, Amer. J. med. Sci., 188: 510–514, Oct. 1934

Kondoleon, Emmanuel. Greek surgeon

OPERATION—for elephantiasis by removal of strips of subcutaneous tissue.

Die Lymphableitung, als Heilmittel bei chronischen Oedemen nach Quetschung. Münch. med. Wsch., 59: 525–526, Mar. 5, 1912

Die chirurgische Behandlung der elefantiastischen Oedeme durch eine neue Methode der Lymphableitung. Ibid., 2726–2729, Dec. 10, 1912

Konrich, Friederich. Berlin bacteriologist

METHOD—of differentiating between tubercle and smega bacillus.

Eine neue Färbung für Tuberkelbazillen. Dtsch. med. Wschr., 46: 741 (only), July 1, 1920

Konzelmann, Frank Williamson. Philadelphia physician. 1894–

MODIFICATION—of Sparkmann technic for quantitative estimation of urobilinogen in feces and urine.
An evaluation of liver function tests. Rev. Gastroenterol., 7: 51–58, Jan.–Feb. 1940
Koontz, Amos Ralph. Baltimore surgeon. 1890–
METHOD—
Dead (preserved) fascia grafts for hernia repair: clinical results. J. A. M. A., 89: 1230–1235, Oct. 8, 1927
Kopaczewski, Wladislas. 1876–
REACTION—
La gélification du sérum par les acides organiques.
C. R. Acad. Sci., 198: 1271–1273, Mar. 26, 1934
Rôle des facteurs physiques dans la lactogélification du sérum. Ibid., 1947–1950, et seq.
Kopetzky, Samuel Joseph. New York otolaryngologist. 1876–
OPERATION—
The suppuration of the petrous pyramid: pathology, symptomatology and surgical treatment with R. Almour, Ann. Otol., Rhin. and Laryng., 39: 996–1016, Dec. 1930
Koplik, Henry. New York pediatrician. 1858–1927
SIGN or SPOTS—
The diagnosis of the invasion of measles from a study of the exanthema as it appears on the buccal mucous membrane. Arch. Pediat., 13: 918–922, Dec. 1896
Kopp, Karl. Freiburg physician
AGAR—thyroid, for cultivation of colon-typhoid group.
Ueber Wachstumsnerschiedenheit einiger Spaltpilze aug Schilddrüsennährboden. Zbl. Bakt., 17: 81–83, Jan. 26, 1895
Koppe, Leonhard. Halle a. S. ophthalmologist
EPITHELIAL PUNCTATE KERATITIS—
Klinische Beobachtungen mit der Nernstspaltlampe und dem Hornhautmikroskop. 8. Mitteilung. Über zwei weitere bisher nicht beschriebene Hornhautveränderungen im Bilde der Nernstspaltlampe. Arch. f. Ophthal., 94: 250–266, Dec. 31, 1917
TUBE—for examination of eye.
Die Mikroskopie des lebenden Augenhintergrundes mit starken Vergrösserungen im fokalen Lichte der Gullstrandschen Nernstsapltlampe. I. Mitteilung. Die Theorie, Apparatur und Anwendungstechnik der Spaltlampenuntersuchung des Augenhintergrundes in fokalen Licht. Ibid., 95: 282–306, Apr. 9, 1918
Koppel, Alice. See W. S. Frei
Koppeschaar, W. F. German chemist
SOLUTION—of bromin, used as a test.
Maassanalytische Bestimmung des Phenols. Z. anal. Chem., 15: 233–245, 1876
Korányi, Alexander von (Sandor). Hungarian physician. 1866–
TREATMENT—of leukemia by benzol.
Die Beeinflussung der Leukämie durch Benzol. Berl. klin. Wschr., 49: 1357–1358, July 15, 1912
Introduced cryoscopy of urine.
A vizelet fagypontjának diagnostikus érteke. Budapesti k. orvosegy, 1894, iki évokonyve, 1895, 74–77
Physiologische und klinische Untersuchungen über den osmotischen Druck thierischer Flüssigkeiten. Z. klin. Med., 34: 1–52, 1898
Korotkoff, Nikolai Sergieyevich. Russian physician. 1874–
METHOD—auscultatory, of determining blood pressure.

(On methods of studying blood pressure.) Izvest. imp. Voyenno-Med. Acad., St. Petersburg, 11: 365, 1905
TEST—if blood pressure in distal part is maintained after main artery is compressed, collateral circulation is adequate. Ibid.
Korsakoff, Sergiee Sergieyevich. Russian psychiatrist. 1853–1900
DISEASE or PSYCHOSIS—
Ob alkoholnom paralichie. Westnik Psychiatrii, 4, 1887
Also: Moskva, Kushnereff, 1887. 462 pp.
Ksaka, T. Peiping physiologist
His work lead to discovery of a hormone inhibiting gastric secretion ("enterogastrone").
Demonstration of the humoral agent in fat inhibition of gastric secretion with R. K. S. Lim, Proc. Soc. exp. Biol., N. Y., 27: 890–891, June 1930
Koschara, W. See P. Ellinger
Koser, Stewart A(rment). American microbiologist. 1894–
METHOD—of examining for food infections.
Suggested laboratory procedures for use in determining the cause of food poisoning. Amer. J. Pub. Health, 24: 203–208, Mar. 1934
SOLUTION—basal ammonium phosphate.
Utilization of the salts of organic acids by the colon-aerogenes group. J. Bact., 8: 493–520 (497), Sept. 1923
SOLUTION—citrate sodium ammonium phosphate, for differentiation of colon-aerogenes group.
Correlation of citrate utilization by members of the colon-aerogenes group with other differential characteristics and with habitat. Ibid., 9: 59–77 (63), Jan. 1924
SOLUTION—glycerol uric acid, for studying B. aerogenes.
The employment of uric acid synthetic medium for the differentiation of B. coli and B. aerogenes. J. infect. Dis.,23: 377–379, Oct. 1918
Koshevnikoff, Alexici Jakovlevich. Russian neurologist. 1836–1902
DISEASE—mild epilepsy. Fischer
Osobaya forma kortikalnei epilepsie. Trudi Obsh. nevropat. i psichiat. Mosk., p. 30, 1893–4
Kossa, Julius von. See Julius von Magyary-Kossa
Kossel, Albrecht. German physiologist. 1853–1927
Awarded Nobel prize in 1910, for his work on chemistry of the cell.
TEST—for histidine.
Zur Analyse der Hexonbasen with A. J. Patten, Z. physiol. Chem., 38: 39–45, May 9, 1903
TEST—for hypoxanthin.
Proved that xanthin bases are derivatives of urine. Garrison
Ueber die Herkunft des Hypoxanthins in den Organismen. Ibid., 5: 152–157, 1881
Did important work on chemistry of cell and its nucleus. Garrison
Ueber die Peptone und ihr Verhältniss zu den Eiweisskörpen. Arch. ges. Physiol., 21: 179–184, 1880
Ueber das Nuclein der Hefe. Z. physiol. Chem., 4: 290–295, 1880
Zur Chemie des Zellkerns. Ibid., 7: 7–22, 1882–3
Weitere Beiträge zur Chemie des Zellkerns. Ibid., 10: 248–264, 1886

The chemical composition of the cell. Harvey Lectures 7: 33–51, 1911
Discovered histinin.
Ueber das Histidin with F. Kutscher, Arb. a d. Physiol. Inst. zu Marburg, 1899, 8: 382–387, 1900
Discovered tymin.
Ueber das Thymin. By H. Steudel and A. Kossel, Z. physiol. Chem., 29: 303–304, 1900

Kossler, A. Prag physician
METHOD—for determination of phenol in urine.
Ueber die maassanalytische Bestimmung der Phenole im Harn with E. Penny, Z. physiol. Chem., 17: 117–139, 1893

Kost, Gotthelf. German physician
TEST—for free hydrochloric acid in gastric juice.
Ueber eine Modification der Methylviolettreaction zum Nachweis freier Salzsäure im Magensaft. Erlangen, Diss., 1887. 21 pp.

Koster, Harry. Brooklyn surgeon. 1893–
APPARATUS—
Physiological transfusion apparatus. Med. J. and Rec., 122: 286–289, Sept. 2, 1925
OPERATION—
Method for preventing or diminishing peritonitis from leakage after intestinal resection or perforation. Proc. Soc. exp. Biol. N. Y., 45: 660–662, Nov. 1940
Also: Amer. J. Surg., 53: 248–254, Aug. 1941
TECHNIC—
Spinal anesthesia with special reference to its use in surgery of the head, neck and thorax. Ibid., 5: 554–570, Dec. 1928

Kosyrew, A. A. Saratow surgeon
OPERATION—
Drainage der Hirnventrikel durch Netzstreifen. Arch. klin. Chir., 141: 691–701, Sept. 16, 1926

Kottmann, Kurt. Bern physician
METHOD—for determination of coagulation time of blood.
Der Koaguloviskosimeter mit spezieller Berücksichtigung seiner klinischen Verwendbarkeit für Gerinnungsbestimmungen des Blutes. Z. klin. Med., 69: 415–430, 1910

Kouwer, Benjamin Jan. Dutch gynecologist. 1861–1933
OPERATION—splenopexy.
Behandeling der wandelende Milt dooe splenopexis. Ned. Tijdschr. Geneesk., 31: 669–673, Oct. 12, 1895
Described ovarian pregnancy.
Een geval van overiaalzwangerschap (zwangerschap in een Graaff'schen follikel). Ned. Tijdschr. v. Verlosk en Gynaec., 8: 157–168, 1897

Kovacs, Nikolaus. Vienna scientist
TEST—for indole in bacterial cultures.
Eine vereinfachte Methode zum Nachweis der Indolbildung durch Bakterien. Z. ImmunForsch., 55: 311–315, Mar. 27, 1928

Kowalewsky, Arnold. Kasan physician
REAGENT—for albuminous substances.
Essigsaures Uranoxyd, ein Reagens auf Albuminstoffe. Z. anal. Chem., 24: 551–556, 1885

Kowalski, H. Vienna army surgeon
AGAR—glycerol lung infusions; culture medium.
Bakteriologische Untersuchungen über die Influenza. Wien. klin. Wschr., 3: 245–247, Mar. 27; 266–270, Apr. 3, 1890 (p. 245)

Kowarsky, Albert. Berlin physician

TEST—of blood for diabetes.
Eine Methode zur Bestimmung des Zuckergehaltes in kleinen Blutmengen (Finger-Blutentnahme). Dtsch. med. Wschr., 39: 1635–1636, Aug. 21, 1913
TEST—for uric acid.
Eine vereinfachte Methode zur quantitativen Bestimmung der Harnsäure im Harn. Dtsch. med. Wschr., 32: 997–998, June 21, 1906
Eine Methode zum Nachweis und zur quantitativen Bestimmung von Harnsäure in relativ kleinen Blutmengen (10 ccm). Ibid., 37: 1112–1113, June 15, 1911

Koziczkowsky, Eugen v. Bad Kissingen physician
TEST—for certain infectious diseases and urobilinogen.
Ueber den klinischen Werth der Ehrlisch'schen Dimethylamidobenzaldehydreaction. Berl. klin. Wschr., 39: 1029–1033, Nov. 3, 1902

Krabbe, Knud H. Copenhagen neurologist. 1885–
CALCIFICATION—
Facial and meningeal angiomatosis associated with calcifications of the brain cortex; a clinical and anatomopathologic contribution. Arch. Neurol. Psychiat., Chicago, 32: 737–755, Oct. 1934
DISEASE—
Beitrag zur Kenntnis der Frühstadien der diffusen Hirnsklerose (die perivasculare Marknekrose). Z. ges. Neurol. Psychiat., Orig. Bd. 20: 108–115, Oct. 25, 1913
A new familiar, infantile form of diffuse brainsclerosis. Brain, 39: 74–114, June 1916

Kraepelin, Emil. German neurologist. 1856–1926
Pioneer in experimental psychiatry; introduced a new, the modern, classification of insanity and concepts "dementia praecox" and manic-depressive insanity. Garrison
Compendium der Psychiatrie. Leipzig, Abel, 1883
Der psychologische Versuch in der Psychiatrie. Psychol. Arb., Leipz., 1: 1–91, 1896

Krafft-Ebing, Richard von. German psychiatrist. 1840–1902
Classified and described various forms of sexual inversion and perversion. Garrison
Psychopathia sexualis. Eine klinisch-forensische Studie. Stuttgart, Enke, 1886

Krainsky, A. Kiev bacteriologist
AGAR—basal starch; for cultivation of actinomyces.
Die Aktinomyceten und ihre Bedeutung in der Natur. Zbl. Bakt., 2 Abt., 41: 649–688 (665), Aug. 29, 1914
SOLUTION—starch ammonium chloride; for isolating actinomyces. Ibid., p. 657

Krajian, Aram A. Los Angeles scientist
STAIN—carbol fuchsin, for mucin.
Histological technic. St. Louis, Mosby, 1940. 272 pp. 124–125
STAIN—congo.
A new elastic tissue stain: rapid method for elastic tissue, connective tissue, fibrin and amyloid, employing congo red. Arch. Path., 18: 378–380, Sept. 1934

Kramer, Richard. Vienna ophthalmologist
DISEASE—
Episkleritis metastatica furunculiformis. Klin. Mbl. Augenheilk., 66: 441–450, Mar.-Apr. 1921

Kramer, Benjamin. Baltimore physician. 1887–
METHOD—
Method for determination of calcium in small quantities

of blood serum with J. Howland, J. biol. Chem., 43: 35–42, Aug. 1920

A simple technique for the determination of calcium and magnesium in small amounts of serum with F. F. Tisdall, Ibid., 47: 475–481, Aug. 1921

METHOD—
Direct quantitative determination of potassium and sodium in small quantities of blood. Ibid., 41: 263–274, Feb. 1920

Kramer, H. See C. A. Good

Kramer, James Gerard. Canton, Ohio physician. 1890–
Showed that sympathetic supply to peripheral vessels is distributed by regional sensory nerves. Homans
The distribution of nerves to the arteries of the arm: with a discussion of the clinical value of results with T. W. Todd, Anat. Rec., 8: 243–255, May 1914

Kramm, William. Berlin physician
REACTION—for creatinine and creatine.
Ueber ein neues Kreatininderivat. Z. med. Wiss., 35: 785–787, Nov. 6, 1897

Krarup, N. B. See H. C. Hagedorn

Kraske, Hans. Freiburg i. Br. surgeon
OPERATION—for hypertrophy of breast.
Die Operation der atrophischen und hypertrophischen Hängebrust. Münch. med. Wschr., 70: 672 (only), May 25, 1923

Kraske, Paul. German surgeon. 1851–1930
OPERATION—for carcinoma of rectum with removal of coccyx.
Die sacrale Methode der Exstirpation von Mastdarmkrebsen und die Resectio recti. Berl. klin. Wschr., 24: 899–904, Nov. 28, 1887
Ueber Resectio recti. Verh. Ges. dtsch. Naturf. u. Aerzte, 1891, Leipzig, 64: 239–242, 1892

Krasnow, Frances. New York biochemist. 1897–
AGAR—meat infusion.
A method of studying the availability of synthetic media for streptococci with Helen Rivkin and Margaret L. Rosenberg, J. Bact., 12: 385–408 (391), Dec. 1926
BROTH—sugar free veal, for cultivation of streptococci. Ibid., p. 389

Kraul, R. See H. Schmalfuss

Kraus, Ida. Chicago scientist
TEST—of liver function; cholesterol-cholesterol ester ratio.
Effect of standing on cholesterol and cholesterol ester values in human blood with Evelyn Kalal, J. Lab. clin. Med., 27: 1208–1211, June 1942

Krauss, Rudolf. Vienna physician. 1868–1932
Demonstrated a hemolysin produced by staphylococci.
Ueber Hämolysine und Antihämolysin with P. Clairmont, Wien. klin. Wschr., 13: 49–56, Jan. 18, 1900

Krause, See K. Herxheimer

Krause, Fedor. German surgeon. 1857–1937
OPERATION—excision of gasserian ganglion for trigeminal neuralgia.
Entfernung des Ganglions Gasseri und des central davon gelegenen Trigeminusstammes. Dtsch. med. Wschr., 19: 341–344, Apr. 13, 1893
OPERATION—skin grafting.
Ueber die Transplantation grosser ungestielter Hautlappen. Arch. klin. Chir., 46: 177–182, 1893
Also: Verh. dtsch. Ges. Chir., 22: 46–51, 1893

OPERATION—approach to pituitary tumor through anterior cranial fossa.
Hirnchirurgie. Dtsch. Klin., 8: 953–1024 (1004), 1909
TUBE—
Subcutane Dauerdrainage der Hirnventrikel beim Hydrocephalus. Verh. Berl. med. Ges., 39: 213–221, June 17, 1909

Krause, Friedrich. Posen physician
AGAR—gelatin urea; for detection of typhoid bacilli.
Beitrag zur kulturellen Typhusdiagnose. Arch. Hyg., Berl., 44: 75–100 (94), 1902

Krause, H. C. See J. E. v. Purkinje

Krause, Wilhelm. German anatomist. 1833–1910
BULBS OF—ovoid glands penetrated by one or more nerve fibers.
CORPUSCLE—round end-bulbs.
Die terminalen Körperchen der einfach sensiblen Nerven. Hannover, Hahn, 1860. 271 pp.

Krauss, Dr.
TEST—for melanin in urine.
Zum Melaninnachweis. Münch. med. Wschr., 71: 1704 (only), Nov. 28, 1924

Krebs, Martin. Leipzig physician. 1895–
LEUKOCYTE INDEX—obtained by dividing percentage of neutrophils by percentage of lymphocytes.
Der Leukocytenindex. Klin. Wschr., 2: 2206–2208, Nov. 26, 1923

Krehbiel, Gustav A. A. New York physician
TEST—for bile pigments in urine.
Nachweisung von Gallenfarbstoff im Harne. Wien. med. Wschr., 33: 9 (only), Jan. 6, 1883

Kreidl, A. See J. P. Karplus

Kretschmer, Ernst. German physician. 1888–
TYPES—
Der Körperbau der Gesunden und der Begriff der Affinität. Z. ges. Neur. Psychiat., 107: 749–757, 1927

Kretschmer, Herman Louis. Chicago surgeon. 1879–
OPERATION—
Transurethral prostatic resection with a report of 551 resections. Southern M. J., 28: 197–205, Mar. 1935

Krida, Arthur. New York surgeon. 1888–
INCISION—
A general utility incision for exploration of the knee joint. J. Bone and Joint Surg., 7: 212–214, Jan. 1925

Krieg, Robert. German surgeon. 1848–1933
OPERATION—on nasal septum.
Beiträge zur Resection der Cartilago quadrangularis narium zur Heilung der Skoliosis septi. Berl. klin. Wschr., 26: 699–701, Aug. 5; 717–720, Aug. 12, 1889

Kriege, Hermann. See Ludwig Heusner

Kries, Johannes Adolf von. German physician. 1853–1928
Wrote on function of retinal rods.
Über die Funktion der Netzhautstächen. Z. Psychol. Physiol. Sinnesorg., 9: 81–123, 1896

Krishaber, Maurice. French physician. 1836–1883
DISEASE—neuropathy affecting nerves of sensation and heart; marked by tachycardia, vertigo, hyperesthesia and sense illusions. Dorland
De la névropathie cérébro-cardiaque. Paris, Masson, 1873. 259 pp.

Krishnaswami, C. S. See A. Whitmore

Krisowski, Max. Berlin physician
SIGN—cicatricial lines radiating from mouth in inherited syphilis.
Ueber ein bisher wenig beachtetes Symptom der hereditären Lues. Berl. klin. Wschr., 32: 893–896, Oct. 14, 1895

Kristeller, Samuel. German obstetrician. 1820–1900
METHOD—of expressing fetus during labor.
Die Expressio foetus. Neues Entbindungsverfahren unter Anwendung äusserer Handgriffe. Mschr. Geburtsk. u. Frauenkr., 29: 337–387, 1867

Krönig, Georg. Berlin physician. 1859–1911
AREA or FIELD—resonance on chest due to apices of lungs.
ISTHMUS—connecting areas, anteriorly and posteriorly.
Zur Topographie der Lungenspitzen und ihrer Percussion. Berl. klin. Wschr., 26: 809–812, Sept. 16, 1889

Krönlein, Rudolf Ulrich. Zürich surgeon. 1847–1910
HERNIA—one partly inguinal and partly properitoneal.
Herniologische Beobachtungen aus der v. Langenbeck'schen Klinik. I. Hernia inguino-properitonealis incarcerata. Arch. klin. Chir., 19: 408–427, 1876
OPERATION—for facial neuralgia.
Ueber eine Methode der Resection des qweiten und dritten Astes des N. trigeminus unmittelbar am Foramen rotundum und ovale. Dtsch. Z. Chir., 20: 484–492, Aug. 25, 1884
OPERATION—modification of Billroth II gastric resection.
Vorstellung einer Patientin, bei welcher wegen Carcinoma pylori die Resectio pylori mit Erfolg ausgeführt worden ist. Abstr.: Cor.-Bl. f. schweis. Aerzte, 18: 316–317, May 15, 1888

Krogh, August. Denmark physiologist. 1874–1920
Awarded Nobel prize in 1920.
(Capillaries.) In Danish, in Videnskabernes Selskabs Biol. Medd., Bd. 1, 1918
The number and distribution of capillaries in muscles with calculations of the oxygen pressure head necessary for supplying the tissue. J. Physiol., 52: 409–415, May 20, 1919
The supply of oxygen to the tissues and the regulation of the capillary circulation. Ibid., 457–474
The anatomy and physiology of capillaries. New Haven, Yale, 1922. 276 pp.
CALORIMETER—
The changes in respiration at the transition from work to rest with J. Linhard, J. Physiol., 53: 431–437, May 18, 1920

Krogius, Frans Ali Bruno. Finland surgeon. 1864–1939
OPERATION—for hemangioma of scalp.
Zur Behandlung des Angioma arteriale racemosum der Schädeldecken. Zbl. Chir., 32: 1025–1029, Sept. 30, 1905
OPERATION—for slipping patella.
Zur operativen Behandlung der habituellen Luxation der Kniescheibe. Ibid., 31: 254–257, 1904

Krokiewicz, Anton. Krakow physician
TEST—for bile pigments in urine.
Eine sehr empfindliche Reaction auf Gallenfarbstoffe im Harne als Modification der Ehrlichschen Methode

mit Diazobensolsulphosäure with J. Batko, Wien. klin. Wschr., 11: 173–174, Feb. 24, 1898

Krompecher, Edmund. Budapest pathologist. 1870–1926
TUMOR—rodent ulcer.
Der drüsenartige Oberflächenepithelkrebs. Beitr. path. Anat., 28: 1–41, 1900

Kronberger, Hans. German physician. 1884–
TEST—for pathological urine.
Das Prinzip der Gramschen Färbung als Grundlage einer prognostische allgemein verwertbaren Urinprobe. Dtsch. med. Wschr., 43: 750–751, June 14; 1363, Oct. 25, 1917

Krückmann, Emil Paul Ernst Olaf Friedrich. Leipzig ophthalmologist. 1865–
BORDER LEAF AND BORDER SKIN OF—optic nerve.
Ueber die Entwicklung und Ausbildung der Stutzsubstanz im Sehnerven und in der Netzhaut. Klin. Mbl. Augenheilk., 44: 162–191, 1917

Krueger, Albert Paul. American bacteriologist. 1901–
METHOD—
A method for the preparation of bacterial antigens. J. infect. Dis., 53: 237–238, Sept.–Oct. 1933

Krüger, Friedrich. German physician. 1862–
Made early studies on fibrinogen content of fetal blood.
Ueber das Verhalten des fötalen Bluts im Momente der Geburt. Arch. path. Anat., 106: 1–21, Oct. 2, 1886

Krüger, Martin. Berlin chemist
REACTION—
Zur Kenntniss des Adenins und Hypoxanthins. Z. physiol. Chem., 18: 423–458 (430), 1894

Krukenberg, Friedrich Ernst. German gynecologist. 1871–
TUMOR—
Ueber das Fibrosarcoma ovarii mucocellulare (carcinomatodes). Arch. Gynaek., 50: 287–321, 1896

Krukenberg, Hermann. German surgeon. 1863–
Described "gall-bladder colic" without stone or infection.
Ueber Gallenblasenkoliken ohne Gallensteine. Berl. klin. Wschr., 40: 667–668, July 20, 1903

Krumbhaar, Edward Bell. Philadelphia pathologist. 1882–
Described case of complete heart block entirely independant of lesion of His bundle. Garrison
Adams-Stokes' syndrome, with complete heart-block, without destruction of the bundle of His. Arch. intern. Med., 5: 583–595, June 1910

Krumwiede, Charles. New York physician. 1879–1930
AGAR—gelatin serum.
ANAEROBIC PLATES—
Fusiform bacilli. Isolation and cultivation with Josephine Pratt, J. infect. Dis., 12: 199–201, Mar. 1913
BRILLIANT GREEN—
The use of brilliant green for the isolation of typhoid and paratyphoid bacilli from feces with Josephine S. Pratt and Helen I. McWilliams, Ibid., 18: 1–13, Jan. 1916
MEDIUM—alkaline egg, for Sp. cholerae.
Cholera with Josephine S. Pratt and Marie Grund, Ibid., 10: 134–141, Mar. 1912
MEDIUM—triple sugar.
A triple-sugar modification of the Russell double-sugar

medium with L. A. Kohn, J. med. Res., 37: 225–227, Nov. 1917

TESTS—absorption, to identify organism of enteric group.

Agglutinin absorption with Georgia Cooper and Dorothy J. Provost, J. Immunol., 10: 55–239, Jan. 1925

TEST—to determine types of pneumococcus.

Determination of the type of pneumococcus in the sputum of lobar pneumonia: a rapid, simple method with E. Valentine, J. A. M. A., 70: 513–515, Feb. 23, 1918

See also W. H. Park

Kruse, Harry Dayton. American biochemist. 1900– Established magnesium as indispensable in diet.

Studies on magnesium deficiency in animals. I. Symptomatology resulting from magnesium deprivation with Elsa R. Orent and E. V. McCollum, J. biol. Chem., 96: 519–539, May 1932

Kruse, Walther. Bonn bacteriologist. 1864–1943

DISEASE—bacillary dysentery of Shiga-Kruse.

Über die Ruhr als Volkskrankheit und ihren Erreger. Dtsch. med. Wschr., 26: 637–639, Oct. 4, 1900

Krýnski, Leon. Cracow surgeon

METHOD—

Zur Technik der Ureterenimplantation in den Mastdarm. Zbl. f. Chir., 23: 73–75, Jan. 25, 1896

Kubeshima, T. Tokio physician

AGAR—

Ueber einen Hämoglobinextrakt-Soda-Agar als Elektionährboden für Choleravibrionen. Zbl. Bakt., 70: 202–208 (203), Aug. 4, 1913

Kubie, Lawrence Schlesinger. New York physician. 1896–

DRAINAGE—forced, of cisterns.

Intracranial pressure changes during forced drainage of the central nervous system. Arch. Neurol. Psychiat., Chicago, 16: 319–328, Sept. 1926

Forced drainage of the cerebro-spinal fluid in relation to the treatment of infections of the central nervous system. Ibid., 19: 997–1005, June 1928

Kuchenbecker, A. German scientist

TEST—for aromatic amino-compounds in urine.

Über den Nachweis aromatischer Amidoverbindungen im Harn. Zbl. Gewerbehyg. Unfallverhut., 8: 68–69, Apr. 1920

Küchler, Heinrich. German physician. 1828–1873 Introduced test-type for examination of vision.

Schriftnummerprobe für Gesichtsleidende. Darmstadt, Diebl, 1843. 4 pp.

Kühne, Willy. German histologist. 1837–1900

PHENOMENON—passage of a continuous current through a living muscle fiber causes an undulation proceeding from positive toward negative pole.

Secundäre Erregung vom Muskel zum Muskel. Z Biologie., 24: 383–422, 1888

Proved that muscle plasma is coagulable (1859) and fluid within living fiber (1863). Garrison

Ueber die gerinnbare Substanz der Muskeln. Mschr. d. k. Akad. d. Wiss. z. Berl., pp. 493–497, 1859

Untersuchungen über Bewegungen und Veränderungen der contraktilen Substanzen. Arch. Anat. Physiol., Lpz., pp. 564–642; 748–835, 1859

Untersuchungen über Protoplasma und die Contractilität. Leipzig, Engelmann, 1864. 158 pp.

Investigated digestion of proteids by pancreatic juice. Garrison

Ueber die Verdauung der Eiweisstoffe durch den Pankreassaft. Arch. path. Anat., 39: 130–174, 1867

Investigated proteolytic enzyme in pancreas, calling it trypsin. Garrison

Über das Trypsin. Verh. d. naturh.-med. Ver. zu Heidlb., n. F., 1: 194–198; 233, 1874–77

Extracted light sensitive substance in retina, visual purple.

Ueber den Sehpurpur. Untersuch. a. d. physiol. Inst., Heidelb., 1: 15–103; Z05; 109; 119; 455, 1877

Chemische Vorgänge in der Netzhaut. Handb. d. Physiol. ed. by L. Hermann, Leipzig, Vogel, 3, pt. 1: 235, 1879

On the photochemistry of the retina and on visual purple. London, Macmillan, 1878. 104 pp.

Investigated intermediate products of peptic and intestinal digestion, isolating many new substances and naming them. Garrison

Ueber die nächsten Spaltungsproducte der Eiweisskörper. Z. Biologie., Munich, 19: 159–208, 1883; 20: 11, 1884; 22: 409; 423, 1886; 25: 358, 1888

Kulz, Rudolph Eduard. German physician. 1845–1895

Studied B-oxybutyric acid in relation to diabetic coma. Garrison

Ueber eine neue linksdrehende Säure (B-Oxybuttersäure). Z. Biologie., 20: 165–178, 1884; 23: 329–339, 1887

Kummell, Hermann. Hamburg surgeon. 1852–1937

DISEASE or SPONDYLITIS or KYPHOSIS—

Die rareficirende Ostitis der Wirbelkörper. Verh. Ges. dtsch. Naturf. u. Aertze, 64: 282–285, 1891

Ueber die traumatischen Erkrankungen der Wirbel säule. Dtsch. med. Wschr., 21: 180–181, 1895

Kunstler, J. See A. Giard

Kuntscher, Gerhard. Kiel surgeon. 1902–

METHOD—steel nail in medullary cavity in treatment of fracture.

Die Technik der Marknagelung des Oberschenkels. Zvl. Chir., 67: 1145–1153, June 22, 1940

Küss, Georges. Paris physician. 1867–1936

Demonstrated that children of consumptives are not born tuberculous but are liable to become so.

De l'hérédité parasitaire de la tuberculose humaine. Paris, Asselin and Hauzeau, .1898. 431 pp.

Kuster, Ernst Georg Ferdinand. German surgeon. 1839–1930

OPERATION—thoracotomy for empyema.

Ueber die Grundsätze der Behandlung von Eiterungen in Staarwandigen Höhlen, mit besonderer Berücksichtigung des Empyems der Pleura. Dtsch. med. Wschr., 15: 185–187, Mar. 7; 254–257, Mar. 28, 1889

OPERATION—on ureter for hydronephrosis.

Ein Fall von Resection des Ureter. Arch. klin. Chir., 44: 850–854, 1892

Kustner, H. See C. W. Prausnitz

Küttner, Hermann. Breslau surgeon. 1870–1932

METHOD—of resection of cancer of rectum, with delayed anastomosis.

Der Mastdarmkrebs und seine chirurgische Behandlung. Med. Klin., 25: 4–8, Jan. 4, 1929

See also O. Förster

Kugelmass, Isaac Newton. New York physician. 1896–

DIET—for patients who have had inadequate intake of protein and foods containing vitamin C.
Clinical control of chronic hemorrhagic states in childhood. J. A. M. A., 102: 204–210, Jan. 20; 287–291 Jan. 27, 1934
See also F. W. Bancroft

Kuhlmann, Frederick. American psychologist. 1876–1941
TEST—
A median mental age method of weighing and scaling mental tests. J. Appl. Psychol., 11: 181–198, 1927–28
A new scale of intelligence test with some new measures. Proc. Amer. Ass. ment. Defic., 62 sess., pt. 1, 47–55, 1938

Kuhn, Dr. German physician
TEST—for diabetes.
Ueber die Formalinreaktion bei Diabetes. Münch. med. Wschr., 54: 1055–1056, May 21, 1907

Kuhn, Charles. Mexico
TEST—
Recherches des pigments biliaires dans l'urine. J. Pharm. Chim., Paris, 8 s., 8: 546–549, Dec. 16, 1928

Kuhn, Ernst. German physician. 1873–
MASK—produces artificial hyperemia, used in treatment of pulmonary tuberculosis.
Die Lungensaugmaske in Theorie und Praxis. Berlin, Springer, 1911. 35 pp.

Kuhn, Franz. German physician. 1866–1929
Introduced intratracheal insufflation method of anesthesia, 1900. Garrison and Morton
Perorale Tubagen mid und ohne Druck. Dtsch. Z. f. Chir., 77: 148–207, Feb. 1905

Kuhnt, Hermann. German surgeon. 1850–1925
OPERATION—on frontal sinus.
Ueber die entzündlichen Erkrankungen der Stirnhöhlen und ihre Folgezustände. Wiesbaden, Bergmann, 1895. 267 pp.

Kukán, Franz. German ophthalmologist
APPARATUS—
Ergebnisse der Blutdruckmessungen mit einem neuen Ophthalmodynamometer. Z. Augenheilk., 90: 166–191, Oct. 1936

Kulenkampff, Dietrich. German surgeon. 1880–
METHOD—of excision of pelvis.
Ueber Resektion einer Beckenhälfte und Exarticulatio interilio-abdominalis. Beitr. klin. Chir., 68: 768–794, 1910

Kull, Harry. Dorpat anatomist
METHOD—for mitochondria.
Eine Modifikation der Altmann'schen Methode zum Färben der Chondriosomen. Anat.,Anz., 45: 153–157, Nov. 22, 1913

Kulp, Walter Leroy. New Haven bacteriologist. 1890–
AGAR—trypsinized casein; culture medium.
Comparative study of bactobacillus acidophilus and bactobacillus bulgaricus with L. F. Rettger, J. Bact., 9: 357–394 (363), July 1924

Kultschitzky, N. Cracow histologist
MODIFICATION—of Weigert method or stain for myelin sheaths.
Über die Färbung der markhaltigen Nervenfasern in den Schnitten des Centralnervensystems mit Hämatoxylin und mit Karmin. Anat. Anz., 5: 519–524, Aug. 22, 1890

Kummer, Ernst. Genf surgeon. 1861–1933

METHOD—
Experimentelles über submucöse Resection von Darm und Magen. Verh. dtsch. Ges. f. Chir., 20: 121–131, 1891

Kummer, R. H. See R. Chodat

Kundrat, Hans. German physician. 1845–1893
DISEASE—
Ueber Lympho-Sarkomatosis. Wien. klin. Wschr., 6: 211–213, Mar. 23; 234–239, Mar. 30, 1893

Kuntz, Albert. St. Louis physician. 1879–
Described—
Distribution of the sympathetic rami to the brachial plexus: its relation to symapthectomy affecting the upper extremity. Arch. Surg., 15: 871–877, Dec. 1927

Kupperman, Herbert S. Augusta, Ga. scientist
TEST—
A two and six-hour pregnancy test with R. B. Greenblatt and C. R. Noback, J. clin. Endocrinol., 3: 548–550, Oct. 1943
The two-hour pregnancy test with R. B. Greenblatt, Sçuth. med. J., 39: 158–165, Feb. 1946

Kupressoff, J. Russian physician
CENTER—spinal c. for sphincter of bladder.
Ke phiziologii joma mochevago puzirja (sphincteris versicae urinariae). St. Petersburg, 1870. 13 pp.

Kurzrok, Raphael. American obstetrician. 1895–
Demonstrated—
The inhibition of lactation during the puerperium by testosterone propionate with C. P. O'Connell, Endocrinology, 23: 467–478, Oct. 1938

Kussmaul, Adolf. German physician. 1822–1902
APHASIA—voluntary refraining from speech, as in insane.
Die Störungen der Sprache. Versuch einer Pathologie der Sprache. Suppl. to Ziemssen: Handb. d. spez. Path. u. Therap., 1877. Vol. 12
BREATHING—hyperpnea in diabetic acidosis.
COMA and SIGN—coma and air-hunger in diabetic acetonuria.
Zur Lehre von Diabetes Mellitus. Ueber eine eigenthümliche Todesart bei Diabetischen, über Acetonämie, Glycerin-Behandlung des Diabetes und Einspirtzungen von Diastase in's Blut bei dieser Krankheit. Dtsch. Arch. klin. Med., 14: 1–46, Aug. 14, 1874
DISEASE or PARALYSIS—ascending spinal paralysis. Garrison
Ueber die fortschreitende Bulbärparalyse und ihr Verhältniss zur progressiven Muskelatrophie. Samml. klin. Vortr., No. 54 (Inn. Med. No. 20), pp. 439–476, 1873
PULSE—paradoxical.
Ueber schwielige Mediastino-Pericarditis und den paradoxen Puls. Berl. klin. Wschr., 10: 433–435, Sept. 15; 445–449, Sept. 22; 461–464, Sept. 29, 1873
SYMPTOM—convulsions and coma due to absorption in disease of stomach.
Ueber die Behandlung der Magenerweiterung durch eine neue Methode mittelst der Magenpumpe. Dtsch. Arch. klin. Med., 6: 455–500, Dec. 23, 1869
First to diagnose mesenteric embolism in living subject. Garrison
Zur Diagnose der Embolie der Arteriae mesentericae. Würz. med. Z., 5: 210, 1864
First accurately described inflammatory disease of medium and small arteries.

Ueber eine bisher nicht beschriebene eigenthümliche Arterienerkrankung (Periarteritis nodosa), die mit Morbus Brightii und rapid fortschreitender allgemeiner Muskellähmung einhergeht with R. Maier, Dtsch. Arch. klin. Med., 1: 484–518, Feb. 1, 1866
Employed thoracentesis.
Sechzehn Beobachtungen von Thoracocentese bei Pleuritis, Empyem und Pyopneumothorax. Ibid., 4: 1–32 Feb. 28, 1868
One of the first users of stomach tube with lavage, for gastric dilatation from pyloric obstruction. See SYMPTOM
Described and coined term word-blindness. Garrison
See APHASIA

Kutscher, F. See A. Kossel

Kutscher, Karl. German physician
GAR—serum placenta.
Ein Beitrag zur Züchtung des Meningococcus. Zbl. Bakt., 45: 286–288, 1908

Kuttner, Arthur. German physician. 1862–
Wrote important work on radiology of accessory nasal sinuses.

Die entzündlichen Nebenhöhlenerkrankungen der Nase im Röntgenbild. Berlin, Wien, Urban und Schwarzenberg, 1908

Kuttner, Theodore. New York physician. 1877–1947
METHOD—for determination of inorganic phosphate.
Micro colorimetric studies. I. A molybdic acid, stannous chloride reagent. The micro estimation of phosphate and calcium in pus, plasma, and spinal fluid with Harriet R. Cohen, J. biol. Chem., 75: 517–531, Nov. 1927
METHOD—modification of.
Micro colorimetric studies. II. Estimation of phosphorus: molybdic acid-stannous chloride reagent with L. Lichtenstein, Ibid., 86: 671–676, Apr. 1930

Kwilecki, Dietrich. Breslau physician
MODIFICATION—of Esbach's method for determination of protein.
Eine Modifikation der Esbachschen Eiweissprobe. Münch. med. Wschr., 56: 1330 (only), June 29, 1909

L

Labarraque, Antoine Germain. French chemist. 1777–1850
SOLUTION—of chlorinated soda, disinfectant.
De l'emploi des chlorures d'oxide de sodium et de chaux. (Paris), Huzard, 1825. 48 pp.
Same, in English. London, Scott, 1826. 36 pp.

Labat, Louis Gaston. French-American surgeon. 1877–1934
Wrote on anesthesia.
Contribution à l'étude de l'anesthésie para-vertébrale en chirurgie gastrique et intestinale. Paris, 1920. 118 pp.
Regional anesthesia: its technic and clinical application. Philadelphia, Saunders, 1922. 496 pp.

Labbé, Ernest Marcel. French physician. 1870–1939
SYNDROME—
Crises solaires et hypertension paroxystique en rapport avec une tumeur surrénale with J. Tinel and Doumer, Bull. Soc. méd. Hôp. Paris, 46: 982–990, June 29, 1922

Laborde, Jean Baptiste Vincent. French physician. 1830–1903
FORCEPS—for grasping tongue in Laborde's respiration.
METHOD—making rhythmic traction movements on tongue to stimulate respiration in asphyxiation.
Application du procédé de traction de la langue, ou procédé de la langue au traitement de l'asphyxie par les gaz égouts, deux succès. La Tribune Méd., 23: 742–744, Nov. 24, 1892
TEST—for death.
Le signe automatique de la mort. .... Paris, Schleicher, 1900. 114 pp.

Labougle, Paul. Bordeaux physician. 1881–
SYMPTOM—
Le dédoublement du 1er temps du coeur dans son rapport avec la fatigue commencante de cet organe. Gaz. hebd. d. Sci. méd. de Bordeaux, 26: 135–138, Mar. 19, 1905

Lacassagne, Antoine Marcelin. French physician. 1884–
Discovered that carcinoma of breast can be induced by estrone benzoate in male mice.

Apparition de cancers de la mamelle chez la souris mâle, soumise à des injections de folliculine. C. R. Acad. Sci., 195: 630–632, Oct. 10, 1932

Chapelle, Mme Marie Louise La. French midwife. 1769–1821
Wrote her experience with 5000 deliveries. Garrison and Morton
Pratique des accouchemens. Paris, Bailliére, 1821–25. 3 vols.

Lackum, H. L. von. See R. A. Hibbs

Lacompte, Dr. Belgian physician
Studied pancreatic secretion.
Observation d'une fistule pancréatique chez l'homme. Ref. in: Bull. Acad. roy. de méd. de Velg., 3 s., 9: 1023, 1875

Lacy, G. R. See Sadie F. Bailey

Ladd, William Edwards. Boston surgeon. 1880–
OPERATION—
Congenital obstruction of the duodenum in children New Engl. J. Med., 206: 277–283, Feb. 11, 1932

Ladd-Franklin, Christine. Baltimore physician. 1847–1930
THEORY—of vision.
Eine neue Theorie der Lichtempfindungen. Z. Psychol. Physiol. Sinnesorg., 206: 274–307, 1881

Ladenburg, Albert. German chemist. 1842–1911
Isolated hyoscine (scopolamine).
Die natürlich vorkommenden mydriatisch wirkenden Alkaloide. Ann. Chim., 206: 274–307, 1881

Ladinski, Louis Julius. New York gynecologist. 1862–
SIGN or TEST—
Diagnosis of early pregnancy with reference to a particular sign. Med. Rec., 71: 597–600, Apr. 3, 1907

Laennec, René Théophile Hyacinthe. French physician. 1781–1826
CATARRH—asthmatic bronchitis, with viscous, pearly expectoration.
CIRRHOSIS or DISEASE—chronic, diffuse interstitial hepatitis.
INFARCT—pulmonary

SIGN—occurrence of rounded, gelatinous masses (Laennec's pearls) in sputum of bronchial asthma. Invented stethoscope; first to discover and describe "anatomic tubercle" (lupus verrucosus) Garrison; is credited for originating term "aneurysma dissecans"; originated terms "egophony", "pectoriloquy", sonorous and sibilant "rales"; first to describe and differentiate bronchiectasis, pneumothorax, hemorrhagic pleurisy, pulmonary gangrene, infarct and emphysema, and esophagitis.

De l'auscultation médiate, ou traité du diagnostic des maladies des poumons et du coeur, fondé principalement sur ce nouveau moyen d'exploration. Paris, Brosson et Chaudé, 1819. 2 vols.

Also, transl. by J. Forbes, Philadelphia, Webster, 1823

Also: 2 ed., Paris, Chaudé, 1826

Also, abstr. in: *Epoch-making contributions to medicine.* . . . by C. N. B. Camac, Philadelphia, Saunders, 1909. pp. 159–203

Also, abstr. in: F. A. Willius and T. E. Keys' *Cardiac classics.* St. Louis, Mosby, 1941. pp. 327–382

Läwen, Arthur. Marburg surgeon. 1876–
DISEASE—of Büdniger, Ludloff and Läwen; torn cartilage of knee.
Knorpelresektion bei fissuraler Knorpeldegeneration der Patella-eine Frühoperation der Arthritis deformans. Beitr. klin. Chir., 134: 265–307, 1925
Made paravertebral injection for angina pectoris.
Paravertebrale Novokaininjektion zur Differentialdiagnose intraabdominaller Erkrankungen. Abstr.: Zbl. Chir., 49: 1510–1512, Oct. 14, 1922

Lafleur, H. A. See W. T. Councilman

Lagrange. French scientist
Maintained, through his pupil J. H. Hassenfratz, that dissolved oxygen of inspired air slowly takes up carbon and hydrogen from tissues as blood courses through them. Garrison
Sur la combinaison de l'oxigène avec le carbone et l'hydrogène du sang, sur la dissolution de l'oxigène dans le sang, et sur la manière dont le calorique se dégage. Ann. d. Chim., Paris, 9: 261–274, 1791

Lagrange, Pierre Felix. French ophthalmologist. 1857–1928
OPERATION—
Traitement du glaucome chronique par l'établissement d'une cicatrice filtrante. Description d'un procédé nouveau. Rev. gén. d'Ophth., 25: 205 (only), May 31; 358 (only), Aug. 31, 1906
On the production of a filtering cicatrix in chronic glaucoma. Transl. by S. Stephenson, Ophthalmoscope, 5: 467–472, Sept. 1, 1907
On the filtering cicatrix in the cure of glaucoma. Transl. by S. Stephenson, Ibid., 6: 363–374, May 1, 1908

Laguna, Andrés. Spanish physician. 1499–1560
Described ileo-cecal valve. Garrison and Morton
Anatomica methodicus, sive de sectione humani corporis contemplatio. Parisiis, 1535
Described treatment of strictures by means of bougies. Garrison and Morton
Methodus cognoscendi extirpandique excrescentes in vesicae collo carunculas. Romae, 1551

Lahey, Frank Howard. Boston surgeon. 1880–
LOCK—
A hemostat for goiter surgery. J. A. M. A., 89: 883 (only), Sept. 10, 1927

METHOD—
The removal of broken spinal anesthesia needles. Ibid., 93: 518–519, Aug. 17, 1929
METHOD—of management of gastrojejunocolic fistula.
METHOD—of taking down a gastro-enterostomy.
METHOD—of transposing short proximal jujunal loop after dismantling of gastro-enterostomy.
The surgical management of some of the more complicated problems of peptic ulcer with S. F. Marshall, S. G. O., 76: 641–648, June 1943
OPERATION—
The technique of the two stage operation for pulsion oesophageal diverticulum. S. G. O., 43: 359–365, Sept. 1926
Esophageal diverticulum. J. A. M. A., 101: 994–997, Sept. 23, 1933
OPERATION—
An operation for pilonidal sinus. S. G. O., 48: 109–111, Jan. 1929
A further suggestion for the operative treatment of pilonidal sinuses. Ibid., 54: 521–523, Mar. 1932
OPERATION—
Two-stage abdominoperineal removal of cancer of the rectum. Ibid., 51: 692–699, Nov. 1930
A two stage abdominoperineal resection of the rectum and rectosigmoid for carcinoma with R. B. Cattell, Amer. J. Surg., 27: 201–213, Feb. 1935
OPERATION—
The surgical management of intrathoracic goiter. S. G. O., 53: 346–354, Sept. 1931
OPERATION—
Strictures of the common and hepatic ducts. Trans. Southern Sur. Soc. 49: 135–160, 1936
OPERATION—
Complete removal of the stomach for malignancy, with a report of five surgically successful cases. S. G. O., 67: 213–223, Aug. 1938
SUTURE—
A new interlocking intestinal stitch. J. A. M. A., 54: 42–45, Jan. 1, 1910
TECHNIC—
Technique of subtotal gastrectomy for ulcer with S. F. Marshall, S. G. O., 69: 498–507, Oct. 1939
TECHNIC—of resection of right colon.
Neoplasms of the cecum and ascending colon. Amer. J. Surg., 46: 3–11, Oct. 1939
See also J. H. Cunningham

Laidlaw, George Frederick. American pathologist. 1871–1937
MODIFICATION—of Bloch's dopa reaction.
Melanoma studies. II. A simple technique for the dopa reaction with S. N. Blackberg, Amer. J. Path., 8: 491–498, Sept. 1932
SILVER STAIN—for silver-negative fibroblastic cells.
Silver staining of the skin and of its tumors. Ibid., 5: 239–248, May 1929

Laidlaw, P. P. See H. H. Dale, W. Smith

Laidley, J. W. S. See R. K. Lee-Brown

Lake, Richard. English otologist. 1861–
OPERATION—for recurrent attacks of vertigo by destruction of labyrinths.
Ménière's disease. Brief note in Lancet, 1: 434; 1057, 1904

Lam, Conrad Ramsey. Detroit surgeon. 1905–

METHOD—
Heparin administration: methods and results in thirty cases. Ann. Surg., 114: 205–211, Aug. 1941

Lamarck, Jean Baptiste Pierre Antoine de Monet. French naturalist. 1744–1829

THEORY—acquired characteristics may be transmitted. Garrison
"Structure follows function."
Philosophie zoölogique. . . . Paris, Baillière, 1809

Lamb, B. H. See W. B. Wherry

Lamb, R. B. See R. N. Harger

Lambert, Adrian Van Sinderen. New York surgeon. 1872–

OPERATION—
Treatment of diffuse dilatation of esophagus by operation; description of a hitherto unpublished method; report of a case. S. G. O., 18: 1–9, Jan. 1914

Lambert, Alexander. New York physician. 1861–1939

TREATMENT—
The obliteration of the craving for narcotics. J. A. M. A., 53: 985–989, Sept. 25, 1909
The treatment of drug addiction. Ibid., 56: 503–504, Feb. 18, 1911

Lambert, Samuel Waldron. American physician. 1859–1942

TREATMENT—
Medical treatment of gastric ulcer. Amer. J. med. Sci., 128: 975–984, Dec. 1904
The Lenzhartz treatment of gastric ulcer. Ibid., 135: 18–25, Jan. 1908

TREATMENT—
Poisoning by mercuric chloride and its treatment with H. S. Patterson. Arch. intern. Med., 16: 865–879, Nov. 1915

Lambl, Wilhelm Dusan. Charkow physician. 1824–1895

First described Entameba histolytica; Giardia lamblia. Osler.
Beobachtungen und Studien aus dem Franz-Joseph-Kinderspital. 1860. Thiel I.

Lambret, Oscar. Lille surgeon. 1872–

OPERATION—for gastroptosis.
Traitement chirurgical de la ptose gastrique par suspension et coulissage de la grande courbure. Pr. méd., 37: 1613–1616, Dec. 11, 1929

OPERATION—reconstruction of thumb.
Résultat élaigné d'une transplantation du gros orteil en remplacement du pouce. Bull. Soc. Chir., 46: 689–695, May 5, 1920

Lambrinudi, Constantine. London surgeon. 1890–1943

OPERATION—
New operation on drop-foot. Brit. J. Surg., 15: 193–200, Oct. 1927

La Motte, Guillaume Mauquest de. French obstetrician. 1665–1737

Extended use of podalic version to head presentations. Garrison
Traité complet des accouchements. Paris, d'Houry, 1721

Lamotte, Joubert. French physician

Wrote first account of fecal concretions in vermiform appendix. H. A. Kelly
Ouverture du cadavre d'une personne morte d'une tympanite. J. de méd., chir. et phar., 24: 65, 1766

Lancaster, Walter Brackett. American ophthalmologist. 1863–

OPERATION—
A satisfactory operation for muscle shortening or advancement. Amer. J. Ophth., 1: 161–168, Mar. 1918
Operation to shorten a rectus muscle with buried sutures. Ibid., 14: 482–488, June 1931

TECHNIC—
Lancaster's technique of cataract extraction. By K. L. Roper, Ibid., 26: 540–550, May 1943

Lancefield, Rebecca Craighill. American bacteriologist. 1895–

METHOD—
A serological differentiation of human and other groups of hemolytic streptococci. J. exp. Med., 57: 571–595, Apr. 1, 1933

REACTION—precipitin, for grouping streptococci.
The antigenic complex of streptococcus haemolyticus. I. Demonstration of a type-specific substance in extracts of Streptococcus haemolyticus. Ibid., 47: 91–103, Jan. 1, 1928, et seq.
See also A. R. Dochez

Lancereau, E. See R. Dalimier

Lancereaux, Étienne. Paris physician. 1829–1910

DIABETES—mellitus with marked emaciation.
De la polyurie (diabète insipide). Paris, Delahaye, 1869. 91 pp.
Notes et réflexions a propos de deux cas de diabète sucré avec altération du pancréas. Bull. Acad. Méd. Paris, 2 s., 6: 1215–1240, Nov. 13, 1877
Le diabète maigre, ses symptômes, son évolution, son pronostic et son traitement; ses rapports avec les altérations du pancréas. Étude comparative du diabète maigre et du diabète gras. Coup d'oeil rétrospectif sur les diabètes. L'Union méd., 3 s., 29: 161–167, Jan. 31, 1880

Lancisi, Giovanni Maria. Italian physician. 1654–1720

He noted hypertrophy and dilatation of heart as causes of sudden death, first described valvular vegetations and gave classification of cardiac diseases. Garrison
De subitaneis mortibus. Romae, Buagni, 1707. 243 pp.
Suggested malaria is transmitted by mosquito. Garrison
De noxiis palundum effluviis. Rome, 1717
Described cardiac syphilis.
De motu cordis et aneurysmatibus. Neapoli, 1738. 219 pp.

Landau, Albin. Sweden physician

METHOD—microsedimentation of erythrocytes.
Microsedimentation (Linzenmeier-Raunert method); its serviceability and significance in pediatrics; use of a modified apparatus with simplified technic, also serviceable in ambulant practice. Amer. J. Dis. Child., 45: 691–734, Apr. 1933

Landau, Wilhelm. German physician

TEST—color t. for syphilis.
Untersuchungen über eine Reaktion luetischer Sera mit einem Jodöl-Reagens. Wien. klin. Wschr., 26: 1702–1705, Oct. 16, 1913

Landerer, Albert Sigmund. German physician. 1854–1904

TREATMENT—injections of cinnamic acid for tuberculosis.

Die Behandlung der Tuberculose mit Zimmtsäure. Leipzig, Vogel, 1892. 96 pp.

Landis, Eugene Markley. Philadelphia physician. 1901–
TEST— (see also J. H. Gibbon, Jr.)
Effects of alternate suction and pressure on circulation in the lower extremities with J. H. Gibbon, Jr., Proc. Soc. exp. Biol., 30: 593–595, Feb. 1933
A simple method of producing vasodilatation in the lower extremities, with reference to its usefulness in studies of peripheral vasocular disease with J. H. Gibbon, Jr., Arch. intern. Med., 52: 785–808, Nov 1933
See also J. H. Gibbon, Jr., T. Lewis

Landmann, G. A. See W. H. Robey

Landois, Leonard. German physician. 1837–1902
TEST—for carbon monoxide in blood.
Verfahren zur Ausmitteilung des Kohlenoxydgases im Blute. Dtsch. med. Wschr., pp. 996–997, Nov. 3, 1892
Discovered that hemolysis of blood cells results when human blood is mixed with blood of other animals in vitro.
Die Transfusion des Blutes. Versuch einer physiologischen Begründung nach eigenen Experimental-Untersuchungen. Mit Berücksichtigung der Geschichte, der Indicationen, der operativen Technik und der Statistik. Leipzig, Vogel, 1875. 358 pp.

Landolt, E. See L. de Wecker

Landouzy, Louis Théophile Joseph. French physician. 1845–1917
ATROPHY—of muscles of face and scapulohumeral region.
De la myopathie atrophique progressive; myopathie sans meuropathie, débutant d'ordinaire dans l'enfance, par la face. Rev. de Med., 5: 81–117, 1885
Contribution à l'étude de la myopathie atrophique progressive (myopathie atrophique progressive, à type scapulo-huméral) with J. J. Dejerine, C. R. Soc. Biol., 8 s., 3: 478–481, Nov. 6, 1886
DISEASE—infectious icterus.
Fièvre bilieuse ou hépatique. Gaz. d. Hôp., Paris, 56: 809–810, Sept. 6, 1883
Typhus hépatique. Ibid., 913–914, Oct. 6, 1883
LAW—
De la déviation conjuguée des yeux et de la rotation de la tête par excitation ou paralysie des 6e et 11e paires; . . . Bull. Soc. anat. de Par., 54: 293–352, 1879
SCIATICA—
De la sciatique et de l'atrophie musculaire qui peut la compliquer. Arch. gén. de méd., Paris, 1: 303–325, Mar.; 424–443, Apr.; 562–578, May 1875

Landry, Jean Baptiste Octave. French physician. 1826–1865
DISEASE—acute ascending paralysis.
Note sur la paralysie ascendante aiguë. Gaz. hebd. de méd., 6: 472–474, July 9; 486–488, Aug. 5, 1859

Landsberg, J. W. See M. M. Wintrobe

Landsteiner, Karl. Austrian-American scientist. 1868–1943
Awarded Nobel prize in 1930.
METHOD—of preparation of alcoholic extract of antigen for Wassermann test.
Zur Frage der Komplementbindungsreaktionen bei Syphilis with O. Pötzl, Wien. klin. Wschr., 20: 1565–1567, Dec. 12, 1907

Established blood grouping.
Zur Kenntniss der antifermentativen, lytischen und agglutinierenden Wirkungen des Blutserums und der Lymphe. Zbl. Bakt., 27: 357–362, Mar. 23, 1900
Ueber Agglutinationserscheinungen normalen menschlichen Blutes. Wien. klin. Wschr., 14: 1132–1134, Nov. 14, 1901
Reported two successful intraperitoneal inoculations of monkeys with spinal cord obtained from two fatal cases of poliomyelitis.
Uebertragung der Poliomyelitis acuta auf Affen with E. Popper, Z. ImmunForsch., 2: 377–390, 1909
Discovered Rh factor.
Agglutinable factor in human blood recognized by immune sera for rhesus blood, with A. S. Wiener, Proc. Soc. exp. Biol., N. Y., 43: 233 (only), Jan. 1940

Lane, Edward F. New Britain, Conn. scientist
METHOD—
A method for the rapid fixation of tissue sections. J. Lab. clin. Med., 9: 653–654, June 1924

Lane, Sir William Arbuthnot. London surgeon. 1856–1943
DISEASE—intestinal stasis.
The operative treatment of chronic constipation. London, Nisbet, 1909
KINK—
The obstruction of the ileum which develops in chronic intestinal stasis. Lancet, 1: 1193–1194, Apr. 30, 1910
The kink of the ileum in chronic intestinal stasis. London, Nisbet, 1910. 12 pp.
OPERATION—for cerebral decompression.
The applicability of the parting tool or angular gouge to the surgery of the skull. Brit. med. J., 2: 1050 (only), Nov. 11, 1893
OPERATION—
Cleft palate. Clin. Jour., 10: 65–72, May 26, 1897
OPERATION—short-circuiting of colon.
Chronic constipation and its medical and surgical treatment. Brit. med. J., 1: 700–702, Apr. 1, 1905
OPERATION—
Excision of a cancerous segment of the oesophagus: restoration of the esophagus by means of skin flap. Ibid., 1: 16–17, Jan. 7, 1911
PLATES—
The operative treatment of fractures. Ibid., 1: 1037–1038, May 4, 1907

Lane-Claypon, Janet Elizabeth. London physiologist. 1877–
Attributed changes in mammary gland during pregnancy to fetus.
An experimental inquiry into the factors which determine the growth and activity of the mammary glands with E. H. Starling, Proc. roy. Soc., S. B., 77: 505–522, Feb. 12, 1906

Lang, A. See J. G. Hopkins

Langdon-Brown, Sir Walter. See Sir Walter Langdon Brown

Lange, Carl Friedrich August. German-American physician. 1883–
AGAR—starch: for diagnosis of cholera.
Ein neuer Nährboden für die Choleradiagnose. Z. Hyg. InfektKr., 81: 138–153, 1916
TEST—
Ueber die Ausflockung von Goldsol durch Liquor cerebrospinalis. Berl. klin. Wschr., 49: 897–901, May 6, 1912

Die Ausflockung kolloidalen Goldes durch Zerebrospinalflüssigkeit bei luetischen Affektion des Zentralnervensystems. Z. f. Chemotherap., 1: 44–78, 1913

Lange, F. Wiesbaden physician

TEST—for acetone in urine.

Eine Ringprobe auf Azeton. Münch. med. Wschr.. 53: 1764–1765, Sept. 4, 1906

Lange, Kurt. New York physician. 1906–

TEST—

The use of fluorescein to determine the adequacy of the circulation with L. J. Boyd, Med. Clin. N. Amer., 26: 943–952, May 1942

Use of fluorescein method in establishment of diagnosis and prognosis of peripheral vascular diseases with L. J. Boyd, Arch. intern. Med., 74: 175–184, Sept. 1944

Lange, Otto. St. Petersburgh ophthalmologist. 1852–1913

SCLERAL LAMP—

Zur Diagnose des intraoculären Sarkoms. Klin. Mbl. Augenheilk., 22: 410–413, 1884

Lagenbeck, Bernard Rudolf Konrad von. German surgeon. 1810–1887

AMPUTATION—

Ueber Resection des Fussgelenks bei Schussgracturen desselben, nebst Vorstellung eines Falles von subperiostaler Resection der Diaphyse der Tibia und Fibula. Berl. klin. Wschr., 15: 29–32, Jan. 23, 1865

OPERATION—for cleft palate.

Operation der angeborenen totalen Spaltung des harten Gaumens nach einer neuen Methode. Dtsch. Klin., 12: 231–232, June 15, 1861

Die uranoplastik mittelst Ablösung des mucös-periostalen Gaumenüberzuges. Arch. f. klin. Chir., 2: 205–287, 1862

Reported transfixion in treatment of fracture of neck of femur.

In discussion of Trendelenburg's:

Vorstellung eines Falles von veraltetem Querbruch der Patella. . . . Verh. dtsch. Ges. f. Chir., 7 Cong., 1: 92–93, 1878

Langenbuch, Carl Johann August. German surgeon. 1864–1901

Performed successful cholecystectomy, July 15, 1882.

Ein Fall von Exstirpation der Gallenblase wegen chronischer Cholelithiasis. Heilung. Berl. klin. Wschr., 19: 725–727, Nov. 27, 1882

Langer, Carl Ritter von Edenberg von. German anatomist. 1819–1887

LINES—of elasticity of skin.

Zur Anatomie und Physiologie der Haut. I. Über die Spaltbarkeit der Cutis. S. B. Akad. Wiss. Wien., 1 Abt., 44: 19–46, 1861

Found lymphatics in periosteum.

Ueber das Gefässsystem der Röhrenknochen, mit Beiträgen zur Kenntniss der Baues und der Entwicklung des Knochengewebes. Ibid., 36, 1875

Also: Wien, Gerold, 1875. 40 pp.

Langer, H. German physician

METHOD—microsedimentation determination of erythrocytes.

Eine Mikromethode zur Bestimmung der Erythrocytensenkungsgeschwindigkeit with W. Schmidt, Z. Kinderheilk., 41: 72–77, 1926

Langerhans, Paul. German pathologist. 1849–1888

CELLS and CORPUSCLES—termination of nerve-fibers in rete mucosum of epidermis.

Zur pathologischen Anatomie der Tastkörper. Arch. f. path. Anat., 45: 413–417, 1869

ISLANDS—in pancreas.

Beiträge zur microkopischen Anatomie der Bauchspeicheldrüse. Inaug. Dissert., Berlin, Lange, 1869. 32 pp.

Also, in German and English transl. by H. Morrison Bull. Inst. Hist. Med., 5: 259–297, Mar. 1937

LAYER—stratum granulosum of skin.

Ueber mehrschichtige Epithelien. Arch. f. path. Anat., 58: 83–92, July 19, 1873

Ueber Tastkörperchen und rete Malpighii. Arch. mikr. Anat., 9: 730–744, 1873

Langhans, Theodore. German pathologist. 1839–1915

CELLS—giant-cells of tubercle.

Die Uebertragbarkeit der Tuberkulose auf Kaninchen Habilitationsschrift. Marburg, Koch, 1867. 66 pp.

METHOD—for obtaining permanent mounts with iodine.

STAIN—iodine, for glycogen.

Ueber Glykogen in pathologischen Neubildungen und den menschlichen Eihäuten. Arch. f. path. Anat., 120: 28–67, Apr. 1, 1890

Described cellular pathology of Hodgkin's disease.

Das maligne Lymphosarkom (Pseudoleukämie). Ibid., 54: 509–537, 1872

Referred to "Hurthle cell tumors."

Ueber die epithelialen Formen der malignen Struma. Ibid., 189: 69–188, 1907

Langley, John Newport. English physiologist. 1852–1925

Studied reflexes from sympathetic ganglion. Garrison

The arrangement of the sympathetic nervous system, based chiefly on observations upon pilo-motor nerves. J. Physiol., 15: 176–244, 1894

On reflex action from sympathetic ganglia. Ibid., 16: 410–440, 1894

Defined "autonomic system."

The autonomic nervous system. Brain, 26: 1–26, 1903

Langworth, H. Virginia. See A. B. Wadsworth

Langworthy, C. F. See W. O. Atwater

Lanken, K. Hamburg physician

SOLUTION—fungus infusion; culture medium.

Ueber den Pilznährboden Much-Pinner with M. Meyer, Zbl. Bakt., 86: 510–512, July 8, 1921

Lannelongue, Odilon Marc. French surgeon. 1841–1911

Transplanted thyroid for cretinism.

Transplantation du corps thyroide sur l'homme. Bull. Méd., Paris, 4: 225, 1890

Lantzounis, Leonidas A. New York surgeon. 1898–

OPERATION—

Congenital subluxation of the fifth toe and its correction by a periosteocapsuloplasty and tendon transplantation. J. Bone and Joint Surg., 22: 147–150, Jan. 1940

Lanz, Otto. Amsterdam surgeon. 1865–1935

OPERATION—for slipping patella.

Sehnenplastik bei habitueller Luxation der Patella. Cor.-Bl. f. schweiz. Aerzte, 34: 270–272, Apr. 15, 1904

POINT—indicating position of appendix; on bispinal line, at junction of outer and middle thirds.

Der McBurney'schen Punkt. Zbl. Chir., 35: 185–190, Feb. 15, 1908

Lanza, Anthony Joseph. American physician. 1884–

CLASSIFICATION—of Lanza and Childs, of stages of silicosis pathology.
Miners' consumption: a study of 433 cases of the disease among zinc miners in Southwestern Missouri: with a chapter on roentgen ray findings in miners' consumption by S. B. Childs. U. S. Pub. Health Bull., No. 85, Jan. 1917, 39 pp.

Lapham, M. E. See M. H. Friedman

Lapicque, Louis. French scientist. 1866–
Defined "chronaxia," duration of excitation of tissue. Définition expérimentale de l'excitabilité. C. R. Soc. Biol., 67: 280–283, July 24, 1909

Laplace, Ernest. Philadelphia surgeon. 1861–1924
FORCEPS—
A new forceps for intestinal anastomosis. Ann. Surg. 29: 297–305, 1899

La Place, P. S. de. See A. L. Lavoisier

Laporte, A. See A. A. Lemierre

Laprade, F. See J. F. Aloy

Laqueur, E. See K. David, E. Dingemanse

Laqueur, Ludwig. German ophthalmologist. 1839–1909
Introduced use of physostigmin in glaucoma. Garrison
Ueber eine neue therapeutische Verwendung des Physostigmin. Zbl. med. Wiss., 14: 421–422, 1876
Ueber Atropin und Physostigmin und ihre Wirkung auf den intraocularen Druck. Arch. Ophthal., 23: 149–176, 1877

Lararjet, André. French surgeon. 1877–
NERVE—presacral.
Le plexus hypogastrique chez l'homme with P. Bonnet, Lyon chir., 9: 619–644, June 1, 1913

Laroche, G. See G. Guillain

LaRoque, George Paul. Richmond, Va. surgeon. 1876–1934
OPERATION—
The permanent cure of inguinal and femoral hernia: a modification of the standard operative procedures. S. G. O., 29: 507–510, Nov. 1919
The intra-abdominal operation for femoral hernia. Ann. Surg., 75: 110–112, Jan. 1922
The intra-abdominal method of removing inguinal and femoral hernia. Arch. Surg., 24: 189–203, Feb. 1932

Laroyenne, Lucien Pierre. French physician. 1831–1902
ICTERUS—neonatal, cyanotic.
Sur une maladie nouvelle des nouveau-nés. Assoc. franc. p. l'avance. d. sci., C. R., 1873, 2: 877–878, 1874
See J. B. A. Chauveau

Larsson, Sven. Stockholm ophthalmologist. 1893–
TREATMENT—
Operative Behandlung von Netzhautabhebung mi t Elektroendothermie und Trepanation: Vorläufige Mitteilung. Acta Ophthalm., København, 8: 172–183, 1930
Electro-endothermy in detachment of the retina. Arch. Ophthal., N. Y., n. s. 7: 661–680, May 1932

Larrey, Domenique Jean. French surgeon. 1766–1842
First to point out contagious nature of Egyptian ophthalmia or granular conjunctivitis. Garrison
Mémoire sur l'ophthalmie régnante en Égypte. Kaire, 1802. 17 pp.

Used a stomach tube, "an elastic esophageal sound of gum."
Relation historique et chirurgicale de l'expédition de l'armée d'orient en Egypte et en Syrie. Paris, Demonville, 1803. 480 pp. p. 286
One of the first to amputate at hip joint. Garrison
Mem. de chir. mil., Paris, 2: 180–195, 1812
Gave first account of trench foot. Garrison, Ibid., 3: 60: 1812

-Larsen, Christian Magnus Falsen Sinding. See Sinding-Larsen

Larson, Hardy William. New York chemist. 1899–
REACTION—
A histochemical method for the detection of cholesterol. J. Lab. clin. Med., 18: 848–849, May 1933

Larsen, L. N. See M. Nordland

Lasègue, Charles Ernest. Paris neurologist. 1816–1883
DISEASE—
Du délire des persécutions. Arch. gén. d. méd., 4 s., 28: 129–150, Feb. 1852
SIGN—in sciatica.
Considérations sur la sciatique. Ibid., 2: 558–580, Nov. 1864
Also in: Études médicales. Paris, Asselin et Cie., 1884. p. 303
Described—
On hysterical anorexia. Med. Times and Gaz., 2: 265–266, Sept. 6; 367–369, Sept. 27, 1873

Lashmet, Floyd Heaton. Ann Arbor physician. 1898–
DIET—
The treatment of nephritic edema by acid. J. A. M. A., 97: 918–919, Sept. 26, 1931
TEST—
An improved concentration test of renal function. II. A simple method for measuring proteinuria with L. H. Newburgh, Ibid., 100: 1328 (only), Aug. 29, 1933
See also A. C. Furstenberg

Lassar, Oskar. German dermatologist. 1849–1908
PASTE—
The treatment of inflammatory diseases of the skin. J. Cutan. and Genito-Urin. Dis., 7: 368–373, Oct. 1889

Lathrop, F. See A. C. Furstenberg

Latzer, Lenore L. See W. J. MacNeal

Latzko, Wilhelm. Vienna obstetrician. 1863–
OPERATION—cesarean section through lower uterine segment in extraperitoneal manner.
Der extraperitoneal Kaiserschnitt. Seine Geschichte, seine Technik und seine Indikationen. Wien. klin. Wschr., 22: 477–482, Apr. 8, 1909
Ueber den extraperitonealen Kaiserschnitt. Zbl. Gynäk., 33: 275–283, 1909

Lauber, Frances U. New York scientist
PROCEDURE—
Microdetermination of blood glucose with Marjorie R. Mattice, J. Lab. clin. Med., 29: 113–116, Jan. 1944

Laughlen, George Franklin. Toronto physician. 1888–
REAGENT and TEST—
A rapid test for syphilis. Canad. med. Ass. J., 33: 179–183, Aug. 1935
Reported lipoid pneumonia.
Studies on pneumonia following nasopharyngeal injections of oil. Amer. J. Path., 1: 407–414, July 1925

Augier, Stanislas. French surgeon. 1799–1872
HERNIA—
Note sur une nouvelle espèce de hernie de l'abdomen à travers le ligament de Gimbernat. Arch. gén. de méd., 2: 27–37, 1833

Launois, Pierre Emile. French physician. 1856–1914
SYNDROME—
Le syndrome hypophysaire adiposo-génital with M. Cleret, Gaz. de hôp., 83: 57–64, Jan. 13; 83–86, Jan. 18, 1910

Laurence, John Zachariah. English physician. 1830–1874
SYNDROME—polydactylism, mental deficiency, pituitary disfunction and visual defect.
Four cases of "retinitis pigmentosa," occurring in the same family, and accompanied by general imperfections of development with R. C. Moon, Ophth. Rev., Lond., 2: 32–41, 1866

Laurens, André du. 1558–1609
Wrote an early historic record of King's Evil, in which contagiousness of scrofula is maintained (struma contagiosus morbus est).
De mirabili strumas sanandi. 1609

Laurent, Emile. French scientist. 1861–1904
SOLUTION—basal ammonium sulphate.
Recherches experimentales sur les maladies des plantes. Ann. Inst. Pasteur, 13: 1–48 (43), Jan. 1899

Laurent, Louis Philippe Eugene. London physician
Introduced—
The influence of large doses of potassium chloride on myasthenia gravis with W. W. Walther, Lancet, 1: 1434–1435, June 22, 1935

Lautenschläger, Ludwig. Freiburg pharmacologist
REACTION—for morphine.
Die Diazoreaktion des Morphiums. Arch. Pharm., 257: 13–18, 1919

Lavater, Johann Caspar Christ. German scientist. 1741–1801
Estimated human character by features.
Von der Physiognomik. Leipzig, 1772
Also: Essay on physiognomy, designed to promote the knowledge and the love of mankind. Transl. by H. Hunter, London, Murray, 1789–92. 3 vol. in 5

Laveran, Charles Louis Alphonse. French Army surgeon. 1845–1922
Awarded Nobel prize in 1907. Discovered on November 6, 1880, malarial parasites in blood cells.
BODIES, CORPUSCLES—
Un nouveau parasite trouvé dans le sang de plusieurs malades atteints de fièvre palustre. Bull. Soc. méd. Hôp. Paris, 2 s., 17: 158–164, 1880
De la nature parasitaire des accidents de l'impaludisme. C. R. Acad. Sci., 93: 627–632, 1881
Also: Paris, Baillière, 1881. 104 pp.

Lavoie, Zenon Annable. Manchester, N. H. surgeon. 1872–
SPLINT—
The Lavoie splint in fracture of the humerus with G. S. Foster. Amer. J. Surg., 17: 444–447, Sept. 1932

Lavoisier, Antoine-Laurent. French chemist. 1743–1794
Discovered oxygen (according to those who claim that Priestley merely isolated it). Garrison
Mémoire sur la nature du principe qui se combine avec les métaux pendant leur calcination et qui en augmente le poids. Hist. Acad. roy. d. sc., 1775, Paris, pp. 520–526, 1778
Also: Transl. by T. Henry, 1777. Clendening
Demonstrated that respiration is in every way the analogue of combustion, the chemical products being carbon dioxid and water. Garrison
Mémoire sur la chaleur with P. S de La Place, Hist. Acad. roy. d. sc. 1780, Paris, pp. 355–408, 1784
See also A. Séquin

Laws, William V. Philadelphia surgeon. 1866–1939
SIGMOIDSCOPE—
A pneumatic sigmoidoscope. Philadelphia med. J., 5: 179–180, Jan. 20, 1900

Lawson, George. English surgeon. 1831–1903
GRAFT—large
On the transplantation of portions of skin for the closure of large granulating surfaces. Trans. Clin. Soc. Lond., 4: 49–53, 1871

Lazarus, A. See P. Ehrlich

Lazear, J. W. See W. Reed

Leadbetter, Guy Whitman. Washington, D. C. surgeon. 1893–1945
PROCEDURE—
A treatment for fracture of the neck of the femur. J. Bone and Joint Surg., 15: 931–940, Oct. 1933
Cervical-axial osteotomy of the femur: a preliminary report. Ibid., 26: 713–720, Oct. 1944

Leahy, Alice D. Rochester, N. Y. scientist
METHOD—
The diagnosis of gonococcal infections by the cultural method with C. M. Carpenter, Amer. J. Syph., Gonor. and Ven. Dis., 20: 347–363, July 1936

Leake, Chauncey Depew. California physiologist. 1896–
Introduced divinyl ether (vinethene).
The anesthetic properties of certain unsaturated ethers with Mei-Yü Chen, Proc. Soc. exp. Biol., N. Y., 28: 151–154, Nov. 1930
See also A. C. Reed

Leake, John. English physician. 1729–1792
Declared puerperal fever is contagious.
Practical observations on the child-bed fever. London, Walter, (1772)

Leake, J. P. See J. F. Anderson

Learmonth, James Rognvald. Rochester, Minn. neurologist. 1895–
OPERATION—
Resection of sensory nerves of perineum in certain irritative conditions of the external genitalia with H. Montgomery and V. S. Counseller, Arch. Surg., 26: 50–63, Jan. 1933
Advocated—
Resection of the presacral nerve in the treatment of cord bladder: preliminary report. S. G. O., 51: 494–499, Oct. 1930
Neurosurgery in the treatment of diseases of the urinary bladder. I. Anatomical and surgical considerations. J. Urol., 25: 531–549, June 1931

Leathes, John Beresford. English biochemist. 1864–
THEORY—of desaturation of fatty acids by liver.
On changes in the amount of higher fatty acids to be obtained from the liver after removal from the body. Arch. exp. Path. Pharmak., Suppl.-Bd., 327–336, 1908

Leber, Theodor. German ophthalmologist. 1840–1917–

DISEASE—hereditary optic atrophy.
Ueber hereditäre und congenital-angelegte Sehnervenleiden. Arch. Ophthal., 17: 249–291, 1871

PLEXUS—venous, in ciliary region connected with Schlemm's canal.
Studien über den Flüssigkeitswechsel im Auge. Ibid., 19: 87–185, 1873
Found how ciliary body excretes intraocular fluid and its method of excretion. Ibid.

Lebert, Hermann. French physician. 1813–1878
Gave first account of microscopic appearance of sulphur bodies in actinomycosis, in 1857; mistook them for hydatid debris. Homans
Traité d'anatomie pathologique. . . . Paris, Baillière, 1857–61. vol. 2, p. 270

Le Boë, Franciscus de. See Sylvius

Leboeuf, F. French bacteriologist
AGAR—egg white liver infusion, for cultivation of gonococci.
Sur les milieux de culture du gonocoque. C. R. Soc. Biol., 90: 768–769, Mar. 17, 1924

Lechelle, P. See G. Guillain

Leclerc, Daniel. Geneva physician. 1652–1728
Wrote first large history of medicine; first edition to Hippocrates, 1696. Garrison
Histoire de la médecine, ou l'on voit l'origine et les progrès de cet art, de siècle en siècle; les sectes, qui s'y sont formées; les noms des médecins, leurs découvertes, leurs opinions, et les circonstances les plus remarquables de leur vie. Amsterdam, Gallet, 1702. Also, 1732

Leclere, A. See W. Beckers, L. L. Grimbert

LeConte, R. G. See H. D. Dakin

Ledderhose, Georg. German physician. 1855–
Discovered glycosamin. Garrison
Ueber Glykosamin. Strassburg, Trübner, 1880. 23 pp.

Ledebt, Suzanne. See A. Frouin

Le Dentu, Jean Francois Auguste. French surgeon. 1841–1926
Reported tuberculosis of clavicle.
(*Résection de l'extrémité interne de la clavicule.*)
(Case report) Soc. de chir., 8: 545 (only) 1882

Lederer, Max. New York pathologist. 1885–
ANEMIA—
A form of acute hemolytic anemia probably of infectious origin. Amer. J. med. Sci., 170: 500–510, Oct. 1925
Three additional cases of acute hemolytic (infectious) anemia. Ibid., 179: 228–236, Feb. 1930

Ledingham, Sir John Charles Grant. English physician. 1875–
DIAGNOSTIC TEST—
Studies on variola, vaccinia, and avian molluscum. J. State Med., 34: 125–143, Mar. 1926

Leduc, Stephane Armand Nicolas. French physicist. 1853–1939
CURRENT—
Traitement des affections cérébrales par le courant continu. Gaz. méd. de Nantes, 18: 318–319, 1900

Lee, Burton James. New York surgeon. 1874–1933
Described—
Traumatic fat necrosis of the female breast and its differentiation from carcinoma with F. Adair, Ann. Surg., 72: 188–195, July 1920

Lee, O. I. See K. M. Vogel

Lee, Pearl. See T. B. Cooley

Lee, Robert. English physician. 1793–1877
GANGLION—
On the nervous ganglia of the uterus. Philos. Trans., 131: 269–275, 1841
POLYP—
Observations on fibro-calcareous tumours and polypi of the uterus. Med.-chir. Trans., 19: 94–133, 1835

Lee, Roger Irving. American physician. 1881–
METHOD—
A clinical study of the coagulation time of blood with P. D. White, Amer. J. med. Sci., 145: 495–503, Apr 1913
TEST—for calcium.
The relation of calcium to the delayed coagulation of blood in obstructive jaundice with B. Vincent, Arch. intern. Med., 16: 59–66, July 15, 1915
Produced—
The effect of antiplatelet serum on blood platelets and the experimental production of purpura hemorrhagica with O. H. Robertson, J. med. Res., 33: 323–336, Jan. 1916

Lee, Walter Estell. Philadelphia surgeon. 1879–
OPERATION—
The surgical treatment of carbuncles with T. McK. Downs, South. Med. and Surg., 89: 425–428, July 1927
See also H. D. Dakin, J. R. Elkington

Lee-Brown, Robert Kingsbury. Sydney urologist.
REFLUX—
The phenomenon of pyelovenous backflow. J. Urol., 17: 105–112, Feb. 1927
Pyelovenous backflow with J. W. S. Laidley, J. A M. A., 89: 2094–2098, Dec. 17, 1927
STAIN—modification of Mallory's aniline blue connective tissue s.
Some observations on the microscopical anatomy of the kidney with J. W. S. Laidley, J. Urol., 21: 259–274, Feb. 1929
See also F. Hinman

Leede, Carl Stockbridge. Seattle, Wash. physician. 1882–
PHENOMENON or TEST—of Rumpel–Leede, of scarlet fever.
Hautblutungen durch Stauung hervorgerufen als diagnostisches Hilfsmittel beim Scharlach. Münch. med. Wschr., 58: 293–295, Feb. 7, 1911

Leeuwen, Willem Storm van. Dutch physician. 1882–1933
Wrote—
Allergic diseases: diagnosis and treatment of bronchial asthma, hay-fever, and other allergic diseases. Philadelphia, Lippincott, 1925. 142 pp.

Leeuwenhoek, Antonius van. Delft naturalist. 1632–1723
The first to describe spermatozoa (originally pointed out to him by the student Hamen in 1674); gave the first complete account of the red blood-corpuscles (1674); discovered striped character of voluntary muscle, the sarcolemma, and the structure of crystalline lens; was the first to see protozoa under microscope (1675); found microorganisms in teeth giving, for the first time, accurate figurations of bacterial chains and clumps as well as of individual spirilla and bacilli (September 17, 1683); and demonstrated capillary anastomosis between arteries and veins. Garrison

Ontledingen en ontdekkingen. Leiden, 1693–1718. 6 vols.

Arcana naturae. Delphis Batavorum, H. a Kroonweld, 1695–1719. 4 vols.

Microscopical observations concerning blood, milk, bones, the brain, spittle, and cuticula, etc. Philos. Trans., Lond., 9: 121–128, 1674

On the circulation of the blood in fishes. . . . Ibid., 5: 461–464, 1703–12 (abridged 1809)

Also in: F. A. Willius and T. E. Keyes' *Cardiac classics.* St. Louis, Mosby, 1941, pp. 120–123

Selected works. London, Nicol. 1798–1807. 2 vol. in 1

Leffman, Henry. Philadelphia scientist. 1847–1930

TEST—for acetone in urine.

Studies of tests for acetone and aldehydes. Amer. J. Pharm., 96: 507–509, July 1924

Le Fort, Léon Clément. French surgeon. 1829–1893

OPERATION—

Nouveau procédé pour la guérison du prolapsus utérin. Bull. gén. de thérap., Paris, 92: 337–344, 1877

Legal, Emmo. Breslau physician. 1859–1922

DISEASE—

Über eine öftere Ursache des Schläfen-und Hinterhauptkopfschmerzes (Cephalalgia pharyngo-tympanica). Dtsch. Arch. f. klin. Med., 40: 201–216, Jan. 20, 1887

TEST—for acetone.

Ueber eine neue Acetonreaction und deren Verwendbarkeit zur Harnuntersuchung. Bresl. ärztl. Z., 5: 25–27, Feb. 10; 38–40, Feb. 24, 1883

Legallois, César Julian Jean. French physiologist. 1770–1814

Showed that bilateral section of vagus nerve may produce fatal bronchopneumonia. Garrison

Expériences sur le principe de la vie, notamment sur celui des mouvemens du coeur, et sur le siége de ce principe: suivies du rapport fait à la première classe de l'Institut sur celles relatives aux mouvemens du coeur. Paris, D' Hautel, 1812. 364 pp.

Also, in English Philadelphia, Thomas, 1813. 328 pp.

Discovered that a lesion of a small circumscribed area of medulla inhibits breathing: first attempt to localize center of respiration. Garrison, *Expériences . . .* p. 37

Legault, R. R. See M. E. Davis

Legg, Arthur Thornton. Boston surgeon. 1874–1939

DISEASE—Legg—Calvé-Perthes' d.: osteochondritis deformans juvenalis.

An obscure affection of the hip-joint. Boston Med. and Surg. J., 162: 202–204, Feb. 17, 1910

OPERATION—for weakness of abductor muscles of thigh in infantile paralysis.

Tensor fascia femoris transplantation in cases of weakened gluteus medius. New Engl. J. Med., 209: 61–62, July 13, 1933

Legg, John Wickham. English physician. 1843–1921

Described multiple hereditary telangiectasis or Rendu—Osler—Weber's disease.

A case of haemophilia complicated with multiple naevi. (Report) Lancet, 2: 856–857, Dec. 16, 1876

Leggett, N. B. See G. E. Brewer

Leggiadro, Vincent Emilio. Port Chester, N. Y. surgeon. 1894–

KNIFE—

A new electric meniscotomy knife. J. Bone and Joint Surg., 19: 246 (only), Jan. 1937

Legroux, Rene. French physician

SOLUTION—formol serum, for enrichment of meningococci.

Succédané du liquide d'ascitie pour quelques cultures bactériennes. C. R. Soc. Biol., 83: 466–467, Apr. 17, 1920

Legueu, Felix. French surgeon. 1863–1939

OPERATION—for vesicovaginal fistula.

De la voie transpéritonéo-vésicale pour la cure de certaines fistules vésico-vaginales opératoires. Arch. urol. Clin. de Necker, 1: 1–11, 1913

Lehman, Edwin Partridge. Charlottesville, Va. surgeon. 1888–

GROUPS—of severity of burns.

The delayed classification of burns. (Editorial). Surgery, 12: 651–653, Oct. 1942

TECHNIC—

The prevention of peritoneal adhesions with heparin: an experimental study with F. Boys, Ann. Surg., 111: 427–435, Mar. 1940

Heparin in the prevention of peritoneal adhesions: report of progress with F. Boys, Ibid., 112: 969–974, Nov. 1940

Lehman, Emmy. See F. W. Bishop

Lehmann, Willem Leopold. Dutch physician

METHOD—iodometric titration m. for glucose.

Hygienische Studien über Kupfer. V. Neue kritische Versuche über quantitative Kupferbestimmung beim Vorhandensein geringer Mengen. Arch. Hyg., Berl., 30: 250–273, 1897

Showed that fasting animals have a glycosuria.

Het arsenigzuur als genusmiddel bij diabetes mellitus. Dissertation Amsterdam, van der Post, 1873. 80 pp.

Lehmann-Facius, Hermann. Mannheim pathologist. 1899–

REACTION—a flocculation test for cancer.

Die Serodiagnostik des Karzinoms durch Präzipitive. Z. ImmunForsch., 48: 397–413, Oct. 15, 1926

Untersuchungen zum Nachweis eines Carcinolysins im Blutserum Krebskranker. Klin. Wschr., 9: 1504 (only), Aug. 9, 1930

Lehndorff, Heinrich. German physician. 1877–

Reported fractures resulting from severe muscular contractions of tetanus.

Verlaufe eines schweren Tetanus Deformitäten der Wirbelsäule und der Rippen. . . . Wien. med. Wschr., 57: 2477–2478, Dec. 14, 1907

Leiboff, S. L. New York biochemist

METHOD—

A simplified method for cholesterol determination in blood. J. biol. Chem., 61: 177–180, Aug. 1924

Leichtenstern, Otto. German physician. 1845–1900

ENCEPHALITIS—of Strumpell and L.

Ueber primäre acute haemorrhagische Encephalitis. Abstr.: Dtsch. med. Wschr., 18: 39–40, Jan. 14, 1892

Described subacute combined degeneration of spinal cord.

Ueber „progressive perniciöse Anämie bei Tabeskranken." Abstr.: Ibid., 10: 849–850, Dec. 25, 1884

Leidy, Joseph. Philadelphia physician. 1823–1891

Discovered trichinella spiralis, in a hog. (No title). Proc. Acad. Nat. Sci., Phila., 3: 107–108, Oct. 1846

Discovered bacterial flora of intestines. (No title), Ibid., 4: 225–233, Oct. 1849

Also: *A flora and fauna within living animals.* Washington, Smithsonian Inst., 1853. 67 pp.

Made first experiments in transplanting malignant tumors. Garrison, Proc. Acad. Nat. Sci., Phila., 5: 212, (only), June 1850

Suggested flies as transmitters of wound infection. Garrison

Flies as a means of communicating contagious diseases. Ibid., 23: 297 (only), 1871

Found hookworm in cat and suggested that it might also be found in man as a cause of pernicious anemia. Garrison

Remarks on parasites and scorpions. Trans. Coll. Phys., Phila., 3 s., 8: 441–443, 1886

Leifer, W. See L. Chargin

Leiner, Carl. Vienna pediatrician. 1871–1930

DISEASE—desquamative erythrodermia of infants. *Über Erythrodermia desquamativa, eine eigenartige universelle Dermatose der Brustkinder.* Arch. f. Derm., 89: 65–76; 163–189, 1908

Leishman, Sir William Bogg. British Army surgeon. 1865–1926

ANEMIA—kala-azar.

BODIES—found in spleen and liver in kala-azar. *On the possibility of the occurrence of trypanosomiasis in India.* Brit. med. J., 1: 1252–1254, May 30, 1903

METHOD—

Note on a method of quantitatively estimating the phagocytic power of the leucocytes of the blood. Ibid., 1: 73–75, Jan. 11, 1902

STAIN—

The application of Romanowsky's stain in malaria. Ibid., 1: 635–637, Mar. 16, 1901

Note on a simple and rapid method of producing Romanowsky staining in malarial and other blood films. Ibid., 2: 757–758, Sept. 1, 1901

See also A. E. Wright

Leistikow, Leo. German bacteriologist. 1847–1917

First reported cultivation of gonococcus. Garrison and Morton

. . . Resultate seiner Untersuchungen über die Tripperbacterien mit. Abstr.: Berl. klin. Wschr., 19: 500 (only), Aug. 7, 1882

Leitch, Archibald. London physician. 1878–1931

Produced cancer experimentally.

Experimental production of cancer by arsenic with E. L. Kennaway, Brit. med. J., 2: 1107–1108, Dec. 9, 1922

Leitch, D. B. See J. B. Collip

Leiter, Joseph. Vienna physician. ?–1892

COIL or TUBE—of metal, placed against body with cold water circulating through it, to reduce temperature.

Ein neuer Wärmeregulator zur Wärmeentziehung und Wärmezufuhr für den erkrankten menschlichen Körper und ein neuer Irrigations-Apparat. Wien, Bräumuller, 1881. 20 pp.

Leland, George H. Dayton, O. electrical engineer

REFRACTOR—

The Leland refractor: a method for refraction under binocular conditions by S. van Wien, Arch. Ophth., 23: 104–111, Jan. 1940

Leloir, Henri Camille Chrysostome. French dermatologist. 1855–1896

DISEASE—lupus vulgaris erythematoides.

Recherches sur l'histologie pathologique et la nature du lupus érythémateux. Ann. d. Dermat., 3 s., 1: 708–709, Aug.–Sept. 1890

Lemaire, François Jules. French physician. 1814–

Pointed out antiseptic properties of carbolic acid. Garrison and Morton

Du coaltar saponiné, désinfectant énergique. Paris, Germer-Baillière, 1860

Lemaire, P. French chemist

REACTION—

Sur une réaction colorée de l'alypine et de divers anesthésiques locaux. Repert. de pharm., 20: 194–195, May 1908

Lembert, Antoine. French surgeon. 1802–1851

SUTURE—for intestine.

Mémoire sur l'entéroraphie, avec la description d'un procédé nouveau pour pratiquer cette opération chirurgicale. Repert. gén. d'anat. et physiol. path., Paris, 100–107, 1826

Le Mesurier, A. B. See W. E. Gallie

Lemierre, André Alfred. Paris physician. 1875–

Isolated streptobacillus moniliformis from case of rat-bite fever.

Sur une nouvelle fièvre par morsure de rat with J. Reilly, A. Laporte and M. Morin, Bull. Acad. Méd. Paris, 3 s., 117: 705–713, June 22, 1937

Lemmon, William Thomas. Philadelphia physician. 1896–

METHOD—

A method for continuous spinal anesthesia. Ann. Surg. 111: 141–144, Jan. 1940

Continuous spinal anesthesia with observations on the first 500 cases with G. W. Paschal, Jr., Pennsylvania Med. J., 44 05–980, May 1941

Lempert, Julius. New York otologist. 1890–

OPERATION—

Improvement of hearing in cases of otosclerosis: a new one stage surgical technic. Arch. Otol., 28: 42–97, July 1938

Fenestra non-ovalis: a new oval window for the improvement of hearing in cases of otosclerosis. Ibid., 34: 880–912, Nov. 1941

Lempert fenestra non-ovalis with mobile stopple: a new advance in the surgical treatment for clinical otosclerosis evolved as a result of a research study of one thousand cases in which fenestration has been performed during the last seven years. Ibid., 41: 1–41, Jan. 1945

Leonard, Philipp. German scientist. 1862–

RAYS—cathode rays after they have issued from a Crookes' tube through a window of platinum foil. *Ueber Kathodenstrahlen. . . .* Berlin, de Gruyter 1920. 120 pp. 2 ed.

Lenhartz, Hermann Albert Dietrich. Hamburg physician. 1854–1910

DIET—for gastric ulcer, abundant.

Eine neue Behandlung des Ulcus ventriculi. Abstr.: Dtsch. med. Wschr., 30: 412–413, Mar. 10, 1904

Lenormant, Charles. French surgeon. 1875–

OPERATION—

Le traitement des mutilations des doigts et en particulier du pouce par les autoplasties et transplantations. Pr. méd., 28: 223–227, Apr. 17, 1920

OPERATION—

Luxation récidivante de l'épaule traitée par le procédé

d'Oudard modifié: résultat après six mois. Bull. et
mém. Soc. nat. de chir., 54: 31–33, Jan. 11, 1928
Le traitement de la luxation récidivante de l'epaule par
la création d'une butée osseuse. Rev. d'orthop., 18:
545–561, Sept. 1931
Lentz, Otto. German bacteriologist. 1873–
AGAR—malachite green infusion, for isolation of
colon-typhoid bacteria from feces.
Eine Anreicherungsmethode für Typhus- und Para-
typhusbacillen with J. Tietz, Münch. med. Wschr.,
50: 2139–2141, Dec. 8, 1903
Lentz, W. See W. Pfeiler
Leo, Hans. German physician. 1854–1927
TEST—for free hydrochloric acid.
Eine neue Methode zur Säurebestimmung im Magenin-
halt. Zbl. med. Wiss., 27: 481–485, June 29, 1889
Leonardo, Richard Anthony. Rochester, N. Y.
surgeon. 1895–
CLAMP—
An improved gastric clamp. J. Internat. Col. Surg., 2:
53–54, Jan.–Apr. 1939
Leonicenus, Nicolaus. Italian physician. 1428–1524
Author of one of the earliest of the Renaissance
tracts on syphilis.
Libellus de epidemia, quam vulgo morbum Gallicum
vocant. Venetiis, Manutii, 1497
Léopold-Levi. E. Paris physician. 1868–1933
SYNDROME—of hyperthyroidism with quiescent
periods.
Sur un travail relatif à l'instabilité thyroidienne et sa
forme paroxystique. Bull. Acad. Méd., Paris, 3 s.,
61: 586–590, May 18, 1909
Lepkovsky, S. See H. McL. Evans
Lereboullet, P. See N. A. Gilbert
Leredde, Laurent Victor Louis Emile. French
physician. 1866–
MODIFICATION—of Wassermann test.
Les erreurs de la syphilimétrie et leurs conséquences.
Bull. de derm. et de syph., 29: 321–326, Nov. 9,
1922
Leri, André. French physician. 1875–1930
Described meolorheostosis, a rare bone disease.
Une affection non décrite des os: hyperostose "en
coulée " sur toute la longeur d'un membre ou "melor-
héostose" with Joanny, Bull. Soc. méd. Hôp. Paris,
46: 1141–1145, July 21, 1922
Leriche, René. French surgeon. 1879–
OPERATION—periarterial sympathectomy.
De la causalgie envisée comme une névrite du sympa-
thique et de son traitement par la dénudation et l'ex-
cision des plexus nerveux péri-artériels. Pr. méd., 24:
178–180, Apr. 20, 1916
De la sympathectomie péri-artérielle. Ibid., 25: 513–
515, Sept. 10, 1917
Some researches on the periarterial sympathetics.
Ann. Surg., 74: 385–393, Oct. 1921
OPERATON—Lumbar sympathectomy by antero-
lateral extraperitoneal approach.
Technique des diverses sympathectomies lombaires with
R. Fontaine, Pr. méd., 41: 1819–1822, Nov. 18, 1933
Résultat, au bout d'une année, d'une ramicotomie
lombaire pour maladie de Little. Lyon chir., 23: 666–
669, June 17, 1926
Leromyez, J. See J. A. Sicard
Lermoyez, M. See G. F. I. Widal
Leroux, Claude Pierre. French accoucher. 1730–1792

METHOD—treatment of placenta previa by tampon-
ade of vagina.
Observations sur les pertes de sang des femmes en
couches, et sur le moyen de les guérir. Dijon, Frantin,
1776. 334 pp.
Leroux, L. See J. Forestier
Lésauvage, Edme. French surgeon. 1778–1852
Described tumors of spermatic cord.
Mémoire sur les tumeurs albumino-gélatineuses (fi-
breuses des auteurs). Arch. gén. de méd., 4 s., 9: 208–
219, Oct. 1845
Leschke, Erich Friedrich Wilhelm. German phy-
sician. 1887–1933
SYNDROME—
Über Pigmentierung bei Funktionsstörungen der
Nebenniere, des sympathischen Nervensystems und
bei der Recklinghausenschen Krankheit. Berl. med.
Ges., June 21, 1922
Abst.: Klin. Klin., 18: 911 (only), July 9, 1922
Abst.: Klin. Wschr., 1: 1433 (only), July 8, 1922
Lesieur, Charles. French physician. 1876–
SIGN—of Lesieur-Privey; presence of albumin in
sputum indicates pulmonary inflammation.
Sur l'albumoptysie, albumino-réaction des crachats de
H. Roner; 190 observations per sonnelles. Bull. Soc.
méd. d. hôp. de Lyon, 9: 312–321, 1910
Le Sodier, Mlle.
FORM—the macrogonococcus.
Les formes atypiques du gonocoque with J. Verge,
C. R. Soc. Biol., 92: 323–324, Feb. 7, 1925
L'Espée, Abbé, Charles Michel de. French priest.
1712–1789
Founded first school for deafmutes, in Paris, in 1755.
Wrote alphabet and several books. Garrison
La véritable manière d'instruire les sourds et muets.
Paris, Nyon l'âiné, 1784
Lespinasse, Victor Darwin. Chicago urologist. 1878–
OPERATION—
Obstructive sterility in the male: treatment by direct
vaso-epididymostomy. J. A. M. A., 70: 448–450, Feb.
16, 1918
Letterer-Siwe, Erich. German physician. 1895–
DISEASE—
Aleukämische Retikulose; (ein Beitrag zu den pro-
liferativen Erkrankungen des Retikuloendothelialap-
parates). Frankfurt. Z. f. Path., München, 30: 377–
394, 1924
Lettsom, John Coakley. Virgin Island physician.
1744–1815
Wrote original account of alcoholism, which is in-
cidentally the first paper on the drug habit; gave
original description of alcoholic multiple neuritis.
Garrison
Some remarks on the effects of lignum quassiae amarae.
Mem. Med. Soc. Lond., 1: 128–165, 1787
Leturc, M. E. French chemist
TEST—for uric acid in sediments or calculi.
Caractérisation rapide de l'acide urique dans les sédi-
ments et dans les calculs organiques. Ann. chim. anal.
12: 194–195, 1907
Leube, Wilhelm Olivier. German physician. 1842–
1912
TEST-MEAL—12 oz. soup, 4 oz. minced steak, 2 oz.
white bread, 6 oz. water.
Beiträge zur Diagnostik der Magenkrankheiten.
Dtsch. Arch. klin. Med., 33: 1–21, Mar. 20, 1883

TREATMENT—of gastric ulcer.
Ueber die Erfolge der internen Behandlung des peptischen Magengeschwürs und die Indikationen zum chirurgischen Eingreifen in dieselbe. Mitt. Grenzgeb. Med. Chir., 2: 1–16, 1897

Leuchs, Karl Julius. Berlin physician
METHOD—
Ueber Malachitgrünnährböden zum Nachweis von Typhus- und Paratyphusbacillen. Dtsch. med. Wschr., 32: 1330–1333, Aug. 16, 1906

Leunbach, Jonathan Hugh. Copenhagen physician. 1884–
PASTE—
Eine neue Form der intrauterinen Therapie mit Einführung einer antiseptischen Paste in den Uterus. Mschr. Geb. u. Gyn., 87: 509–520, 1931

Levaditi, Constantin. Paris physician. 1874–1928
METHOD—for Spirochaeta pallida in sections.
A propos de l'imprégnation au nitrate d'argent des Spirochètes sur coupes. C. R. Soc. Biol., 1: 67–68, Jan. 13, 1906
Nouvelle méthode rapide pour la coloration des spirochètes sur coupes. Ibid., 134–136, Jan. 20, 1906
See also R. Sazerac

Levasseur, Paul. French physician
SIGN—of death.
De la catalepsie au point de vue du diagnostic de la mort apparente. Rouen, Boissel, 1866. 31 pp.

Levene, Phoebus Aaron Theodore. American biochemist. 1869–
REAGENT—for amino acids.
Über die Fällbarkeit der Aminosäuren durch Phosphorwolframsäure with W. Beatty, Z. phys. Chem., 47: 149–150, 1906
See also A. L. Raymond

Lever, John Charles Weaver. London physician. 1811–1858
Found albuminous urine in connection with puerperal convulsions. Garrison
Cases of puerperal convulsions, with remarks. Guy's Hosp. Rep., 2 s., 1: 495–517, 1843

Levert, Henry S. Alabama surgeon
EXPERIMENTS—
Experiments on the use of metallic ligatures, as applied to arteries. Amer. J. med. Sci., 4: 17–23, 1829

Levin, Abraham Louis. New Orleans physician. 1880–1940
TUBE—
A new gastroduodenal catheter. J. A. M. A., 76: 1007 (only), Apr. 9, 1921

Levin, William. Portland, Ore. scientist, 1879–
METHOD—
The intradermal test as an aid in the diagnosis of undulant fever. J. Lab. clin. Med., 16: 275–281, Dec. 1930

Levine, Max. American bacteriologist. 1889–
AGAR—rosolic acid china blue peptone.
Dysentery and allied bacilli. J. infect. Dis., 27: 31–39, July 1920
MEDIUM—
Differentiation of B. coli and B. aerogenes on a simplified eosin—methylene blue agar. Ibid., 23: 43–47, July 1918
SOLUTION—crystal violet peptone.
Notes on Bact. coli and Bact. aerogenes. Amer. J. Pub. Health, 11: 21–23, Jan. 1921

Levine, Milton. Minnesota physician
TEST—
Skin sensitivity to human plasma with D. State, Science, 96: 68–69, July 17, 1942

Levine, Philip. American pathologist. 1900–
METHOD—of determining compatibility of blood specimens.
A dangerous "universal donor" detected by the direct matching of bloods with Jennie Mabee, J. Immunol. 8: 425–431, Nov. 1923

Levine, S. A. See H. L. Blumgart

Levine, Victor Emanuel. American biochemist. 1891–
TEST—
A new test for sugar in the urine. Science, 52: 391 (only), Oct. 22, 1920
TEST—
A general test for carbohydrates. Proc. Soc. exp. Biol. N. Y., 27: 830–831, May 1930
TEST—
A test for cholesterol based upon the use of sulphuric acid containing selenious acid with E. Richman, Ibid., 27: 832–833, May 1930
TEST—
A color reaction for carotene with G. E. Bien, Ibid. 31: 581–582, Feb. 1934
Reaction of trichloracetic acid and of chloral hydrat with carotene. Ibid., 32: 335–337, Nov. 1934
TEST—
*Differentiation of ergosterol from cholesterol with Frances M. McKay, Ibid., 33: 546–549, Jan. 1936
See also A. Sachs

Levinson, S. A. See W. F. Petersen
Levison, L. A. See E. Fuld

Levitt, Walter Montague. London physician. 1900–
METHOD—
Regional x-ray baths in the treatment of lymphadenoma Brit. J. Radiol., n. s., 11: 183–188, Mar. 1938

Levret, André. French accoucheur. 1703–1780
FORCEPS—
Observations sur les causes et les accidens de plusieur accouchemens laborieux, avec des remarques sur ce qui a été proposé ou mis en usage pour les terminer, et de nouveaux moyens pour y parvenir plus aisément Paris, Delaguette, 1747. 427 pp.

Levy, Fernand. French neurologist
TECHNIC—of injection of mandibular and maxillar branches of fifth nerve.
Les injections profondes dans le traitement de la névralgie facile rebelle with A. Baudouin, Pr. méd., 14 108–109, Feb. 17, 1906

Levy, R. See J. Morgenroth
Levy, Robert Louis. New York physician. 1888–
METHOD—
A simple method for determining variations in t hydrogen-ion concentration of the blood with L. G. Rowntree and W. M. Marriott, Arch. intern. Med 16: 389–405, Sept. 1915
METHOD—
Effects of induced oxygen want in patients with cardi pain with A. L. Barach and H. G. Bruenn, Amer. Heart J., 15: 187–200, Feb. 1938

Levy Simpson, Samuel. See S. L. Simpson
Lewandowsky, Felix. Bern and Hamburg dermato ogist. 1879–1921
CULTURE METHOD—
Über Impetigo contagiosa s. vulgaris, nebst Beiträg

zur Kenntnis der Staphylo- und Streptokokken bei Hautkrankheiten. Arch. Derm. Syph., Wien, 94: 163–226, 1909
Zur Impetigofrage. Ibid., 138: 438–445, 1922

Lewin, Georg Richard. German surgeon. 1820–1896
Removed a tumor from larynx by aid of laryngoscope.
Die Laryngoscopie. Beiträge zu ihrer Verwerthung für praktische Medicin. Berlin, Hirschwald, 1860. 24 pp. Abstr.: Allg. Med. Zbl. Zeitung, 7: 652–655, Oct. 12, 1861

Lewin, Louis. German physician. 1850–1929
REACTION—for proteins.
Eine Farbenreaktion auf Eiweisskörper. Ber. dtsch. chem. Ges., 46: 1796–1798, June 7, 1913

Lewin, Philip. Chicago surgeon. 1888–
SYMPTOM—differential, of Paget's disease.
Osteitis deformans (Paget's disease), with a report of three cases. J. Bone and Joint Surg., 20: 45–67, Jan. 1922
See also J. L. Miller

Lewis, D(avid) Sclater. Montreal physician. 1886–
TEST—for amylase in blood.
The diastatic ferments of the blood with E. H. Mason, J. biol. Chem., 44: 455–463, Nov. 1920

Lewis, Dean DeWitt. American surgeon. 1874–1941
INCISION—
Bleeding nipple, with plastic operation upon the breast. Surg. Clin. Chicago, 1: 117–124, Feb. 1917
OPERATION—arterial ligation in thromboangiitis obliterans.
Spontaneous gangrene of the extremities. Arch. Surg., 15: 613–626, Oct. 1927
OPERATION—for deltoid paralysis.
Trapezius transplantation in the treatment of deltoid paralysis. J. A. M. A., 55: 2211–2213, Dec. 24, 1910
See also C. F. Geschickter

Lewis, Lloyd Griffith. Baltimore urologist. 1902–
CYSTOMETER—
A new clinical recording cystometer. J. Urol., 41: 638–645, Apr. 1939

Lewis, M. J. See S. W. Mitchell

Lewis, P. A. See J. Auer, C. W. Duval, S. Flexner

Lewis, Robert Curtis. New York biochemist. 1888–
METHOD—
A method for the estimation of sugar in small quantities of blood with S. R. Benedict, J. biol. Chem., 20: 61–72, Jan. 1915
See also A. R. Peebles

Lewis, Robert Morton. New Haven obstetrician. 1886–
Advocated—
A study of the effects of theelin on gonorrheal vaginitis in children. Amer. J. Obstet. Gynaec., 26: 593–599, Oct. 1933

Lewis, Sir Thomas. English physician. 1881–1945
TEST—for acidosis.
Observations on respiration and metabolism in cardio-renal patients, with special reference to acid intoxication with J. H. Ryffel, C. G. L. Wolf, T. Cotton, G. L. Evans and J. Barcroft, J. Physiol., 46: liii–liv, June 28, 1913
THEORY—of cardiac pain in coronary occlusion.
Pain in muscular ischaemia: its relation to anginal pain. Arch. intern. Med., 49: 713–727, May 1932
Coined term auricullar fibrillation.

Auricular fibrillation: a common clinical condition. Brit. med. J., 2: 1528 (only), Nov. 27, 1909
Auricullar fibrillation and its relation to clinical irregularity of the heart. Heart, 1: 306–372, 1909–10
Named sino-auricular node "the pace-maker of the heart."
Galvanometric curves yielded by cardiac beats generated in various areas of the auricular musculature. The pace-maker of the heart. Ibid., 2: 23–40, 1910–11
Described arterial changes in Raynaud's disease.
Experiments relating to the peripheral mechanism involved in spastic arrest of the circulation in the fingers, a variety of Raynaud's disease with W. J. Kerr, Ibid., 15: 7–101, Aug. 3, 1929
Described acrocyanosis.
Observations upon the vascular mechanism in acrocyanosis with E. M. Landis, Ibid., 15: 229–246, Dec. 12, 1930
Studied—
Vasodilatation in the limbs in response to warming the body; with evidence for sympathetic vasodilator nerves in man with G. W. Pickering, Ibid., 16: 33–51, Oct. 7, 1931

Lewis, Warren Harmon. Baltimore anatomist, 1870–
First noted that dorsal lip of blastopore is center and starting point of cell differentiation and regulation of form in embryo. Garrison
Experiments on the origin and differentiation of the optic vesicle in amphibia. Amer. J. Anat., 7: 259–277, Aug. 1, 1907
See also C. R. Bardeen

Lewis, William Bevan. English pathologist. 1847–1929
Described giant cells of precentral convolution.
On the comparative structure of the cortex cerebri. Brain, 1: 79–96, Apr. 1878

Lewisohn, Richard. New York surgeon. 1875–
METHOD—
A new and greatly simplified method of blood transfusion: a preliminary report. Med. Rec., 87: 141–142, Jan. 23, 1915
Blood transfusion by the citrate method. S. G. O., 21: 37–47, July 1915

Lexer, Erich. German surgeon. 1867–1937
OPERATION—rhinoplasty.
Zur Gesichtsplastik. Arch. f. klin. Chir., 92: 749–793, 1910
OPERATION—esophagojejunogastrostomosis.
Vollständiger Ersatz der Speiseröhre. Münch. med. Wschr., 58: 1548–1550, July 18, 1911
OPERATION—for ptosis.
Ptosisoperation, Herstellung der Oberlidfalte und Herstellung des Unterlides durch Faszienzügel. Klin. Mbl. Augenheilk., 70: 464–467, Apr. 1923

Leyden, Ernst Victor von. German physician. 1832–1910
ATAXIA—pseudotabes.
Ueber acute Ataxie. Z. klin. Med., 18: 576–587, 1891
DISEASE—a form of periodic vomiting.
Ueber periodisches Erbrachen (gastrische Krisen) nebst Bemerkungen über nervöse Magenaffectionen. Ibid., 4: 605–615, 1882
NEURITIS—lipomatous n.
Ueber Poliomyelitis und Neuritis. Ibid., 1: 387–434, 1879–80

PARALYSIS—hemiplegia alterans superior.
Klinik der Rückenmarkskrankheiten. Berlin, 1875.
Vol. 2, p. 65
TYPE—of muscular dystrophy; Leyden—Möbius.
Ibid., p. 525
Leydig, Franz von. German anatomist. 1821–1908
CELLS—interstitial c. of testes.
Zur Anatomie der männlichen Geschlechtsorgane und Analdrüsen der Säugethiere. Z. wiss. Zool., 2: 1–57 (47–48), 1850
Li, C. P. New York physician
METHOD—
Cultivation of vaccine virus with T. M. Rivers, J. exp. Med., 52: 465–470, Oct. 1, 1930
Libman, Emanuel. New York physician. 1872–1946
DISEASE or ENDOCARDITIS—verucous, atypical.
SYNDROME—
A hitherto undescribed form of valvular and mural endocarditis with B. Sachs, Trans. Ass. Amer. Phys., 38: 46–61, 1923
Also: Arch. intern. Med., 33: 701–737, June 1924
Described subacute bacterial endocarditis.
On some experiences with blood-cultures in the study of bacterial infections. Johns Hopk. Hosp. Bull., 17: 215–228, July 1906
Liborius, Paul. Kronstadt bacteriologist
METHOD—for making anaerobic cultures.
Beiträge zur Kenntniss des Sauerstoffbedürfnisses der Bacterien. Z. Hyg. InfektKr., 1: 115–177, 1886
Lichtenberg, Alexander von. Berlin urologist. 1880–
OPERATION—for hydronephrosis.
Plastic surgery of the renal pelvis and ureter. J. A. M. A., 93: 1706–1708, Nov. 30, 1929
Introduced uroselectan.
Klinische Prüfung des Uroselectans with M. Swick, Klin. Wschr., 8: 2089–2091, Nov. 5, 1929
Lichtenstein, L. See T. Kuttner
Lichtenstein, M. E. See R. W. McNealy
Lichtenstein, Stefanie. Berlin physician
AGAR—blood clot infusion; culture medium.
Ueber die Herstellung des Blutnährbodens. Zbl. Bakt., 77: 362–363, Jan. 31, 1916
SOLUTION—cenovis; culture medium.
Hefenährböden aus einem Hefepräparet der Fabrik Cenovis im München. Ibid., 90: 389–391, June 28, 1923
Lichtenstern, Otto. German physician. 1845–1900
SYNDROME—
Ueber progressive perniciose Anämie bei Tabeskranken. Dtsch. med. Wschr., 10: 849–850, Dec. 25, 1884
Lichtheim, Ludwig. Bern physician. 1845–1915
APHASIA, SIGN—in subcortical aphasia, although patient cannot speak, he is able to indicate with his fingers the number of syllables in the word he is thinking of.
On aphasia. Brain, 7: 433–484, Jan. 1885
Ueber Aphasie. Dtsch. Arch. f. klin. Med., 36: 204–268, Feb. 19, 1885
Lichtman, Sol Sydney. New York physician. 1898–
TEST—
Origin and significance of tyrosinuria in disease of the liver. Arch. intern. Med., 53: 680–688, May 1934
Liébeault, Ambroise Auguste. Nancy physician. 1823–1904
Wrote important works on hypnotism. Garrison
Du sommeil et des états analogues, considérés sur tout

ou point de vue de l'action du moral sur le physique. Paris, Masson, 1866. 535 pp.
Thérapeutique suggestive. Paris, Doin, 1891
Lieberkühn, Johann Nathanael. German anatomist. 1711–1756
AMPULLA, CRYPTS, FOLLICLES, GLANDS— in mucous membrane of intestine.
De fabrica et actione villorum intestinorum tenuium hominis. Lugd. Bat., Wishof, 1745. Diss. anat.-med. 36 pp.
Liebermann, C. German chemist
TEST—for ethyl sulfide in urine.
Ueber die Thiophrenreaction mit nitrosehaltigen Schwefelsäure. Ber. dtsch. chem. Ges., 20: 3231–3234, 1887
Liebermann, Leo von Szentlörinez. Hungarian physician. 1852–1926
TEST—for proteins.
Zur Eiweissreaction mit Salzsäure. Zbl. med. Wiss., 25: 450 (only), June 18, 1887
Liebermeister, Carl von. German physician. 1833–1901
FURROWS or GROOVES—on liver.
Beiträge zur pathologischen Anatomie und Klinik der Leberkrankheiten. Tübingen, Laupp u. Siebeckm 1864. 378 pp.
RULE—in febrile tachycardia, pulse increases about eight to every degree centigrade of temperature. Dorland
Ueber Wärmeregulirung und Fieber. Samml. klin. Vortr., No. 19 (Inn. Med., No. 7), 115–138, 1871
Liebers, Dr. German physician
TEST—for albumin in urine.
Zum Eiweissnachweis im Urin. Dtsch. med. Wschr., 42: 323 (only), Mar. 16, 1916
Liebig, Justus von. German chemist. 1803–1873
REAGENT—for urea.
Reagens auf Harnstoff. Ann. d. Chem., 80: 123–124, 1852
Über einige Harnstoffverbindungen und eine neue Methode zur Bestimmung von Kochsalz und Harnstoff im Harn. Ann. d. Pharm., 85: 289–328, 1853
Prepared chloral and chloroform.
Ueber die Verbindungen, welche durch die Einwirkung des Chlors auf Alcohol, Aether, ölbildendes Gas und Essiggeist entstehen. Ibid., 1: 182–230, 1832
Liebreich, Mathias Eugenius Oscar. Berlin physician. 1839–1908
Introduced chloral and demonstrated its value.
Das Chloralhydrat, ein neues Hypnoticum und Anaestheticum, und dessen Anwendung in der Medicin. Eine Arzeneymittel-Untersuchung. Berlin, Müller, 1869. 60 pp.
Abstr.: Arch. dtsch. Ges. f. Psychiat., 16: 237–238, 1869
Liebreich, Richard. Königsberg ophthalmologist. 1830–1917
Introduced lateral illumination in microscopic investigation of living eye. Garrison
Seitliche Beleuchtung und mikroskopische Untersuchung am lebenden Auge. Arch. f. Ophthal., Berl., 1, 2 Abth., 351–356, 1855
Published first atlas of ophthalmoscopy. Garrison
Atlas der Ophthalmoscopie. Dartstellung des Augen-

*rundes im gesunden und krankhaften Zustande en-
haltend.* Berlin, Hirschwald, 1863
Also: Paris, Germer-Baillière 1863
epmann, Hugo Karl. Berlin neurologist. 1863–
1925
RAXIA—
*Das Krankheitsbild der Apraxie („motorischen
Asymoblie") auf Grund eines Falles von einseitiger
Apraxie.* Mschr. Psychiat. Neurol., 8: 15–44, July;
102–132, Aug.; 182–197, Sept. 1900
eske, Rudolf. Heidelberg physician. 1886–
LUTION—ammonium sulphate, for cultivation of
eptothrix ochracea.
ur Ernährungsphysiologie der Eisenbakterien. Zbl.
Bakt., 2 Abt., 49: 413–425 (422), Oct. 22, 1919
utaud, Joseph. French physician. 1703–1780
DY, TRIANGLE, UVULA—of bladder.
Essais anatomiques. Paris, Huart, 1742
schutz, J. German chemist
CACTION—for cholesterol.
Eine Farbenreaktion auf Cholesterin durch Oxydation.
Ber. dtsch. chem. Ges., 41: 252–255, Jan. 20, 1908
gnières, Joseph Léon Maral. Buenos Aires phy-
ician. 1868–1933
Discovered actinobacillus.
Actinobacilosis with J. Spitz, Semana Méd., 9: 207–
215, Mar. 27, 1902
lenfeld, A. See I. S. Wright
ienthal, Howard. New York surgeon. 1861–1946
CISION—
Surgical approach to the posterior mediastinum. In
his: *Thoracic surgery.* Philadelphia, Saunders, 1926.
.: 266–280
OBE—for metal foreign bodies. In his: *Imperative
urgery.* New York, Macmillan, 1901. pp. 33–35
ERATION—multiple stage resection of esophagus.
*Carcinoma of thoracic oesophagus extrapleural resec-
ion and plastic; description of an original method with
eport of a successful case without gastrostomy.* Ann.
Surg., 74: 259–279, Sept. 1921
ienthal, J. L., Jr. See A. Blalock
Iie, R. D. See C. Armstrong, J. Goldberger
n, R. K. S. See T. Kosaka
aberg, Boris E. Russian surgeon
ERATION—(devised by Tikhoff in 1922).
*nterscapulo-thoracic resection for malignant tumors of
he shoulder joint region.* J. Bone and Joint Surg.,
0: 344–349, Apr. 1928
ad, James. Scottish physician. 1716–1794
Founder of naval hygiene in England. Garrison
Treatise on the scurvy. Edinburgh, Sands, Murray
.nd Cochran, 1753
*An essay on the most effectual means of preserving the
.ealth of seamen in the royal navy. Containing cau-
ions necessary for those who reside in or visit unhealthy
ituations; with directions proper for the security of all
uch as attend sick persons in fevers, and an appendix
f observations on the treatment of diseases in hot
limates.* London, Millar, 1757, 119 pp.
adau, Arvid. Swedish pathologist. 1892–
SEASE—angioreticuloma or hemangioblastoma of
Cushing and Bailey.
*tudien über Kleinhirncysten. Bau, Pathogenese, und
Beziehungen zur Angiomatosis retinae.* Acta path. u.
microbiol. Scandinav., suppl. 1: 1–128, 1926
ademan, Edward. New York surgeon. 1797–1919

METHOD—
*Simple syringe transfusion with special cannulas. A
new method applicable to infants and adults. Prelimin-
ary report.* Amer. J. Dis. Child., 6: 28–32, July 1913
*Blood transfusion: report of 135 transfusions by the
syringe-cannula system.* J. A. M. A., 62: 993–996,
Mar. 28, 1914
Lindemann, Ludwig. München physician
TEST—for acetoacetic acid in urine.
Zum Nachweis der Azetessigsäure im Harn. Münch.
med. Wschr., pp. 1386–1388, July 18, 1905
Lindhard, Johannes. Copenhagen physiologist. 1870–
METHOD—
*Dye-methods for determining the blood-volume tested in
vitro.* Amer. J. Physiol., 76: 497–507, May 1, 1926
*A dye-method for determining the blood-volume in
man.* Ibid., 77: 669–679, Aug. 1, 1926
Lindner, Karl David. Vienna ophthalmologist. 1883–
OPERATION—
Ueber die Ptosisoperation nach Blaskovics. Klin.
Mbl. Augenheilk., 93: 1–12, July 1934
Lindo, David. British chemist
REACTION—for morphine.
Morphia reactions. Chem. News, 38: 65–66, Aug. 9,
1878
REACTION—for saccharin.
*Tests for so-called saccharine, antipyrine, and anti-
febrine.* Ibid., 58: 51–52, July 27, 1888
Lindsay, Janvier Whitton. Washington, D. C. path-
ologist. 1881–
METHOD—
Frozen sections prepared by use of "dry ice." with
E. C. Rice and M. A. Selinger, J. A. M. A., 96:
773 (only), Mar. 7, 1931
Lindstedt, A. F. Swedish surgeon
Described volvulus.
*Volvulus flexurae sigmoideae coli—Laparo-colotomia
—Helsa* with J. A. Waldenström, Upsala Läkaref.
Förhandl., 14: 513–527, 1878–79
Lindt, Wilhelm, Jr. Bern physician. 1860–1916
METHOD—for direct inspection of nasopharyngeal
space, with his palate hook.
*Die direkte Besichtigung und Behandlung der Gegend
der Tonsilla pharyngea und der Plica salpingo-
pharyngea in ihrem obersten Theil.* Arch. f. Laryngol.,
6: 47–56, 1897
Ling, Per Henrik. Swedish physician. 1776–1839
Introduced gymnastics for therapeutic purposes,
about 1813. Garrison
Gymnastikens allmänna Grunder. Üpsala, Palmblad,
1834. 239 pp. In English, Boston, 1853
Linhard, J. See A. Krogh
Links, Rudolf. German physician
REACTION—chemical, for cancer.
Chemische Frühdiagnose maligner Tumoren. Med.
Klin., 30: 165–168, Feb. 2, 1934
Linné, Carolus von. Swedish physician. 1707–1778
Originated binomial nomenclature in science, calling
each definite natural object by a generic or family
name and a specific or given name. Garrison
Systema naturae. Lugduni Batavorum, 1735
Genera plantarum. Lugduni Batavorum, Wishoff,
1737
Linser, Paul. Tübingen physician. 1871–
Advocated injection treatment of varicose veins.

Ueber die konservative Behandlung der Varicen.
Med. Klin., Berlin, 12: 897–898, Aug. 20, 1916
Lint, K. de. See W. Einthoven
Lintner, C. J. German chemist
METHOD—of preparation of soluble starch.
Studien über Diastase. J. prakt. Chem., 34: 378–394,
Oct. 13, 1886
Linton, Robert Ritchie. Boston surgeon. 1900–
TECHNIC—
*The communicating veins of the lower leg and the opera-
tive technic for their ligation.* Ann. Surg., 107: 582–
593, Apr. 1938
Linzenmeier, Georg. German physician. 1882–
METHOD—microsedimentation.
*Eine Mikromethode zur Messung der Senkungsge-
schwidigkeit der roten Blutkörperchen* with Raunert,
Zbl. Gynäk., 48: 786–790, Apr. 12, 1924
TEST—sedimentation t. of erythrocytes.
*Eine neue Schwangerschaftsreaktion und ihre theore-
tische Erklärung.* Ibid., 44: 816–820, July 24, 1920
*Die Blutkörperchensenkrungsgeschwindigkeit als dif-
ferentialdiagnostisches Hilfsmittel bei Adnexerkrank-
ungen.* Ibid., 46: 535–542, Apr. 8, 1922
Lipliawsky. Semjou. Berlin physician. 1873–
TEST—for diacetic acid in urine.
*Eine neue Methode zum sichern Nachweis von Acetes-
sigsäure im Harn.* Dtsch. med. Wschr., 27: 151–153,
Mar. 7, 1901
Lipp, Dr. Von. Munich bacteriologist
TEST—for protein in urine.
*Eine ungemein praktische, genügend genaue portative
Probe zum Eiweissnachweis im Harn.* Münch. med.
Wschr., 81: 1469 (only), Sept. 21, 1934
Lippich, Friedrich. German chemist. 1875–
TEST—for amino acids and leucine in urine.
*Über analytische Anwendungen der Uramidosäure-
reaktion.* Z. physiol. Chem., 90: 124–144, Apr. 4,
1914
Lipschitz, Werner Ludwig. Frankfurt pharmacolo-
gist. 1892–
TEST—for determining death or viability of tissues.
*Über den Mechanismus der Zelloxydationen und der
Blausäurewirkung.* Arch. ges. Physiol., 196: 463–502,
Nov. 11, 1922
Lipschütz, Benjamin. Vienna physician. 1878–1931
BOUILLON—egg albumin, for cultivation of gon-
ococci.
Ueber einen einfachen Gonokokkenährboden. Zbl.
Bakt., 36: 743–747, Aug. 26, 1904
ERYTHEMA—
Zur Kenntnis des "Erythema chronicum migrans."
Acta derm. vener., Stockh., 12: 100–102, 1931
ULCER—
Ueber Ulcus vulvae acutum. Wien. klin. Wschr., 31:
461–464, Apr. 25, 1918
*Die Reinzüchtung des Bacillus crassus und die Frage
der Nomenklatur des „ Ulcus vulvae acutum."* Arch.
Dermat. u. Syphil., 134, Orig., 370–373, July 20,
1921
Lisbonne, M. See C. A. Fleig
Lisfranc, Jacques. French surgeon. 1790–1847
AMPUTATION—of arm at shoulder joint.
*Nouveau procédé opératoire pour l'amputation du bras
dans son articulation scapulo-humérale.* Paris, Cro-
chard, 1815. 64 pp.

AMPUTATION—tarso-metatarsal disarticulation.
*Nouvelle méthode opératoire pour l'amputation pa
tielle du pied dans son articulation tarso-métatarsienn
méthode précédée des nombreuses modifications qu
subies celle de Chopart.* Paris, Gabon, 1815. 50 pp.
JOINT—tarso-metatarsal. Ibid.
LIGAMENT—from first cuneiform to second met
tarsus. Ibid.
OPERATION—excision of cancer of rectum.
*Mémoire de l'excision de la partie inférieure du rectu
devenue carcinomateuse.* Mem. Acad. roy. de Méd.,
291–302, 1833
Lison, Lucien. Brussels scientist. 1907–
TEST—for hemoglobin.
*Une technique de détection histochimique de l'hém
globine.* C. R. Soc. Biol., 103: 36–38, Jan. 10, 19
Lissauer, Heinrich. German neurologist. 1861–18
COLUMN, TRACT or ZONE—marginal bundle
cord.
*Beitrag zur pathologischen Anatomie der Tabes do
salis und zum Faserverlauf in menschlichen Rücke
mark.* Neurol. Zbl., 4: 245–246, June 1, 1885
PARALYSIS or TYPE—of dementia paralytica.
*Ueber einige Falle atypischen progressiver Paraly
By E. Storch. Nach einem hinterlassenen Man
script Dr. H. Lissauer's.* Mschr. Psychiat. Neuro
9: 401–434, June 1901
List, Carl Felix. Ann Arbor physician. 1902–
TEST—starch and iodine.
*Sweat secretion in man. I. Sweat responses in norm
persons* with M. M. Peet, Arch. Neurol. Psychia
39: 1228–1237, June 1938
Lister, Lord Joseph. English surgeon. 1827–1912
DRESSING—phenol, linseed oil and white cha
sufficient to make a soft paste. See antiseptic tec
nic.
OPERATION—
Excision of wrist for caries. Lancet, 1: 308–312: 3
338; 362–364, 1865
Confirmed von Kölliker's observation that contra
tile tissues of iris consist of smooth muscle. Ga
first correct account of mechanism of dilating pu
Garrison
Observations on the contractile tissue of the iris. Qua
J. micr. Sci., London, 1: 3–11, 1853
Introduced antiseptic technic.
*On a new method of treating compound fracture, a
cess, etc., with observations on the conditions of s
puration.* Lancet, 1: 326–329; 352–359; 387–3
507–509; 2: 95–96, 1867
Also: Medical classics, 2: 28–71, Sept. 1937
*On the antiseptic principle in the practice of surge
Lancet, 2: 353–356, 1867
Also: Medical classics, 2: 72–83, Sept. 1937
*On the effects of the antiseptic system of treatment u
the salubrity of a surgical hospital.* Lancet, 1: 1
200, 1870
Also: Medical classics, 2: 84–101, Sept. 1937
Lister, Joseph Jackson. English physician. 178
1869
Devised improved achromatic lenses of the compou
microscope.
*On some properties in achromatic object-glasses ap
cable to the improvement of the microscope.* Phi
Trans., 120: 187–200, Jan. 21, 1830

Listing, Johann Benedict. German physiologist. 1808–1882

LAW—of eyeball motions.

PLANE—containing center of motion of eyes.
Beitrag zur physiologischen Optik. Göttingen, Vandenhoeck und Rupprecht, 1845. 61 pp.

Liston, Robert. Scottish surgeon. 1794–1847
Described method of exploring larynx with mirror. In his: *Practical surgery.* London, 1837. p. 350

Liston, William Glen. Bombay physician. 1873–
AGAR—trypsinized casein blood.
A note on the preparation of two media for the growth of B. influenzae (Pfeiffer). Ind. J. Med. Res., 6: 418–421 (419), Jan. 1919

Litchfield, J. T. Jr. See E. K. Marshall, Jr.

Litten, Moritz. German physician. 1845–1907
ENDOCARDITIS—malignant.
Casuistische Beobachtungen. Chaité Ann., 3: 135–190, 1878

PHENOMENON or SIGN—diaphragm p.
Ueber die normaliter bei jeder Respiration am Thorax sichtbaren Zwerchfellsbewegungen. Dtsch. med. Wschr. 18: 273–275, Mar. 31, 1892
Das „Zwerchfellphänomen" und seine Bedeutung vom physiologischen und klinischen Standpunkte aus. Verh. d. Kong. f. inn. Med., 13: 309–319, 1895

THEORY—of spread of carcinoma; "paradoxical metastasis"; (patent foramen ovale).
Ueber embolische Muskelveränderung und die Resorption todler Muskelfasern. Ein Beitrag zur Frage von der Ueberwanderung embolischen Materials bei offen gebliebenem Foramen ovale. Arch. f. path. Anat., 80: 281–295, May 10, 1880

Little, Sir Ernest Gordon Graham. English physician. 1867–
Described condition now known as Waterhouse-Friderichsen syndrome (Aegerter).
Cases of purpura, ending fatally, associated with hemorrhage into the suprarenal capsules. Brit. J. Derm., 13: 445–467, Dec. 1901

Little, Mary F. See W. D. Frost

Little, W. D. See W. D. Gatch

Little, William John. English physician. 1810–1894
DISEASE or PARALYSIS—cerebral spastic p. of childhood.
Course of lectures on the deformities of the human frame. Lancet, 1: 350–354, Dec. 16, 1843
Established relation between difficult labor and disorders of nervous system.
On the influence of abnormal parturition, difficult labors, premature births, and asphyxia neonatorum, on the mental and physical conditions of the child, especially in relation to deformities. Trans. Obstet. Soc., Lond., 3: 293–344, 1862

Littlewood, Harry. English surgeon. 1861–1921
MODIFICATION—of Senn's plates.
A successful case of ileo-sigmoidostomy (Senn's method) for intestinal obstruction due to malignant disease of the hepatic flexure of the colon; with some remarks on intestinal anastomosis and a description of a modification of Senn's bone plates. Lancet, 1: 864–866, Apr. 16, 1892

OPERATION—interscapulothoracic amputation.
Amputations at the shoulder and at the hip. Brit. med. J., 1: 381–383, Mar. 11, 1922

Littré, Alexis. French surgeon. 1658–1725

GLANDS—in urethra.
Description de l'urèthre de l'homme. Hist. Acad. roy. d. sci., Paris, 311–316, 1700

HERNIA—of Meckel's diverticulum.
Observation sur une nouvelle éspece de hernie. Ibid., 1700, 300–310, 1719

Litzmann, Carl Conrad Theodor. German obstetrician. 1815–1890
CLASSIFICATION—of pelves.
Die Formen des Beckens, insbesondere des engen weiblichen Beckens. Berlin, Reimer, 1861

OBLIQUITY—inclination of fetal head so that posterior parietal bone presents to parturient canal.
Das schräge-ovale Becken, mit besonderer Berücksichtigung seiner Entstehung im Gefolge einseitiger Coxalgie. Keil, Buchhandlung, 1853. 33 pp.

Lium, Rolf. Boston surgeon. 1907–
TUBE—
A suction tube for ileostomy. New Engl. J. Med., 216: 345 (only), Feb. 25, 1937

Livingood, L. E. See H. W. Cushing

Livingston, Edward Meakin. New York surgeon. 1895–
SIGN or TRIANGLE—
The skin signs or viscerosensory phenomena in acute appendicitis. Arch. Surg., 7: 83–95, July 1923
The skin triangle of appendicitis: a discussion of its significance and its diagnostic value as observed in more than four hundred cases of acute appendicitis. Ibid. 13: 630–643, Nov. 1926

Lizars, John. Edinburgh surgeon. 1787?–1860
Performed first ovariotomy in Great Britain. Garrison and Morton
Observations on extraction of diseased ovaria. Edinburgh, Lizard, 1825

Ljungren, Gustaf. Norwegian physician. 1894–
REAGENT—for carbon monoxide.
Die Entdeckung von Kohlenoxyd in gesundheitsschädlicher Menge. Skand. Arch. Physiol., 55: 277 (only), Mar. 1929

Lloyd, Wray Devere Marr. American physician. ?–1936
Cultivated yellow fever virus.
Modification of the virulence of yellow fever virus by cultivation in tissues in vitro with M. Theiler and N. I. Ricci, Trans. Roy. Soc. Trop. Med. and Hyg., London, 29: 481–529, Feb. 1936
See also W. A. Sawyer

Lloyd-Davies, O. V. London surgeon
OPERATION or TECHNIC—
Lithotomy—Trendelenburg position for resection of rectum and lower pelvic colon. Lancet 2: 74–76, July 8, 1939
See also J. P. Lockhart-Mummery

Lobstein, Jean Georges Chrétien Frédéric Martin. Strassburg surgeon. 1777–1835
DISEASE—osteopsathyrosis or osteogenesis imperfecta.
De la fragilité des os ou de l'ostéopsathyrose. In his: Traité de l'anatomie pathologique. Paris, 1833. Vol. 2, pp. 204–212
First suggested term arteriosclerosis. Ibid., p. 550

Lochelongue, Joseph. French physician
ESTIMATION—of protein content of cerebrospinal fluid.

Le liquide céphalorachidien et ses anomalies....
Paris, Maloine, 1918. 281 pp.
De quelques anomalies constatées au cours d'une série de 250 examens de liquide céphalo-rachidien. Bull. Soc. méd. Hop. Paris, 43: 238–241, Mar. 7, 1919
Lochte, Eduard Heinrich Theodore. Göttingen physician. 1864–
TEST—for carbon monoxide in blood.
Über den Nachweis des Kohlenoxyds im Blute mittels Schwefelammonium und Wasserstoffsuperoxyd. Therap. Mschr., 25: 608–609, Oct. 1911
Locke, E. A. See W. B. Castle
Locke, Frank Spiller. American scientist
FLUID or SOLUTION—
Notiz über den Einfluss physiologischer Kochsalzlösung auf die elektrische Erregbarkeit von Muskel und Nerv. Zbl. Physiol., 8: 166–167, June 2, 1894
On a supposed action of distilled water as such on certain animal organisms. J. Physiol., 18: 319–331, 1895
Lockemann, George. Berlin physician
SOLUTION—citrate ammonium sulphate, for cultivation of tubercle bacilli.
Welche Nährstoffe sind für des Washstum der Tuberkelbazillen unbedingt notwendig? Zbl. Bakt., 83: 420–425, Sept. 27, 1919
Lockhart-Mummery, John Percy. English surgeon. 1875–
HYPOTHESIS—of Crile-Mummery; exhaustion theory of shock.
The Hunterian lectures on the physiology and treatment of surgical shock and collapse. Lancet, 1: 696–703, Mar. 18; 776–782, Mar. 25; 846–854, Apr. 1, 1905
OPERATION—
Excision of the rectum for cancer. Amer. J. Cancer, 18: 1–14, May 1933
The treatment of cancer of the rectum. S. G. O. 66: 527–533, Feb. 15, 1938
OPERATION—for fistula in ano.
In his: *Diseases of the rectum and anus.* Baltimore, Wood, 1934. 2 ed. pp. 193–231 (210–231)
OPERATION—excision and suture of hemorrhoids. Ibid., pp. 64–109 (88–95)
OPERATION—for prolapse of rectum. Ibid., pp. 110–129 (122–126)
OPERATION—
The operative treatment of fibrous stricture of the rectum: with the description of a new technique with O. V. Lloyd-Davies, Brit. J. Surg., 23: 19–24, July 1935
Lockwood, Ambrose Lorne. Rochester, Minn. surgeon. 1888–
METHOD—of preventing retraction in amputation stump.
Amputations. J. A. M. A., 79: 1490–1496, Oct. 28, 1922
Lockwood, Charles Barrett. English surgeon. 1858–1914
LIGAMENT—suspensory l. of globe of eye.
The anatomy of the muscles, ligaments and faciae of the orbit, including an account of the capsule of Tenon, the check ligaments of the recti, and of the suspensory ligament of the eye. J. Anat., London, 20: 1–25, Oct. 1885
OPERATION—

The radical cure of femoral and inguinal hern Lancet, 2: 1297–1302, Nov. 25, 1893
Lockwood, John Salem. Philadelphia physicia 1907–
THEORY—peptone, of sulfonamide action.
Studies on the mechanism of the action of sulfani mide. III. The effect of sulfanilamide in serum a blood on hemolytic streptococci in vitro with H.] Lynch, J. Immunol., 35: 155–190, Sept. 1938
Locock, Sir Charles. English physician. 1799–187 Recommended use of bromides in epilepsy. (N title) In discussion of paper by E. H. Sievekin Lancet, 1: 528 (only), 1857
Loeb, Jacques. German-American scientist. 185 1924
Founded theory of tropisms.
Der Heliotropismus der Thiere und seine Übereinsti mung mit dem Heliotropismus der Pflanzen. Würzbu Hertz, 1890
THEORY—mechanistic, of life. The father-nucle can be dispensed with in fertilization of ovum.
Die chemische Entwicklungserregung des tierisch Eies.... Berlin, Springer, 1909. 259 pp.
The dynamics of living matter. New York, Macmilla 1906
The mechanistic conception of life. Chicago, 1922
Loeb, Leo. American pathologist. 1869–
Showed that carcinoma and sarcoma can be tran planted and retransplanted in mice and rats.
On transplantation of tumors. J. med. Res., 1: 28–8 July 1901
Ueber den Krebs der Thiere. Arch. f. klin. Chir., 7 845–847, 1903
Produced uterine tumors in animals by using secr tions of corpus luteum.
Ueber die experimentelle Erzeugung von Knoten v Decidua-gewebe in dem Uterus des Meerschweinche nach stattgefundener Copulation. Zbl. allg. Path. path. Anat., 18: 563–565, July 31, 1907
Noted that incidence of hereditary mammary canc in mice could be reduced by oophorectomy.
Further investigation on the origin of tumors in mi VI. Internal secretion as a factor in the origin tmors. J.med.Res., 40: 477–496, Sept. 1919
Loeb, Robert Frederick. NewYork physician. 189 Recognized—
Chemical changes in the blood in Addison's diseas Science 76: 420–421,Nov. 4, 1932
Effect of sodim chloride in treament of a patient w Addison's disease. Proc. Soc. exp. Biol., N. Y., 3 808–812, Mar. 1933
See also J. W. Ferrebee
Loebisch, Wilhelm Franz. Vienna physician. 183 FORMULA—multiply last two figures of specifi gravity of urine by 2.2; product gives number grains of solids in 100 c.c. of urine.
Anleitung zur Harn-Analyse für praktisch Aerzt Apotheker und Studirende. Wien, Urban und Schwar enberg, 1878. 238 pp.
Löffl, K. Munich physician
SOLUTION—trypsinized blood; culture medium.
Plasma Nährstoff für Massenkulturen. Zbl. Bakt., 7 108–110, Sept. 8, 1915
Loffler, Friederich August Johann. German ba teriologist. 1852–1915

BACILLUS—Klebs-Löffler b., B. diphtheriae.
METHYLENE BLUE—for staining bacteria.
MEDIUM—for B. diphtheriae.
Untersuchungen über die Bedeutung der Mikroorganismen für die Entstehung der Diphtherie beim Menschen, bei der Taube und beim Kalbe. Mitth. a. d. k· Gesundh., 2: 421–499, 1884
MEDIUM—for B. diphtheriae.
Untersuchungen über die Diphtherie-Bacillen. Zbl. Bakt., 2: 105–106, 1887
MEDIUM—malachite green, for typhoid-paratyphoid group.
Der kulturelle Nachweis der Typhusbacillen in Faeces, Erde und Wasser mit Hilfe des Malachitgrüns und die Verwendung von Malachitgrün-Nährböden zum Nachweise und zur Differentialdiagnose der Typhusbacillen und verwandter Bakterienarten. Dtsch. med. Wschr., 32: 289–295, Feb. 22, 1906
METHOD—for staining flagella.
Eine neue Methode zum Färben der Mikroorganismen, im besonderen ihrer Wimperhaare und Geisseln. Zbl. Bakt., 6: 209–224, Aug. 18, 1889
Discovered bacteria of glanders.
Einige Bemerkungen betreffend die Entdeckung des Rotzbacillus with Schütz, Dtsch. med. Wschr., 9: 197–198, Apr. 4, 1883
Discovered ultra-virus causing disease in animals (foot and mouth disease).
Summarischer Bericht über die Ergebnisse der Untersuchungen der Commission zur Erforschung der Maul-und Klauenseuche. Ibid., 23: 617 (only), Sept. 23, 1897

Loeffler, W. Zurich physician
SYNDROME—fleeting infiltration of infraclavicular portion of lungs with high blood eosinophilia.
Zur Differential-Diagnose der Lungeninfiltrierungen. I. Frühinfiltrate unter besonderer Brücksichtigung der Rückbildungszeiten. Beitr. z. Klin. d. Tuberk., 79: 338–367, Feb. 22, 1932
(Same) II. Über flüchtige Succedan-Infiltrate (mit Eosinophilie). Ibid., 368–382
Die flüchtigen Lungeninfiltrate mit Eosinophilie. Schweiz. med. Wschr., 66: 1069–1078, Nov. 7, 1936

Löhlein, Christian Adolph. German gynecologist. 1847–1901
DIAMETER—
Ueber die Kunsthülfe bei der durch allgemeine Beckenenge erschwerten Geburt. Berlin, Schade, 1870. 36 pp.

Löhlein, Max Hermann Friedrich. German physician. 1877–1921
FOCAL NEPHRITIS OF—
Über die entzündlichen Veränderungen der Glomeruli der menschlichen Nieren und ihre Bedeutung für die Nephritis. Leipzig, Hirzel, 1907

Löhr, Wilhelm. German surgeon. 1889–
TREATMENT—cod liver oil externally.
Über ein neuartiges Prinzip in der Behandlung der akuten und chronischen Osteomyelitis. Zbl. Chir., 60: 1611–1613, July 8, 1933
Über die Lebertransalbenbehandlung (mit und ohne Gipsverband) bei frischen Verletzungen, Verbrennungen und phlegmonösen Entzündungen. Ibid., 61: 1686–1695, July 21, 1934

Lösch, Friedrich. German physician
Discovered Entamoeba histolytica.

Massenhafte Entwickelung von Amöben im Dickdarm. Arch. f. path. Anat., 65: 196–211, Nov. 10, 1875
Loevenhart, Arthur Salomon. American pharmacologist. 1878–1929
METHOD—for estimating lipase.
On the relation of lipase to fat metabolism—lipogenesis. Amer. J. Physiol., 6: 331–350, Feb. 1, 1902
METHOD—
The determination of the circulation time in rabbits and dogs and its relation to the reaction time of the respiration to sodium cyanide with B. H. Schlomovitz and E. G. Seybold, J. Pharmacol., 19: 221–238, Apr. 1922
See also J. H. Kastle

Löwe, Julius. German chemist
REAGENT and TEST—for glucose.
Ueber die Anwendung des Glycerin-Kupferoxyd-Natrons zur Nachweisung und Bestimmung des Traubenzuckers. Z. anal. Chem., 9: 20–24, 1870

Loewe, Leo. Brooklyn physician. 1896–
TREATMENT—
Combined penicillin and heparin therapy of subacute bacterial endocarditis; report of seven consecutive successfully treated patients with P. Rosenblatt, H. J. Greene and M. Russell, J. A. M. A., 124: 144–149, Jan. 15, 1944
Studied encephalitis.
Etiology of epidemic (lethargic) encephalitis; preliminary note with I. Strauss, Ibid., 73: 1056–1057, Oct. 4, 1919
Isolated Riakettsia prowazeki from blood.
Cultivation of rickettsia-like bodies in typhus fever. with S. Ritter and G. Baehr, Ibid., 77: 1967–1969, Dec. 17, 1921

Löwenberg, Benjamin Benno. German surgeon. 1836–
CANAL—part of cochlear c.
SCALA—cochlear canal; contains organ of Corti.
La lame spirale du limaçon de l'oreille de l'homme et des mammiféres; recherches d'anatomie microscopique. Paris, 1866. 55 pp.
FORCEPS—for removing adenoids.
Les tumeurs adénoides du pharynx nasal, leur influence sur l'audition, la respiration et la phonation, leur traitement. Paris, Delahaye, 1879. 75pp.
Sarcina—pathogenic form from case of ozena.
First to consider nature and treatment of ozena. Garrison
De la nature et du traitement de l'ozène. Paris, Alcan-Lévy, 1884. 19 pp.
Die Natur und die Behandlung der Ozaena. Dtsch. med. Wschr., 11: 5–8, Jan. 1; 22–24, Jan. 8, 1885
Le microbe de l'ozène. Ann. Inst. Pasteur, 8: 292–317, May 1894

Loewenfeld, Leopold. Munich physician. 1847–
Recognized significance of cataplexy as a symptom.
Ueber Narkolepsie. Münch. med. Wschr., 40: 1041–1045, June 24, 1902

Loewenhardt, Sigismund Eduard. German physician. 1796–1875
Described tabes dorsalis.
De myelophthisi chronica vera et notha. Berolini, typ. Haynianis, (1817)

Löwenstein, Ernest. German bacteriologist. 1878–
SOLUTION—glycerol ammonium carbonate.

LÖWENSTEIN, ERNEST   260   LORENZ, ADOLF

Beitrag zur Chemie des Tuberkelbacillus. Zbl. Bakt.,
68: 591–593, Apr. 23, 1913

Löwenthal, J. German chemist
REAGENT—for glucose.
Ein empfindliches Reagens auf Traubenzucker. J.
prakt. Chem. 73: 71–72, 1858

Loewi, Otto. German physician. 1873–
SIGN and TEST—dilation of pupil by adrenalin in
conjunctival sac, in pancreatic insufficiency, diabetes,
and hyperthyroidism.
*Über eine neue Funktion des Pankreas und ihre
Beziehung zum Diabetes melitus.* Arch. exp. Path.
Pharmak., 59: 83–94, June 19, 1908
Awarded Nobel prize in 1936, with H. H. Dale, for
work "on transmission of nerve impulse."
*Über humorale Übertragbarkeit der Herznervenwir-
kung.* Arch. ges. Physiol., 189: 239–242, Aug. 17,
1921
(Same) *II Mitteilung.* Ibid., 193: 201–213, Dec. 24,
1921
The humoral transmission of nervous impulse. Harvey
Lectures, 1932–33, pp. 218–233, 1934

Lofaro, F. French surgeon
OPERATION—
*Gastrostomie par dédoublement du muscle droit suivant
son épaisseur.* Arch. gen. de chir., 6: 1026–1034, Oct.
25, 1910

Lohnstein, Theodor. Berlin physician. 1866–1918
SACCHARIMETER—
*Ueber Gährungs-Sacchaoometer nebst Beschreibung
eines neuen Gährungs-Saccharometers für unverdünnte
Urine.* Münch. med. Wschr., No. 50: 1671–1675,
Dec. 12, 1899

Loiseau, G. See L. Martin

Lombard, Henri Clermond. Geneva physician. 1803–
1895
Drew attention to radical differences between typhus
and typhoid fevers.
*Observations suggested by a comparison of the post
mortem appearances produced by typhus fever in
Dublin, Paris, and Geneva.* Dublin J. med. Sci., 10:
17–24, Sept. 1, 1836

Lombard, Warren Plimpton. Würzburg physiologist. 1855–1939
Studied skin.
*The blood pressure in the arterioles, capillaries, and
small veins of the human skin.* Amer. J. Physiol., 29:
335–362, Jan. 1912

Lombardo, C. Modena physician
TEST—for mercury in urine.
*La micro ed isto-chimica nella ricerca tossicologica del
mercurio.* Arch. farmacol. sper., 7: 400–420, 1908

Lombroso, Cesare. Italian scientist. 1836–1909
Inaugurated doctrine of a criminal type. Garrison
and Morton
*L'uomo delinquente, studiato in rapporto alla antro-
pologia, alla medicina legale ed alle discipline car-
cerarie.* Milano, Hoepli, 1876

London, E. S. See S. W. Goldberg

Long, Crawford Williamson. Danielsville, Ga. physician. 1815–1878
Used ether in surgical operation, March, 1842. Did
not publish any reports. Abstract of paper read in
1852 in Trans. Georgia Med. and Surg. Ass., 1853
Also in: L. Clendening's *Source book of medical history.* New York, Hoeber, 1942. pp. 356–358

Long, Joseph Abraham. American zoologist. 1879–
SIGN—placental s.; microscopic bleeding.
*The oestrous cycle in the rat and its associated phe-
nomena* with H. M. Evans, Mem. Univ. California,
6: 1–148, 1922
See also H. M. Evans

Long, Perrin Hamilton. American physician. 1899–
Made first American report on therapeutic value of
sulfanilamide.
*Para-amino-benzene-sulfonamide and its derivatives.
Experimental and clinical observations on their use in
the treatment of beta-hemolytic streptococci infections:
a preliminary report* with Eleanor A. Bliss, J. A. M.
A., 108: 32–37, Jan. 2, 1937
See also E. K. Marshall, Jr.

Longcope, Warfield Theobald. American physician.
1877–
Made early study in America of eosinophils in
Hodgkin's disease.
*On the pathological histology of Hodgkin's disease,
with a report of a series of cases.* Bull. Ayer Clin.
Lab. Penn. Hosp., Phila., No. 1, pp. 4–77, Oct. 1903
*A study of the distribution of the eosinophilic leuko-
cytes in a fatal case of Hodgkin's disease with general
eosinophilia.* Ibid., No. 3 pp. 86–95, June 1906

Longworth, Stephen G. English physician
TEST—for glucose.
Ambiguous reactions in sugar testing. Brit. med. J.,
2: 19–20, July 6, 1907

Looney, Joseph Michael. Boston biochemist. 1896–
TEST—for cystine in urine.
The colorimetric estimation of cystine in urine. J.
biol. Chem., 54: 171–175, Oct. 1922

Looss, Arthur. Cairo physician. 1861–1923
Discovered that hookworms can penetrate skin,
1898.
*Ueber das Eindringen der Ankylostomalarven in die
menschliche Haut.* Zbl. Bakt., 1 Abt., 29: Orig., 733–
739, May 31, 1901

Lorain, Paul Joseph. French physician. 1827–1875
TYPES—of dwarfism and sexual infantilism.
*Lettre préface de Faneau de la Cour. Du féminisme et
de l'infantilisme chez les tuberculeux.* Thèse de Paris,
1871

Lóránd, Sandor. Budapest gynecologist. 1892–
TOCOGRAPH—for measuring uterine contractions.
Erfahrungen mit dem modifizierten Tokograph.
Mschr. Geburtsch. u. Gynäk., 103: 137–145, Sept.
1936

Lord, J. W. Jr. See A. H. Blakemore

Lorente de Nó, Rafael. New York scientist
THEORY—of internuncial pool in syndrome of reflex
sympathetic dystrophy.
*Analysis of the activity of the chains of internuncial
neurons.* J. Neurophysiol., 1: 207–244, May 1938

Lorenz, Adolf. Austrian surgeon. 1854–1946
OPERATION—
*Die blutige Reposition der angeborenen Hüftverren-
kung (Luxat, coxae congenita).* Samml. klin. Vortr.,
No. 117 (Chir., No. 32, pp. 169–188), 1895
*The operative treatment of congenital dislocation of the
hip-joint.* Trans. Amer. Ortho. Ass., 7: 99–103, 1895
*A new method of treatment of irreducible, acquired or
congenital hip dislocations.* New York med. J., 117:
130–136, Feb. 7, 1923
OPERATION—for fracture of neck of femur.

Ueber die Behandlung der irreponiblen angeborenen Huftluxationen und der Schenkelhals pseudoarthrosen mittels Gabelung (Bifurkation des oberen Femurendes). Wien. klin. Wschr., 32: 997–999, Oct. 9, 1919
SIGN—ankylotic rigidity of spine in incipient phthisis.
Die Behandlung der tuberculösen Spondylitis. Wien. Klinik, 15: 127–164, May 1889
Lorenzini, Stephan.
AMPULLAE—
Osservazioni intorno alle Torpedini. Florence, 1678
Loretz, Wilhelm. Frankfurt a. M. physician
Described ganglioneuroma.
Ein Fall von gangliösem Neurom (Gangliom). Arch. f. path. Anat., 49: 435–437, Feb. 21, 1870
Loring, Edward Greely. American oculist. 1837–1888
OPHTHALMOSCOPE—
A new modification of the ophthalmoscope. Amer. J. med. Sci., 67: 114–116, Jan. 1874
Loring, H. S. See W. M. Stanley
Lorry, Antoine Charles. Paris physician. 1726–1783
Drew attention to skin eruptions (allergy) from various aromatic medicines, essential oils, etc.
Tractatus de morbis cutaneis. Parisiis, Cavelier, 1777. 704 pp.
Lorthioir, Jules. Brussels surgeon. 1864–1931
OPERATION—
Huit cas d'arthrodèse du pied avec extirpation temporaire de l'astragale. J. de Chir. et Ann. Soc. belg. de Chir., 11: 184–187, June 24, 1911
Lossen, Hermann. German surgeon. 1864–1910
OPERATION—
Neurectomie des II Astes des V nach osteoplastischer Resection des Jochbeins, nebst Vorschlag zu einer neuen Schnittführung. Zbl. Chir., 5: 65–70, Feb. 2, 1878
Lotheissen, Georg. German surgeon. 1868–
OPERATION—for femoral hernia.
Zur Radikaloperation der Schenkelhernien. Zbl. Chir., 25: 548–550, 1898
OPERATION—
Zur operativen Behandlung der Dupuytren'schen Kontraktur. Ibid., No. 30, pp. 761–763, July 28, 1900
Lothrop, Howard Augustus. Boston surgeon. 1864–1928
OPERATION—
Fractures of the superior maxillary bone caused by direct blows over the malar bone. A method for the treatment of such fractures. Boston Med. and Surg., J., 154: 8–11, Jan. 4, 1906
Lotsch, Fritz Wilhelm. Magdeburg surgeon. 1879–
OPERATION—transposition of nipple.
Ueber Hängebrustplastik. Klin. Wschr., 7: 603–606, Mar. 25, 1928
Lough, W. G. See V. C. Myers
Louis, Pierre Charles Alexander. French physician. 1787–1872
LAW—pulmonary tuberculosis generally begins in left lung.
LAW—tuberculosis of any part is attended by localization in lungs.
Recherches anatomico-physiologiques sur la phthisie. Paris, Gabon, 1825. 560 pp.
Same, in English. Boston, Butts, 1836
Same, transl. by W. H. Walshe, London, Sydenham Soc. 1844. Same, 1876
Invented term typhoid fever.
Recherches anatomiques, pathologiques et thérapeutiques

sur la maladie connue sous les noms de gastro-entérite fièvre putride, adynamique, ataxique, typhoïde, etc., etc., comparée avec les maladies aigues les plus ordinaires. Paris, Baillière, 1829. 2 vols.
Advocated statistics in study of disease.
Recherches sur les effets de la saignée dans quelques maladies inflammatoires, et sur l'action de l'émetiqué et des vésicatoires dans la pneumonie. Paris, Baillière, 1835
Louyer-Villermay, Jean Baptiste. French physician. 1776–1837
Wrote classic paper on appendicitis.
Observations pour servir à l'histoire des inflammations de l'appendice du caecum. Arch. gén. de méd., Paris, 5: 246–250, 1824
Love, J. Grafton. Rochester, Minn. surgeon. 1903–
OPERATION—
Protruded intervertebral disks: with a note regarding hypertrophy of ligamenta flava. J. A. M. A., 113: 2029–2035, Dec. 2, 1939
Intraspinal protrusion of intervertebral disks with M. N. Walsh, Arch. Surg., 40: 454–484, Mar. 1940
Lovelace, W. R. See W. M. Boothby
Lovell, J. See W. Beaumont
Loven, Otto Christian. German physician. 1835–1904
REFLEX—vasodilatation of an organ when its afferent nerve is stimulated.
Veranderungen im Herzschlag und Blutdruck, welche eintreten während der Reizung eines sensiblen Nerven, der mit dem Hirn und dem Rückenmark in Verbindung steht. Ber. Sächs, Ges. Wiss., 18: 85–110, May 30, 1866
Lovett, Beatrice Russell. Chicago pediatrician. 1898–
TEST—
The percutaneous tuberculin reaction. Amer. J. Dis. Child., 37: 918–922, May 1929
Lovett, R. W. See E. H. Bradford, R. Jones
Lowden, May M. See Anna W. Williams
Lowe, Franklin Alexander. San Francisco surgeon. 1890–
KNIFE—
A new knife for use in removing semilunar cartilages with L. W. Breck, J. Bone and Joint Surg., 20: 220–221, Jan. 1938
Lowe, Peter. English surgeon. 1552–1612
Made first English translation of Hippocrates; gave first reference in English to ligation of arteries in amputation. Garrison
A discourse of the whole course of chirurgerie. 1597
Lower, Richard. English physician. 1631–1691
RINGS—of tendon around four orifices of heart.
TUBERCLE—an eminence within right auricle of heart.
Tractatus de corde, item de motu, et colore sanguinis et chyli in eum transitu. Londini, Allestry, 1669. 220 pp.
The first to perform direct tranfusion of blood from one animal to another, February, 1665. Garrison
The method observed in transfusion blood out of one animal into another. Philos. Trans., 1: 353–358, Dec. 17, 1666
An account of the experiment of transfusion, practiced upon a man in London with Sir E. King, Ibid., 2: 557–564, 1667
Overthrew, with Schneider, old Galenic idea that nasal secretions originate in pituitary body, 1672. Garrison This discovery localized catarrh in air-

passages and did away with endless recipes for "purging the brain." Neuburger, quoted by Garrison
Dissertatio de origine catarrhi in qua ostenditur illum non pronenire a cerebro. In his: *Tractatus de corde.* London, edition of 1670, pp. 221–239; edition of 1680, pp. 163–175

Lowsley, Oswald Swinney. New York urologist. 1884–
METHOD—
A new method of repairing kidney wounds with C. Bishop, S. G. O., 57: 494–500, Oct. 1933
OPERATION—
A three-stage operation for the repair of hypospadias: report of cases with C. L. Begg, J. A. M. A., 110: 487–493, Feb. 12, 1938

Lozner, E. L. See R. Kark

Lubarsch, Otto. German pathologist. 1860–1933
Originated term hypernephroma.
Beiträge zur Histologie der von Nebennierenkeimen ausgehenden Nierengeschwülste. Arch. f. path. Anat., 135: 149–223, Feb. 5, 1894

Lubash, Samuel. New York urologist. 1896–
OPERATION—for hydronephrosis.
Uretero-pyeloneostomy for hydronephrosis: a new operative technique. A preliminary report. J. Urol., 34: 222–229, Sept. 1935
Uretero-pyeloneostomy for hydronephrosis, with case and experimental reports with A. Madrid, Ibid., 38: 634–642, Dec. 1937

Lubenau, C. Berlin physician
AGAR—lactose caffeine; for detection of typhoid bacteria.
Das Koffeinanreicherungsverfahren zum Typhusnachweis im Stuhl. Arch. Hyg., Berl., 61: 232–249 (249), 1907
MEDIUM—glycerin egg.
Der Eigelbnährboden als Ersatz des Serums zur Kultur von Diphtherie- und Tuberkelbacillen. Hyg. Rundschau., 17: 1455–1463, Dec. 15, 1907

Lubinski, Ws. Kiew pathologist
MEDIUM—
Zur Kultivierungsmethode, Biologie und Morphologie der Tuberkelbacillen. Zbl. Bakt., 18: 125–128 (126), Aug. 8, 1895

Lubowski, R. See M. Neisser

Lubs, H. A. See W. M. Clark

Luc, Henry. French surgeon. 1855–1925
OPERATION—of Caldwell-Luc.
Des abcès du sinus maxillaire. . . . Paris, Steinheil, 1889. 46 pp.

Lucae, Johann Constantin August. Berlin otologist. 1835–1911
First studied transmission of sounds through cranial bones in diagnosis of aural diseases. Garrison
Die Schalleitung durch die Kopfknochen und ihre Bedeutung für die Diagnostik der Ohrenkrankheiten. Eine physiologisch-klinische Studie. Würzburg, Stahel, 1870. 48 pp.

Lucas, George Herbert William. Toronto pharmacologist. 1894–
Used cyclopropane (trimethylene) experimentally for anesthesia in animals.
A new anesthetic gas: cyclopropane. A preliminary report with V. E. Henderson, Canad. med. Ass. J., 21: 173–175, Aug. 1929

Lucas, Richard Clement. English surgeon. 1848–1915

INCISION—for nephrectomy.
On surgical diseases of the kidney, and the operations for their relief. Brit. med. J., 2: 611–615, Sept. 29, 1883

Lucas-Championnière, Just Marie Marcellin. French surgeon. 1843–1913
Introduced antisepsis in France.
Chirurgie antiseptique. Paris, Baillière, 1876
Wrote classic work on hernia.
Cure radicale des hernies. Paris, Delahaye et Lecrosnier, 1887. 128 pp.

Luce-Clausen, Ethel M. See Augusta B. McCoord

Luck, James Vernon. Los Angeles surgeon. 1906–
SAW and DRILL—
An electric bone saw and drill. Amer. J. Surg., 54 505–507, Nov. 1941
See also A. Steindler

Luckett, William Henry. New York surgeon. 1872–
OPERATION—
A new operation for prominent ears based on the anatomy of the deformity. S. G. O., 10: 635–637, June 1910

Luckhardt, Arno Benedict. Chicago surgeon. 1885–
Applied ethylene (C_2H_4) to clinical use.
The physiological effects of ethylene, a new gas anesthetic with J. B. Carter, J. A. M. A., 80: 765–770 Mar. 17, 1923
Ethylene as a gas anesthetic: preliminary communication with J. B. Carter, Ibid., 80: 1440–1442, May 19 1923

Lucy, R. H. English surgeon
METHOD—of gastrostomy.
The after-treatment of cases of gastrostomy. Edinburg med. J., 5: 46–50, Jan. 1899

Ludington, Nelson Amos. New Haven surgeon 1879–
SIGN—failure to contract biceps with hands on head
Rupture of the long head of the biceps flexor cubii muscle. Ann. Surg., 77: 358–363, Mar. 1923

Ludloff, Konrad. German surgeon. 1867–
DISEASE—torn cartilage of knee.
Zur Pathologie des Kniegelenkes. Abstr.: Verh. dtsch Ges. f. Chir., 39: 223–225, Apr. 2, 1910

Ludwig, Carl Friedrich Wilhelm. German physiologist. 1816–1895
NERVE—see Elie de Cyon
THEORY—of formation of lymph, by diffusion fluids from blood through vessel walls. Garrison
Ueber den Lymphstrom in den Lymphgefässen und d wesentlichsten anatomischen Bestandtheile der Lympl drüsen By F. W. Noll, Z. rat. Med., Heidelb., 52–93, 1850
THEORY—of urinary secretion, by filtration and r absorption.
Beiträge zur Lehre vom Mechanismus der Harnsecr tion. Marburg, Elwert, 1843
Introduced graphic method with new instrument like the kymograph and blood-pump. Garrison
Beiträge zur Kenntniss des Einflusses der Respira tions bewegungen auf den Blutlauf im Aortensysten Arch. f. Anat., Physiol. u. wiss. Med., 6: 242–30 1847
Discovered ganglionic cells of interauricular septur Garrison
Ueber die Herznerven des Frosches. Ibid., pp. 13 143, 1848

Discovered innervation of submaxillary glands. Garrison

Neue Versuche über die Beihilfe der Nerven zur Speichelabsonderung with E. Becher and C. Rahn, Z. rat. Med., n. F., 1: 225–292, (254–277), 1851

Studied effect of spinal cord on blood current. Garrison

Über den Einfluss des Halsmarkes auf den Blutstrom with L. Thiry, S. B. Akad. Wiss. Wien, 49: 2 Abth., 421–454, 1864

Introduced idea of keeping excised portions of an organism active by an artificial circulation or perfusion. Garrison

Die physiologischen Leistungen des Blutdrucks. Leipzig Inaugural, 1865. 24 pp.

Invented stromuhr for measuring amount of blood passing in unit time. Garrison

Die Ausmessung der strömenden Blutvolumina with J. Dogiel, Arb. a. d. physiol. Anst. zu Leipz., 2: 196–271, 1867

Discovered depressor nerve of heart and "nervi erigentes" of peripheral vessels. Garrison

Die Reflexe eines der sensiblen Nerven des Herzens auf die motorischen der Blutgefässe. Ibid., 2: 128–149, (1867) 1868

See also E. de Cyon

Ludwig, Wilhelm Friedrich von. German surgeon. 1790–1865

ANGINA—acute inflammation of floor of mouth.

(. . . *ueber eine in neuerer Zeit wiederholt hier vorgekommene Form von Halsentzündung* . . .) Med. Cor.-Bl. d. Württemb. ärztl. Ver., Stuttgart, 6: 21–25, Feb. 5, 1836

Also, English transl. by J. Burke in Bull. Hist. Med., 7: 1115–1123, Nov. 1939

Lueders, Charles Williamson. Philadelphia physician. 1883–

SYSTEM—for estimation of duodenal enzymes.

Quantitative estimation of enzyme concentration in duodenal fluids: a practical clinical method. Amer. J. Digest. Dis., 2: 224–229, June 1935

Lüttge. Leipzig physician

TECHNIC—for serological identification of sex.

Serologische Alkoholextraktreaktion with v. Mertz, Dtsch. med. Wschr., 52: 1677–1678, Oct. 1, 1926

Lugol, Jean Guillaume Auguste. Paris physician. 1786–1851

SOLUTION—

Mémoire sur l'emploi de l'iode dans les maladies scrofuleuses, lu à l'Académie royale des sciences, dans la séance du 22 juin 1829. . . . Paris, Baillière, 1829. 78 pp.

Luikart, Ralph Herbert. Omaha, Neb. obstetrician. 1889–

FORCEPS—obstetrical.

A new forceps possessing a sliding lock, modified fenestra, with improved handle and axis traction attachment. Amer. J. Obstet. Gynaec., 40: 1058–1060, Dec. 1940

Luisinus. See A. Luvigni

Luithlen, Friedrich. German physician. 1869–1927

Introduced autoemotherapy and autoserotherapy in treatment of skin diseases.

Veränderungen der Hautreaktion bei Injektion von Serum und kolloidalen Substanzen. Wien. klin. Wschr., 26: 653–658, Apr. 24, 1913

Lukens, Marguerite. See F. Boerner

Lull, Clifford Bell. Philadelphia obstetrician. 1893–

METHOD—of tubal sterilization: Pomeroy-Lull m.

A resume of 223 cases of surgical sterilization. Amer. J. Obstet. Gynaec., 31: 101–105, Jan. 1936

Lum, E. A. English pharmacologist

TEST—for glucose.

Differentiation of sucrose, glucose, and lactose. Pharm. J., 129: 371 (only), Oct. 29, 1932

See also C. L. M. Brown

Lumsden, Thomas William. English physician

Introduced conception of subsidiary respiratory centers in brain stem.

The regulation of respiration. J. Physiol., 58: 81–91, Oct. 22; 111–126, Dec. 28, 1923

Lund, Edward. English surgeon. 1823–1898

HOOKS—for picking up the bowel in colotomy.

On air-inflation of the bowel as a rule of practice in the operation of left lumbar colotomy. Lancet, 1: 588–589, Apr. 7, 1883

Lund, Frederick Bates. Boston surgeon. 1865–

SWATHE—to support arm and shoulder.

The treatment of old dislocations of the shoulder. Boston Med. and Surg., J. 136: 397–402, Apr. 29, 1897

Lundblad, R. A. See H. O. McPheeters

Lundborg, Herman Bernhard. Swedish physician. 1868–

Called attention to bone lesions in disease of parathyroid glands.

Spielen die Glandulae parathyreoideae in der menschlichen Pathologie eine Rolle? Dtsch. Z. Nervenheilk., 27: 217–238, Nov. 9, 1904

Lunde, G. See J. M. Holst

Lundsgaard, C. See K. A. Hasselbalch

Lunin, Nikolay Ivanovich. Russian chemist. 1854–

Did early work on vitamins.

Ueber die Bedeutung der anorganischen Salz fur die Ernährung des Thieres. Z. phys. Chem., 5: 31–39, 1881

Luschka, Hubert von. German anatomist. 1820–1875

BURSA—b. pharyngea.

CARTILAGE—in anterior part of true vocal cord.

Der Kehlkopf des Menschen. Tübingen, Laupp, 1873. 199 pp.

DUCTS—tubular structures in wall of gallbladder.

Die Drüsen der Gallenblase des Menschen. Z. rat. Med., 4: 189–192, 1858

GLAND—coccygeal.

In: *Die Anatomie des Menschen.* . . . Tübingen, Laupp, 1863–69. Vol. 2, pt. 2, p. 208

LACUNAE—cyst-like cavities in urachal canal.

Ueber den Bau des menschlichen Harnstranges. Arch. f. path. Anat., 23: 1–7, 1862

TONSIL—lymph glands between nasopharyngeal orifices of Eustachian tubes.

Der Schundkopf des Menschen. Tübingen, Laupp, 1868. 221 pp. p. 110

Described chordoma (tumors arising from remnants of fetal notochord).

Die Altersveränderungen der Zwischenwirbelknorpel. Arch. f. path. Anat., 9: 311–327, 1856

Lusk, Graham. American biochemist. 1866–1932

Made extensive studies of diabetes. Garrison

Ueber den Einfluss der Kohlenhydrate auf den Eiweisserfall. Z. Biologie., 27: 459–481, 1890

Influence of the carbohydrates on proteid catabolism, with special reference to diabetes. New York med. J., 54: 628–630, Dec. 5, 1891

Lusk, William Thompson. New York physician. 1838–1897
RING—thickening of uterus, just above internal os, during labor; Bandl's r.
The etiology and indications for treatment of irregular uterine action during labor. New York med. J., 17: 561–577, June 1873

Lustgarten, Sigmund. Austrian and New York physician. 1857–1911
BACILLUS—once thought to be cause of syphilis.
Die Syphilisbacillen. Wien, Braumüller, 1885. 2 ed.

Lustig, Allesandro. Italian physician. 1857–1938
SERUM—antitoxic and bacterial plague serum.
Sieroterapia e vaccinazioni preventive contro la peste bubbonica. Torino, Rosenberg and Sellier, 1899. 150 pp.

Lutembacher, René. French physician
SYNDROME—interarterial septal defect and mitral stenosis.
De la sténose mitrale avec communication interauriculaire. Arch. d. mal. du coeur, 9: 237–260, June 1916

Luther, Ernst. German physician
TEST—for glucose in urine.
Methoden der Untersuchung des Harns auf Zucker und über das Verkommen von Koblenhydraten im normalen Harn. Abstr.: Prager med. Wschr., 15: 479–480, Sept. 17, 1890
Ueber das Verkommen von Kohlenhydraten im normalen Harn. Berlin, Simon, 1890. 57 pp.

Lutz, Henri Charles. French physician
Described keratosis follicularis.
De l'hypertrophie générale du système sebacé. Paris, 1860. Thèse No. 65

Luvigni, Aloisio. Venetian physician
Wrote on syphilis.
De morto gallico omnia quae extant. Venetiis, apud J. Zilettum, 1566–67. 2 vols.

Luys, Georges. French urologist. 1870–
OPERATION—prostectomy.
"Le forage de la prostate" dans le traitement de l'hypertrophie de la prostate. Bull. Acad. de Med. Paris, 3 s., 79: 141–144, 1918
Same, in English: J. Urol., 3: 17–24, Feb. 1919
SEGREGATOR—an instrument for collecting urine from each kidney separately.
La séparation de l'urine des deux reins. Paris, Masson, 1904. 298 pp.

Luys, Jules Bernard. French physician. 1828–1897
BODY or NUCLEUS—hypothalamus.
Recherches sur le système nerveux cérébro-spinal; sa structure, ses fonctions et ses maladies. Paris, Baillière, 1865
Noted degeneration of anterior horn cells in progressive muscular atrophy.
Atrophie musculaire progressive. Lésions histologiques de la substance grise de la moelle épinière. Abstr.: Gaz. méd. de Paris, 3 s., 15: 505 (only), Aug. 11, 1860

Luzet, Charles. French physician
DISEASE—pseudoleukenia, of Jaksch-Hayem-Luzet.
L'anémie infantile pseudo-leucémique. Arch. gén. de méd., 1: 579–592, May 1891

Lyall, Harold William. Brooklyn bacteriologist. 1888–
BOUILLON—carbonate ascitic fluids to determine hemolysis by streptococci.
On the classification of the streptococci. J. med. Res., 30: 487–513 (497), July 1914

Lyerly, James Gilbert. Jacksonville, Fla. surgeon. 1893–
TECHNIQUE—
Prefrontal lobotomy in involutional melancholia. J. Florida Med. Ass., 25: 225–229, Nov. 1938
Transsection of the deep association fibers of the prefrontal lobes in certain mental disorders. South. Surg., 8: 426–434, Oct. 1939

Lyle, Henry Hamilton Moore. New York surgeon. 1875–1947
OPERATION—
Deformity of hand—formation of a new thumb from stump of first metacarpal. Ann. Surg., 74: 120 (only), July 1921
OPERATION—
The operative treatment of thenar paralysis. Ibid., 84: 288–294, Aug. 1926
OPERATION—
Ombrédanne's pouch operation for hypospadias. Ibid., 98: 513–519, Oct. 1933

Lyle, William Gordon. New York physician. 1892–
TEST—
The catalytic reactions of blood. I. A study of some of the factors involved in the benzidine test for occult blood with L. J. Curtman and J. T. W. Marshall, J. biol. Chem., 19: 445–451, Dec. 1914
A new method for the detection of occult blood in stools with L. J. Curtman, Ibid., 33: 1–6, Jan. 1918

Lyman, Henry. Boston biochemist
METHOD—
A rapid method for determining calcium in urine and feces. J. biol. Chem., 21: 551–556, July 1915
A rapid method for determining calcium in blood and milk. Ibid., 29: 169–178, Mar. 1917

Lynah, Henry Lowndes. New York City otolaryngologist. 1879–1922
Studied bronchiectasis.
Roentgenographic studies of bronchiectasis and lung abscess after direct injection of bismuth mixture through the bronchoscope with W. H. Stewart, Amer. J. Röntgenol., 8: 49–61, Feb. 1921

Lynch, Frank Worthington. San Francisco obstetrician. 1871–
Introduced gas-oxygen anesthesia in child birth.
Eutocia by means of nitrous oxid gas analgesia; a safe substitute for the Freiburg method. J. A. M. A., 64: 1187–1189, Apr. 3, 1915

Lynch, H. M. See J. S. Lockwood

Lynch, J. See H. Goldblatt

Lynch, Kenneth Merrill. American pathologist. 1887–
Reported first fatal case of uncomplicated asbestosis in United States.
Pulmonary asbestosis. II. Including the report of a pure case with W. A. Smith, Amer. Rev. Tuberc. 23: 643–660, June 1931

Lynch, Robert Clyde. New Orleans otolaryngologist. 1880–

TECHNIC—
Technic of a pan-sinus operation. South. med. J., 17: 289–292, Apr. 1924

Lyon, Bethuel Boyd Vincent. Philadelphia physician. 1880–
SIGMOIDOSCOPE—
A new type sigmoidoscope with H. J. Bartle, J. A. M. A., 79: 1135–1136, Sept. 30, 1922
TEST—of biliary pathology.
Diagnosis and treatment of diseases of the gallbladder and biliary ducts: preliminary report on a new method. Ibid., 73: 980–983, Sept. 27, 1919
TIP—for Rehfuss tube.
A new metal tip possessing obvious advantages for use on gastric or duodenal tubes. Ibid., 74: 246 (only), Jan. 24, 1920

Lyon, George Marshall. Huntington, W. Va. physician. 1895–
METHOD—"substitution".
Serum therapy in meningococcus meningitis. Amer. J. Dis. Child., 43: 572–576, Mar. 1932

Lyons, Albert Brown. American pharmacist. 1841–1926
TEST—
Improved phenylhydrazine test for formaldehyde. J. Amer. Pharm. Ass., 13: 7–9, Jan. 1924
TEST—
Notes on the phenylhydrazine test for sugar. Pharm. Rev., 20: 155–158, Apr. 1902

Lyster, William John L. U. S. Army surgeon. 1869–1947
BAG—
Present status of artificially treated drinking water in the field. Military Surg., 40: 401–410, Apr. 1917

Lyttle, John Dooley. New York physician. 1889–
MODIFICATION—of Addis count.
The Addis sediment count in normal children. J. clin. Invest., 12: 87–93, Jan. 1933
The Addis sediment count in scarlet fever. Ibid., pp. 95–103

M

Mabee, Jennie. See P. Levine
Macadie, W. English scientist
TEST—
A rapid and delicate method of detecting bile-pigments in urine. Pharm. J., 26: 686 (only), May 23, 1908
MacAllum, A. B. See O. K. O. Folin
MacArthur, C. G. See F. A. Hartman
McArthur, Janet. See H. A. Davenport
McArthur, Lewis Linn. Chicago surgeon. 1858–1934
OPERATION—for inguinal hernia, in which a fascial strip from aponeurosis of external oblique, left attached at its lower end, is imbricated between conjoined tendon and Poupart's ligament.
Autoplastic suture in hernia, and other diastases—preliminary report. J. A. M. A., 37: 1162–1165, Nov. 2, 1901
Autoplastic sutures in hernia and other diastases. Final report. Ibid., 43: 1039–1048, Oct. 8, 1904
OPERATION—hypophysectomy.
An aseptic surgical access to the pituitary body and its neighborhood. Trans. Sect. Surg., A. M. A., 1912, pp. 78–86
MacAusland, William Russell. Boston surgeon. 1882–
OPERATION—
Recurrent dislocation of the patella with A. F. Sargent, S. G. O., 35: 35–41, July 1922
McBride, Earl Duwain. Oklahoma City surgeon. 1892–
OPERATION—
A conservative operation for bunion. J. Bone and Joint Surg., 10: 735–739, Oct. 1928
The conservative operation for "bunions:" end results and refinements of technic. J. A. M. A., 105: 1164–1168, Oct. 12, 1935
McBryde, C. N. See M. Dorset
McBurney, Charles. New York surgeon. 1845–1913
INCISION—muscle splitting.
The incision made in the abdominal wall in cases of appendicitis, with a description of a new method of

operating. Ann. Surg., 20: 38–43, July 1894
Also: Med. Classics, 2: 533–538, Jan. 1938
MANEUVER—with hooks.
Dislocation of humerus complicated by fracture at or near the surgical neck, with a new method of reduction with C. N. Dowd, Ann. Surg., 19: 399–415. Apr. 1894
OPERATION—
The radical cure of hernia, with special reference to open treatment of the operation wound. New York med. J., 47: 57–61, Jan. 21, 1888
POINT or SIGN—of tenderness in appendicitis.
Experience with early operative interference in cases of disease of the vermiform appendix. Ibid., 50: 676–684 (678), Dec. 21, 1889
Also: Med. Classics, 2: 506–531, Jan. 1938
McCallig, John James. Rochester, Minn. surgeon. 1911–
TEST—tight bandage t., to detect localized deep obstruction to veins of leg.
A basic understanding of varicose veins with W. W. Heyerdale, J. A. M. A., 115: 97–100, July 13, 1940
MacCallum, William George. Baltimore pathologist. 1874–1944
METHOD—
A stain for influenza bacilli in tissues; a combination of Goodpasture's and Weigert's stains. J. A. M. A., 72: 193 (only), Jan. 18, 1919
MODIFICATION—of Cowdry's copper hematoxylin stain, for pituitary gland.
Relation of the Cushing syndrome to the pars intermedia of the hypophysis with T. B. Futcher, G. L. Duff and R. Ellsworth, Johns Hopk. Hosp. Bull., 56: 350–365, June 1935
Observed conjugation of organisms (of malaria) in birds and thus explained their flagellate form. Garrison
On the haematozoan infections of birds. Ibid., 8: 235–236, Nov. 1897
On the flagellated form of the malarial parasite. Lancet, 2: 1240–1241, Nov. 13, 1897

Showed relation of tumors of parathyroid glands with disease of kidneys.
Tumor of the parathyroid gland. Johns Hopk. Hosp. Bull., 16: 87–89, Mar. 1905
Demonstrated—
On the relation of the parathyroid to calcium metabolism and the nature of tetany with C. Voegtlin, Ibid. 19: 91–92, Mar. 1908
Suggested—
On the relation of the islands of Langerhans to glycosuria. Ibid., 20: 265–268, Sept. 1909

McCarrison, Sir Robert. India physician. 1878–
Showed that urinary calculi could follow a diet deficient in vitamin A.
The experimental production of stone-in-the-bladder with a note on pernicious anaemia and epidemic dropsy. (Preliminary note). Ind. J. med. Res., 14: 895–899, Apr. 1927 et seq.

MacCarty, William Carpenter. Rochester, Minn. pathologist. 1880–
THEORY—cancer of stomach frequently develops on chronic benign ulcer.
Chronic gastric ulcer and its relation to gastric carcinoma: review of six hundred eighty-four specimens with A. C. Broders, Arch. intern. Med., 13: 208–223, Feb. 1914
Coined term strawberry gallbladder.
The pathology of the gall-bladder and some associated lesions. A study of specimens from 365 cholecystectomies. Ann. Surg., 51: 651–669 (656), May 1910
The frequency of "strawberry" gall-bladders. Ibid., 69: 131–137, Feb. 1919

McCaughan, John Milton. St. Louis surgeon. 1899–
TECHNIC—
Subtotal pancreatectomy for hyperinsulinism: operative technic. Ann. Surg., 101: 1336–1341, June 1935

McClellan, U. S. See R. R. Hannon

M'Clintock, Alfred Henry. Irish physician. 1822–1881
SIGN—pulse rate exceeding 100 an hour or more after childbirth points to postpartem hemorrhage.
On secondary hemorrhage after parturition. Dublin Q. J. M. Sci., 11: 257–300, May 1, 1851

McClung, Clarence Erwin. Philadelphia zoologist. 1870–
Identified chromosomes as determinants of sex.
The accessory chromosome: sex determination. Biol. Bull., Boston, 3: 43–48, 1902

McGuire, Roy Donaldson. Baltimore surgeon. 1882–
OPERATION—
Hydrocephalus treated by drainage into a vein of the neck. Johns Hopk. Hosp. Bull., 20: 110–113, Apr. 1909
See also H. N. Harkins

McClure, William Bradbury. Chicago physician
TEST—for occult edema.
Time required for disappearance of intradermally injected salt solution. Preliminary report of observations with special reference to cases of edema with C. A. Aldrich, J. A. M. A., 81: 293–294, July 28, 1923
See also C. A. Aldrich

MacCollum, Donald Wieting. Boston surgeon. 1908–
OPERATION—
Webbed fingers. S. G. O., 71: 782–789, Dec. 1940

McCollum, Estel Bertrum. Detroit physician. 1903–

TUBE—
McCollum tube for sinus drainage. J. A. M. A., 112: 1821 (only), May 6, 1939

McCollum, Elmer Verner. American biochemist. 1879–
Discovered vitamin A.
The necessity of certain lipins in the diet during growth with Marguerite Davis, J. biol. Chem., 15: 167–175, July 1913
See also H. D. Kruse, H. J. Prebluda

McConghan, J. M. See R. Elman

MacConkey, Alfred Theodore. London bacteriologist. 1861–1931
AGAR and TEST—basal bile salt peptone.
Note on a new medium for the growth and differentiation of the Bacillus coli communis and the Bacillus typhi abdominalis. Lancet, 2: 20 (only), July 7, 1900
METHOD—
Note on staining the capsules of pneumococcus and of the bacillus of Friedländer. Ibid., 2: 1262 (only), Nov. 12, 1898

McCool, Joseph Lettelle. Portland, Ore. ophthalmologist. 1879–
OPERATION—
Graduated tenotomy of the inferior oblique muscle as an aid in the correction of certain forms of squint. Trans. Amer. Acad. Ophthal., pp. 163–170, 1922

McCoord, Augusta B. American scientist
METHOD—for determination of vitamin A.
The storage of vitamin A in the liver of the rat with Ethel M. Luce-Clausen, J. Nutrition, 7: 557–572, May 10, 1934

McCord, Carey Pratt. American physician. 1886–
PARADOX—
The pineal gland: the influence of the pineal gland upon growth and differentiation with particular reference to its influence upon prenatal development. S. G. O., 25: 250–260, Sept. 1917
TEST—
The basophilic aggregation test in lead poisoning: preliminary report with Dorothy K. Minster and Mathilde Rehm, J. A. M. A., 82: 1759–1763, May 31' 1924

McCordock, H. A. See R. S. Mackenfuss

MacCormac, Sir William. Irish surgeon. 1836–1901
OPERATION—
Some observations on rupture of the urinary bladder, with an account of two cases of intra-peritoneal rupture successfully treated by abdominal section and subsequent suture of the vesical rent. Lancet, 2: 1118–1122, Dec. 11, 1886

MacCormick, Sir Alexander. Australian surgeon. 1856–
OPERATION—suture of common bile duct after exploration.
Choledocholithotomy with intraduodenal drainage and closure of the common duct: MacCormick's technique by Douglas Miller, Aust. and New Zealand J. Surg., 3: 265–269, Jan. 1934

McCormick, Charles Owen. Indianapolis physician. 1886–
APPARATUS—for rectal instillation of ether in oil.
Popularizing ether-oil rectal analgesia in obstetrics. J. Indiana State Med. Ass., 25: 454–456, Oct. 1932
See also J. T. Gwathmey

MacCorquodale, Donald William. St. Louis chemist. 1898–

Isolated estradiol.

The isolation of the principle estrogenic substance of liquor folliculi with S. A. Thayer and E. A. Doisy, J. biol. Chem., 115: 435–448, Sept. 1936

See also R. W. McKee

McCoy, George Walter. American physician. 1876–

Described tularaemia.

I. Studies upon plague in ground squirrels. II. A plague-like disease of rodents. Bull. Hyg. Lab., U. S. Pub. Health Service, No. 43, Apr. 1911. pp. 71

Further observations on the plague-like disease of rodents with a preliminary note on the causative agent, Bacterium tularense with C. W. Chapin, J. infect. Dis., 10: 61–72, Jan. 1912

McCrae, John. Johannesburg scientist

REAGENT—

Kobert's reagent as a test for salicylic acid. Analyst, 36: 540–541, Nov. 1911

McCrearry, Charles. Kentucky surgeon. 1785–1826

First to successfully excise clavicle, 1811, Garrison *Osteo-sarcoma. Professor Mott and Dr. McCrearry.* By J. H. Johnson, New Orleans Med. and Surg. J., 6: 474–476, Jan. 1850

(Successful excision of clavicle at its articulation, 1813). Trans. Kentucky Med. Soc., 1852, 2: 276, 1853

McCreary, J. F. See C. D. May

McCrudden, Francis Henry. Boston physician. 1879–

METHOD—

The quantitative separation of calcium and magnesium in the presence of phosphates and small amounts of iron devised especially for the analysis of foods, urine and feces. J. biol. Chem., 7: 83–100, Jan. 1910

McCullagh, D(ouglas) Roy. Cleveland biochemist. 1903–

METHOD—

A new method for the determination of iodine. J. biol. Chem., 107: 35–44, Oct. 1934

McCurdy, James Huff. Boston physician. 1866–

RISE—

The effect of maximum muscular effort on blood-pressure. Amer. J. Physiol., 5: 95–103, Mar. 1, 1901

McCurdy, U. F. See K. M. Vogel

McDaniel, O. See F. F. Westbrook

McDermott, Katherine. See J. T. Freund

McDill, John Rich. Milwaukee surgeon. 1860–1934

METHOD—of hemostasis of liver.

Bloodless surgery of the liver: an experimental study of the possibility of excision of maximum amounts of liver tissue, with the usual instruments at hand in any hospital. J. A. M. A., 59: 1283–1286, Oct. 5, 1912

MacDonagh, James Eustace Radclyffe. English physician. 1881–

TEST—

A new test for syphilis (the emulsoid gelation, or the "gel" test). Brit. J. Dermat., 38: 114–119, 1916

McDonald, Ellice. American surgeon. 1876–

SOLUTION—

Disinfection of the hands and abdominal skin before operation. S. G. O., 21: 82–86, July 1915

A new McDonald's solution. Ibid., 66: 246 (only), Feb. 1, 1938

McDonald, H. P. See E. G. Ballenger

MacDonald, Katherine. See Florence Hulton-Frankel

McDonald, W. See J. B. Cleland

Macdonald, William Dean. St. Catharines, Ont. physician. 1905–

METHOD—of testing liver function.

Some observations on the disappearance of bromsulphalein dye from the blood: its relation to liver function. Canad. med. Ass. J., 39: 556–560, Dec. 1938

McDonnell, C. H. See R. M. Nesbit

McDowell, Ephraim. American surgeon. 1771–1830

OPERATION—ovariotomy.

Three cases of extirpation of diseased ovaria. Eclectic Repertory and Anal. Rev., 7: 242–244, 1817

Also: Med. Classics, 2: 651–653, Mar. 1938

Observations on diseased ovaria. Eclectic Repertory and Anal. Rev., 9: 546–553, 1819

Also: Med. Classics, 2: 654–661, Mar. 1938

McDowell, M. M. See Bullis

McElroy, W. S. See O. K. O. Folin

Macewen, Sir William. Glasgow surgeon. 1848–1924

OPERATION, OSTEOTOMY—supracondyloid division of femur for genu valgum.

Lecture on antiseptic osteotomy for genu valgum, genu varum, and other osseous deformities. Lancet, 2: 911–914, 1878; 1: 586–587, 1879

OPERATION—

Radical cure of hernia: ligature of internal inguinal ring by chromic acid sutures. Glasgow med. J., 13: 54–60, 1880

On the radical cure of oblique inguinal hernia by internal abdominal peritoneal pad, and the restoration of the valved form of the inguinal canal. Ann. Surg., 4: 89–119, Aug. 1886

OPERATION—

An address on aneurism: its cure by inducing the formation of white thrombi within the sac. Brit. med. J., 2: 1107–1109, Nov. 15; 1164–1168, Nov. 22, 1890

SIGN—cracked-pot note on percussion in fracture of skull.

Pyogenic infective diseases of the brain and spinal cord. Glasgow, Maclehose, 1893. 354 pp. pp. 148–149

TUBES—drainage.

Clinical lectures on some points connected with the treatment of wounds. Brit. med. J., 1: 185–187, Feb. 5, 1881

McFarland, Joseph. Philadelphia pathologist. 1868–1945

INSTRUMENT—

The nephelometer: an instrument for estimating the number of bacteria in suspensions used for calculating the opsonic index and for vaccines. J. A. M. A., 49: 1176–1178, Oct. 5, 1907

MacFarlane, Robert Gwyn. London physician

Wrote—

The haemostatic possibilities of snake-venom with B. Barnett, Lancet, 2: 985–987, Nov. 3, 1934

MacFee, William Frank. New York surgeon. 1890–

OPERATION—

Pilonidal cysts and sinuses: a method of wound closure: review of 230 cases. Ann. Surg., 116: 687–699, Nov. 1942

McFetridge, Elizabeth M. See F. F. Boyce

McGarry, R. A. See M. F. Engman

McGee, Lemuel Clyde. American biochemist. 1902–

Made successful preparations of male hormone.

The effect of the injection of a lipoid fraction of bull testicle in capons. Proc. Inst. Med., Chicago, 6: 242–244, 1927

McGee, W. Ambrose. Richmond physician. 1899–
METHOD—rapid Giemsa stain for blood.
The value of the Schilling differential blood count in pediatrics. South. med. J., 25: 484–489, May 1932

Macgill, George. Maryland surgeon. 1838–1867
First to successfully tie both primitive carotids in continuity, within a months' interval, 1823. Garrison
Account of a case in which both carotids were successfully tied by Dr. Macgill, Maryland, in a letter from Dr. Joshua I. Cohen of Baltimore, to Dr. J. Kearny Rodgers of New York. New York Med. and Phys. J., 4: 576 (only), 1825

McGlannon, Alexius. Baltimore surgeon. 1872–1940
OPERATION—for umbilical hernia.
Massive umbilical and ventral hernias. S. G. O., 20: 700–704, June 1915

McGrath, Bernard Francis. American surgeon. 1869–1933
APPARATUS—
A simple apparatus for transfusion by the aspiration-injection method. S. G. O., 18: 376–377, Mar. 1914

McGraw, Theodore A. Detroit surgeon. 1839–1921
LIGATURE—
Upon the use of the elastic ligature in the surgery of the intestines. J. A. M. A., 16: 685–694, May 16, 1891

McGregor, Leone. Canadian physician. 1900–
METHOD—
The finer histology of the normal glomerulus. Amer. J. Path., 5: 545–557, Nov. 1929

MacGregor, William Wilbur. Detroit surgeon. 1886–
OPERATION—
The demonstration of a true internal inguinal sphincter and its etiologic role in hernia. S. G. O., 49: 510–515, Oct. 1929
The fundamental operative treatment of inguinal hernia. Ibid., 50: 438–440, Feb. 1930

McGuigan, H. See C. L. von Hess

McGuire, Hunter Holmes. Richmond surgeon. 1835–1900
Ligated aorta.
Surgical cases. I. Aneurism of the external iliac of the left side, both common iliacs, and lower end of aorta; ligation of the aorta; death; . . . Amer. J. med. Sci., 56: 415–418, Oct. 1868

Machell, T. Scottish surgeon
SAW—circular bone cutting.
Description of an annular saw. Edinburgh Med. and Surg. J., 1: 273–279, July 1815

Machek, Dr. Lemberg surgeon
OPERATION—for ptosis.
Eine Ptosisoperation mit Bildung einer Deckfalte am oberen Lid. Arch. Augenheilk., 76: 8–14, Jan. 1914

McHenry, E. W. See C. H. Best

Machin, John. English physician. ?–1751
Made original observation of ichthyosis hystrix. Garrison
An uncommon case of a distempered skin. Philos. Trans., 1731–1732, 37: 299–301, 1733

Machol, Alfred. German surgeon
OPERATION—formation of new thumb.
Beitrag zur Daumenplastik. Beitr. klin. Chir., 114: 181–188, 1919

Macht, David Israel. American pharmacologist. 1882–
Introduced—
A pharmacological and therapeutic study of benzyl alcohol as a local anesthetic. J. Pharmacol., 11: 263–279, Apr. 1918
See also J. J. Abel

McIndoe, Archibald Hector. London surgeon
CRITERIA—for delayed rupture after splenic injury.
Delayed hemorrhage following traumatic rupture of the spleen. Brit. J. Surg., 20: 249–268, Oct. 1932
OPERATION—
The treatment of hypospadias. Amer. J. Surg., 38: 176–185, Oct. 1937
OPERATION—
An operation for the cure of congenital absence of the vagina with J. B. Banister, J. Obstet. Gynaec. Brit. Emp., 45: 490–494, June 1938

McIntosh, J. F. See E. Möller

McIntosh, James. English physician
METHOD—
A new apparatus for the isolation and cultivation of anaerobic micro-organisms with P. Fildes, Lancet, 1: 768–770, Apr. 8, 1916

McIntosh, R. L. See O. H. Foerster

Macintyre, John. Glasgow physician. 1869–
Wrote—
Roentgen rays. Photography of renal calculus; description of an adjustable modification in the focus tube. Lancet, 2: 118 (only), July 11, 1896
X-ray records for the cinematograph. Arch. clin. Skiagraphy, London, 1: 37 (only), Apr. 1897

McIver, Robert Boyd. Jacksonville, Fla. urologist. 1892–
OPERATION—for hydronephrosis.
Plastic surgery of the renal pelvis. J. Urol., 42: 1069–1083, Dec. 1939

McJunkin, Frank Adam. Milwaukee pathologist. 1882–
METHOD—for recognition of monocytes.
A simple technic for the demonstration of a phagocytic mononuclear cell in peripheral blood. Arch. intern. Med., 21: 59–65, Jan. 15, 1918
STAIN—
A benzidine-polychrome stain for blood. J. A. M. A., 74: 17–19, Jan. 3, 1920
Peroxydase staining with benzidin in paraffin sections of human tissue: sixth report of studies on the mononuclear leukocytes of the blood. Anat. Rec., 24: 67–76, Sept. 20, 1922

McKay, F. S. See G. V. Black

McKay, Frances M. See V. E. Levine

McKay, Robert Witherspoon. Charlotte, N. C. urologist. 1875–
DISLODGER—
A urethreal stone dislodger. J. A. M. A., 95: 794 (only), Sept. 13, 1930

Mackay, William John Stewart. English physician. 1866–
METHOD—
The blood-platelet: its clinical significance. Quart. J. Med., 24: 285–328, Apr. 1931

McKee, Clara M. New Jersey scientist
TEST—
Complement fixation test in lymphogranuloma ve-

nereum with G. Rake and M. F. Shaffer, Proc. Soc. exp. Biol., N. Y., 44: 410–413, June 1940

McKee, Ralph Wendell. St. Louis biochemist. 1912– Isolated vitamin K.
The isolation of vitamins K_1 and K_2 with S. B. Binkley, D. W. MacCorquodale, S. A. Thayer and E. A. Doisy, J. Amer. Chem. Soc., 61: 1295 (only), May 1939
See also E. A. Doisy

Mackenfuss, Ralph S. St. Louis physician
Isolated St. Louis encephalitis virus.
Encephalitis: studies on experimental transmission with C. Armstrong and H. A. McCordock, Pub. Health Rep., Washington, 48: 1341–1443, Nov. 3, 1933

McKenna, Charles Morgan. Chicago urologist. 1880–
OPERATION—
Hypospadias: observations on its surgical correction. J. A. M. A., 113: 2138–2143, Dec. 9, 1939

Mackenrodt, Alwin Karl. German gynecologist. 1859–1925
LIGAMENT—uterosacral.
Ueber die Ursachen der normalen und pathologischen Lagen des Uterus. Arch. f. Gynaek., 48: 393–421, 1895
OPERATION—plastic reformation of vagina.
Ueber den künstlichen Ersatz der Scheide. Zbl. Gynack., 20: 546–550, 1896
Ueber den hinteren Scheidenbauchschnitt. Samml. klin. Vortr., No. 156 (Gynaek., No. 56, pp. 569–596, 1896

McKenzie, B. F. See E. C. Kendall

MacKenzie, Hector Graham Gordon. English physician
TREATMENT—
A case of myxedema treated with great benefit by feeding with fresh thyroid glands. Brit. med. J., 2: 940–941, Oct. 29, 1892

Mackenzie, James. English physician. 1853–1925
First investigated multiform arrhythmias and differentiated "nodal rhythm" or auricular fibrillation. Garrison
Diseases of the heart. London, Fromde, 1908

MacKenzie, Kenneth Alexander J. Portland, Ore. surgeon. 1859–1920
OPERATION—
Surgical treatment of fistula in ano without mutilation of the sphincter. Trans. Amer. Surg., Ass., pp. 160–173, 1911

Mackenzie, Richard James. Edinburgh surgeon. 1821–1854
AMPUTATION—
On amputation at the ankle-joint by internal lateral flap. Month. J. med. Sci., 9: 951–954, Aug. 1849

MacKenzie, Sir Stephen. London physician. 1844–1909
SYNDROME—
Two cases of associated paralysis of the tongue, soft palate, and vocal cord on the same side. Trans. clin. Soc. Lond., 19: 317–319, 1886

Mackenzie, William. Scottish oculist. 1791–1868
Wrote on catoptrics.
On the vision of objects on and in the eye. Edinburgh med. and Surg., J., 64: 38–97, July 1, 1845

McKesson, Elmer Isaac. Toledo, O. physician. 1881–1935
APPARATUS—
Nitrous oxid-oxygen anaesthesia: with the description of a new apparatus. S. G. O., 13: 456–462, Oct. 1911

McKhann, C. F. See P. Drinker

McKibben, P. S. See L. H. Weed

Mackid, Ludwig Stewart. Calgary surgeon. 1882–
OPERATION—for sliding hernia.
Inguinal hernia: with special reference to sliding hernia and a new treatment. Canad. med. Ass. J., 34: 269–271, May 1926

Mackie, T. J. See C. H. Browning

Mackie, Thomas Turlay. New York physician. 1895–
Emphasized frequency and importance of deficiency states in chronic ulcerative colitis. Haden
Ulcerative colitis: II. The factor of deficiency states. J. A. M. A., 104: 175–178, Jan. 19, 1935

McKinlay, C. A. See H. Downey

McKinlay, Leland Murray. Grand Rapids, Mich. urologist. 1893–
CYSTOMETER—
A valveless cystometer delivering an uninterrupted stream. J. Urol., 28: 727–730, Dec. 1932

McKinney, Marion. See E. F. Hirsch

McKinnon, Neil E. Toronto physician. 1894–
DIAGNOSTIC TEST—
The reaction in the skin of the normal rabbit following intradermal injection of material from small pox lesions: the specificity of this reaction and its application as a diagnostic test with R. D. Defries, Amer. J. Hyg., 8: 93–106, Jan. 1928

McKittrick, Leland Sterling. Boston surgeon. 1893–
CRITERIA—for amputation.
The operative treatment of lesions of the lower extremities in diabetes mellitus with T. C. Pratt, Arch. Surg., 21: 555–581, Oct. 1931

Maclachlan, W. W. G. See O. Klotz

Maclagan, N. F. English pathologist
TEST—
The thymol turbidity test as an indicator of liver dysfunction. Brit. J. exp. Path., 25: 234–241, Dec. 1944

Maclagan, Thomas John. Edinburgh physician. 1838–1903
Introduced salicylate treatment for rheumatism.
Rheumatism; its nature, its pathology, and its successful treatment. London, Pickering, 1881. 333 pp.

MacLean, A. R. See B. T. Horton

McLean, Franklin Chambers. American physician. 1888–
FORMULA-INDEX—of kidney function.
Urea and total non-protein nitrogen in normal human blood: relation of their concentration to rate of elimination with L. Selling, J. biol. Chem., 19: 31–38, Sept. 1914
The numerical laws governing the rate of excretion of urea and chlorides in man. I. An index of urea excretion and the normal excretion of urea and chlorides. J. exp. Med., 22: 212–236, 1915
Clinical determination of renal function by an index of urea excretion. J. A. M. A., 66: 415–421, Feb. 5, 1916
METHOD—
A method for the determination of chlorides in small

amounts of body fluids with D. D. Van Slyke, J. biol. Chem., 21: 361–370, June 1915

MacLean, Hugh. London pathologist. 1879–
TEST—
The estimation of sugar tolerance with O. L. de Wesselow. Quart. J. Med., 14: 103–119, Jan. 1921
TEST—urea concentration.
On the testing of renal efficiency, with observation on the "urea coefficient" with O. L. de Wesselow, Brit. J. exp. Path., 1: 53–65, Feb. 1920

McLean, Jay. Baltimore scientist. 1890–
First isolated naturally occurring anticoagulant (heparin).
The thromboplastic action of cephalin. Amer. J. Physiol., 41: 250–257, Aug. 1, 1916

McLean, John Milton. Baltimore ophthalmologist. 1909–
SUTURE—
A new corneoscleral suture. Arch. Ophthal., 23: 554–559, Mar. 1940

MacLean, R. M. See V. J. Harding

McLean, Regina. See C. C. Franseen

MacLenathen, Elizabeth. See I. S. Wright

MacLennan, Alexander. Scottish surgeon
OPERATION—
The radical cure of femoral hernia in children. Glasgow med. J., 96: 83–87, Aug. 1921
SKIN GRAFTING—
"Tunnel" skin-grafting: a new method of covering raw surfaces with epithelium. Ibid., 78: 86–90, Aug. 1912

MacLeod, A. G. See J. L. Morris

MacLeod, C. M. See F. L. Horsfall, Jr.

McLeod, James Walter. British bacteriologist. 1887–
METHOD—
Cultivation of the gonococcus as a method in the diagnosis of gonorrhea with special reference to the oxydase reaction and to the value of air reinforced in its carbon dioxide content with J. C. Coates, H. C. Happold, D. P. Priestley and B. Wheatley, J. Path. Bact., 39: 221–231, July 1934
See also J. S. Anderson

MacLeod, John James Richard. Canadian physiologist. 1876–1935
Awarded, with F. G. Banting, Nobel prize in 1923, for work on diabetes and insulin.
Diabetes; its pathological physiology. London, Arnold, 1913. 224 pp.
The antidiabetic functions of the pancreas and the successful isolation of the antidiabetic hormone—insulin with F. G. Banting, St. Louis, Mosby, 1924. 69 pp.
See also F. G. Banting

MacLeod, Roderick. Scottish physician. 1795–1852
RHEUMATISM—
On rheumatism in its various forms, and on the affections of internal organs, more especially the heart and brain, to which it gives rise. London, Longman, 1842. 164 pp.

McMaster, P. D. See R. Elman, F. P. Rous

McMichael, William. English physician. 1784–1839
Author of—
The gold-headed cane. London, Murray, 1827; also, ed. 1828, 1884, 1915, 1926, 1932.

McMillen, Robert M. Wheeling, W. Va. surgeon. 1862–1935
SUTURE—on-end mattress.

A new suture. West Virginia med. J., 4: 90–91, Sept. 1909

McMurray, Thomas Porter. Liverpool surgeon. 1887–
OPERATION—
Ununited fractures of the neck of the femur. J. Bone and Joint Surg., 18: 319–327, Apr. 1936

McNally, William Duncan. Chicago physician. 1882–
TECHNIC—for testing for silicon in lungs.
Silicon dioxide content of lungs in health and disease. J. A. M. A., 101: 584–587, Aug. 19, 1933

Macnaughton, Eric Alexander. Montreal surgeon. 1901–
SUCTION—to remove intestinal secretions from intestinal fistula.
The treatment of external fistulas of the proximal small bowel; a means of temporary mechanical anastomosis Surgery, 9: 372–380, Mar. 1941

Macnaughton, F. G. English physician
BROTH—blood infusion.
A simple emergency medium for the primary growth of the gonococcus. J. Path. Bact., 26: 297 (only), Apr. 1923

MacNeal, Ward J. American pathologist. 1881–1946
ADAPTATION—of Strasburger procedure, for quantitative determination of fecal bacteria.
The fecal bacteria of healthy men. Part I. Introduction and direct quantitative observations with Lenore L Latzer and Josephine E. Kerr, J. infect. Dis., 6 123–169, Apr. 1, 1909
AGAR—blood infusion, for isolation of Trypanosomes
The life-history of Trypanosoma Lewisi and Trypanosoma Brucei. Ibid., 1: 517–543, Nov. 5, 1904
AGAR—gelatin, culture medium for Bacillus abortus
Bacillus abortus of Bang, the cause of contagious abortion in cattle with Josephine E. Kerr, Ibid., 7 469–475, May 20, 1910
METHOD—
A rapid and simple method of staining spirocheta pallida. J. A. M. A., 48: 609–610, Feb. 16, 1907
STAIN—
Tetrachrome blood stain: an economical and satisfactory imitation of Leishman's stain. Ibid., 78: 1122–1123, Apr. 15, 1922
See also F. G. Novy

McNealy, Raymond William. Chicago surgeon 1886–
METHOD—of duodenal tamponade.
Problems with duodenal stump in gastric resections Surgery, 12: 207–215, Aug. 1942
OPERATION—
Simple technique for cecostomy with M. E. Lichtenstein, Amer. J. Surg., 36: 620–622, June 1937
TECHNIC—
Surgery of carotid body tumors with R. I. Hedin, J Internat. Col. Surg., 2: 285–294, Oct. 1939

M'Nee, John William. Glasgow pathologist. 1887–
Studied icterus and showed that bile pigment formation is not a function of liver cells alone.
Experiments on haemolytic icterus. J. Path. Bact. 18: 325–342, Jan. 1914

McNeil, Ethel. See C. A. Kofoid

MacPhail, F. L. See J. R. Goodall

McPheeters, Herman Oscar. Minneapolis surgeon 1891–

SPONGE HEART—
  Varicose ulcers: treatment with "the rubber sponge or venous heart" and supportive bandage with C. E. Merkert, S. G. O., 52: 1164–1169, June 1931
TEST—pulse percussion from varicose vein to saphenous vein.
  Causes of failure in injection treatment of varicose veins with C. E. Merkert and R. A. Lundblad, J. A. M. A., 96: 1114–1117, Apr. 4, 1931
McReynolds, John Oliver. Dallas, Texas otolaryngologist. 1865–1942
OPERATION—
  The nature and treatment of pterygia. Trans. Sect. Ophthal., A. M. A., pp. 47–55, 1902
McVay, Chester Bidwell. Ann Arbor, Mich. surgeon. 1911–
OPERATION—
  An anatomic error in current methods of inguinal herniorrhaphy. Ann. Surg., 113: 1111–1112, June 1941
McWhorter, Golder Lewis. Chicago urologist. 1888–1938
APPROACH—posterior, to shoulder.
  Fracture of the greater tuberosity of the humerus with displacement. Report of two operated cases with author's technic of shoulder incision. Surg. Clin. N. Amer., 5: 1005–1017, Aug. 1925
OPERATION—
  Operative treatment for extensive hypospadias. Ibid., 10: 275–282, Apr. 1930
MacWilliam, John Alexander. Aberdeen physician. 1857–1937
  Produced, experimentally, extrasystoles, ventricular fibrillation and auricular flutter.
  Fibrillar contraction of the heart. J. Physiol., 8: 296–310, 1887
  Also, in F. A. Willius and T. E. Keys' *Cardiac classics.* St. Louis, Mosby, 1941 pp. 666–678
  Described death from ventricular fibrillation.
  Cardiac failure and sudden death. Brit. med. J., 1: 6–8, Jan. 5, 1889
McWilliams, Helen I. See C. Krumwiede
Madden, R. J. See C. A. Elvehjem
Maddock, Walter Grierson. Ann. Arbor, Mich. surgeon. 1901–
INDEX—of water metabolism.
  Water balance in surgery with F. A. Coller, J. A. M. A., 108: 1–6, Jan. 2, 1937
  See also F. A. Coller
Maddox, Ernest Edmund. English ophthalmologist. 1860–1933
PRISM—used in testing for torsion of eyeball.
  The clinical use of prisms, and the decentering of lenses. Bristol, Wright, 1889. 113 pp.
RODS—used in testing for heterophoria.
  Tests and studies of the ocular muscles. Bristol, Wright, 1898. 422 pp.
Madelung, Otto Wilhelm. German surgeon. 1846–1926
DISEASE or DEFORMITY—
  Die spontane Subluxation der Hand nach vorne. Verh. dtsch. Ges. f. Chir., 7: 259–276, 1878
  Also: Arch. f. klin. Chir., 23: 395–412, 1879
DISEASE or FAT NECK.
  Ueber den Fetthals (diffuses Lipom des Halses). Ibid., 37: 106–130, 1888

OPERATION—lumbar colotomy.
  Über eine Modifikation der Colotomie wegen Carcinoma recti. Zbl. Chir., 11: 68–69, June 7, 1884
OPERATION—for varicose veins.
  Ueber die Ausschälung cirsoider Varicen an den unteren Extremitäten. Abstr.: Verh. dtsch. Ges. f. Chir., 13: 114–118, Apr. 19, 1884
SUTURE—to close intestinal wound, with small discs from costal cartilage from calf.
  Ueber circuläre Darmnaht und Darmresection. Verh. dtsch. Ges. f. Chir., 10: 415–464, 1881
Madlener, Max. German gynecologist
METHOD—of tubal sterilization.
  Ueber sterilisierende Operationen an den Tuben. Zbl. Gynaek., 40: 380–384, May 17, 1919
Madrid, A. See S. Lubach
Maechling, E. H. New York City scientist
METHOD—
  Calorimetric determination of small amounts of arsenic in biologic material with F. B. Flinn, J. Lab. clin. Med., 15: 779–782, May 1930
Maes, Urban. New Orleans surgeon. 1878–
TECHNIC—for leg amputation.
  The surgery of diabetes as it concerns gangrene of the lower extremities and carbuncles. S. G. O., 51: 700–704 Nov. 1930
Maffucci, Angelo. Italian physician. 1845–1903
  Isolated avian tubercle bacillus (B. Gallinaceous).
  Ricerche sperimentali sull'azione dei bacilli della tuberculosi dei Gallinacci e dei mammiferi nella vita embrionale ed adulta del pollo. Rif. med., Napoli, 5: 1251; 1257; 1263; 1268, 1275, 1889
Magath, T. B. See B. T. Horton, A. H. Sanford
Magendie, Francois. French physiologist. 1783–1855
FORAMEN—connecting fourth ventricle with subarachnoid space.
  Recherches physiologiques et cliniques sur le liquide céphalorachidien ou cérébro-spinal. Paris, Méquignon-Marvis, 1842
LAW—anterior spinal roots are motor, posterior are sensory.
  Expériences sur les fonctions des racines des nerfs rachidiens. J. de Physiol. expér., Paris, 2: 276–279; 366–371, 1822
  Also, English transl. in J .F. Fulton's *Selected readings in the history of physiology.* 1930, pp. 258–265
SOLUTION—of morphine.
  Formulaire pour la préparation et l'emploi de plusieurs nouveaux médicamens, tels que la noix vanique, la morphine, etc. Paris, Méquignon-Marvis, 1822
  Also, in English, 1824
  Described mechanism of act of deglutition. Garrison
  Mémoire sur l'usage de l'épiglotte dans la déglutition. . . . Paris, Méquignon-Marvis, 1813. 36 pp.
  Mémoire sur le vomissement. Paris, Crochard, 1813
  Also, English transl.: Ann. Phil., London, 1: 429–438 1813
  Demonstrated that absorption of fluids is function of blood vessels as well as of lymphatics.
  Mémoires sur le mécanisme de l'absorption chez les animaux à sang rouge et chaud. J. de Physiol. expér., 1: 1–31, 1821
  Described cerebrospinal fluid.
  Mémoire sur un liquide qui se trouve dans le crâne et le canal vertébral de l'homme et des animaux mammifères. Ibid., 5: 27–37, 1825; 7: 1–29, 1827

Experimentally produced purpura.
Précis élementaire de physiologie. Paris, 1833. ed 3, Vol. 2, p. 417
Also, transl. by J. Revere. N. Y., Harper, 1844
Made first experiments in anaphylaxis. Garrison
In: *Lectures on the blood, and on the changes which it undergoes during disease.* Philadelphia, Harrington et al., 1839, 276 pp. pp. 244–249
Showed that digested food is carried to liver in portal blood. Homans
Treatise on human physiology. N. Y., Harper, 1844. pp. 368–369
See also P. J. Pelletier

Magill, Ivan Whiteside. English physician
TUBE—
Endotracheal anaesthesia. Proc. roy. Soc. (Sect. Anaesth.), 22: 1–6, Dec. 1928
See also E. S. Rowbotham

Magitot, Emile. Paris surgeon. 1833–1897
DISEASE—
Sur l'ostéo-périostite alvéolo-dentaire. Arch. gén. de méd., Paris, 6 s., 10: 35–49, July 1867

Magnus, Gustav. German physician. 1802–1870
"Showed, with aid of a Sprengel's air-pump, that venous and arterial blood both contain oxygen as well as CO_2, demonstrating that all tissues respire in sense of assimilating oxygen and giving up CO_2." Garrison
Ueber die im Blute enthaltenen Gase, Sauerstoff, Stickstoff und Kohlensäure. Ann. d. Phys. u. Chem., Leipz., 12: 583–606, 1837
Also, transl.: Ann. de chim., Paris, 65: 169–192, 1837

Magnuson, Paul Budd. Chicago surgeon. 1884–
OPERATION—
The repair of ununited fracture of the neck of the femur. J. A. M. A., 98: 1791–1794, May 21, 1932
OPERATION—
Recurrent dislocation of the shoulder with J. K. Stack, Ibid., 123: 889–892, Dec. 4, 1943

Magnus-Levy, Adolf. German physician. 1865–
Introduced experimental method of determining thyroid disturbances.
Ueber den respiratorischen gaswechsel unter dem Einfluss der Thyreoidea sowie unter verschiedenen pathologische Zuständen. Berl. klin. Wschr., 32: 650–652, July 29, 1895
Studied relationship of B-oxybutyric acid and diabetic coma. Garrison and Morton
Die Oxybuttersäure und ihre Beziehungen zum Coma diabeticum. Arch. exp. Path. Pharmak., 42: 149–237, May 16, 1899
Untersuchungen über die Acidosis im Diabetes melitus und die Säureintoxication im Coma diabeticum. Ibid., 45: 389–434, Apr. 19, 1901

Magoun, H. W. See S. W. Ranson

Magyary-Kossa, Julius von. Budapest physician
METHOD—silver nitrate, for staining calcium.
Ueber die im Organismus künstlich erzeugbaren Verkalkungen. Beitr. path. Anat., 29: 163–202, 1901
REACTION—for blood.
Ein Verfahren zum Nachweiss von Blut. Dtsch. med. Wschr., 35: 1469–1470, Aug. 26, 1909

Maher, Frank Thomas. Chicago scientist. 1909–

TEST—
A qualitative test for bile in the urine. Science, 94: 398 (only), Oct. 24, 1941

Mahler, Richard A. German obstetrician
SIGN—steady increase of pulse rate without corresponding elevation of temperature indicates thrombosis.
Thrombose, Lungenembolie und plötzlicher Tod. 1895

Mahomed, Frederick Henry Horatio Akbar. English physician. 1849–1884
Discovered pre-albuminuric stage of hypertension.
Chronic Bright's disease without albuminuria. Cambridge, 1881. 106 pp.

Mahoney, John Friend. Staten Island, N. Y. physician. 1889–
TREATMENT—
Penicillin treatment of early syphilis: a preliminary report with R. C. Arnold and A. Harris, Ven. Dis. Inform., 24: 355–357, Dec. 1943
(Same) II with R. C. Arnold, B. L. Sterner, A. Harris and M. R. Zwally, J. A. M. A., 126: 63–67, Sept. 9, 1944
See also J. E. Moore

Mahorner, Howard Raymond. New Orleans surgeon. 1903–
TEST—
A new test for evaluating circulation in the venous system of the lower extremity affected by varicosities with A. Ochsner, Arch. Surg., 33: 479–492, Sept. 1936
See also E. W. A. Ochsner

Maier, R. See A. Kussmaul

Maingot, Rodney Honor. London surgeon
TECHNIC—
Resection of head of pancreas and duodenum for carcinoma. Lancet, 2: 798–800, Dec. 27, 1941

Maissonneuve, Jacquer Gilles Thomas Francois. French surgeon. 1809–1897
FRACTURE—lateral dislocation of foot with high fibular fracture.
Recherches sur la fracture du péroné. Arch. gén. de méd., 1: 165–187; 433–473, 1840
Introduced a hair catheter.
Mémoire sur un moyen très-simple et très-sûr de pratiquer le cathétérisme dans les cas même les plus difficiles. C. R. Acad. Sci., Paris, 20: 70–72, Jan. 6, 1845

Maitland, Hugh Bethune. Toronto bacteriologist
MEDIUM—
Cultivation of vaccinia virus without tissue culture with Mary C. Maitland, Lancet, 2: 596–597, Sept. 22, 1928

Maitland, Sir H. L. Sydney surgeon
OPERATION—
A radical method of extirpating malignant growths in the neck, secondary to mouth carcinoma. Australasian Med. Gaz., 25: 497–503, Oct. 20, 1906

Majocchi, Domenico. Italian dermatologist. 1849–1929
DISEASE—purpura telangiectoides annularis.
Sopra una dermatosi telangiectode non ancora descritta "Purpura annularis." G. ital. d. mal. ven. e d. mal. d. pelle, 31: 263–264, 1896

Major, Johann Daniel. German physician. 1634–1693
Made first successful intravenous injection in man, in 1662. Garrison
Chirurgia infusoria. Kiloni, Reumannus, 1667. 328 pp.

Major, Randolph Thomas. Westfield, N. J. chemist. 1901–
Introduced mecholyl.
Preparation and properties of Alpha- and Beta-methylcholine and Gamma-homocholine with J. K. Cline, J. Amer. Chem. Soc., 54: 242–249, Jan. 1932
See also W. L. Ruigh

Makgill, R. H. New Zealand physician
BOUILLON—
The neutral-red reaction as a means of detecting Bacillus coli in water supplies. J. Hyg., 1: 430–436 (431), Oct. 1901

Makins, George Henry. English surgeon. 1853–
CLAMP—for resection of intestine.
A case of artificial anus treated by resection of the small intestine. St. Thomas' Hosp. Rep., 13: 81, 1884

Makkas, M. Bonn surgeon
OPERATION—for ectopia of bladder.
Zur Behandlung der Blasenektopie. Umwanglung des ausgeschalteten Coecum zur Blase und der Appendix zur Urethra. Zbl. Chir., 37: 1073–1076, Aug. 13, 1910

Makuen, George Hudson. Philadelphia laryngologist. 1855–1917
METHOD—of lengthening palate.
Cleft palate and its relation to speech. Amer. Med., 2: 532–533, Oct. 5, 1901

Malaquin, Paul. French pharmacologist
REACTION—for strychnine.
Nouvelle réaction pour la caractérisation de la strychnine. J. pham. chim., 6 s., 30: 546–549, 1909

Malassez, Louis Charles. Paris physiologist. 1842–1909
DISEASE—cyst of testicle.
Note sur un cas de maladie kystique du testicule. Arch. Physiol. norm. path., 2 s., 2: 122–135, Jan. 1875
Designed first harmocystometer. Garrison and Morton.
Nouvelle méthode de numération des globules rouges et des globules blancs du sang. Ibid., 2 s., 1: 32–52, Jan. 1874

Malcolm, John David. English surgeon
Showed that in shock there is a constriction of peripheral vessels.
The physiology of death from traumatic fever; a study in abdominal fever. London, Churchill, 1893. 129 pp. p. 22 ff.

Malcolmson, John Grant. English physician. ?–1844
Wrote classic account of beri-beri. Garrison and Morton
A practical essay on the history and treatment of beri-beri. Madras, Govt. Press, 1835

Malerba, Pasquale. Naples physician. 1849–1917
TEST—for acetone.
Réactif pour l'acétone et l'acide urique. Abstr.; Arch. ital. biol., 22: LXXXVI–LXXXVII, 1895

Malfatti, Hans. German chemist

METHOD—of determination of ammonia in urine.
Eine klinische Methode zur Bestimmung des Ammoniaks im Harne. Z. anal. Chem., 47: 273–278, 1908

Malgaigne, Joseph Francois. French surgeon. 1806–1865
FRACTURE—bilateral of pelvis.
Traité des fractures et des luxations. Paris, Baillière, 1847. Vol. 1, pp. 650–656
Also, in German. Stuttgart, 1850. Vol. 1, p. 635

Maliner, Martin M. Brooklyn physician. 1896–
TEST—
An adrenalin chloride test for murmurs in children. Arch. Pediat., 49: 305–313, May 1932

Maliniac, Jacques W. New York surgeon. 1889–
OPERATION—
The pendulous hypertrophic breast: comparative values of present-day methods of repair and the procedure of choice. Arch. Surg., 31: 587–600, Oct. 1935

Mall, Franklin Paine. Baltimore anatomist. 1862–1917
FORMULA—for age of embryo.
OVUM—
A human embryo of the second week. Anat. Anz., Jena, 8: 630–633, Aug. 5, 1893
Contributions to the study of the pathology of early human embryos. Baltimore, 1899–1908. 3 pts.
Studied peristalsis.
A study of the intestinal contractions. Johns Hopk. Hosp. Rep., 1: 37–75, 1896
Reversal of the intestine. Ibid., 93–110

Mallory, Franklin Burr. Boston pathologist. 1863–1941
METHOD—for actinomyces.
A case of actinomycosis. Med. and Surg. Rep. Boston City Hosp., 6 s., 179–189, 1895
PHOSPHO-MOLYBDIC HAEMOTOXYLIN—
Phospho-molybdic acid haematoxylon. Ana. Anz., pp. 375–376, July 18, 1891
STAIN—
On certain improvements in histological technique. I. A differential stain for amoeba coli. . . . J. exp. Med., 2: 529–533, Sept. 1897
STAIN—
(Same) *III A method of fixation for neuroglia fibers.* Ibid.
STAIN—for elastic fibers.
A contribution to staining methods. . . . Ibid., 5: 15–20, Oct. 1, 1900
STAIN—for connective tissue. Ibid.
STAIN—eosin and methylen blue.
Scarlet fever. Protozoon-like bodies found in four cases. J. med. Res., 10: 483–492, Jan. 1904
STAINS—haematoxylin.
In: *Pathological technique.* Philadelphia, Saunders, 1897. pp. 239–244
STAIN—for tubercle bacilli in sections. Ibid., p. 285. Ed., 1938, p. 413
STAIN—iron chloride (ferric) hematoxylin. See
STAIN—*A contribution to* . . .
STAIN—phosphotungstic acid hematoxylin. Ibid.
STAIN— *
A lead hematoxylin stain for axis cylinders. Amer. J. Path., 12: 569–571, July 1936

Named mononuclear phagocytes of typhoid fever "endothelial leucocytes."

A histological study of typhoid fever. J. exp. Med., 3: 611–638, Nov. 1898

Established causal relation of specific bacillus of whooping cough to the disease.

The relation of the Bordet-Gengou bacillus to the lesion of pertussis with A. A. Homer and F. F. Henderson, J. med. Res., 27: 391–397, Mar. 1913

Malmros, H. See O. K. O. Folin

Malmstem, Peter Henrik. Swedish physician. 1811–1883

Discovered Balantidium coli, the first parasitic protozoon to be discovered and recognized as such. Garrison

Infusorier, sosom intestinaldjur hos menniskon. Hygiea, Stockholm, 19: 491–501, 1857

Also: Allg. med. Zbl.-Ztg., Berlin, 27: 81–89, 1858

Malpighi, Marcello. Italian anatomist. 1628–1694

BODIES or GLOMERULI—in kidney.

CANAL or TUBULES—uriniferous t.

CAPSULE—same as Bowman's c., beginning of uriniferous tubule in kidney.

CORPUSCLE or TUFTS—of blood vessels in kidney; same as bodies.

LAYER—in kidney.

PYRAMID—of kidney.

De viscerum structura exercitatio anatomica. Bononiae, Montii, 1666. 172 pp.

Also, abstr. transl. by J. M. Hayman, Jr. Ann. Med. Hist., 7: 245–263, Sept. 1925

Discovered capillary anastomosis in lungs, which supplied missing link in Harvey's demonstration. Garrison

De pulmonibus observationes anatomicae. Bologna, 1661

Transl. by J. Young. Proc. Roy. Soc. Med., Pt. 1, 23: 7–11, 1929–30

Also, in F. A. Willius and T. E. Keys' *Cardiac classics.* St. Louis, Mosby, 1941. pp. 92–97

"The first account of those lymphadenomatous formations (general enlargement of lymphatics with nodules in spleen) which were fully described by Hodgkin in 1832. . . ." Garrison

De viscerum structura exercitatio anatomica. Bononiae, Montii, 1666. pp. 125–126

"The founder of description or iconographic embryology, surpassing all other contemporary workers on the subject in the accurate notation of such minutiae as the aortic arches, the headfold, the neural groove, the cerebral and optic vesicles." Garrison

De formatione pulli in ovo. Londini, Martyn, 1673

De ovo incubato observationes. Londini, Martyn, 1673

Noticed "cells" in plants.

Anatome plantarum. Cui subjungitur appendix iteratus et auctas ejusdem authoris de ovo incubato observationes continens. Londini, Martyn, 1675–1679. 2 pts.

Described leontiasis ossea.

Opera posthuma. Amstelodami, Gallet, 1700. p. 68

Maltaner, Elizabeth. F. Maltaner. See A. B. Wadsworth

Maltby, E. J. See G. W. Howland

Man, Evelyn B(rower). New Haven biochemist. 1904–

PROCEDURE—of lipid determination.

A note on the stability and quantitative determination of phosphatides. J. biol. Chem., 117: 183–187, Jan. 1937

Manalang, C. See H. W. Wade

Manceaux, L. See C. J. H. Nicolle

Manchester,

OPERATION—of Manchester, England. See Archibald Donald

Mandach, Friedrich von. Swiss physician

TEST—

Eosin, als Reagens auf Gallenfarbstoff im Urin. Cor.-Bl. f. schweiz. Aerzte, 37: 422–423, July 1, 1907

Mandel, E. See H. Popper

Mandelbaum, Frederick Samuel. New York pathologist. 1867–

TEST—

The diagnosis of malignant tumors by paraffin sections of centrifuged exudates. J. Lab. clin. Med., 2: 580 (only), Apr. 1917

Mandelbaum, Martin. Munich physician. 1881–

AGAR—basal rosolic acid, to differentiate members of colon typhoid group.

Veränderung zweier Nährböden—(Rosolsäure- und Blutager)—durch Säure bzw. Alkali bildende Bakterien. Münch. med. Wschr., 56: 2475–2476, Nov. 30, 1909

AGAR—lactose blood, for isolation of colon typhoid group.

Eine neue Platte zur Züchtung von Bakterien der Typhuskoligruppe aus Fäces. Ibid., 59: 306–307, Feb. 6, 1912

REACTION—for detection of typhoid carriers.

Eine neue einfache Methode zur Typhusdiagnose. Ibid., H. 4: 178–181, Jan. 25, 1910

Mandl, Felix. Vienna surgeon. 1892–

Removed an adenomatous parathyroid gland and thus alleviated metabolic abnormalities in a case of generalized osteitis fibrosa.

Therapeutischer Versuch bei Ostitis fibrosa generalisata mittels Exstirpation eines Epithelkörperchentumors. Abstr.: Wien. klin. Wschr., 38: 1343–1344, Dec. 10, 1925

Therapeutischer Versuch bei einem Falle von Ostitis fibrosa generalisata mittels Exstirpation eines Epithelkörperchentumors. Zbl. Chir., 53: 260–264, Jan. 30, 1926

Klinisches und Experimentelles zur Frage der lokalisierten und generalisierten Ostitis fibrosa. Unter besonderer Berücksichtigung der Therapie der letzteren. Arch. klin. Chir., 143: 1–46, Oct. 18, 1926

Artificially produced renal pelvic stones in guinea pigs by injecting parathyroid extract and intermittentingly obstructing flow of urine.

Parathormon—Ostitis fibrosa—Nierenstein (Experimentelle Studie). Zbl. Chir., 60: 68–70, Jan. 14, 1933

See also F. Brunn

Mangold, O. See H. Speman

Mankowski, Abraham. Kiew physician

AGAR—fungus infusion peptone.

Ein Verfahren zum schnellen und leichten Unterscheiden von Kulturen des Typhus bacillus vom Bacterium coli. Zbl. Bakt., 27: 21–23, Jan. 6, 1900

Mann, E. See L. Danielson

Mann, Frank Charles. Rochester, Minn. surgeon. 1887–

OPERATION—

The experimental production of peptic ulcer with C. S. Williamson, Ann. Surg., 77: 409–423, Apr. 1923

See also E. S. Judd

Mann, James. U. S. Army surgeon. 1759–1832
First to successfully excise at elbow joint. Garrison
Observations on amputation at the joints: Med. Repository, N. Y., n. s., 7: 14–20, 1822
Mann, Ludwig. Breslau neurologist. 1866–
TYPE—of Wernicke-Mann, of paralysis.
Klinische und anatomische Beiträge zur Lehre von der spinalen Hemiplegie. Dtsch. Z. Nervenheilk., 10: 1–66, Dec. 31, 1896
Manning, Helen M. See Maud L. Menten
Manoilow, E. O. St. Petersburg scientist
TEST—chemical, for determining sex.
Eine chemische Blutreaktion der Geschlechtsbestimmung bei menschen und Tieren. Wratschebnaja Gaseta (russ), 15: 345, 1923
Weitere Erfahrungen über meine chemische Blutreaktion zur Geschlechtsbestimmung bei Menschen, Tieren und durch Chlorophyll bei Pflanzen. Münch. med. Wschr., 71: 1784–1789, Dec. 19, 1924
Manson, Sir Patrick. British physician. 1844–1922
"Father of modern tropical medicine."
Tropical diseases. A manual of the diseases of warm climates. London, Cassell, 1898
Proved that mosquito is vector of Filaria sanguinis hominis.
On the development of filaria sanguinis hominis, and on the mosquito as a nurse. J. Linnaean Soc., Lond., 14: 304–311, 1879
Manson-Bahr, Philip Henry. London physician
Reported Weil's disease in England.
A case of Weil's disease occurring in London with C. Wenyon and H. C. Brown, Lancet, 2: 1056–1059, Nov. 18, 1922
Mansour, M. See G. Milian
Manteaux, Charles. French physician. 1877–
TEST—for tuberculosis.
Intradermo-réactions de la tuberculine. C. R. Acad. Sci., 149: 355–357, 1908
Manwaring, Joshua George Ross. Flint, Mich. surgeon. 1877–1935
OPERATION—
Replacing depressed fractures of the malar bone. J. A. M. A., 60: 278–279, Jan. 25, 1913
Manzullo, Alfred. Buenos Aires physician
TEST—a rapid clinical t. for diphtheria.
Nuevo método para el cultivo del "Corynebacterium diphtheriae" y nuevo método para el diagnostico de la difteria en el hombre. Bol. Acad. nac. de med. de Buenos Aires, pp. 160–169, June 1938
Marbais, Salomon. French physician. 1875–
SOLUTION—lactose serum.
Diagnostic differentiel du bacille typhique, des paratyphiques et du Colibacillus, cultives dans du serum dilue lactose et tournesole. C. R. Soc. Biol., 81: 602–604, June 8, 1918
Marbel, Meyer M. Chicago surgeon. 1886–
TROCAR—for paracentesis abdominis.
A trocar with perforations. Illinois med. J., 69: 375–376, Apr. 1936
Marburg, Otto. German neurologist. 1878–
Described "leukoencephalitis concentrica" or concentric sclerosis.
Die sogenannte „akute multiple Sklerose" (Encephalomyelitis periaxialis scleroticans). Jb. Psychiat. Neurol., 27: 211–312, 1906
Marcet, Alexander John Gaspard. Scottish physician. 1770?–1822

Described alcaptonuria.
Account of a singular variety of urine, which turned black soon after being discharged; with some particulars respecting its chemical properties. Med.-chir Trans., 12: 37–45, 1823
Marcet, William. English physician. 1829–1900
Described coprosterol.
On the immediate principles of human excrements in the healthy state. Philos. Trans., 147: 403–413, 1858
Marchbanks, S. S. See R. P. Ball
Marchi, Vittorio. Italian physician. 1851–1908
FLUID—for fixation. Mallory
Sulle degenerazioni discendenti consecutive a lesioni della corteccia cerebrale with G. Algeri, Riv. sperim. fren., 11: 492–494, 1885
STAINING METHOD—for degenerated nerve fibers.
REACTION—failure of myelin sheath to become discolored when treated with osmic acid.
Sulle degenerazioni consecutive all'estirpazione totale e parziale del cervelletto. Ibid., 12: 50–56, 1886
Marchiafava, Ettore. Italian pathologist. 1847–1916
Accurately described hemacytozoa of malaria. Garrison
Die Veranderung der rothen Blutscheiben bei Malaria-Kranken with A. Celli, Fort. d. Med., 1: 573–575, Sept. 15, 1883
Neue Untersuchungen über die Malaria-Infection with A. Celli, Ibid., 3: 339–354, June 1, 1885
Weitere Untersuchungen über die Malariainfection with A. Celli, Ibid., 787–806, Dec. 15, 1885
Nuove ricerche sulla infezione malarica. Roma, Botta, 1885. 32 pp.
See also G. Baccelli
Marchoux, Émile Gabriel. French physician. 1862–
STAIN—of thionin for malarial parasites.
Le paludisme au Sénégal. Ann. Inst. Pasteur, 11: 640–662, Aug. 1897
Employed yellow fever convalescent serum.
Le fièvre jaune with Salimbeni and P. L. Simond, Ibid., 17: 665–731, Nov. 1903
Introduced use of stovarsol.
Le stovarsol guérit rapidement la dysenterie ambiene Bull. Soc. Path. Exot., Paris, 16: 79–81, Feb. 14, 1923
Marcy, Henry Orlando. Boston surgeon. 1837–1924
OPERATION—for inguinal hernia.
The radical cure of hernia by the antiseptic use of the carbolized catgut ligature. Trans. Amer. med. Ass., 29: 295–305, 1878
The cure of hernia by the antiseptic use of animal ligature. Trans. Internat. Med. Cong., 7 sess., 2: 446–448, 1881
OPERATION—myomectomy.
The histology and surgical treatment of uterine myoma. Ibid., 9 sess., 2: 835–844, 1887
Maréchal, Louis Eugene. French physician
TEST—for bile pigments in urine.
Étude chimique de l'urine. Paris, Parent, 1868. 86 pp.
Maresch, Rudolf. Vienna pathologist
METHOD—of silver impregnation for collagen and reticulum.
Ueber Gitterfasern der Leber und die Verwendbarkeit der Methode Bielschofskys zur Darstellung feinster Bindegewebsfibrillen. Zbl. allg. Path. u. path. Anat., 16: 641–649, Sept. 7, 1905
Marey, Étienne Jules. French physiologist. 1830–1904

LAW—a pulse of high tension is slow.
Loi qui préside à la fréquence des battements du coeur.
C. R. Acad. Sci., 53: 95–98, July 15, 1861
Invented sphygmograph and did early work with cardiac galvanometer.
Recherches sur le pouls au moyen d'un nouvel appareil enregistreur, le sphygmographe. Paris, Thunot, 1860
See also J. B. A. Chauveau

Marfan, Bernard Jean Antonin. French physician. 1858–1942
DISEASE—
Un cas de déformation congénitale des quartre membres, plus prononcée aux extrémités, charactérisee par l'allongement des os avec un certain degré d'amincissement. Bull. Soc. méd. Hôp Paris, 3 s., 13: 220–226, Feb. 28, 1896
Described "acetonemic vomiting." Garrison
Nouvelle contribution à l'étude des vomissements paroxystiques avec acétonémie. Bull. Soc. de pédiat. de Paris, 7: 41–52, 1905

Marie, Pierre. French neurologist. 1853–1940
ATAXIA—
Sur l'hérédo-ataxie cérébelleuse. Semaine m d., 13: 444–447, 1893
CLASSIFICATION—of aphasia.
Revision de la question de l'aphasie: la troisième circonvolution frontale gauche ne joue aucun rôle spécial dans la fonction du langage. Ibid., 26: 241–247, May 23, 1906
DISEASE—(1)—acromegaly.
Sur deux cas d'acromégalie; hypertrophie singuliere non congénitale des extrémitiés supérieures, inférieures et céphalique. Rev. de méd., 6: 297–333, Apr. 1886
Anatomie pathologique de l'acromégalie. Nouv. Icon. de la Salp., Paris, 2: 139–145; 188–195; 224–240; 327–341, 1889
Essays on acromegaly with Souza-Leite, Transl. by P. S. Hutchinson. London, New Sydenham Soc., 1891. 182 pp.
DISEASE—(2)—of Bamberger-Marie;
De l'ostéo-arthropathie hypertrophiante pneumique. Rev. de Méd., 10: 1–36, Jan. 1890
DISEASE—(3)—Strümpell-Marie type of spinal arthritis deformans.
Sur la spondylose rhizomélique. Ibid., 18: 285–315, 1898
DISEASE—(4)—Charcot-Marie-Tooth d.
Sur une forme particulière d'atrophie musculaire progressive souvent familiale débutant par les pieds et les jambes et atteignant plus tard les mains By J. M. Charcot, with P. Marie, Ibid., 6: 97–138, 1886
SIGN—tremor of body or extremities in exophthalmic goiter.
Sur la nature et sur quelques-uns des symptomes de la maladie de Basedow. Arch. d. Neurol., 6: 79–85, 1883
See also J. M. Charcot

Marina, Allesandro. Rome neurologist
PHENOMENA—movements of eye.
Sul restringimento pupillare, che si osserva ai movimenti laterali dei bulbi, nell'occhio che va all'interno. Policlinico, (sez. med.), 11: 162–165, Apr. 1904

Marine, David. Cleveland physician. 1880–
Gave iodine by mouth to eradicate simple goiter in regions where water and soil are deficient in iodine.
The prevention of simple goiter in man. Part I. A survey of the incidence and types of thyroid enlargements in the schoolgirls of Akron (Ohio), from the 5th to the 12th grades, inclusive—the plan of prevention proposed with O. P. Kimball, J. Lab. clin. Med 3: 40–48, Oct. 1917
Same, Part II By Kimball and Marine Arch. intern. Med., 22: 41–44, July 1918

Marinesco, Gheorghe. Bucharest neurologist. 1863–1938
HAND—
Main succulente et atrophie musculaire dans la syringomyélie. Paris, 1897. 44 pp.
TEST—for thyrotoxicosis.
Sur la réaction de fixation de l'alexine dans la maladie de Basedow. Dtsch. Z. Nervenheilk., 41: 268–270, Feb. 7, 1911

Marjolin, Jean Nicholas. French surgeon. 1780–1850
ULCER—carcinomatous ulcers originating in old degenerating scars.
Ulcère. Dictionnaire de Medecine pratique. Paris, 1828. 2 ed., 1846

Mark, Leonard Portal. English physician. 1855–1930
Described—
Acromegaly: a personal experience. London, Baillière, 1912

Markoe, Thomas Masters. New York surgeon. 1819–1901
ABSCESS—chronic sinuous a. of bone.
A treatise on diseases of the bones. New York, Appleton, 1872. 416 pp.

Marks, Heine. St. Louis surgeon. 1859–
Operated on wound of heart.
Two cases of stab wound of the heart. Med. Fortnightly, 3: 44–46, Jan. 16, 1893

Marmier, Louis. French physician
SOLUTION—glycerol protease, for production of anthrax toxin.
Sur la toxine charbonneuse. Ann. Inst. Pasteur, 9: 533–574 (537), July 1895

Marmorek, Alexandre. Paris physician. 1865–1923
SERUM—
La streptocoque et la sérum antistreptococcique. Ann. Inst. Pasteur, 9: 593–620, July 1895

Marple, Wilbur Boileau. American ophthalmologist. 1855–1916
INSTRUMENT—
An improved electric ophthalmoscope. Trans. Amer. Ophth. Soc., 11: 225–229, 1907

Marpmann, Georg. German physician
AGAR—flour casein, for cultivation of tubercle bacilli.
Ueber die Herstellung eines Bakterienpräparates aus Kulturen von Tuberkelbacillen. Zbl. Bakt., 33: 634–637, Apr. 4, 1903

Marrian, Guy Frederic. London biochemist
Obtained crystalline oestrin.
The chemistry of oestrin. III. An improved method of preparation and the isolation of active crystalline material. Biochem. J., 24: 435–445, 1930

Marriott, Hugh Leslie. London physician
Introduced—
Continuous drip blood transfusion, with case records of very large transfusions with A. Kekwick, Lancet, 1: 977–981, Apr. 27, 1935

Marriott, W(illiams) McKim. American physician. 1885–1936

METHOD—
The determination of small quantities of iron with
C. G. L. Wolf, J. biol. Chem., 1: 451–461, June 1906
METHOD—
*Nephelometric determination of minute quantities of
acetone.* Ibid., 16: 289–291, Nov. 1913
METHOD—
*The determination of B-oxybutyric acid in blood and
tissues.* Ibid., 16: 293–298, Nov. 1913
METHOD—
*The determination of alveolar carbon dioxid tension by
a simple method.* J. A. M. A., 66: 1594–1596, May 20,
1916
METHOD—
*A method for the determination of the alkali reserve of
the blood plasma.* Arch. intern. Med., 17: 840–851,
June 15, 1916
METHOD—
*A micro method for the determination of calcium and
magnesium in blood serum* with J. Howland, J. biol.
Chem., 32: 233–239, Nov. 1917
TREATMENT—
*The food requirements of malnourished infants, with
a note on the use of insulin.* J. A. M. A., 83: 600–603,
Aug. 23, 1924
See also J. Howland, R. L. Levy, P. A. Shaffer
Marrus, J. See D. I. Abramson
Marsh, Sir Henry. Irish physician. 1790–1860
DISEASE—exophthalmic goiter.
*Dilatation of the cavities of the heart. Enlargement of
the thyroid gland.* Abstr.: Dublin J. Med. Sci., 20:
471–474, 1842
Marsh, James. English chemist. 1794–1846
TEST—for arsenic.
*Account of a method of separating small quantities of
arsenic from substances with which it may be mixed.*
Edinburgh N. Phil. J., 21: 229–236, 1836
Marshall, Eli Kennerly, Jr. Baltimore pharmacol-
ogist. 1889–
METHOD—
*Para-aminobenzenesulfonamide absorption and ex-
cretion: method of determination in urine and blood*
with E. K. Kendall, Jr., K. Emerson and W. C.
Cutting, J. A. M. A., 108: 953–957, Mar. 20, 1937
Determination of sulfanilamide in blood and urine.
J. biol. Chem., 122: 263–273, Dec. 1937
TEST—
*A rapid clinical method for the estimation of urea in
urine.* Ibid., 14: 283–290, Apr. 1913
A new method for the determination of urea in blood.
Ibid., 15: 487–494, Sept. 1913
The determination of urea in urine. (Second communi-
cation.) Ibid., 15: 495–496, Sept. 1913
Noted increase in non-protein nitrogen in blood of
adrenalectomized animals.
The influence of the adrenals on the kidneys with
D. M. Davis, J. Pharmacol., 8: 525–550, Sept. 1916
Introduced—
The intravenous use of sodium sulfapyridine with
P. H. Long, J. A. M. A., 112: 1671–1675, Apr. 29,
1939
Introduced—
*Sulfanilylguanidine: a chemotherapeutic agent for
intestinal infections* with A. C. Bratton, H. J. White
and J. T. Litchfield, Jr., Johns Hopk. Hosp. Bull.,
67: 163–188, 1940
See also A. C. Bratton

Marshall, George Morley. Philadelphia laryngolo-
gist. 1859–1935
OPERATION—
*Correction of nasal deformities, particularly external
lateral deflections and depressions with obstructing de-
viations of the septum.* J. A. M. A., 60: 179–181,
Jan. 18, 1913
Marshall, H. T. See P. Ehrlich
Marshall, J. T. W. See W. G. Lyle
Marshall, John. English surgeon. 1818–1891
OPERATION—
Clinical lecture on colectomy. Lancet, 1: 721–722,
May 6; 771–773, May 13, 1882
Marshall, John. American physician. 1855–1925
METHOD—of detecting mercury in urine.
In: *Mercurial nephritis.* By J. M. Swan, Trans. Coll.
Phys. Phila., 25: 77–89 (81), 1903
Marshall, S. F. See F. H. Lahey
Marston, Jeffery Allen. English physician. 1831–
1911
Differentiated Malta fever from other fevers. Garri-
son and Morton
Report on fever (Malta). Army Med. Dept. Statist.
Rep., 1861, London, 3: 486–521, 1863
Marten, Benjamin. English physician. 1704–1782
Considered a parasitic micro-organism to be the cause
of tuberculosis, thus forecasting the existence of
the tubercle bacillus 162 years before its discovery.
Garrison and Morton
*A new theory of consumptions, more especially of a
phthisis, or consumption of the lungs.* London, Knap-
lock, 1720
Martin, A. L. F. J. See P. P. E. Roux
Martin, Alfred. Zürich physician
MODIFICATION—of Gumprecht's manometer.
*Technisches über das Riva-Roccische Sphygmoma-
nometer und Gärtners Tonometer.* Münch. med. Wschr.,
50: 1021–1024, June 16; 1072–1075, June 23, 1903
Martin, August Eduard. Berlin gynecologist. 1847–
1933
OPERATION—
*Zur Enucleation der intraparietalen Myome des corpus
uteri.* Z. Geburtsh. u. Frauenkr., 1: 143–167, 1876
Martin, C. E. See A. W. Elting
Martin, Sir Charles James. Sydney physiologist.
1866–
METHOD—
*A simple and rapid method of desiccating serum
and keeping it sterile during the process.* J. Path. Bact.,
3: 507–509, Jan. 1896
Martin, E. See W. G. Spiller
Martin, E. D. See F. W. Parham
Martin, F. A. See R. W. G. Owen
Martin, Franklin H. Chicago surgeon. 1857–1935
TABLE—
A new operating table. Chicago Med. J. and Examiner,
47: 34–36, July 1883
Martin, Hayes Elmer. New York surgeon. 1892–
MODIFICATION—of Janeway gastrostomy.
The original Janeway gastrostomy with W. L. Wat-
son, S. G. O., 56: 72–78, Jan. 1933
Martin, Henry Austin. American surgeon. 1824–
1884
BANDAGE—for varicose veins.
*A new adhesive plaster especially adapted to the re-
quirements of modern surgery.* Boston Med. and Surg.
J., 97: 407–411, Oct. 11, 1877

Martin, Henry Newell. Baltimore biologist. 1848–1896
METHOD—
On a method of isolating the mammalian heart. Science, 2: 228 (only), May 14, 1881
Studied—
On the respiratory function of the internal intercostal muscles with E. M. Hartwell, J. Physiol., 2: 24–27, 1879–80

Martin, Louis. French bacteriologist. 1864–1946
AGAR—glucose litmus, for differentiation of diphtheria and pseudo-diphtheria bacillus.
Les pseudo-diphthériques with G. Loiseau, Bull. Acad. Méd. Paris, 81: 73–78 (73), Jan. 21, 1919
AGAR—peptic digest, for isolation of diphtheria bacillus.
Culture du bacille de la diphthérie en tubes de veillon with G. Loiseau, C. R. Soc. Biol., 79: 677–680 (678), July 22, 1916
PEPTONE or SOLUTION—stomach digest, for cultivation of diphtheria bacilli.
Production de la toxine diphthérique. Ann. Inst. Pasteur, 12: 26–48 (32), Jan. 1898
SOLUTION—liver digest, for cultivation of typhoid bacilli.
Le bouillon panse-foie pour le culture du bacille typhique. C. R. Soc. Biol., 78: 261–263, May 15, 1915
SOLUTION—sérum.
Culture du Spirochaeta icterohemmorragiae with A. Pettit and A. Vandremer, Ibid., 80: 197–200 (197), Feb. 17, 1917

Martin, S. J. See L. W. Gorham

Martine, George. Scottish physician. 1702–1741
Wrote first scientific treatise on clinical thermometry. Garrison
Essays, medical and philosophical. London, Millar, 1740. 376 pp.

Martzloff, Karl Henry. Portland, Ore. surgeon. 1890–
CLAMP and TECHNIC—for intestinal anastomosis.
The closed intestinal loop. III. Antiseptic end-to-end intestinal anastomosis and a method for making a closed intestinal loop suitable for physiologic studies with G. E. Burget, Arch. Surg., 23: 26–37, July 1931

Marwedel, Georg. German surgeon
INCISION—for diaphragmatic hernia.
Die Aufklappung des Rippenbogens zur Erleichterung operativer Eingriffe im Hypochondrium und im Zweichfellkuppelraum. Zbl. Chir., 30: 938–941, Aug. 29, 1903
OPERATION—a method of gastrostomy.
Zur Technik der Gastrostomie. Beitr. klin. Chir., 17: 56–74, Oct. 1896

Marx, H. See S. von Horoszkiewicz

Marx, Hellmut. Bonn physician. 1901–
DRINKING TEST OF—for glaucoma.
Untersuchungen über den Wasserhaushalt. V. Mitteilung. Die Blutverdünnung nach Flüssigkeitaufnahme. Klin. Wschr., 4 (2): 2339–2342, Dec. 3, 1925
(Same) *II. Mitteilung. Die psychische Beeinflussung des Wasserhaushaltes.* Ibid., 5 (1): 92–94, Jan. 5, 1926

Maryan, Harry Oliver. Chicago gynecologist. 1895–
COLPOSCOPE—
A new colposcope. Amer. J. Obstet. Gynaec., 30: 148–150, July 1935

Mascagni, Paolo. Italian physician. 1752–1815
Wrote on lymphatics. Garrison and Morton
Vasorum lymphaticorum corporis humani historia et iconographia. Senis, Carli, 1787

Maschke, O. German chemist
REACTION—for creatinine.
Ueber eine neue Kreatinin-Reaction. Z. anal. Chem., 17: 134–141, 1888

Mason, E. H. See D. S. Lewis

Mason, Francis. London surgeon. 1837–1886
OPERATION—
Case of cleft palate; novel procedure for improving the voice after the operation of staphyloraphy. Lancet, 2: 198 (only), Aug. 7, 1869

Mason, Harold Lawrence. American chemist. 1901–
Isolated corticosterone.
Chemical studies of the suprarenal cortex. II. The identification of a substance which possesses the qualitative action of cortin; its conversion into a diketone closely related to androstenedione with C. S. Myers and E. C. Kendall, J. Biol. Chem., 116: 267–276, Nov. 1936
See also E. C. Kendall

Mason, J(ames) Tate. Seattle surgeon. 1882–1936
INCISION—
A new abdominal incision. Arch. Surg., 19: 129–142, July 1929

Mason, Michael Livingood. Chicago surgeon. 1895–
SUTURE—for tendon.
Primary and secondary tendon suture: a discussion of the significance of technique in tendon surgery. S. G. O., 70: 392–402, Feb. 15, 1940
Described—
Tumor of a subcutaneous glomus: tumeur glomique; tumeur du glomus neuromyo-artériel; subcutaneous painful tubercle; angio-myo-neurone; subcutaneous glomal tumor with A. Weil, Ibid., 58: 807–816, May 1934
See also S. L. Koch

Mason, V. R. See G. H. Whipple

Massa, Niccolò. Italian physician. ?–1569
Described neurological manifestations of syphilis.
Liber de morbo gallico. Venetiis, 1532. n. p.

Masselin, E. J. See L. H. Thoinot

Massini, Rudolf. Swiss physician. 1880–
AGAR—triple dye lactose, for detection of typhoid and dysentery.
Dreifarbennährboden zur Typhusruhdiagnose. Cor.-Bl., f. schweiz. Aerzte, 48: 887 (only), June 29, 1918

Massol, L. See L. C. A. Calmette

Masson, C. L. Pierre. Montreal pathologist. 1880–
METHOD—trichrome staining for nerve tissue.
METHOD—gelatin, for attaching paraffin sections to slides.
Carcinoids (argentaffin-cell tumors) and nerve hyperplasia of the appendicular mucosa. Amer. J. Path., 4: 181–212, May 1928
Trichrome stainings and their preliminary technique. J. Tech. Methods and Bull. Int. Ass. Med. Mus., 12: 75–90, Mar. 1929

Masson, James Carruthers. Rochester, Minn. surgeon. 1881–
FASCIA STRIPPER—
A new instrument for securing fascia lata for repair of hernia. Proc. Staff Meet., Mayo Clinic, 8: 528–530, Aug. 30, 1933

Masson, Paul. French surgeon

OMPLEX—musculonervous, of appendix.
Les névromes sympathiques de l'appendicite oblitérante.
Lyon Chir., 18: 281–299, May–June 1921
Identified source of glomus tumor or angioneuroma.
Le glomus neuromyo-artériel des régions tactiles et ses tumeurs. Ibid., 21: 257–280, May–June 1924

Master, Arthur Morris. New York physician. 1895–
EST—
A simple exercise tolerance test for circulatory efficiency, with standard tables for normal individuals with E. T. Oppenheimer, Amer. J. med. Sci., 177: 223–243, Feb. 1929
The two-step test of myocardial function. Amer. Heart J., 10: 495–510, Apr. 1935

Masucci, P. See F. McE. Huntoon

Matas, Rudolph. New Orleans surgeon. 1860–
AND—
Occlusion of large surgical arteries with removable metallic bands to test the efficiency of the collateral circulation; experimental and clinical observations with C. W. Allen, J. A. M. A., 56: 233–239, Jan. 28, 1911
MODIFICATION—of O'Dwyer's intubating apparatus with anesthesia attachment.
Intralaryngeal insufflation, for the relief of acute surgical pneumothorax: its history and methods with a description of the latest devices for this purpose. Ibid., 34: 1371–1375, June 2: 1468–1473 (1470), June 9, 1900
OPERATION—for radical cure of aneurism; endoaneurysmorrhaphy.
Traumatic aneurism of the left brachial artery. Failure of direct and indirect pressure; ligation of the artery immediately above tumor; return of pulsation on the tenth day; ligation immediately below tumor; failure to arrest pulsation; incision and partial excision of sac; recovery. Med. News, 53: 462–466, Oct. 27, 1888
An operation for the radical cure of aneurism based upon arteriorrhaphy: with the report of four cases successfully operated upon by the author. Trans. Amer. Surg. Ass., 20: 396–434, 1902
Operation for the radical cure of aneurism based upon arteriorrhaphy. Ann. Surg., 37: 161–196, Feb. 1903
OPERATION—
Fracture of the zygomatic arch: a simple method of reduction and fixation, with remarks on the prevalence, symptomatology and treatment of this fracture. New Orleans Med. and Surg. J., 49: 139–157, Sept. 1896
OPERATION—
Local and regional anesthesia with cocain and other analgesic drugs, including the subarachnoid method, as applied in general surgical practice. Philadelphia Med. J., 6: 820–843, Nov. 3, 1900
TEST—
Some of the problems related to the surgery of the vascular system: testing the efficiency of the collateral circulation as a preliminary to the occlusion of the great surgical vessels. Trans. Amer. Surg. Ass., 28: 4–54, 1910
Tests to determine the efficiency of the collateral circulation before attempting the permanent occlusion of the great surgical arteries. Abstr.: Ann. Surg., 52: 126–130, July 1910
Testing the efficiency of the collateral circulation as a preliminary to the occlusion of the great surgical arteries: further observations, with special reference to

the author's methods, including a review of other tests thus far suggested. J. A. M. A., 63: 1441–1447, Oct. 24, 1914

Mather, Cotton. American clergyman. 1662–1728
Wrote on inoculation.
An account of the method and success of inoculating the small pox in Boston in New England. London, 1722

Mathes, Paul. Innsbruck obstetrician. 1871–1923
MASTITIS—
Eine typische Form der Brustentzündung im Wochenbett. Münch. med. Wschr., 68: 15 (only), Jan. 7, 1921

Mathews, Albert Prescott. Cincinnati biochemist. 1871–
TEST—
An easy method for the distinction and estimation of lactose and glucose in urine. J. A. M. A., 75: 1568–1569, Dec.4, 1920

Mathieu, A. See H. D. Haskins

Mathieu, Albert. Paris physician. 1855–1917
DISEASE—infectious jaundice; same as Lancereaux or Weil's disease.
L'ictère grave d'après les travaux récents au point de vue de sa nature et de sa pathogénie. Arch. gén. de méd., 7 s., 6, 1880
Typhus hépatique bénin; rechute—guérison. Rev. d. méd., 6: 633–639, July 1886
PROCEDURE—for determining quantity of stomach contents.
Note sur un moyen de déterminer la quantité de liquide contenu dans l'estomac et la quantité de travail chlorhydropeptique effectué par cet organe with Rémond, C. R. Soc. Biol., pp. 591–593, Nov. 8, 1890

Mathijsen, Anthonius. Brabant surgeon. 1805–1878
Introduced Plaster-of-Paris bandages in 1852. Garrison
Nieuwe wijze van oonwending van het gips-verband bij heenbreuken. Eene bijdrage tot de militaire chirurgie. Haarlem, van Loghem, 1852
Du bandage plâtré et de son application dans le traitement des fractures. Liége, Grandmont-Donders, 1854

Matson, Ralph Charles. Portland, Ore. physician. 1880–1945
TECHNIC—
Der Vergleicherungswert einiger neuerer Methoden der Sputumuntersuchung auf Tuberkelbazillen des Ziehlschen und Muchschen Typus. Beitr. z. Klin. d. Tuberk., 24: 193–216, 1912

Matsuzaki, H. See T. Ito

Mattei, Vittorio. Milan physician
TEST—for urobilin in urine.
Un metodo semplice e sensibile per la ricerca dell'urobilina nelle urine. Osped. magg., 10: 198–199, July 31, 1922

Matteucci, Carlo. Italian scientist. 1811–1868
Established difference of potential between injured nerve and its muscle.
Sur le courant électrique ou propre de la grenouille; second mémoire sur l'électricité animale faisant suite à celui sur la torpille. Ann. d. Chim., Paris, 68: 93–106, 1838
Demonstrated rheoscopic frog effect (contraction of muscle by stimulation of its nerve by another contracting muscle).
Électricité animale. Sur le courant électrique de la

grenouille et des animaux à sang chaud. C. R. Acad.
Sci., 14: 315–316, 1842
*Sur le courant électrique des muscles des animaux
vivants ou récemment tués* with F. H. Humboldt,
Extrait d'une Lettere: Ibid., 16: 197–200, Jan. 23,
1843

Matthews, John. English physician
AGAR—trypsinized blood.
*On a method of preparing medium for the culture of
Pfeiffer's influenza bacillus that gives profuse growth
and is to a marked degree selective for this organism.*
Lancet, 2: 104 (only), July 27, 1918

Matthieu, Albert. Paris physician
METHOD—use of fat in test-meal to determine motility of stomach.
*Ueber ein neues Mittel, die motorische Kraft des Magens
und den Durchgang der Flussigkeiten durch denselben
zu messen.* Arch. VerdauKr., 1: 345–354, 1896

Mattics, Marjorie R. See Frances U. Lauber

Mattill, Henry Albright. American chemist. 1883–
METHOD—
*A method for the quantitative determination of fecal
bacteria* with P. B. Hawk, J. exp. Med., 14: 433–444,
Oct. 1, 1911

Mattioli, Pietro Andrea. Venetian physician. 1501–
1577
Considered mercury a specific in treatment of syphilis. Garrison and Morton
De morbo gallico curatione dialogus. Venetiis, 1535

Matzger, Edward. San Francisco physician. 1898–
Described allergy to liver extract.
*Bronchial asthma caused by liver and liver extract
diet in a patient suffering from primary anemia.*
J. A. M. A., 96: 110 (only), Jan. 10, 1931

Matzuschita, Teisi. Japanese physician
AGAR—basal sodium chloride peptone: for cultiva-
tion of intestinal bacteria.
*Untersuchungen über die Mikroorganismen des men-
schlichen Kotes.* Arch. Hyg., Berl., 41: 211–255
(214), 1902
AGAR—glucose peptone: for cultivation of tubercle
bacilli.
*Ueber die Wachstumsunterschiede des Bacillus der
Hühnertuberkulose und der menschlichen Tuberkulose
auf pflanzeichen, Gelatine- und Agarnährboden.* Zbl.
Bakt., 26: 125–135 (128), July 31, 1899
SOLUTION—glucose peptone: for cultivation of spore
forming bacilli.
*Zur Physiologie der Sporenbildung der Bacillen,
nebst Bemerkungen zum Wachstum einiger Anaëroben.*
Arch. Hyg., Berl., 43: 267–376 (287), 1902

Mauck, H(enry) Page. Richmond, Va. surgeon.
1891–
OPERATION—for laxity of internal lateral ligament of
knee.
A new operative procedure for instability of the knee.
J. Bone and Joint Surg., 18: 984–990, Oct. 1936

Maugaret, Reine. French physician. 1860–
THEORY—of acute pancreatitis by lymph channels
from gall bladder.
Cholécysto-pancréatite; essai de pathogénie. Paris,
1908. 150 pp.

Maumené, Edme Jules. French chemist. 1818–
TEST—for glucose.
*Sur un nouveau réactif pour distinguer la présence du
sucre dans certains liquides.* C. R. Acad. Sci., 30:
314–316, 1850

Maunoir, Jean Pierre. French surgeon. 1768–1861
HYDROCELE—cervical h.
*Mémoires sur les amputations, l'hydrocèle du cou e
l'organisation de l'iris.* Genève et Paris, Paschoud
1825. 159 pp.

Maunsell, H(enry) Widenham. New Zealand sur
geon. 1847–1895
METHOD—
A new method of intestinal surgery. Amer. J. med
Sci., s 2., 103: 245–257, Mar. 1892

Mauriac, Charles Marie Tamarelle. French syphi
lologist. 1832–1905
DISEASE—erythema nodosum syphiliticum.
Pathologie générale de la syphilis tertiaire. Paris
Capiomont et Renault, 1886. 112 pp.

Mauriceau, Francois. French obstetrician. 1637-
1709
LANCE—pointed knife used in embryotomy. "H
was the first to correct the ancient view that th
pelvic bones are separated in normal labor, and tha
the amniotic discharge is an accumulation of men
strual blood or milk; he was also the first to refe
to tubal pregnancy, difficult labor from involvemen
of the umbilical cord, and epidemic puerperal fever."
Garrison
*Traité des maladies des femmes grosses et de celles qu
sont accouchées.* . . . Paris, Houry, 1668. Also, 1675
501 pp. Also, 1694

Maury, Francis F. American surgeon. 1840–1879
GASTROSTOMY—
*Case of stricture of the oesophagus in which gastros
tomy was performed.* Amer. J. med. Sci., 59: 365-
371, Apr. 1870

Maury, John William Draper. New York surgeon
1871–
LETHAL LINE OF—
*Death in acute intestinal obstruction and kindred con
ditions is due to physiologic disturbance. Study I
Has the duodenum a toxic internal secretion?* J. A
M. A., 54: 5–9, Jan. 1, 1910

Mautz, F. R. See C. S. Beck

Maxcy, Kenneth Fuller. American physician. 1889
DISEASE—murine typhus.
*Clinical observations on endemic typhus (Brill's dis
ease) in southern United States.* U. S. Public Healtl
Rep., 41: 1213–1220, June 18, 1926
*An epidemiological study of endemic typhus (Brill'
disease) in the southeastern United States, with specia
reference to its mode of transmission.* Ibid., 2967–
2995, Dec. 24, 1926

Maxeiner, Stanley Robert. Minneapolis surgeon
1885–
OPERATION—
*The present surgical management of esophageal divertic
ula with presentation of a new (?) method.* Trans
West. Surg. Ass., 49: 365–377, 1939

Maximow, Alexander A. Russian-American phy
sician. 1874–1928
METHOD—of serial sections by celloidin method.
*Über zweckmässige Methoden für cytologische un
histogenetische Untersuchungen am Wirbeltierembryc
mit spezieller Berücksichtigung der Celloidinschnitt
serien.* Z. wiss. Mikr., 26: 177–190, Sept. 21, 1909
METHOD—of tissue culture.
*Über das Mesothel (Deckzellen der serösen Häute
und die Zellen der serösen Exsudate. Untersuchunge*

an entzündetem Gewebe und Gewebskulturen. Arch. exper. Zellforsch., 4: 1–42, 1927

TAINS—azur II eosin and alum hematoxylin. See METHOD, 1909

THEORY—of blood regeneration.
Relation of blood cells to connective tissues and endothelium. Physiol. Rev., 4: 533–563, Oct. 1924

Maxwell, John Preston. English physician in China. 1871–
Showed osteomalacia to be due to lack of vitamin D.
Further studies in osteomalacia. Proc. R. Soc. Med., London, 23: 639–562, Mar. 1930

May, Charles Davidson. Boston physician. 1908–
MODIFICATION—of Carr-Price method of determination of vitamin A.
Clinical studies of Vitamin A in infants and in children with K. D. Blackfan, J. F. McCreary and F. H. Allen, Jr., Amer. J. Dis. Child., 59: 1167–1184, June 1940

May, Charles Henry. American ophthalmologist. 1861–1943
OPERATION—
Restoration of the conjunctival cul-de-sac in a case of total symblepharon, by means of Thiersch skin grafts. Arch. Ophthal., 28: 182–190, 1899

May, Hans. Philadelphia surgeon. 1902–
OPERATION—
A plastic operation on the breast. Arch. Surg., 38: 113–117, Jan. 1939
See also G. C. Engel

May, R. Munich physician
STAINING SOLUTION—
Über Blutfärbungen with L. Grünwald, Zbl. inn. Med., 23: 265–270, Mar. 15, 1902

Maydl, Karl. Vienna surgeon. 1853–1903
HERNIA—strangulated.
Die Lehre von den Unterleibsbrüchen (Hernien). Wien, Safar, 1898. 517 pp.
OPERATION—colostomy.
Zur Technik der Kolotomie. Zbl. Chir., 15: 433–439, June 16, 1886

Mayer, A. See P. F. Armand-Delille

Mayer, Emil. Rochester, N. Y. rhinologist. 1854–
OPERATION—
Deviation of the cartilaginous nasal septum: its cure. New York Med. J., 62: 748–750, Dec. 14, 1895

Mayer, Erich. Munich physician
REACTION—for detecting increase of leukocytes in blood.
Ueber den Nachweis der Leukocytenvermehrung im Blute mittelst chemischer Reagentien. Abstr.: Klin.-therap. Wschr., 10: 1267 (only), Nov. 1, 1903

Mayer, Georg. Würzburg physician
BOUILLON—mucin; culture medium.
Ueber das Wachstum von Mikroorganismen auf Speicheldrüsen- und Mucin-Nährböden. Zbl. f. Bakt., 25: 815–826 (818), June 10, 1899

Mayer, Helene. See H. Popper

Mayer, Julius Robertson. German scientist. 1814–1878
Demonstrated principle of conservation of energy in physiological processes.
Bemerkungen über die Kräfte der unbelebten Natur. Ann. d. Chem. u. Pharm., Lemgo, Heidelberg, 42: 233–240, 1842

Mayer, K. See E. Waldschmidt-Leitz

Mayer, Leo. New York surgeon. 1884–

OPERATION—
The operative treatment of paralytic deformities of the foot. Amer. J. Surg., 7: 80–88, July 1929
See also K. Biesalski

Mayer, Paul. German-Italian scientist. 1848–1923
HEMALUM—
Über das Färben mit Hämatoxylin. Mitt. a. d. Zool. Stat. Neapel, 10: 170–186, July 21, 1891
METHOD—
Einfache Methode zum Aufkleben mikroskopischer Schnitte. Ibid., 4: 521–522, Dec. 21, 1883
SOLUTION—glycerin-alum-hematein.
Über Schleimfärbung. Ibid., 12: 303–330 (310), Apr. 25, 1896
STAINS—mucicarmine; muchematein. Ibid.
STAIN—carmalum alcoholic carmine (paracarmine). Mallory
Über das Färben mit Carmin, Cochenille und Hämatëin-Thonerde. Ibid., 10: 480–501, 1891–93

Mayer-Gross, Willy. German neurologist. 1889–
APRAXIA—
Some observations on apraxia. Proc. R. Soc. Med., 28: 1203–1212, July 1935

Mayo, Charles Horace. Rochester, Minn. surgeon. 1865–1939
ENTEROSTOMY—
Enterostomy and the use of the omentum in the prevention and healing of fistula. Ann. Surg., 66: 568–570, Nov. 1917
OPERATION—
Treatment of varicose veins. S. G. O., 2: 385–388, Apr. 1906
OPERATION—
The surgical treatment of bunion. Ann. Surg., 48: 300–302, Aug. 1908
OPERATION—
Diagnosis and surgical treatment of oesophageal diverticula. Ibid., 51: 812–817, June 1910
TECHNIC—of vaginal hysterectomy.
Uterine prolapse with associated pelvic relaxation. S. G. O., 20: 253–260, Mar. 1915
Removed successfully a pheochromocytoma.
Paroxysmal hypertension with tumor of retroperitoneal nerve: report of case. J. A. M. A., 89: 1047–1050, Sept. 24, 1927

Mayo, Charles William. Rochester, Minn. surgeon. 1898–
MODIFICATION—of Moschcowitz operation.
Complete rectal prolapse: a fascial repair. Trans. West. Surg. Ass., pp. 166–169, 1937

Mayo, E. W. See W. M. Boothby

Mayo, Herbert. English physician. 1796–1852
Described functions of facial nerves and reflex action.
Anatomical and physiological commentaries. London, Underwood, 1822–23. 2 pts.

Mayo, William James. Rochester, Minn. surgeon. 1861–1939
BAND—attaching first loop of jejunum to transverse mesocolon.
The relation of the mesocolic band to gastroenterostomy. Ann. Surg., 47: 1–3, Jan. 1908
INCISION—
The incision for lumbar exposure of the kidney. Ibid., 55: 63–65, Jan. 1912
METHOD—reconstruction of common duct by direct implantation into duodenum.
Some remarks on cases involving operative loss of

continuity of the common bile duct: with the report of a case of anastomosis between the hepatic duct and the duodenum. Ibid., 43: 90–96, July 1905

Restoration of the bile passage after serious injury to the common or hepatic ducts. S. G. O., 22: 1–6, Jan. 1916

LINE—of incision on stomach wall for subtotal gastrectomy. See Operation 2

PYLORIC VEIN—See Operation 2

OPERATION—(1).

An operation for the radical cure of umbilical hernia. Ann. Surg., 34: 276–280, Jan. 1901

OPERATION—(2); partial gastrectomy.

Malignant diseases of the stomach and pylorus. Trans. Amer. Surg. Ass., 18: 97–123, 1900

A review of three hundred and three operations upon the stomach and first portion of the duodenum. Ann. Surg., 38: 30–46, July 1903

Ulcer of the duodenum, with report of two hundred and seventy-two operations. J. A. M. A., 51: 556–558, Aug. 15, 1908

OPERATION—(3).

Removal of the rectum for cancer: statistical report of 120 cases. Ann. Surg., 51: 854–862, June 1910

The radical operation for the relief of cancer of the rectum and rectosigmoid. Ibid., 56: 241–256, Aug. 1912

Suggested ligation of splenic artery.

Principles underlying surgery of the spleen, with a report of ten splenectomies. J. A. M. A., 54: 14–18, Jan. 1, 1910

Mayor, Matthias Louis. French surgeon. 1775–1847

SCARF—a triangular bandage.

Nouveau système de déligation chirurgicale, ou exposé des moyens simples et faciles de ramplacer avec avantage les bandes et la charpie; . . . Paris, Cherbuliez, 1832. 319 pp.

Mayo Robson, Sir Arthur. See Robson

Mayou, Marmaduke Stephen. English ophthalmologist. 1876–

DISEASE—Batten-Mayou d.: juvenile amaurotic idiocy.

Cerebral degeneration, with symmetrical changes in the maculae, in three members of a family. Trans. Ophthal. Soc. U. King., 24: 142–145, 1904

Mayow, John. English physiologist. 1643–1679

Showed that respiration in fetus is effected by placenta; located seat of animal heat in muscles; gave first account of substance now known as oxygen. Garrison

Tractatus quinique medico-physici. Oxonii, Sheldoniano, 1674

Mazzini, L. Y. Indianapolis scientist

TEST—

A reliable, sensitive, simple, and rapid slide flocculation test for syphilis. Amer. J. clin. Path., 9: 163–175, Mar. 1939

Mead, Richard. English physician. 1673–1754

Wrote first book of epidemiological advice produced by a medical practitioner at request of the State. Riesman. (Plague active in Marseilles)

A short discourse concerning pestilential contagion, and the methods to be used to prevent it. London, Buckley and Smith, 1719. 59 pp.

Meader, P. D. See G. H. Robinson

Means, P. H. See C. M. Jones

Meckel, Johann Friedrich. German anatomist. 1724–1774

CAVITY—between two layers of dura mater at end of petrous portion of temporal bone. Dorland

GANGLION—in sphenomaxillary fossa.

SPACE—intradural cavity containing gasserian ganglion.

De quinto pare nervorum cerebri. Gottingae, Vandenhoeck, 1748. 136 pp. Inaug. Dis.

De ganglio secundi rami quinti paris nervorum cerebri nuper detecto, deque vera gangliorum nervosorum utilitate. Berolini, 1749

Meckel, Johann Friedrich. German anatomist. 1781–1833

DIVERTICULUM—of ileum.

Ueber die Divertikel am Darmkanal. Arch. f. Physiol. 9: 421–453, 1809

Also in: *Manual of descriptive and pathological anatomy.* Transl. by A. S. Doane, London, Henderson, 1838. p. 375

Medalia, Leon Samuel. American physician. 1881–

STAIN—

Staining for the spirochaeta pallida in smear preparations. J. A. M. A., 70: 914–915, Mar. 30, 1918

Medes, Grace. American physiochemist. 1887–

TEST—

The determination of ascorbic acid in urine with phospho-18-tungstic acid. Biochem. J., 29: 2251–2255, Oct. 1935

See also C. C. Farahaugh

Medin, Oskar. Swedish physician. 1847–1928

DISEASE—acute anterior or epidemic poliomyelitis.

En epidemi af infantil paralysi. Hygiea, 52: 657–668, Sept. 1890

Über eine Epidemie von spinaler Kinderlähmung. Verh. d. X Internat. Kongr., Berlin, pp. 37–46, 1891

Om den infantila paralysien, med särskild hänsyn till dess akuta stadium. Nord. med. Ark., Stockholm, n. F., 6: 1–84, 1896

Medlar, Edgar Matthias. New York physician. 1887–

FORMULA or RATIO—

An evaluation of the leucocytic reaction in the blood as found in cases of tuberculosis. Amer. Rev. Tuberc. 20: 312–346, Sept. 1929

Reported case of chromoblastomycosis.

A cutaneous infection caused by a new fungus, Phialophora Verrucosa, with a study of the fungus. J. med. Res., 32: 507–521, July 1915

Meduna, Ladislaus von. Budapest psychiatrist

Originated treatment of schizophrenia with camphor, metrazol.

Versuche über die biologische Beinflussung des Ablaufe der Schizophrenie: Campher- und Cardiazolkrämpfe. Z. ges. Neurol. Psychiat., 152: 235–262, Jan. 24, 1935

Also: Arch. Neurol. u. Psychiat., 35: 361–363, 1936

Die Konvulsionstherapie der Schizophrenie. Berlin, 1937

Medvei, C. V. See O. Weltmann

Meeh, K. Tübingen physiologist

FORMULA—to obtain calories per square meter per hour.

Oberflächenmessungen des menschlichen Körpers. Z. Biol., 15: 425–458, 1879

Meekeren, Job Janszoon van. Dutch surgeon. ?–1666

First to successfully transplant piece of bone from dog's skull to cranial defect of soldier, but Church ordered him to remove it. Garrison and Morton

Heel—en geneeskonstige aanmerkingen. Amsterdam, Commelijin, 1668
Also, in German, 1675

Mehring, Joseph von. Cologne pathologist. 1848–1908
Experimentally produced diabetes by exhibition of phlorizin. Garrison
Ueber künstlichen Diabetes. Zbl. med. Wiss., 23: 531 (only), July 25, 1885
Ueber experimentelle Diabetes. (Einwirkung des Phloridzin.) Verh. Cong. f. inn. Med., Wiesb., 5: 185–189, 1886
Depancreatized dogs and produced diabetes.
Diabetes mellitus nach Pankreasexstirpation with O. Minkowski. Arch. exp. Path. Pharmak., 26: 371–387, Jan. 17, 1890

Méhu, Camille Jean Marie. French physician. 1835–1887
TEST—for albumin.
Ueber die Bestimmung des Eiweisses, namentlich im Harne. Chem. Zbl., 40: 236–238, Apr. 14, 1869

Meibomius, Heinrichs. German anatomist. 1638–1700
CYST—chalazion.
GLANDS—sebaceous follicles of eyelids.
De vasis palpebrarum novis epistola. Helmstädi, Mulleri, 1666

Meier, G. See O. Porges

Meige, Henry. French physician. 1866–
DISEASE—
Le trophoedème chronique héréditaire. N. Iconog. de la Salpêtriere, Paris, 12: 453–480, 1889
Sur le trophoedème. Ibid., 14: 465–472, Nov.–Dec. 1901
Chronic hereditary trophoedema. Abstr.: Brit. J. Dermat., 12: 372–376, Oct. 1900

Meigs, Arthur Vincent. Philadelphia surgeon. 1850–1912
CAPILLARY—
The microscopical anatomy of the human heart, showing the existence of capillaries within the muscular fibers. Amer. J. med. Sci., 101: 583–591, June 1891
FORMULA—for preparation of milk for infant feeding.
Proof that human milk contains only about one per cent of casein, with remarks upon infant feeding. Proc. Phila. Co. Med. Soc., pp. 92–108, 1883
Milk analysis and infant feeding. A practical treatise on the examination of human and cows' milk, cream, condensed milk, etc., and directions as to the diet of young infants. Philadelphia, Blakiston, 1885. 102 pp.

Meigs, Charles DeLucena. American physician. 1792–1869
Described embolism as cause of sudden death.
The heart-clot. Med. Exam., Phila., 5: 141–152, Mar. 1849

Meigs, Edward Browning. American scientist. 1879–
TEST—
The quantitative determination of phosphorus by the nephelometric method. J. biol. Chem., 36: 335–346, Nov. 1918

Meigs, Joe Vincent. Boston surgeon. 1892–
SYNDROME—
In his: *Tumors of the female pelvic organs.* New York, Macmillan, 1934
Fibroma of the ovary with ascites and hydrothorax;

with a report of seven cases with J. W. Cass, Amer. J. Obstet.Gynaec., 33: 249–267, Feb. 1937
Fibroma of the ovary with ascites and hydrothorax; a further report. Ann. Surg., 110: 731–754, Oct. 1939
A further contribution to the syndrome of fibroma of the ovary with fluid in the abdomen and chest: Meigs' syndrome. Amer. J. Obstet Gynaec., 46: 19–37, July 1943

Meinicke, Ernst. German scientist. 1878–
SEROREACTION—for tuberculosis.
Zur Serologie der Tuberkulose. Klin. Wschr., 13: 258–260, Feb. 17, 1934
Eine neue Serumreaktion auf Tuberkulose. III Mitteilung. Ibid., 833–838, June 9, 1934
TESTS—for syphilis.
Ueber eine neue Methode der serologischen Luesdiagnose. Abstr.: Berl. klin. Wschr., 54: 613–614, June 18, 1917
Neue serologische Syphilis-Diagnose. Abstr.: Dtsch. med. Wschr., 43: 797 (only), June 21, 1917
Ueber die dritte Modifikation meiner Luesreaktion. Münch. med. Wschr., 66: 932–933, Aug. 15, 1919
Ein neues Trübungsreaktion für Syphilis. Dtsch. med. Wschr., 48: 384–385, Mar. 24, 1922
Meinickes Trübungsreaktion auf Syphilis (M. T. R.) mit cholesterinfreien Balsamextrakten with E. Grün, Ibid., 49: 43–45, Jan. 12, 1923
Ein neue Syphilisreaktion (MKR.). Klin. Wschr., 8: 112–113, Jan. 15, 1929
Meine Klärungsreaktion auf Syphilis. Münch. med. Wschr., 76: 1965–1968, Nov. 22, 1929

Meldrum, Norman Urquhart. English chemist. 1907–1933
Isolated—
Carbonic anhydrase. Its preparation and properties with F. J. W. Roughton, J. Physiol., 80: 113–142, Dec. 5, 1933

Meleney, Frank Lamont. New York surgeon. 1889–
TEST—
The sterility of catgut in relation to hospital infections, with an effective test for the sterility of catgut with Mabel Chatfield, S. G. O., 52: 430–441, Feb. 15, 1931
TREATMENT—
Zinc peroxide in the treament of microaërophilic and anaërobic infections with special reference to a group of chronic, ulcerative, burrowing, non-gangrenous lesions of the abdominal wall apparently due to a microaërophilic haemolytic streptococcus. Ann. Surg., 101: 997–1011, Apr. 1935

Meleney, H. E. See W. H. Robey

Melhado, Gerald C. Montreal obstetrician. 1890–
MANEUVER—
The occipitoposterior position: a method of management, with an analysis of 976 cases. Amer. J. Obstet. Gynaec., 26: 696–704, Nov. 1933

Melick, Clark Owen. Chicago physician. 1886–
SOLUTION—lactate asparagin; culture medium.
The preparation of bacterial antigens. J. med. Res., 43: 405–417 (408), Aug.–Oct. 1922

Mélier, Francois. French surgeon. 1798–1866
Wrote important description of appendicitis.
Mémoire et observations sur quelques maladies de l'appendice coecale. J. gén. de méd., 100: 317–345, July 1827

Mellanby, Sir Edward. English physiologist. 1884–

WROTE—
The part played by an "accessory factor" in the production of experimental rickets. J. Physiol., 52: XI-XII, Jan. 26, 1918
A further demonstration of the part played by accessory food factors in the etiology of rickets. Ibid., LII-LIV, Dec. 14, 1918

Mellanby, John. English physiologist. 1878–
TECHNIC—
Prothrombase—its preparation and properties. Proc. roy. Soc. London, s. B., 107: 271–285, Dec. 2, 1930

Meller, Josef. Vienna ophthalmologist
PERIVASCULITIS—sympathetic.
Chronische Iridocyclitis und Neuritis retrobulbaris. Arch. f. Ophthal., 105: 299–332, June 14, 1921

Mellon, Ralph Robertson. American pathologist. 1883–
BROTH—serum veal infusion, for cultivation of diphtheroids.
A study of the diphtheroid group of organisms with special reference to their relation to the streptococci. Part I. Characteristics of a peculiar pleomorphic diphtheroid. J. Bact., 2: 81–107 (84), Mar. 1917
THEORY—
New observations on mechanism of sulfanilamide's action; phenomenon of potentiation. Med. Rec., 146: 247–248, Sept. 15, 1937

Melnick, P. See A. C. Ivy

Meltzer, Samuel James. New York physician. 1851–1920
ANESTHESIA or METHOD—
The method of respiration by intratracheal insufflation, its scientific principle and its practical availability in medicine and surgery. Med. Rec., 77: 477–483, Mar. 19, 1910
Intratracheal insufflation. J. A. M. A., 57: 521–525, Aug. 12, 1911
TEST—adrenalin mydriasis in suprarenal disease.
Über die Einwirkung von subkutanen Einspritzungen von Adrenalin auf das Auge von Katzen, deren Sympathikus reseziert oder deren oberes Halsganglion entfernt ist. Zbl. Physiol., 17: 652–653, Jan. 30, 1904
Same, abstr. in English: Amer. J. Physiol., 10: XXXVII (only), 1904
Studies on the "paradoxical" pupil-dilatation caused by adrenalin. I. The effect of subcutaneous injections and instillations of adrenalin upon the pupils of rabbits with Clara Meltzer Auer, Ibid., 11: 28–51, Apr. 1, 1904
TEST—for biliary pathology, by giving magnesium sulphate per duodenum.
The disturbance of the law of contrary innervation as a pathogenetic factor in the diseases of the bile ducts and gall-bladder. Amer. J. med. Sci., 153: 469–491, Apr. 1917
THEORY—of shock; inhibition t.
The nature of shock. Arch. intern. Med., 1: 571–588, July 1908
TREATMENT—
The effects of intraspinal injection of magnesium salts upon tetanus with J. Auer, J. exp. Med., 8: 692–706, Dec. 21, 1906

Melville, R. Saunders. Dundee, Scotland surgeon
OPERATION—
A modification of Lotheison's operation: utilization of the sac in the radical cure of femoral hernia. Brit. med. J., 1: 467–468, Mar. 9, 1935

Ménard, M. C. See N. C. Foot

Mendel, Felix. German physician. 1862–1912
TEST—tuberculin.
Die von Pirquetsche Hautreaktion und die intravenöse Tuberkulinbehandlung. Med. Klin., 4: 402–404 Mar. 22, 1908
Introduced fibrolysin. Garrison
Fibrolysin, eine neue Thiosinaminverbindung. Therap Mschr., 19: 93–103, Feb. 1905

Mendel, Gregor Johann. Abbot of the Augustinia monastery at Brünn. 1822–1884
LAW—mathematical law governing dominant ar recessive characters in hybrids.
Versuche über Pflanzen-Hybriden. Verh. d. natur Ver. in Brünn, 1865, 4: 3–270, 1866
Also, Ibid., 49: 3–47, 1911

Mendel, Johann. Dresden physician
SOLUTION—basal peptone, for studying decomp sition of sugars.
Über Umsetzung verschiedener Zucherarten dur Bakterien. Zbl. Bakt., 2 Abt., 29: 290–330 (297 Mar. 2, 1911

Mendel, Kurt. German neurologist. 1874–
REFLEX—plantar flexion of toes on percussing do sum of foot.
Ein Reflex am Fussrücken. Neurol. Zbl., 23: 197–19 Mar. 1, 1904

Mendel, Lafayette Benedict. New Haven physi chemist. 1872–1935
TEST—for zinc in tissues.
Experimental studies on the physiology of the molluscs-second paper with H. C. Bradley, Amer. J. Physio 14: 311–327 (320), 1905
See also T. B. Osborne

Mendeleff, Mlle P. French biologist
TEST—for cancer by blood coagulation.
Le pouvoir coagulant de tissus cancéreux de cobaye C. R. Soc. Biol., 118: 196–198, Dec. 15, 1935
Action coagulante des extraits de tissus, chez les cobay cancéreux. Ibid., 364–369, Dec. 22, 1935

Mendelsohn, Martin. Berlin physician. 1860–
TEST—of heart function.
Die Erholung als Mafs der Herz-Function. XI Kongr. f. inn. Med., pp. 200–212, 1901

Mendelssohn, Arnoldus. German physician. 181
Advanced idea that atelectasis is of great importan in causing pneumonia.
Der Mechanismus der Respiration und Cirkulatic oder das explicirte Wesen der Lungenhyperämie ... Berlin, Behrs, 1845. 384 pp.

Mendelssohn, Edwin. Philadelphia surgeon. 191
METHOD—
Submucous hemorrhoidectomy: a modification of Calman method. Amer. J. Surg., 71: 676–680, M 1946

Mendenhall, W. L. See W. B. Cannon

Menees, Thomas Orville. Grand Rapids physici 1890–1937
Introduced—
Amniography: preliminary report with J. D. Mil and L. E. Holly, Amer. J. Roent., 24: 363–366, O 1930

Menges, K. See K. Franke

Ménière, Prosper. French physician. 1799–1862
DISEASE or SYNDROME—aural vertigo.
Sur une forme particulière de surdité grave dépende

d'une lésion de l'oreille interne. Abstr.: Gaz. méd. de
Paris, 16: 29 (only), Jan. 12, 1861
  Nouveau documents relatifs aux lésions de l'oreille interne caractérisées par des symptômes de congestion cérébrale apoplectiforme. Ibid., 239–240, Apr. 13, 1861
  Observations de maladies de l'oreille interne caractérisees par des symptômes de congestion cérébrale apoplectiforme. Ibid., 379–380, June 15, 1861
  Mémoire sur des lésions de l'oreille interne donnant lieu a des symptômes de congestion cérébrale apoplectiforme. Ibid., 597–601, Sept. 1, 1861

Menk, W. See P. Mühlens

Menkin, Valy. American physician. 1901–
NTINECROSIN—
  Dynamics of inflammation; an inquiry into the mechanism of infectious processes. New York, Macmillan, 1940. 244 pp.
  Chemical basis of injury in inflammation. Arch. Path., 36: 269–288, Sept. 1943
  Chemical basis of fever with inflammation. Ibid., **39**: 28–36, Jan. 1945

Menten, Maud Lenore. Pittsburgh physician. 1879–
OLUTION—lactose bile infusion.
  Relationship of enteritidis-paratyphoid B infections to hyperglycemia in rabbits with Helen M. Manning, J. infect. Dis., 37: 400–410 (401), Nov. 1925

Mentzel, C. See C. Arnold

Menzer, Arthur August Ludwig. German bacteriologist. 1872–
ERUM—for treating rheumatic fever.
  Die Aetiologie des akuten Gelenkrheumatismus, nebst kritischen Bemerkungen zu seiner Therapie. Berlin, Hirschwald, 1902. 126 pp.

Mercer, Walter. Edinburgh surgeon
NIFE—
  A new knife for the removal of the meniscus. J. Bone and Joint Surg., 21: 474 (only), Apr. 1939

Mercier, Louis Auguste. French urologist. 1811–1882
ATHETER—
  Mémoire sur le cathétérisme de l'urèthre dans les cas difficiles. Gaz. d. hôp., 31: 314–315, July 8, 1858
ALVE—
  Troisième série d'observations et remarques sur le traitement de la rétention d'urine causée par les valvules du col de la vessie. (Paris, le Normant, 1850). 79 pp.

Meredith, J. M. See C. C. Coleman

Méricourt, Alfred LeRoy de. French physician. 1825–1901
eported chromidrosis.
  Sur la coloration partielle en noir ou en bleu de la peau chez les femmes. Abstr. by Lasègue: Bull. Acad. Méd., Paris, 23: 1141–1144, Aug. 31, 1858

Merkel, Friedrich Siegmund. German anatomist. 1845–1919
ORPUSCLES—tactile.
  Ueber die Endigungen der sensibilen Nerven in der Haut der Wirbelthiere. Rostock, Schmidt, 1880. 214 pp.
CHEME—of deformities of face and lip. In: Hand. d. top. Anat., Braunschweig, Vieweg, Bd. 1: 341, 1885–90

Merkert, C. E. See H. O. McPheeters

Mermingas, K. Athens surgeon
PERATION—for inguinal hernia.
  Neueres zur Operationsmethodik der Leistenbrüche. Zbl. Chir., 63: 2050–2055, Aug. 29, 1936

Merseburg. city in Germany
TRIAD—goiter, exophthalmos, and tachycardia; three cardinal symptoms of Basedow's disease. Dorland

Mertens, Victor E. Munich surgeon. 1875–
REACTION—intradermic, for cancer.
  Über die diagnostische Anwendung des Serums von bestrahlten Krebskranken und über die Wirkungsweise der Röntgenstrahlen. Dtsch. Z. Chir., 179: 216–225, May 1923

Mertz, V. See Lüttge

Méry, Jean. Paris anatomist. 1645–1722
GLAND—same as Cowper's g. in urethra.
  Observations anatomiques. Journal des Scavans, June 1684. Amsterdam, 12: 228–229, 1685

Merzbacher, Ludwig. German physician in Buenos Aires. 1875–
DISEASE—of Pelizaeus-Merzbacher; familial centrolobar sclerosis.
  Weitere Mitteilungen über eine eigenartige hereditär-familiäre Erkrankung des Zentralnervensystems. Med. Klin., 4: 1952–1955, Dec. 20, 1908

Mesmer, Friederich Anton. Swiss physician. 1733–1815
MESMERISM—
  Mémoire sur la découverte du magnétisme animal. Genevà, Paris, Didot, 1779. 85 pp.

Messerschmidt, Theodor Albert Heinrich. Strassburg physician. 1886–
TEST—
  Zum klinischen Nachweis von Blut in den Fäzes. Münch. med. Wschr., 56: 388–389, Feb. 23, 1909

Mester, A. J. Cracow, Poland physician
TEST—for rheumatic disease.
  Nowy kierunek w leczeniu pewnych schorzen reumatyeznych. Polska gaz. lek., 11: 388–393, May 22, 1932
  A specific reaction in acute rheumatism and rheumatoid arthritis. Ann. Rheumat. Dis., 2: 266–268, Dec. 1941

Mestivier. French surgeon
Described appendicitis in 1759.
  Observations sur une tumeur située proche la région ombilicale, du côté droit, occasionée par une grosse épingle trouvée dans l'appendice vermiculaire du cecum. J. de Méd., Chir. et Phar., 10: 441–442, 1759

Metchnikoff, Elie Ilya Illyich. Russian physiologist. 1845–1916
Awarded, with P. Ehrlich, Nobel prize in 1908.
Discovered phagocytes and phagocytosis.
  Ueber eine Sprosspilzkrankheit der Daphnien. Beitrag zur Lehre über den Kampf der Phagocyten gegen Krankheitserreger. Arch. path. Anat., 96: 177–195, May 5, 1884
  Ueber die Beziehung der Phagocyten zu Milzbrandbacillen. Ibid., 97: 502–526, Sept. 8, 1884
  Lektsii o sravnitelnoi patologii vospaleniy. St. Petersburg, Rikker, 1892. 162 pp.
  Also, in French Paris, Masson, 1892. 239 pp.
  Also, English transl. by F. A. and E. H. Starling. London, Kegan Paul et al., 1893. 218 pp.
LAW—whenever body is attacked by bacteria, polynuclear leukocytes and large mononuclear leukocytes quickly become protective phagocytes. Dorland
  Sur la lutte des cellules de l'organisme contre l'invasion des microbes. Ann. Inst. Pasteur, 1: 321–336, July 1887
THEORY—of effect of lactic acid on bacteria.

Quelques remarques sur le lait aigri. Paris, Maloine, 1906
Gave accurate description of tubercle.
Ueber die phagocytäre Rolle der Tuberkelriesenzellen. Arch. path., Anat., 113: 63–94, July 2, 1888
Showed that higher apes can be inoculated with syphilis.
Etudes experimentales sur la syphilis with E. Roux, Ann. Inst. Pasteur, 17: 809–821, Dec. 1903; 18: 1–6, Jan. 1904
Mettauer, John Peter. Virginia surgeon. 1787–1875
OPERATION—
On staphyloraphy. Amer. J. med. Sci., 21: 309–332, 1837
Operated successfully for—
Vesico-vaginal fistula. Boston Med. and Surg. J., 22: 154–155, Apr. 15, 1840
Meulengracht, Einar. Swedish physician. 1887–
DIET—
Behandling af haematemese og melaena med mad. Ugeskr. Laeg., 95: 1257–1259, Nov. 23, 1933
Treatment of hematemesis and melaena with food. Acta med. Scand., suppl. 59, pp. 375–385, 1934
Treatment of haematemesis and melaena with food: the mortality. Lancet, 2: 1220–122, Nov. 30, 1935
ICTERUS INDEX OF—
Die klinische Bedeutung der Untersuchung auf Gallenfarbstoff im Blutserum. Dtsch. Arch. f. klin. Med., 132: 285–300, July 13, 1920
Ein Bilirubinkolorimeter behufs klinischer Bestimmung der Bilirubinmenge im Blute. Ibid., 137: 38–46, Aug. 12, 1921
METHOD—
Die klinische Bedeutung der Untersuchung auf Gallenfarbstoff im Blutserum. Dtsch. Arch. f. klin. Med., 132: 285–300, July 13, 1920
REGIMEN—in gastric hemorrhage from ulcer.
Weitere Erfahrungen über die Behandlung massiver Magenblutungen ohne Beschränkung der Nährungszufuhr. Münch. med. Wschr., 84: 1565–1569, Oct. 1, 1937
Meunier, Henri. French physician
Employed gastric lavage to establish diagnosis of tuberculosis in infants.
Bacilloscopie des crachats extraits de l'estomac pour le diagnostic de la tuberculose pulmonaire de l'enfant. Pr. méd., 2: 81–82, Aug. 13, 1898
Meyer, A. H. See Ingeborg Chievitz
Meyer, Arthur Woldemar. Berlin surgeon. 1885–
MODIFICATION—of Trendelenburg operation for pulmonary embolus.
Trendelenburgsche Lungenembolie-Operation. Med. Klin., 24: 1436–1437, Sept. 14, 1928
The operative treatment of embolism of the lungs. Proc. Staff Meet. Mayo Clin., 4: 258–260, Aug. 28, 1929
(Same title) S. G. O., 50: 891–898, May 1930
Meyer, Georg Hermann von. Zurich anatomist. 1815–1892
LINE—in normal foot line of great toe when prolonged backward should pass through center of heel. Dorland
Die richtige Gestalt der Schuhe. . . . Zürich, Meyer und Zeller, 1858. 30 pp.
Also, in English, Edinburgh, Edmonston and Douglas, 1864. 55 pp.

Meyer, Hans Wilhelm. Copenhagen physician. 1824–1895
DISEASE—
Om adenoide Vegetationer i Naesesvaelgrummet. Hospitalstid, Kjobenh., 11: 171–181, 1868
On adenoid vegetations in the naso-pharyngeal cavity: their pathology, diagnosis, and treatment. Med.-Chir. Trans., 53: 191–215, 1870
Meyer, Herbert Willy. New York City surgeon. 1896–
OPERATION—
Intrathoracic esophagojejunostomy for total gastrectomy with lower esophagectomy for carcinoma. Surgery, 12: 115–127, July 1942
Meyer, J. See F. W. Co-Tui, L. Ruzicka
Meyer, Karl Friedrich. San Francisco pathologist. 1884–
AGAR—sulphite gential violet infusion, for cultivation of B. pestis.
Selective mediums in the diagnosis of rodent plague with A. P. Batchelder, J. infect. Dis., 39: 370–385 (385), Nov. 1926
See also Bertha J. Dubovsky, J. E. Stickel
Meyer, Lothar. German physician. 1830–1895
Investigated blood gases.
Die Gase des Blutes. Z. f. rat. Med., 8: 256–316, 1857
De sanguine oxydo carbonico infesto. Wratislaviae, typ. Grasii, Barthii et Soc., 1858
Meyer, M. See K. Lanken
Meyer, R. K. See F. L. Hisaw
Meyer, Robert. Berlin gynecologist 1864–1947
Described arrhenoblastoma and described relation to sex characteristics.
Beitrage zur Frage der Funktion von von Tumoren der Ovarien, insbesondere solcher, die zur Entweiblichung und zur Vermännlichung führen. Arrhenoblastome. Zbl. Gynäk., 54: 2374–2389, Sept. 30, 1930
The pathology of some special ovarian tumors and their relation to sex characteristics. Amer. J. Obstet. Gynaec., 22: 697–713, Nov. 1931
Meyer, Victor. German scientist. 1848–1897
Discovered mustard gas.
Ueber Thiodiglykolverbindungen. Ber. dtsch. chem Ges., 19: 3259–3266, 1886
Meyer, Willy. New York surgeon. 1859–1932
MODIFICATION—of Sauerbruch negative pressure chamber.
Pneumectomy with the aid of differential air pressure an experimental study: the new type of apparatus used J. A. M. A., 53: 1978–1987, Dec. 11, 1909
OPERATION—
An improved method of the radical operation for carcinoma of the breast. Med. Rec., 46: 746–749, Dec 15, 1894
OPERATION—
Impermeable cardiospasm successfully treated by thoracotomy and esophagoplication. Abstr.: Ann Surg., 53: 293–294, Feb. 1911
Also: J. A. M. A., 56: 1437–1438, May 20, 1911
While a pupil of Trendelenburg, first described Trendelenburg's position.
Ueber die Nachbehandlung des hohen Steinschnitte sowie über Verwendbarkeit desselben zur Operation vo Blasenscheidenfisteln. Arch. f. klin. Chir., 31: 494 525, 1884
See also K. G. A. Bier, F. Trendelenburg
Meyerhof, Otto. Hannover biochemist. 1884–
Awarded, with A. V. Hill, Nobel prize in 1922.

Über das Vorkommen des Coferments des alkoholischen Hefegärung im Muskelgewebe und seine muttmassliche Bedeutung im Atmungsmechanismus. Z. physiol. Chem., 101: 165–175, Jan. 26, 1918
Die Energieumwandlungen im Muskel I. Über die Beziehungen der Milchsäure zur Wärmebildung und Arbeitsleistung des Muskels in der Anaerobiose. Arch. Physiol., 182: 232–283, Aug. 18, 1920
(Same) *II. Das Schicksal der Milchsäure in der Erhohlungsperiode des Muskels.* Ibid., 284–317, Aug. 18, 1920
Chemical dynamics of life phenomena. Philadelphia, Lippincott, 1924
Meyers, V. C. See I. H. Einsel
Meyerstein, Wilhelm. Cologne bacteriologist. 1881–
MEDIUM—bile; culture m. for typhoid bacilli.
Ueber Typhusanreicherung. Münch. med. Wschr., 53: 1864–1865, Sept. 18, 1906
Meymott, Charles. See C. M. Tidy
Meynert, Theodor. French physician. 1833–1892
AMENTIA—polyneuritis psychosis; same as Korsakoff's psychosis.
Klinische Vorlesungen über Psychiatrie. Wien, 1890. p. 92
BUNDLE, CELLS, COMMISSURE, FIBERS, LAYER, RADIATION—
Der Bau der Gross-Hirnrinde und seine örtliche Verschiedenheiten, nebst einem pathologisch-anatomischen Corollarium. Viertl. f. Psychiat., 1: 77–93; 125–217, 1867; 1: 381–403; 2: 88–113, 1868
Also: Neuwied, Heuser, 1872. 68 pp.
Mialhe, Louis. French scientist. 1807–1886
Isolated ptyalin. Garrison
De la digestion et de l'assimilation des maitères sucrées et amiloides. Abstr.: C. R. Acad. Sci., 20: 954–959, 1845
Mibelli, Vittorio. Italian dermatologist. 1860–1910
DISEASE—angiokeratoma.
D'une nouvelle forme de keratose "angio-kératome." Congr. intern. de dermat. et de syph., 1889, Paris, p. 899, 1890
L'angiokeratoma. Gior. ital. di mal. ven., Milano, 26: 159–180, 1891
DISEASE—porokeratosis.
Contributo allo studio della ipercheratosi dei canali sudoriferi (porokeratosis). Ibid., 28: 313–355, 1893
Michaëlis, Gustav Adolf. German obstetrician. 1798–1848
Applied name "rachitic or pseudo-osteomalacic" pelvis. Garrison
Das enge Becken: nach eigenen Beobachtungen und Untersuchungen. Hrsg. von C. C. T. Litzmann, Leipzig, Wigand, 1851. 440 pp.
Michaelis, Leonor. German-American biochemist. 1875–
STAIN—for chromatin.
Das Methylenblau und seine Zersetzungsprodukte. Zbl. Bakt., 29: 763–769, June 5, 1901
TEST—for syphilis.
Präcipitinreaktion bei Syphilis. Berl. klin. Wschr., 44: 1477–1478, Nov. 18, 1907
Michelsen, J. See J. H. Talbott
Middeldorpf, Albrecht Theodor von. Breslau surgeon. 1824–1868
OPERATION—for excision of cancer of tongue.
Die Galvanokaustik. Breslau, Max, 1854

Performed first operation for esophageal tumor. Garrison
De polypis oesophagi atque de tumore ejus generis primo prospere exstirpato. Vratislaviae, Max, 1857. 24 pp.
Performed first operation for gastric fistula. Garrison
Commentatio de fistulis ventriculi externis et chirurgica earum sanatione, accedente historia fistulae arte chirurgorum plastica prospere curatae. Vratislaviae, Grassii, 1859. 33 pp.
Middleton, George Stevenson. Glasgow physician
Described erythema elevatum diutinum.
A case of subcutaneous nodules in the hands of a rheumatic patient. Amer. J. Med. Sci., 94: 433–436, Oct. 1887
Middleton, Peter. American physician. ?–1781
Wrote first American contribution to medical history. Garrison
A medical discourse, or an historical inquiry into the ancient and present state of medicine. New York, Gaine, 1769
Middleton, W. S. See J. W. Gale
Miescher, Friedrich. Swiss scientist. 1844–1893
Discovered nuclein. Garrison
Die Spermatozoen einiger Wirbelthiere. Ein Beitrag zur Histochemie. (Nuclein). Verh. d. naturf. Ges. in Basel, 6: 138–208, 1874
Mignon, Alfred. French surgeon. 1854–
Described synovectomy.
Synovectomie du genou. Bull. et mem. Soc. d. Chirurg. de Paris, 26: 1113–1116, Dec. 12, 1899
Migula, Walter. German scientist. 1863–
SOLUTION—glucose nitrate, for differentiation of typhoid bacilli from B. coli.
Compendium der bakteriologischen Wasseruntersuchung. Wusbaden, Memnich, 1901. p. 20
SOLUTION—hay infusion; culture medium. Ibid.
Mikulicz-Radecki, Johann von. Austrian surgeon. 1850–1905
ANGLE—of declination, of femur.
Ueber individuelle Formdifferenzen am Femur und an der Tibia des Menschen. Arch. Anat. Physiol. (Anat. abth.), pp. 351–404, 1878
Die seitlichen Verkrümmungen am Knie und deren Heilungsmethoden. Arch. klin. Chir., 23: 671–770, 1879
CELLS—"foam cells".
Ueber das Rhinosclerom (Hebra). Ibid., 20: 485–534, 1876
DICTUM—it is highly dangerous to give a general anesthesia to a patient whose hemoglobin in below 30.
Ueber den Hämoglobingehalt des Blutes bei chirurgeschen Erkrankungen, mit besonderer Rücksicht auf den Wiederersatz bei Blutverlusten. Wien. med. Wschr., 40: 803–804, May 10, 1890
DISEASE or SYNDROME—chronic, hypertrophic enlargement of lacrymal and salivary glands.
Über eine eigenartige symmetrische Erkrankung der Thränen- und Mundspeicheldrüsen. Beitr. z. Chir., Festschrift f. Theodor Billroth. Stuttgart, 1892. pp. 610–630
Also, in German with English transl. by W. deRouville. Med. Classics, 2: 137–186, Oct. 1937
DRAIN—
Ueber die Anwendung der Antisepsis bei Laparoto-

mieen, mit besonderer Rücksicht auf die Drainage der Peritonealhöhle. Arch. klin. Chir., 26: 111–150, 1881

KENTOTRIBE—an instrument for crushing intestinal spur.
Illust. in Handb. d. prak. Chir., 2 Aufl., Bd. III, p. 193, 1903

LINE—on stomach, for gastric resection. Illust. in Ibid., Bd. IV, p. 173

OPERATION—for carcinoma of esophagus.
Ein Fall von Resection des carcinomatösen Oesophagus mit plastischen Ersatz des excidierten Stückes. Prag. med. Wschr., 11: 93–94, Mar. 10, 1886

OPERATION—for stricture of esophagus.
Zur Pathologie und Therapie des Cardiospasmus. Dtsch. med. Wschr., 30: 17–19, Jan. 1; 50–54, Jan. 7, 1904

OPERATION—on foot.
Eine neue osteoplastische Resectionsmethode am Fusse. Arch. klin. Chir., 26: 494–501, 1881

OPERATION—gastroenterostomy.
Die chirurgische Behandlung des chronischen Magengeschwürs. Ibid., 55: 84–119, 1897
Also: Zbl. Chir., 24: 69–98, 1897

OPERATION—hip dislocation, reduction.
Die unblutige Reduktion der angeborenen Hüftverrenkung. Arch. klin. Chir., 49: 368–386, 1894

OPERATION—intestine, resection of, by two stage or exteriorization method.
Chirurgische Erfahrungen über das Darmcarzinom. Chirurgenkongress, 1902
Also: Arch. klin. Chir., 69: 28–47, 1903
Also, in German with English transl. by W. deRouville: Med. Classics, 2: 188–229, Oct. 1937
Small contributions to the surgery of the intestinal tract. . . . Boston Med. and Surg. J., 148: 608–611, June 4, 1903
Also: Trans. Amer. Surg. Ass., 21: 124–134 (132–134), 1903

OPERATION—on nasal lobule.
Przycznki do plastycznej chirurgii nosa. Gaz. lekarska, Warszawa, 2 s., 3: 429; 453, 1883
Also: Arch. klin. Chir., 30: 106–118, 1884

OPERATION—on nasal sinuses.
Zur operativen Behandlung des Empyems der Highmorshöhle. Ibid., 34: 626–634, 1886

OPERATION—pharyngotomy, for exposure of tonsillar tumors.
Zur Operation des Tonsillarkarzinoms; ein Beitrag zur Pharyngotomie. Dtsch. med. Wschr., 10: 33–35, 1884
Die seitliche Pharyngotomie behufs Exstirpation maligner Geschwülste der Tonsillargegend. Ibid., 12: 157–158, Mar. 11; 178–180, Mar. 18, 1886

OPERATION—pyloroplasty.
Zur operativen Behandlung der Pylorusstenose. Chirurgenkongress, 1887
Zur operativen Behandlung des stenosirenden Magengeschwüres. Arch. klin. Chir., 37: 79–90, 1888

OPERATION—for rectal prolapse.
Invagination und Prolaps des Dickdarms durch den Mastdarm; Resektion eines 76 cm. langen Darmstückes; Heilung. Wien. med. Pr., 50: 1565–1567, Dec. 16; 1597–1601, Dec. 23, 1883
Zur operativen Behandlung des Prolapsus recti et coli invaginati. Verh. d. dtsch. Ges. Chir., 17: 294–317, 1888

Also: Arch. klin.Chir., 38: 74–97, 1889

Introduced gastroscopy. Garrison
Uebe Gastroskopi und Oesophagoskopie. Wien. med. Pr., 22: 1405–1408, Nov. 6; 1437–1443, Nov. 13; 1473–1477, Nov. 20; 1505–1507, Nov. 27; 1537–1541, Dec. 4; 1573–1577, Dec. 11; 1629–1631, Dec. 25, 1881

Miles, Catharine C. See L. M. Terman

Miles, H. S. See F. M. Wilson

Miles, J. A. R. See E. G. L. Bywaters

Miles, William Ernest. English surgeon. 1869–1947
OPERATION—
A method of performing abdomino-perineal excision for carcinoma of the rectum and of the terminal portion of the pelvic colon. Lancet 2: 1812–1813, Dec. 19, 1908
The pathology of the spread of cancer of the rectum, and its bearing upon the surgery of the cancerous rectum. S. G. O., 52: 350–359, Feb. 15, 1931

Milian, Gaston. French dermatologist
ERYTHEMA—biotropic.
Erythème polymorphe photobiotropique avec localisation présternale with M. Mansour, Bull. Soc. fr. derm. syph., 39: 651–652, June 9, 1932

Milkman, Louis Arthur. Scranton roentgenologist. 1895–
SYNDROME—multiple, spontaneous, idiopathic, symmetrical fractures.
Pseudofractures (hunger osteopathy, late rickets, osteomalacia): report of a case. Amer. J. Roent., 24: 29–37, July 1930

Millar, John. British physician. 1733–1805
ASTHMA—laryngismus stridulus.
Observations on the asthma and on the hooping cough. London, Cadel, 1769. 207 pp.

Miller, A. See R. D. Carman

Miller, Alexander. Scottish surgeon
Wrote on psoas abscess.
A probationary essay on lumbar, or psoas abscess, submitted, by authority of the President and his council, to the examination of the Royal College of Surgeons of Edinburgh. . . . Edinburgh, Millar, 1831. 16 pp.
Also, Edinburgh, Ballantyne, 1831. 17 pp.

Miller, Benjamin Frank. American physician. 1907–
METHOD—
A direct microtitration method for blood sugar with D. V. Van Slyke, J. biol. Chem., 114: 583–595, July 1936

Miller, C. W.

Miller, Douglas. See A. MacCormick

Miller, Edwin Morton. Chicago surgeon. 1888–
METHOD—of controlling hemorrhage from spleen.
Temporary complete control of the main blood supply as a preliminary step in difficult splenectomies. J. A. M. A., 112: 229 (only), Jan. 21, 1939

Miller, J. D. See T. O. Menees

Miller, Joseph Leggett. Chicago physician. 1867–1937
Considered migraine and idiopathic hydrarthrosis as sensitization diseases.
Treatment of migraine with peptone: evidence of the anaphylactic character of the seizure with B. O. Raulston, J. A. M. A., 80: 1894–1896, June 30, 1923
Evidence of the anaphylactic character of intermittent hydrarthrosis with P. Lewin, Ibid., 82: 1177–1179, Apr. 12, 1924

Miller, M. W. See M. M. Wintrobe

Miller, Thomas Grier. Philadelphia physician. 1886–
TUBE—
Intestinal intubation: a practical technique with W. O. Abbott, Amer. J. Med. Sci., 187: 595–599, 1934

Miller, Willoughby Dayton. American physician. 1853–1907
BACILLUS—from carious teeth.
The micro-organisms of the human mouth. Phila., White Dental Manuf. Co., 1890

Milligan, E. T. C. London surgeon
TECHNIC—
Surgical anatomy of the anal canal, and the operative treatment of haemorrhoids with C. N. Morgan, L. E. Jones and R. Officer, Lancet, 2: 1119–1124, Nov. 13, 1937

Millon, Auguste Nicholas Eugène. French chemist. 1812–1867
TEST—for proteins.
Sur un réactif propre aux composés protéiques. C. R. Acad. Sci., 28: 40–42, 1849

Mills, Charles Karsner. Philadelphia neurologist. 1845–1931
DISEASE—
A case of unilateral progressive ascending paralysis, probably representing a new form of degenerative disease. J. nerv. ment. Dis., 27: 195–200, Apr. 1900
Unilateral ascending paralysis and unilateral descending paralysis. Their clinical varieties and their pathologic causes. J. A. M. A., 47: 1638–1645, Nov. 17, 1906

Milne, A. D. See P. H. Ross

Milne, Robert. English physician. 1849–1922
METHOD—of prophylaxis.
A plea for the home treatment and prevention of scarlet fever. London, Nisbet, 1910. 80 pp.

Milroy, John Alexander. Belfast scientist
REAGENT—
A method for the estimation of glucose in blood. Biochem. J., 19: 746–749, 1925

Milroy, William Forsyth. Omaha physician. 1855–
DISEASE—(name supplied by Sir W. Osler)
An undescribed variety of hereditary edema. New York Med. J., 16: 505–508, Nov. 5, 1892
Chronic hereditary edema: Milroy's disease. J. A. M. A., 91: 1172–1175, Oct. 20, 1928

Milton, John Laws. English physician. 1820–1898
Described—
On giant urticaria. Edinburgh Med. J., 22: 513–526, Dec. 1876

Minami, Seigo. Tokio physician
Described crush syndrome.
Über Nierenveränderungen nach Verschüttung. Arch. path. Anat., 245: 247–267, Sept. 19, 1923

Mines, George Ralph. Cambridge scientist
Described isolated electrical alternans in electrograms of frog's heart.
On dynamic equilibrium in the heart. J. Physiol., 46: 349–383, July 18, 1913

Mink, Owen Joseph. U. S. Army surgeon. 1879–1936
METHOD—
A method for the preparation of flatworms for study with A. H. Ebeling, U. S. Naval Med. Bull., 3: 267–268, July 1909

Minkman, D. C. J. See M. W. Beijerinck

Minkowski, Oscar. Russian pathologist. 1858–1931
SYNDROME—of Minkowski-Chauffard.
Ueber eine hereditäre, unter dem Bilde eines chronischen Icterus mit Urobilinurie, Splenomegalie und Nierensiderosis verlaufende Affection. Verh. d. dtsch. Cong. f. inn. Med., 18: 316–319, 1900
Studied B-oxybutyric acid in relation to diabetic coma.
Ueber das Vorkommen von Oxybuttersäure im Harn bei Diabetes mellitus. Arch. exp. Path. Pharmak., 18: 35–48, June 5, 1884
Noted relationship between pituitary enlargement and acromegaly.
Über einen Fall von Akromegalie. Berl. klin. Wschr., 24: 371–374, 1887
Studied production of diabetes by excision of pancreas with J. von Mehring.
De l'extirpation du pancréas chez les animaux et du diabète expérimental. Lettres. Semaine méd., 175–176, May 22, 1889
Untersuchungen über den Diabetes mellitus nach Exstirpation des Pankreas. Arch. exp. Path. Pharmak., 31: 85–189, Apr. 11, 1893
See also J. von Mehring

Minor, Lazar Salomovitsch. Moscow neurologist. 1855–
DISEASE—
Central Hämatomyelie. Arch. Psychiat., 24: 693–729, 1892

Minor, Victor. Moscow physician
TEST—for sweating.
Eines neues Verfahren zu der klinischen Untersuchung der Schweissabsonderung. Dtsch. Z. f. Nervenh., 101: 302–308, Jan. 1928

Minot, A(nnie) Stone. Nashville physiologist. 1894–
Introduced—
The response of the myasthenic state to guanidine hydrochloride with Katharine Dodd and S. S. Riven, Science, 87: 348–350, Apr. 15, 1938
See also J. C. Aub

Minot, Francis. American physician. 1821–1899
Described hemorrhagic disease of newborn.
On hemorrhage from the umbilicus in newborn infants, with an analysis of forty-six cases. Amer. J. Med. Sci., 24: 310–320, Oct. 1852

Minot, George Richards. Boston physician. 1885–
Awarded, with W. P. Murphy and G. H. Whipple, Nobel prize in 1934 for work on liver therapy in pernicious anemia.
Treatment of pernicious anemia by a special diet with W. P. Murphy, J. A. M. A., 87: 470–476, Aug. 14, 1926
The development of liver therapy in pernicious anemia: Nobel Lecture. Lancet, 1: 361–364, Feb. 16, 1935
METHODS—
Methods for testing donors for transfusion of blood and consideration of factors influencing agglutination and hemolysis. Boston Med. and Surg. J., 174: 667–674, May 11, 1916
TREATMENT—
Lymphatic leukemia: age incidence, duration and benefit derived from irradiation with R. Isaacs, Ibid., 191: 1–9, July 3, 1924
Lymphoblastoma (malignant lymphoma); age and sex incidence, duration of disease, and the effect of roentgen-ray and radium irradiation and surgery

with R. Isaacs, J. A. M. A., 86: 1185–1189, Apr. 17, 1926
See also W. P. Murphy

Minster, Dorothy K. See C. P. McCord

Mintz. S. Warsaw physician
METHOD—for free hydrochloric acid.
Eine einfache Methode zur quantitativen Bestimmung der freien Salzsaure in Mageninhalt. Wien. klin. Wschr., 2: 400 (only), May 16, 1889

Mirault, Germanicus. French surgeon. 1796–1879
OPERATION—for excision of cancer of tongue.
Mémoire sur la ligature de la langue, et sur celle de l'artère linguale en particulier; precédé d'une observation de cancer de la langue guéri par la ligature de cat organe. Mém. Acad. de Méd., 1833–34, Paris, 4, 1835

Mirsky, A. E. See M. L. Anson

Mitchell, A. Philip. Edinburgh surgeon
TECHNIC—of securing bone graft in position.
Ununited fractures due to war injuries: with end-results of operative treatment in 100 cases. Brit. J. Surg., 10: 259–289 (264), Oct. 1922

Mitchell, Clifford. Chicago physician. 1854–1939
TEST—
Nickel sulphate as a test for alkalies (a useful reagent in urine analysis). Clin. Med., 35: 167 (only), Mar. 1928

Mitchell, John Kearsley. Philadelphia physician. 1798–1858
First to describe neurotic spinal arthropathies. Garrison
On a new practice in acute and chronic rheumatism. Amer. J. Med. Sci., 8: 55–64, 1831
Wrote early essay on parasitic etiology of disease. Garrison
On the cryptogamous origin of malarious and epidemic fevers. Philadelphia, Lea and Blanchard, 1849. 137 pp.

Mitchell, Silas Weir. Philadelphia neurologist. 1829–1914
DISEASE—erythromelalgia.
Clinical lecture on certain painful affections of the feet. Philadelphia Med. Times, 3: 81–82, Nov. 9; 113–115, Nov. 23, 1872
On a rare vaso-motor neurosis of the extremities, and on the maladies with which it may be confounded. Amer. J. Med. Sci., 76: 17–36, July 1878
TREATMENT—rest t.
Wear and tear, or hints for the overworked. Philadelphia, Lippincott, 1871. 59 pp.
On rest in the treatment of nervous disease. New York, Putnam's, 1875. 20 pp.
Made early investigations of serpent venoms. Garrison
Researches upon the venom of the rattlesnake; with an investigation of the anatomy and physiology of the organs concerned. Smithson. Contrib. Knowl., Washington, 12, 1860. 145 pp.
Researches upon the venoms of poisonous serpents with E. T. Reichert, Washington, Smithsonian Inst., 1886
First to describe causalgia and make exhaustive study of traumatic neuroses. Garrison
Reflex paralysis, the result of gunshot wounds, and other injuries of nerves, founded chiefly upon cases observed in the United States General Hospital,

Christian Street, Philadelphia with G. R. Morehouse and W. W. Keen, Philadelphia, Lippincott, 1864
Pointed out coördinating functions of cerebellum. Garrison
Researches on the physiology of the cerebellum. Amer. J. Med. Sci., 57: 320–338, Apr. 1869
Wrote early account of ascending neuritis and of treatment of neuritis by cold and splint rests. Garrison
Injuries of nerves, and their consequences. Philadelphia, Lippincott, 1872. 377 pp.
Noted relation of eye-strain (asthenopia) and astigmatism to headaches and other neurotic symptoms. Garrison
Headaches, from heat-stroke, from fevers, after meningitis, from over use of brain, from eye strain. Med. and Surg. Reporter, Phila., 31: 67–70, July 25; 81–84, Aug. 1, 1874
First to describe—(Garrison)
Post-paralytic chorea. Amer. J. Med. Sci., 68: 342–352, Oct. 1874
Wrote on—
The relations of pain to weather, being a study of the natural history of a case of traumatic neuralgia. Ibid., 73: 305–329, Apr. 1877
Demonstrated that knee-jerk can be reenforced by sensory stimulation. Garrison
Physiological studies of the knee-jerk, and of the reactions of muscles under mechanical and other excitants with M. J. Lewis, Med. News, Phila., 48: 169–173, Feb. 13; 198–203, Feb. 20, 1886

Miura, Kinnosuke. Japanese physician. 1864–
Discovered Trichomonas vaginalis in voided urine of a man.
Trichomonas vaginalis im frischgelassenen Urin eines Mannes. Zbl. Bakt., 16: 67–73, July 9, 1894

Mixter, Charles Galloupe. Boston surgeon. 1882–
Wrote—
Total ablation of the thyroid for angina pectoris and congestive heart failure: results of eighteen months' experience with H. L. Blumgart and D. D. Berlin, Trans. Amer. Surg. Ass., pp. 10–17, 1934

Mixter, Samuel Jason. American surgeon. 1855–1926
TREATMENT—swallowing silk thread in stricture of esophagus.
Symposium on the surgery of the esophagus. First paper. From the standpoint of the general surgeon. Trans. Amer. Laryng. Ass., pp. 342–348, 1909

Mixter, W. J. See J. C. White

Miyata, T. See A. Fujita

Moczutkowsky, Osip Osipovich. Odessa physician. 1845–1903
Demonstrated communicability of relapsing fever and specific pathogenic significance of spirochaete.
Materialien zur Pathologie und Therapie des Rückfallstyphus. Dtsch. Arch. klin. Med., 24: 80–97, July 1, 1879

Modinos, P. Egyptian physician
TREATMENT—of drug addict, by blister fluid.
La guérison des toxicomanes. Bull. Acad. méd., Paris, 3 s., 102: 283–285, Nov. 5, 1929

Möbius, Paul Julius. German neurologist. 1853–1907
DISEASE— ophthalmoplegic migraine.
Ueber periodisch wiederkehrende Oculomotoriuslähmung. Berl. klin. Wschr., 21:6 04–608, Sept 22, 1884

SIGN—inability to keep eyeballs converged in exophthalmic goiter.
In a review of P. Marie's *Contribution à l'étude et au diagnostic des formes frustes de la maladie de Basedow.* Jb. d. inn. Med. u. ausl. ges. Med., 200: 98–100, 1883
Die Basedow'sche Krankheit. Wien, Hölder, 1896. 121 pp.

Moeckel, Kurt. Wiesbaden scientist
METHOD—of determination of blood amylase.
Über den Ursprung und die Bedeutung des amylolytischen Blutferments with F. Rost, Z. physiol. Chem., 67: 433–485, Aug. 15, 1910

Möller, Eggert. New York scientist
TEST—
Studies of urea excretion. II. Relationship between urine volume and the rate of urea excretion by normal adults with J. F. McIntosh and D. D. Van Slyke, J. clin. Invest., 6: 427–504, Dec. 1928

Moeller, H. Greifswald botanist
METHOD—for spore staining.
Ueber eine neue Methode der Sporenfärbung. Zbl. Bakt., 10: 273–277, Sept. 14, 1891

Möller, Hans Ulrik. Copenhagen ophthalmologist
HEREDITY—of angiomatosis of retina.
Familial angiomatosis retinae et cerebelli-Lindau's disease. Acta ophthal., 7: 244–260, 1929
See also C. Edmund

Moeller, Julius Otto Ludovicus. Königsberg surgeon. 1813–1887
DISEASE—subperiosteal hematoma in rickets.
Über akute Rachitis. Königsb. med. Jahrb., 1: 377, 1859
GLOSSITIS—exfoliativa.
Klinische Bemerkungen über einige wenigen bekannte Krankheiten der Zunge. Dtsch. Klinik, 3: 273–275, June 28, 1851

Müller, Sam. Berlin physician. 1880–
TEST—
Zur Azetonbestimmung im Harn. Z. klin. Med., 64: 207–210, 1907

Mönckeberg, Johann Georg. German physician. 1877–1925
SCLEROSIS—
Ueber die reine Mediaverkalkung der Extremitätenarterien und ihr Verhalten zur Arteriosklerose. Arch. path. Anat., 171: 141–167, Jan. 2, 1903

Mörner, Carl Axel Hampus. Swedish physician. 1854–1917
BODY—nucleo-albumin.
Untersuchungen über die Proteinstoffe und die eiweissfällenden Substanzen des normalen Menschenharns. Skand. Arch. f. Physiol., 6: 332–437, 1895
METHOD—for determination of urea in urine.
Eine Harnstoffbestimmungsmethode with J. Sjöqvist, Ibid., 2: 438–487, 1891
TEST—for acetoacetic acid in urine.
Kleinere Mittheilungen. Ibid., 5: 271–276 (276), 1895

Mörner, Carl Thore. Upsala physician
METHOD—for determination of free hydrochloric acid in stomach contents.
Einfache Methode zur Untersuchung der Fähigkeit des Magens, Salzsäure abzusondern. Salzsäurebestimmung des Mageninhaltes von Gesunden und Kranken. Maly's Jber. Fortschr. d. Thierchemie, 19: 253–254, 1890

Also: Upsala Läkareför. Förhandl., 24, 483–491
TEST—for cysteine.
Beitrag zur Kenntniss einiger Eigenschaften des Glutins. Z. physiol. Chem., 28: 471–523, Nov. 14, 1899
TEST—for homogentistic acid in urine.
Zur Chemie des Alkaptonharns bezw. der Homogentisinsäure (nebst einigen ihrer Verwandten). Ibid. 69: 329–365, Nov. 18, 1910
Showed cystin to be a decomposition product of protein.
See TEST—for cysteine.

Moersch, H. J. See W. McK. Craig

Moffat, Dean Alexander. American physician. 1907–
TECHNIC—of capillary study.
The modern apparatus and technic for the study of diseases of the peripheral vascular system. Med. Clin. N. Amer., 17: 1457–1465, Mar. 1934

Moffatt, M. R. German scientist
TEST—for lead in water.
Einfache kolorimetrische Bestimmung des Bleies in Trinkwasser with H. S. Spiro, Apoth.-Ztg., Berl., 22: 559, 1907

Mohr, Bernhard. Würzburg physician
Described tumor of pituitary with obesity. Garrison
Mittheilungen für neuropathologische Studien. 4. Hypertrophie (markschwammige Entartung?) der Hypophysis cerebri und dadurch bedingter Druck auf die Hirngrundfläche, insbesondere auf die Sehnerven das Chiasma derselben und den linkseitigen Hirnschenkel. Wschr. f. d. ges. Heilk., 6: 565–571, Aug. 29, 1840

Mohrschulz, Wilhelm. German physician
TEST—for barbituric acid in urine.
Ueber den toxikologischen Nachweis von Schlafmitteln der Barbitursäurereihe im ärztlichen Laboratorium. Münch. med. Wschr., 81: 672–763, May 4, 1934

Mohs, Frederic Edward. Madison, Wis. surgeon. 1910–
Introduced—
Pre-excisional fixation of tissues in the treatment of cancer in rats with M. F. Guyer, Cancer Res., 1: 49–51, Jan. 1941
Chemosurgery: a microscopically controlled method of cancer excision. Arch. Surg., 42: 279–295, Feb. 1941
Chemosurgical treatment of cancer of the lip: a microscopically controlled method of excision. Ibid., 48: 478–488, June 1944

Moir, Chassar. English surgeon
APPARATUS—
Nitrous oxide analgesia in obstetrics. Lancet, 1: 615–618, Mar. 13, 1937
See also H. W. Dudley

Moleschott, Jacob. Heidelberg physician. 1822–1893
TEST—for cholesterol.
Notes sur une réaction microchimique de la cholestérine et les corpuscules amyloides. C. R. Acad. Sci., 40: 361–362, Feb. 12, 1855

Molisch, Hans. Vienna chemist. 1856–
SOLUTION—basal nutrient.
Die Purpurbakterien nach neuen Untersuchungen. Jena, Fischer, 1907. p. 68
TEST—for sugars.
Zwei neue Zuckerreactionen. Mschr. f. Chem., 7: 198–209, 1886

Moloney, Paul Joseph. Canadian physician. ?–1939

TEST—of immunity to diphtheria.
Immunization with diphtheria toxoid (anatoxine Ramon) with C. J. Fraser, Amer. J. Pub. Health, 17: 1027–1030, Oct. 1927

Moloy, H. C. See W. E. Caldwell

Molsberry, J. M. See C. S. O'Brien

Momberg, Fritz, August. Berlin physician. 1870–1939
ANEMIA, BELT or TUBE—passed around waist to arrest bleeding in postpartum hemorrhage.
Die künstliche Blutleere der unteren Körperhälfte. Zbl. Chir., 35: 697–699, June 6, 1908

Mommsen, Dr. Frankfurt a. M. physician
NEUTROPHIL—toxic, granulation.
Über das Verhalten der neutrophilen Granula im Verlauf akuter Infektionskrankheiten. Mschr. Kinderheilk., 34: 624 (only), Dec. 1926
Über die neutrophilen Granulationen der Leukozyten und ihre gesetzmässige Veränderung bei Scharlach und lobärer Pneumonie. Jb. Kinderheilk., 3 F., 66: 293–309, July 1927

Monakow, Konstantin von. Zürich neurologist. 1853–1930
Described mechanism of red nucleus. Garrison
Der rote Kern, die Haube und die Regio hypothalamica bei einigen Säugetieren und beim Menschen. Arb. a. d. hirnanat. Inst. in Zürich, Wiesb., 3 Heft., 49–267, 1909; 5 Gft., 103–225, 1910

Monaldi, V. Rome physician
DRAINAGE—transpleural aspiration, of tuberculous cavities.
Procedimento di aspirazione endocavitaria delle caverne tubercolari del polmone. (Basi teoriche.) Ann. Inst. Carlo Forlanini, 16: 665–682, Oct. 1938

Monasterio, Gabriel. Italian physiologist. 1903–
TEST—
Neue Reaktionen des Bilirubins im Blutserum. Klin. Wschr., 9: 1772–1773, Sept. 20, 1930

Mondiére, Julien Théophile. Vienne physician
Described cancer of pancreas.
Récherches pour servir à l'histoire pathologique du pancréas. Arch. gén. de méd., 2 s., 11: 36–58; 265–294; 12: 133–163, 1836

Monfet, M. L. French scientist
TEST—for indican in urine.
Méthode de dosage de l'indican. C. R. Soc. Biol., 55: 1251–1252, Oct. 31, 1903

Monfort, W. F. See Esther A. Wagner

Moñge, Carlos. Lima, Peru physician. 1884–
DISEASE—chronic mountain sickness.
La enfermedad de los Andes (Sindromes Eritrémicos). An. Facultad de Medicina, Lima, 1928
High altitude disease. Arch. intern. Med., 59: 32–40, Jan. 1937

Moniz, Antonio Caetano de Abreu Freire Egas. See under Egas Moniz

Monks, George Howard. Boston surgeon. 1853–1933
METHOD—of intestinal localization.
Intestinal localization. A study on the cadaver for the purpose of determining to what extent the various parts of the small intestine may be identified through an abdominal wound. Ann. Surg., 38: 574–592, Oct. 1903
Intestinal localization. A review of certain studies (on the cadaver) in the surgical anatomy of the small intestine and its mesentery. S. G. O., 49: 213–219, Aug. 1929

OPERATION—
The restoration of a lower eyelid by a new method. Boston Med. and Surg., J., 139: 385–387, Oct. 20, 1898

Monneret, Jules Edouard Auguste. Paris physician. 1810–1868
PULSE—full, slow and soft, characteristic of jaundice.
Études cliniques sur la maladie qui a reçu le nom de cirrhose du foie. Arch. gén. de Méd., 4 s., 29: 385–404, Aug.; 30: 56–70, Sept. 1852

Monro, Alexander. Scottish anatomist. 1697–1767
BURSA—intratendinous b. of olecranon.
Osteology; or a treatise on the anatomy of the bones, to which are added a treatise of the nerves. Edinburgh, 1726

Monro, Alexander. Scottish anatomist. 1733–1817
HYPOTHESIS—skull and spinal column form a rigid container for central nervous system.
Observations on the structure and functions of the nervous system. Edinburgh, Creech and Johnson, 1783
Used stomach tube.
De dysphagia. Edinburgh, Neill, 1767. p. 83

Monro, Alexander. Scottish anatomist. 1773–1859
Described—
Observations on crural hernia; to which is prefixed a general account of the other varieties of hernia. Edinburgh, Laing, 1803

Montesano, G. See C. Fermi

Monteverde, Angelo. Italian physician
SIGN—of death; failure of any response to subcutaneous injection of ammonia.
Note sur un moyen simple, facile, prompt et certain de distinguer la mort vraie de la mort apparente de l'homme. Crémone, Ronzi & Signori, 1874. 20 pp.

Montgomery, H. See J. R. Learmonth

Montgomery, J. C. See W. C. C. Cole

Montignie, E. French chemist
REACTION—for sterols.
Nouvelle réaction de coloration des stérols. Bull. Soc. Chim., 51: 690 (only), May 1932
TEST—for ergosterol.
De l'action de l'anhydride sélénieux sur les stérols. Ibid., 144 (only), Jan. 1932

Monto, Raymond Walter. Detroit physician. 1913–
METHOD—
The determination of sulfanilamide and related compounds in body fluids by a simple, rapid method. Amer. J. clin. Path., Tech. Supp., 5: 165–167, Nov. 1941

Moon, R. C. See J. Z. Laurence

Moon, Virgil Holland. American pathologist. 1879–
MEDIUM—brain, for cultivation of Negri bodies.
The organism of rabies and experiments in its artificial cultivation. J. infect. Dis., 13: 232–235 (233), Sept. 1913

Moore, A. British scientist
STAIN—night-blue, for capsules.
Capsule staining. Trans. Jenner Inst. Prevent. Med., London, 2 ser., p. 244 (only), 1899

Moore, Alexander Berkeley. Rochester, Minn. roentgenologist. 1883–
CRITERIA—
A roentgenologic study of benign tumors of the stomach. Amer. J. Roent., 11: 61–66, Jan. 1924

Moore, Anna C. See A. B. Wadsworth

Moore, Austin Talley. Columbia, S. C. surgeon. 1899–

OPERATION and PINS—
Fracture of the hip joint—a new method of treatment.
Internat. Surg. Digest, 19: 323–330, June 1935
Fracture of the hip joint; treatment by extraarticular fixation with adjustable nails. S. G. O., 64: 420–436, Feb. 15, 1937
Moore, Carl Richard. Chicago zoologist. 1892–
Investigated physiological action of testicular extracts.
On the prevention of castration effects in mammals by testis extract injection with T. F. Gallagher, Amer. J. Physiol., 89: 388–394, July 1, 1929.
Moore, Charles Hewitt. English surgeon. 1821–1870
PRINCIPLES—of surgical treatment of cancer.
On the influence of inadequate operations on the theory of cancer. Med.-chir. Trans., 50: 245–280, 1867
TREATMENT—
On a new method of procuring the consolidation of fibrin in certain incurable aneurisms. Ibid., 47: 129–149, 1864
Described intermittent hydrarthrosis.
Periodical inflammation of the knee-joint. Lancet, 1: 485–486, Apr. 30, 1864
Moore, Edward Mott. American surgeon. 1814–1902
FRACTURE—
A luxation of the ulna not hitherto described, with a plan of reduction and mode of after-treatment; including the management of Colles' fracture. Albany, Weed, 1872. 12 pp.
Moore, George Colton. Boston anesthetist. 1876–
INTRODUCER—a guide for flexible, soft intraspinous needle.
In: *Spinal anesthesia: factors influencing its success.* By L. V. Hand, J. A. M. A., 121: 32–35, Jan. 2, 1943
Moore, J. W. See H. Noguchi
Moore, Joseph Earle. Baltimore physician. 1892–
TREATMENT—
The treatment of early syphilis with penicillin: a preliminary report of 1,418 cases with J. F. Mahoney, W. Schwartz, T. Sternberg and W. B. Wood, J. A. M. A., 126: 67–73, Sept. 9, 1944
Moore, Norman Slawson. Ithaca physician. 1901–
FORMULA—
The relationships between plasma specific gravity, plasma protein content and edema in nephritis with D. D. Van Slyke, J. clin. Invest., 8: 337–355, Apr. 20, 1930
Moore, Robert Foster. London ophthalmologist. 1878–
PSEUDO-ARGYLL ROBERTSON PUPIL—
In discussion of: *Physiology and pathology of the pupil reactions.* Trans. Ophthal. Soc. U. Kingdom, 44: 38–43, 1924
The non-luetic Argyll-Robertson pupil. Ibid., 51: 203–209, 1931
TREATMENT—
Choroidal sarcoma treated by the intraocular insertion of radon seeds. Brit. J. Ophthal., 14: 145–152, Apr. 1930
Moore, Thomas. English chemist. 1881–
TECHNIC—for measuring concentration of vitamin A in biopsied liver tissue.
Vitamin A and carotene: the vitamin A reserve of the adult human being in health and disease. Biochem. J., 31: 155–164, 1937

Proved that carotene is precursor to vitamin A in animal body.
The distribution of vitamin A and carotene in the body of the rat. Ibid., 25: 275–286, 1931
Moore, William O. Leningrad chemist
REACTION—urea.
Über das Vorkommen einer bis jetzt unbekannten Form des Harnstoffs im menschlichen Harn. Biochem. Z., 149: 575–584, July 26, 1924
Moorhead, C. L. D. See A. V. Partipilo
Moorhead, John Joseph. New York surgeon. 1874–
LOCATOR—
A foreign body finder: the locator. J. A. M. A., 121: 123–125, Jan. 9, 1943
Metallic foreign bodies and the electromagnetic locator. Amer. J. Surg., 69: 306–317, Sept. 1945
SAW—
An electric cable driven bone instrument. J. A. M. A., 84: 1333–1334, May 2, 1925
Moots, Charles William. Toledo surgeon. 1869–1933
INDEX or TEST—of operability.
PRESSURE RATIO—
Observation on blood pressures during operations. Trans. Amer. Ass. Ostet. Gynaec., 29: 74–80, 1916
Evaluation of risk, blood pressure protection, and nitrous oxyde—oxygen anesthesia as vital factors in safer gastric surgery. Brit. med. J., 295–297, Aug. 14, 1926
Reported case of arrhenoblastoma.
Lateral partial glandular hermaphroditism. Amer. J. Obstet. Gynaec., 1: 864–867, May 1921
Moppett, Warnford. Sydney physician
TEST—
A serological test for cancer. Med. J. Australia, 21: 681–684, May 26, 1934
Morand Sauveur Francois. French surgeon. 1697–1773
Successfully operated on abscess of brain.
Opuscules der chirurgie. Paris, Desprez et Le Prieur, 1768. Pt. 1, p. 161
Morau, Henry. French physician. 1860–
Observed structural changes in vaginal epithelium of rodents under influence of estrus and ovulation.
Des transformations épithéliales de la muqueuse du vagin de quelques rongeurs. J. Anat., Paris, 25: 277–297, 1889
Successfully transplanted tumors.
Inoculation en série d'une tumeur épithéliale de la souris blanche. C. R. Soc. Biol., 9 s., 3: 289–290, May 2, 1891
Morawitz, Paul Oskar. German physiochemist. 1879–1936
THEORY—of coagulation of blood.
Zur Kenntnis der Vorstufen des Fibrinferments. Beitr. chem. Physiol. Path., 4: 381–420, Nov. 1903
Beiträge zur Kenntnis der Blutgerinnung. Dtsch. Arch. klin. Med., 79: 1–28, Dec. 29, 1903; 79: 215–233, Feb. 18, 1904; 79: 432–442, Mar. 15, 1904
Morax, Victor. Paris physician. 1866–1935
BACILLUS or DIPLOCOCCUS; CONJUNCTIVITIS—
Note sur un diplobacille pathogène pour la conjonctivite humaine. Ann. Inst. Pasteur, 10: 337–345, June 1896
Moreau, P. F. French surgeon
Described excision of elbow, 1786. Garrison

Observations pratiques relatives à la résection des articulations affectées de carie. Paris, Farge, 1803. 87 pp. Thesis

Moorehouse, G. R. See S. W. Mitchell

Morel, Benedict Augustin. French alienist. 1809-1873

DELIRIUM—
Traité des maladie mentales. Paris, 1860. p. 400

EAR—deformed.
Traité des dégénerescences physiques, intellectuelles et morales de l'éspéce humaine, etc. Paris, 1857

Morel, Ch. See D. Anglade, M. Chavassieu

Moreland, Randall B. Illinois surgeon. 1904-

TECHNIC—
Two-stage resection of carcinoma of the ampulla of Vater with B. S. Freeman, Surgery, 9: 712-719, May 1941

Moreno y Maiz, Thomas.
Suggested use of cocaine as local anesthetic. Garrison and Morton
Recherches chimiques et physiologiques sur l'erythroyxlum coca du Pérou et la cocaine. Paris, Leclerc, 1868

Moreschi, Carlo. Pavia physician. 1876-1921
Studied effects of underfeeding in modifying growth of tumor transplants in mice.
Beziehungen zwischen Ernährung und Tumorwachstum. Z. ImmunForsch., 2: 651-685, 1909

Moretti, Giulio. Italian surgeon
Described theca cell tumors of ovary.
Contributo alla conoscenza dei tumori solidi dell'ovaria with P. Arrigoni, Folia gynaec. (Genova), 24: 33-48, 1927

Morgagni, Giovanni Battista. Italian anatomist. 1682-1771
Founder of modern pathologic anatomy.
De sedibus et causis morborum per anatomen indagatis libri quinque. Dissectiones, et animadversiones, nunc primum editats complectuntur propemodum innumeras, medicis, chirurgis, anatomicis profuturas. Venetiis, ex typog. Remondiniana, 1761
The seats and causes of diseases investigated by anatomy; in five books, containing a great variety of dissections, with remarks. Transl. by B. Alexander. London, Millar and Cadell, 1769
Recorded first case of heart block. Garrison
In: *De sedibus. . . .* Vol. 1, p. 70
Described angina pectoris. Ibid., p. 282
Described mitral stenosis. Ibid., Letter 3
Described silicosis. Ibid., Letter 15, Par. 17
Also, selections in: R. H. Major's *Classic descriptions of disease.* Springfield, Ill., Thomas, 1932, pp. 293-296
E. C. Kelly's *Medical classics.* Baltimore, Williams & Wilkins Co., 4: 640-839. Mar. 1940
F. A. Willius and T. E. Keyes' *Cardiac classics.* St. Louis, Mosby, 1941. pp. 179-182

Morgan, C. N. See E. T. C. Milligan

Morgan, John. American physician. 1735-1789
Wrote first American contribution to medical education. Garrison
A discourse upon the institution of medical schools in America . . . with a preface containing, amongst other things, the author's apology for attempting to introduce the regular mode of practicing physic in Philadelphia. Philadelphia, Bradford, 1765. 63 pp.
Also: Baltimore, Johns Hopkins Press, 1937. 63 pp.

Morgan, John. English physician. 1797-1847
Wrote on action of poisons on living body.
An essay on the operation of poisonous agents upon the living body with T. Addison, London, Longmans, 1829. 91 pp.

Morgan, Parry. London physician
Described—
On the possibility of achieving by partial pneumothorax the advantages of complete pneumothorax in the treatment of pulmonary tuberculosis. Lancet, 2: 18-19, July 5, 1913

Morgan, Thomas Hunt. American biologist. 1866-1945
Awarded Nobel prize in 1933 for work on genetics.
Heredity and sex. New York, Columbia Univ. Press, 1913. 282 pp.
The mechanism of Mendelian heredity with A. H. Sturtevant, H. J. Muller and C. B. Bridges, New York, Holt, 1915. 262 pp.
Sex-linked inheritance in Drosophila with C. B. Bridges, Washington, Carnegie Inst., 1916. 87 pp.

Morgenroth, Julius. German physician. 1871-1924
Introduced optochin. Garrison
Chemotherapie der Pneumokokkeninfektion with R. Levy, Berl. klin. Wschr., 48: 1560-1561, Aug. 21, 1911
Discovered high potency of eucupin as a local anesthetic.
Zur chemotherapeutischen Desinfektion durch Chinaalkaloide un ihre Abkömmlinge with E. Bumke, Dtsch. med. Wschr., 44: 729-733, July 4, 1918
See also P. Ehrlich

Morin, M. See A. A. Lemierre

Morishima, Kan-Ichiro. Washington, D. C. scientist
SOLUTION—
Phenol red—china blue as an indicator in fermentation tests of bacterial cultures. J. infect. Dis., 26: 43-44, 43-44, Jan. 1920
SOLUTION—nutrose peptone.
Variations in typhoid bacilli. J. Bact., 6: 275-323 (277), May 1921
See also J. J. Bronfenbrenner

Morison, J. Rutherford. English surgeon. 1853-1939
METHOD, PASTE—
The treatment of infected suppurating war wounds. Lancet, 2: 268-272, 1916
Same title but not same paper in: Brit. J. Surg., 4: 659-678, Apr. 1917
"Bipp" treatment of war wounds. London, Oxford Press, 1918. 72 pp.
OPERATION—epiplopexy or omentopexy.
A case of ascites due to cirrhosis of the liver, cured by operation. By D. Drummond and R. Morison, Brit. med. J., 2: 728-729, 1896
SPACE—
The anatomy of the right hypochondrium relating especially to operations for gall stones. Ibid., 2: 968-971, Nov. 3, 1894

Moritz, Friedrich. German physician. 1861-1938
METHOD—of determining venous pressure.
Ueber eine Methode, beim Menschen den Druck in oberflächlichen Venen exakt zu bestimmen with D. Tabora, Dtsch. Arch. klin. Med., 98: 475-505, Feb. 16, 1910
Introduced orthodiagraphy of heart.

Ueber orthodiagraphische Untersuchungen am Herzen.
Münch. med. Wschr., 49: 1–8, Jan. 7, 1902
Moritz, Fritz. Munich physician
TEST—for glucose in urine.
*Ueber die Kupferoxyd-reducirenden Substanzen des
Harns unter physiologischen und pathologischen
Verhältnissen.* Dtsch. Arch. klin. Med., 46: 217–272,
(265), May 23, 1890
Morner, See Mörner
Moro, Ernst. Graz pediatrician. 1874–
OINTMENT and REACTION—
*Zur Pathogenese gewisser Integumentveränderungen
bei Skrofulose* with A. Doganoff, Wien. klin. Wschr.,
20: 933–936, Aug. 1, 1907
*Ueber eine diagnostisch verwertbare Reaktion der
Haut auf Einreibung mit Tuberkulinsalbe.* Münch.
med. Wschr., 55: 216–218, Feb. 4, 1908
Isolated L. acidophilus.
*Ueber die nach Gram färbbaren Bacillen des Säuglings-
stuhles.* Wien. klin. Wschr., 13: 114–115, Feb. 1,
1900
Morquio, Luio. Uruguay physician. 1867–1935
DISEASE—
Sur une forme de dystrophe osseuse familiale. Bull.
Soc. pediat. de Paris, 27: 145–152, Feb. 19, 1929
Also: Arch. de méd. d. enf., 32: 129–140, Mr. 1929
Morris, J(ames) Lucien. American biochemist. 1885–
METHOD—
*A new salt of uric acid and its application to the an-
alysis of uric acid and phenol.* J. biol. Chem., 25:
205–210, June 1916
*New titration method for the determination of uric
acid in urine.* Ibid., 37: 231–238, Feb. 1919
*Calorimetric determination of uric acid. Estimation of
0.03 to 0.5 mg. quantities by a new method* with A. G.
MacLeod, Ibid., 50: 55–63; 65–75, Jan. 1922
Morris, Robert Tuttle. New York City surgeon.
1857–1945
INCISION—
*The inch-and-a-half incision and week-and-a-half
confinement in appendicitis.* Med. News, 64: 375–
377, Apr. 7, 1894
POINT—of tenderness in appendicitis.
SIGN—of chronic appendicitis, tenderness an inch
and a half to the right of umbilicus and a little below
that point.
Appendicitis. N. Engl. Med. Month., 12: 327–333,
Apr. 1892
*McBurney's point and another point in appendix
diagnoses.* J. A. M. A., 50: 278 (only), Jan. 25, 1908
*Metaplasia of the appendix vermiformis and a new
diagnostic point.* Abstr.: New York Med. J., 87:
1060–1062, May 30, 1908
See also C. H. Cargile
Morris, Roger Sylvester. American physician. 1877–
1934
STAGE—anerythremic, of erythremia.
Anerythraemic erythraemia (?). Johns Hopk. Hosp.
Bull., 21: 37–40, Feb. 1910
TREATMENT—for pernicious anemia.
*A specific hematopoietic hormone in normal gastric
juice: preliminary note* with L. Schiff, G. Burger and
J. E. Sherman, J. A. M. A., 98: 1080–1081, Mar. 26,
1932
Morrison, G. M. See F. J. Cotton

Morrow, Howard. San Francisco dermatologist. 1874–
1941
TREATMENT—
Treatment of impetigo contagiosa. J. A. M. A., 69:
176–178, July 21, 1917
Morse
FINGER—deformity of finger due to constant use of
Morse telegraph key.
Morson, A. C. See B. H. Wedd
Mortimer's
DISEASE—
Cases of Mortimer's malady. (*Lupus vulgaris multi-
plex non-ulcerans et non-serpiginosus* by Sir Jona-
than Hutchinson, Arch. Surg., 9: 307–314, 1898
(Patient was a Mrs. Mortimer)
Morton, C. J. See A. F. Hertz
Morton, Charles A. Bristol surgeon
OPERATION—
*The inguinal operation for the radical cure of femoral
hernia.* Brit. med. J., 1: 418–420, Feb. 24, 1912
Morton, John Jamieson. Rochester, N. Y. surgeon.
1886–
DERMATHERM—
*The measurement of sympathetic vasoconstriction ac-
tivity in the lower extremities* with W. J. M. Scott,
J. clin. Invest., 9: 235–246, Oct. 20, 1930
METHODS—
*Methods for estimating the degree of sympathetic vaso-
constriction in peripheral vascular diseases* with
W. J. M. Scott, New Engl. J. Med., 204: 955–962,
May 7, 1931
OPERATION—sympathetic neurectomy for mega-
colon.
*Studies of the activity of the lumbar sympathetic nervous
system* with W. J. M. Scott, Ann. Surg., 92: 919–930,
Nov. 1930
Morton, Richard. English physician. 1635–1698
"His most important contribution was his proof that
tubercles in the lungs produced one of the most wide-
spread types of consumption that afflicted the human
body." Major
*Phthisiologia, seu exercitationes de phthisi tribus libris
comprehensae. Totumque opus variis historiis illus-
tratum.* London, Smith, 1689. 411 pp.
Also: Francofurti & Lipsiae, Kühn, 1691. 455 pp.
Also, English transl. by S. Smith and B. Wolford.
London, 1694
Morton, Thomas George. American physician. 1835–
1903
DISEASE or METATARSALGIA—
*A peculiar and painful affection of the fourth metatarso-
phalangeal articulation.* Amer. J. med. Sci., n. s.,
71: 37–45, 1876
Reported treatment of purpura by transfusion of
defibrinated blood.
On transfusion of blood. . . . Ibid., 68: 110–118 (116),
July 1874
Morton, William James. New York physician. 1848–
1920
Introduced dental radiography.
The x-ray and its application to dentistry. Dental
Cosmos, Phila., 38: 478–486, June 1896
Morton, William Thomas Green. Boston physician.
1819–1868
Discovered ether anesthesia, first used at Massa-
chusetts General Hospital, Oct. 16, 1846

Insensibility during surgical operations by inhalation.
by H. J. Bigelow, Boston Med. and Surg. J., 35:
309–317, Nov. 18, 1846
Circular. *Morton's letheon.* Boston, Dutton and
Wentworth, (1846)
*Remarks on the proper mode of administering sulphuric
ether by inhalation.* Boston, Dutton and Wentworth,
1847. 44 pp.
Also in: *Epoch-making contributions to medicine,
surgery and the allied sciences.* By C. N. B. Camac,
Phila., Saunders, 1909. pp. 313–332
*On the physiological effects of sulphuric ether, and its
superiority to chloroform.* Boston, Clapp, 1850. 24 pp.
Also in: Camac, pp. 361–375
Comparative value of sulphuric ether and chloroform.
Boston Med. and Surg. J., 43: 111–119, Sept. 11,
1850

Morvan, Augustin Marie. French physician. 1819–
1897
CHOREA—
De la chorée fibrillaire. Gaz. hebd. de méd., 2 s., 27:
173–176, Apr. 12; 186–189, Apr. 19; 200–202, Apr.
26, 1890
DISEASE or SYNDROME—
*De la parésie analagésique à panaris des extrémités
supérieures ou paréso-analgésie des extrémitiés supérieures.* Ibid., 20: 580–583, Aug. 31; 590–594, Sept.
7; 624–626, Sept. 21, 1883

Moschcowitz, Alexis Victor. New York surgeon.
1865–1933
OPERATION—
Femoral hernia: a new operation for the radical cure.
New York State J. Med., 7: 396–400, Oct. 1907
OPERATION—
*The pathogenesis, anatomy, and cure of prolapse of
the rectum.* S. G. O., 15: 7–21, July 1912
OPERATION—
"Pudendal hernia." Amer. J. med. Sci., 156: 394–404,
Sept. 1918

Moschcowitz, Eli. New York physician. 1879–
THEORY—
The psychogenic origin of organic disease. Abstr.:
Arch. Neurol. Psychiat., 32: 903, Oct. 1934

Moschutkowsky, Osip Osipovich. See Moczutkowsky

Mosenthal, Herman Otto. American physician. 1878–
TEST—
*Kidney fatigue with diuretics in experimental nephri-
tis.* Boston Med. and Surg. J., 170: 245 (only),
Feb. 12, 1914
*Renal function as measured by the elimination of
fluids, salt and nitrogen, and the specific gravity of the
urine.* Arch. intern. Med., 16: 733–774, Nov. 1915

Moser, Paul. Vienna pediatrician. 1865–1924
SERUM—
*Ueber die Behandlung der Scharlachs mit einem
Scarlachstreptococcenserum.* Wien. klin. Wschr., 15:
1053–1055, Oct. 9, 1902

Mosetig-Moorhof, Albert von. Vienna surgeon.
1838–1907
BONE–WAX, FILLING or PLUGS—
Die Jodoformknochenplombe. Zbl. Chir., 30: 433–438,
Apr. 18, 1903
Introduced iodoform dressing.
Der Jodoform-Verband. Samml. klin. Vortr., Leipz.,
No. 211 (Chir., No. 68), 1811–1864, 1882

Mosher, Eliza Maria. Brooklyn physician. 1846–1928
SIGN—short sternum.
An anatomical cause for enteroptosis and the V colon.
Arch. Pediat., 41: 422–426, June 1924

Mosher, Harrison Peyton. American surgeon. 1867–
INSTRUMENT—
*Stenosis of the esophagus, anatomy, anomalies, instru-
ments, and technique.* Trans. Amer. Laryngol., Rhinol.
and Otol. Soc., 20: 179–202, June 1914
BASKET—
*The paraffin basket mould for applying a skin graft
to the radical mastoid cavity.* Trans. Amer. Otol.
Soc., 17: 283–295, May 1925

Moskowicz, Ludwig. see Moszkowicz

Moss, William Lorenzo. Baltimore physician. 1876–
CLASSIFICATION—of blood groups.
METHOD—for direct matching of blood specimens.
TEST—for hemolysis.
Studies on iso-agglutinins and iso-hemolysins. Johns
Hopk. Hosp. Bull., 21: 63–70, Mar. 1910
*Classification and treatment of the anemias and hemor-
rhagic diseases.* In: Forchheimer's *Therapeusis of
internal diseases.* Ed. by Billings and Irons. New
York, Appleton, 1914. Vol. 5, pp. 804–824 (813–814)

Mosse, Max. Berlin physician. 1873–
TYPE—of erythremia.
*Ueber Polycythämie mit Urobilinkterus und Milz-
tumor.* Dtsch. med. Wschr., 33: 2175–2176, Dec. 26,
1907

Mosso, Angelo. Italian physiologist. 1846–1910
ERGOGRAPH—for recording force and frequency of
flexion of fingers.
Le leggi della fatica studiate nei muscoli dell'uomo.
Atti d. r. Accad. d. Lincei, Cl. disc. fis., matemat.
nat., Roma, 4 s., 5, 1888–89
SPHYGMOMANOMETER—
*Sphygmomanomètre pour mesurer la pression du sang
chez l'homme.* Arch. ital. de biol., 23: 177–179, 1895
THEORY—acapnia.
Studied respiration at high altitudes.
*Fisiologia del l'uomo sulle Alpi. Studii fatti sul Mont
Rosa.* Milano, frat. Treves, 1897
Demonstrated reflex character of deglutition.
Ueber die Bewegungen der Speiseröhre. In: Mole-
schott's Untersuch. z. Naturlehre d. Mensch. u. d.
Thiere, Frankf., 11: 331–349; 327–349, 1876
Studied cerebral pulsations and counted duration and
degree of sensation transmitted to brain from with-
out. Garrison
*Introduzione ad una serie di esperienze sui movimenti
del cervello nell'uomo.* Arch. p. l. sci. med., Turin,
1: 206–244, 1876–77
Showed fatigue is due to a toxic product of muscular
contraction. Garrison
*Le sang des animaux fatigués, alors même qu'il est
privé du Co_2, fait augmenter la fréquence de la respiration et la pression du sang si l'on opère sa transfusion
un autre animal.* Trans. Internat. Med. Cong., 1890,
Berlin, 2, 2 Abth., 13–14, 1891
La fatica. Milano, frat. Treves, 1891

Mosny, Ernest. French surgeon. 1861–1918
Described first successful embolectomy by G.
Labey, Nov. 16, 1911. Garrison and Morton
*Embolie fémorale au cours d'un rétrécissement mitral
pur. Arteriotomie. Guérison* with J. Dumont, Bull.
Acad. de méd., 3 s., 66: 358–361, Dec. 19, 1911

Moszkowicz, Ludwig. Vienna pathologist. 1873–
EST—reactive hyperemia t.
*Die Diagnose des Arterienverschlusses bei Gangraena
pedis.* Mitt. Grenzgeb. Med. Chir., 17: 216–228,
1907
Described relation of breast to hormones.
Ueber den monatlichen Zyklus der Brustdrüse. Arch.
klin. Chir., 142: 374–418, 1926
*Sexualzyklus, Mastopathie und Geschwulstwachstum
der Mamma.* Ibid., 144: 138–161, Jan. 29, 1927

Motais, Ernst. French ophthalmologist. ?–1913
PERATION—for ptosis.
*Nouvelle méthode opératoire du ptosis par la suppléance
du muscle droit supérieur.* Bull. Soc. d'ophth. de
Paris, 11: 105–113, Nov. 8, 1898

Mott, Frederick Walker. English physician. 1853–
1926
EST—
The physiological action of choline and neurine with
W. D. Halliburton, Philos. Trans., s. B., 191: 211–
267, 1899

Mott, Valentine. New York surgeon. 1785–1865
First to ligate arteria innominata. Garrison
*Reflections on securing in a ligature the arteria in-
nominata, to which is added a case in which this artery
was tied by a surgical operation.* Med. and Surg.
Register, N. Y., 1: 9–54, 1818
Excised mandible.
*Case of osteo sarcoma, in which the right side of the
lower jaw was removed successfully after tying the
carotid artery.* New York Med. and Phys. J., 1: 385–
393, Oct. Nov. Dec., 1822
Amputated at hip joint.
Successful amputation at the hip-joint. Philadelphia
J. Med. and Phys. Sci., 14: 101–104, 1827
Excised clavicle.
*An account of a case of osteo-sarcoma of the left clavicle,
in which exsection of that bone was successfully per-
formed.* Amer. J. med. Sci., 3: 100–108, 1828

Moty, F. French surgeon
Reported successful operation for rupture of in-
testine.
Laparotomie pour rupture traumatique de l'intestin.
Bull. Soc. chir. Paris, n. s., 16: 428–429, June 4, 1890

Motz, B. See J. Albaran y Dominguez

Mouchet, Albert. French surgeon. 1869–
PERATION—for slipping patella.
*Traitement opératoire de la luxation congénitale com-
plète et irréductible de la rotule* with J. Durand, J.
de Chir., 18: 225–233, Sept. 1921

Mount, Lester Adran. New York physician. 1910–
SYNDROME—
*Familial paroxysmal choreoathetosis: preliminary re-
port on a hitherto undescribed clinical syndrome* with
S. Reback, Arch. Neurol. Psychiat., Chicago, 44:
841–847, Oct. 1940

Moussu, Gustav. French physician. 1864–
Demonstrated functional independence of parathyroid glands and thyroid.
*Recherches sur les fonctions thyroïdienne et para-
thyroïdienne.* Paris, 1897

Moynihan, Sir Berkeley George Andrew. Leeds
surgeon. 1866–1936
UNGER PAIN—three or more hours after eating,
indicative of duodenal ulcer.

In his: *Duodenal ulcer.* Philadelphia, Saunders, 1910.
379 pp. p. 19
OPERATIONS—I and II, modifications of Billroth
II gastric resection.
In his: *Abdominal operations.* Philadelphia, Saunders,
1905. pp. 195–215
SCHEME—of intestinal localization; same as Monks.
Ibid., pp. 251–258
TEST—for hour-glass stomach; after giving two parts
of Seidlitz powder separately, sound can be heard
with stethoscope at constriction two to three inches
to left of midline.
Remarks on hour-glass stomach. Brit. med. J., 1:
413–416, Feb. 20, 1904

Much, Hans C. R. German physician. 1880–1932
BACILLUS, GRANULES, STAINING—
*Ueber die granuläre nach Ziehl nicht färbbare Form
des Tuberkulosevirus.* Beitr. Klin. d. Tuberk., 8:
85–99, 1907
REACTION—
Eine Reaktion im Blute von Geisterskranken with W.
Holzmann, Munch. med. Wschr., 56: 1001-1003,
May 18, 1909
TREATMENT—
Tuberkulosebehandlung mit Partigenen. Dermat.
Wschr., 64: 433–441, 1917
Spezifische Kur und völliger Immunkörpermangel.
Beitr. z. Klin. d. Tuberk., Berl., 46: 414–416, 1920

Mudd, S. See F. Boerner, E. W. Flosdorf

Mühlens, Peter. German physician. 1874–1943
METHOD—of cultivation of—
Über Bacillus fusiformis und Spirochaeta dentium
with M. Hartmann, Z. Hyg., InfektKr., 55: 81–111,
1906
Introduced yatren.
*Ueber Behandlungsversuche der chronischen Amoeben-
ruhr mit Yatren* with W. Menk, Münch. med. Wschr.,
68: 802–803, June 30, 1921

Mühlmann, Moissey. Odessa chemist. 1867–
REACTION—for epinephrine.
Zur Physiologie der Nebenniere. Münch. med. Wschr.,
43: 623 (only), June 30, 1896

Mühlpfordt, H. Allenstein physician
REACTION—
Zum Nachweis des Cholesterins. Dermat. Wschr., 97:
1651–1653, Nov. 25, 1933

Müller, Eduard. German physician. 1876–1928
SIGN—loss of abdominal reflexes in multiple sclerosis.
*Ueber einige weniger bekannte Verlaufsformen der
multiplen Sklerose.* Neurol. Zbl., 24: 593–601, July
1, 1905
TEST—for tuberculous pus.
*Zur Kenntnis des proteolytischen Leukocytenfermentes
und seines „Antifermentes." (Demonstration einer
einfachen Methode zum Nachweise proteolytischer
Fermentwirkungen)* with Jochmann, 24. Cong. f. inn.
Med., pp. 566–577, 1907
TEST—for trypsin in stools.
*Ueber das Verhalten des proteolytischen Leukocyten-
fermentes und seines „Antifermentes" in den normalen
und krankhaften Ausscheidungen des menschlichen
Körpers.* Arch. klin. Med., 92: 199–216, Jan. 30,
1908

Müller, Ernst. German surgeon
OPERATION—for flat foot.
Sehnentransplantation und Verhalten der Sehnen beim

Plattfusse. Zbl. Chir., 30: 40–42, Jan. 10, 1903
Described slipping of upper femoral epiphysis.
Ueber die Verbiegung der Schenkelhalses im Wachstumsalter; ein neues Krankheitsbild. Beitr. klin. Chir., 4: 137–148, Nov. 1888

Müller, Friedrich von. Marburg physician. 1858–
Noted increase of metabolism in exophthalmic goiter.
Beiträge zur Kenntniss der Basedow'schen Krankheit. Dtsch. Arch. f. klin. Med., 51: 335–412, June 27, 1893

Müller, Heinrich. German anatomist. 1820–1864
FIBERS—in retina.
MUSCLE—circular part of ciliary m.
Anatomische Beiträge zur Ophthalmologie. Arch. Ophthal., 4: 363–388, 1858
FLUID—fixation. Mallory
Anatomische Untersuchung eines Mikrophthalmus. H. Müller's gesammelte und hinterlassene Schriften zur Anatomie und Physiologie des Auges. Leipzig, Engelmann, 1872. 1: 380–386
Discovered visual purple.
Zur Histologie der Netzhaut. Z. wiss. Zool., 3: 234–237, 1851
Suggested that chordoma has its origin in notochordal remains.
Ueber das Vorkommen von Resten der Chorda dorsalis bei Menschen nach der Geburt und über ihr Verhaltniss zu den Gallertgeschwülsten am Clivus. Z. rat. Med., 3 s., 2: 202–229, 1858
See also R. A. von Kölliker

Müller, J. See W. Ebstein

Müller, Johannes. German physiologist. 1801–1858
DUCTS—
Über die Entwicklung der Eier im Eierstock bei den Gespenstheuschrecken. Nova acta Acad. Nat. Curios., Bonnae, pt. 2, 565–672, 1825
Coined phrase "doctrine of specific nerve energies."
Ueber die phantastischen Gesichtserscheinungen.... Coblenz, Holscher, 1826. 117 pp.
Zur vergleichenden Physiologie des Gesichtssinnes des Menschen und Thiere.... Leipzig, 1826. 462 pp.
Explained color sensations ("pressure-phosphenes") produced by pressure on retina. Ibid., p. 73
Worked our whole finer anatomy of glandular and cartilaginous tissues. Garrison
De glandularum secernentium structure penitiori. Lipsiae, Vossii, 1830
Proved conclusively with frogs that anterior spinal roots are motor and posterior are sensory. (Bell-Magendie law)
Bestätigung des Bell'schen Lehrsatzes. Notiz. a. d. Geb. d. Nat. u. Heilk., Weimar, 30: 113–122, 1831
Discovered lymph-hearts in frog.
On the existence of four distinct hearts, having regular pulsations, connected with the lymphatic system, in certain amphibious animals. Philos. Trans., London, pt. 1, 89–94, 1833
Über die Lymphherzen den Schildkröten. Berlin, Druckerei d. k. Akad., 1840
Isolated chondrin and glutin.
Über Knorpel und Knochen. Ann. Pharm., Heidelb., 21: 277–282, 1837
Wrote monumental work on tumors. Garrison
Ueber den feinern Bau und die Formen der krankhaften Geschwülste. Berlin, Reimer, 1838
Also: *On the nature and structural characteristics of*

cancer and of those morbid growths which may be confounded with it. Transl. by C. West, London, Sherwood et al., 1840. 182 pp.

Mueller, J(ohn) Howard. American pathologist. 1891–
SOLUTION—glucose peptone salt.
Studies on cultural requirements of bacteria. J. Bact. 7: 309–338 (317), May 1922
SOLUTION—heart infusion aminoid. Ibid., p. 331

Müller, Otto Friedrick. German physician. 1730–1784
First to classify bacteria. Garrison
Vermium terrestrium et fluviatilium.... Havniae Heineck et Faber, 1773–74. 3 vols.

Müller, Rudolf. Vienna physician. 1877–1934
DIAGNOSIS, REACTION—complement fixation test for gonorrhea.
Ueber den Nachweis von Antikörpern im Serum eine an Arthritis gonorrhoica Erkrankten mittels Komplementablenkung with M. Oppenheim, Wien. klin. Wschr., 19: 894–895, July 19, 1906
TEST—flocculation for syphilis.
Die Ballungsreaktion bei Lues (M. B. R. II) und ihre Verwendbarkeit bei nichtluischen Infektionen (Immuno-Ballungs-Reaktion (Im. B. R.)). Klin. Wschr., 11: 1916–1918, Nov. 12, 1932

Müller, Walther. Marburg surgeon. 1888–
OPERATION—plastic on thumb.
Anatomische Studien zur Frage des Daumenersatzes. Beitr. klin. Chir., 120: 595–598, 1920

Müller, Wilhelm. Aachen surgeon. 1855–1937
OPERATION—skull flap for repair of cranial defect.
Zur Frage der temporären Schädelresektion an Stelle der Trepanation. Zbl. Chir., 17: 65–66, Jan. 25, 1890

Münchmeyer
DISEASE—
Ueber Myositis ossificans progressiva. Z. rat. Med. Leipzig u. Heidelberg, 3 R., 34: 9–41, 1869

Münter, F. Halle chemist
SOLUTION—basal ammonium nitrate.
Über Actionmyceten des Bodens. I. Mitteilung. Zbl. Bakt., 2 Abt., 36: 365–381 (368; 371), Jan. 11, 1917
SOLUTION—basal salt. Ibid., p. 373
SOLUTION—basal galactose salt. Ibid., p. 377

Muer, Theodore C. Brooklyn scientist
SOLUTION—
Value of brilliant-green in eliminating errors due to the anaerobes in the presumptive test for B. coli with R. L. Harris. Amer. J. Pub. Health, 10: 874–875 Nov. 1920
See also D. D. Jackson

Muir, M(atthew) M(oncrieff) Pattison. English chemist. 1848–
REAGENT—
On a method of detecting small quantities of bismuth. Chem. News, 35: 176 (only), Apr. 27, 1877

Muir, Robert. English bacteriologist. 1864–
STAINING METHOD—for capsules.
In: *Manual of bacteriology* with S. Ritchie, Edinburgh, Pentland, 1910. 5 ed., p. 110
STAINING METHOD—for flagella. Ibid., 1897. ed., p. 103
STAINING METHOD—for spores. Ibid., p. 103

Muirhead, Archibald Laurence. Omaha pharmacologist. 1863–1921

TREATMENT—for Addison's disease by epinephrin to tolerance.
An autograph history of a case of Addison's disease. J. A. M. A., 76: 652–653, Mar. 5, 1921

Mulder, Gerardus Johann. Dutch chemist. 1802–1880
Coined word protein for substance he separated and believed to be fundamental constituent of tissues.
Action de l'acide hydrochlorique sur la protéine. Bull. d. sc. phys. et nat., Leyde, p. 153, 1838

Mules, Philip Henry. Manchester oculist. 1843–1905
OPERATION—
On the surgical, physiological, and aesthetic advantages of the artificial vitreous body. Brit. med. J., 2: 1153–1155, Dec. 9, 1885
Entire freedom from pain and undue reaction after evisceration and introduction of the glass vitreous. Ibid., 1: 1213 (only), June 4, 1886
OPERATION—
New operation for relief of ptosis. Eighth Int. Ophthalmol. Cong., pp. 57–60, 1894

Muller, George Paul. Philadelphia surgeon. 1877–1947
OPERATION—with permanent rubber tube.
Cholecyst-duodenostomy. Ann. Surg., 84: 95–99, July 1926

Muller, Hermann Joseph. American biologist. 1890–
Awarded Nobel prize in 1946 for work on effect of roentgen rays on genes and chromosomes.
Artificial transmutation of the gene. Science, 66: 84–87, July 22, 1927
The treatment of gene mutation rate in Drosophila, its high variability, and its dependence upon temperature. Genetics, 13: 279–357, July 1928
Cytological expression of changes in gene alignment produced by x-rays in Drosophila with T. S. Painter, Amer. Naturalist, 63: 193–200, May–June 1929
See also T. H. Morgan

Muller, L. Liege scientist
BOUILLON—iodine.
Un nouveau milieu d'enrichissement pour la recherche du bacille typhique et des paratyphiques. C. R. Soc. Biol., 89: 434–437 (435), June 30, 1923

Mullins, C. R. See A. O. Whipple

Mulsow, Frederick William. Iowa City pathologist. 1882–
TECHNIC—
Culture mediums for the gonococcus. J. infect. Dis., 36: 419–423, Apr. 1925

Munch-Petersen, Carl. Jul. Copenhagen physician
ENCEPHALOMYELITIS—
Encephalo-myelitis disseminata (Redlich) og encephalo-myelitis funicularis infektiosa. Bibl. Laeger. 126: 97–132, Mar.; 137–183, Apr. 1934

Munk, Fritz. German physician. 1879–
Introduced term "lipoid nephrosis."
Klinische Diagnostik der degenerativen Nierenerkrankungen. I. Sekundär-degenerative—primär-degenerative Nierenerkrankung. II. Degenerative Syphilisniere. Z. klin. Med., 78: 1–52, 1913

Munk, Hermann. German neurologist. 1839–1912
Investigated functions of temporal lobes.
Über die Functionen der Grosshirnrinde. Berlin, Hirschwald, 1881

Munro, Donald. Boston surgeon. 1889–
APPARATUS and METHOD—
Tidal drainage of the urinary bladder. A preliminary

report of this method of treatment as applied to "cord bladders" with a description of the apparatus with J. Hahn, New Engl. J. Med., 212: 229–239, Feb. 7, 1935

Munson, Edward Lyman. American hygienist. 1868–1947
LAST—
The soldier's foot and the military shoe. Menasha, Wis., Banta, 1917. 147 pp.

Murat, Dr. French physician
SIGN—
Un signe nouveau pour le diagnostic précoce de la tuberculose pulmonaire. Gaz. hebd. de Méd., 46: 221 (only), Mar. 5, 1899

Murchison, Charles. English physician. 1830–1879
Described hemolytic jaundice.
Clinical lectures on diseases of liver. London, Longmans, Green, 1868; 1877; 1885

Muret, Dr. See E. A. V. A. Quene

Murlin, J. R. See S. R. Benedict, T. M. Carpenter

Murphy, Elizabeth A. See H. McL. Evans

Murphy, James Bumgardner. New York pathologist. 1884–
Wrote—
Transplantability of malignant tumors to the embryos of a foreign species. J. A. M. A., 59: 874–875, Sept. 14, 1912
A source of defense to heteroplastic tissue grafting. Ibid., 62: 199 (only), Jan. 17, 1914
See also H. D. Taylor

Murphy, John Benjamin. Chicago surgeon. 1857–1916
BUTTON—
Cholecysto-intestinal, gastro-intestinal, entero-intestinal anastomosis, and approximation without sutures. (Original research.) Chicago Med. Recorder, 3: 803–840, 1892
Also: Med. Rec., 42: 665–676, Dec. 10, 1892
DRIP—
Perforative peritonitis, general, free, suppurative. S. G. O., 6: 565–598 (593), June 1908
Proctoclysis in the treatment of peritonitis. J. A. M. A., 52: 1248–1250, Apr. 17, 1909
OPERATION—
Diverticulum of esophagus—conservative treatment. Surg. Clin. of J. B. Murphy, 5: 391–395, June 1916
OPERATION—for slipping patella.
Luxation of the patella and fracture of the internal semilunar cartilage; description of Dr. Murphy's operation for luxation of the patella. Ibid., 3: 151–160, Feb. 1914
Congenital luxation of the patella,—reduction. Excavation of a groove in the femur for its lodgement. Plastic operation and imbrication of joint capsule to hold it in its new position. Ibid., 817–838, Aug. 1914
PERCUSSION—piano p.
SIGN—inability to take a deep breath when examiner's fingers are held under right costal arch, in gall bladder disease.
Five diagnostic methods of John B. Murphy. Surg. Clin. of J. B. Murphy, 1: 459–466, June 1912
TREATMENT—of peritonitis. See DRIP, first reference.
TREATMENT—of pulmonary tuberculosis by artificial pneumothorax.
Surgery of the lungs. J. A. M. A., 31: 151–165, July

23; **203-216**, July **30**; 281-297, Aug. 6; 341-356, Aug. 13, 1898
Performed first successful circular suturing of blood vessels in man. Garrison
Surgery of arteries and veins injured in continuity— end-to-end suture—experimental and clinical research. Med. Rec., 51: 73-88, Jan. 16, 1897

Murphy, William Parry. American physician. 1892–
Awarded, with G. R. Minot and G. H. Whipple, Nobel prize in 1934 for work on liver therapy in pernicious anemia.
A special diet for patients with pernicious anemia with G. R. Minot, Boston Med. and Surg. J., 195: 410-411, Aug. 26, 1926
See also G. R. Minot

Murray, Everitt George Dunne. English bacteriologist. 1890–
AGAR—heart infusion.
Observations on the growth of meningococci in vitro in relation to virulence with R. Ayrton, J. Hyg., 23: 23-63 (49), Sept. 1924

Murray, George Redmayne. English physician. 1865-1939
TREATMENT—
Note on the treatment of myxedema by hypodermic injections of an extract of the thyroid gland of a sheep. Brit. med. J., 2: 796-797, Oct. 10, 1891

Murray, S. E. See L. M. Randall

Murray, William Smith. American scientist. 1899–
Produced mammary cancer in male mice by ovarian implantation after removal of testes.
Ovarian secretion and tumor incidence. J. Cancer Res., 12: 18-25, Mar. 1928

Murrell, William. English physician. 1853-1912
Introduced—
Nitro-glycerine as a remedy for angina pectoris. Lancet, 1: 80-81, Jan. 18; 113-115, Jan. 25; 151-152, Feb. 1; 225-227, Feb. 15, 1879
Also, in: F. A. Willius and T. E. Keys' *Cardiac classics*, St. Louis, Mosby, 1941, pp. 642-650

Muscovitz, A. N. See E. E. Osgood

Muskens, Louis Jacob Josef. German neurologist. 1872–
TONOMETER—for measuring tonicity of Achilles tendon.
Muskeltonus und Sehnenphänomene. Neurol. Zbl., 18: 1074-1086, Dec. 1, 1899

Muss, J. See J. R. Di Palma

Mussey, R. D. See L. M. Randall

Mutch, Nathan. English physician. 1886–
RULE—multiples of 15 for remembering percentages of oxygen furnished by different methods.
Some methods of oxygen administration—essential data. Guy's Hosp. Gaz., 54: 189-192, June 29, 1940

Myers, Arthur Bowen Richards. English physician. 1838-1921
Described "effort syndrome" of heart.
On the etiology and prevalence of disease of the heart among soldiers. London, Churchill, 1870

Myers, C. S. See E. C. Kendall, H. L. Mason

Myers, Victor Caryl. American biochemist. 1883–
COLORIMETER—test-tube c.
A simple colorimeter for clinical purposes. J. Lab. clin. Med., 1: 760-761, July 1916
METHOD—
The colorimetric estimation of cholesteral in blood, with a note on the estimation of coprosterol in feces with Emma L. Wardell, J. biol. Chem., 36: 147-156, Oct. 1918
SIGN—
The creatinin of the blood in nephritis: its diagnostic value with W. G. Lough, Arch. intern. Med., 16: 546-546, Oct. 1915
TEST—starch-digestion t. for serum amylase.
Studies on animal diastases. I. The increased diastatic activity of the blood in diabetes and nephritis with J. A. Killian, J. biol. Chem., 29: 179-189, Mar. 1917
WEIGHING BOTTLE—for total solids of blood.
Chemical composition of the blood in health and disease. VI. Total solids, total nitrogen and chlorides. Post.- Graduate, 30: 35-39, Jan. 1915
See also F. G. Benedict

Myerson, M. C. See E. J. Browder

Mylius, F. German chemist
REACTION—for cholic acid.
Ueber die Cholsäure. Ber. dtsch. chem. Ges., 20: 683-688, Mar. 14, 1887
TEST—for bile acids.
Zur Kenntniss der Pettenkofer'schen Gallensäurereaction. Z. physiol. Chem., 11: 492-496, 1887

Mynter, Hermann. Buffalo surgeon
OPERATION—
Excision of the wrist-joint by a new method. Amer. Orthop. Ass., 7: 253-255, 1894

N

Nachlas, Israel William. Baltimore physician. 1894–
SIGN—
The knee-flexion test for pathology in the lumbosacral and sacro-iliac joints. J. Bone and Joint Surg., 18: 724-725, July 1936

Naegele, Franz Karl. German obstetrician. 1777-1851
OBLIQUITY or PELVIS—
Das schräg verengte Becken, nebst einem Anhange über die wichtigsten Fehler des weiblichen Beckens überhaupt. Mainz, Zabern, 1839. 118 pp.
Also, transl. by A. M. Hellman and G. Musa, New York, Pynson, 1939

Naegell, A. See H. R. A. Schridde

Nägeli, Carl Wilhelm von. Swiss botanist. 1817-1891

First to investigate chemical nature of protoplasm. Garrison
Über die Reaction von Jod auf Stärkekörner und Zellmembranen. S. B. d. k. Bayer. Akad. d. Wiss., Munchen. 2: 280-312, 1862; 1: 161-199; 483-546, 1863

Nägeli, Otto. Zurich physician. 1871-1938
LAW—presence of eosinophils must incite caution in diagnosis of typhoid fever. Dorland
Blutkrankheiten und Blutdiagnostik. Leipzig, Veit, 1907. 519 pp.
METHOD—
Zur Acidität bestimmung des Urins. Z. physiol. Chem., 30: 313-349, Sept. 22, 1900

Naffziger, Howard Christian. San Francisco surgeon. 1884–
METHOD—
A method for the localization of brain tumors—the pineal shift. S. G. O., 40: 481–484, Apr. 1925
OPERATION—
The surgical treatment of progressive exophthalmos following thyroidectomy with O. W. Jones, Jr., J. A. M. A., 99: 638–642, Aug. 20, 1932
OPERATION—
Progressive exophthalmos following thyroidectomy; its pathology and treatment. Ann. Surg., 94: 582–586, Oct. 1931
REACTION or TEST—
Dermoid tumors of the spinal cord. Report of four cases, with observations on the clinical test for the differentiation of the source of radicular pains with O. W. Jones, Arch. Neurol. Psychiat., Chicago, 33: 941–958, May 1935

Nagel, Wilibald A. German physiologist. 1870–1911
TEST—of color vision.
Tafeln zur Diagnose der Farbenblindheit. Wiesbaden, Bergmann, 1898

Nagelschmidt, Karl Franz. German physician. 1875–
First used high-frequency currents in electrocoagulation and diathermy. Garrison
Ueber Diathermie (Transthermie, Thermopenetration). Münch. med. Wschr., 56: 2575–2576, Dec. 14, 1909
Lehrbuch der Diathermie. . . . Berlin, Springer, 1913. 328 pp. 2 ed., 1921

Nageotte, Jean. French scientist
THEORY—of nature and origin of connective tissue.
Les substances conjonctives sont des coagulums albuminoides du milieu intérieur. C. R. Soc. Biol., 79: 833–839, Oct. 21, 1916
See also J. F. F. Babinski

Nagle, John Michael. Agnew, Cal. physician. 1902–
TEST—endermic, for tolerance to alcohol.
Alcohol susceptibility test. Abstr.: J. Allergy, 10: 179–180, Jan. 1939

Nagler, F. P. O. Sydney bacteriologist
METHOD—of identification of Clostridium welchii.
Observations on a reaction between the lethal toxin of Cl. welchii (type A) and human serum. Brit. J. exp. Path., 20: 473–485, Dec. 1939

Naiman, Barnet. New York chemist. 1900–
REAGENT—
A reagent for vitamin B_1. Science, 85: 290 (only), Mar. 19, 1937

Nakanishi, K. Tokio physician
VITAL STAINING—of bacteria.
Vorläufige Mittheilung über eine neue Färbungsmethode zur Darstellung des feineren Baues der Bacterien. Münch. med. Wschr., 47: 187–188, Feb. 6, 1900

Nakayama, M. Japanese chemist
TEST—for bile in urine.
Ueber eine Modification der Huppert'schen Gallenfarbstoffreaction. Z. phys. Chem., 36: 398–400, Oct. 1, 1902

Nansen, Fridtjof. Norwegian scientist. 1861–1930
Showed that posterior root fibers divide on entering spinal cord into ascending and descending branches. Garrison and Morton
The structure and combination of the histological ele-

ments of the central nervous system. Bergens Mus. Aarsberetning, 29–214, 1886

Narath, Albert. Utrecht surgeon. 1864–1924
OPERATION—omentopexy in hepatic cirrhosis.
Ueber die subkutane Verlagerung des Omentum. Zbl. Chir., 32: 833–836, Aug. 12, 1905

Nash, Thomas Palmer, Jr. New York biochemist. 1890–
METHOD—
The ammonia content of the blood, and its bearing on the mechanism of acid neutralization in the animal organism with S. R. Benedict, J. biol. Chem., 48: 463–488, Oct. 1921

Nasmyth, Alexander. London dentist. ?–1847
MEMBRANE—covering enamel of an unborn tooth.
Researches on the development, structure, and diseases of the teeth. London, Churchill, 1839

Nasse, Christian Friedrich. German physician. 1788–1851
LAW—of inheritance of hemophilia, only in males and only through females.
Von einer erblichen Neigung zu tödtlichen Blutungen. Arch. f. med. Erfahr. (Horn), 1: 385–434, 1820

Nasse, Hermann. German physician. 1807–1892
Noticed sedimentation of erythrocytes in certain diseases.
Das Blut in mehrfacher Beziehung physiologisch und pathologisch untersucht. Bonn, Habicht, 1836. 370 pp.

Nasse, Otto. German physician
REAGENT—for albumin.
Ueber die Verwendbarkeit des Millon'schen Reagens. Arch. f. Physiol., 83: 361–368, Feb. 2, 1901

Nassonov, Dimitry N. St. Petersburg histologist
MODIFICATION—of Kopsch's osmic acid method, for Golgi's apparatus.
Das Golgische Binnennetz und seine Beziehungen zu der Sekretion. Untersuchungen über einige Amphibiendrüsen. Arch. f. mikr. Anat., 97: 136–186, Jan. 15, 1923
Das Golgische Binnennetz und seine Beziehungen zu der Sekretion. Morphologische und experimentelle Untersuchungen an einigen Säugetierdrüsen. Ibid., 100: 433–472, 1924

Nather, Carl. Vienna surgeon
OPERATION—
Retroperitoneal operation for subphrenic abscess: with the report of two cases with A. Ochsner, S. G. O., 37: 665–678, Nov. 1923

Nau, Pierre. French physician
Mentioned deformity of platyspondyly.
Les scolioses congénitales. Thèse de Paris, No. 446, 1904. 114 pp.

Naumann, Hans Norbert. English scientist
TEST—
Studies on bile pigments. II. A new test for bilirubin in the urine and its use for detection of bilirubin in normal urine. Biochem. J., 30: 762–764, 1936

Naunyn, Bernard. Strassburg physician. 1839–1925
MITRAL INSUFFICIENCY—
Ueber den Grund, weshalb hin und wieder das systolische Geräusch bei der Mitralinsufficienz am lautesten in der Gegend der Pulmonalklappe zu vernehmen ist. Berl. klin. Wschr., 5: 189–190, Apr. 27, 1868
SIGN—of cholecystitis; deep tenderness beneath costal arch at end of full inspiration. In his: Klinik der Cholelithiasis. Leipzig, Vogel, 1892. 187 pp.

Same, in English London, New Sydenham Soc., 1896. 192 pp.
Believed cholesterine is a product of gall bladder and ducts. Garrison Ibid.
Introduced term acidosis. In his: *Der Diabetes mellitus.* Wien, Hölder, 1898. 526 pp. 2 ed., 1906. New York, Appleton, 1909

Navderleck, J. See F. C. Harrison

Nawiasky, P. German scientist
SOLUTION—basal salt.
Über die Umsetzung von Aminosäuren durch Bac. proteus vulgaris. Arch. Hyg., 66: 209–243, 1908

Neefe, John R. American physician
MODIFICATION—of Hanger's test, for liver function.
Photosensitivity as cause of falsely positive cephalin-cholesterol flocculation tests with J. G. Reinhhold Science, 100: 83–85, July 28, 1944
TEST—thymol flocculation.
Results of hepatic tests in chronic hepatitis without jaundice: correlation with the clinical course and liver biopsy findings. Gastroenterology, 7: 1–19, July 1946

Neelson, Friedrich Carl Adolf. German physician. 1854–1894
STAINING METHODS—
Grundriss der pathologisch-anatomischen Technik für praktische Aerzte und Studierende. Stuttgart, Enke, 1892. 94 pp.

Neff, W. B. See J. A. Stiles

Negri, Adelchi. Italian physician. 1876–1912
BODIES—related to hydrophobia.
Contributo allo studio dell'eziologia della rabbia. Atti. r. Ist. Lomb. di sc. e lett., 1903–04, Milano, 19, 1905
Also: Boll. Soc. Med.-Chir., Pavia, p. 88; 229, 1903; p. 22, 1904; p. 321, 1905
Beitrag zum Studium der Aetiologie der Tollwuth. Z. Hyg. InfektKr., 43: 507–527, 1903
Zur Aetiologie der Tollwuth. Die Diagnose der Tollwuth auf Grund der neuen Befunde. Ibid., 44: 519–540, 1903

Neill, J. M. See D. D. Van Slyke

Neill, John. American surgeon. 1819–1880
SPLINT—straight-leg.
New means for making extension and counter-extension in fractures of the leg and thigh. Philadelphia, Merrihew and Thompson, 1855. 7 pp.

Neisser, Albert Ludwig Siegmund. German physician. 1855–1916
Discoverer of the gonococcus.
Ueber eine der Gonorrhoe eigenthümliche Micrococcusform. Zbl. med. Wiss., 17: 497–500, July 12, 1879
See also A. von Wassermann

Neisser, Max. German bacteriologist. 1869–1938
PHENOMENON—deviation of complement.
Lässt sich durch Einspritzung von agglutinierten Typhusbacillen eine Agglutinproduktion hervorrufen with R. Lubowski, Zbl. Bakt., 30: 483–491, Oct. 15, 1901
STAIN—for metachromatic granules in diphtheria bacilli.
Zur Differentialdiagnose des Diphtheriebacillus. Z. Hyg. InfektKr., 24: 443–469, 1897
TEST—for living and dead cells.
Ueber eine neue einfache Methode zur Beobachtung von Schädigungen lebenden Zellen und Organismen (Bioskopie). Münch. med. Wschr., 47: 1261–1262, Sept. 11, 1900

Nélaton, Auguste. French surgeon. 1807–1873
DISEASE—central tumor of bone.
Elémens de pathologie chirurgicale. Paris, 1847–48. 5 vols. Vol. 2, p. 46
LINE—from anterior superior process of ilium to tuberosity of ischium. Ibid., p. 441
OPERATION—for ankylosis of wrist.
Du traitement de l'ankylose du poignet d'origine blennorragique. Rev. d'orthop., 2 s., 5: 39–43, 1905
Described pelvic hematocele and hemorrhage from ruptured graafian follicle.
Leçons sur l'hématocèle rétro-utérine. Gas. d. Hôp., Paris, 3 s., 3: 573; 578–579, 1851; 4: 45–46; 66–67, 1852

Neller, James Locke. Madison, Wis. surgeon. 1914–
METHOD—
Wheal-fluorescence: a new method of evaluating peripheral vascular diseases. Preliminary report with E. R. Schmidt, Ann. Surg., 121: 328–337, Mar. 1945
The use of fluorescent wheals in determining extent and degree of peripheral vascular insufficiency: further observations. Ibid., 122: 898–901, Nov. 1945

Nelms, W. F. See E. Bishop

Nelson, Casper Irving. Chicago bacteriologist. 1886–
AGAR—ammonium succinate, for cultivation of colon-typhoid group.
The intracellular proteins of bacteria. I. Globulins. J. infect. Dis., 38: 371–377 (373), Apr. 1926

Nelson, J. W. See G. F. Cartland

Nelson, M. C. See N. K. Jensen

Nencki, Marcellus von. Polish physician. 1847–1901
TEST—for urobilin in urine.
Ueber das Urorosein, einen neuen Harnfarbstoff. J. prakt. Chem., 26: 333–336, Oct. 23, 1882

Nepveu, Gustave. Marseille surgeon. 1841–1903
Found trypanosomes in human blood.
Etude sur les parasites du sang chez les paludiques. C. R. Soc. Biol., 43: 39–50, 1891

Néri, V. See A. Serra

Nesbit, Reed Miller. American surgeon. 1898–
DIET—
A low calorie ketogenic diet for the treatment of chronic urinary tract infections with C. H. McDonnell and Genevieve C. Rourke, J. Michigan Med. Soc., 34: 347–349, June 1935

Nesset, N. See W. L. Tatum

Nessler, Julius. German chemist. 1827–
REAGENT and TEST—for ammonia.
Verhalten des Iodquecksilbers zu Ammoniak und eine neue Reaction auf Ammoniak. Chem. Zbl., 27: 529–541, July 19, 1856

Nettleship, Edward. English dermatologist. 1845–1913
DISEASE—urticaria pigmentosa.
"... chronic urticaria, leaving brown stains: nearly two years' duration." Brit. med. J., 2: 435 (only), Oct. 23, 1869

Neubauer, Otto. Munich physician
TEST—for carcinoma of stomach.
Über das Vorkommen eines peptidspaltenden Fermentes im carcinomatösen Mageninhalt und seine diagnostische Bedeutung with H. Fischer, Dtsch. Arch. f. klin. Med., 97: 499–507, Nov. 2, 1909

Neuber, (Carl) Ernest. Budapest surgeon. 1885–
TECHNIC—
Technique of gastric resection. S. G. O., 45: 204–208, Aug. 1927

euber, Gustav Adolf. Kiel physician. 1850–1932
UBES—drainage t. of bone.
*Ein antiseptischer Dauerverband nach gründlicher
Blutstillung.* von Langenbeck's Archiv, 24: 314–
330, 1879
Attempted asepsis.
*Die aseptische Wundbehandlung in meinen chirurgis-
chen Privat-Hospitälern.* Kiel, Lipsius u. Tischer,
1886

euberg, Carl. Berlin biochemist. 1877–
METHOD—of preparation of osazone.
*Ueber Vorkommen und Nachweis von Fruchtzucker
in den menschlichen Körpersäften* with H. Strauss,
Z. physiol. Chem., 36: 227–238, Sept. 6, 1902
TEST—for levulose.
Ueber die Farbenreactionen von Zuckern. Ibid., 31:
564–573, Feb. 21, 1901

euendorf
TREATMENT—of rheumatoid arthritis by mud-
baths of Neuendorf, Germany.

eufeld, Alonzo J. Los Angeles surgeon. 1906–
FEMORAL NAIL, PLATE—
See G. M. Taylor

eufeld, Ferdinand. German bacteriologist. 1869–
REACTION—capsular swelling in typing of pneumo-
coccus.
*Ueber die Agglutination der Pneumokokken und über
die Theorien der Agglutination.* Z. Hyg. InfektKr.,
40: 54–72, 1902
Named and described bacteriotropins.
*Über die Antikörper des Streptokokken-und Pneumo-
kokken-Immunserums* with W. Rimpau, Dtsch. med.
Wschr., 30: 1458–1460, 1904

euhaus, Dr. Hagen i. W. chemist
TEST—for santonin in urine.
Eine neue Harnprobe auf Santonin. Dtsch. med.
Wschr., 32: 466 (only), Mar. 22, 1906

euhof, Harold. New York surgeon. 1884–
METHOD—
*Abdominal puncture in the diagnosis of acute intra-
peritoneal disease* with I. Cohen, Ann. Surg., 83:
454–462, Apr. 1926

eumann, Albert. Berlin chemist
METHOD—for determination of iron in urine.
*Einfache Verasuchungsmethode (Säuregemisch-Veras-
chung) und Vereinfachte Bestimmungen von Eisen,
Phosphorsäure, Salzsäure und anderen Aschenbestand-
theilen unter Benutzung dieser Säuregemisch-Veras-
chung.* Z. phys. Chem., 37: 115–142, Dec. 20, 1902
TEST—for carbohydrates.
Neue Farbenreactionen der Zucker. Berl. klin. Wschr.,
41: 1073–1074, Oct. 10, 1904

eumann, Ernst. German pathologist. 1834–1918
Described myelogenous leukaemia.
*Leukaemia mit Erkrankung des Knochenwarks (Mye-
logene Leukaemia).* Arch. d. Heilk., 11: 1–14, 1870
Described "fibrinoid" in wall of arteries.
*Die Picrocarminfärbung und ihre Anwendung auf die
Entzündungslehre.* Arch. mikr. Anat., 18: 130–150,
1880

eumann, Isidor. Vienna dermatologist. 1837–1906
DISEASE—pemphigus vegetans.
Ueber Pemphigus vegetans (frambosiodes). Viertelj.
f. Dermat., 13: 157–178, 1886
Described porokeratosis (Mibelli).

*Über eine seltene Hautkrankheit (Dermatitis circum-
scripta herpetiformis).* Ibid., 2: 41–52, 1875

Neve, Ernest Frederic. Kashmir surgeon. 1861–
CANCER—
Kangri-burn cancer. Brit. med. J., 2: 1255–1256,
Dec. 29, 1923
Squamous celled epithelium due to Kangri burn.
Indian med. Gaz., 59: 341–344, July 1924

Nevin, Mary. American bacteriologist. 1880–
METHOD—of isolation of B. botulinus.
Botulism from cheese. J. Infect. Dis., 28: 226–231,
Mar. 1921

New, Gordon Balgarnie. Rochester, Minn. surgeon.
1885–
METHOD—of treating fractures of nose.
Fractures of the nasal and malar bones. Surg. Clin. N.
Amer., 15: 1241–1250, Oct. 1935
TECHNIC—of total laryngectomy.
A two-stage laryngectomy. S. G. O., 47: 826–830, Dec.
1928
The surgical treatment of carcinoma of the larynx.
Ibid., 68: 462–466, Feb. 15, 1939

Newburger, Robert Anton. New York physician.
1911–
METHOD—
Determination of the icteric index by the acetone method.
J. Lab. clin. Med., 22: 1192–1195, Aug. 1937

Newburgh, L. H. See F. H. Lashmet

Newcomer, Harry Sidney. New York physician.
1887–
METHOD—of determining hemoglobin.
*Absorption spectra of acid hematin, oxyhemoglobin,
and carbon monoxide hemoglobin. A new hemoglobinometer.* J. biol. Chem., 37: 465–496, Mar. 1919
*A new optical instrument for the determination of
hemoglobin.* Ibid., 55: 569–574, Apr. 1923
See also H. S. Gasser

Newton, Sir Isaac. English scientist. 1642–1727
Proposed corpuscular theory of light.
*Opticks; or a treatise of the reflexions, refractions, in-
flexions and colours of light. . . .* London, Smith and
Walford, 1704

Ney, Karl Winfield. New York surgeon. 1882–
OPERATION—
A tendon transplant for intrinsic hand muscle paralysis.
S. G. O., 33: 342–348, Oct. 1921

Neymann, Clarence Adolph. Chicago neurologist.
1887–
METHOD—
*A new method for making Wassermann antigens from
normal heart tissue* with L. T. Gager, J. Immunol.,
2: 573–583, Oct. 1917
Introduced electropyrexia.
*Artificial fever produced by high-frequency currents:
preliminary report* with S. L. Osborne, Illinois med.
J., 56: 199–203, Sept. 1929
*The treatment of dementia paralytica with hyperpyrexia
produced by diathermy.* J. A. M. A., 96: 7–13, Jan.
3, 1931

Nicholls, E. E. See R. L. Cecil

Nicholson, Jesse Thompson. Philadelphia surgeon.
1903–
METHOD—
Spontaneous reduction of cervical spine dislocations.
J. A. M. A., 115: 2063–2069, Dec. 14, 1940

Nicola, Toufick. New York surgeon. 1894–

OPERATION—
Recurrent anterior dislocation of the shoulder. A new operation. J. Bone and Joint Surg., 11: 128–132, Jan. 1929
Recurrent dislocation of the shoulder: its treatment by transplantation of the long head of the biceps. Amer. J. Surg., 6: 815 (only), June 1929
Nicoladoni, Carl. German surgeon. 1847–1902
OPERATION—plastic on finger.
Daumenplastik und organischer Ersatz der Fingerspitze (Anticheiroplastik und Dactyloplastik). Arch. klin. Chir., 61: 606–614, 1900
Nicolaier, Arthur. Berlin physician. 1862–
BACILLUS—B. tetani.
Ueber infectiösen Tetanus. Dtsch. med. Wschr., 10: 842–844, Dec. 25, 1884
Introduced urotropin.
Ueber die therapeutische Verwendung des Hexamethylentetramin. Zbl. med. Wiss., 32: 897–900, Dec. 22, 1894
Introduced cinchophen, using trade name of atophan.
Ueber die Wirkung von Chinolincarbonsäure und ihrer Derivate auf die Ausscheidung der Harnsäure. Dtsch. Arch. klin. Med., 93: 331–355, June 18, 1908
Nicolas, A. See E. Gley
Nicolas, Joseph. French physician. 1878–
See J. Durand
Nicolas, Marie Eugène. French scientist. 1879–
TEST—for indican in urine.
(No title) Bull. Soc. chim., 3 s., 33: 743–744, 1905
Nicolaysen, Johan. Christiania surgeon. 1860–
OPERATION—transfixion of fracture of neck of femur.
Lidt om Diagnosen og Behandlingen av Fr. colli femoris. Nord. med. arvik., 8: No 16, pp. 19, 1897
Nicoll, James H. Scottish surgron. 1864–1921
OPERATION—
Case operated on for femoral hernia, with an account of the operation carried out. Glasgow Path. and Clin. Soc., 9: 82–83, 1902
OPERATION—(advocated in 1898)
Case of hydrocephalus in which peritoneo-meningeal drainage has been carried out. Glasgow med. J., 63: 187–191, Mar. 1905
PASTE—a feeding form for pyloric spasm.
Congenital hypertrophic stenosis of the pylorus; with special reference to the treatment. Practitioner, Lond., 85: 659–664, 1910
Nicolle, Charles Jules Henri. French physician. 1866–1936
Awarded Nobel prize in 1928 for studies of typhus.
La géographie actuelle de la peste. Rev. med. de Normandie, 1: 23–27, Jan. 10, 1900
La peste. Ibid., 413–425, Sept. 25, 1900
Sur les résultats de la sérothérapie dans le traitement du typhus exanthématique. Bull. Acad. de méd., 76: 95–101, Aug. 1, 1916
Contribution nouvelle à la connaissance du typhus expérimental chez les muridés. Arch. Inst. Pasteur de Tunis, 15: 267–275, Sept. 1926 (et seq.)
MODIFICATION—of Gram's stain.
Pratique des colorations microbiennes (Méthode de Gram modifiée et méthode directe). Ann. Inst. Pasteur, 9: 664–670, Aug. 1895
SOLUTION—peptone.
Études sur le bacilli d'Eberth et les bacilles parathy-

phiques with A. Raphael and E. Debains. Ibid., 31: 372–387 (380), Aug. 1917
First observed toxoplasma, a genus of protozoan parasites, in gondi.
Sur une infection à corps de Leishman (ou organismes voisins) du gondi with L. Manceaux, C. R. Acad Sci., 147: 763–766, Oct. 26, 1908
Described—
Le kala azar infantile. Ann. Inst. Pasteur, 23: 361–401, May; 441–471, June 1909
Proved that relapsing fever is conveyed by body louse.
Étiologie de la fièvre récurrente, son mode de transmission par les poux with L. Blaizot and E. Conseil, Inid., 27: 204–225, Mar. 25, 1913
Nicolle, Maurice. French physician. 1862–
Demonstrated "passive" anaphylaxis.
Contribution à l'étude du "phénomène d'Arthus." Ann. Inst. Pasteur, 21: 128–137, Feb. 1907
Niedner. See W. Hesse
Niehans, Paul. Zürich urologist. 1882–
OPERATION—modification of Steinach o.
Modern views on hypertrophy of the prostate. Lancet, 1: 307–311, Feb. 8, 1936
Nielsen, Holger. Copenhagen physician
METHOD—"arm lift," in resuscitation.
En oplivningsmethode. Ugeskr. Laeger, 94: 1201–1203, Dec. 15, 1932
Niemann, Albert. German scientist
Isolated cocaine from coca leaves.
Ueber eine neue organische Base in den Cocablättern. Göttingen, Huth, 1860. 52 pp.
Niemann, Albert. German surgeon. 1880–1921
DISEASE—form of xanthomatosis.
Ein unbekanntes Krankheitsbild. Jb. f. Kinderh., 79: 1–10, Jan. 6, 1914
Niessen, Max Alexander von. German physician
BACILLUS—
Der Syphilisbacillus. Wiesbaden, Bergmann, 1896. 92 pp.
Niewenglowski, Gaston Henri. French physician
RAYS—luminous rays given out by substances which have been exposed to the sun. Dorland
L'objectif photographique. . . . Paris, 1892. 59 pp.
Nigg, Clara. American bacteriologist. 1897–
Grew Rickettsia, with living tissue as medium.
On the preservation of typhus fever Rickettsiae in cultures. J. exp. Med., 61: 17–26, Jan. 1935
Nikiforoff, Mikhaïl Nikiforovich. Russian dermatologist. 1858–
METHOD—of fixing blood-films.
Mikroskopisch-technische Notizen. Z. wiss. Mik., 8: 189–190, 1891
Niles, W. B. See M. Dorset
Nippe, Martin O. H. Königsberg physician. 1883–
TEST—for blood.
Eine Vereinfachung der Häminkristallprobe. Dtsch. med. Wschr., 38: 2222–2223, Nov. 21, 1912
Nirenstein, Edmund. Vienna physician
DETERMINATION—of peptic activity.
Ueber die Pepsinbestimmung nach Mette und die Notwendigkeit ihrer Modifikation für klinische Zwecke. with A. Schiff, Arch. VerdauKr., 8: 559–604, 1902
Nisbet, William. English physician. 1759–1822
CHANCRE—
First lines on the theory and practice in venereal diseases. Edinburgh, Elliot, 1787. 453 pp.

ssl, Franz. Heidelberg neurologist. 1860–1919

DIES, GRANULES, METHOD, STAIN—
Ueber eine neue Untersuchungsmethode des Central-
organs speciell zur Feststellung der Localisation der
Nervenzellen. Abstr.: Neurol. Zbl., 13: 507–508,
July 1, 1894
Ueber die sogenannten Granula der Nervenzellen.
Ibid., 781–789, Nov. 1, 1894

tze, Max. German surgeon. 1848–1906
Introduced use of cystoscope, urethroscope and recto-
scope.
Eine neue Beleuchtungs- und Untersuchungsmethode
für Harnröhre, Harnblase und Rectum. Wien. med.
Wschr., 29: 779–782, July 19; 806–810, July 26, 1879
Lehrbuch der Kystoskopie. Ihre Technik und klinische
Bedeutung. Wiesbaden, Bergmann, 1889. 329 pp.

oback, C. R. See H. S. Kupperman

obel, Alfred Bernard. Swedish scientist. 1833–1896
Established Nobel prizes; one of the five is awarded
annually in field of Physiology and Medicine.
For biography see: *Nobel: dynamite and peace.* By
R. Sohlman and H. Schuck; English transl. by B.
and B. Lunn, New York, Cosmopolitan Book Corp.,
1929. 353 pp.

obl, Gabor. Vienna dermatologist. 1864–1938
Used dextrose in injection of varicose veins.
Die Calorose als Verödungsmittel varikös entarteter
Venen. Wien. klin. Wschr., 39: 1217–1219, Oct. 14,
1926

oble, George Henry. American gynecologist. 1860–
PERATION—
A flap operation for atresia of the vagina. Trans.
South. Surg. and Gynec. Ass., 13: 78–83, 1900

oble, Thomas Benjamin. Indianapolis surgeon.
1867–
PERATION—
A good way to treat femoral hernia. Amer. J. Obstet.,
67: 512–519, Mar. 1913

ocard, Edmund Isidore Étienne. French veterinar-
ian. 1850–1903
ACILLUS—of psittacosis; Nocardiosis.
Note sur la maladie des boeufs de la Guadeloupe connue
sous le nom de farcin. Ann. Inst. Pasteur, 2: 293–302,
June 1888
Recognized an avian tubercle bacillus.
Tuberculose; transmission de l'homme aux volailles et
aux chiens. Bull. et mém. Soc. centr. de méd. vet.,
Paris, n. s., 3: 98–101, 1885
Made early study of filtrable virus.
Le microbe de la péripneumonie with P. P. E. Roux,
Ann. Inst. Pasteur, 12: 240–262, Apr. 1898

ocht, Bernhard Albrecht Eduard. German physician. 1857–
TAIN—
Zur Färbung der Malariaparasiten. Zbl. Bakt., 24:
839–843, Dec. 15, 1898

oeggerath, Emil Jacob. American physician. 1827–
1895
PERATION—
On epicystotomy. New York, J. Med., s 3., 4: 9–24,
1858
Emphasized importance of latent gonorrhea in
women.
Die latente Gonorrhoe in weiblichen Geschlecht. Bonn,
Cohen, 1872. 125 pp.

Latent gonorrhea, especially with regard to its influence
on fertility in women. Trans. Amer. Gynec. Soc., 1:
268–300, 1876

Noguchi, Hideyo. Japanese pathologist in New York.
1876–1928
MEDIUM—ascitic fluid tissue.
Pure cultivation of Spirochaeta refrigens. J. exp. Med.,
15: 466–469, May 1, 1912
The pure cultivation of Spirochaeta duttoni, Spirochaeta
kochi, Spirochaeta obermeieri, and Spirochaeta novyi.
Ibid., 16: 199–210 (201), Aug. 1, 1912
MEDIUM—for leptospira Icteroides: original.
Etiology of yellow fever. VI. Cultivation, morphology,
virulence, and biological properties of leptospira icter-
oides. Ibid., 30: 13–29, July 1, 1919
(Same) improved.
Experimental studies of yellow fever in northern Brazil.
Monogr. Rockefeller Inst. Med. Res., No. 20, Aug.
9, 1924. 36 pp.
METHOD—
A method for the pure cultivation of pathogenic tre-
ponema pallidum (spirochaeta pallida). J. exp. Med.,
14: 99–108, Aug. 1, 1911
METHOD—
Contribution to the cultivation of the parasite of rabies.
Ibid., 18: 314–316, Sept. 1, 1913
METHOD—of staining Treponema pallida in brain
tissue.
A demonstration of Treponema pallidum in the brain
in cases of general paralysis with J. W. Moore, Ibid.,
17: 232–238, Feb. 1, 1913
Additional studies on the presence of spirochaeta
pallida in general paralysis and tabes dorsalis. J. cutan.
Dis., 31: 547–549, Aug. 1913
REACTION—
The relation of protein, lipoids and salts to the Wasser-
mann reaction. J. exp. Med., 11: 84–99 (92), Jan. 9,
1909
REACTION—
A cutaneous reaction in syphilis. Ibid., 14: 557–568,
Dec. 1, 1911
TEST—
The butyric reaction for syphilis in man and in the
monkey. Proc. Soc. exp. Biol., N. Y., 6: 51–54, Dec.
16, 1908
Discovered bacterial agent of yellow fever and named
it.
Spirochaeta icterohaemorrhagiae in American wild
rats and its relation to the Japanese and European
strains. J. exp. Med., 25: 755–763, May 1917
Morphological characteristics and nomenclature of
leptospira (Spirochaeta) icterohaemorrhagiae (Inada
and Ida). Ibid., 27: 575–592; 593–608; 609–625,
May 1918
Isolated Bact. granulosis.
Experimental production of a trachoma-like condition
in monkeys by means of a micro-organism isolated from
American Indian trachoma. J. A. M. A., 89: 739–742,
Sept. 3, 1927
The etiology of trachoma. J. exp. Med., 48, suppl. 2,
July 1, 1928, 53 pp. 31 pl.
See also T. Ohira

Nolf, Pierre. Belgian physician. 1873–
METHOD—
De l'action antithermique et antiinfectieuse des injec-

tions intraveineuses de peptone. C. R. Soc. Biol., 79: 649–651, July 22, 1916

Noll, Friedrich Guil. German physiologist

THEORY—of lymph formation by diffusion of fluids from blood through vessel walls.

De cursu lymphae in vasis lymphaticis. Marburgi Cattorum, Elwerti, 1849. 36 pp.

See also C. F. W. Ludwig

Nonne, Max. Hamburg neurologist. 1861–

HEREDITARY LYMPHEDEMA—of Nonne-Milroy-Meige.

Vier Fälle von Elephantiasis congenita hereditaria. Arch. path. Anat., 125: 189–196, July 6, 1891

REACTION—of cerebrospinal fluid.

Ueber fractionirte Eiweissausfällung in der Spinalflüssigkeit von Gesunden, Luetikern, functionell- und organisch-Nervenkranken und über ihre Verwerthung zur Differentialdiagnose der Dementia paralytica, Tabes dorsalis, tertiären und abgelaufenen Syphilis with F. Alpert, Arch. Psychiat. Nervenkr., 43: 433–460, Oct. 1907

SYNDROME—cerebellar agenesis—

Über das Vorkommen von starker Phase I-Reaction bei fehlender Lymphocytose bei 6 Fällen von Rückenmarkstumor. Dtsch. Z. Nervenheilk., 40: 161–167, Oct. 12, 1910

Described loss of deep reflexes in trichiniasis.

Klinische und anatomische Beiträge zur Pathologie der Trichinenerkrankung with Hoepfner, Z. klin. Med., 15: 455–474, 1889

Noorden, Carl Harko von. Vienna physician. 1858–1944

Studied albuminuria in health. Garrison

Ueber Albuminurie bei gesunden Menschen. Dtsch. Arch. klin. Med., 38: 205–247, Jan. 20, 1886

Made dietetic studies of diabetes and introduced oatmeal diet for diabetes.

Die Zuckerkrankheit und ihre Behandlung. Berlin, Hirschwald, 1910

See also G. Honigmann

Nordau, Max Simon. German scientist. 1849–1923

DISEASE—degeneracy.

Dégénérescence. Paris, Alcan, 1894. 2 vols.

Same, in English. New York, Appleton, 1895

Nordentoft, O. Denmark physician

Successfully treated gliomas.

Rontgenbehandlede Tumores cerebri. Ugeskr. Laeg., 79: 775–788, May 17, 1917

Nordland, Martin. Minneapolis surgeon. 1889–

TECHNIC—for ligation of inferior thyroid arteries.

Advantages and technic of preliminary hemostasis in thyroidectomy with L. N. Larson, West. J. Surg., 41: 485–496, Sept. 1933

Nordrach Treatment

of consumption by fresh air, rest, and an abundance of nourishing food. Dorland. At Nordrach Ranch, Colorado, U. S. A.

Normand, A. French physician

Described strongyloidiasis.

Sur la maladie dite diarrhée de Cochinchine. C. R. Acad. Sci., 5: 316–318, July 31, 1876

Also: Paris, Baillière, 1877. 86 pp., reprint from: Arch. de méd. nav., Paris, 27, 1877

Norris, Charles. New York scientist. 1867–1935

Isolated spirochaete causing American variety of relapsing fever.

AGAR—blood peptone, for cultivation of spirochete

Study of a spirocheta obtained from a case of relapsing fever in man, with notes on morphology, animal reactions, and attempts at cultivation with A. M. Pappenheimer and T. Flournoy, J. infect. Dis., 3: 266–29 (281), May 18, 1906

Norris, Dorothy. Punjab scientist

SOLUTION—trypsinized caselnogen; culture medium

The preparation of a simplified culture medium for field workers. Ind. J. med. Res., 7: 704–709 (706 Apr. 1920

Norris, Richard. English physiologist. 1831–1916

CORPUSCLES—disks in blood serum.

On the origin and mode of development of the morphological elements of mammalian blood. Birmingham Corns, et al., 1879

Norris on the discovery of an invisible or third corpuscular element in the blood. Abstr., with critical note. London med. Rec., 8: 2–4, Jan. 15, 1880

North, Elisha. Connecticut physician. 1771–1843

Published book on cerebrospinal meningitis.

A treatise on a malignant epidemic commonly called spotted fever; interspersed with remarks on the nature of fever in general, etc.; with an appendix in which republished a number of essays written by different authors on this epidemic, with the addition of original notes; containing also a few original and selected cases with critical remarks. New York, Swords, 1811. 249 pp

Northrop, John Howard. New York biochemist 1891–

Crystallized enzymes.

Crystalline pepsin; I. Isolation and tests of purity J. gen. Physiol., 13: 739–766, July 20, 1930

Crystalline pepsin; II. General properties and experimental methods. Ibid., 767–780, July 20, 1930

Northrup, Zoe. Michigan bacteriologist

AGAR—peptone bile.

The influence of the products of lactic organisms upon Bacillus typhosus. Zbl. Bakt., 61: 417–442 (120) Dec. 30, 1911

Norton, Arthur Trehern. English surgeon. 1841–191

OPERATION—

A new and reliable operation for the cure of webbed fingers. Brit. med. J., 2: 931–932, Dec. 10, 1881

Norton, J. F. See N. S. Ferry

Norwood, Wesley U. American physician. 1806–188

TINCTURE—of veratrum viride.

The therapeutical powers and properties of Veratrum viride. New York, Kneeland, 1854. 40 pp.

Nosik, William André. Cleveland physician. 1911–

IRRIGATOR—

A neurosurgical suction-irrigator with W. J. Gardner Amer. J. Surg., 44: 477–478, May 1939

Nothnagel, Hermann. German physician. 1841–190

SIGN—paralysis of facial muscles, especially in respect of movements connected with emotions. Dorland

Zur Lehre von den vasomotorischen Neurosen. Dtsch Arch. klin. Med., 2: 173–191, Sept. 7, 1866

SYNDROME—unilateral oculomotor paralysis with cerebellar ataxia and crossed paralysis. Dorland

Topische Diagnostik der Gehirnkrankheiten. Berlin Hirschwaldm, 1879. p. 220

Described—

Angina pectoris vasomotoria. Dtsch. Arch. klin. Med. 3: 309–322, Aug. 2, 1867

Nott, Josiah Clark. Mobile, Ala. physician. 1804–1873
One of the first to suggest "mosquito theory" in
reference to transmission of yellow fever. Garrison
*Sketch of the epidemic of yellow fever of 1847, in
Mobile.* Charleston med. J. and Rev., 3: 1–21, Jan.
1848
*Yellow fever contrasted with bilious fever—reasons for
believing it a disease sui generis—its mode of propagation—remote cause—probable insect or animalcular
origin, etc.* New Orleans med. J., 4: 563–601, Mar.
1848

Novak, Milan. Minneapolis bacteriologist. 1907–
SOLUTION—for skin sterilization.
TEST—for skin sterility.
*A method for determining the efficiency of preoperative
skin sterilization* with H. Hall, Surgery, 5: 560–566,
Apr. 1939

Nové-Josserand, Gabriel. French surgeon
OPERATION—
Traitement de l'hypospadias; nouvelle méthode. Lyon
méd., 85: 198–200, June 6, 1897
OPERATION—
"Artrorise" of the foot. J. Bone and Joint Surg., 10:
261–267, Apr. 1928

Novy, Frederick George. American bacteriologist.
1864–
MEDIA—
On the cultivation of trypanosoma brucei with W. J.
McNeal, J. infect. Dis., 1: 1–30, Jan. 2, 1904
Discovered spirochete of American variety of re-
lapsing fever.
Studies on Spirillum obermeieri and related organisms
with R. E. Knapp, Ibid., 3: 291–393, May 18, 1906

Nowicki, Witold. Polish bacteriologist. 1878–
TEST—
*Ueber eine Modifikation der Ehrlichschen Indolreak-
tion in Bakterienkulturen.* Wien. klin. Wschr., 30:
983 (only), Aug. 2, 1917

Noyer, Rondeau du. French scientist
MIXTURE—lanolin-colophony, for mounting.
Nouveau lut pour préparations microscopiques. C.
R. Soc. Biol., 81: 741–742, July 20, 1918

Noyes, Harry Alfred. American chemist. 1890–
AGAR—asparaginate; culture medium.
Media for soil bacteria. J. Bact., 1: 93–94, Jan. 1916

Noyes, Henry Dewey. American ophthalmologist.
1832–1900
Described—
Retinitis in glycosuria. Trans. Amer. Ophthal. Soc.,
1867–68, pp. 71–75, 1869

Nuck, Antonius. Dutch anatomist. 1650–1742
CANAL or DIVERTICULUM—
Adenographia curiosa et uteri foeminei anatome nova.
. . . Lugd. Bat., Luchtmans, 1691. 152 pp.
GLAND—near apex of tongue.
*De ductu salivali novo, saliva, ductibus oculorum
aquosis, et humore oculi aqueo.* Leyden, vander Aa,
1685. 175 pp.

Nuhn, Anton. German anatomist. 1814–1889
GLAND—near tip of tongue.
*Ueber eine bis jetzt noch nicht näher beschriebene
Drüse im Innern der Zungenspitze.* Mannheim, Basser-
mann, 1845. 8 pp.

Nussbaum, Johann Nepomuk von. Munich surgeon.
1829–1890

PROCEDURE—stretching fifth nerve for trigeminal
neuralgia.
*Blosslegung und Dehnung der Rückenmarksnerven;
eine erfolgreiche Operation.* Dtsch. Z. Chir., 1: 450–
465, Sept. 10, 1872

Nussbaum, Moritz. German histologist. 1850–1915
EXPERIMENT—ligation of renal arteries in order to
isolate glomeruli of kidneys from the circulation.
Ueber die Secretion der Niere. Arch. ges. Physiol.,
16: 139–143, 1878
*Fortgesetzte Untersuchungen über die Secretion der
Niere.* Ibid., 17: 580–591, 1878

Nutt, John Joseph. American surgeon. 1870–
OPERATION—
*Intra-perineural neurotomy. An operation for infan-
tile cerebral hemiplegia: with report of two cases.*
Amer. J. Orthop. Surg., 7: 151–156, Nov. 1909
*Further observations on intra-perineural neurotomy
in spastic conditions.* J. Bone and Joint Surg., 4:
453–458, July 1922

Nuttall, George Henry Falkiner. American physician. 1862–1937
BULB—for collecting blood-serum under antiseptic
precautions.
Einige Beiträge zur bakteriologischen Technik. Zbl.
Bakt., 11: 538–540, Apr. 23, 1892
TEST—for blood stains.
*Progress report upon the biological test for blood as
applied to over 500 bloods from various sources, together with a preliminary note upon a method for
measuring the degree of reaction.* Brit. med. J., 1:
825–827, Apr. 5, 1902
Demonstrated bactericidal power of defibrinated
blood of certain animals. Garrison and Morton
*Experimente über die bacterienfeindlichen Einflüsse
des thierischen Körpers.* Z. Hyg. InfektKr., 4: 353–
394, 1888
Proved that healthy life and perfect digestion are
possible without presence of bacteria in digestive
tract. Garrison and Morton
*Thierisches Leben ohne Bakterien im Verdauungs-
kanal* with H. Thierfelder, Z. physiol. Chem., 21:
109–121, 1895; 22: 62–73, 1896; 23: 231–235, 1897
Summarized role of insects as transmitters of diseases.
Garrison
*On the role of insects, arachnids, and myriapods, as
carriers in the spread of bacterial and pasasitic diseases of man and animals. A critical and historical
study.* Johns Hopk. Hosp. Rep., 8: 1–154, 1899
Established identification of different kinds of blood
by precipitin test. Garrison
*Blood immunity and blood relationship; a demonstra-
tion of certain blood relationships amongst animals
by means of the precipitin test for blood.* Cambridge,
Univ. Press, 1904. 444 pp.
See W. H. Welch

Nuttall, H. C. W. Liverpool surgeon
OPERATION—
Rectus transplantation for midline incisional herniae.
Brit. J. Surg., 25: 344–350, Oct. 1937

Nyiri, Wilhelm. German physician
TEST—functional, of kidney.
*Die Thiosulfatprobe; eine neue Methode des Nieren-
funktionsprüfung.* Wien u. Leipzig, Deuticke, 1923.
157 pp.

Die Thiosulfatprobe im Dienst des Praktikers. Aerztl. Rdsch., 36: 146–149, 1926
Nylander, Emil. Swedish chemist. 1835–1907
REAGENT—for glucose in urine.
Ueber alkalische Wismuthlösung als Reagens auf Traubenzucker im Harne. Z. physiol. Chem., 8: 175–185, 1883–4
Nyström, Erik Gunnar. Swedish surgeon. 1877–

TECHNIC—
Experiences with the Trendelenburg operation for pulmonary embolism. Trans. Amer. Surg. Ass., 48: 18–52, 1930
Same: Ann. Surg., 92: 498–532, Oct. 1930
Contributions to the technic of pulmonary embolectomy: an experimental study with A. Blalock, J. Thoracic Surg., 5: 169–188, Dec. 1935

O

Ober, Frank Roberts. Boston surgeon. 1881–
INCISION—for drainage of hip.
Posterior arthrotomy of the hip joint. J. A. M. A., 83: 1500–1502, Nov. 8, 1924
OPERATION—fasciotomy.
Back strain and sciatica. Ibid., 104: 1580–1583, May 4, 1935
OPERATION—
Slipping patella or recurrent dislocation of the patella. J. Bone and Joint Surg., 17: 774–779, July 1935
SIGN or TEST—for tense fascia lata.
The role of the iliotibial band and fascia lata as a factor in the causation of low-back disabilities and sciatica. Ibid., 18: 105–110, Jan. 1936
TECHNIC—
Tendon transplantation in the lower extremity. New Engl. J. Med., 209: 52–59, July 13, 1933
Obermayer, Fritz. Vienna chemist. 1861–1925
TEST—for albumin.
Studien zur Kenntniss der Eiweissfäulniss with R. Kerry, Zbl. Physiol., 7: 806–810, 1893–4
TEST—for indican in urine.
Ueber eine Modification der Jaffe'schen Indicanprobe. Wien. klin. Wschr., 3: 176 (only), Feb. 27, 1890
Obermeier, Otto Hugo Franz. German physician. 1843–1873
SPIRILLUM—recurrentis, of relapsing fever.
Vorkommen feinster, eine Eigenbewegung zeigender Fäden im Blute von Recurrenskranken. Zbl. med. Wiss., 11: 145–147, 1873
Obermüller, Kuno. German physician. 1861–
TEST—for cholesterin.
Beiträge zur Kenntnis der Cholesterine und ihre quantitation Bestimmung in den Fetten. Berlin, Francke, 1892. 69 pp.
Oberst, Max. German surgeon. 1849–1925
METHOD—of local anesthesia. See Ludwig Pernice
Oberstadt, Dr. Berlin scientist
BOUILLON—egg albumin; culture medium.
Über einen neuen Eiernährboden. Z. Hyg. InfektKr., 79: 134–143 (137), Dec. 10, 1914
Obrastzow, W. P. Kiew physician
Described coronary thrombosis.
Zur Kenntniss der Thrombose der Koronararterien des Herzens with N. D. Straschesko, Z. klin. Med., 71: 116–132, 1910
O'Brien, Cecil Starling. Iowa City ophthalmologist. 1889–
SNOW-FLAKE CATARACT OF—
Diabetic cataract: incidence and morphology in 126 young diabetic patients with J. M. Molsberry and J. H. Allen, J. A. M. A., 103: 892–897, Sept. 22, 1934
METHOD—
Akinesis during cataract extraction. Arch. Ophthal., 1: 447–449, Apr. 1929

O'Brien, J. R. See H. W. Kinnersley
Occo, Adolph. Augsburg physician. 1524–1606
Wrote pharmacopoeia.
Enchiridion, sive ut vulgo vocant dispensatorium, compositorum medicamentorum, pro Reipub. Augsburgensis pharmacopoeia. Augsburg, 1564
Also, several subsequent editions. Also, in facsimile, ed. by T. Husemann, State Hist. Soc., Wisconsin, 1928
Ochsner, Albert John. Chicago surgeon. 1858–1925
OPERATION—
Femoral herniotomy. J. A. M. A., 47: 751–754, Sept. 8, 1906
TREATMENT—
The cause of diffuse peritonitis complicating appendicitis and its prevention. Ibid., 36: 1747–1754, June 22, 1901
Also: Med. Classics, 4: 600–626, Feb. 1940
TROCAR—
Technique of gall-bladder operations. S. G. O., 2: 204–208, Feb. 1906
Ochsner, Edward William Alton. New Orleans surgeon. 1896–
OPERATION—
Subphrenic abscess: an analysis of 3,372 collected and personal cases with A. M. Graves, Ann. Surg., 98: 961–990, Dec. 1933
TEST—comparative tourniquet t.
The modern treatment of varicose veins, with a review of 235 cases with H. R. Mahorner, Surgery, 2: 889–902, Dec. 1937
THEORY—of thrombophlebitis.
Therapeutic considerations of thrombophlebitis and phlebothrombosis with M. E. DeBakey, New Engl. J. Med., 225: 207–227, Aug. 7, 1941
See also H. R. Mahorner, C. Nather
O'Connell, C. P. See R. Kurzrok
O'Connor, G. B. See G. W. Pierce
O'Connor, Roderic P. American ophthalmologist. 1878–
OPERATION—
Shortening and advancement methods without employing sutures under tension. J. A. M. A., 58: 626–627, Mar. 2, 1912
Further experience with the writer's method of shortening ocular muscles without employing sutures under tension. Arch. Ophthal., 43: 368–376, July 1914
Transplantation of portions of vertical recti for abducens paralysis with successful result. Amer. J. Ophthal., 2: 197–199, Mar. 1919
Ocular tendon transplantations: three new methods. Arch. Ophthal., 5: 209–211, Feb. 1931
O'Connor, William. English physician. ?–1880
Introduced—
Cases of epilepsy, associated with amenorrhoea an

vicarious menstruation, successfully treated with the iodide of potassium. Lancet, 1: 525 (only), May 23, 1857

'Conor, V. J. See B. C. Corbus

ddi, Ruggero. Italian surgeon
PHINCTER—at duodenal termination of bile and pancreatic ducts.
D'une disposition à sphincter spéciale de l'ouverture du canal cholédoque. Arch. ital. Biol., 8: 317–322, 1887
Di una speciale disposizione a sfintere allo sboceo del coledoco. Perugia, Santucci, 1887. 18 pp.
Sulla tonicità dello sfintere del coledoco. Arch. per le sci. med., 12: 333–339, 1888

driozola, E. See D. A. Carrion

'Dwyer, Joseph P. Cleveland physician. 1841–1898
'UBES—
Intubation of the larynx. New York med. J., 42: 145–147, Aug. 8, 1885
Analysis of fifty cases of croup treated by intubation of the larynx. Ibid., 47: 33–37, Jan. 14, 1888

ehler, Johannes. German physician. 1879–
YMPTOM—coldness and pallor of feet in intermittent claudication.
Über einen bemerkenswerten Fall von Dyskinesia intermittens brachiorum. Arch. klin. Med., 92: 154–165, Nov. 19, 1907

ertel, Max Joseph. Munich physician. 1835–1897
REATMENT—of heart and circulatory diseases.
Therapie der Kreislaufs-Störungen, Kraftabnahme des Herzmuskels, ungenügender Compensationen bei Herzfehlern, Fettherz und Fettsucht, Veränderungen im Lungenkreislauf, etc. Leipzig, Vogel, 1884. 304 pp.

ffer, Th. R. Vienna chemist
EST—for uric acid.
Phosphormolybdänsäure als Reagens auf Harnsäure. Zbl. Physiol., 8: 801–802, Mar. 9, 1895

fficer, R. See E. T. C. Milligan

gata, Masaki. Tokyo physician
ROTH—porphyra infusion, for isolation and cultivation of protozoa (infusoria).
Ueber die Reinkultur gewisser Protozoen (Infusorien). Zbl. Bakt., 14: 165–169 (168), Aug. 7, 1893
Proved that flea is vector of buobonic plague.
Ueber die Pestepidemie in Formosa. Ibid., 1 Abt., 21: 769–777, June 24, 1897
Transmitted rat-bite fever to guinea pigs by causing rats to bite them.
Über die Aetiologie der Rattenbisskrankheit. Mitt. a. d. med. Fakult. d. k. Univ. z. Tokyo, 8: 287–326, 1909

gata, Tonrosaburo. Tokyo physician
ETHOD—silver, for chromaffin cells.
Über die Henle'sche Chromreaktion der sogenannten chromaffinen Zellen und den mikrochemischen Nachweis des Adrenalins with A. Ogata, Beitr. z. path. Anat. u. z. allg Path., 71: 376–387, 1923

gino, Kyusaku. Japanese gynecologist
HEORY—of "safe Period" for intercourse.
Ovulationstermin und Konzeptionstermin. Zbl. Gynäk., 54: 464–479, Feb. 22, 1930
Über den Konzeptionstermin des Weibes und seine Anwendung in der Praxis. Ibid., 56: 721–732, Mar. 19, 1932
Conception periods of women. Harrisburg, Pa., Med. Arts Pub. Co., 1934

Ogston, Sir Alexander. Aberdeen surgeon. 1844–1929
OPERATION—
The operative treatment of genu valgum. Edinburgh med. J., 22: 782–784, Mar. 1877
OPERATION—
On flat-foot, and its cure by operation. Bristol med.-chir. J., 2: 1–20, Mar. 1884
A new principle of curing club-foot in severe cases in children a few years old. Brit. med. J., 1:1524–1526, June 21, 1902
OPERATION—
Trephining the frontal sinuses for catarrhal diseases. Med. Chronicle, 1: 235–238, Dec. 1884

Oguro, Y. Japanese physician
TEST—for albumin in urine.
Neue Proben zum Nachweis von Eiweiss im Harn. Z. exp. Path. Ther., 7: 349–351, 1909

Ohara, Hachiro. Japanese physician
DISEASE—tularemia.
Über Identität von „Yato-Byo" (Ohara's disease) und „Tularämie", sowie ihren Erreger. Zbl. Bakt., 1 Abt., 117: 440–450, July 28, 1930

O'Hara, Michael. Philadelphia gynecologist. 1869–1926
CLAMP—
A method of performing anastomosis of hollow viscera by means of a new instrument. Amer. J. Obstet., 42: 81–90, July 1900

Ohira, Tokuzo. Japanese physician. 1882–
SOLUTION—glucose ascitis fluid; culture medium.
The cultivation of trichomonas of the human mouth (Tetratrichomonas hominis) with H. Noguchi, J. exp. Med., 25: 341–347, Feb. 1, 1917

Ohlmacher, Albert Philip. Cleveland physician. 1865–1916
PROCESS—formaldehyde, for nuclear staining.
Some notes on the use of formalin as a mordant in anilin-staining. Med. News, 66: 184–185, Feb. 16, 1895
SOLUTION—alcohol of sublimate, for fixing.
STAIN—acid fuchsin, for myelin.
Technical note. I. A modified fixing fluid for general histological and neuro-histological purposes. II. A staining combination of gentian violet and picro-acid fuchsin. J. exp. Med., 2: 671–676, Nov. 1897

Oka, Mitsutoma. Japanese physician
Introduced thorium dioxide. ("Thorotrast").
Eine neue Methode zur röntgenologischen Darstellung der Milz (kienographie). Fort. a. d. Geb. d. Röntgenstr., Leipzig, 40: 497–501, Sept. 1929

Okada, Seizaburo. Tokyo physician
TEST—
On the estimation of amino-acid nitrogen in the blood. J. biol. Chem., 33: 325–331, Feb. 1918

Oken, Lorenz. German physiologist. 1779–1851
THEORY—vertebral, of skull.
Über die Bedeutung der Schädelknochen. Jena, 1807

Oldekop, A. Dorpat physician
AGAR—neutral red glucose extract; for differentiation between coli and typhoid bacteria.
Eine Modifikation des Rotherger-Schefferschen Neutrolrotnährbodens. Zbl. Bakt., 35: 120–124, Nov. 5, 1903

O'Leary, J. L. See H. G. Schwartz

Olef, Isadore. Boston physician. 1897–
METHOD—
Blood platelets: an improved indirect method for their

Der Sehnen und die Nebenhöhlen der Nase. . . .
Wien, Hölder, 1907. 69 pp.
Die Nebenhöhlen der Nase beim Kinde. . . . Würzburg, Katitzsch, 1911. 102 pp.
Onslow, H. See S. W. Cole
Ophüls, W. See P. K. Brown
Opie, Eugene Lindsay. Baltimore pathologist. 1873–
Demonstrated sexual conjugation in malarial parasites.
On the haemocytozoa of birds. J. exp. Med., 3: 79–101, Jan. 1898
Did important work on pancreatic diabetes.
On the relation of chronic interstitial pancreatitis to the islands of Langerhans and to diabetes mellitus. Ibid., 5: 397–428, Jan. 15, 1901
The relation of diabetes mellitus to lesions of the pancreas. Hyaline degeneration of the islands of Langerhans. Ibid., 5: 527–540, Mar. 25, 1901
Wrote—
The influence of diet on hepatic necrosis and toxicity of chloroform with L. B. Alford, J. A. M. A., 62: 895–896, Mar. 21, 1914
Opitz, Hans. Breslau pediatrician. 1888–
Syndrome—
Zur Kenntnis der thrombophlebitischen Splenomegalie. Jb. Kinderheilk., 107: 211–222, Nov. 1924
Oppenheim, Hermann. Berlin neurologist. 1858–1919
DISEASE or SYNDROME—congenital myotonia.
Ueber allgemeine und localisierte Atonie der Muskulatur (Myatonie) in frühen Kindesalter. Mschr. Psychiat. Nrurol., 8: 232–233, Sept. 1900
DISEASE—dystonia musculorum deformans.
Über eine eigenartige Krampfkrankheit des kindlichen und jugendlichen Alters (Dysbasia lordotica progressiva, Dystonia musculorum deformans). Neurol. Zbl., 30: 1090–1107, Oct. 1, 1911
REFLEX or SIGN—
Zur Pathologie der Hautreflexe an den unteren Extremitäten. Mschr. Psychiat. Neurol., 12: 421–423, 1902
Oppenheim, Moritz. Vienna dermatologist. 1876–
Described necrobiosis lipoidica diabeticorum.
Über eine bisher nicht beschriebene, mit eigentümlicher lipoider Degeneration der Elastica und des Bindegewebes einhergehende chronische Dermatose bei Diabetes mellitus. Arch. Dermat. Syphil., 166: 576–583, Oct. 21, 1932
See also R. Müller
Oppenheimer, E. T. See A. M. Master
Oppenheimer, G. D. See B. B. Crohn
Oppler, Bruno. Berlin physician
BACILLUS—
Zur Kenntniss des Mageninhalts beim Carcinoma ventriculi. Dtsch. med. Wschr., 21: 73–75, Jan. 31, 1895
Ord, William Miller. English surgeon. 1834–1902
Gave name myxedema.
On myxedema, a term proposed to be applied to an essential condition in the "cretinoid" affection occasionally observed in middle-aged women. Med.-chir. Trans., 2 s., 43: 57–78, 1878
Ordway, Thomas. Albany, N. Y. physician. 1877–
Reported—
Occupational injuries due to radium: report of cases. J. A. M. A., 64: 1–6, Jan. 1, 1916

Reported—
Remissions in leukemia produced by radium in 'cases completely resistant to x-ray and benzol treatment. Boston M. and S. J., 176: 490–503, Apr. 5, 1917
See also V. C. Jacobsen
Oré, Pierre Cyprien. French physician
TRANSFUSION—
Thèses . . . 1. *Recherches expérimentales sur la transfusion du sang.* Bordeaux, Gounouilhou, 1865. 57 pp.
Études historiques et physiologiques sur la transfusion du sang. Paris, Baillière, 1868. 189 pp.
Orent, Elsa R. See H. D. Kruse
Orr, Hiram Winnett. Lincoln, Neb. surgeon. 1877–
TREATMENT—
A new method of treatment for infections of bone. Trans. Sect. Orthop. Surg., Amer. Med. Ass., pp. 138–144, 1923
The treatment of osteomyelitis and other infected wounds by drainage and rest. S. G. O., 45: 446–464, Oct. 1927
Orr, Paul Frederick. American physician. 1898–
BOUILLON—glucose heart.
Studies on Bacillus botulinus. J. med. Res., 42: 127–136 (128), Nov. 1920–Jan. 1921
Orr, Thomas Grover. Kansas City surgeon. 1884–
TECHNIC—
Resection of duodenum and head of pancreas for carcinoma of the ampulla. S. G. O., 73: 240–243, Aug. 1941
TECHNIC—(one stage procedure)
In discussion of paper by S. C. Harvey and A. W. Oughterson: *The surgery of carcinoma of the pancreas and ampullary region.* Ann. Surg., 115: 1066–1090 (1087), June 1942
Pancreaticoduodenectomy for carcinoma of the ampulla and ampullary region. Surgery, 18: 144–158, Aug. 1945
Orr-Ewing, J. See E. Chain
Orskov, J. Denmark bacteriologist
METHOD—
Method for the isolation of bacteria in pure culture from single cells and procedure for the direct tracing of bacteriological growth on a solid medium. J. Bact., 7: 537–549, Nov. 1922
Orth, Johannes J. Berlin pathologist. 1847–1923
SOLUTION—histologic fixation s.
Ueber die Verwendung des Formaldehyd im pathologischen Institut in Göttingen. Berl. klin. Wschr., 33: 273–275, Mar. 30, 1896
STAIN—(Mallory)
(Lithium carmine.) In: *Pathologisch-anatomische Diagnostik.* Berlin, Hirschwald, 1900. 6 Ed., p. 25
Orthmann, Ernst Gottlob. German physician. 1858–1922
TUMOR—same as Brenner's t.; oophoroma folliculare.
Ueber die Entstehungsweisen der Sactosalpingen und Tubo-Ovarialcysten. Arch. path. Anat., 155: 220–234, 1899
Ortmayer, Maris. See R. Schindler
Ortolff, Bayrlant von. circa 1400
Wrote first German pharmacopoeia.
Ein artzbuch. Nürenberg, Koburger, 1477
Osborne, Earl Dorland. Rochester, Minn. physician. 1895
Introduced—
Roentgenography of urinary tract during excretion of sodium iodid with C. G. Sutherland, A. J. Scholl and

L. G. Rowntree, J. A. M. A., 80: 368–373, Feb. 10, 1923

Osborne, S. L. See C. A. Neymann

Osborne, Thomas Burr. New Haven biochemist. 1859–

Discovered vitamin A.

The influence of butter-fat on growth with L. B. Mendel, J. biol. Chem., 16: 423–437, Dec. 1913

The incidence of phosphatic calculi in rats fed on experimental rations with L. B. Mendel and E. L. Ferry, J. A. M. A., 69: 32–33, July 7, 1917

Osgood, Edwin Eugene. Portland, Ore. physician. 1899–

METHOD—

A new permanent standard for estimation of hemoglobin by the acid hematin method with H. D. Haskins, J. biol. Chem., 57: 107–110, Aug. 1923

A simplification of the Osgood-Haskins hemoglobin method with H. D. Haskins and F. E. Trotman, J. Lab. clin. Med., 16: 482–486, Feb. 1931

METHOD—for staining reticulocytes.

Reticulocytes with Mable M. Wilhelm, Ibid., 19: 1129–1135, July 1934

Reported—

Culture of human bone marrow. Preliminary report with A. N. Muscovitz, J. A. M. A., 106: 1888–1890, May 30, 1936

Culture of human bone marrow; a simple method for multiple cultures with Inez E. Brownlee, Ibid., 107: 123 (only), July 11, 1936

See also H. D. Haskins

Osgood, Robert Bayley. Boston surgeon. 1873–

DISEASE—

Lesions of the tibial tubercle occurring during adolescence. Boston Med. and Surg. J., 148: 114–117, Jan. 29, 1903

OPERATION—

A method of osteotomy of the lower end of the femur in cases of permanent flexion of the knee-joint. Amer. J. Orthop. Surg., 11: 336–346, Oct. 1913

OPERATION—

Radiohumeral bursitis, epicondylitis, epicondylalgia (tennis elbow). A personal experience. Arch. Surg., 4: 420–433, Mar. 1922

See also J. E. Goldthwait

O'Shaughnessy, Laurence. English surgeon. 1900–1940

Performed cardioomentopexy.

An experimental method of providing a collateral circulation to the heart. Brit. J. Surg., 23: 665–670, Jan. 1936

Surgical treatment of cardiac ischaemia. Lancet, 1: 185–194, Jan. 23, 1937

See also E. F. Sauerbruch

Osler, Sir William. Canadian, American and English physician. 1849–1919

DISEASE—

Chronic cyanosis, with polycythemia and enlarged spleen: a new clinical entity. Amer. J. med. Sci., 126: 187–201, Aug. 1903

Also: Trans. Ass. Amer. Phys., 18: 299–325, 1903

Also: Med. Classics, 4: 254–275, Nov. 1939

DISEASE—Rendu-Osler-Weber's d.

On a family form of recurring epistaxis, associated with multiple telangiectases of the skin and mucous

membranes. Johns Hopk. Hosp. Bull., 12: 333–337 Nov. 1901

Also: Med. Classics, 4: 243–253, Nov. 1939

On multiple hereditary telangiectases with recurring hemorrhages. Quart. J. Med., 1: 53–58, Oct. 1907

Also: Med. Classics, 4: 276–283, Nov. 1939

NODES, SIGNS or SPOTS—small, painful, erythematous swellings in skin of hands and feet in malignant endocarditis.

The Gulstonian lectures on malignant endocarditis. Brit. med. J., 1: 467–470, 1885

Chronic infectious endocarditis. Quart. J. Med., 2: 219–230, 1909

Also, abstr. in F. A. Willius and T. E. Keys' *Cardiac Classics.* St. Louis, Mosby, 1941. pp. 807–811

PHENOMENON—aggregation of blood platelets which takes place as soon as blood is withdrawn from body. 1881

On certain problems in the physiology of the blood-corpuscles. I. The blood-plaque or third corpuscle. II. Degeneration and regeneration of the corpuscles. III. The relation of the corpuscles to coagulation and thrombosis. The Cartwright Lectures. Med. News, 48: 365–370; 393–399; 421–424, 1886

Also: Med. Rec., 29: 377–381; 405–410; 433–436, 1886

Also: Med. Classics, 4: 178–225, Nov. 1939

SYNDROME—

On some of the effects of the chronic impaction of gallstones in the bile-passages, and on the "fièvre intermittente hépatique" of Charcot. Med. Times and Gaz., 2: 111–114, 1881

A clinical lecture on the ball-valve gall-stone in the common duct. Lancet, 1: 1319–1323, 1897

Also: Med. Classics, 4: 226–242, Nov. 1939

Discovered blood platelets, Oct. 6, 1873

An account of certain organisms occurring in the liquor sanguinis. Proc. roy. Soc., 22: 391–398, 1873–4

Described—

On the visceral complications of erythema exudativum multiforme. Amer. J. med. Sci., 110: 629–646, 1895

On the surgical importance of the visceral crises in the erythema group of skin diseases. Ibid., 127: 751–754, May 1904

Osnato, Michael. New York neurologist. 1883–

Showed that diffuse parenchymatous degeneration of brain following head injury may closely resemble lesion of encephalitis, of whatever cause.

Postconcussion neuritis—traumatic encephalitis: a conception of postconcussion phenomena with V. Giliberti, Arch. Neurol. Psychiat., 18: 181–214, Aug. 1927

Ost, Hermann. German chemist

REAGENT—for determining glucose.

Die Bestimmung der Zuckerarten mit Kupferkaliumcarbonatlösung. Ber. dtsch. chem. Ges., 23: 3003–3011, 1890

Osterberg, Arnold Erwin. Rochester, Minn. biochemist. 1894–

METHOD—

A modification of the electrolytic Gutzeit apparatus for the estimation of arsenic in biological material. J. biol. Chem., 76: 19–22, Jan. 1928

See also S. B. Harper, A. H. Sanford, B. Sepulveda, A. M. Snell

Ostwalt, Dr. Paris surgeon
INJECTION—for tic douloureux.
  Traitement des névralgies rebelles par les injections profondes d'alcool. Pr. méd., No. 101, 812–813, Dec. 16, 1905

Osumi, S. See K. Futaki

Oszacki, Alexander. Polish physician. 1883–
REAGENT—for dealbuminating blood serum.
  Über Enteiweissung und Reststickstoffbestimmung des Blutes und seröser Flüssigkeiten mittels Uranilazetat. Zbl. inn. Med., 33: 1165–1168, Nov. 23, 1912

Otaki, Ikusaburo. Japanese physician
SOLUTION—sodium citrate blood extract.
  A new medium for the cultivation of the typhoid group of organisms in blood with C. Akimoto, Kitasato Arch. Exper. Med., 5: 101–108, Nov. 1922

Otis, Arthur Sinton. California scientist. 1886–
TEST—of intelligence.
  A criticism of the Yerkes-Bridges point scale, with alternative suggestions. J. Educ. Psychol., 8: 129–150, Mar. 1917

Otis, Fessenden Nott. New York urologist. 1825–1900
OPERATION—
  Remarks on strictures of the urethra of extreme calibre, with cases, and a description of new instruments for their treatment. New York med. J., 15: 152–174, Feb. 1872
  Used local anesthesia in urology.
  The hydrochlorate of cocaine in genito-urinary procedures. Ibid., 40: 635–637, Dec. 6, 1884

Ott, Adolf. Prag chemist
TEST—
  Ueber Nucleoalbumin im menschlichen Harne. Verh. XIII Kong. Inn. Med., pp. 496–502, 1895

Ott, Isaac A. American physiologist. 1847–1916
Wrote—
  The relation of the nervous system to the temperature of the body. J. nerv. ment. Dis., 11: 141–152, Apr. 1884

Ott, L. H. See I. Friedman

Ott, W. O. See A. W. Adson

Otten, Max. German physician. 1877–
Diagnosed primary carcinoma of lung by means of Roentgen rays.
  Zur Röntgen-Diagnostik der primären Lungencarcinome. Fort. a. d. Geb. d. Röntgenstrah., 9: 369–376, 1905–06

Ottenberg, Reuben. New York physician. 1882–
Developed clinical methods for typing human blood.
  Studies in isoagglutination. I. Transfusion and the question of intravascular agglutination. J. exp. Med., 13: 425–438, Apr. 1, 1911
  Accidents in transfusion; their prevention by preliminary blood examination: based on an experience of one hundred twenty-eight transfusions with D. J. Kaliski, J. A. M. A., 61: 2138–2140, Dec. 13, 1913
  Established jurisprudence of paternity by blood groupings.
  Medicolegal application of human blood grouping. J. A. M. A., 77: 682–683, Aug. 27, 1921
  (Same) *Second communication.* Ibid., 78: 873–877, Mar. 25, 1922
  (Same) *Third communication: sources of error in blood group tests, and criteria of reliability in investigations on heredity of blood groups.* Ibid., 79: 2137–

2143, Dec. 23, 1922
  See also A. A. Epstein

Otto, John Conrad. Philadelphia physician. 1774–1844
Described hemophilia.
  An account of an hemorrhagic disposition existing in certain families. Med. Repository, N. Y., 61: 1–4, 1803

Otto, Richard Ernst Wilhelm. German pathologist. 1868–
See Theobald Smith
METHOD—modified Koch m., for potency of old tuberculin.
  Die staatliche Prüfung der Heilsera und des Tuberkulins with H. Hetsch, Arb. a. d. Staatsinst. f. exp. Therapie, No. 13, 1921. 116 pp. p. 107
Described—
  Das Theobald Smithsche Phänomen der Serum-Überfindlichkeit. In: Gedenkschr. f. d. verstorb. Generalstabsarzt . . . von Leuthold. Berlin, 1: 153–172, 1906

Ottolenghi, Donato. Italian physician. 1874–
SOLUTION—nitrate bile; culture medium for cholera vibrio.
  Ueber eine neue Methode zur Isolierung der Choleravibrionen aus den Faeces. Zbl. Bakt., 58: 369–375 (370), Apr. 19, 1911

Oudard, P. French surgeon
OPERATION—for recurrent dislocation of shoulder.
  La luxation récidivante de l'épaule (variété antérointerne). Pr. méd., 1: 201–202, Feb. 15, 1928

Oughterson, A. W. See I. Friedman

Ould, Sir Fielding. Irish obstetrician. 1710–1789
Wrote—
  A treatise of midwifery. Dublin, Nelson and Connor, 1742. 203 pp.

Overholt, Richard Hollis. Boston surgeon. 1901–
TECHNIC—
  Extrapleural pneumothorax in the treatment of pulmonary tuberculosis: a preliminary report with O. S. Tubbs, J. Thoracic Surg., 7: 591–604, June 1938
TREATMENT—
  The treatment of pulmonary abscess by peripheral lung fixation and regional thoracoplasty. Ibid., 3: 134–152, Dec. 1933
  Thoracoplasty with lung mobilization. Part I. The first-stage operation. Part II. The second- and subsequent stage operations. Amer. Rev. Tuberc., 35: 411–442, Apr. 1937

Owen, C. A. See H. P. Smith, S. E. Ziffren

Owen, D. R. See E. D. Adrian

Owen, Edmund Blackett. English surgeon. 1847–1915
OPERATION—
  Cleft-palate and hare-lip; the earlier operation on the palate. London, Baillière et al., 1904. 111 pp.

Owen, Sir Isambard. London physician. 1850–1927
Described—
  A case of extreme dilatation of the left auricle of the heart with W. J. Fenton, Clin. Soc. Trans., Lond., 34: 183–188, 1901

Owen, Sir Richard. English physician. 1804–1892
THEORY—vertebrate, of origin of skull.
  On the archetype and homologies of the vertebrate skele-

ton. London, Van Vorst, 1848
Described Trichina spiralis.
Description of a microscopic entozoon (Trichina spiralis) infesting the muscles of the human body.
Trans. Zool. Soc., Lond., 1: 315–324, 1835
Also: London Med. Gaz., 16: 125–127, 1834–5
Introduced distinction between serial homologies (organs of similar structure and development) and morphologic analogies (different organs of similar function).
Lectures on the comparative anatomy and physiology

of the invertebrate animals. London, Longma*
1843. 392 pp.
Owen, Robert W. Goldsborough. Detroit bacter
ologist. 1882–
TRYPSIN BEEF TEA—
*Trypsin broth—an ideal medium for making bloo
cultures* with F. A. Martin and W. G. Pitts, J. La*
clin. Med., 2: 198–199, Dec. 1916
Owens, F. M., Jr. See L. R. Dragstedt, H. P. Jenkin
Oxford
UNIT—of penicillin; same as Florey unit, q. v.

P

Pacchioni, Antonius. Italian anatomist. 1665–1726
BODIES—
DEPRESSIONS—for bodies.
Diss. epistolaris de glandulis conglobatis durae meningis humanae. Rome, 1705
Pachon, Michel Victor. French physiologist. 1867–1939
OSCILLOMETER—
Sur la méthode des oscillations et les conditions correctes de son emploi en sphygmomanométrie clinique. C. R. Soc. Biol., 66: 733–735, May 8, 1909
Paci, Agostino. Pisa surgeon
OPERATION—for congenital dislocation of hip.
Della lussazione iliaca commune congenita del femore— Illustrazione clinica e anatomo-patologica— Ana razionale ortopedica. Trans. 11. Internat. Med. Cong., Rome, 378–411, 1894
Della lussazione commune congenita del femore e della sua cura razionale incruenta. Arch. di ortop., 13, 1896
Pacini, A. E. Chicago chemist
TEST—
An improved color test for vitamin A with M. H. Taras, J. Amer. Pharm. Ass., 26: 721–723, Aug. 1937
Pacini, Filippo. Italian anatomist. 1812–1883
FLUID or SOLUTION—used in microscopic examination of blood.
Sur quelques methodes de preparation et de conservation des elements microscopiques des tissus animaux et vegetaux. J. Mikr., 4: 136–142, Apr.–May; 191–196, June–July; 235–236, Aug.–Sept. 1880
Pack, G. T. See F. P. Underhill
Padgett, Earl Calvin. Kansas City surgeon. 1893–1946
METHOD—
Calibrated intermediate skin grafts. S. G. O., 69: 779–793, Dec. 1939
Skin grafting. Springfield, Ill., Thomas, 1942. 149 pp.
OPERATION—
Total reconstruction of the auricle. S. G. O., 67: 761–768, Dec. 1938
Padlewsky, Leon. Polish microbiologist. 1870–
AGAR—malachite green bile; for detection of typhoid group bacilli.
Eine neue Anwendungsmethode des Malachitgrünagars zum Nachweis von Bacillen der Typhusgruppe. Zbl. Bakt., 47: 540–544 (543), 1908
Page, A. B. See C. M. Carpenter
Page, Charles Max. English surgeon. 1882–
OPERATION—for Volkman's ischemic contracture.
An operation for the relief of flexion-contracture in the

forearm. J. Bone and Joint Surg., 5: 233–234, Ap*
1923
Page, F. J. M. See J. S. Burdon-Sanderson
Page, Herbert William. London surgeon. 1845–192
DISEASE—nervous shock.
Railway injuries. London, 1891
Page, Irvine Heinly. American physician. 1901–
TEST—
A simple test for plasma protein contents belo
the edema-producing level* with D. D. Van Slyke
J. A. M. A., 99: 1344 (only), Oct. 15, 1932
See also A. C. Corcoran, E. Kirk
Pagenstecher, Alexander. German ophthalmo*
ogist. 1828–1879
OPERATION—
*Ueber die Extraktion des grauen Staares bei uneröf
neter Kavsel durch den Srleralschnitt.* (1866). 37 pp
Pagès, C. See N. M. Arthus
Paget, Sir James. English surgeon. 1814–1899
ABSCESS—
On residual abscesses. St. Bartholomew's Hosp. Rep.
5: 73–79, 1869
DISEASE—of bone; osteitis deformans.
*On a form of chronic inflammation of bones—osteiti
deformans.* Med.-chir. Trans., 60: 37–64, 1877
Also: Gaz. d. hop., Paris, 52: 705–708, 1879
Also: *Selected essays.* London, New Sydenham Soc.
1901. pp. 199–223
Also: Med. classics, 1: 29–59, Sept. 1936
Additional cases of osteitis deformans. Ibid., 65: 225–236, 1882
Also: Med. classics, 1: 60–71, Sept. 1936
DISEASE—of nipple; (CELLS)—found in this con
dition, but not described by Paget.
On disease of the mammary areola preceding cancer o
the mammary gland.* St. Bartholomew's Hosp. Rep.
10: 87–89, 1874
Also: *Selected essays.* London, New Sydenham Soc.
1901. pp. 195–197
Also: Med. classics, 1: 75–78, Sept. 1936
TUMOR—
Recurring fibroid and fibro-nucleated tumors. In
Lectures on surgical pathology. London, Longman
1853. vol. 2, p. 155
Made early note on erythromelalgia (Weir Mitchell's
disease).
Clinical lecture on some cases of local paralysis. Med
Times and Gaz., 1: 331–332, Mar. 26, 1864
Discovered Trichina spiralis.
Account of the trichina spiralis. Trans. Abernethian
Soc., 1835

See note in St. Bartholomew's Hosp. Rep., 4: 276–277, 1868

agniez, Philippe. French physician
Demonstrated connection between clot retraction and number of platelets.
Aperçu sur l'état actuel de la question des plaquettes sanguines. Arch. d. mal. du coeur, 2: 1–33 (18–21), Jan. 1909

aine, A. See F. J. Poynton

aine, J. R. See O. H. Wangensteen

aine, S. G. See H. G. Plimmer

ainter, Charles Fairback. Boston surgeon. 1869–
APPROACH—to sacro-iliac joint.
OPERATION—
Excision of the os innominatum. Arthrodesis of the sacro-iliac synchondrosis. Boston Med. and Surg. J., 159: 207–208, Aug. 13, 1908
See also J. E. Goldthwait

ainter, T. S. See H. J. Muller

ajot, Charles. French obstetrician. 1816–1896
HOOK—for decapitating fetus.
De la présentation de l'épaule dans les rétrécissements extrêmes du bassin, et d'un nouveau procédé d'embryotomie. Paris, Osselin, 1865. 15 pp.

al, Jakob. Vienna physician. 1863–1936
METHOD or STAIN—for myelin sheath. Mallory.
Ein Beitrag zur Nervenfärbetechnik. Med. Jahrb., Wien, 233; 619–631, 1886
Advocated use of papaverine for relief of smooth muscle spasm.
Das Papaverin als Gefässmittel und Anästheticum. Dtsch. med. Wschr., 40: 164–168, Jan. 22, 1914

alladin, Vladimir Ivanovitch. St. Petersburg physician. 1859–1922
SOLUTION—basal ammonium phosphate.
Ueber normale und intramolekulare Atmung der einzelligen Alge Chlorothecium saccharophilum. Zbl. Bakt., 2 Abt., 11: 146–153, Nov. 11, 1903

allen, Montrose Anderson. American gynecologist. 1836–1890
Performed immediate trachelorrhaphy.
On some of the accidents of parturition requiring surgical treatment. Richmond and Louisville J., 17: 544–571, May 1874

almer, Walter Lincoln. Chicago physician. 1896–
ACID TEST—
The "acid test" in gastric and duodenal ulcer: clinical value of experimental production of the typical distress. J. A. M. A., 88: 1778–1780, June 4, 1927
See also L. R. Dragstedt

almer, Walter Walker. New York physician. 1882–
DETERMINATION—
The colorimetric determination of hemoglobin. J. biol. Chem., 33: 119–126, Jan. 1918
See also L. J. Henderson

altauf, Richard. Vienna pathologist. 1858–1924
DISEASE—
Lymphosarkom (Lymphosarkomatose, Pseudoleukämie, Myelom, Chlorom). Ergebn. d. allg. Path. u. path. Anat., 3, 1: 652–691, 1897

anas, Photinos. Greek surgeon. 1832–1903
PERATION—
Du traitement des rétrécissements du rectum par la rectotomie externe. Gaz. des Hôp., 45: 1148–1149, Dec. 1872

OPERATION—
D'un nouveau procédé opératoire applicable au ptosis congénital et au ptosis paralytique. Arch. Ophthal., 6: 1–14, 1886

Panayotatou, A. See Maud Crendiropoulo

Pancoast, Henry Khunrath. Philadelphia roentgenologist. 1875–1939
SYNDROME—
Importance of careful roentgen ray investigation of apical chest tumors. J. A. M. A., 83: 1407–1411, Nov. 1, 1924
Superior pulmonary sulcus tumor; tumor characterized by pain, Horner's syndrome, destruction of bone and atrophy of hand muscles. Ibid., 99: 1391–1396, Oct. 22, 1932

Pancoast, Joseph. New Jersey surgeon. 1805–1882
Performed, successfully, in February, 1858–
(Plastic operation for exstrophy of the bladder in the male.) Reported by S. D. Gross, North Amer. Med.-Chir. Rev., Philadelphia, 3: 710–711, 1859
Advocated—
New operation for the relief of persistent facial neuralgia. Reported by F. Woodbury, Philadelphia med. Times, 2: 285–287, May 1, 1872

Pander, Heinrich Christian von. German anatomist. 1794–1865
Recognized three germ layers.
Dissertatio sistens historiam metamorphoseos, quam ovum incubatum prioribusque quinque diebus subit. Wirceburgi, Nitribitt, 1817. 69 pp.

Pandy, K. Budapest physician. 1868–
TEST—
Über eine neue Eiweissprobe für die Cerebrospinalflüssigkeit. Neurol. Zbl., 29: 915–919, Sept. 1, 1910

Pane, Nicola. Naples physician
SERUM—antipneumococcic.
Richerche sull'immunizzazione del conigli contro il bacillo setticoemico dello sputo mediante inoculazione batterio virulento. Riv. Clin. e Therapeut., 14: 641–655, Nov. 1892

Paneth, Josef. German anatomist. 1857–1890
CELLS—in crypts of Lieberkühn.
Ueber die secernirenden Zellen des Dünndarm-Epithels. Arch. mikr. Anat., 31: 113–191, 1888

Panizza, Bartolomeo. Italian physician. 1785–1867
Localized visual function in posterior part of cerebellum and noted relation of optic thalamus to opposite-sided sensation, especially in eye. Garrison
Osservazioni sul nervo ottico. Giorn. R. Ist. Lomb. di Sci., Milano, 7: 237–252, 1855

Pansa, Martin. German physician
Wrote on occupational diseases. Garrison and Morton
Consilium peripneumoniacum. Leipzig, Schürer, 1614

Pansch, Adolf. German anatomist. 1841–1887
FISSURE—
De sulcis et gyris in cerebris simiarum et hominum. Kiliae, Mohr, 1866. 42 pp.

Panum, Peter Ludwig. Swedish physician. 1820–1885
Wrote classical paper on measles.
Iagttagelser, anstillede under Maeslinge-Epidemien paa Faeroene i Aaret 1846. Bibliothek for Laeger, Copenhagen, 3 R., 1: 270–344, 1847
Also, transl. by Ada S. Hatcher: Med. Classics, 3: 828–886, May 1939

Also, transl. by Ada S. Hatcher: New York, Delta Omega Soc., 1940

Precipitated protein by neutral salts.

Neue Beobachtungen über die eisweissartigen Körper. Arch. path. Anat., 4: 419–467, 1852

Investigated chemical products of putrefaction.

Bidrag til Laeren om den saakaldte putride eller septiske Infection. Bibl. f. Laeger, Kjobenhavn, 4 R., 8: 253–285, 1856

Also, abstr.: Jahrb. f. inn. u. ausland. ges. Med. Leipzig, 101: 213–217, 1859

Studied experimental pathology of embolism.

Experimentelle Beiträge zur Lehre von der Embolie. Arch. path. Anat., 25: 308–338; 433–530, 1862

Also: *Experimentelle Untersuchungen zur Physiologie und Pathologie der Embolie, Trasnfusion, und Blutmenge.* Berlin, Reimer, 1864. 286 pp.

Advised transfusion of defibrinated blood.

Experimentelle Untersuchungen ueber die Transfusion, Transplantation oder Substitution des Blutes in theoretischer und practischer Beziehung. Arch. path. Anat., 27: 240–295; 433–459, 1863

Papanicolaou, George Nicholas. New York physician. 1883–

METHOD—vaginal smear.

SOLUTION—

The sexual cycle in the human female as revealed by vaginal smears. Amer. J. Anat., (suppl.), 52: 519–616, May 15, 1933

Action of ovarian follicle hormone in ovarian insufficiency in women as indicated by vaginal smears with E. Shorr, Proc. Soc. exp. Biol., N. Y., 32: 585–587, Jan. 1935

The action of ovarian follicular hormone in the menopause, as indicated by vaginal smears with E. Shorr, Amer. J. Obstet. Gynaec., 31: 806–831, May 1936

See also C. R. Stockard

Papin, Denis. French physicist. 1647–1710

DIGESTER—apparatus for subjecting substances to action of water at a heat greater than boiling-point. Dorland.

La manière d'amolir les os, et de faire cuire toutes sortes de viandes en fort peu de temps, et à peu de frais; avec une description de la machine dont il se faut servir pour cet effet, ses propriétez et ses usages, confirme: par plusieurs expériences. Nouvellement inventé. Paris, Michallet, 1682. 164 pp.

Pappenheim, Artur. German physician. 1870–1917

STAIN—for differentiating between basophilic granulations of red cells and nuclear fragments.

Eine panoptische Triazidfärbung. Dtsch. med. Wschr., 27: 798–799, Nov. 14, 1901

STAIN—for plasma cells.

Vergleichende Untersuchungen über die elementare Zusammensetzung des rothen Knochenmarkes einige Säugethiere. Arch. path. Anat. u. Physiol., 157: 19–76, Aug. 10, 1899

STAIN—for tubercle bacilli.

Befund von Smegmabacillen im menschlichen Lungenauswurf. Berl. klin. Wschr., 35: 809–814, Sept. 12, 1898

Grundriss der Farbchemie zum Gebrauch bei mikroskopischen Arbeiten. Berlin, Hirschwald, 1901. 476 pp.

Paquelin, Claude André. French physician. 1836–1905

CAUTERY—

Du cautère Paquelin. Bull. gén. de thérap., 93: 145–158, 1877

Paquin, Paul. American physician. 1860–1916

SERUM—

Anti-tubercle serum: the treatment of consumption by serotherapy—report and presentation of cases treated—exhibition of serum, etc. J. A. M. A., 24: 341–346, Mar. 9, 1895

Observations on some criticisms of serum therapy. The action of serum on the blood. The results of serum therapy in tuberculosis. New York med. J., 63: 732–738, June 6, 1896

Papacostas, G. See J. Gaté

Pappenheim See J. E. v. Purkinje

Pappenheimer, A. M. See C. Norris

Paraf, J. See J. A. Sicard

Pardee, Harold Ensign Bennett. New York physician. 1886–

SIGN—

An electrocardiographic sign of the coronary artery obstruction. Arch. intern. Med., 26: 244–257, Aug. 1920

Paré, Ambroise. French surgeon. 1509–1590

Father of French surgery, reformed treatment of gun-shot wounds, substituted ligation of arteries for cauterization, etc.

La methode de traicter les playes faictes par hacquebutes et aultres bastons à feu; . . . Paris, Ches viuan Gaulterot, 1545

Also: *The method of curing wounds made by gun-shot. Also by arrowes and darts, with their accidents.* Transl. by W. Hamond, London, Iaggard, 1617

Les oeuvres. Paris, Chez G. Buon, 1575

Also: *The workes . . .* transl. by Th. Johnson, London, Cotes and Young, 1634

Parham, Frederick William. New Orleans surgeon. 1856–1927

BAND—

A new device for the treatment of fracture with E. D. Martin, New Orleans Med. and Surg. J., 66: 451, 465–467, 1913–14

Device for treatment of fractures with E. D. Martin Mod. Hosp., 6: 75, 1916

Circular constriction in treatment of fractures of long bones. S. G. O., 23: 541–544, 1916

Wrote—

Thoracic resection for tumors growing from the bony wall of the chest. New Orleans, 1899. 147 pp.

Parinaud, Henri. French ophthalmologist. 1844–1905

CONJUNCTIVITIS—

Conjonctivite infectieuse paraissant transmise l'homme par les animaux. Rev. d'Ophth., 3 s., 1: 176–180, 1889

OPERATION—

Nouveau procédé opératoire du ptosis. Ann. d'Ocul. 117: 12–17, July 1897

Paris, John Ayrton. English physician. 1785–1856

Described arsenic cancer.

Pharmacologia; or the history of medicinal substances with a view to establish the art of prescribing. . . London, Phillips, 1822. p. 208

Also: New York, Lockwood, 1822. 428 pp. p. 20

Paris, M. French surgeon

Described coarctation of aorta.

Rétrécissement considérable de l'aorte pectorale, o

servé à l' Hôtel Dieu de Paris. J. de chir. de Desault,
2: 107–110, 1791

ºark, William Hallock. New York bacteriologist.
1863–1939
ßROTH—glycerol veal infusion, for cultivation of B.
mallei.
   In: *Pathogenic microorganisms* with Anna W.
Williams and C. Krumwiede, New York, Lea and
Febiger, 1924. p. 122
ßROTH—stomach digest infusion; culture medium.
Ibid., p. 118.
MEDIUM—meat, for culture. Ibid., p. 125.
OLUTION—asparagin salt; culture medium. Ibid.,
p. 122.
OLUTION—whey peptone; culture medium. Ibid.,
p. 134.
OLUTION—litmus glycerol milk; for cultivation of
tubercle bacilli.
   *The relative importance of the bovine and human types
of tubercle bacilli in the different forms of human tu-
berculosis* with C. Krumwiede, Jr., J. med. Res.,
23: 205–368 (215), Oct. 1910
Did valuable work on immunization against diph-
theria. Cecil
   *Duration of antitoxic immunity in man and animals
after diphtheria toxin-antitoxin injections* with A.
Zingher, Arch. Pediat., 34: 278–282, Apr. 1917
   See also M. Brodie
arker, C. H. See J. Dunlop
ºarker, Edward Mason. Washington, D. C. surgeon.
1860–1941
ℝESECTION—
   *Intestinal anastomosis without open incisions by means
of basting stitches* with H. H. Kerr, Johns Hopk.
Hosp. Bull., 19: 132–137, May 1908
arker, Willard. New York surgeon. 1800–1884
NCISION—over area of dullness in appendiceal
abscess.
First, after Hancock of London, to operate for ap-
pendicitis. Garrison
   *An operation for disease of the appendix vermiformis
caeci.* Med. Rec., 2: 25–27, Mar. 1, 1867
Performed cystotomy for inflammation and rupture
of bladder. Garrison
   *Cystitis; lateral operation on the bladder, death; tu-
berculous kidney.* New York Med. J., n. s. 7: 83–86,
July 1851
   Cystitis with rupture of the bladder treated by cystotomy.
Trans. Med. Soc. New York, pp. 345–349, 1867
arkes, A. S. London scientist
Produced abortion in animals with excessive doses of
estrogenic material.
   *Studies on the internal secretions of the ovary: II. The
effects of injection of the oestrus-producing hormone
during pregnancy* with C. W. Bellerby, J. Physiol.,
62: 145–155, Dec. 10, 1926
   See also R. Deanesly
arkinson, J. See L. Wolff
arkinson, James. English surgeon. 1755–1824
ºISEASE—paralysis agitans.
ACIES or SIGN—in paralysis agitans.
   An essay on the shaking palsy. London, Whittingham
and Rowland, 1817. 66 pp.
Also, facsimile ed. Chicago, Amer. Med. Ass. Press,
1917
Also: Arch. Neur. and Psychiat., 7: 681–710, 1922

Also: Med. classics, 2: 964–997, June 1938
Reported the first case of appendicitis in English,
this case being also the first in which perforation was
recognized as the cause of death. H. A. Kelly
   Case of diseased appendix vermiformis. By John
Parkinson, communicated by James Parkinson,
Med.-chir. Trans., 3: 57–58, 1812
Parona, C. and E. See B. Grassi
Parrish, B. F. American surgeon
Performed successful tendon transplantation.
   *A new operation for paralytic talipes valgus, and the
enunciation of a new surgical principle.* New York
med. J., 66: 402–403, Oct. 8, 1892
Parrot, Joseph Marie Jules. French physician. 1829–
1883
ATROPHY—primary, infantile.
   L'arthrepsie. Paris, Masson, 1877. 450 pp.
DISEASE—syphilitic pseudoparalysis in infants.
   *Sur une pseudo-paralysie causée par une altération du
système osseux chez les nouveau-nés atteints de syphilis
héréditaire.* Arch. de Physiol., 4: 319–333: 470–490;
613–623, 1871–72
NODE or SIGN—on outer table of skull of syphilitic
infants.
   Lésions du crâne, causées par la syphilis héréditaire.
Progres med., Paris, 7: 268, 1879
Recognized that involvement of lymph nodes is com-
ponent of primary tuberculous infection. (No title)
C. R. Soc. Biol., 28: 308 (only), 1876
   See also L. Pasteur
Parry, Caleb Hillier. English physician. 1756–1822
DISEASE—exophthalmic goiter.
   *Diseases of the heart. Enlargement of the thyroid gland
in connection with enlargement or palpitation of the
heart.* In: *Collected works.* London, 2: 111–128, 1825
Also, abstr. in R. H. Major's *Classic descriptions of
disease.* Springfield, Ill., Thomas, 1939. 2 ed., pp.
294–297
Also, abstr.: Medical classics, 5: 8–20, Sept. 1940
Also, abstr. in F. A. Willius and T. E. Keys' *Cardiac
classics.* St. Louis, Mosby, 1941. pp. 387–391
Described condition now known as histaminic cephal-
gia.
   *On the effects of compression of the arteries in various
diseases, and particularly in those of the head; with
hints towards a new mode of treating nervous disorders.*
Mem. M. Soc. London, 3: 77–113, 1792
Described first recorded case of congenital idiopathic
dilatation of colon. Garrison
   Affections of the bowels. In: *Collected works.* London,
2: 375–440, 1825
Described first recorded cases of facial hemiatrophy,
1814. Garrison
   *Hemiplegia, chiefly, to all appearance, of the secreting
arteries of the left side.* In: Ibid., 1: 478–480, 1825
Parry, John S. Philadelphia gynecologist. 1843–1876
Wrote first authoritative treatise on extra-uterine
pregnancy. Garrison
   *Extra-uterine pregnancy; its causes, species, patho-
logical anatomy, clinical history, diagnosis, prognosis,
and treatment.* Philadelphia, Lea, 1876. 276 pp.
Parry, R. H. Glasgow surgeon
OPERATION—
   Radical cure of femoral hernia. Brit. med. J., 2: 1136–
1138, Oct. 19, 1901
Parsons, Elizabeth I. See C. E. A. Winslow

Parsons, J. W. See I. R. Trimble
Parsons, T. R.: Parsons, W. See J. Barcroft
Parsons, W. B. See A. O. Whipple
Part, J. Shepley. English surgeon
Wrote—
Novocaine in minor surgery. Lancet, 2: 1473 (only),
Nov. 24, 1906
Partipilo, Anthony Victor. Chicago surgeon. 1900–
METHOD—
*A closed aseptic and quick method of gastrointestinal
anastomosis; a preliminary report.* Amer. J. Surg.,
6: 362–363, Mar. 1929
*A closed aseptic and quick method of gastrointestinal
anastomosis* with C. L. D. Moorhead and W. J.
Pickett, Illinois med. J., 57: 345–348, May 1930
Partsch, Fritz. Duisburg surgeon
METHOD—of gastrostomy.
Zur Indikation und Technik der Magenfistel. Zbl. f.
Chir., 62: 1449–1454, June 22, 1935
Pascal, Blaise. French scientist. 1623–1662
LAW—pressure applied to a liquid at any point is
transmitted equally in all directions.
*Traitez de l'équilibre des liqueurs, et de la presanteur de
la masse de l'air.* . . . Paris, Desprez, 1673. 232 pp.
Paschal, G. W., Jr. See W. T. Lemmon
Pascheff, C. Sofia ophthalmologist
CONJUNCTIVITIS—
*Ueber eine besondere Form von Bindehaut-Entzündung
(Conjunctivitis necroticans infectiosa).* Klin. Mbl.
Augenheilk., 57: 517–529, Dec. 16, 1916
*Weitere Mitteilung über meine besondere Bindehaut-
Entzündung.* Ibid., 58: 97–99, Dec. 27, 1916
*The differential diagnosis between Parinaud's con-
junctivitis and conjunctivitis necroticans infectiosa.*
Brit. J. Ophthal., 8: 25–32, Jan. 1924
·FOLLICULOMA—
*Researches on the follicular diseases of the conjunctiva:
their relation to the laws of true trachoma, its etiology,
and unification of conception.* Amer. J. Ophthal., 15:
690–708, Aug. 1932
Paschen, Enrique. Hamburg pathologist. 1860–1936
ELEMENTARY BODIES—minute granules in cells
of tissues in variola and vaccinia.
Was wissen wir über den Vakzineerreger? Münch.
med. Wschr., 53: 2391–2393, Dec. 4, 1906
Paschkis, Rudolf. Vienna surgeon
APPLICATOR—cystoscopic radium a.
Radiumbehandlung von Blasengeschwülsten. Wien.
klin. Wschr., 24: 1562–1564, Nov. 9, 1911
Pascoe, T. A. See R. L. Gregory
Passavant, Phipippus Gustavus. Frankfurt a. M.
surgeon. 1815–1893
CUSHION—in nasopharynx.
*Zweiter Artikel über die Operation der angeborenen
Spalten des harten Gaumens und der damit complicirten
Hasenscharten.* Arch. d. Heil., 3: 305–338, 1862
*Ueber die Beseitigung der näselnden Sprache bei an-
geborenen Spalten des harten und weichen Gaumens
(Gaumensegel-Schlundnach und Rücklagerung des
Gaumensegels).* Arch. f. klin. Chir., 6: 333–349, 1865
Passey, R. D. See H. E. Harding
Pasteur, Louis. French chemist. 1822–1895
AVIAN SEPTICEMIA—
THEORY—immunity secured by an attack of a disease
is caused by exhaustion of material needed for growth
of organism of that disease. Dorland

*Sur les maladies virulentes et un particulier sur le
maladie appelée vulgairement choléra des poules.* C. R
Acad. Sci., 90: 239–248, Feb. 9, 1880
Also: Bull. de l'Acad. de méd., 2 s., 9: 121–134, Feb
10, 1880
*De l'atténuation des virus et de leur retour à la viru-
lence* with Chamberland and Roux, C. R. Acad
Sci., 92: 429–435, Feb. 28, 1881
TREATMENT—protective t. against rabies, firs
used on man on July 6, 1885.
Méthode pour prévenir la rage après morsure. Ibid.
101: 765–772, Oct. 26, 1885
VIBRION—organism of malignant edema.
*Recherches sur l étiologie et la prophylaxie de la maladi
charbonneuse dans le département d'Éure-et-Loire*
Rec. de méd. vet., Paris, p. 193, 1879
Studied fermentation.
Mémoire sur la fermentation appelée lactique. C. R
Acad. Sci., 45: 913–916, Nov. 30, 1857
*Nouveaux faits pour servir à l'histoire de la levûr
lactique.* Ibid., 48: 337–338, Feb. 14, 1859
Established germ theory of disease and thereby re
futed experiments on spontaneous generation
showed that fermentation and putrefaction depen
on living organisms.
*Mémoire sur les corpuscules organisés qui existent dan
l'atmosphere, examen de la doctrine des génération
spontanées.* Ann. sci. Nat., (zool.), 16: 5–98, 1861
Discovered Vibrion septique.
Charbon et septicémie with Joubert, C. R. Acad. Sci
85: 101–145, July 16, 1877
Cultivated streptococcus of puerperal sepsis.
Sépticémie puerpérale. Bull. Acad. de Med., 2 s., 8
505–508, 1879
First used attenuated bacterial virus for therapeuti
purposes. Garrison and Morton
Sur l'étiologie du charbon with C. Chamberlan an
P. P. E. Roux, C. R. Acad. Sci., 91: 86–94, July 12
1880
Described pneumococcus.
*L'organism microscopique trouvé dans la maladie nou
velle provoquée par la salive d'un enfant mort de l
rage* with J. Parrot, Bull. Acad. de Méd., 2 s., 10
379, 1881
Demonstrated rabies virus in blood.
Nouvelle communication sur la rage with C. Chambe
land and P. P. E. Roux, C. R. Acad. Sci., 98: 457
463, Feb. 25, 1884
Sur la rage with C. Chamberland and P. P. E. Rou
Ibid., 1229–1231, May 19, 1884
Pasteur, William. English physician. 1855–
Described—
*Respiratory paralysis after diphtheria as a cause
pulmonary complications, with suggestions as to trea
ment.* Amer. J. med. Sci., 100: 242–257, Sept. 189
Described—
Massive collapse of the lung. Lancet, 2: 1351–135
Nov. 7, 1908
Patch, Frank Stewart. Montreal urologist. 1878–
OPERATION—for hydronephrosis.
*The treatment of hydronephrosis secondary to aberra
renal vessels* with J. T. Codnere, Canad. med. Ass. .
45: 495–499, Dec. 1941
Patrick, Hugh Talbot. Chicago neurologist. 186(
1939

SIGN—outward rotation of semiflexed thigh may be limited and painful in lesions of hip joint.
Brachial neuritis and sciatica. J. A. M. A., 69: 2176–2179, Dec. 29, 1917

SOLUTION—
The technic and results of deep injections of alcohol for trifacial neuralgia. Ibid., 58: 155–163, Jan. 20, 1912

Patten, A. J. See A. Kossel

Patterson, D. R. Cardiff otolaryngologist
SYNDROME—Patterson-Kelly or Plummer-Vinson s.
A clinical type of dysphagia. Laryng., Rhin. and Otol., 34: 289–291, Aug. 1919

Patterson, H. S. See S. W. Lambert

Patterson, Robert Lee, Jr. New York surgeon. 1907–
METHOD—
Treatment of acute bursitis by needle irrigation with W. Darrach, J. Bone and Joint Surg., 19: 993–1002, Oct. 1937

Patton, James McDowell. Omaha ophthalmologist. 1876–1930
Described—
Agricultural conjunctivitis with S. R. Gifford, Amer J. Ophthal., 5: 623–637, Aug. 1922

Pauchet, Victor. Paris surgeon. 1869–1936
METHOD—of closure of colostomy.
Fermeture d'un anus artifiel gauche consecutif a une colectomie gauche segmentaire. In: *La pratique chirurgicale illustrée.* Ed. by V. Pauchet, Paris, Doin, 1934. vol. 19, p. 130

OPERATION—excision of rectum for stricture. In: *Practical surgery illustrated.* London, Benn, 1925 Vol. 4, p. 195

Paul, Benjamin Horatio. English chemist. 1828–1902
Obtained emetine in pure form.
The chemistry of ipecacuanha with A. J. Cownley, Pharm. J., London, 54: 111–115, Aug. 11; 373–374, Nov. 10, 1894; 690–692, Feb. 16, 1895

Paul, Frank Thomas. English surgeon. 1851–1941
OPERATION, TUBE—
Colectomy. Liverpool med.-chir. J., 15: 374–388, 1895
Remarks on excision of the rectum, with a report of fourteen cases, and a new rectal truss. Brit. med. J., 1: 519–522, Mar. 9, 1895
Two cases of colectomy. Liverpool med.-chir. J., 20: 55–60, Feb. 1900
See also R. Caton

Paul, Gustav. Vienna physician. 1859–1935
TEST—for variola.
Zur Differentialdiagnose der Variola und der Varicellen. Die Erscheinungen an der variolierten Hornhaut des Kaninchens und ihre frühzeitige Erkennung. Zbl. Bakt., Abt. 1, Orig., 75: 518–524, Mar. 13, 1915

Paul, John Rodman. New Haven physician. 1893–
TEST—
The presence of heterophile antibodies in infectious mononucleosis with W. W. Bunnell, Amer. J. med. Sci., 183: 90–104, Jan. 1932

Paul, Milroy. English surgeon
TOURNIQUET—
A simpler tourniquet. Lancet, 2: 686 (only), Nov. 30, 1940

Paul, R. W. English scientist

JACKET—
The Bragg-Paul pulsator: an apparatus for prolonged artificial respiration by Sir William Bragg's method. Proc. R. Soc. Med., 28: 436–438, Feb. 1935

Paulesco, Nicholas C. Bucharest surgeon
First to point out that removal of anterior lobe of pituitary is fatal and removal of posterior lobe negative. Garrison
L'hypophyse du cerveau. Paris, Vigot Frères, 1908. 144 pp.

Pauli, Ruth H. See A. F. Coburn

Pauly, Hermann. Heidelberg physiologist. 1870–
Determined structure of histidine.
Über die Konstitution des Histidins. Z. physiol. Chem., 42: 508–518, Aug. 17, 1904

Pauwels, Friedrich. Aachen surgeon
RECLINATION—physiological reconstruction for non-united fracture of neck of femur.
Eine neue Methods zur operativen der Schenkelhalspseudarthrose. Z. orthop. Chir., 51: 125–134, 1929

Pauzat, Jean Eugène. French physician
DISEASE—
De la périostite ostéoplasique des métatarsiens à la suite des marches. Arch. de méd. et pharm. mil., Paris, 10: 337–353, 1887

Pavlov, Ivan Petrovich. Russian physiologist. 1849–1936
Awarded Nobel prize in 1904.
CONDITIONED REFLEXES—
DOGS—
METHOD—study of changes in salivary reflex produced by psychic influence.
STOMACH—isolated portion, opening on abdominal wall through fistula, for studying gastric secretion.
Lektsii o rabotie glavnikh pishtshevaritelnikh zheyloz. St. Petersburg, Kushnereff, 1897. 223 pp.
(Same, in French) Paris, 1901
(Same) *The work of the digestive glands.* Transl. by W. H. Thompson, London, Griffin, 1902. 196 pp.
Conditioned reflexes; an investigation of the physiological activity of the cerebral cortex. Transl. by G. V. Anrep, London, Milford, 1927. 430 pp.
(Same) Transl. by W. H. Gantt, New York, Internat. Pub., 1928. 414 pp.

Pavlovsky, A. D. Russian physician
Studied effects of mixed infection or bacterial symbiosis. Garrison
(*Study on etiology of pyaemia.*) Russk. Med., St. Petersb., 5: 51–54, 1887

Pavy, Frederick William. English physician. 1829–1911
DISEASE—
On cyclic albuminuria (albuminuria in the apparently healthy). Lancet, 2: 706–708, Oct. 17, 1885
BLUE FLUID—substitution of ammonia for caustic potash in Fehling's solution, which, as Pavy's pellets, was one of the first preparations to be made in tabloid form. Garrison
PELLETS—
REAGENT, SOLUTION, TEST—
Volumetric estimation of sugar by an ammoniated cupric test giving reduction without precipitation. Chem. News, 39: 77–79, Feb. 21, 1879
Studied diabetes.
Researches on the nature and treatment of diabetes. London, Churchill, 1862. 210 pp.

Pawlik, Karl J. Prague gynecologist. 1849–1914
FOLDS, TRIANGLE, TRIGONE—
*Ueber Harnleitersondirung beim Weibe und ihre
praktische Verwendung.* Wien. med. Presse, 27:
1425–1430, Oct. 31; 1462–1465, Nov. 7; 1492–1495,
Nov. 14; 1557–1560, Nov. 28: 1615–1620, Dec. 12,
1886
Performed successful cystectomy, 1889.
Ueber Blasenexstirpation. Wien. med. Wschr., 41:
1814–1815, Nov. 7, 1891
Paxton, Francis Valentine. English physician. ?–
1924
DISEASE—tinea nodosa or trichorrhexis nodosa.
*On a diseased condition of the hair of the axilla, prob-
ably of a parasitic origin.* J. Cutan. Med., London, 3:
133–136, 1869–70
Payen, Anselme. French physiologist. 1795–1871
Isolated diastase.
*Memoire sur la diastase, les principaux produits de
ses reactions, et leurs applications aux arts industriels*
with Persoz, Ann. Chim. (Phys.), 53: 73–92, 1833
Payne, Robert Lee. Norfolk, Va. surgeon. 1882–
OPERATION—
*Femoral hernia: operative repair by living fascial su-
tures.* J. A. M. A., 104: 276–278, Jan. 26, 1935
TECHNIC—of implantation of ureter into bladder.
*Uretero-vesical implantation: a new method of anasto-
mosis, with report of cases.* Ibid., 51: 1321–1325,
Oct. 17, 1908
Payr, Erwin. Leipzig surgeon. 1871–
DISEASE—kinking at hepatic and splenic colonic
flexures.
*Über eigentümliche, durch abnorm starke Knickungen
und Adhäsionen bedingte gutartige Stenosen an der
Flexura lienalis und hepatica coli.* Verh. dtsch. Kongr.
f. inn. Med., Wiesbaden, 27: 276–305, 1910
METHOD—use of absorbable cylinders of magnesium
for performing suture of blood vessels.
*Weitere Mittheilungen über Verwengung des Magne-
siums bei der Naht der Blutgefässe.* Arch. klin. Chir.,
64: 726–740, 1901
*Zur Frage der circulären Vereinigung von Blutgefäs-
sen mit resorbirbaren Prothesen.* Ibid., 72: 32–54, 1904
METHOD or OPERATION—for hydrocephalus.
*Drainage der Hirnventrikel mittelst frei transplantirter
Blutgefässe: Bemerkungen über Hydrocephalus.* Ibid.,
87: 831–885, 1908
OPERATION—on external ear.
*Plastische Operationen an den Ohren (Stellungsverbes-
serung, Verkleinerung).* Ibid., 78: 918–928, 1905
Paz, D. de la. See W. B. Cannon
Peabody, Francis Weld. Boston physician. 1881–
1927
BROTH—
*On the value of malachite green media in differentiat-
ing typhoid and colon bacilli with the description of a
new method for isolating typhoid bacilli from feces.*
Boston Med. and Surg. J., 158: 213–217, Feb. 13,
1908
TEST—alkali tolerance.
*Clinical studies on the respiration. II. The acidosis of
chronic nephritis.* Arch. intern. Med., 16: 958–966,
Dec. 1915
Peacock, Thomas Bevill. English physician. 1812–
1882
Noted congenital anomaly of heart later called
tetralogy of Fallot.

On malformations of the human heart. London
Churchill, 1858. 2 ed., 1866
Péan, Jules Émile. French surgeon. 1830–1898
FORCEPS—
*Clinique chirurgicale. De la forcipressure ou de l'appli-
cation des pinces à l'hémostasie chirurgicale.* Paris
Germer-Baillière, 1875. 72 pp.
Performed pylorectomy on April 9, 1879.
*De l'ablation des tumeurs de l'estomac par la gastrec
tomie.* Gaz. d. hôp., 52: 473–475, May 27, 1879
Pearce, Louise. New York City physician. 1886–
Introduced—
*Studies on the treatment of human trypanosomiasi
with tryparsamide (the sodium salt of N-phenylgly
cineamide-p-arsonic acid).* J. exp. Med., 34, suppl
1–104, Dec. 1, 1921
Pearl, Felix Lyzwa. San Francisco surgeon. 1897–
OPERATION—
*Muscle-splitting extraperitoneal lumbar ganglionec
tomy.* S. G. O., 65: 107–112, July 1937
Pearse, Herman Elwyn. Rochester, N. Y. surgeon
1899–
DILATOR—
Modified Bakeš common duct dilators. Ann. Surg., 123
1120–1121, June 1946
OPERATION—
*Benign stricture of the bile ducts treated with a vitalliun
tube.* Surgery, 10: 37–44, July 1941
TECHNIC—
*A simplified anastomosis for resection of the duodenun
and head of the pancreas.* S. G. O., 75: 333–336
Sept. 1942
Pechey, John. English physician. 1655–1716
Wrote important pediatric treatise. Garrison
General treatise on the diseases of infants. . . . London
1679
Peck, E. C. See O. K. O. Folin
Peck, Samuel Mortimer. New York dermatologist
1900–
TEST—
*The value of the prognostic venom reaction in thrombo
cytopenic purpura* with N. Rosenthal and L. A. Erf
J. A. M. A., 106: 1783–1891, May 23, 1936
Peck, S. N. See B. Bloch
Pecker, Henri. French biologist
TEST—
Sur la diazoréaction "picramique" dans l'urine. J
Pharm. Chim., Paris, s. 7, 13: 268–269, 1916
Pecquet, Joannes. French anatomist. 1622–1674
CISTERN or RESERVOIR—receptaculum chyli.
DUCT—thoracic.
Experimenta nova anatomica. . . . Paris, 1651
Pedersen, O. C. See J. M. Holst
Pedersen, S. See F. A. Coller
Pedley, F. G. See A. T. Shohl
Peebles, Alvin R. Colorado physician
COLORIMETER—
A simple and accurate colorimeter for clinical use with
R. C. Lewis, J. A. M. A., 70: 679–680, Mar. 9, 191
Peer, Lyndon A(rthur). Newark, N. J. surgeon
1899–
METHOD—of preserving cartilage.
*Diced cartilage grafts; new method for repair of skul
defects, mastoid fistula and other deformities.* Arch
Otolaryng., 38: 156–165, 1943
Peet, Max Minor. Ann Arbor neurosurgeon. 1885–

OPERATION—for hypertension.
Splanchnic resection for hypertension: a preliminary report. Univ. Hosp. Bull., Ann Arbor, 1: 17–18, June 1935
The surgical treatment of hypertension. Proc. California Acad. Med., 5: 58–90, 1935–36
See also C. F. List
Pégurier, Gaston. Nice pharmacologist
TEST—for albumin.
Dosage pondéral pratique de l'albumine urinaire. Rep. de pharm., 3 s., 32: 225–227, 1920
Peightal, T. C. See G. H. Whipple
Pel, Pieter Klazes. Amsterdam physician. 1852–1919
CRISES—ophthalmic.
Augenkrisen bei Tabes dorsalis (Crises ophthalmiques). Berl. klin. Wschr., 35: 25–27, Jan. 10, 1898
PYREXIA, SYMPTOM or SYNDROME—chronic relapsing pyrexia of Hodgkin's disease.
Zur Symptomatologie der sog. Pseudo-Leukämie. Ibid., 22: 3–7, Jan. 5, 1885
Pseudoleukaemie oder chronisches Rückfallsfieber? Ibid., 24: 644–646, Aug. 29, 1887
Peligot, Eugène Melchior. French physician. 1812–
Proved that sugar of diabetic urine is grape-sugar.
Recherches sur la nature et les propriétés chimiques des sucres with A. Bouchardat, Ann. Chim. et Pharm., 67: 113–177 (140), 1838
Pelizaeus, Fredrich. German neurologist. 1850–
DISEASE—familial centrolobar sclerosis.
Über eine eigentümliche Form spastischer Lähmung mit Cerebralerscheinungen auf hereditärer Grundlage (Multiple Sklerose). Arch. f. Psych., 16: 698–710, 1885
Pelkan, K. F. See W. R. Bloor
Pellegrini, Augusto. Florence surgeon
DISEASE—calcification of tibial collateral ligament following injury.
Ossificazione traumatica del legamento collaterale tibiale dell'articolazione del ginocchio sinistro. La clinica moderna, 11: 433–439, 1905
Per la storia delle ossificazioni post-traumatiche della regione laterale interna del ginocchio. Chir. d. org. di movimento, 16: 283–288, July 1931
Pelletier, Pierre Joseph. French chemist. 1788–1842
Isolated emetine. Garrison and Morton
Recherches chimiques et physiologiques sur l'ipéca-cuanha with F. Magendie, Ann. Chim. (Phys.), 4: 172–185, 1817
Isolated strychnine.
Mémoire sur un nouvel alcali (la strychnine) trouvé dans la fève de Saint-Ignace, la noix vomique, etc. with J. B. Caventou, J. Pharm. et Sci. acces., 5: 142–174, 1819
Isolated quinine.
Recherches chimiques sur les quinquinas with J. B. Caventou, Ann. Chim. (Phys.), 15: 289–318; 337–365, 1820
See also J. B. Caventou
Pellissier, M. French physician
TEST—
Recherche rapide de la bile dans l'urine with Schaibéle, Abstr.: Repert. de pharm., 3 s., 21: 214 (only), Apr. 1909
Pellizzi, G. B. Pisa physician

SYNDROME—progeria or Hasting Gilford's disease.
La sindrome epifisaria "macrogenitosomia precoce". Riv. ital. di neuropat., psichiat. e elettroterap., Catania, 3: 193–207, e continua, 1910
Pelouze, Percy Starr. Philadelphia urologist. 1876–1947
AGAR—brain veal infusion.
A new medium for gonococcus culture with L. E. Viteri, J. A. M. A., 86: 684–685, Mar. 6, 1926
Penada, Jacopo. Italian physician. 1748–1828
Described perforating duodenal ulcer. Garrison and Morton
Saggio d'osservazioni, e memorie sopra alcuni casi sigolari riscontrati nell'esercizio della medicina, e della anatomia pratica. Padova, Penada, 1793
Pende, Nicolo. Italian physician. 1880–
Coined term endocrinology.
Sistema nervoso simpatico e glandole a secrezione interna; distrofie endocrino-simpatiche. Il Tommasi, Napoli, 4: 732–738, Nov. 10, 1909
Penfield, Wilder Graves. Montreal surgeon. 1891–
METHOD—
A method of staining oligodendroglia and microglia (combined method). Amer. J. Path., 4: 153–157, Mar. 1928
MODIFICATION—of Cajal's uranium nitrate method.
Alterations of the Golgi apparatus in nerve cells. Brain, 43: 290–305, Nov. 1920
OPERATION—
Spina bifida and cranium bifidum: results of plastic repair of meningocele and myelomeningocele by a new method with W. Cone, J. A. M. A., 98: 454–461, Feb. 6, 1932
TREATMENT—
Chronic meningeal (post-traumatic) headache and its specific treatment by lumbar air insufflation; encephalography. S. G. O., 45: 747–759, Dec. 1927
Pénières, L. Toulouse surgeon
OPERATION—
De la gastrostomie par la méthode de la valvule ou du plissement de la muqueuse stomacale. Arch. prov. de Chir., 2: 284–293, May 1893
Pennington, John Rawson. Chicago surgeon. 1858–1927
PROCEDURE—
Treatment of hemorrhoids by the open method. J. A. M. A., 64: 1136–1138, Apr. 3, 1915
Etiology and treatment of hemorrhoids. Med. Rec., 92: 225–229, Aug. 11, 1917
Pennock, Caspar Wistar. American physician. 1801–1867
Reported—
Case of anomalous aneurysm of the aorta resulting from effusion of blood between the laminae composing the middle coat of that vessel. Amer. J. med. Sci., 23: 2–19, Nov. 1838
Penny, E. See A. Kossler
Penrose, Charles Bingham. Philadelphia surgeon. 1862–1925
DRAIN—
Drainage in abdominal surgery. J. A. M. A., 14: 264–268, Feb. 22, 1890
Penrose, Clement Abdariese. Baltimore surgeon. 1874–1919
APPARATUS—
A new apparatus designed for the support and safe

anaesthetization of patients while in the knee-chest position. Johns Hopk. Hosp. Bull., 10: 209–211, Nov. 1899

Penrose, F. G. See T. Barlow

Penzoldt, Franz. Erlangen physician. 1849–1927
TEST—for acetone.
Beiträge zur Lehre von der Acetonurie und von verwandten Erscheinungen. Dtsch. Arch. f. klin. Med., 34: 127–142, Oct. 31, 1883
TEST—for glucose in urine.
Ueber die Resorptionsfähigkeit der menschlichen Magenschleimhaut und ihre diagnostische Verwerthung with Faber, Berlin klin. Wschr., 19: 313–315, May 22, 1882
Neue Reaktion der Aldehyde with E. Fischer, Ber. d. dtsch. chem. Ges., 16: 657–658, 1883
TEST—for stomach absorption. (Alvarez)
Beiträge zur Lehre von der menschlichen Magenverdauung unter normalen und abnormen Verhältnissen. Dtsch. Arch. f. klin. Med., 51: 535–582, July 27, 1893

Pepper, William. American physician. 1843–1898
Described bone-marrow changes in—
Progressive pernicious anaemia, or anaematosis. Amer. J. med. Sci., 70: 313–347, Oct. 1875

Pepper, William. Philadelphia physician. 1874–1947
TYPE—of adrenal medullary tumor.
A study of congenital sarcoma of the liver and suprarenal: with report of a case. Amer. J. med. Sci., 121: 287–299, Mar. 1901

Peppler, August. Erlangen bacteriologist. 1873–
STAIN—for flagella.
Ein einfaches Verfahren zur Darstellung der Geisseln. Zbl. Bakt., 29: 345–355, Mar. 14, 1901

Percival, John. English plant bacteriologist
AGAR—basal litmus extract; culture medium.
SOLUTION—basal.
Agricultural bacteriology. London, Duckworth, 1920

Percival, Thomas. English physician. 1740–1804
Collector of public health statistics.
Proposals for the establishment of more accurate and comprehensive bills of mortality. 1770
Introduced cod liver oil into therapeutics. Garrison and Morton
Observations on the medical uses of the oleum jecoris aselli, or cod liver oil, in the chronic rheumatism, and other painful disorders. London med. J., 3: 392–401, 1782
Wrote—
Medical ethics. London, Johnson, 1803
(Same) Ed. by C. D. Leake, Baltimore, Williams and Wilkins, 1927, 291 pp.

Percy, James Fulton. Galesburg, Ill. surgeon. 1864–
CAUTERY or METHOD or TREATMENT—
A method of applying heat both to inhibit and destroy inoperable carcinoma of the uterus and vagina. S. G. O., 17: 371–376, Sept. 1913

Percy, Nelson Mortimer. Chicago surgeon. 1875–
METHOD—modification of Kimpton-Brown m.
A simplified method of blood transfusion with report of six cases of pernicious anemia treated by massive blood transfusion and splenectomy. S. G. O., 21: 360–365, Sept. 1915

Péró, M. A. French pharmacist
SOLUTION—basal ammonium sulphate.
Mécanisme de la combustion des corps ternaires par

un groupe de microbes aerobies. Ann. Inst. Pasteur, 10: 417–448 (421), Aug. 1896

Pereira, Antonio de Sousa. Porto surgeon
OPERATION—for arterial hypertension.
Résection des nerfs splanchiniques par voie sous-diaphragmatique. Pr. méd., 37: 620–622, May 11, 1929
Nervi splanchnici. Porto, Portugal, Tipografia Porto Medico, Ltd., 1929, p. 331

Perelstein, M. Bern biochemist
TEST—for mercury in urine.
Ueber eine empfindliche klinische Methode zum Nachweis des Quecksilbers im Urin with J. Abelin, Münch. med. Wschr., 62: 1181–1183, Aug. 31, 1915

Perényi, Josef. Budapest scientist
SOLUTION—chromo-nitric acid; an embryologic fixing s.
Über eine neue Erhärtungsflüssigkeit. Zool. Anzeig., 5: 459–460, Aug. 28, 1882

Perez, Fernand. Spanish physician. 1863–1935
Isolated Coccobacillus foetidus ozaenae.
Recherches sur la bactériologie de l'ozène. Ann. Inst. Pasteur, 13: 937–950, Dec. 1899

Pergola, M. Rome physician
AGAR—tellurite egg yolk: for diagnosis of diphtheria.
Contributo alla diagnosi batteriologica della difterite. Ann. d'igiene, Roma, 28: 101–110, Mar. 31, 1918
INFUSION—mussel; for cultivation of typhoid and cholera bacillus.
Bakterizides Vermögen der organischen Säfte der Weichtiere. Bedeutung der Mollusken in der Epidemiologie der infektiösen Krankheiten intestinalen Typus und besonders der Cholera. Zbl. Bakt., 65: 171–183 (171), July 3, 1912
SOLUTION—nitrate peptone; to enrich cholera vibrio.
Die rasche bakteriologische Choleradiagnose. Beobachtungen über das Dieudonnesche Blutalkaliagar. Ibid., 59: 83–96 (85), June 10, 1911

Perkins, Elisha. Connecticut physician. 1740–1799
TRACTOR—metallic; used in attempted cure of many diseases.
Certificates of the efficacy of Doctor Perkins' patent metallic instruments. Newburyport, Blunt, 1796. 24 pp.

Perkins, John Walter. Kansas City surgeon. ?1860–1923
OPERATION—
Complete dislocation of patella, reduced by arthrotomy after six years. Ann. Surg., 18: 654–657, Dec. 1893

Pernice, Ludwig. Halle a. S. surgeon
METHOD—of M. Oberst.
Über Cocainanänsthesie. Dtsch. med. Wschr., 16: 287–289, Apr. 3, 1890

Peronnet, Marcel. French scientist
REACTIONS—for amino acids and uric acid.
Sur les réactions de coloration fournies par la méta dinitrobenzène en milieu alcalin with R. Truhaut, J Pharm. Chim., Paris, 8 s., 18: 339–343, 1933

Persoz. See A. Payen

Perthes, George Clemens. Leipzig surgeon. 1869–1927
DISEASE—
Ueber Arthritis deformans juvenilis. Dtsch. Z. Chir., 107: 111–159, Oct. 1910
Ueber Osteochondritis deformans juvenilis. Arch. klin. Chir., 101: 779–807, June 17, 1913

OPERATION—
  Zur Pathologie und Operation der habituellen Luxation der Patella. Zbl. Chir., 44: 233–235, Mar. 24, 1917
OPERATION—plastic to form thumb.
  Ueber plastischen Daumenersatz insbesondere bei Verlust des ganzen Daumenstrahles. Arch. f. orthop. u. Unfall., 19: 198–214, July 18, 1921
TEST—of deep circulation of a limb.
  Ueber die Operation der Unterschenkelvaricen nach Trendelenburg. Dtsch. med. Wschr., 21: 253–257, Apr. 18, 1895
  Originator of deep x-ray therapy. Garrison
  Ueber den Einfluss der Röntgenstrahlen auf epitheliale Gewebe, insbesondere auf das Carcinom. Arch. f. klin. Chir., 71: 955–1000, 1903
  Versuch einer Bestimmung der Durchlässigkeit menschlicher Gewebe fur Röntgenstrahlen mit Rücksicht auf die Bedeutung der Durchlässigkeit der Gewebe für die Radiotherapie. Fort. a. d. Geb. d. Röntgenstrahlen, 8: 12–25, 1904–05

Perutz, Alfred. Vienna physician
REACTION or TEST—
  Die klinische Bedeutung der Serodiagnose der Syphilis mittels der Ausflockungsreaktion für die Prognose und Therapie der Lues. Wien. klin. Wschr., 32: 953–955, Sept. 9, 1919
  See also O. Hermann

Peter, Luther Crouse. Philadelphia ophthalmologist. 1869–1942
OPERATION—
  The use of the superior oblique as an internal rotator in third-nerve paralysis. Amer. J. Ophthal., 17: 297–300, Apr. 1934

Peterfi, Tibor. Jena biologist. 1883–
METHOD—of embedding tissue.
  Eine beschleunigte Celloidin-Paraffin-Einbettung mit Nelkenöl- oder Methylbenzoatcelloidin. Z. f. wiss. Mikr., 38: 342–345, 1921

Peters, Amos William. Boston biochemist. 1866–
METHOD—for determination of glucose in urine.
  A critical study of sugar analysis by copper reduction methods. J. Amer. Chem. Soc., 34: 928–954, July 1912

Peters, George Armstrong. Canadian surgeon. 1859–1907
OPERATION—
  Transplantation of ureters into rectum by an extraperitoneal method for exstrophy of bladder, and a new operation for procidentia recti in the same patient. Brit. med. J., 1: 1538–1542, June 22, 1901

Peters, Hubert. Vienna obstetrician
OVUM—one which was obtained 5 or 6 days after impregnation.
  Ueber die Einbettung des menschlichen Eies und das früheste bisher bekannte menschliche Placentationsstadium. Leipzig, Deuticke, 1899. 143 pp.

Peters, John Punnett. American physician. 1887–
MODIFICATION—of Peters and Van Slyke, of Howe's method of determination of total proteins and albumin.
  In: *Quantitative clinical chemistry.* By J. P. Peters and D. D. Van Slyke, Baltimore, Williams and Wilkins, 1932, Vol. 2, pp. 691–693

Peters, R. A. See C. W. Carter, H. W. Kinnersley

Petersen, William Ferdinand. Chicago pathologist. 1887–

Suggested terms parasympathetic status and sympathetic status.
  Studies in endothelial permeability: I. The effect of epinephrine on endothelial permeability with S. A. Levinson and T. P. Hughes, J. Immunol., 8: 323–348, Sept. 1923
  See also E. R. Whitmore

Petri, Richard Julius. German bacteriologist. 1852–1922
METHOD—sand-filter for bacteria in air.
  Eine neue Methode Bacterien und Pilzsporen in der Luft nachzuweisen und zu zählen. Z. Hyg. InfektKr., 3: 1–145, 1888

Petroff, Strashimis Alburtus. American bacteriologist. 1882–
MEDIUM—gentian-violet egg.
  A new and rapid method for the isolation and cultivation of tubercle bacilli directly from the sputum and feces. J. exp. Med., 21: 38–42, Jan. 1, 1915
  Some cultural studies on the tubercle bacillus. Johns Hopk. Hosp. Bull., 26: 276–279, Aug. 1915

Pettenkofer, Max Joseph von. Munich chemist. 1818–1901
METHOD—for demonstration of arsenic by means of Marsch apparatus.
  Sichere und einfache Methode das Arsenik mittelst des Marsh'schen Apparates entwickelt von allen andern ähnlichen Erscheinungen augenfällig zu unterscheiden. Buchner's Repert. f. Pharm., 77: 289, 1842; 82: 328, 1844
METHOD—of estimating carbon dioxide in air and water.
  Ueber die Bestimmung des Kohlensäuregehalts der atmosphärischen Luft. Abhandl. d. naturw.-techn. Comm. bei d. Münch. Akad., 2: 1, 1858
TEST—for bile acids in urine.
  Notiz über eine neue Reaction auf Galle und Zucker. Ann. de Chem. u. Pharm., Heidelb., 52: 90–96, 1844
THEORY—of epidemics.
  Untersuchungen und Beobachtungen über die Verbreitungsart der Cholera. München, Cotta, 1855
  Demonstrated hippuric acid, creatin and creatinin in urine. See TEST
  Showed that saliva contains sulphocyanic acid.
  Ueber den Schwefelcyangehalt des menschlichen Speichels. Buchner's Repert. f. Pharm., 91: 289, 1846
  Prepared a copper amalgam for use as a dental filling material.
  Ueber den amorphen und krystallinischen Zustand eines Kupfer-Amalgams. Münch. Gelehrt. Anzeig., 27: 409, 1848
  Made classical investigations of metabolism in respiration. Garrison
  Ueber Bestimmung des in der Respiration ausgeschiedenen Wasserstoff, und Grubengases with C. von. Voit, Sitzber. Münch. Akad., 2: 162, 1862
  Über die Respiration. Ann. d. Chem. u. Pharm., Suppl. 2: 1–52, 1862–63
  Untersuchungen über die Respiration with C. von Voit, Ibid., 52–70, 1862–63

Petters, Wilhelm. Prague physician
  Discovered acetone in diabetic urine. Garrison
  Untersuchungen über die Honigharnruhr. (Entdeckung des Acetons im diabetischen Urin.) Vrtljschr. f. prakt. Heilk., Prag. 55: 81–94, 1857

Pettersson, Alfred. Stockholm physician. 1867–

AGAR—brain ascitic fluid.
Ein neuer, besonders für die Züchtung von Gonokokken geeigneter Gehirnnährboden. Dtsch. med. Wschr., 46: 1385 (only), Dec. 9, 1920

Petteruti, G. Italian physician
SYMPTOM—murmur beneath left clavicle.
Sull'espirazione sistolica. Lavori d. Cong. di med. int. 1888, Milano, 1: 324–330, 1889

Pettey, George E. Memphis, Tenn. physician. 1857–1920
TREATMENT—of drug addiction.
The narcotic drug diseases and allied ailments. . . . Philadelphia, Davis, 1913. 516 pp.

Pettit, A. See L. Martin

Petz, Aladár de. Hungarian surgeon
CLAMP—
Aseptic technique of stomach resections. Ann. Surg., 86: 385–392, Sept. 1927

Peyer, Johann Corad. Swiss anatomist. 1653–1712
GLANDS, PATCHES—lymphatic glands, chiefly of ileum.
Exercitatio anatomico-medica de glandulis intestinorum, earumque usu et affectionibus. Cui subjungitur anatome ventriculi gallinacei. Schaffhausen, Onophrius et Waldkirch, 1677. 136 pp.
Wrote on physiology of rumination. Garrison
Merycologia, sive de ruminantibus et ruminatione commentarius. Basileae, Koenig, 1685. 288 pp.

Peyrilhe, Bernard. French physician. 1735–1804
Did first experimental work on cancer; injected fluid from human mammary cancer into a dog. Garrison and Morton
Dissertation académique sur le traitement du cancer par la compression méthodique. Paris, Gabon, 1829. 2 vols.

Pezard, A. French physician
Introduced use of capon as a quantitative biological test animal for androgens.
Sur la détermination des caractères sexuels secondaires chez les gallinacés. C. R. Acad. Sci., 153: 1027–1029, Nov. 20, 1911

Pezzi, Cesare. Pavia physician
Called attention to electrical alternans.
Signification de l'onde T du groupe ventriculaire de l'électrocardiogramme. Arch. d. mal. du coeur, 15: 378–386, June 1922

Pfaff, Philippe. German dentist. 1715–1767
First to describe casting of models for false teeth. Garrison and Morton
Abhandlung von den Zähnen des menschlichen Körpers und deren Krankheiten. Berlin, Haude und Spener, 1756

Pfannenstiel, Hermann Johannes. Breslau gynecologist. 1862–1909
INCISION—abdominal.
Ueber die Vortheile des suprasymphysären Fascienquerschnitts für die gynäkalogischen Koeliotomien, zugleich ein Beitrag zu der Indikationsstellung der Operationswege. Samml. klin. Vortr., No. 268, (Gynäkol., No. 97, pp. 1735–1756), 1900

Pfau, Hermann. Basel chemist
TEST—for free iodine in urine.
Zum Nachweis von Jod im Urin. Korrespond. f. schweiz. Ärzte, 44: 273–274, Feb. 28, 1914

Pfaundler, Meinhard von. German pediatrician. 1872–

REACTION—for detection of typhoid carriers.
Eine neue Form der Serumreaktion auf Coli- und Proteusbacillosen. Zbl. Bakt., 23: 9–15, Jan. 8; 71–79, Jan. 19; 131–138, Jan. 31, 1898
SYNDROME—congenital, multiple symmetrical skeletal deformaties with disturbance of lipoid metabolism.
Demonstrationen über einen Typus kindlicher Dysostose. Jb. f. Kinderh., 92: 420–421, 1920

Pfeffer, Wilhelm Friedrich Philipp. German scientist. 1845–1920
Studied osmotic pressure.
Osmotische Untersuchungen. Leipzig, Engelmann, 1877

Pfeifer, Viktor. German physician
SYNDROME—relapsing, febrile, nodular, non-suppurative panniculitis.
Ueber einen Fall von herdweiser Atrophie des subcutanen Fettgewebes. Dtsch. Arch. klin. Med., 50: 438–449, 1892

Pfeiffer, Damon Beckett. Philadelphia surgeon. 1878–
TECHNIC—of closure of gastrojejunocolic fistula.
The value of preliminary colostomy in the correction of gastrojejunocolic fistula with E. M. Kent, Ann. Surg., 110: 659–668, Oct. 1939
The surgical treatment of gastrojejunocolic fistula. S. G. O., 72: 282–289, Feb. 15, 1941

Pfeiffer, Emil. Wiesbaden physician. 1846–1921
DISEASE—infectious mononucleosis; glandular fever.
Drüsenfieber. Jb. f. Kinderh., n. F., 29: 257–264, 1889

Pfeiffer, Richard Friedrich Johannes. Breslau bacteriologist. 1858–
BACILLUS—influenza.
Vorläufige Mittheilungen über die Erreger der Influenza. Dtsch. med. Wschr., 18: 28 (only), Jan. 14, 1892
BLOOD AGAR—for cultivating bacteria.
Die Aetiologie der Influenza. Z. Hyg. InfektKr., 13: 357–386, 1893
PHENOMENON, REACTION—bacteriolysis.
Ueber die specifische Bedeutung der Choleraimmunität (Bakteriolyse) with V. I. Isayeff, Ibid., 17: 355–400, 1894
Weitere Untersuchungen über das Wesen der Choleraimmunität und über specifisch bactericide Processe. Ibid., 18: 1–16, 1894
Reported immunization of men against typhoid fever.
Ueber die specifische Immunitätsreaction der Typhus bacillen with W. Kolle, Dtsch. med. Wschr., 20: 898 (only), Nov. 29, 1894

Pfeiler, W. German bacteriologist
AGAR—ringer solution a.; culture medium.
Ueber die Herstellung von festen Nährböden ohne Verwendung des Fleischwassers und der Fleischbrühe. Ein Vorschlag zur Vereinfachung der Herstellungsweise und Verbilligung des Kulturmaterials with W. Lentz, Zbl. Bakt., 68: 122–126 (123), Feb. 12, 1913

Pfiffner, Joseph John. American biochemist. 1903–
Prepared a potent cortical extract of adrenal gland.
The preparation of an active extract of the suprarenal cortex with W. W. Swingle, Anat. Rec., 44: 225 (only), Dec. 25, 1929
Studies on adrenal cortex; revival of cats prostrate from

adrenal insufficiency with aqueous extract of cortex
with W. W. Swingle, Amer. J. Physiol., 96: 180–190,
Jan. 1931
See also W. W. Swingle

Pflüger, Eduard Friedrich Wilhelm. Bonn physiologist. 1829–1910
Law—a nerve tract is stimulated when catelectrotonus develops or anelectrotonus disappears. Dorland
Untersuchungen über die Physiologie des Electrotonus.
Berlin, Hirschwald, 1859. 500 pp.
METHOD—of determination of glycogen.
Das Glykogen und seine Beziehungen zur Zuckerkrankheit. 2. Aufl. Bonn, Hager, 1905. 528 pp.
Showed that stimulation of splanchnic nerves inhibits intestinal movements. Garrison
Ueber das Hemmungs-Nervensystem für die peristaltischen Bewegungen der Gedärme. Berlin, Hirschwald, 1857. 75 pp.
Proved that essential seat of respiration is in tissues, and not in blood. Garrison
Zur Gasometriedes Blutes. Zbl. med. Wiss., 4: 305–308, 1866

Phaer, Thomas. English physician. 1510–1560
Wrote first work on diseases of children. Garrison and Morton
The regiment of life, whereunto is added a treatise of the pestilence, with the boke of children. London, 1545

Pheasant, H. C. See H. C. Pitkin

Phelps, Abel Mix. New York surgeon. 1851–1902
BOX—
The wood corset, with improvements, for the treatment of lateral curvature and Pott's disease of the spine. New Engl. med. Month., 11: 195–202, Feb. 1892
OPERATION—
The treatment of double talipes equino varus by open incision and fixed extension. Trans. Med. Soc. New York, pp. 269–276, 1881

Philip, Sir Robert William. Edinburgh physician. 1857–1912
GLANDS—above clavicle, seen in children with tuberculosis.
Address on the presence and prevalence of tuberculosis in childhood. Edinburgh med. J., 9: 293–299 (296), Oct. 1912
Also in his: *Collected papers.* London, Oxford Univ. Press, 1937. pp. 193–202 (196)
Tuberculosis of the lymphatic system. Trans. Tuberculosis Soc. of Scotland, Nov. 1921
Also in his: *Collected papers.* pp. 259–270 (264–265)

Phillips, Francis James. Columbus, Ohio physician. 1904–
METHOD—
Blood iodine studies. IV. The clinical determination of iodine in blood, urine and feces with G. M. Curtis, Amer. J. clin. Path., 4: 346–353, July 1934

Phillips, James McIlvaine. Columbus, Ohio physician. 1874–
METHOD—dilution, of preventive inoculation against rabies.
Prophylactic treatment for rabies by means of standardized glycerinated virus. J. Immunol., 7: 409–421, Sept. 1922

Phillips, John Roberts. Houston surgeon. 1904–

TECHNIC—
Excision of the duodenum and head of the pancreas for carcinoma of the ampulla: method of anastomosing pancreatic duct to the jejunum. Amer. J. Surg., 60: 137–139, Apr. 1943

Phillips, Robert Allan. New York physician. 1906–
METHOD—of calculation of plasma protein concentration.
The copper sulfate method for measuring specific gravities of whole blood and plasma with D. D. Van Slyke, V. P. Dole, K. Emerson, Jr., P. B. Hamilton and R. M. Archibald, Burned News Letter, 1: No. 9, June 25, 1943
Also: Bull. U. S. Army Med. Dept., 71: 66–83, Dec. 1943
Noted increase in number of platelets following viosterol.
The effect of irradiated ergosterol on thrombocytes and the coagulation of the blood with D. F. Robertson, W. C. Corson and G. F. Irwin, Ann. intern. Med., 4: 1134–1143, Mar. 1931

Physick, Philip Syng. Philadelphia surgeon. 1768–1837
OPERATION—
Extracts from an account of a case in which a new and peculiar operation for artificial anus was performed. Philadelphia J. Med. and Phys. Sci., 13: 199–202, 1826
The first in America to wash out the stomach with syringe and tube in a case of poisoning. Garrison
Account of a new mode of extracting poisonous substances from the stomach. Eclect. Repertory and Ana. Rev., Phila., 3: 111–113, 381–382, 1813
Introduced—
(*Buck-skin and kid ligatures.*) Ibid., 6: 389, 1816
Invented tonsillotome.
Description of a forceps, employed to facilitate the extirpation of the tonsil. Amer. J. med. Sci., 2: 116–117, 1828

Pic, Adrien. French physician. 1863
SYNDROME—see Louis Bard

Piccoli, E. Lendinara surgeon
OPERATION—for umbilical hernia.
Zur Radikalbehandlung der Nabelhernien. Zbl. f. Chir., 27: 37–38, Jan. 13, 1900

Pichevin, R. See J. A. Doléris

Pick, Arnold. Prague neurologist. 1851–1924
DISEASE or SYNDROME—circumscribed atrophy of cerebral cortex.
Über die Beziehungen der senilen Hirnatrophie zur Aphasie. Prag. med. Wschr., 17: 165–167, Apr. 20, 1892
Described agrammatism. Garrison
Die agrammatischen Sprachstörungen.... Berlin, Springer, 1913. 291 pp.

Pick, Friedel. German physician. 1867–1926
SYNDROME—
Über chronische, unter dem Bilde der Lebercirrhosverlaufende Pericarditis (pericarditische Pseudolebercirrhose) nebst Bemerkungen über die Zuckergusslebere (Curschmann). Z. klin. Med., 29: 386–410, 1896

Pick, Louis. Königsburg ophthalmologist. 1872–
RETINITIS CACHETICORUM—
Netzhautveränderungen bei chronischen Anämieen. Klin. Mbl. Augenheilk., 39 (1): 177–192, 1901

Pick, Ludwig. German physician. 1868–

DISEASE—
Zur pathologischen Anatomie des Morbus Gaucher.
Med. Klin., 18: 1423–1424, Oct. 29, 1922
Der Morbus Gaucher und die ihm ähnlichen Erkrank-
ungen (die lipoidzellige Splenohepatomegalie Typhus
Niemann und die diabetische Lipoidzellenhypoplasie
der Milz). Ergebn. inn. Med. u. Kinderh., 29: 519–
627, 1926
Niemann-Pick's disease and other forms of so-called
xanthomatosis. Amer. J. med. Sci., s 2., 185: 601–616,
May 1933
Described testicular tubular adenoma (arrhenoblas-
toma).
Ueber Adenome der männlichen und weiblichen Keim-
drüse bei Hermaphroditismus verus und spurius;
nebst Bemerkungen ueber das endometriumähliche
Adenom am innern weiblichen Genitale. Berl. klin.
Wschr., 42: 502–509, Apr. 24, 1905
Pickering, George White. English scientist
TEST—
On the clinical recognition of structural disease of the
peripheral vessels. Brit. med. J., 2: 1106–1110, Dec.
16, 1933
See also T. Lewis
Pickett, W. J. See A. V. Partipilo
Pickerell, Kenneth LeRoy. Baltimore surgeon. 1910–
SOLUTION—3.5% sulfadiazine in triethanolamine.
A new treatment for burns: preliminary report. Johns
Hopk. Hosp. Bull., 69: 217–221, Aug. 1941
TECHNIC—
The surgical treatment of carcinoma of the common
bile duct with A. Blalock, Surgery 15: 923–937,
June 1944
Picque, Robert. French surgeon. 1877–1927
OPERATION—
Du traitement de la sacro-coxalgie par la résection sacro-
iliaque. Bull. Soc. Chir., Paris, 35: 1107–1116, Nov.
17, 1909
Pierce, George Warren. San Francisco surgeon.
1889–
METHOD—of preserving rib cartilage for transplant.
Reconstruction surgery of the nose with G. B. O'Con-
nor, Ann. Otol., Rhin. and Laryng., 47: 437–452,
June 1938
OPERATION—
Reconstruction of thumb after total loss. S. G. O., 45:
825–826, Dec. 1927
OPERATION—
Reconstruction of the external ear. Ibid., 50: 601–605,
Mar. 1930
Pieri, Gino. Belluno surgeon
OPERATION—for arterial hypertension.
La resezione dei nervi splancnici. Contributo tecnico
alla chirurgia del sistem a nervoso vegetativo. Ann. ital.
di chir., 6: 678–684, July 1927
Performed sympathectomy for relief of pain in
urinary bladder.
Enervation ou ramisection? Pr. méd., 34: 1141–1142,
Sept. 8, 1926
Pijper, Adrianus. Pretoria, South Africa, pathologist
METHOD—
An improved diffraction method for diagnosing and
following the course of pernicious and other anemias.
Brit. med. J., 1: 635–638, Apr. 6, 1929

TREATMENT—with arsenicals.
The treatment of human anthrax. Lancet, 1:88–89,
Jan. 9, 1926
Pilon, P. Tübingen physician
AGAR—alkaline blood.
Blut-Soda-Agar als Elektivnährboden für Cholera-
vibrionen. Zbl. Bakt., 60: 330–333, Sept. 21, 1911
Pinard, Adolphe. French obstetrician. 1844–1934
SIGN—pain on pressure over fundus uteri, after sixth
month, indicates breech presentation.
Traité du palper abdominale au point de vue obstétri-
cal. Paris, Lauwereyns, 1878
(Same) Treatise on abdominal palpation, as applied
to obstetrics. New York, Vail, 1885. 101 pp.
Pinel, Philippe. French alienist. 1745–1826
SYSTEM—management of insane without use of
forcible restraint.
Founder of the "open door" school of psychiatry
Garrison
Traité médico-philosophique sur l'aliénation mentale,
ou la manie. Paris, Richard, Caille-Ravier, an IX
1801. 318 pp.
Pineles, Friedrich. German physician. 1868–1936
Differentiated forms of creatinism.
Ueber Thyreoaplasie (kongenitales Myxoedem und
infantiles Myxoedem). Wien. klin. Wschr., 15: 1129–
1136, Oct. 23, 1902
Pinerua Alvarez, E. French chemist
REAGENT—for cholic acid.
Observations sur la diphénylamine, comme réactif des
nitrites, nitrates, chlorates et utilité de son emploi
quand elle est mélangée avec la résorcine et le naphthol B.
Bull. Soc. Chim., 33: 717–719, 1905
REAGENT and TEST—
On some chromatic reactions produced by organic acids,
principally tartaric, citric, and malic acids. Chem.
News, 75: 61, Feb. 5, 1897
Pinkus, Felix. German dermatologist, 1868–
DISEASE—
Ueber eine neue knötchenförmige Hauteruption: Lichen
nitidus. Arch. f. Dermat. u. Syph., 85: 11–36, 1907
Pinoff, E. Göttingen chemist
TEST—for levulose.
Ueber einige Farben- und Spectral-Reactionen der
wichtigsten Zuckerarten. Ber. dtsch. chem. Ges., 38:
3308–3309, Oct. 9, 1905
Pinto's
DISEASE—discoloration of skin, with positive Wasser-
mann reaction.
El mal del pinto. By E. del Pinto, Crón. méd. mexi-
caca, México, 15: 57; 93, 1912
Piorkowski, Max. German bacteriologist. 1859–
MEDIUM—
Ein einfaches Verfahren zur raschen Sicherstellung der
Typhusdiagnose. Dtsch. med. Wschr., 25: 39–40,
Feb. 16, 1899
METHOD—of staining for metachromatic granules.
(Über eine Modifikation der Diphtheriebacillenfär-
bung.) Zbl. Bakt., 29: 63–64, Jan. 25, 1901
TEST—for typhoid bacilli.
Ueber die Differenzierung von Bacterium coli commune
und Bacillus typhi abdomini auf Harnnährsubstraten.
Ibid., 19: 686–694, May 9, 1896
Piorry, Pierre Adolphe. French physician. 1794–
1879
Pioneer of mediate percussion.

De la percussion médiate et des signes obtenus à l'aide de ce nouveau moyen d'exploration, dans les maladies des organes thoraciques et abdominaux. Paris, Chaudé, 1828. 336 pp.

(Same) *Die mittelbare Percussion.* Würzburg, 1828
Invented pleximeter.

Traité de plessimétrisme et d'organographisme; anatomie des organes sains et malades établie pendant la vie au moyen de la percussion médiate et du dessin à l'effet d'éclairer le diagnostic. Paris, Delahaye, 1866. 752 pp.

Iotrowski, Zygmunt A. New York psychiatrist
IGNS—of organic brain disease.
The Rorschach inkblot method in organic disturbances of the central nervous system. J. nerv. ment. Dis., 86: 525–537, Nov. 1937

iper, Hans Edmund. Berlin physiologist. 1877–1915
Measured dark adaptation.
Ueber Dunkeladaptation. Z. Psychol. Physiol. Sinnesorg., 31: 161–214, 1903

iria, Raffaele. French scientist. 1815–1865
Isolated salicin.
Recherches sur la salicine et les produits qui en dérivent. C. R. Acad. Sci., 8: 479–485, 1839

irogoff, Nicolai Ivanovich. Russian surgeon. 1810–1881
MPUTATION—of foot.
Kostno-plasticheskoye udlineniye kostei goleni pri vilushtshenii stopi. Voyenno-med. Jour., St. Petersburg, 63, Sect. 2, 83–100, 1854
Also, in German. Leipzig, 1854
Described ether anesthesia per rectum.
Recherches pratiques et physiollgogie sur l'éthérisation. St. Petersbourg, Bellizard, 1847. 109 pp.

ironneau. See G. Variot

irquet, Clemens Peter. Austrian pediatrician. 1874–1929
REACTION—cutaneous tuberculin.
Tuberkulindiagnose durch cutane Impfung. Berl. klin. Wschr., 44: 644–645, May 20, 1907
Die Allergieprobe zur Diagnose der Tuberkulose im Kindersalter. Wien. med. Wschr., 57: 1369–1374, July 6, 1907
Der diagnostische Wert der kutanen Tuberkulinreaktion bei der Tuberkulose des Kindesalters auf Grund von 100 Sektionen. Wien. klin. Wschr., 20: 1123–1128, Sept. 19, 1907
Studied serum disease.
Die Serumkrankheit with B. Schick, Leipzig und Wien, Deuticke, 1905
Suggested term allergy.
Klinische Studien über Vakzination und vakzinale Allergie. Leipzig und Wien, Deuticke, 1907
Introduced concept of allergy in tuberculosis.
Allergie. Ergebn. d. inn. Med. u. Kinderh., 1: 420–464, 1908
Invented new kind of isolation bed for new-born babies.
Isolierbetten. Z. f. d. ges. Krankenhausw., 24: 741–743, Dec. 17, 1928

Piso, Gulielmus Le Pois. 1611–1678
Described yaws and separated it from syphilis. Garrison
De lue Indica. In his: *Historia naturalis Brasiliae, in qua non tantum plantae et animalia, sed et indigenarum morbi, ingenia et mores describuntur et iconibus*

supra quingenits illustrantur. Lugd. Bat., Hackium, 1648

Pitfield, Robert Lucas. Philadelphia physician. 1870–1942
METHOD—
A new method of staining flagella. Med. News, 67: 268 (only), Sept. 7, 1895

Pitkin, Horace Collins. San Francisco surgeon. 1898–
METHOD—
Sacrarthrogenetic telalgia: I. A study of referred pain with H. C. Pheasant, J. Bone and Joint Surg., 18: 111–133, Jan. 1936

Pitt, R. Margaret. See A. Felix

Pittarelli, Emilio. Italian scientist
REACTION—for creatinine.
Una reazione cromatica della creatina e dell'urea. Arch. farmacol., sper., 45; 173–186, 1928
TEST—for ascorbic acid.
Ricerche sull'analisi della Vitamina C (acid ascorbico) with M. Pittarelli, Biochem. terap. sper., 22: 100–106, Mar. 31, 1936
TEST—for glucose.
Intorno a due reazioni nuove per la ricerca delle minime quantita di glucosio negli umori dell'organismo. Ibid., 17: 272–274, June 30, 1930

Pitts, W. G. See R. W. G. Owen

Pitzman, Marsh. St. Louis surgeon. 1882–
OPERATION—
A fundamentally new technic for inguinal herniotomy. Ann. Surg., 74: 610–619, Nov. 1921

Pize, Paul Louis. French physician
TREATMENT—of purpura by perchloride of iron.
Memoire sur l'action thérapeutique et physiologique du perchlorure de fer. Monit. des Hôp., 5: 140–142, Feb. 10, 1857

Place, Edwin Hemphill. Boston pediatrician. 1880–
See Haverhill Fever.

Placido, A. Porto ophthalmologist
Invented keratoscope. (No title). Zbl. f. prakt. Augenh., Leipzig, 6: 30–31, 1882

Plaignaud. French surgeon
Successfully operated on tumor of maxillary sinus. Garrison and Morton
Observation sur un fongus du sinus maxillaire. J. de Chir., 1: 111–116, 1791

Plass, E. D. See E. L. DeGowin

Platner, Joh. Zacharian. German physician. 1694–1747
Wrote on tuberculous nature of gibbous spine. Garrison
De iis, qui ex tuberculis gibberosi fiunt. Leipzig. Langenhemiana, 1744

Plato, Julius. Breslau dermatologist
VITAL STAINING—of gonococci.
Ueber Gonokokkenfärbung mit Neutralroth in lebenden Leukocyten. Berl. klin. Wschr., 36: 1085–1086, Dec. 4, 1899

Platter, Felix. Swiss physician. 1536–1614
Made first attempt at systematic classification of disease. Garrison
Praxeos seu de cognoscendis, praedicendis, praecavendis curandisque affectibus homini-incommodantibus. Basileae, Waldkirchius, 1602–03. 2 vols.
Reported first known case of death from hypertrophy of thymus gland in an infant. Garrison

Observationum in hominis affectibus. Basileae, König 1614. p. 172
Also, in: J. Ruhräh: *Pediatrics of the past.* New York, 1925. p. 239
Plaut, F. See A. von Wassermann
Plaut, Hugo Carl. Leipzig physician. 1858–1928
ANGINA or ULCER—Vincent's angina.
Studien zur bacteriellen Diagnostik der Diphtherie und den Anginen. Dtsch. med. Wschr., 20: 920–923, Dec. 6, 1894
Playfair, William Smoult. English physician. 1835–1903
TREATMENT—by rest and feeding.
The systematic treatment of nerve prostration and hysteria. Philadelphia, Lea, 1883. 111 pp.
Plenck, Joseph Jakob von. Vienna physician. 1738–1807
SOLUTION—
A new and easy method of giving mercury to those affected with the venereal disease. Transl. from Latin by W. Saunders, London, Dilly, 1767. 55 pp.
Classified skin diseases. Garrison
Doctrina de morbis cutaneis, qua hi morbi in suas classes, genera et species rediguntur. Viennae, Graeffer, 1776. 2 ed., 1783
Plesch, Johann. German physiologist
METHOD—of collecting alveolar air.
Hämodynamische Studien. Z. exp. Path. Ther., 6: 380–618, June 10, 1909
Plesch, Johann von. Budapest surgeon
INSTRUMENT—for obtaining specimens of tissue from living subject.
Probebohrung als diagnostisches Hilfsmittel. Dtsch. med Wschr., 32: 721 (only), May 3, 1906
Pleth, Valdemar. Chicago surgeon
METHOD—
A simple and practical method of performing anastomosis by means of two knitting needles. Amer. J. Surg., 20: 170–172, June 1906
Plimmer, Henry George. London pathologist. 1856–1918
BODIES—vesicular structures found in malignant growths.
On the aetiology and histology of cancer, with special reference to recent work on the subject. Practitioner, 62: 430–455, Apr. 1899
BROTH—tartaric acid infusion.
Vorläufige Notiz über gewisse vom Krebs isolierte Organismen und deren pathogene Wirkung in Tieren. Zbl. Bakt., 25: 805–809 (806), June 10, 1899
METHOD—
A new method for the staining of bacteria flagella with S. G. Paine, J. Path. Bact., 24: 286–288, July 1921
Introduced antimony in—
Further results of the experimental treatment of trypanosmiasis in rats with J. D. Thomson, Proc. roy. Soc., S. B., 80: 1–10, Dec. 1908
Plimmer, Robert Henry Aders. English chemist. 1877–
METHOD—
The quantitative estimation of urea, and indirectly of allantoin, in urine by means of urease with Ruth F. Skelton, Biochem. J., 8: 70–73, Feb. 1914
Plombières, France
DOUCHE- SYSTEM, TREATMENT—by rectal irrigation.

Plotz, Harry. New York physician. 1890–1947
BACILLUS—
The etiology of typhus fever (and of Brill's disease): preliminary communication. J. A. M. A., 62: 1556 (only), May 16, 1914
The etiology of typhus exanthematicus with P. K. Olitsky and G. Baehr, J. Infect. Dis., 17: 1–68, July 1915
Plucker, See B. Bardenhauer
Plummer, Henry Stanley. Rochester, Minn. physician. 1874–1937
SYNDROME—of Plummer-Vinson; hypochromic anemia, achlorhydria, atrophic gastritis, dysphagia and glossitis.
Diffuse dilatation of the esophagus without anatomic stenosis (cardiospasm): a report of ninety-one cases. J. A. M. A., 58: 2013–2015, June 29, 1912
TEST—silk thread t. to differentiate stricture from diverticulum of esophagus.
Cardiospasm, with report of cases. J. Minnesota State Med. Ass., 26: 419–424,Oct. 1, 1906
Also: Coll. Papers . . . Mayo Clinic, 1905–09, pp. 21–32, 1911
Diverticulum of the esophagus, with a report of six cases. J. Minnesota State Med. Ass., 29: 270–274, June 15, 1909
Also: Coll. Papers . . . Mayo Clinic, 1905–09, pp. 11–20, 1911
TREATMENT—
Cardiospam; with a report of forty cases. J. A. M. A., 51: 549–554, Aug. 15, 1908
Advocated—
The value of iodine in exophthalmic goiter with W. M. Boothby, Coll. Papers Mayo Clinic, 15: 565–576, 1923
Plummer, William Ward. Buffalo surgeon. 1877–
OPERATION—
Two cases of recurrent anterior dislocation of the shoulder with F. N. Potts, J. Bone and Joint Surg., 7: 190–198, Jan. 1925
Poehl, Alexander Vasilyevich von. Russian chemist 1850–1898
Isolated spermin from testis.
(On spermin.) J. Russk. fis.-chim. Obsh., St. Petersburg, 23: 151–155, 1891
Pötzl, O. See K. Landsteiner
Poirot, G. See L. Cuny
Poiseuille, Jean Léonard Marie. Paris physiologist. 1799–1869
LAW—speed of currents in capillary tubes is proportional to square of their diameter; fundamental principle in determining viscosity of blood. Dorland
Recherches expérimentales sur le mouvement des liquides dans les tubes de très petits diamètres. C. R. Acad. Sci., 11: 961–967; 1041–1048, 1840; 12; 112–115, 1841
Devised first mercury manometer; called it hemodynamometer. Garrison
Recherches sur la force du coeur aortique. Paris Thèse No. 166. 1828. 45 pp.
Also: Arch. gén. de méd., 18: 550–554, 1828
Also: J. de physiol. expér., Paris, 8: 272–305, 1828
Pol, B. Douchy surgeon
Wrote on "caisson sickness."
Memoire sur les effects de la compression de l'ai

with T. J. J. Watelle, Ann. d'Hyg. publ., Paris, 2 s., 1: 241–279, 1854

Polocki, B. See J. E. v. Purkinje

Politzer, Adam. Hungarian otologist. 1835–1920

BAG—for inflating middle ear.

TREATMENT—of disease of middle ear by inflation.
Beiträge zur Ohrenheilkunds. Allg. Wien. med. Ztg., 8, 1863
Über ein neues Heilverfahren gegen Schwerhörigkeit in Folge von Unwegsamkeit der Eustachischen Ohrtrompte. Wien. med. Wschr., 13: 84–87; 102–104; 117–119; 148–152, 1863
Die Beleuchtungsbilder des Trommelfells im gesunden und kranken Zustande- Klinische Beiträge zur Erkenntniss und Behandlung der Ohren-Krankheiten. Wien, Braumüller, 1865. 143 pp.
Same, in English, New York, Wood, 1869. 183 pp.
Described otosclerosis.
On a peculiar affection of the labyrinthine capsule as a frequent cause of deafness. Trans. PanAmerican Med. Congr., 1893, Washington, pt. 2, 1607–1608, 1895

Poljak, G. D. Kiew ophthalmologist

OPERATION—dacryostomy.
Beiträge zur Behandlung unwegsamer tränenableitender Wege. Klin. Mbl. Augenheilk., 83: 510–515, Nov. 19, 1929

Pollender, Franz Aloys Antoine. Wipperfürth physician
Discovered B. anthracis, in 1849.
Mikroskopische und mikrochemische Untersuchung des Milzbrandblutes, so wie über Wesen und Kur des Milzbrandes. Viert. f. gerichtk. u. öff. Med. Berlin, 8: 103–114, 1855

Pollitzer, Sigmund. New York dermatologist. 1859–1937

DISEASE—
Hydradenitis destruens suppurativa. J. cutan. Dis., 10: 9–24, Jan. 1892
Described—
Acanthosis nigricans with V. Janowsky, Internat. Atlas f. seltene Hautkr., Hamburg, pt. 4, Plates 10, 11, 1890
Reported—
Rhinoscleroma cured by x-ray treatment. J. cutan. Dis., 28: 388–390, Aug. 1910

Polowe, David. Paterson, N. J. surgeon. 1893–

TEST—
Measurement of blood amylase activity by cuprous oxide precipitation with H. D. Ratish and J. G. M. Bullowa, Amer. J. clin. Path., Tech. Supp., 6: 62–64, Sept. 1942
Blood amylase. Amer. J. clin. Path., 13: 288–301, June 1943

Pólya, Eugen Alexander. Budapest surgeon. 1876–1944?

OPERATION—for femoral hernia.
Ein neues Verfahren zur Radikaloperation grosser Schenkelbrüche. Zbl. Chir., 32: 489–494, May 6, 1905

OPERATION—
Zur Strumpfversorgung nach Magenresektion. Ibid., 38: 892–894, July 1, 1911

Pommer, Gustav. German pathologist

BONE CYST—of Haberer and Pommer. See H. von Haberer
Zur Kenntnis der progressiven Hämatom- und Phleg-

masieveränderungen der Röhrenknochen auf Grund der mikroskopischen Befunde am neuen Knochenzystenfalle H. v. Haberers. Arch. f. orth. Chir., 17: 17–69, 1920

Poncet, Antonin. Lyon surgeon, 1849–1913

DISEASE—tuberculous rheumatism.
Faits de polyarthrite tuberculeuse simulant des lésions rheumatismales chroniques déformantes. La Lancette franc., gaz. d. hôp. civ. et milit., 70: 1219 (only), Oct. 30, 1897
OPERATION—
De l'uréthrostomie périnéale ou création méthodique au périnée d'un méat contre nature, dans les rétrécissements incurables de l'urèthre. Arch. prov. de chir., 4: 81–96, Feb. 1895

Pond, G. P. See W. S. Haines

Ponder, E. See W. E. Cooke

Ponflick, Emil. German pathologist. 1844–1913
Established that ray funges (actinomycosis) in man and cattle are identical. Garrison
Die Actinomykose des Menschen, eine neue Infectionsktrankheit auf vergleichend-pathologischer und experimenteller Grundlage geschildert. . . . Berlin, Hirschwald, 1882. 132 pp.
Also, abstr.: Berl. klin. Wschr., 17: 660–661, 1880

Ponndorf, Wilhelm Hermann Friedrich. Weimar physician. 1864–
TREATMENT—of pulmonary tuberculosis with vaccine.
Beitrage zur Heilung der Tuberkulose. Münch med. Wschr., 61: 750–752, Apr. 7: 826–830, Apr. 14, 1914
Meine Tuberkulosebehandlung. Beitr. z. Klin. d. Tuberk., Berlin, 48: 248–249, 1921

Pool, Eugene Hillhouse. New York surgeon. 1874–
PHENOMENON or SIGN—leg, in tetany.
Tetany parathyreopriva: a case report, with a brief discussion of the disease and of the parathyroid glands. Ann. Surg., 46: 507–540 (510), Oct. 1907

Pool, James Lawrence. New York neurologist. 1906–
MENINGOSCOPE—
Myeloscopy; intraspinal endoscopy. Surgery, 11: 169–182, Feb. 1942

Poole, L. T. See J. Barcroft

Pope, Charles Evans. American surgeon. 1899–
OPERATION—
New and successful closed operative procedure for pilonidal sinus: gluteus maximus mobilization: a sliding muscle graft procedure. Arch. Surg., 62: 701–712, June 1946

Popoff, Nicholas Wasil. Rochester, N. Y. pathologist. 1889–
TUMORS—glomus.
The digital vascular system with reference to the state of glomus in inflammation, arteriosclerotic gangrene, diabetic gangrene, thrombo-angiitis obliterans and supernumerary digits in man. Arch. Path., 18: 295–330, Sept. 1934

Poppen, James Leonard. Boston surgeon. 1903–
TECHNIC—
Exophthalmos: diagnosis and surgical treatment of intractable cases. Amer. J. Surg., 64: 64–79, Apr. 1944

Popper, E. See K. Landsteiner

Popper, Hans. Vienna physician
METHOD—of determining creatinine.
Zur Kreatininbestimmung im Blute with E. Mandel

and Helene Mayer, Biochem. Z., 291: 354–367, Aug. 2, 1937

See also Z. Dische

Popper, J. L. See G. Horrax

Porak, R. See H. Claude

Porcher, Charles. French chemist. 1877–1933

TEST—

Über Harnindican with Ch. Hervieux, Z. physiol. Chem., 39: 147–154, July 31, 1903

Porges, Otto. Vienna physician. 1879–

REACTION or TEST—

Ueber die Rolle der Lipoide bei der Wassermann'schen Syphilis-Reaktion with G. Meier, Berl. klin. Wschr., 45: 731–735, Apr. 13, 1908

Abstr.: Wien. klin. Wschr., 21: 206, 1908

Demonstrated hypoglycemia in patients with Addison's disease.

Ueber Hypoglykämie bei Morbus Addison sowie bei nebennierenlosen Hunden. Z. klin. Med., 69: 341–349, 1909

Introduced—

Über Gastrophotographie. Abstr.: Wien. klin. Wschr., 42: 89, Jan. 17; 889, June 27, 1929

See also D. Aldersberg

Porro, Edoardo. Milan surgeon. 1842–1902

OPERATION—

Dell'amputazione utero-ovarica come complemento di taglio cesareo. Ann. univ. de med., 237: 291–350, 1876

Also: Milano, Rechiedei, 1876. 83 pp.

Porta, Giovanni Battista della. Naples physician. 1536–1615

A forerunner of Lavater in estimating human character by features. Garrison

De humana physiognomia. Sorrento, 1586; 1593

One of the principal founders of optics. Garrison

De refractione, optices parte, libri novem. Neapoli, Carlinum, 1593. 230 pp.

Portal, Paul. Montpellier obstetrician. 1630–1703

Taught that version can be done by one foot and that face presentations usually run a normal course. Garrison

La pratique des accouchemens soutenue d'un grand nombre d'observations. Paris, Martin, 1685. 368 pp.

Porter, Charles Allen. Boston surgeon. 1866–

TREATMENT—

Avulsion of the scalp. Review of the literature and the report of a case with W. M. Shedden, Boston M. and S. J., 186: 727–730, June 1, 1922

Porter, Charles Burnham. Boston surgeon. 1840–1909

HOOK MANEUVER—

Some surgical cases. Fracture of the surgical neck of the humerus, complicated by dislocation of the head beneath the coracoid process. . . . Trans. Amer. Surg. Ass., 12: 287–289, 1894

Porter, T. C. English scientist

LAW—of Ferry-Porter.

Contributions to the study of 'flicker'. Proc. roy. Soc., 63: 347–356, 1898

(Same) Paper II. Ibid., 70: 313–329, 1902

Porter, William Henry. Irish physician. 1790–1861

SIGN—tracheal tugging, of aneurysm of aorta.

In his: Observations on the surgical pathology of the larynx and trachea. . . . Dublin, Hodges and M'Arthur, 1826. 283 pp.

Porter, William Henry. New York physician. 1853–1933

TEST—for uric acid in urine.

In his: A practical treatise on renal diseases and urinary analysis. New York, Wood, 1887. 349 pp. p. 265

Porter, William Townsend. Boston physician. 1862–

THEORY—fat embolism t. of shock.

Traumatic shock. Harvey Lectures, 13: 21–43, 1917

Portes, Louis. French obstetrician

OPERATION—

Césarienne suivie d'extériorisation temporaire de l'utérus et de réintégration secondaire dans le bassin. Bull. Soc. d'Obstet. et de Gynéc., 13: 171–176, Mar. 10, 1924

Porteus, Stanley David. Hawaii psychiatrist. 1883–

TEST—maze t. for intelligence; a non-language performance t.

Test interpretation. Training School Bull., 17: 68–72, 1920–21

Studies in mental deviation. Vineland, N. J., 1922. 276 pp.

Maze tests and social adaptability. Lancet, 1: 1152–1153, May 28, 1927

Portier, Paul Jules. French physician. 1866–

Described anaphylaxis; named by Richet. Garrison and Morton.

De l'action anaphylactique de certains venins with Ch. Richet, C. R. Soc. Biol., 54: 170–172, Feb. 15, 1902

Post, Anna L. See F. B. Kingsbury

Post, Wright. New York surgeon. 1766–1822

First to tie primitive carotid in its continuity with success. Garrison

A case of carotid aneurism successfully treated. Amer. Med. and Phil. Register, N. Y., 4: 366–377, 1814

First in America to ligate femoral artery successfully for popliteal aneusysms, according to John Hunter's method. Garrison

A case of inguinal aneurism. Ibid., 443–453

The second in America to ligate external iliac artery successfully. Garrison. Ibid.

First to ligate subclavian artery outside scaleni. Garrison, Trans. Phys. Med. Soc., N. Y., 1: 387–394, 1817

Potain, Pierre Carl Edouard. French physician. 1825–1901

AIR SPHYGMOMANOMETER—

Du sphygmomanomètre et de la mesure de la pression artérielle chez l'homme, a l'état normal et pathologique. Arch. Physiol. norm. path., 1: 556–569, 1880

Described movements and murmurs of jugular veins.

Des mouvements et des bruits qui se passent dans les veines jugulaires. Bull. Soc. méd. Hôp. Paris, 4: 3–27, 1867

Also, transl. by J. P. Wozencraft in: F. A. Willius and T. E. Keys' Cardiac classics. St. Louis, Mosby, 1941. pp. 533–556

Poth, Edgar Jacob. American surgeon. 1899–

CLAMP—

Intestinal clamps: a new structural principle. Amer. J. Surg., 61: 449–450, Sept. 1943

MODIFICATION—

An aseptic uretero-enterostomy. S. G. O., 60: 875–878, Apr. 1935

TECHNIC—
A new technique for cutting skin grafts, including description of new instruments. Surgery, 6: 935–939, Dec. 1939
TECHNIC—
The implantation of the pancreatic duct into the gastrointestinal tract: experimental and clinical study. Ibid., 15: 693–704, May 1944
Potjan. German medical student
TEST—for albumin in urine.
Eiweissnachweis mit Chlorkalklösung und Salzsäure with Steffenhagen, Dtsch. med. Wschr., 43: 530 (only), Apr. 26, 1917
Pototsknig, Giorgio. Prague pathologist. 1892–
Reported chordoma with metastases.
Ein Fall von malignem Chordom mit Metastasen. Beitr. path. Anat., 65: 356–361, 1919
Pott, Percival. English physician. 1714–1788
CURVATURE, DISEASE, PARALYSIS or PARA-
PLEGIA—
Remarks on that kind of palsy of the lower limbs which is frequently found to accompany a curvature of the spine and is supposed to be caused by it, together with its method of cure. London, Johnson, 1779. 84 pp.
Also, in Dutch. Leyden, de Pecker, 1779
Also, in French. Paris, Mequignon, 1783
Also, in German, Leipzig, Jacobaer, 1786
Also in: *Surgical works.* London, 1808, 3: 229–258
Also in: *Medical classics,* 1: 281–297, Dec. 1936
Further remarks on the useless state of the lower limbs, in consequence of a curvature of the spine; being a supplement to a former treatise on that subject. London, Johnson, 1782. 64 pp.
Also in: *Surgical works.* London, 1808, 3: 259–296
Also in: *Medical classics,* 1: 298–328, Dec. 1936
FRACTURE—of ankle.
Some few general remarks on fractures and dislocations. London, Howes, 1769. 126 pp. pp. 57–64
Also, in French. Paris, Didot, 1771
Also, in Italian. Venezia, Bassaglia, 1784
Also in: *Surgical works.* London, 1808, 1: 325–331
Also in: *Medical classics, 1: 331–337,* Dec. 1936
GANGRENE—senile.
Chirurgical observations relative to the cataract, the polypus of the nose, the cancer of the scrotum, the different kinds of ruptures, and the mortification of the toes and feet. London, Hawes, 1775. 208 pp.
PUFFY TUMOR—associated with osteolyelitis of skull.
Observations on the nature and consequences of wounds and contusions of the head, fractures of the skull, concussions of the brain, etc. London, Hitch and Howes, 1760. 182 pp.
First to describe cancer due to industrial trauma, epitheliomata of chimney sweeps. See GANGRENE
Wrote—
A treatise on ruptures. London, Hitch and Hawes, 1756
Wrote—
Practical remarks on the hydrocele, or watry rupture. London, Hitch and Hawes, 1762
Pottenger, Frances Marion. American physician. 1869–
SIGN—
Muscle spasm and degeneration in intrathoracic inflammations. . . . St. Louis, Mosby, 1912. 105 pp.

Pottenger, Joseph Elbert. Monrovia, Calif. physician. 1878–
METHOD—
The demonstration of rare tubercle bacilli in sputum by the dilution-flotation method in conjunction with picric acid. Amer. Rev. Tuberc., 24: 583–595, Nov. 1931
Potter, Caryl Ashby. St. Joseph, Mo. surgeon. 1886–1933
METHOD—
The treatment of duodenal fistula: report of a case. J. A. M. A., 88: 899–901, Mar. 19, 1927
Treatment of duodenal and fecal fistula: further observations. Ibid., 92: 359–363, Feb. 2, 1929
Potter, Irving White. Buffalo obstetrician. 1868–
OPERATION—
Version. Amer. J. Obstet. Gynaec., 1: 560–573, Mar. 1921–
Potts, F. N. See W. W. Plummer
Potts, Willis John. Oak Park, Ill., surgeon. 1895–
OPERATION—
Anastomosis of the aorta to a pulmonary artery: certain types in congenital heart disease with S. Smith and S. Gibson, J. A. M. A., 132: 627–631, Nov. 16, 1946
VEIN OCCLUDER—
Chemical obliteration of varicose veins: improved technic. Ann. Surg., 92: 475–477, Sept. 1930
Poullet, J. French surgeon. 1870–1915
OPERATION—
Cure radicale des hernies; même chez les vieillards, par méthode à lambeau fibro-périostique. Arch. prov. de Chir., Paris, 3: 310–313, 1894
Poupart, Francois. French anatomist. 1661–1709
LIGAMENT—inguinal.
(Oral communication on inguinal ligaments before Royal Academy of Sciences.) Histoire de l'Academie Royale des Sciences, 1705, p. 51, 1796
Also: Amsterdam, Kuyper, 1707. p. 64
Pouteau, Claude. French surgeon. 1725–1775
FRACTURE—of distal end of radius, similar to Colles'.
Oeuvres posthumes de M. Pouteau. Paris, Pierres, 1783. Vol. 2, p. 251
Povitzky, Olga R. See Anna W. Williams
Powell, C. B. See W. Snow
Power, M. H. See R. M. Wilder
Power, R. Wood. English surgeon
OPERATION—
The treatment of mid-line ventral hernia. Brit. med. J., 1: 958–960, May 8, 1937
Poynton, Frederick John. English physician. 1869–
Concluded that streptococcus is cause of acute rheumatism.
Researches on rheumatism with A. Paine, London, Churchill, 1913. 461 pp.
Pratt, Gerald Hillary. New York surgeon. 1903–
TEST—
Test for incompetent communicating branches in the surgical treatment of varicose veins. J. A. M. A., 117: 100–101, July 12, 1941
Pratt, Josephine. See C. Krumwiede
Pratt, T. C. See L. S. McKittrick
Praun, Eduard. German surgeon
OPERATION—on frontal sinus.
Die Stirnbeinhöhleneiterung und deren Operativbehandlung. Würzburg, Röhrl, 1890. 46 pp.

Prausnitz, Carl Willy. Breslau bacteriologist. 1876–
REACTION—demonstrates transferability and skin
sensitizing ability of a specific antibody.
Studien über die Ueberempfindlichkeit with H.
Küstner, Zbl. Bakt., 86: 160–169, Apr. 1, 1921

Pravaz, Charles Gabriel. French surgeon. 1791–1853
Invented modern galvanocautery.
*Sur un nouveau moyen d'opérer la coagulation du sang
dans les artères, applicable à la guérison des aneurismes.*
C. R. Acad. Sci., 36: 88–90, Jan. 10, 1853

Prebluda, Harry Jacob. Baltimore biochemist. 1911–
REAGENT—
*A chemical reagent for the detection and estimation of
vitamin B_1* with E. V. McCollum, Science, 84: 488
(only), Nov. 27, 1936

Pregl, Fritz. Graz chemist. 1871–1931
SOLUTION—of iodine, used in infections.
*Ueber eine in der praktischen Medizin verwendbare
Jodlösung.* Wien. klin. Wschr., 34: 288–289, June
21, 1921

Preiser, George Karl Felix. Hamburg surgeon. 1879–
1913
DISEASE—rarefaction of carpal scaphoid.
*Zur Frage der typischen traumatischen Ernährungs-
störungen der kurzen Hand- und Fusswurzelknochen.*
Fort. Geb. d. Roentgenstr., 17: 360–362, 1911

Presch, W. Berlin physician
TEST—for thiosulfate in urine.
*Ueber das Verhalten des Schwefels im Organismus und
den Nachweis der unterschwefligen Säure im Men-
schenharn.* Arch. path. Anat., 119: 148–167, Jan. 2,
1890

Prevost, Jean Louis. French physician. 1790–1850
Used defibrinated blood in animal transfusion.
*Examen du sang et de son action dans les divers
phénomènes de la vie* with J. B. A. Dumas, Ann. de
Chim., Paris, 18: 280–297, 1821
Described segmentation of frog's egg.
Mémoire sur la développement du poulet dans l'oeuf
with J. B. A. Dumas, Ann. d. sci. nat., Paris, 12:
415–443, 1827

Prevost, Jean Louis. Swiss physician. 1838–1927
LAW and SIGN—
*De la déviation conjuguée des yeux et de la rotation de la
tête dans certains cas d'hémiplegie.* Paris, 1868. 144 pp.

Preyer, Wilhelm Thierry. German chemist
TEST—for carbon monoxide in blood.
Beiträge zur Kenntniss des Blutfarbstoffs. Zbl. med.
Wiss., 5: 259–260, Apr. 13, 1867

Pribram, Bruno Oskar. Berlin surgeon. 1887–
METHOD—of dissolving gallstones in common duct
by use of ether and amyl nitrite.
New methods in gall-stone surgery. S. G. O., 60: 55–64,
Jan. 1935
OPERATION—excision of cardia followed by esopha-
gogastrostomy.
Zur Pathologie und Chirurgie der spastischen Neurosen.
Arch. klin. Chir., 120: 207–261, July 21, 1922

Price, C. W. R. English surgeon
METHOD—
*Removal of plaster casts: a modification of Bickford's
method.* Brit. med. J., 2: 772 (only), Nov. 29, 1941

Price, E. A. See F. H. Carr

Price-Jones, Cecil. London pathologist
CURVE and METHOD—of measurement of size of
blood cells.

The variation in the sizes of red blood cells. Brit. med.
J., 2: 1418–1419, Nov. 5, 1910
*Anisocytosis with special reference to pernicious
anemia.* Guy's Hosp. Rep., 74: 10–22, Jan. 1924

Prichard, James Cowles. Edinburgh physician. 1786–
1848
First described moral insanity. Garrison
*A treatise on insanity, and other disorders affecting the
mind.* London, Sherwood, 1835. 483 pp.

Priestley, D. P. See J. W. McLeod

Priestley, J. G. See J. S. Haldane

Priestley, James Taggart. Rochester, Minn. surgeon.
1903–
OPERATION—for hydronephrosis.
*The conservative surgical treatment of non-calculous
hydronephrosis.* S. G. O., 68: 832–841, Apr. 1939

Priestley, Joseph. English naturalist. 1733–1804
Discovered oxygen.
Observations on different kinds of air. Philos. Trans.,
62: 147–264, 1772
*Experiments and observations relating to various
branches of natural philosophy, with a continuation of
the observations on air.* London and Birmingham,
1779–1786, 3 vols.

Priestley, Sir William Overend. Scottish gynecol-
ogist. 1829–1901
Wrote—
Cases of intermenstrual or intermediate dysmenorrhea.
Brit. med. J., 2: 431–432, Oct. 19, 1872

Primavera, Arturo. Naples physician
TEST—for indican in urine.
*Un nuovo metodo per la ricerca dell'indicamo nelle
urine in presenza di clorato di potassio e ioduri.* Giorn.
intern. sci. med., 30: 163–170, Feb. 29, 1908

Prince, Arthur E. Springfield, Ill. ophthalmologist.
1853–1930
OPERATION—
*Section and exsection of the rectus muscles for cosmetic
effect in cases of squint inoperable by tenotomy and advancement.* Amer. J. Ophthal., 19: 259–276, Aug.
1902

Pringle, James Hogarth. Glasgow surgeon
METHOD—
Notes on the arrest of hepatic hemorrhage due to trauma.
Ann. Surg., 48: 541–549, Oct. 1908

Pringle, Sir John. Scottish physician. 1707–1782
Founder of modern military medicine and originator
of the Red Cross idea. Garrison
Named influenza.
*Observations on the diseases of the army, in camp and
garrison.* London, Millar and Wilson, 1752. 431 pp.
*A discourse upon some late improvements of the means
for preserving the health of mariners.* London, Roy.
Soc., 1776

Pringle, John James. London dermatologist. 1855–
1922
DISEASE—nevus sebaceus.
Über einen Fall von kongenitalen Adenoma sebaceum.
Mschr. f. prakt. Dermat., 10: 197–211, Mar. 1, 1890

Prior, J. See D. Finkler

Privey, Paul. French physician. 1885–
SIGN—Lesieur-Privey s.
*De l'albumoptysie, albumino-réaction des expectora-
tions. . . .* Lyon, 1911. 113 pp.

Proca, G. French physician

SOLUTION—spleen infusion.
Milieux de culture simplifiés. C. R. Soc. Biol., 90:
1164–1165, Feb. 21, 1924
STAIN—to distinguish living from dead bacteria.
Sur une coloration différentielle des bactéries mortes.
Ibid., 67: 148–149, June 18, 1909
Prochaska, Georg. Prague physiologist. 1749–1820
Introduced idea of sensorium commune.
*Adnotationum academicarum fasciculi tres. III. De
functionibus systematis nervosi.* Prague, Gerle, 1784
Proetz, Arthur Walter. St. Louis otolaryngologist.
1888–
DISPLACEMENT SUCTION—
*Displacement irrigation of nasal sinuses; a new pro-
cedure in diagnosis and conservative treatment.* Arch.
Otolaryngol., Chicago, 4: 1–13, July 1926
Profeta, Giuseppe. Italian physician. 1840–1911
IMMUNITY or LAW—a non-syphilitic child born of
syphilitic parents is immune. Obs.
Sulla sifilide per allattamento. Lo Sperimentale, 4 s.,
15: 328–338; 339–418, 1865
Transl. by H. Maccarini in: Semana medica, May 1,
1941
Profichet, Georges Charles. French ohysician. 1873–
DISEASE or SYNDROME—
*Sur une variété de concrétions phosphatiques sous-
cutanées (pierres de la peau).* Paris, 1900. 79 pp.
Pros. E. Warschau bacteriologist
TEST—for acetone in urine.
*Über eine neue quantitative Acetonbestimmung in
Harn.* Klin. Wschr., 9: 2039–2040, Oct. 25, 1930
Proskauer, Bernhard. Berlin physician. 1851–1915
MEDIUM—protein-free.
*Beiträge zur Ernahrungsphysiologie des Tuberkel-
bacillus* with M. Beck, Z. Hyg. InfektKr., 18: 128–
152 (146), 1894
See also A. Capaldi, O. Vosges
Proske, H. O. American scientist
TEST—
*The protein tyrosin reaction: a biochemical diagnostic
test for malaria.* Pub. Health Rep., 54: 158–172, Feb.
3, 1939
Prosser, Thomas. English physician
Introduced use of powder containing calcined sponge
(iodine). Garrison and Morton
*An account and method of cure of the bronchocele or
Derby neck.* London, Owen, 1769
Proust, Robert. French surgeon. 1873–
MODIFICATION—
La technique de l'opération de Kraske. Pr. méd., No.
105, pp. 845–847, Dec. 28, 1907
Prout, William. English chemist. 1785–1850
Proved that gastric juice contains free hydrochloric
acid.
*On the nature of the acid and saline matters usually
existing in the stomachs of animals.* Philos. Trans.,
114:45–49, 1824
Provost, Dorothy J. See C. Krumwiede
Prudden, T. M. See F. Delafield
Pryce, Daniel Merlin. London pathologist
METHOD—
*A simplification of the "halo" method of measuring the
diameter of red blood corpuscles.* Lancet, 2: 275–276,
Aug. 10, 1929
Pryde, J. See R. C. Jordan

Pryor, William Rice. New York gynecologist. 1858–
1904
POSITION—
*An improved position of examining the female bladder,
admitting intravesical operations and treatment of the
ureters.* Med. Rec., 59: 327–329, Mar. 2, 1901
Przewalski, B. Charkow physician
SIGN—
Ein sehr frühes Symptom der Pleuritis exsudativa.
Zbl. Chir., 1: 377–378, Apr. 5, 1902
Puchot, Ed. French scientist
REACTION—for albumin.
Observations sur l'iode réactif de l'amidon. C. R. Acad.
Sci., 83: 225–226, July 17, 1876
Pugh, Benjamin. English obstetrician
Introduced curved forceps in 1740. Garrison
*A treatise on midwifery, chiefly with regard to the
operation, with several improvements in that art; to
which is added some cases and descriptions, with
plates of several new instruments, both in midwifery
and surgery.* London, Buckland, 1754. 152 pp.
Pugh, Winfield Scott. New York surgeon. 1879–
OPERATION—
Circumcision. Surg. Clin. North Amer., 15: 461–470,
Apr. 1935
Punnett, R. C. See W. Bateson
Pupin, Michael Idvorsky. New York engineer, 1858–
Introduced intensifying screen.
A few remarks on experiments with Röntgen rays.
Electricity, N. Y., 10: 68–69, 1896
Purdy, Charles Wesley. American physician. 1846–
1901
FLUID, METHOD, REAGENT, SOLUTION—
Quantitative testing for sugar in the urine. Chicago,
1891
Practical urinalysis and urinary diagnosis. Phila-
delphia, Davis, 1894. 357 pp.
Purjesz, Béla von. German physician
TEST—
*Eine einfache Reaktion zum Nachweis von Bilirubin
im Harn.* Med. Klin., 33: 1271 (only), Sept. 17,
1937
Purkinje, Johannes Evangelista von. Hungarian
physiologist. 1787–1869
CELLS or CORPUSCLES—large branching neurons
in middle layer of cortex cerebelli. (No title, but
plate has legend *Purkinje's mikrosc. Untersuchungen
II.*) Ber ü. d. Versamml. dtsch. Naturf. u. Aerzte,
1837, Prague, 15: 174–175; 178–180, 1838. Fig. 18
FIBERS and NETWORK—in subendocardial tissue
of ventricles.
De musculari cordis structura. In student's dissertation by Bogislaus Policki. Breslau, 1839
FIBERS—of uterus.
De structura fibrosa uteri nongravidi. In student's
dissertation by Wilhelm Kasper. Breslau, 1840
FIGURES—produced by retinal vessels.
IMAGE—on retina, produced by shadow of blood
vessels.
IMAGE—three pairs of images of one object seen in
observing pupil.
*Commentatio de examine physiologico organi visus et
systematis cutanei.* Breslau, 1823. 58 pp.
PHENOMENON—fields of equal brightness but
different color become unequally bright if intensity
of illumination is decreased.

Beiträge zur Kenntniss des Sehens in subjectiver Hinsicht. Prag, Calve, 1823. 176 pp. (Graduation dissertation)

VESICLE—germinal, of embryo.

Subjectae sunt symbolae ad ovi avium historiam ante incubationem cum duobus lithographis. Vratislaviae, typ. Universitatis, (1825) 22 pp.

". . . the starting-point of modern work on vestibular and cerebellar nystagmus." Garrison

De cerebri laesi ad motum voluntarium relatione, certaque vertiginis directione ex certis cerebri regionibus laesis pendente. In student's dissertation by Heinrich Carl Krause, Breslau, 1824

Beiträge zur Kenntniss des Schwindels aus heantognostischen Daten. Med. Jahrb., Wien, 6: 79–125, 1820

Also: Rust's Mag. f. d. ges. Heilk., Berl., 23: 284–310, 1825

Pointed out importance of finger-prints and gave accurate figuration. See FIGURES—

Discovered sudoriferous glands of skin with their excretory ducts.

In student's dissertation, *De epidermide humana*, by Adolph Wendt. Breslau, 1833

Wrote on ciliary epithelial motion.

De phaenomeno generali et fundamentali motus vibratorii continui in membranis cum externis tum internis animalium plurimorum et superiorum et inferiorum ordinum obvii with G. G. Valentin, Vratislaviae, Schulz, 1835. 95 pp.

Pointed out probable identity of structure in animal and plate cells. See CELLS

Discovered lumen of axis-cylinder of nerves. Ibid.

Wrote on artificial digestion. Garrison

Ueber künstliche Verdauung with Pappenheim, Müller's Arch., Berlin, 1838. pp. 1–4

Coined term protoplasm.

De formatione granulosa in nervis aliisque partibus organismi animalis. In student's dissertation by Joseph Rosenthal. Breslau, 1839

Purtscher, Otmar. German ophthalmologist. 1852–1927

DISEASE—

Angiopathia retinae traumatica. Lymphorrhagien des Augengrundes. Arch. f. Ophthal., 82: 347–371, June 25, 1912

Pusey, William Allen. American dermatologist. 1865–1940

METHOD—

The use of carbon dioxid snow in the treatment of nevi and other lesions of the skin: a preliminary report. J. A. M. A., 49: 1354–1356, Oct. 19, 1907

Advocated—

Roentgen-rays in the treatment of skin diseases and for the removal of hair. J. Cutan. Dis., 18: 302–315, July 1900

Pussep, Lyudvig Martinovich. German surgeon. 1876–

OPERATION—

Operative Behandlung des Hydrocephalus internus bei Kindern. Arch. f. Kinderh., 59: 172–198, 1912

Putnam, James Jackson. Boston neurologist. 1846–1918

SYNDROME—

A group of cases of system sclerosis of the spinal cord, associated with diffuse collateral degeneration; occurring in enfeebled persons past middle life, and especially in women; studied with particular reference to etiology. J. nerv. ment. Dis., 18: 69–110, Feb. 1891

TREATMENT—

The treatment of a form of painful periarthritis of the shoulder. Boston M. and S. J., 107: 509–512, Nov. 30; 536–539, Dec. 7, 1882

Putnam, Tracy Jackson. Boston neurologist. 1894–

TREATMENT—

Treatment of hydrocephalus by endoscopic coagulation of the choroid plexus. New Engl. J. Med., 210: 1373–1376, June 28, 1934

Putti, Vittorio. Bologna surgeon. 1880–1940

TREATMENT—

Early treatment of congenital dislocation of the hip. J. Bone and Joint Surg., 11: 798–809, Oct. 1929

Coined word platyspondyly and was first to describe deformity.

Die angeborenen Deformitäten der Wirbelsäule. Fort. a. d. Geb. d. Röntgenst., 15: 65–92 (70), 1910

Puzos, Nicholas. Paris accoucheur. 1686–1753

METHOD—early rupture of membranes in placenta previa.

Traité des accouchemens, contenant des observations importantes sur la pratique de cet art; . . . Paris, Desaint et Saillant, 1759. 419 pp.

Pyl, Theodorus

Noted existence of elastic fluid in labyrinth and its rôle in transmission of sound. Neuburger and Garrison

Dissertatio medica de auditus in genere et de illo que fit per os in specie. Greifswald, 1742. p. 20

Pylarino, James. 1659–1715

Accredited with "medical" discovery of variolation. Garrison and Morton

Nova et tuta variolas excitandi per transplantationem methodus. Venetiis, Hertz, 1715

Pyle, Eleanor. See Florence Hulton-Frankel

Pyle, John Sherman. Canton, Ohio surgeon. 1865–

OPERATION—

Opening the cranial cavity with a new set of instruments: the operation illustrated from an interesting case, with a report. Med. Rec., 45: 163–165, Feb. 10, 1894

Q

Quain, Eric Peer. Bismarck, N. D. surgeon. 1870–

METHOD—

The application of the sewing machine stitch in gastric and intestinal anastomoses. S. G. O., 23: 489 (only), Oct. 1916

A new instrument for the application of the sewing machine stitch in gastric and intestinal surgery. Amer. J. Surg., 31: 262–267, Oct. 1917

Quatrefages de Breau, Jean Louis Armand de. French naturalist. 1810–1892

ANGLE—parietal a.

Crania ethnica; les crânes des races humaines décrits et figurés d'après les collections du Muséum d'histoire naturelle de Paris, de la Société d'anthropologie de Paris, et les principales collections de la France et de l'étranger with E. T. J. Hamy, Paris, Baillière, 1872–82. 2 vols.

Queckenstedt, Hans. Rostock physician. ?–1918

JUGULAR SIGN or TEST—of spinal block.

Zur Diagnose der Rückenmarkskompression. Dtsch. Z. Nervenheilk., 55: 325–333, Dec. 28, 1916

Quenu, Edouard André Victor Alfred. Paris surgeon. 1852–

OPERATION—for cancer of rectum.

Chirurgie du rectum. Paris, Steinheil, 1895 & 1899 2 vols.

SIGN—if blood flows from a puncture at the periphery after main artery is compressed, collateral circulation is adequate.

Sur la traitement moderne des anéurismes poplités with Muret, Rev. de Chir., 41: 282–294, Feb. 10, 1910

Quervain, Fritz de. Swiss surgeon. 1868–

DISEASE—fibrosis of sheath of a tendon of finger.

Ueber eine Form von chronischer Tendovaginitis. Cor.-Bl. f. schweiz. Aerzte, Basel, 25: 389–394, July 1, 1895

Quesada, Fortunato. Lima surgeon

TREATMENT—of fractures.

Aparato fenestrado y periostiorrafía en las fracturas de irreductibilidad transversal. La Crónica méd., Lima, 53: 89–108, Mar. 1936

Quetelet, Lambert Adolphe Jacques. French physician. 1796–1874

INDEX—of constitution; weight-stature.

Anthropométrie, ou mesure des différentes facultés de l'homme. Paris, Bailliere, 1871. 479 pp.

Queyrat, Auguste. French physician. 1872

ERYTHROPLASIA of—a precancerous lesion.

Érythroplasie du gland. Bull. Soc. franc. de Dermat. et Syph., Paris, 22: 378–382, Nov. 9, 1911

Quick, Armand James. American physician. 1894–

METHOD—of determining prothrombin clotting time of blood; a test for control of vitamin K therapy.

The prothrombin in hemophilia and in obstructive jaundice. J. biol. Chem., 109: LXXIII–LXXIV, May 1935

A study of the coagulation defect in hemophilia and in jaundice with Margaret Stanley-Brown and F. W. Bancroft, Amer. J. med. Sci., 190: 501–511, Oct. 1935

METHOD—of preparation of thromboplastin.

The nature of the bleeding in jaundice. J. A. M. A., 110: 1658–1662, May 14, 1938

TEST—hippuric acid, of liver function.

The synthesis of hippuric acid: a new test of liver function. Amer. J. med. Sci., 185: 630–635, May 1933

Clinical value of the test for hippuric acid in cases of disease of the liver. Arch. intern. Med., 57: 544–556, Mar. 1936

MODIFICATION—

Intravenous modification of the hippuric acid test for liver function. Amer. J. Digest. Dis., 6: 716–717, Dec. 1939

Quigley, B. See W. K. Smith

Quimaud, J. See A. Borrel

Quincke, Heinricus Iranaeus. German physician. 1842–1922

DISEASE or EDEMA—angioneurotic e.

Über akutes umschriebenes Hautädem. Mschr. f. prakt. Dermat., 1: 129–131, 1882

Also, in English in R. H. Major's

Classic descriptions of disease. Springfield, Ill., Thomas, 1939. 2 ed., pp. 682–683

OPERATION, PUNCTURE—spinal.

Ueber Hydrocephalus. Verh. Kongr. inn. Med., 10 Kongr., pp. 321–340, 1891

Die Lumbalpunction des Hydrocephalus. Berl. klin. Wschr., 28: 929–933, Sept. 21; 965–968, Sept. 28, 1891

Die Technik der Lumbalpunktion. Berlin und Wien, 1902. 15 pp.

PULSE or SIGN—of aortic insufficiency; blanching of finger nails at each diastole of heart.

Described capillary and venous pulse.

Beobachtungen über Capillar- und Venenpuls. Berl. klin. Wschr., 5: 357–359, Aug. 24, 1868

Also, abstr. in English in R. H. Major's

Classic descriptions of disease. Springfield, Ill., Thomas, 1939 pp. 393–397

Also, abstr. in English in F. A. Willius and T. E. Keys' *Cardiac classics.* St. Louis, Mosby, 1941. pp. 569–573

Reported chylous effusion in chest from traumatic rupture of thoracic duct.

Ueber fetthaltige Transsudate. Hydrops chylosus und Hydrops adiposus. Dtsch. Arch. f. klin. Med., 16: 121–139, Sept. 1875

Reported carcinoma cells in smears from pleural and abdominal fluids.

Ueber die geformten Bestandtheile von Transsudaten. Ibid., 30: 580–588, Apr. 25, 1882

Distinguished Entamoeba histolytica from E. coli.

Über Amöben-Enteritis with E. Roos, Berl. klin. Wschr., 30: 1089–1094, Nov. 6, 1893

Quinquand, Charles Eugène. French physician. 1841–1894

DISEASE—purulent folliculitis of scalp.

Folliculite destructive des régions velues. Bull. Soc. méd. Hôp. Paris, 5: 395–398, Aug. 10, 1888

See also N. Gréhant

Quint, H. See G. de Takats

Quintin, Réné. French physician

SERUM or TREATMENT—subcutaneous injection of sea-water for malnutrition, etc.

L'eau de mer; milieu organique; constance du milieu marin originel, comme milieu vital des cellules à travers la série animale. Paris, Masson, 1904. 503 pp.

Quittenbaum, Carl Friedrich. German surgeon. 1793–1852

Advocated splenectomy.

Commentatio de splenis hypertrophia et historia extirpationis splenis hypertrophici cum fortuna adversa. Rostochii, typ. Adlerianis, (1836)

R

Raab, Wilhelm. Prag pathologist. 1895–
THEORY—of fat metabolism.
Das hormonal-nervöse Regulationssystem des Fett-
stoffwechsels. Z. ges. exp. Med., 49: 179–269, Mar. 3,
1926
Rabello, Eduardo, Jr. Brazil physician
CLASSIFICATION—of leprosy on basis of pathology.
Uma classificacao clinica-epidemiologica das formas da
lepra. Rev. brasil. de leprol., (Spec. no.), 4: 375–
410, 1936
Rabl, Carl. Vienna anatomist. 1853–1917
SOLUTION—chromoformic acid.
Über Zelltheilung. Morph. Jb., 10: 215–330, 1885
THEORY—of formation of branchial cysts or fistulas.
Zur Bildungsgeschiechte des Halses. Prag. med.
Wschr., 11: 497–499, Dec. 29, 1886; 12: 3–4, Jan.
5, 1887
Rabl, Carl R. H. Berlin surgeon. 1894–
TEST—for dissolved lime in growing bones.
Über die Kalkablagerung bei der Knochenentwick-
lung. Klin. Wschr., 2: 1644–1646, Aug. 27, 1923
Racely, C. A. See J. A. Gius
Rademaker, Gijsbertus Godefriedus Johannes.
Utrecht neurologist
Demonstrated rôle of red nucleus.
Die Bedeutung der roten Kerne und des übrigen Mit-
telhirns für Muskeltonus, Körperstellung und Laby-
rinthreflexe. Monog. a. d. Geb. d. Neurol. u. Psychiat.,
Heft 94, 1926. 340 pp.
Raffel, S. See G. H. Bailey
Ragan, C. See J. W. Ferrebee
Rahn, C. See C. F. W. Ludwig
Rajasingham, A. S. Ceylon surgeon
OPERATION—
A new technique for the repair of umbilical and mid-
line incisional herniae. J. Ceylon Br., Brit. med. Ass.,
36: 123–125, Mar. 1939
Rake, Geoffrey William. New Brunswick, N. J.
scientist. 1904–
METHOD—
A rapid method for estimation of penicillin with
Helen Jones, Proc. Soc. exp. Biol., N. Y., 54 : 189–
190, Nov. 1943
See also Clara M. McKee
Ramazzini, Bernardino. Padua physician. 1633–
1714
Wrote first book on trade diseases and industrial hy-
giene. Garrison
De morbis artificium diatriba. Mutinae, Capponi,
1700. 360 pp.
Opera omnia, medica et physica. Genevae, Cramer &
Perachon, 1716. 864 pp.
A treatise on the diseases of tradesmen: showing the
various influence of particular trades upon the state of
health; with the best methods to avoid or correct it, and
useful hints proper to be minded in regulating the cure
of all diseases incident to tradesmen. London, Bell,
1705. 274 pp.
Also, transl. by W. C. Wright from Latin test of
1713. Chicago, Univ. Chicago Press, 1940
Rammelkamp, Charles Henry. American physician.
1911–

METHOD—
A method for determining the concentration of penicilli
in body fluids and exudates. Proc. Soc. exp. Biol.
N. Y., 51: 95–97, Oct. 1942
Ramon, Gaston. French physician
ANATOXIN—in American called formol toxoid.
REACTION—
Sur la toxine et sur l'anatoxine diphthériques pouvoi
floculant et propriétés immunisantes. Ann. Inst. Pas-
teur, 38: 1–10, Jan. 1924
Sur l'anatoxine diphtérique et sur les anatoxines er
général. Ibid., 39: 1–21, Jan. 1925
Introduced tetanus toxoid.
Sur la valeur et la durée de l'immunité conférée pai
l'anatoxine tétanique dans la vaccination de l'homme
contre le tétanos with C. Zoeller, C. R. Soc. Biol., 112
347–350, Jan. 28, 1933
Ramond, Felix. French physician. 1871–
AGAR—rubine acid lactose, for detection of typhoid
bacilli.
Nouveau milien pouvant servir a differencier le bacille
d'Eberth du Bacterium coli (2). C. R. Soc. Biol., 48
883–885, Nov. 7, 1896
Ramón y Cajal, Santiago. Spanish histologist. 1852–
1934
Awarded Nobel prize in 1906, with C. Golgi.
CELL—in cerebral cortex.
Nuevo concepto de la histologia de los centros nerviosos.
Rev. de Cien. Méd., Barcel., 18: 457–476, 1892
METHOD—gold chloride and sublimate, for neuroglia.
Sobre un nuevo proceder de impregnación de la neuro-
glia y sus resultados en los centros nerviosus del hombre
y animales. Trab. Lab. Invest. Biol., Madrid, 11:
219–237, 1913
Contribución al conocimiento de la neuroglia del
cerebro humano. Ibid., 255–315.
METHOD—for nerve-endings.
Une formule pour colorer dans les coupes les fibres
amédullées et les terminaisons centrales et périphériques.
Ibid., 23: 237–240, Nov. 1925
METHOD—for sections of cortex cerebelli.
Una formula de impregnación argéntica especialmente
aplecable a los cortes del cerebelo, y algunas considera-
ciones sobre la teoria de Liesegang, acerca del principio
del método del nitrato de plata reducido. Ibid., 19:
71–87, 1921
METHOD—uranium nitrate, for Golgi apparatus.
Mallory
Fórmula defijación para la demonstración fácil del
aparato reticular de Golgi y apuntes sobre la disposi-
ción de dicho aparato lu la retina, en los nervios y
algunos estados patológicos. Ibid., 10: 209–220, 1912
METHOD—gold chloride sublimate, for astrocytes.
Mallory
Quelques méthodes simples pour la coloradion de la
névroglie. Schweiz. Arch. f. Neurol. y. Psychiat., 13:
187–193, 1923
PROCESS—double impregnation.
Sur la structure de l'écorce cérébrale de quelques mammi-
feres. La Cellule, 7: 125–176, 1891
STAIN—improvement of Golgi's chrome-silver s.
Garrison
Manual de histologia normal y técnica micrográfica.
Valencia, Aguilar, 1889. 692 pp.

Worked on minute anatomy of nervous system.
Estudios anatómicas. Observaciones microscópicas sobre las terminationes nerviosas en las músculos voluntarios. Zaragosa, 1881. 50 pp.
Described vertebrate retina. Garrison and Morton *Die Retina der Wirbelthiere.* Wiesbaden, Bergmann, 1894

Ramos, Raoul Leon. American surgeon. 1906–
OPERATION—
Inguinal hernia: application of cardinal principles in the repair of inguinal hernia with C. C. Burton, S. G. O., 69: 688–693, Nov. 1939

Ramsey, Thomas LeRoy. Toledo pathologist. 1885–
METHOD—for titration of saline solution for colloidal gold test.
The preparation of colloidal gold solution with H. J. Eilmann, J. Lab. clin. Med., 18: 298–300. Dec. 1932

Ramstedt, William Conrad. German surgeon. 1867–
OPERATION—
Zur Operation der angeborenen Pylorusstenose. Med. Klin., 8: 1702–1705, 1912

Rand, G. See C. E. Ferree

Rand, R. Frank. English surgeon
TEST—
On a mode of identifying the upper and lower ends of any given piece of small intestine. Lancet, 2: 1083–1084, Dec. 22, 1883

Randall, Alexander. Philadelphia urologist. 1883–
CALCIUM PLAQUES—
The origin and growth of renal calculi. Ann. Surg., 105: 1009–1027, June 1937
The etiology of primary renal calculus. Intern. Abstr. Surg., S. G. O., 71: 209–240, Sept. 1940

Randall, E. L. See A. A. Christman

Randall, Lawrence Merrill. Rochester, Minn. obstetrician. 1895–
TEST—
The "cold test" in pregnancy. A preliminary report of its use in prenatal care with S. E. Murray and R. D. Mussey, Amer. J. Obstet. Gynec., 29: 362–365, Mar. 1935

Ranges, H. A. See A. Cournand

Rankin, Fred Wharton. Rochester, Minn. surgeon 1886–
DOUBLE CLAMP METHOD—of extirpation of lesion of colon.
In his: *Cancer of the colon and rectum; its diagnosis and treatment* with A. S. Graham, Springfield, Ill. Thomas, 1939. 358 pp. pp. 273–275
OPERATION—
The technique of anterior resection of the rectosigmoid S. G. O., 46: 537–546, Apr. 1928
The colon, rectum and anus with J. A. Bargen and L. A. Buie, Philadelphia, Saunders, 1932. pp. 714–811
VACCINE—
Carcinoma of the colon; intraperitoneal vaccination by mixed vaccine of colon bacilli and streptococci with J. A. Bargen, Arch. Surg., 19: 906–914, Nov. 1929
Advised raminectomy for Hirschsprung's disease.
Section of the sympathetic nerves of the distal part of the colon and the rectum in the treatment of Hirschsprung's disease and certain types of constipation. Ann. Surg., 92: 710–720, Oct. 1930

Ranque, A. See A. Besson

Ransohoff, Joseph Louis. Cincinnati surgeon. 1853–1921
OPERATION—
Discussion of the pleura in the treatment of chronic empyema. Ann. Surg., 43: 502–511, Apr. 1906
TEST—
Anaphylaxis in the diagnosis of cancer. J. A. M. A., 61: 8–10, July 5, 1913
Performed gastroenterostomy. (No title), Med. News, 45: 578–579, Nov. 22, 1884

Ranson, Stephen Walter. Chicago neurologist. 1880–
STAIN—pyridine-silver, for non-myelinated nerve fibers.
The structure of the vagus nerve of man as demonstrated by a differential axon stain. Anat. Anz., 46: 522–525, June 12, 1914
Demonstrated nerve pathways from hypothalamus to pituitary.
Autonomic responses to electrical stimulation of hypothalamus, preoptic region and septum with H. Kabat and H. W. Magoun, Arch. Neurol. Psychiat., Chicago, 33: 467–477, Mar. 1935

Rantzman, Eli. Greensboro, N. C. chemist
TEST—for acetone in urine.
A modification of the Lange acetone test. J. Lab. clin. Med., 16: 1217–1218, Sept. 1931

Ranvier, Louis Antoine. French pathologist. 1835–1929
CROSSES, NODES or SEGMENTS—
Lecons sur l'histologie du système nerveux. Paris, Savy, 1878
DISKS—tactile.
Lecons d'anatomie générale faites au College de France. Année 1877–78. Appareils nerveux terminaux des muscles de la vie organique; . . . Paris, Baillière, 1880 530 pp.
FLUID—macerating.
In: *Traité technique d'histologie.* Paris, Savy, 1875. pp. 241
MASS—
Masse au carmin. Ibid., pp. 116–118
MASS—
Masse au bleu de Prusse soluble. Ibid., pp. 119–121
METHOD—of decalcifying bone.
Tissu osseux. Ibid., pp. 297–325
METHOD—lemon juice, for nerve endings. Ibid., pp. 813–814
STAIN—picrocarmin.
Technique microscopique. Acide picrique (Acide phénique trinitré; acide carbazotique; amer de Welter). Arch. d. Physiol., 1: 319–321, 1868

Ranzi, E. See P. Clairmont

Rao, R. S. See H. E. Shortt

Raphael, Alexander. Latvia physician
TEST—for bile pigments.
Ueber eine empfindliche Methode zum Nachweis von Gallenfarbstoff im Harn. St. Petersburger med. Wschr., 2 F., 22: 128 (only), Apr. 9 (22), 1905
See also C. J. H. Nicolle

Rappaport, F. See F. Silberstein

Raskin, Marie. St. Petersburg bacteriologist
AGAR—whey peptone; culture medium.
Zur Züchtung der pathogenen Mikroorganismen auf aus Milch bereitenen festen und durchsichtigen Nährböden. St. Petersburg. med. Wschr., n. F. 4, 12: 357–360 (358), Oct. 24, 1887

Rasmussen, Fritz Vald. Danish physician. 1834–1877

ANEURYSM—dilatation of terminal artery in tuberculous cavity.

Om haemoptyse novnlig den lethale, i anatomisk og klinisk henseende. Hosp. Tid. Kjobenh., 11: 33; 45; 49, 1868

Same, transl. by W. D. Moore: On hemoptysis, especially when fatal, in its anatomical and clinical aspects. Edinburgh med. J., 14: 385–401, Nov.; 486–503, Dec. 1868

Rathke, Martin Heinrich. German anatomist 1793–1860

POCKET or POUCH—diverticulum from embryonic buccal cavity.

Ueber die Entstehung der Glandula pituitaria. Arch. f. Anat., Physiol. u. wiss. Med., No. 5, pp. 482–485, 1838

Ratish, H. D. See D. Polowe

Rattone, G. See A. Carle

Rauchfuss, Charles Carl Andreyevich. St. Petersburg physician. 1835–1915

TRIANGLE—same as Grocco's.

Die paravertebrale Dämpfung auf der gesunden Brustseite bei Pleuraergüssen. Verh. Ges. f. Kinderh Breslau, 1904, 21: 202–211, 1905

Raulston, B. O. See J. L. Miller

Raunert. See G. Linzenmeier

Rausche, C. See H. Bock

Ravaton, Hughes. French surgeon

Wrote on military surgery.

Chirurgie d'armée. Paris, Didot, 1768

Ravaut, Paul. French physician. 1872–

Introduced sodium thiosulfate for treatment of arsenical dermatitis.

L'importance des traitements internes en dermatologie.

L'emploi du cacodylate de soude a hautes doses et de l'hyposulfite de soude. Pr. méd., 28: 73–75, Jan. 28 1920

Ravdin, I. S. See A. Stengel, Jr.

Ravenel, Mazyck Porcher. Columbia, Mo. physician. 1861–1946

Isolated bovine tubercle bacilli from tuberculous children.

The intercommunicability of human and bovine tuberculosis. Univ. Penn. Med. Bull., 15: 66–87, May 1902

Raw, Robert. English scientist

TEST—

Note on the detection of acetone by means of the reaction with O-nitrobenzaldehyde. J. Soc. Chem. Ind., 51: 276T (only), Aug. 12, 1932

Rawles, Lyman Talmage. Huntertown, Ind. physician. 1877–

American discoverer of cause of grain itch.

Dermatitis ditropenotus aureoviridis; synonym, grain itch. J. Indiana med. Ass., 2: 337–340, Aug. 15, 1909

Rawlinson, Christopher. English physician

Reported—

A praeturnatural perforation found in the upper part of the stomach, with the symptoms it produced. Philos. Trans., 35: 361–362, 1727

Rawls, Reginald McCreary. New York gynecologist. 1873–1936

OPERATION—

Cystocele: a review of the literature with a further preliminary report of an operation for its relief. Amer J. Obstet., 78: 328–347, Sept. 1918

Rawson, A. J. See W. O. Abbott

Ray, H. See W. H. Robey

Ray, Isaac. Massachusetts psychiatrist. 1807–1881

MANIA—moral insanity.

A treatise on the medical jurisprudence of insanity. London, Henderson, 1839. 436 pp.

Raybin, Harry W. New York chemist

REACTION—

A new color reaction with sucrose. J. Amer. Chem. Soc., 55: 2603–2604, June 1933

Reaction—

A new color reaction of vitamin B_1 (thiamin). Science, 88: 35 (only), July 8, 1938

Rayer, Pierre Francois Olive. French dermatologist. 1793–1867

Described pituitary obesity.

Observations sur les maladies de l'appendice sussphenoidal (glande pituitaire) de cerveau. Arch. gén. de Méd., Paris, 3: 350–367, 1823

First to describe adenoma sebaceum and xanthoma. Garrison

Traité theorique et pratique des maladies de la peau fondé sur de nouvelles recherches d'anatomie et de physiologie pathologiques. Paris, Baillière, 1826–27. 2 vols. Also, English ed., 1835

First described glanders in man.

De la morve et du farcin chez l'homme. Mem. Acad. de Méd., 6: 625–873, 1837. Also: Paris, Baillière, 1837. 251 pp.

Pointed out causal relationship of anomalous renal arteries to hydronephrosis.

Traité des maladies des reins et des altérations de la sécrétion urinaire. . . . Paris, Baillière, 1839–40. 3 vols et atlas

Same, in English. Philadelphia, Carey and Hart, 1845. 494 pp.

Raymond, Albert L. New York biochemist. 1901–

METHOD—for determination of inorganic phosphate.

Hexose phosphates and alcoholic fermentation with P. A. Levene, J. biol. Chem., 79: 621–635 (628), Oct. 1928

Raymond, Fulgence. Paris neurologist. 1844–1910

SYNDROME—

Sur un cas d'endothéliome épithéloide du noyau rouge with R. Cestan, Rev. neurol., 10: 463–464, May 30, 1902

Raynaud, A. G. Maurice. Paris physician. 1834–1881

DISEASE or GANGRENE—

De l'asphyxue locale et de la gangrène symétrique des extrémités. Thèse de doct., Paris, Rignoux, 1862. 177 pp. Also, in English. London, New Sydenham, Soc., 1888. 150 pp.

Nouvelles recherches sur la nature et le traitement de l'asphyxie locale des extrémités. Arch. gén. de méd. 5: 189–206, Feb. 1874

Read, Alexander. English surgeon. 1586?–1641

Reported lingual cancer.

The chirurgicall lectures of tumors and ulcers. London, 1635. Treat. 2, lect. 26, p. 313

Read, Grantly Dick. English obstetrician. 1890–

PROCEDURE—of labor, with minimum of pain.

Revelation of childbirth; the principles and practice

of natural childbirth. London, Heinemann, 1942. 262 pp.
Published in United States under title:
Childbirth without fear. New York, Harper, 1945

Read, Jay Marion. San Francisco physician. 1889–
FORMULA—
Correlation of basal metabolism rate with pulse rate and pulse pressure. J. A. M. A., 78: 1887–1889, June 17, 1922
Basal pulse rate and pulse pressure changes accompanying variations in the basal metabolic rate. Arch. intern. Med., 34: 553–565, Oct. 1924
New formulae for prediction of basal metabolism from pulse rate and pulse pressure. Proc. Soc. exp. Biol. N. Y., 31: 723–725, Mar. 1934

Réaumur, René Antoine Ferchault de. French scientist. 1683–1757
Isolated gastric juice and demonstrated its solvent effect on foods. Garrison
Sur la digestion des oiseaux. Hist. Mém. Acad. roy. d. Sci., 1752, Paris, pp. 266–307, 1756

Reback, S. See L. A. Mount

Recalde, Juan F. Brazil surgeon
OPERATION—sympathectomy.
Sabre um caso de "mal de engasgo", curado circurgicamente: apresentacao do doente. Bol. Soc. de med. e cirurg. de Sao Paulo, pp. 78–81, July–Oct. 1924

Récamier, Joseph Claude Anthelm. French gynecologist. 1774–1852
Coined term "metastasis" and described spread of cancer.
Recherches sur le traitement du cancer par la compression méthodique, et sur l'histoire générale de la même maladie. . . . Paris, Gabon, 1829. 2 vols., 731 pp.
Invented a vaginal speculum.
Invention du speculum plein et brisé. Bull. Acad. de Méd., Paris, 4 s., 8: 661–668, 1842–43

Recklinghausen, Friedrich Daniel von. German pathologist. 1833–1910
CANALS—small lymph-channels.
Die Lymphgefässe und ihre Beziehung zum Bindegewebe. Berlin, Hirschwald, 1862. 98 pp.
DISEASE—
Über die Acromegalie. Arch. f. path. Anat., 119: 36–53, Jan. 2, 1890
DISEASE—
Ueber die multiplen Fibrome der Haut und ihre Beziehung zu den multiplen Neuromen. . . . Festschrift 25 Jährig. Inst. R. Virchow. Berlin, Hirschwald, 1882. 138 pp.
DISEASE—
Demonstration von Knochen mit tumorbildender Ostitis deformans. Tagebl. d. Naturf., 1889, Heidelberg, p. 321, 1890
Die fibröse oder deformirende Osteitis, die Osteomalacie und die osteoplastische Carcinose, in ihren gegenseitigen Beziehungen. Festschr. z. Rudolf Virchow. Berlin, Reiner, 1891. 89 pp.
HYPOTHESIS—cancer metastases to bone are by blood stream.
Ueber die venöse Embolie und den retrograden Transport in den Venen und in den Lymphgefässen. Arch. f. path. Anat., 100: 503–539, June 8, 1885
Described—
Ueber Haemochromatose. Berl. klin. Wschr., 26: 925 (only), Oct. 21, 1889

Ueber Hämochromatose. Tagebl. d. Naturf., 1889, Heidelberg, p. 324, 1890

Reclus, Paul. French surgeon. 1847–1914
DISEASE—
La maladie kystique des mammelles. Bull. Soc. anat., de Paris, 4 s., 8: 428–433, Nov. 1883
DISEASE—
Phlégmon ligneux du cou. Rev. chir., 16: 522–531, 1896
METHOD—
La cocaine en chirurgie. Paris, Masson, 1895. 192 pp.
L'anesthésie localisée par la cocaine. Paris, Masson, 1903. 275 pp.

Redewill, F. H. See F. Hinman

Redi, Francesco. Italian naturalist. 1626–1697
Wrote first methodical work on snake poison. Garrison and Morton
Osservazioni intorno alle vipere. Firenze, Stella, 1664
Dealt "the first hard blow to doctrine of spontaneous generation." Garrison
Esperienze intorno alla generazione degl'insetti. . . . Firenze, Stell, 1668
Experimenta circa generationem insectorum. . . . Amsterdam, Frisii, 1671. 330 pp.

Redisch, Walter. Prague pathologist
TECHNIC—of capillary study.
Zur Kapillarmikroskopie und Kapillarphotographie. Z. KreislForsch., 22: 561–564, Sept. 1, 1930

Reed, Alfred Cummings. San Francisco physician. 1884–
Introduced—
Carbarsone in the treatment of amebiasis with H. H. Anderson, N. A. David and C. D. Leake, J. A. M. A., 98: 189–194, Jan. 16, 1932

Reed, Dorothy M. Baltimore pathologist
CELLS—
On the pathological changes in Hodgkin's disease, with especial reference to its relation to tuberculosis. Johns Hopk. Hosp. Rep., 10: 133–196, 1906

Reed, John. English physician
Invented a stomach pump. (No title). Lancet, 1: 276–277, Nov. 23, 1823
Advertisement. To the editor of the Lancet. Ibid., 7: 158–159, May 7, 1825

Reed, Walter. American physician. 1851–1902
Demonstrated mode of transmission of yellow fever.
The etiology of yellow fever: a preliminary note with J. Carroll, A. Agramonte and J. W. Lazear, Philadelphia med. J., 6: 790–796, Oct. 27, 1900
The etiology of yellow fever: an additional note. J. A. M. A., 36: 431–440, Feb. 16, 1901

Rees, Clarence Edwin. San Diego, Cal. surgeon. 1892–
OPERATION—
Single incision, transabdominal, extraperitoneal approach to lumbar ganglia. Amer. J. Surg., 32: 234–237, May 1936
TREATMENT—
Dried milk as a dressing for intestinal fistula: report of a case. California and West. Med., 30: 419 (only), June 1929

Reese, Robert Grigg. New York ophthalmologist 1866–1926
OPERATION—
A new muscle resection operation for squint. New York med. J., 95: 60–62, Jan. 13, 1912

OPERATION—

An operation for blepharoptosis with the formation of a fold in the lid. Trans. Amer. Ophthal. Soc., 21: 71–78, 1923

OPERATION—

Technic of iridectomy done under a conjunctival flap for glaucoma, using a broad keratome. J. A. M. A., 82: 614–619, Feb. 23, 1924

Reeser, Hendrick E. Rotterdam bacteriologist

BROTH—potato veal infusion.

Das Tuberkulin. Zbl. Bakt., 46: 149–167 (152), 1908

Reeves, E. B. See A. A. Weech

Regaud, Claude. French radiologist. 1870–

FLUID—fixation.

METHOD—for mitochondria.

Études sur la structure des tubes séminifères et sur la spermatogénèse chez les mammifères. Arch. d'anat. micr., 11: 291–431, Mar. 31, 1910

METHOD—Paris m. of radium treatment of cancer of uterus.

Considérations sur la radiothérapie des cancers cervico-uterus, d'après l'expérience et les résultats acquis à l'Institut du Radium de Paris. Radiophysiol. et Radiothrap., 3: 155–170, Dec. 1934

Regele, Heinz. Vienna surgeon

METHOD—for reduction of old shoulder dislocation.

Ein neuer Handgriff zur Einrenkung veralteter Schulterverrenkungen. Münch. med. Wschr., 83: 1345 (only), Aug. 14, 1936

Regnault, Henri Victor. French scientist. 1810–1878 Determined respiratory quotient.

Recherches chimiques sur la respiration des animaux des diverses classes with J. Reiset, Ann. Chim. (Phys.), 3 s., 26: 299–519, 1849

Regniers, P. See C. Heymans

Rehberg, Poul Brandt. Copenhagen physiologist

FUNCTIONAL TEST—of kidneys.

Determined glomerular filtration rate in man.

Studies on kidney function. I. The rate of filtration and reabsorption in the human kidney. Biochem. J., 20: 447–482, 1926

Rehfuss, Martin Emil. Philadelphia physician. 1887–

METHOD, TEST, TUBE—

A new method of gastric testing, with a description of a new method for the fractional testing of the gastric juice. Amer. J. med. Sci., 173: 848–855, June 1914

Rehm, Mathilde. See C. P. McCord

Rehn, Eduard. German surgeon. 1880–

TEST—functional, of kidney.

Über die Grundlagen und den jetzigen Stand der Säurealkaliausscheidungsprobe zur Funktionsdiagnose kranker Nieren. Z. Urol., 19: 27–37, 1926

Rehn, Ludwig. German surgeon. 1849–1930

Performed thyroidectomy for exophthalmic goiter in 1880.

Ueber die Exstirpation des Kropfs bei Morbus Basedowii. Berl. klin. Wschr., 21: 163–166, Mar. 17, 1884

Reported aniline cancer in a dye worker.

Blasengeschwülste bei Fuchsin-Arbeitern. Arch. f klin. Chir., 50: 588–600, 1895

Performed successful suture of heart.

Fall von penetrirender Stichverletzung des rechten Ventrikel's. Herznaht. Abstr.: Zbl. Chir., 22: 1048–1049, Oct. 31, 1896

Üeber penetrirende Herzwunden und Herznaht. Arch. f. klin. Chir., 55: 315–329, 1897

Reich, Adolph. New York gynecologist. 1864–

First to obtain cholangiograms. Garrison and Mortor

Accidental injection of bile ducts with petrolatum and bismuth paste. J. A. M. A., 71: 1555 (only), Nov. 9, 1918

Reichard, C. German chemist

REACTION—for nicotine.

Beiträge zur Kenntnis der Alkaloidreaktionen, Nikotin und Koniin. Pharm. Zentralhalle, 46: 252–256 Mar. 30; 309–313, Apr. 20, 1905

Reichel, Friedrich Paul. German surgeon. 1858–

OPERATION—

Modification of Billroth II. Technik der Magenresektion Verh. dtsch. Ges. f. Chir., 37: 211–212, Apr. 23, 1908 Described chondromatosis.

Chondromatose der Kniegelenkkapsel. Ibid., 29: 332–339, 1900

Reichert, E. T. See S. W. Mitchell

Reichert, Frederick Leet. San Francisco surgeon 1894–

METHOD—

In discussion of *Pain low in the back and "sciatica."* By J. S. Barr, A. O. Hampton and W. J. Mixter J. A. M. A., 109: 1270, Oct. 16, 1937

The injection of air for localization of lesions in the spinal canal—pneumomyelography. West. J. Surg. 47: 297–300, June 1939

Reichert, Karl Bogislaus. German anatomist, 1811–1884

CARTILAGE—of hyoid arch in embryo.

De embryonum arcubus sic dictis branchialibus Berolini, Nietackianis, 1836. 26 pp.

Demonstrated visceral arches in vertebrata.

Ueber die Visceralbogen der Wirbelthiere im Allgemeinen und deren Metamorphose bei den Sängethieren und Vögeln. Berlin, Sittenfeld, 1837. 115 pp.

Reichmann, F. See K. Goldstein

Reichmann, Mikola. Warsaw physician. 1851–1918

DISEASE or SYNDROME—continuous secretion of gastric juice.

Przypadek chorobowo wzmozonego wydzielania sokc zoladkowego. Gaz. Lek., Warszawa, 2 s., 2: 516–522 1882

Ein Fall von krankhaft gesteigerter Absonderung de Magensaftes. Berl. klin. Wschr., 19: 606–608, Oct. 2 1882

SIGN—presence of organic acid food residues in fasting stomach, in pyloric stenosis.

Ueber sogenannte „Dyspepsia acida." Ibid., 21: 768–771, Dec. 1, 1884

Reichstein, Tadeus. Zurich chemist. 1897–

Synthesized vitamin C.

Synthese der d- und l-Ascorbinsäure (C- vitamin with A. Grüssner and R. Oppenauer, Helvet. Chim Acta, Basel, 16: 1019–1033, 1933

See also Marguerite Steiger

Reid, Alexander. English physician

Described—

A remarkable case of a person cut for the stone in the new way, commonly called the lateral, by William Cheselden. Philos. Trans., 1746, pp. 33–35, 1748

Reid, Douglas G. English anatomist

REID, DOUGLAS G. 341 REITER, HANS

FOLD—genitomesenteric.
Studies of the intestine and peritoneum in the human foetus. J. Anat. and Physiol., 45: 73–84, Jan. 1911
Reid, John. Scottish physician. 1809–1849
Drew attention to cervical tumor pressing on sympathetic fibers causing myosis. Argyll Robertson
On the effects of lesion of the trunk of the ganglionic system of nerves in the neck upon the eyeball and its appendages. Edinburgh M. and S. J., 52: 36–43, July 1839
Reid, Mont Rogers. Cincinnati surgeon. 1889–1943
APPARATUS—
Treatment of obliterative vascular diseases by means of an intermittent negative pressure environment with L. G. Herrmann, J. Med., Cincinnati, 14: 200–204, June 1933
See L. G. Herrmann
Reid, Robert William. English anatomist. 1851–
BASE-LINE—
Observations on the relation of the principal fissures and convolutions of the cerebrum to the outer surface of the scalp. Lancet, 2: 539–540, Sept. 27, 1884
Reid, William W. Rochester, N. Y. physician. 1799–1866
REDUCTION—
Dislocation of the femur on the dorsum ilii, reducible without pulleys, or any other mechanical power. Buffalo med. J., 7: 129–143, Aug. 1851
Re'f, Georges Joseph Eugene. Berlin chemist. 1883–
TEST—for uric acid in milk and blood.
Über eine neuartige Anwendung der Phosphorwolfram- und Phosphormolybdänsaure zur Bestimmung der Harnsäure im Milch und Blut. Biochem. Z., 161: 128–138, Aug. 11, 1925
Reifenstein, E. C. See H. F. Klinefelter
Reifer, I. See F. Silberstein
Reil, Johann Christian. Dutch anatomist. 1759–1813
ANSA, FISSURE, ISLAND, SULCUS—
Exercitationum anatomicarum fasciculus primus. De structura nervorum. Halle, Venalis, 1796. 32 pp.
Untersuchungen über den Bau des grossen Gehirns im Menschen. Arch. f. Physiol., 9: 136–146, 1809
Advanced doctrine of the life-force as chemical expression of physiologic function. Garrison
Von der Lebenskraft. Ibid., 1: 8–162, 1796
Wrote early work on psychic (humane) treatment of insane.
Rhapsodieen über die Anwendung der psychischen Curmethode auf Geisteszerrüttungen. Halle, Curt, 1803. 504 pp.
Founded first journal of psychiatry. Garrison
Magazin für psychische Heilkunde. 1805
Reilly, H. Christine. See S. A. Waksman
Reilly, J. See A. A. Lemierre
Rein, C. R. See F. Wise
Rein, Friedrich Hermann. Freiburg i. B. physiologist. 1898–
THERMOSTROMUHR—for measuring blood volume flow.
Die Thermo-Stromuhr. Ein Verfahren zur fortlaufenden Messung der mittleren absoluten Durchflussmengen in uneröffneten Gefässen in situ. Z. Biologie, 87: 394–418, June 25, 1928
Reinbold, R. Rumania physiologist

TEST—for sugars.
Über die Molisch-Udránszky'sche a-Naphtol-Schwefelsäure-Reaction. Arch. ges. Physiol., 103: 581–617, July 21, 1904
Reinhart, W. H. See W. P. Yant
Reinhold, John Gunther. Philadelphia biochemist. 1900–
METHOD—
The determination of blood cholesterol. I. A comparison of standard colorimetric methods and a modified method with gravimetric determination of digitonin precipitates with Ethel M. Shiels, Amer. J. clin. Path., 6: 22–30, Jan. 1936
See also J. R. Neefe
Reinke, Friedrich Berthold. German anatomist. 1862–1919
CRYSTALLOIDS—in interstitial cells of testis.
Beiträge zur Histologie des Menschen. I. Ueber Krystalloidbildung in den interstitiellen Zellen des menschlichen Hodens. Arch. mikr. Anat., 47: 34–44, 1896
STAIN—orange method, for plasma.
Zellstudien. Ibid., 44: 259–284 (262), 1894
Re'nl, C. See A. Hegar
Reinsch, Adolf. German physician. 1862–1916
MEDIUM—milk; culture m.
Auf kaltem Wege sterilisirte eiweisshaltige Nährböden. Zbl. Bakt., 12: 30–32, July 5, 1892
Reiset, J. See H. V. Regnault
Reisinger, Franz. German ophthalmologist. 1787–1855
Used hyoscyamin and atropin in eye examinations.
Ophthalmologische Versuche bey Thieren mit dem Hyoscyamin und Atropin. Med.-chir. Ztg., Innsbruck, 1: 237; 253, 1825
Also: *On the effects of hyoscyamine and atropia.* Edinburgh M. and S. J., 26: 276–279, Oct. 1, 1826
Reisinger, Gottlieb. Mainz surgeon. 1866–1917
OPERATION—for dilatation of esophagus (suggested by Jaffé).
Ueber die operativ Behandlung der Erweiterung des Oesophagus mit Krankervorstellung. Verh. dtsch. Ges. f. Chir., 36: 26–27, 1907
Reisseisen, Franz Daniel. German anatomist. 1773–1828
MUSCLES—muscular elements of bronchi.
De pulmonis structura. Argentorati, 1803. 42 pp.
Über die Struktur, die Verrichtung und den Gebrauch der Lungen with S. T. Soemmerring, Berlin, Voss, 1808
Reissner, Ernst. Riga anatomist. 1824–1878
CANAL—of cochlea.
MEMBRANE—vestibular.
De auris internae formatione. Inaug. Diss. Univ. Dorpat, 1851. 53 pp.
FIBER—in central canal of spinal cord.
Der Bau das centralen Nervensystemes der ungeschwänzten Batrachier, untersucht und Leschrieben. Dorpat, Karow, 1864. 118 pp.
Reissner, Otto. Bad Nauheim physician
MODIFICATION—of Martius and Lüttke m. for determination of free hydrochloric acid in gastric contents.
Zur Methodik der Salzsäurebestimmung am Mageninhalt. Z. klin. Med., 48: 101–119, 1903
Reiter, Hans. Berlin physician. 1881–

DISEASE or SYNDROME—urethritis, conjunctivitis and arthritis.
Ueber eine bisher unerkannte Spirochäteninfektion (Spirochaetosis arthritica). Dtsch. med. Wschr., 42: 1535–1536, Dec. 14, 1916
Reith, Allen F (under). Chicago bacteriologist. 1890–
SOLUTION—plant infusion; culture medium.
Growth of Pfeiffer bacillus in mixed culture in blood-free medium. J. infect. Dis., 32: 243–246, Mar. 1923
Remak, Ernest Julius. German neurologist 1848–1911
PARALYSIS—of extensor muscles of fingers and wrist, as in lead poisoning.
Zur Pathogenes der Bleilähmungen. Arch. f. Psychiat., 6: 1–56, 1875
Remak, Robert. German neurologist. 1815–1865
BAND—an axis-cylinder.
FIBER—non-medullated nerve-fibers.
Observationes anatomicae et microscopicae de systematis nervosi structura. Berolini, Reimerianis, 1838. 30 pp.
Produced favus experimentally; called fungus Achorion Schonleini.
Diagnostische und pathogenetische Untersuchungen. . . . Berlin, Hirschwald, 1845. 242 pp. p. 196–208
First defined three categories, ectoderm, mesoderm and endoderm. Garrison
Untersuchungen über die Entwickelung des Wirbelthieres. Berlin, Reimer, 1851. 194 pp.
Pointed out that proliferation of cells to form tissue is accomplished by cell division.
Ueber extracellulare Entstehung thierischer Zellen und über Vermehrung derselben durch Theilung. Arch. f. Anat., Physiol. u. wiss. Med., Berlin, pp. 47–57, 1852
Pioneer of electrotherapy, substituting galvanic for induced current.
Galvanotherapie der Nerven- und Muskelkrankheiten. Berlin, Hirschwald, 1858. 461 pp.
Remen, Lazar. Münster i. W. physician. 1907–
Introduced prostigmine in treatment of myasthenia gravis.
Zur Pathogenese und Therapie der Myasthenia gravis pseudoparalytica. Dtsch. Z. Nervenheilk., 128: 66–78, Sept. 15, 1932
Remington, Roe Eugene. American biochemist. 1881–
DIET—goitrogenic; low in iodine.
Improved growth in rats on iodine deficient diets. J. Nutrition, 13: 223–233, Feb. 10, 1937
Rémond, A. See G. M. Débove, A. Mathieu
Remy, L. Liege bacteriologist
GELATIN—phenolated lactose peptone, for isolation of typhoid bacillus.
Contribution a l'étude de la fièvre typhoide et de son bacille. Ann. Inst. Pasteur, 14: 555–570 (561), Aug. 1900
Renault, Joseph Louis. French physician. 1844–1917
BODIES—found in nerve-bundles.
Recherches sur quelques points particuliers de l'histologie des nerfs. Arch. Physiol. norm. path., 2 s., 8: 161–190, 1881
Rendu, Henri Jules Louis Marie. French physician. 1844–1902
DISEASE—of Rendu-Osler; multiple hereditary telangiectasis.
Epistaxis répétées chez un sujet porteur de petits an-

giomes cutanés et muqueux. Bull. Soc. méd. Hôp Paris, 3 s., 13: 731–733, Oct. 23, 1896
Rennie, Alexander. Canton physician. 1859–1940
THEORY—of plague transmission by rats.
The plague in the East. . . . Brit. med. J., 2: 615–616, Sept. 15, 1894
Renon, Louis. French neurologist. 1863–1922
SYNDROME—
Insuffisance thyro-ovarienne et hyperactivité hypophysaire (troubles acroméqaliques). Amélioration par l'opthérapie thyro-ovarienne augmentation de l'acromegalie par la médication hypophysaire with A. Delille, Bull. Soc. méd. hôp. Paris, 3 s., 25: 973–979, June 19, 1908
Renucci, Simon François. French physician
Rediscovered Acarus scabiei and proved origin of disease.
Sur la découverte de l'insecte qui produit la contagion de la gale, du prurigo et du phlyzacia. Paris, Thèse No. 83: 1835. 41 pp.
Reschad, Hassan. Hamburg physician
Described monocytic leukemia.
Ueber eine neue Leukämie durch echte Uebergangsformen (Splenozytenleukämie) und ihre Bedeutung für die Selbstständigkeit dieser Zellen with V. Schilling-Torgau, Münch. med. Wschr., 60: 1981–1984, Sept. 9, 1913
Respighi, Emilio. Italian physician
Described hyperkeratosis.
Di una ipercheratosi non ancora descritta. Gior. ital. di mal. ven., Milano, 28: 356–386, 1893
Sull'ipercheratosi eccentrica. . . . Milano, Rivera, 1895 15 pp.
Retan, George Matthew. Syracuse pediatrician. 1889–
TECHNIC—
The development of the therapeutic use of forced perivascular (spinal) drainage. J. A. M. A., 105: 1333–1340, Oct. 26, 1935
Rettger, Leo Frederick. New Haven bacteriologist. 1874–
BASAL SOLUTION—
Further studies on bacterial nutrition: the utilization of proteid and non-proteid nitrogen with N. Berman and W. S. Sturges, J. Bact., 1: 15–33, Jan. 1916
See also N. Berman, W. L. Kulp, H. C. Robinson
Retzius, Magnus Gustav. Swedish histologist. 1842–1919
FORAMEN, GYRUS—
Das Menschenhirn. Stockholm, Norstedt, 1892. 2 vols.
Reuter, Karl Otto. Hamburg physician. 1873–
METHOD—of staining for chromatin.
Ueber den färbenden Bestandteil der Romanowsky-Nochtschen Malariaplasmodien-färbung, seine Reindartstellung und praktische Verwendung. Zbl. Bakt., 30: 248–256, Aug. 26, 1901
Reported spirochetes in aortic lesions.
Ueber Spirochaete pallida in der Aortenwand bei Hellerscher Aortitis. Münch. med. Wschr., 53: 778 (only), Apr. 17, 1906
Reverdin, Auguste. Geneva surgeon. 1849–1908
TABLE—operating.
Nouvelle table d'opérations en usage a la clinique des Docteurs Reverdin. Rev. Chir., 8: 592–598, July 1888
Reverdin, Jacques Louis. Swiss surgeon. 1842–1929

OPERATION—skin grafting.
Greffe épidermique. Expérience faite dans la service de M. le docteur Guyon, à l'hôpital Necker. Bull. Soc. imp. de chir., Paris, 1869, 2 s., 10: 511–515, 1870
Greffes épidermiques. D'une qualite particulière des ilots développes autour des greffes. Gaz. méd. de Paris, 26: 544–545, 1871
Reported a syndrome as of myxedema following complete thyroidectomy.
(Accidents consécutifs à l'ablation totale du goitre). Rev. méd. de la Suisse romande, Genève, 2: 539–540, Oct. 15, 1882
Contribution a l'étude du myxoèdeme consécutif à l'extirpation totale ou partielle du corps thyroide. Ibid., 7: 275–291, May 15; 318–330, June 15, 1887

Revis, Cecil. London bacteriologist. 1875–
SOLUTION—glycerol ammonium chloride, for studying colon bacilli.
The stability of the physiological properties of coliform organisms. Zbl. Bakt., 2 Abt., 26: 161–178 (173), 1910

Reybard, Jean Francois. Lyons surgeon. 1790–1863
Performed intestinal resection for cancer.
Mémoire sur une tumeur cancéreuse affectant l'S iliaque du colon; ablation de la tumeur et de l'intestin; réunion directe et immédiate des deux bouts de cet organe. Guérison. Abstr.: Bull. Acad. Méd., 9: 1031–1043, July 30, 1844

Reynals, Francesc Duran. French-American physician
SPREADING FACTOR—extracts of normal rabbit testicle, added to an injection fluid, will greatly facilitate spread of vaccine virus through dermal tissues and enhance its infectivity and pathogenicity.
Exaltation de l'activité du virus vaccinal par les extraits de certains organes. C. R. Soc. Biol., 99: 6–7, June 2, 1928
The effect of extracts of certain organs from normal and immunized animals on the infecting power of vaccine virus. J. exp. Med., 50: 327–340, Sept. 1, 1929

Reynolds, F. H. K. See J. S. Simmons
Reynolds, James Emerson. Edinburgh physician. 1844–1920
TEST—for acetone.
Research on a new group of colloid bodies containing mercury, and certain members of the series of fatty ketones. Proc. roy. Soc., 19: 431–442, Apr. 20, 1871

Reynolds, R. P. See M. O. Cantor
Reynolds, Samuel Robert Means. American physiologist. 1903–
Inhibited estrus motility in rabbits with progestin.
The effect of progestin-containing extracts of corpora lutea on uterine motility in the unanesthetized rabbit with observations on pseudopregnancy with W. M. Allen, Amer. J. Physiol., 102: 39–55, Oct. 1, 1932

Reznikoff, P. See J. C. Aub, R. Chambers
Rhazes. Persian physician. 850?–923
Differentiated measles from small-pox.
De variolis et morbilis. Venetiis, per Simonem Papiensem, 1498
Also, transl. by W. A. Greenhill. London, Sydenham Soc., 1848
Also in: Medical classics, 4: 22–84, Sept. 1939

Rhoads, Cornelius Packard. New York physician. 1898–

METHOD—
A method for explantation of the kidney. Amer. J. Physiol., 109: 324–328, Aug. 1, 1934
See also L. A. Erf

Ribbert, Moritz Wilhelm Hugo. Zurich pathologist. 1855–1920
METHOD—for staining films on coverslips and for capsules.
Zur Färbung der Pneumoniekokken. Dtsch. med. Wschr., 11: 136 (only), Feb. 26, 1885
THEORY—a tumor is formed from development of cell rests owing to reduced tension in surrounding tissues.
Geschwulstlehre für Arzte und Studierende. Bonn, Cohen, 1904
Die Entstehung des Carcinoms. Bonn. Cohen, 1905
Das Karzinom des Menschen, sein Bau, sein Wachstum, seine Entstehung. Bonn, Cohen, 1911. 526 pp.
Applied name chordoma and established their origin from notochordal tissue.
Ueber die Ecchondrosis physalifora sphenooccipitalis. Zbl. allg. Path., 5: 457–461, June 1, 1894

Ricard, Alfred Louis. French surgeon. 1858–
Performed cholecystoduodenostomy.
Sur une observation de cholécystentérostomie, déposée par M. Ricard. Bull. Soc. Chir. Paris, 20: 572–578, July 11, 1894

Ricci, N. I. See W. D. M. Lloyd
Rice, C. O. See O. H. Wangensteen
Rice, E. C. See J. W. Lindsay
Rich, Arnold Rice. Baltimore pathologist. 1893–
CLASSIFICATION—
The pathogenesis of the forms of jaundice. Johns Hopk. Hosp. Bull., 47: 338–377, Dec. 1930

Richards, Alfred Newton. American pharmacologist. 1876–
PREPARATION—of elastin.
Chemical studies of elastin, mucoid, and other proteids in elastic tissue, with some notes on ligament extractives with W. J. Gies, Amer. J. Physiol., 7: 93–134, Apr. 1, 1902
Showed that only a fraction of glomeruli of kidney work at same time.
Kidney function. Harvey Lectures, 16: 163–187, 1920–21
Kidney function: glomeruli function and the modes of its regulaton. Amer. J. med. Sci., 163: 1–19, Jan. 1922
See also H. H. Dale, J. T. Wearn

Richards, J. T. See Bullis
Richards, Theodore William. Cambridge, Mass. chemist. 1868–1928
NEPHELOMETER—
Neubestimmungs des Atomgewichts von Strontium. Transl. by A. Rosenheim, Z. anorg. Chem., 8: 253–273 (269), 1895
The nephelometer, an instrument for detecting and estimating opalescent precipitates with R. C. Wells, Amer. Chem. J., 31: 235–243, Mar. 1904

Richardson, Edward Henderson. Baltimore gynecologist. 1877–
OPERATION—
An efficient composite operation for uterine prolapse and associated pathology. Amer. J. Obstet., 34: 814–827, Nov. 1937

Richardson, F. S. See E. C. Kendall

Richerand, Baron Anthelme Balthasar. French surgeon. 1779–1840
Resected ribs. Garrison
Histoire d'une résection des côtes et de la plèvre; lue à l'Académie royale des sciences de l'Institut de France. Paris, Caille et Ravier, 1818. 22 pp.
Richet, Charles Robert. French physiologist. 1850–1913
Awarded Nobel prize in 1913 for work on anaphylaxis, a word which he coined. See Paul Portier
De l'anaphylaxis ou sensibilité croissante des organismes à des doses successives de poison. Arch. di fisiol., Firenze, 1: 129–142, 1903–04
De l'anaphylaxie en général et de l'anaphylaxie par la mytilo-congestive en particulier. Ann. Inst. Pasteur, Paris, 21: 497–524, July 1907
De l'anaphylaxie et des toxogénines. Ibid., 22: 465–495, June 1908
L'anaphylaxie. Paris, Alcan, 1911. 286 pp.
Also, transl. by J. M. Bligh, Liverpool, Univ. Press, 1913. 266 pp.
See also J. Héricourt, P. J. Portier
Richman, E. See V. E. Levine
Richmond, John Lambert. Newton, Ohio surgeon. 1785–1855
Performed and reported first cesarean section done in United States, on April 22, 1827. Garrison
History of a successful case of casearean operation. West. J. Med. and Phys. Sci., Cincinnati, 3: 485–489, Jan. Feb. Mar. 1830
Richter A. German bacteriologist
AGAR—meat infusion wine; culture medium for anthrax and other bacteria.
Agar-Agar-Nährsubstanz für Bakterienculturen. Berl. klin. Wschr., 24: 600 (only), Aug. 8, 1887
SOLUTION—ammonium nitrate, for growing Aspergillus niger.
Zur Frage über den Tod von Pflanzen infolge niedriger Temperatur. (Kälteresistenz von Aspergillus niger.) Zbl. Bakt., 2 Abt., 28: 617–624 (619), 1910
Richter, Augustus Gottlieb. German surgeon. 1742–1812
HERNIA—only a part of caliber of gut is involved.
Abhandlung von den Brüchen. Göttingen, Dietrich, (1777–1779) 1785, Ch. 24, pp. 596–597
Richter, Eduard. Hamburg physician
REACTION—for reducing substances in urine.
Neue kolloid-chemische Harnreaktion. Med. Klin., 15: 689–691, July 13, 1919
Richter, P. F. See L. Casper
Rickards, Burt Ranson. American bacteriologist. 1876–
METHOD—for concentrating tubercle bacilli.
An apparatus and method for rapidly staining large numbers of sputum specimens. K. Boston Soc. med. Sci., 5: 391–394, Mar. 19, 1901
Ricketts, Howard Taylor. American pathologist. 1871–1910
RICKETTSIAE—
RICKETTSIA prowazeki, specific organism of typhus; isolated by Ricketts.
Contributions to medical science by Howard Taylor Ricketts. Chicago, Univ. Chicaro Press, 1911. 497 pp.
Demonstrated—
The transmission of Rocky Mountain spotted fever by

the bite of the wood-tick (Dermacantor occidentalis). J. A. M. A., 47: 358 (only), Aug. 4, 1906
Ricord, Phillippe. French physician. 1799–1889
CHANCRE—initial lesion of syphilis.
TREATMENT—of syphilis.
Differentiated gonorrhea from syphilis and divided latter into three stages.
Traité pratique des maladies vénériennes. . . . Paris, Rauvier et Le Bouvier, 1838. 808 pp.
Same: *Lectures on venereal and other diseases.* Philadelphia, Barrington and Haswell, 1840
Riddle, Oscar. American scientist. 1877–
Wrote—
The preparation, identification and assay of prolactin —a hormone of the anterior pituitary with R. W. Bates and S. W. Dykshorn, Amer. J. Physiol., 105: 191–216, July 1, 1933
Riddoch, George. English physician. 1888–
MASS REFLEX—
The reflex functions of the completely divided spinal cord in man, compared with those associated with less severe lesions. Brain, 40: 264–402, Nov. 1917
Rideal, Samuel. English physician. 1863–
COEFFICIENT—
Standardization of disinfectants with J. T. A. Walker, J. Sanitary Inst. London, 24: 424–441, Oct. 1903
Riedel, Bernhard Moritz Karl Ludwig. Jena surgeon. 1846–1916
DISEASE or STRUMA—ligneus thyroiditis.
Die chronische, zur Bildung eisenharter Geschwülste führende Entzündung der Schilddrüsse. Verh. dtsch. Ges. f. Chir., 25: 75–76, 1896
LOBE or PROCESS—of liver.
Ueber den zungenförmigen Fortsatz des rechten Leberlappens und seine pathognostische Bedeutung für die Erkrankung der Gallenblase nebst Bemerkungen über Gallensteinoperationen. Berl. klin. Wschr., 25: 577–581, July 16; 602–607, July 23, 1888
TUMOR—of chronic pancreatitis.
Über entzündliche der Rückbildung fähige Vergrösserungen des Pankreaskopfes. Ibid., 33: 1–5, Jan. 6; 32–35, Jan. 13, 1896
Riedel, Gustav. Frankfurt surgeon
OPERATION—subtrochanteric osteotomy in coxa vara.
Haltelochplatte für Schanz'sche Schrauben. Zb. Chir. 57: 84–86, Jan. 11, 1930
Rieder, Hermann. German physician. 1858–1932
LYMPHOCYTE—
Beiträge zur Kenntniss der Leukocytose und verwandter Zustände des Blutes. Leipzig, Vogel, 1892. 220 pp.
MOVEMENT—of colon, large pendular.
Die physiologische Dickdarmbewegung beim Menschen. Fort. geb. Roentgen., 18: 85–121, 1911–12
PARALYSIS—of brachial plexus.
Die „Steinträger-Lähmung." Münch. med. Wschr., 40: 121–123, Feb. 14, 1893
Riegel, E(mil) Raymond. Buffalo chemist. 1882–
REACTION—
A new color reaction for procaine and some cther local anesthetics, and its application to the determination of procaine with J. F. Williams, J. Amer. Chem. Soc., 48: 4871–4878, Nov. 1926
Riegel, Franz. German physician. 1843–1904

PULSE—diminished in size during expiration.
Ueber die diagnostische Bedeutung des Venenpulses.
Samml. klin. Vortr., No. 227 (Inn. Med., No. 78),
2051–2082, Mar. 13, 1883
SYMPTOM—"alternating mydriasis" in neurasthenia.
Ueber die springende Mydriasis. Z. Nervenheilk.,
17: 169–170, May 17, 1900
Distinguished between respiratory and phonatory
paralysis of larynx.
Über respiratorische Paralysen. Samml. klin. Vortr.,
No. 95 (Inn. Med., No. 33), 761–796, 1875
Riegler, E. Jassy chemist
TEST—for acetoacetic acid in urine.
Neuere Reaktionen auf Azetessigsäure. Münch. med.
Wschr., 53: 448–449, Mar. 6, 1906
TEST—for bile pigments in urine.
Eine neue empfindliche Reaction auf Gallenpigmente.
Wien. med. Bl., 22: 271–272, Mar. 23, 1899
TEST—for blood coloring matter.
*Ein neues Reagens zum Nachweis der verschiedenen
Blutfarbstoffe oder der Zersetzungsprodukte derselben.*
Z. anal. Chem., 43: 539–547 (541), 1904
TEST—for glucose in urine.
Eine neue empfindliche Zuckerprobe. Dtsch. med.
Wschr., 27: 40 (only), Jan. 17, 1901
TEST—for iodine in urine.
TEST—for indican in urine.
*Ein neues Verfahren, um Jod in seinen Verbindungen
mit metallen nachzuweisen.* Pharm. Zentralhalle, n.
F., 24: 565–567, Aug. 27, 1903
TEST—for urea.
*Eine leicht und rasch ausführbare Methode zur Bestim-
mung des Harnstoffs, beruhend auf der Zerlegung
desselben durch Millon's Reagens.* Z. anal. Chem.,
33: 49–53, 1894
TEST—for uric acid.
Eine neue Reaction auf Harnsäure. Wien. med. Bl.,
20: 431 (only), July 1, 1897
Riehl, Gustav. German physician. 1855–
Advocated blood transfusion for shock after burns.
Garrison and Morton
Zur Therapie schwerer Verbrennungen. Wien. klin.
Wschr., 38: 833–834, July 23, 1925
Riemer, Pieter de. 1760–1831
Used frozen sections.
*Afbeeldingen van de juiste plaatsing der inwendige
deelen van het menschelijk ligchaam.* s'Gravenhage,
Allart, 1818
Rienhoff, William Francis, Jr. Baltimore surgeon.
1894–
OPERATION—
The surgical technic of total pneumonectomy. Arch.
Surg., 32: 218–231, Feb. 1936
*A two-stage operation for total pneumonectomy in the
treatment of carcinoma of the lung, demonstrating a
new technique for closure of the bronchus.* J. Thoracic
Surg., 8: 254–271, Feb. 1939
Ries, Emil. Chicago surgeon. 1865–1939
OPERATION—
Eine neue Operationsmethode des Uteruscarcinoms.
Z. f. Geburtsh. u. Gynäk., 32: 266–274, 1895
Reported benign tumor of placenta.
Angioma of the placenta. Amer. J. Obstet., 50: 84–
85, July 1904
Suggested mammography with intraductal injection.
Diagnostic lipiodol injection into milk-ducts followed

by abscess formation. Amer. J. Obstet. Gynec., 20:
414–416, Sept. 1930
Riesman, David. Philadelphia physician. 1867–1940
SIGN—
Soft eyeball in diabetic coma. J. A. M. A., 66: 85
(only), Jan. 8, 1916
SIGN—
Bruit over the eyeball in exophthalmic goiter. Ibid.,
1381–1382, Apr. 29, 1916
SIGN—transdigital auscultation, over apex beat.
Some points in physical diagnosis. Trans. Ass. Amer.
Phys., pp. 4–6, May 1922
Rieux, Léon. French surgeon
HERNIA—retrocecal.
*Considérations sur l'étranglement de l'intestin dans la
cavité abdominale et sur un mode d'étranglement non
décrit par les auteurs.* Paris, Thèse, 1853. No. 128
Rigby, Edward. English physician. 1747–1821
Wrote on placenta previa.
An essay on the uterine hemorrhage. London, Johnson,
1775
Riggs, John M. American dentist. 1810–1885
DISEASE—alveolar pyorrhea.
*Suppurative inflammation of the gums, and absoption
of the gums and alveola process.* Pennsylvania J. Dent.
Sci., 3: 99–104, Mar. 1876
Rigler, L. G. See E. A. Boyden
Riley, H. A. See F. Tilney
Rimington, Claude. English scientist
Described—
*Porphyrinuria following sulfanilamide: sulfanilamide
dermatitis* with A. W. Hemmings, Lancet, 1: 770–
776, Apr. 2, 1938
Rimpau, W. See F. Neufeld
Ring, John. English surgeon. 1752–1821
Described hernia into supravesical fossa of Cooper.
A case of internal inguinal hernia. London med.
Reposit., 2: 204–205, Sept. 1, 1814
Ringer, Sydney. English physiologist. 1834–1910
MIXTURE or SOLUTION—
*Regarding the action of hydrate of soda, hydrate of
ammonia, and hydrate of potash on the ventricle of the
frog's heart.* J. Physiol., 3: 195–202, 1880–82
Ringier, B. H. See P. Karrer
Rinne, Friedrich Heinrich. Göttingen otologist.
1819–1868
TEST—
Beiträge zur Physiologie des menschlichen Ohres.
Vrtljschr. f. d. prakt. Heilk., Prague, 1: 71–123;
2: 45–72, 1855
Rio-Hortega, Pio del. Spanish scientist
METHOD—silver carbonate, for oligodendroglia.
La glia de escasas radiaciones (oligodendroglia). Arch.
de neurobiol., 2: 16–43, 1921
METHOD—silver carbonate, for microglia.
*Histogénesis y evolución normal; éxodo y distribución
regional de la microglia.* Ibid., pp. 212–255
MODIFICATION—of silver carbonate method for
pineal body.
*Constitution histologique de la glande pinéale. I. Cel-
lules parenchymateuses.* Trab. Lab. Invest. biol.
Univ. Madr., 21: 95–141, 1923
STAIN—carbonate of silver, for nerve.
*Noticia de un nuevo y fácil método para la coloración de
la neuroglia y del tejido conjuntivo.* Ibid., 15: 367–378
1917

Estudios sobre la neuroglia. La microglia y su trans-formación en células en bastoncito y cuerpos gránul-adiposos. Ibid., 18: 37–82, Jan. 1920

Ripault, Louis Henry Antoin. French physician. 1807–1856

SIGN—eye, of life.

Remarques sur divers phénomènes de la vie organique qui persistent pendant quelque temps après la mort. Paris, Baillière, 1841. 22 pp.

Risley, Samuel Doty. Philadelphia ophthalmologist. 1845–1920

PRISM—

A new apparatus for detecting and measuring the anomalies of ocular muscles. Med. and Surg. Reporter s 2., 65: 884–886, Dec. 5, 1891

Risser, Joseph Charles. New York surgeon. 1892–

METHOD—turn-buckle cast, for scoliosis. See R. A. Hibbs

Ritchie, Charles. English physician. ?–1878

Introduced term "enteric fever."

Practical remarks on the continued fevers of Great Britain, and on the generic distinctions between enteric fever and typhus. Monthly J. med. Sci., 7: 247–258, 1846–47

Ritchie, S. See R. Muir

Ritchie, William Thomas. English physician. 1873–

Recognized auricular flutter.

Complete heart-block, with dissociation of the action of the auricles and ventricles. Proc. roy. Soc. Edinb., 25: 1085–1091, 1905–06

Auricular flutter. Edinburgh and London, Green, 1914. 144 pp.

Ritgen, Ferdinand August Marie Franz von. German obstetrician. 1787–1867

OPERATION—a substitute for cesarean section.

Die Anzeigen der mechanischen Hülfen bei Entbind-ungen, nebst Beschreibung einiger, in neuerer Zeit empfohlenen geburtshülflichen Operationen und einer verbesserten Geburtszange. Giessen, Heyer, 1820. 470 pp.

Geschichte eines mit ungünstigem Erfolge verrichteten Bauchscheidenschnitts und Folgerung daraus. Heidelb. klin. Ann., 1: 263–277, 1825

Ritter, Jacob. Uster, Switzerland physician

Described psittacosis in man.

Beitrage zur Frage des Pneumotyphus. Eine (Haus-epidemie in Uster (Schweiz) betreffend). Dtsch. Arch. f. klin. Med., 25: 53–96, Dec. 10, 1879

Ritter, S. See L. Loewe

Rittershain, Gottfried Ritter von. German physician. 1820–1883

DISEASE—dermatitis exfoliativa infantum or neona-torum.

Dermatitis erysipelatosa; Gangraena; Enkephalitis. Österr, Jahrb. f. Pädiat., Wien, 1: 23–24, 1870

Die exfoliative Dermatitis die jungeren Säuglinge. Zentral-Zeit. f. Kinderheilk., 2: 3–23, Oct. 1878

Rittman, G. E. See M. J. Romansky

Rivalta, Sebastiano. 1852–

DISEASE—actinomycosis. Fischer

Del cose detto farcino o moccio dei bovini e della detta tuberculosi o mal del raspo (Trutta) della lingua dei medisemi animali. G. anat. fisiol. e pat. d'animali, Pisa, 7: 198, 1875

REACTION—

Su di una nuova reazione per la diagnosi chimica

differenziale fra gli essudati sierosi ed i semplici trans-udati. Rif. med., 2: 242–245, 1895

Riva-rocci, Scipione. Italian physician

SPHYGMOMANOMETER—

Un nuovo sfigmomanometro. Gaz. med. di Torino, 47 981–996; 1001–1017, 1896

Rivas, Damoso. Nicaragua physician. 1874–

BOUILLON—glucose.

Ein Beitrag zur Anaërobenzuchtung. Zbl. Bakt., 32 831–841 (836), Nov. 17, 1902

Rivat, G. Lyon physician

REACTION—for oxyhemoglobin.

Les causes d'erreurs possibles dans la recherche du sang par les procédés classiques; nouvelle réaction d l'oxyhémoglobine par l'albuminate de manganèse Lyon Med., 11: 813–818, Oct. 15, 1911

Riven, S. S. See Annie S. Minot

Rivers, Thomas Milton. New York physician. 1888–

METHOD—of intradermal injection against small pox. See Alexia Carrel

Cultivation of vaccine virus for Jennerian prophylaxi in man. J. exp. Med., 54: 453–461, Oct. 1, 1931

METHOD—

Diagnosis of psittacosis in man by means of injection of sputum into white mice with G. P. Berry, Ibid., 61 205–212, Feb. 1, 1935

SOLUTION—blood cell peptone.

The biological and the serological reactions of influenze bacillis producing meningitis. Ibid., 34: 477–49 (479), Nov. 1921

See also A. Carrel, C. P. Li

Rivers, William Halse Rivers. English physician 1864–1922

Wrote, after experimentation on H. Head—

A human experiment in nerve division with Henry Head, Brain, 31: 323–450, 1908

Riviere, Clive. London physician. 1872–1929

SIGN—"saddle" and "collar" dullness, in pulmonary tuberculosis.

In his: *The early diagnosis of tubercle.* London, Ox-ford, 1921. 3 ed., pp. 34–36

Rivière, Lazare. French physician. 1589–1655

Described aortic stenosis. Garrison and Morton

Opera medica universa. Francofurti, Zubrodt, 1674 p. 638

Rivinus, Augustus Quirinus. Leipsic anatomist 1652–1723

CANALS or DUCTS—of sublingual gland.

GLAND—sublingual.

INCISURE or NOTCH—groove in osseous tympanic ring filled with Shrapnell's membrane.

(De anatomia.) (Lipsiae), Colerianis, 1691

Rivkin, Helen. See Frances Krasnow

Rixford, Emmet. California surgeon. 1865–

Described coccidioidal granuloma.

A case of protozoic skin disease with W. S. Thorne Abstr.: Occidental med. Times, 8: 326 (only), Dec 1894

Two cases of protozoan (coccidioidal) infection of the skin and other organs with T. C. Gilchrist, Johns Hopk. Hosp. Rep., 1: 209–268, 1896

Riza, Ali. French chemist

TEST—for cystine in urine.

Nouveau réactif de la cystine. Bull. Soc. Chim. biol. Paris, 3 s., 249–250, 1903

Rizzatti, E. See A. M. Fiamberti

Roaf, Herbert Eldon. London physiologist. 1881–
THEORY—of vision.
On the measurement of colour-blindness in terms of wave-lengths. Quart. J. exp. Physiol., 14: 151–159, Apr. 1924
The relation of wave-length and light intensity to colour discrimination in normal and hypochromatic (colourblind individuals. Ibid., 16: 379–392, Jan. 29, 1927

Robb, George Porter. New York physician. 1898–
METHOD—
A practical method of visualization of the chambers of the heart, the pulmonary circulation, and the great blood vessels in man with I. Steinberg, J. clin. Invest., 17: 507 (only), July 1938
Visualization of the chambers of the heart, the pulmonary circulation, and the great blood vessels in man: a practical method with I. Steinberg, Amer. J. Roentgenol., 41: 1–17, Jan. 1939

Roberts, Dudley DeVore. Brooklyn physician. 1874–1940
ENEMATOR—
A new rectal enemator. J. A. M. A., 47: 273 (only), July 28, 1906

Roberts, John Bingham. Philadelphia surgeon. 1852–1924
OPERATION—
Excision of the lumbar lymphatic nodes and spermatic vein in malignant disease of the testicle. Ann. Surg., 36: 539–549, 1902

Roberts, Percy Willard. New York surgeon. 1867–1937
OPERATION—
An operation for dislocation of the shoulder. J. Bone and Joint Surg., 15: 233–234, Jan. 1933

Roberts, Robert Edward. Liverpool obstetrician
METHOD—
Internal pelvimetry by x rays. Brit. J. Radiol., 32: 11–14, Jan. 1927

Roberts, Sam Earl. Kansas City, Mo. otolaryngologist. 1887–
OPERATION—
Fracture of the malar zygomatic arch—review of the literature—a simplified operative technic—case reports. Ann. Otol., Rhin. and Laryngol., 37: 826–838, Sept. 1928

Roberts, Sir William. Manchester physician. 1830–1899
TEST—
On a new test for albumin in urine. Lancet, 2: 613–614, Oct. 14, 1882
Acidulated salt solution as a test for albumin and peptone in urine. New Remedies, 12: 17–18, Jan. 1883

Robertson, Andrew. London protozoologist
Wrote—
Observations on the causal organism of rat-bite fever in man. Ann. Trop. Med. and Parasitol., Liverpool, 18: 157–175, Aug. 2, 1924

Robertson, D. F. See R. A. Phillips

Robertson, Douglas Moray Cooper Lamb Argyll. Scottish physician. 1837–1909
OPERATION—
A new operation for ectropion. Edinburgh Clin. and Path. J., 1: 201–203, Dec. 15, 1883
PUPIL—miotic and responds to accommodation but not to light.

On an interesting series of eye symptoms in a case of spinal disease, with remarks on the action of belladonna on the iris, etc. Edinburgh med. J., 14: 696–708, Feb. 1869
Four cases of spinal myosis; with remarks on the action of light on the pupil. Ibid., 15: 487–493, Dec. 1869
Also, both papers in: Medical classics, 1: 851–876, May 1937

Robertson, H. E. See R. M. Wilder

Robertson, Muriel. London scientist
MEDIUM—cooked beef heart.
Notes upon certain anaerobes isolated from wounds. J. Path. Bact., 20: 327–349, Jan. 1916

Robertson, Oswald Hope. American physician. 1886–
Described use of preserved blood and blood banks.
Transfusion with preserved red blood cells. Brit. med. J., 1: 691–695, June 22, 1918
See also I. J. Kligler, R. I. Lee

Robey, William Henry. Boston physician. 1870–
AGAR—glucose serum, for isolation of meningococci.
Clinical and epidemiological studies on epidemic meningitis with H. L. Saylor, H. E. Meleney, H. Ray and G. A. Landmann, J. infect. Dis., 23: 317–336 (324), Oct. 1918

Robin, Edouard Charles Albert. Paris physician. 1847–1928
TYPHUS—abdominal. Fischer
Essai d'urologie clinique; la fièvre typhoïde. Paris, Thèse, No. 77, 1877

Robin, Charles Philippe. French anatomist. 1821–1885
MYELOPLAX—osteoclasts.
Observations sur l'ostéogénie. Paris, Martinet, 1851. 16 pp.

Robin, M. L. Paris physician
SOLUTION—lactose peptone, for differentiation of colon and typhoid group.
Note sur un nouveau milieu coloré pour la différenciation du colibacille et du bacille d'Eberth. C. R. Soc. Biol., 49: 49–51, Jan. 16, 1897

Robineau. See R. Sicard

Robins, Charles Russell. Richmond, Va. surgeon 1868–
OPERATION—
Direct inguinal hernia: presentation of an operation for its cure. Ann. Surg., 108: 389–410, Sept. 1938

Robinson, Andrew Rose. New York dermatologist. 1845–1924
DISEASE—hidrocystoma.
Milaria and sudamina. Trans. Amer. Dermat. Ass., 14–16, 1884
Hidrocystoma. J. Cutan. Dis., 11: 293–303, Aug. 1893

Robinson, F. H. See Alice C. Evans

Robinson, Fred Byron. American surgeon. 1857–1910
ABDOMINAL BRAIN—ganglion coeliacum.
The abdominal brain and automatic visceral ganglia. Chicago, Clin. Pub. Co., 1899. 261 pp.
CIRCLE—
Arteria uterina ovarica. The utero-ovarian artery, or the genital vascular circle.... Chicago, Colegrove, 1903. 182 pp.
PLATE—
The rawhide plate: a new plate for intestinal anastomosis. New York med. J., 52: 429–433, Oct. 18, 1890

SUTURE—
Circular enterorrhaphy by a new method. Ann. Surg., 13: 81–95, Feb. 1891

Robinson, George Henry. American bacteriologist. 1989–
SOLUTION—basal azolitmin peptone.
Isolation, identification, and serum reactions of typhoid and paratyphoid bacilli. J. med. Res., 32: 399–418 (407), July 1915
TISSUE BROTH—
The use of tissue in broth in the production of diphtheria toxin with P. D. Meader, J. infect. Dis., 27: 106–114, Aug. 1920

Robinson, Harold Cunningham. American bacteriologist. 1889–
AGAR—glycerol opsine; culture medium.
The growth of bacteria in protein-free enzyme and acid-digestion products with L. F. Rettger, J. Bact., 3: 209–230 (212), May 1918
MODIFICATION—
Studies on the use of brilliant green and a modified Endo's medium in the isolation of Bacillus typhosus from feces with L. F. Rettger, J. med. Res., 34: 363–376, July 1916
SOLUTION—basal opsine; culture medium. See AGAR
SOLUTION—opsine, for cultivation of B. diphtheriae.
The part played by protein-free digestion products and by meat infusion in diphtheria toxin production with L. F. Rettger, J. Med. Res., 36: 357–376 (363), July 1917

Robinson, Samuel. Rochester, Minn. surgeon. 1877–
OPERATION—
The treatment of chronic non-tuberculous empyema. S. G. O., 22: 557–571, May 1916

Robinson, W. L. See G. W. Howland

Robinson, William. Washington, D. C. entomologist. 1890–
APPARATUS—
Surgical maggots in the treatment of infected wounds: recent apparatus and methods in maggot production and research with S. W. Simmons, J. Lab. clin. Med., 19: 339–343, Jan. 1934

Robiquet, Pierre Jean. French physician. 1780–1840
Isolated codeine.
Nouvelles observations sur les principaux produits de l'opium. Ann. Chim. (Phys.), Paris, 51: 225–267, 1832

Robison, Robert. English biochemist. 1883–1941
Indicated important role of phosphatase and conversion of blood calcium into insoluble calcium in process of ossification.
The possible significance of hexosephorphoric esters in ossification. Biochem. J., 17: 286–293, 1923
(Same) *Part II. The phosphoric esterase of ossifying cartilage* with Katharine M. Soames, Ibid., 18: 740–754, 1924

Robscheit-Robbins, Frieda Saur. San Francisco scientist. 1893–
METHOD—
A comparative study of hemoglobin determination by various methods. J. biol. Chem., 41: 209–226, Feb. 1920
Did basic work on liver therapy. See G. H. Whipple
(Also) *Blood regeneration in severe anaemia. II. Favorable influence of liver, heart, and skeletal muscle*

in diet with G. H. Whipple, Amer. J. Physiol., 7: 408–418, May 1925
See also G. H. Whipple

Robson, Sir Arthur William Mayo. English surgeo 1853–1933
BONE ROBBIN—
Two cases of pylorectomy and one of jejunostomy, wi remarks, and with a suggested modification of the form operation. Med.-chir. Trans., 75: 407–420, 1892
A method of performing intestinal anastomosis means of decalcified bone bobbins. Brit. med. J., 688–689, Apr. 1, 1893
CATGUT PREPARATION—
A simple and effectual method of sterilizing catg Lancet, 2: 874 (only), Oct. 1, 1898
INCISION—for operations on biliary tract.
The surgical treatment of obstruction in the comm bile-duct by concretions, with especial reference to t operation of choledochotomy as modified by the auth illustrated by 60 cases. Ibid., 1: 1023–1027, Apr. 1902
OPERATION—
A series of cases of spina bifida treated by plastic oper tion. Trans. clin. Soc. London, 18: 210–220, 1885
POINT—of greatest tenderness in gall bladder inflam mation.
The surgery of the gall bladder and bile ducts, with br notes of 78 cases. Brit. med. J., 1: 901–904, Apr. 1894
Lectures on diseases of the gall bladder and bile duc Ibid., 1: 641–646, Mar. 13, 1897
POSITION—for operations on gall bladder.
A series of cases of choledochotomy, including three duodenocholedochotomy. Ibid., 2: 1404–1406, Nov. 1898
See also INCISION
SIGN—coin test for subphrenic abscess.
An address on the diagnosis and treatment of ac inflammations of the upper abdomen. Ibid., 1: 61– Jan. 8, 1910
Reported—
Actinomycosis of the gall-bladder. Trans. Med.-ch Soc., London, 88: 225–228, 1905

Rochaix, Jean Anthelme. French scientist
AGAR—carrot.
Nouveau milieu végétal pour cultures microbien (Agar au jus de carotte). C. R. Soc. Biol., 74: 60 606, Mar. 15, 1913
See also G. Roux

Rocha-Lima, Henrique da. Berlin physician. 187 Isolated cause of typhus, Rickettsia prowaze and named it after two workers who died of disea Garrison and Morton
Zur Aetiologie des Fleckfiebers. Berl. klin. Wschr., 567–569, May 22, 1916

Rocher, Henri Gaston Louis. French surgeon. 187 OPERATION—for slipping patella; costal graft inserted into external condyle of femur.
Butee rotulienne par greffon costal dans un cas luxation congenitale des deux torules. Résultat eloi de 4 ans. Bordeaux chir., 4: 365–369, Oct. 1933

Rochon-Duvigneaud, André. French ophthalm ogist. 1863–
SCLERO-CORNEAL TRABECULA—
SCLERAL SINUS—
Recherches anatomiques sur l'angle de la chambre

térieure et le canal de Schlemm. Arch. d'Ophthal., 12: 732–744, Dec. 1892

Rodda, Frederick C. Minneapolis pediatrician. 1880–
METHOD—
Studies with a new method for determining the coagulation time of the blood in the new-born. Amer. J. Dis. Child., 11: 269–276, Apr. 1920

Roddenbery, S. A. See C. S. Stone

Roddy, John Augustus. Philadelphia physician. 1884–
BOUILLON—bile; culture medium.
In his: *Medical bacteriology.* Philadelphia, Blakiston, 1917. p. 42

Rodgers, John Kearney. New York surgeon. 1793–1851
Wired ununited fractures successfully.
Case of un-united fracture of the os brachii, successfully treated. New York Med. and Phys. J., 6: 521–523, 1827
First to tie left subclavian artery within scaleni for aneurysm, 1845, but with fatal result. Garrison
Ligature of the left subclavian artery within the scalenus muscle, for aneurism. Amer. J. med. Sci., n. s. 11: 541–545, Apr. 1846
Also: New York J. Med., 6: 219–227, Mar. 1846

Rodis, I. See H. Shay

Rodman, William Louis. Philadelphia surgeon. 1858–1916
OPERATION—radical mastectomy.
Diseases of the breast, with special reference to cancer. Philadelphia, Blakiston, 1908. 385 pp.
Also, London, Appleton, 1908. 385 pp. pp. 259–326
THEORY—of ulcer-bearing area of stomach.
Pylorectomy and partial gastrectomy or excision of the ulcer-bearing area in the treatment of gastric ulcer. S. G. O., 20: 25–30, Jan. 1915

Roe, Joseph Hyram. Washington, D. C. biochemist. 1892–
METHOD—
The colorimetric determination of blood calcium with B. S. Kahn, J. biol. Chem., 81: 1–8, Jan. 1929
TEST—
A colorimetric method for the determination of fructose in blood and urine. Ibid., 107: 15–22, Oct. 1934

Römer, Carl. German physician
TREATMENT—of parkinson syndrome with massive doses of atropine.
Zur Atropinbehandlung der enzephalitischen Folgezustände. Münch. med. Wschr., 77: 2156–2157, Dec. 12, 1930

Römer, Paul. German physician. 1873–1937
EXPERIMENT, SERUM—
Experimentelle und klinische Grundlagen für die Serumtherapie der Pneumokokkeninfektion der menschlichen Cornea (Ulcus serpens). Wiesbaden, Bergmann, 1909. 218 pp.

Rönne, Henning Kristian Trappaud. Copenhagen ophthalmologist. 1878–
NASAL STEP—
Ueber das Gesichtsfeld beim Glaukom. Klin. Mbl. Augenheilk., 47 (1): 12–33, Jan. 1909

Röntgen, Wilhelm Conrad von. Munich physicist. 1845–1923
RAY—x-ray.
Über eine neue Art von Strahlen. S. B. d. phy.-med. Ges. zu Würzb., pp. 132–141, 1895

A new form of radiation. Science, n. s., 3: 227–231, Feb. 14; 726–729, May 15, 1896

Röpke, W. German surgeon
OPERATION—temporary laminectomy.
Zur Technik der Laminektomie in der Behandlung von Rückenmarkstumoren. Zbl. Chir., 37: 1076–1077, Aug. 13, 1910
Credited with first performance of Beck-Jianu gastrostomy on man.
Ein neues Verfahren für die Gastrostomie und Ösophagoplastik. Ibid., 39: 1569–1571, Nov. 16, 1912

Rössler, Carl. German physician
TEST—for skatol red in urine.
Über skatolroth und ähnliche Harnfarbstoffe. Zbl. inn. Med., 22: 847–855, Aug. 31, 1901

Rösslin, Eucharius. ?–1526
Wrote earliest printed textbook for midwives.
Der swangern frawen und lebammen roszgarten. Hagenau, Gran, 1513
Also, transl. by R. Jonas
The byrth of mankynde. London, T. R., 1540

Roethlisberger, Paul. Geneva physician
TEST—for uric acid in blood.
Notiz über eine klinische Methode der quantitativen Bestimmung der Harnsäure im Blutserum. Münch. med. Wschr., 57: 344–347, Feb. 15, 1910

Roffo, Angel H. Argentina physician. 1882–1947
TEST—for cancer.
Reacción celular en el cáncer. Presna méd. argentina, 3: 114–117, 1916–17
On a reaction for the diagnosis of cancer. Cancer, 3: 294–300, July 1926

Roger, Georges Henri. French physiologist. 1860–1946
REFLEX—
Le réflexe oesophago-salivaire. Pr. méd., 100: 793–794, Dec. 14, 1904
Le rôle du réflexe oesophago-salivaire dans la déglutition. Ibid., 19: 145–146, Mar. 8, 1905

Roger, Henri Louis. Paris physician. 1811–1892
DISEASE—congenital communication between ventricles of heart.
Recherches cliniques sur la communication congénitale des deux coeurs, par inocclusion du septum interventriculaire. Bull. Acad. Méd. Paris, 2 s., 8: 1074–1094; 1189–1191, 1879
Also, English transl. by J. P. Wozencraft in: F. A. Willius and T. E. Keys' *Cardiac classics.* St. Louis, Mosby, 1941. pp. 624–636; 637–638

Rogers, G. See M. E. Davis

Rogers, Horatio. Boston surgeon. 1897–
OPERATION—
Pilonidal sinus. S. G. O., 57: 803–810, Dec. 1933
Pilonidal sinus: surgical treatment and pathologic structure with M. G. Hall, Arch. Surg., 31: 742–766, Nov. 1935
Pilonidal sinus: observations on one hundred forty cases treated by cautery excision with R. W. Dwight, Ann. Surg., 107: 400–418, Mar. 1938

Rogers, L. M. See J. Goldberger

Rogers, Sir Leonard R. English physician. 1868–
TREATMENT—of cholera.
Cholera and its treatment. London, Oxford, 1913. 236 pp.
Advocated—
The rapid cure of amoebic dysentery and hepatitis by

hypodermic injections of soluble salts of emetine.
Brit. med. J., 1: 1424–1425, June 22, 1912
Demonstrated—
Note on the occurrence of Leishman-Donovan bodies in "cachexial fevers," including kala-azar. Ibid., 1: 1249–1251, May 28, 1904
Rogers, Lore Alford. Washington, D. C. physician. 1875–
BROTH—basal extract, for studying fermentation by bacteria.
The colon group of bacteria with W. M. Clark and B. J. Davis, J. infect. Dis., 14: 411–475, May 1914
Rogers, William Alexander. Boston surgeon. 1892–
FRAME—
An extension frame for the reduction of fracture of the vertebral body. S. G. O., 50: 101–104, Jan. 1930
Rogoff, Julius Moses. Cleveland physician. 1884–
Obtained cortical hormone.
The influence of adrenal extracts on the survival period of adrenalectomized dogs with G. N. Stewart, Science, s. 2., 66: 327–328, Oct. 7, 1927
Used—
Suprarenal cortical extracts in suprarenal insufficiency (Addison's disease) with G. N. Stewart, J. A. M. A., 92: 1569–1571, May 11, 1929
Rohde, Erwin. Munich physician. 1881–1915
REACTION—for albumins.
Die Farbenreaktionen der Eiweisskörper mit p-Dimethylaminobenzaldehyd und anderen aromatischen Aldehyden. Z. physiol. Chem., 44: 161–170, May 6, 1905
Rokitansky, Carl Freiherr von. Vienna pathologist. 1804–1878
DISEASE—acute yellow atrophy of liver.
Hat zuerst die gelbe Leberatrophie als eine besondere anatomisch charakterisierte Krankheitsform aufgestellt. Handb. d. path. Anatomie, 3: 269; 313, 1842–46
PELVIS—spondylolisthetic.
Beitrag zur Kenntniss der Rückgrathskrümmungen, und der mit denselben zusammentreffenden Abweichungen des Brustkorbes und Beckens. Med. Jahrb. d. öster. Staates, Vienna, 19: 41; 195, 1839
Differentiated between lobar and lobular pneumonia.
In: Handb. d. path. Anatomie, 1842
Also in: *A manual of pathological anatomy.* Philadelphia, Blanchard, and Lea, 1855. Vol. 4, p. 65
Wrote on defects of septum of heart.
Die Defecte der Scheidewände des Herzens. Wien, Braumüller, 1875
Rolando, Luigi. Italian anatomist. 1773–1831
ANGLE, CELLS, COLUMN, FASCICULUS, FIBERS, FOSSA, LINE, POINT, TUBERCLE, etc.
Saggio sopra la vera struttura del cervello dell'uomo e degl'animali e sopra le funzioni del sistema nervoso. Sassari, Stamp. Privileg., 1809
Ricerche anatomiche sulla struttura del midollo spinale. Dizionario periodico di med., 1824. Also: Torino, 1824. 118 pp.
Osservazioni sul cervelletto. Mem. r. Accad. d. sci. di Torino, 29: 163–188, 1825
Rolland. See M. L. Thevenon
Roller, Christian Friedrich Wilhelm. Strassburg neurologist. 1802–1878

NUCLEUS—
Der centrale Verlauf des Nervus accessorius Willisii. Allg. Z. f. Psychiat., 37: 469–489, 1881
Rolleston, H. D. See F. L. Golla
Rollett, Joseph Pierre Martin. French dermatologist 1824–1894
CHANCRE—mixed.
Coincidence du chancre syphilitique primitif avec la gale, la blénorrhagie, le chancre simple, et la vaccina. Gaz. méd. de Lyon, 18: 160–163, 1866
Rollier, Auguste. Switzerland physician. 1874–
TREATMENT—of tuberculosis by exposure to sun.
Die Heliotherapie der Tuberkulose mit besonderer Berücksichtigung ihrer chirurgischen Formen. Berlin Springer, 1913. 119 pp.
Rollo, John. English physician. ?–1809
Reported on diabetes.
An account of two cases of the diabetes mellitus, with remarks as they arose during the progress of the cure. London, Dilly, 1797
Rolly, Frederick. Leipzig physician
RESPIRATION CALORIMETER—
Ein nach dem Regnault-Reiset'schen Prinzip für klinische Gaswechseluntersuchungen gebauter modifizierter Benedict'scher Respirationsapparat with J Rosiewicz, Dtsch. Arch. f. klin. Med., 103: 58–92 June 9, 1911
Same Verh. dtsch. Kong. inn. Med., 28: 512–519 1911
Romanowsky, Dmitriy Leonidovich. Russian physician. 1861–1921
METHOD—contrast-stain for malarial parasite.
K voprosu o parazitologii i terapii bolotnoi likhoradki St. Petersburg, Skovokhodoff, 1891
Romansky, Monroe James. American physician 1911–
FORMULA—
A method of prolonging the action of penicillin with G. W. Rittman, Science, 100: 196–198, Sept. 1, 194
Penicillin. I. Prolonged action in beeswax-peanut o mixture. II. Single injection treatment of gonorrhe with G. E. Rittman, Bull. U. S. Army Med. Dept. 2: 43–49, Oct. 1944
Romberg, Moritz Heinrich. Berlin physician. 1795 1873
DISEASE or TROPHONEUROSIS—facial hemia trophy.
In: *Klinische Ergebnisse.* Berlin, Förstner, 1846. p. 7
SIGN—
Tabes dorsalis. In his: *Lehrbuch der Nerven-Krank heiten des Menschen.* Berlin, Duncker, 1846. 85 pp. p. 795
Same 1851. vol. 2, p. 185
Also, transl. by E. H. Sieveking. London, Sydenhar Soc., 1853
SPASM—masticatory.
Neuralgiae nervi quinti specimen. Berolini, Duncker 1840. 14 pp.
Wrote early thesis on achondroplasia. Garrison
De rachitide congenita. Berlin, Plateni, 1817. 58 pp
Romero, Francisco. Barcelona surgeon
Did first successful pericardiocentesis. Garrison an Morton
Sur l'hydrothorax et l'hydropéricarde. Bull. Fac. d Méd. de Paris, 4: 373–376, 1814–15
Romieu, Marc. Toulouse histologist

REACTION—phosphoric acid, for determination of protein. Garrison
Sur la détection histochimique des substances protéiques. Bull. d'histol. appliq. à la physiol., Lyon, 2: 185-191, June 1925
Romijn, G. German chemist
REAGENT—for glucose.
Ueber eine jodometrische Zuckerbestimmung. Z. anal. Chem., 36: 349-359 (351), 1897
Rona, Peter. German chemist. 1871-
FORMULA—
Beitrag zur Frage nach dem Verhalten des Calciums im Serum with D. Takahashi, Biochem. Z., 49: 370-380, Mar. 27, 1913
Ronchèse, A. French physician
TEST—of ammonia in urine.
Nouveau procédé de dosage de l'ammoniaque. Bull. Soc. Chim. de France, 4 s., 1: 900-905, July 12, 1907
Methodes de dosage de quelques composés azotés ammoniaque, urée, acide urique. Paris, Lehure, 1908. 72 pp.
Rones, B. See W. H. Wilmer
Ronsseus, Balduinus. Dutch physician. 1525-1597
Described in 1564 use of orange and lemon juice by Dutch sailors, for scurvy. Garrison
De magnis Hippocratis lienibus Pliniique stomacace, ac sceletyrbe, seu vulgo dicto scorbuto libellus. Antverpiae, apud viduam Martini Nutii, 1564
Roonhuyze, Hendrik van. Dutch surgeon. 1622-1672
Wrote on operative gynecology.
Heel-konstige aanmerkkingen betreffende de gebreeken der vrouwen. Amsterdam, Jacobsz, 1663
Roos, E. See H. I. Quincke
Roper, K. L. See W. B. Lancaster
Roques, Henri. French biologist
REAGENT—
Sur un nouveau procédé de recherche du glycogène. C. R. Soc. Biol., 95: 575-576, July 6, 1926
Rorschach, Hermann. German psychiatrist. 1884-1922
TEST—ink blots, for intelligence.
Psychodiagnostik. . . . Arb. z. ang. Psychiat., Vol. 2, 1921. 174 pp.
Same: Bern, Bircher, 1921. 174 pp.
Rose, E. B. See W. O. Atwater
Rose, Anton Richard. American biochemist. 1877-
METHOD—
A micro-urease method for the determination of urea with Katherine R. Coleman, Biochem. Bull., 3: 411-415, Apr. and July 1914
See also W. G. Exton
Rose, Edmund. Zurich surgeon. 1836-1914
POSITION—head dependent; used in certain operations on air-passages.
Vorschlag zur Erleichterung der Operationen am Oberkiefer. Arch. f. klin. Chir., 17: 454-471 (459), 1874
Rose, Ferdinand. German scientist
TEST—biuret, for albumen.
Ueber die Verbindungen des Eiweiss mit Metalloxyden. Ann. d. Physik, 28: 132-142, 1833
Rose, William. English surgeon. 1847-1910
OPERATION—gasserectomy.
The Lettsomian Lectures: Surgical treatment of tri-geminal neuralgia. Trans. Med. Soc., London, 15: 157-230, 1892
The surgical treatment of neuralgia of the fifth nerve (tic douloureux). London, Bailliere, 1892. 85 pp.
OPERATION—for hare-lip.
In: Rose and Carless, *Manual of surgery.* New York, Wood, 1922. 10 ed., pp. 888-891
Rose, William Cumming. New Haven biochemist. 1887-
MODIFICATION—
A modified method for the clinical estimation of pepsin. Arch. intern. Med., 5: 459-465, May 1910
Rosenbach, Anton Julius Frederick. German pathologist. 1842-1923
BACILLUS—saprogenes.
Mikro-Organismen bei den Wund-Infektions-Krankheiten des Menschen. Wiesbaden, Bergmann, 1884. 122 pp.
Applied term "erysipeloid" to skin infection caused by Erysipelothrix rhusiopathiae.
Über das Erysipeloid. Arch. klin. Chir., 36: 346-350, 1887
Rosenbach, Ottomar. German physician. 1851-1907
DISEASE—with Heberden's nodes.
Die Auftreibung der Endphalangen der Finger—eine bisher noch nicht beschriebene tropische Störung. Zbl. Nervenheilk., 13: 199-205, Aug. 1890
LAW—governing site of immobilization of vocal cords. Garrison
Zur Lehre von der doppelseitigen totalen Lähmung des Nerv. laryngeus inferior (recurrens). Breslau. Aerztl. Z., 2: 14-16, 1880
SYNDROME—paroxysmal tachycardia with gastric and respiratory complications.
Beitrag zur Lehre von den Krankheiten des Verdauungsapparates. I. Über einen wahrscheinlich auf einer Neurose des Vagus beruhenden Symptomenkomplex. Dtsch. med. Wschr., 5: 535-538, Oct. 18; 555-557, Oct. 25, 1879
TEST—for bile pigments.
Zur Untersuchung des Harns auf Gallenfarbstoff. Zbl. med. Wiss., 14: 5-6, Jan. 1, 1876
Die Chromsäure als Reagens auf Eiweiss und Gallenfarbstoff. Dtsch. med. Wschr., 18: 381 (only), Apr. 28, 1892
TEST—for glucose.
Eine Reaktion auf Traubenzucker. Zbl. klin. Med., 13: 257-261, Apr. 2, 1892
Rosenberg, Ludwig. German physician
TEST—for bile pigments in urine.
Eine neue Methode zur Feststellung von Gallenfarbstoffen im Harne. Münch. med. Wschr., 63: 887 (only), June 13, 1916
Rosenberg, Margaret L. See Frances Krasnow
Rosenberg, Mat. Berlin physician. 1887-
TEST—functional, of kidney.
Das Alkaliausscheidungsvermögen der Niere als Nierenfunktionsprüfung with A. Hellfors, Münch. med. Wschr., 74: 926-929, June 3, 1927
Rosenblatt, P. See L. Loewe
Rosenblueth, A. See W. B. Cannon
Rosenfeld, Georg Ernst. Breslau physician. 1861-
Suggested administration of glucose in prevention and treatment of hepatic necrosis due to chloroform.
Zur Lehre von der Fettwanderung. Abstr.: Allg. med. Zbl. Zeitung, 89: 1051 (only), Nov. 7, 1900

Fettbildung. Ergebn. Physiol., 2: 50–94, 1903
Der Process der Verfettung. Berl. klin. Wschr. 41:
587–590, May 30; 617–620, June 6, 1904
Rosenheim, Max Leonard. English physician
Introduced—
Mandelic acid in the treatment of urinary infections.
Lancet, 1: 1032–1037, May 4, 1935
Rosenheim, Otto. London scientist
METHOD—
*A volumetric method for the estimation of ethereal and
inorganic sulphates in urine* with J. C. Drummond,
Biochem. J., 8: 143–151, Apr. 1914
REACTION—for choline.
New tests for choline in physiological fluids. J. Physiol.,
33: 220–224, Dec. 19, 1905
REACTION—for proteins.
*A colour reaction for formaldehyde with proteids and
its relation to the Adamkiewicz reaction.* Biochem. J.,
1: 233–240, Apr. 1906
REACTION—for sterol.
A specific colour reaction for ergosterol. Ibid., 23: 47–
53, 1929
TEST—for vitamin A.
A delicate colour reaction for the presence of vitamin A
with J. C. Drummond, Ibid., 19: 753–756, 1925
Rosenheim, Theodor. German physician. 1860–
Developed a new type of gastroscope.
*Ueber die Besichtigung der Cardia nebst Bemerkungen
über Gastroskopie.* Dtsch. med. Wschr., 21: 740–744,
Nov. 7, 1895
Rosenmüller, Johannes Christianus. Leipzig an-
atomist. 1771–1820
GLAND—
*Organorum lachrymalium partiumque externarum
oculi humani descriptio anatomica.* Lipsiae, Krameria,
1797. 56 pp.
Rosenoff-Saloff, Mme. See A. Souques
Rosenow, Edward Carl. American bacteriologist.
1875–
AGAR—glucose ascitic fluid; culture medium.
*The etiology of acute rheumatism, articular and
muscular.* J. infect. Dis., 14: 61–80, Jan. 1914
STAIN—
*A new stain for bacterial capsules with special reference
to pneumococci.* Ibid., 9: 1–8, July 1911
Protagonist of doctrine of variability and selectivity
of microorganisms.
*Transmutations within the streptococcus-pneumococcus
group.* Ibid., 14: 1–32, Jan. 1914
Elective localization of streptococci. J. A. M. A., 65:
1687–1691, Nov. 13, 1915
*The etiology of cholecystitis and gall stones and their
production by the intravenous injection of bacteria.*
J. infect. Bis., 19: 527–556, Oct. 1916
*Results of experimental studies on focal infection and
elective localization.* Med. Clin. N. Amer., 5: 573–592,
Sept. 1921
See also J. A. Bargen
Rosenthal, Eugen. Hungarian chemist
TEST—
*Eine neue Reaktion zum Nachweis und zur kolorim-
etrischen Bestimmung des Vitamins A* with J.
Erdélyi, Biochem. Z., 267: 119–123, Dec. 12, 1933
A new color test for the determination of vitamin A
with J. Erdélyi, Biochem. J., 28: 41–44, 1934
Rosenthal, Felix. Breslau physician. 1885–

TEST—bromsulfalein, of liver function.
*Zur polarimetrischen Gallensäurenbestimmung in
Körperflüssigkeiten und Organen.* Arch. exp. Path.
Pharmak., 157: 165–177, Dec. 1930
Rosenthal, Isidor. German physiologist. 1838–1915
Studied action of vagus on respiration.
*Die Athembewegungen und ihre Beziehungen zum
Nervus vagus.* Berlin, Hirschwald, 1862. 272 pp.
Rosenthal, J. See J. E. v. Purkinje
Rosenthal, Lazar. Brooklyn bacteriologist. 1874–
METHOD—for preparing type sera.
*The staining of blood-grouping sera for preservation and
identification.* J. Lab. clin. Med., 16: 1123–1124,
Aug. 1931
Rosenthal, N. See N. E. Brill, S. M. Peck
Rosenthal, Sanford M. American physician. 1897–
REAGENT—
*An improved method for using phenoltetrachlorphthal-
ein as a liver function test.* J. Pharmacol., 19: 385–
391, June 1922
*Clinical application of the bromsulphalein test for
hepatic function* with E. C. White, J. A. M. A., 84:
1112–1114, Apr. 11, 1925
TECHNIC—for production of standardized shock from
burns and from trauma.
*Experimental chemotherapy of burns and shock. I.
Methods. II. Effects of local therapy upon mortality
from shock.* Pub. Health Rep., 57: 1923–1935, Dec.
18, 1942
(Same) *III. Effects of systemic therapy on early
mortality.* Ibid., 58: 513–522, Mar. 26, 1943
(Same) *IV. Production of traumatic shock in mice. V.
Therapy with mouse serum and sodium salts.* Ibid.,
1429–1436, Sept. 24, 1943
(Same) *VI. Standardized hemorrhage in the mouse.
VII. Therapy of experimental hemorrhage.* Ibid., 59:
637–658, May 19, 1944
Rosen von Rosenstein, Nils Sweden physician. 1706–
1773
Founder of modern pediatrics.
*Underrättelser om barns Sjukdomar och deras brote-
medel.* Stockholm, 1764
Roseo, Italo Giuseppe. Rome physician
TEST—for thyrotoxicosis.
*Sulla deviazione del complemento nel morbo di Flajani-
Basedow.* Biochem. e terap. sper., Milan, 4: 1–4,
Aug.–Sept. 1912
Rosiewicz, J. See F. Rolly
Rosin, Heinrich. Berlin physician. 1855–
TEST—for bile-pigments in urine.
*Eine empfindliche Probe für den Nachweis von Gallen-
farbstoff im Harn.* Berl. klin. Wschr., pp. 106–107,
Jan. 30, 1893
Rosin, Joseph. New Jersey chemist. 1886–
TEST—
Detection of dextrose and sucrose in lactose with F. C.
Hitchcock, J. Amer. Pharm. Ass., 21: 1282–1286,
Dec. 1932
Ross, Cecil John. Portland, Ore. surgeon, 1898–
TECHNIC—
New and improved method of circumcision. Western
J. Surg., Obstet. and Gynec., 48: 755–756, Dec.
1940
Circumcision by ligation. Northwest Med., 41: 170–
171, May 1942

Ross, Sir George William. Toronto physician. 1841–1941
TEST—for excess of globulin in spinal fluid.
On the use of certain new chemical tests in the diagnosis of general paralysis and tabes with E. Jones, Brit. med. J., 1: 1111–1113, May 8, 1909
Ross, J. P. See G. E. Gask
Ross, Philip Hedgeland. Uganda bacteriologist. 1876–1929
Discovered causative agent in African variety of relapsing (tick) fever.
"Tick fever" with A. D. Milne, Brit. med. J., 2: 1453–1454, Nov. 26, 1904
Ross, Sir Ronald. English physician. 1857–1932
Awarded Nobel prize in 1902 for work in India about 1890 in proving that mosquito plays part of an intermediary host in transmission of malaria.
Some objections to haematozoic theories of malaria. Med. Reporter, India., 2: 65–71, Mar. 1, 1893
The third element of the blood and the malaria parasite Indian med. Gaz., 29: 5–14, Jan. 1894
Some observations on the crescent-sphere-flagella metamorphosis of the malaria-parasite within the mosquito. Indian Lancet, 7: 227–230, Mar. 1; 259–262, Mar. 16, 1896
Rossbach, Michael Joseph. German physician. 1842–1894
DISEASE—hyperchlorhydria.
Nervöse Gastroxynsis, als eine eigene, genau charakterisirbare Form der nervösen Dyspepsie. Dtsch. Arch. f. klin. Med., 35: 383–401, Sept. 24, 1884
Rossel, Otto. Swiss physician. 1875–1911
TEST—for blood.
Beitrag zum Nachweis von Blut bei Abwesenheit anderer anorganischer und organischer Substanzen in klinischen und gerichtlichen Fällen. Naumburg, Pätz, 1903. 15 pp.
Rossenbeck, H. See R. Feulgen
Rossi, Ferdinando. Padova surgeon
OPERATION—for arterial hypertension.
La resezione del tronco simpatico toracico e dei nervi splancnici nello spatium inframediastinale posterius. Arch. ital. di chir., 21: 729–740, 1928
Rossolimo, Grigoriy Ivanovich. Moscow physician. 1860–1928
Suggested term "myotonia atrophica."
De la myotonie atrophique: contribution a la théorie des myopathies. Nouv. inconog. de la Salpêtrière, 15: 63–77, 1902
Rossy, C. S. See R. M. Yerkes
Rost, Ernest Reinhold. English physician in India. 1872–
Prepared Leprolin and was successful in—
The cultivation of the Bacillus leprae. Indian med. Gaz., Calcutta, 39: 167–169, 1904
Rost, F. See K. Moeckel
Rostan, Léon Louis. French physician. 1790–1866
ASTHMA—cardiac.
Mémoire sur cette question, l'asthme des vieillards est-il une affection nerveuse? Nouv. J. de Méd., Chir. Pharm., Paris, 3: 3–30, 1817
Described softening of brain. Garrison
Recherches sur le ramollissement du cerveau; ouvrage dans lequel on s'efforce de distinguer les diverses affections de ce viscère par des signes caractéristiques. Paris, Béchet jeune, 1823. 2 ed., 503 pp.

Rotch, Thomas Morgan. Boston pediatrician. 1849–1914
SIGN—
Absence of resonance in the fifth right intercostal space diagnostic of pericardial effusion. Boston M. and S. J., 99: 421–429, Oct. 3, 1878
Introduced method of percentage feeding of fat, sugar or protein. Garrison
The artificial feeding of infants. Arch. Pediat., 4: 458–480, Aug. 1887
Roth, Emil. Berlin physician. 1850–1917
MEDIUM—culture, for typhoid bacilli.
Versuche über die Einwirkung des Coffeins auf das Bacterium typhi and coli. Hyg. Rundschau, 13: 489–491, May 15, 1903
Versuche über die Einwirkung des Trimethylxathins auf das Bacterium typhi und coli. Arch. Hyg., Berl., 49: 199–228, 1904
Roth, Moriz von. Basel pathologist. 1839–1914
SPOT—purulent and hemorrhagic foci in retina.
Über Netzhautaffectionen bei Wundfiebern. I. Die embolische Pahophthalmitis. Dtsch. Z. f. Chir., 1: 471–484 (475), 1872
Roth, Paul. American physiologist. 1871–
TECHNIC—
The value of acetone determination in expired air in correlation with alveolar carbon dioxide tension; practical methods, technic, and apparatus. J. Lab. clin. Med., 11: 275–288, Dec. 1925
Roth, Vladimir Karlovich. Russian neurologist. 1848–1916
DISEASE—
(Meralgia paraesthetica.) Med. Obozr., Mosk., 43: 678–688, 1895
Also: *Meralgia paraesthetica.* Berlin, Karger, 1895
Rothberg, W. See C. E. A. Winslow
Rothberger, Carl Julius. German bacteriologist. 1871–
AGAR—indicator; for differentiation between typhoid and colon bacilli.
Differentialdiagnostische Untersuchungen mit gefärbten Nährböden. Zbl. Bakt., 24: 513–518, Oct. 15, 1898
Rothberger, J. See H. Eppinger
Rothenberg, R. E. See W. L. Wolfson
Rothera, Arthur Cecil Hamel. Melbourne biochemish. 1880–1915
TEST—for acetone bodies in urine.
Note on the sodium nitro-prusside reaction for acetone. J. Physiol., 37: 491–494, Dec. 15, 1908
A new and delicate test for acetone. Australas. Med. Cong. Trans., Victoria, 2: 232, 1909
Rothmund, August. Munich ophthalmologist. 1830–1906
DISEASE or SYNDROME—poikiloderma strophicans.
Ueber Cataracten in Verbindung mit einer eigenthümlichen Hautdegeneration. Arch. f. Ophthal., 14: 159–182, 1868
Rothschild, Otto. Frankfurt a. M. surgeon
OPERATION—for paralysis of trapezius muscle.
Über funktionelle Heilung der Cucullarislähmung mittels freier Fascienplastik. Zbl. Chir., 37: 1441–1442, Nov. 5, 1910
Rothwell, Carmen S. New Haven chemist

METHOD—
   Direct precipitation of calcium in cows' milk. J. biol.
   Chem., 65: 129–133, Aug. 1925
Rotter, Josef. Berlin surgeon. 1857–1924
NODES—lymph n. between pectoralis major and
   minor.
   *Günstigere Dauererfolge durch ein verbessertes Opera-
   tionsverfahren der Mammacarcinome.* Berl. klin.
   Wschr., 33: 69–72, Jan. 27; 99–101, Feb. 3, 1896
OPERATION—for fracture of patella.
   *Eine neue Operationsmethode für Heilung veralteter
   Kniesscheibenbrüche.* Zbl. Chir., 35: 540–541, Apr.
   25, 1908
Rouanet, Joseph R. French physician. 1797–1865
   Advanced theory that all heart sounds are purely
   valvular.
   Analyse des bruits du coeur. Thèse de Paris, 1832.
   28 pp.
Rouelle, Hilaire Marie. French physician. 1718–
   1779
   Discovered urea.
   Observations sur l'urine humaine. J. de Med., Chir.
   Pharm., Paris, 40: 451–468, 1773
Roughton, F. J. W. See N. U. Meldrum
Rougnon de Magny, Nicolas Francois. Besançon
   physician. 1724?–1799
DISEASE—angina pectoris.
   *Lettre de M. Rougnon à M. Lory, touchant les causes
   de la mort de feu Monsieur Charles, etc.* Besançon,
   Charmet, 1768
Rouiller, C. A. See J. J. Abel
Rourke, Genevieve C. See R. M. Nesbit
Rourke, M. Dorothy. Boston scientist
METHOD—
   *A method for correcting the erythrocyte sedimentation
   rate for variations in the cell volume percentage of
   blood* with A. C. Ernstene, J. clin. Invest., 8: 545–
   559, June 20, 1930
Rous, Francis Peyton. New York physician. 1879–
METHOD—
   *A method for the permanent sterile drainage of intra-
   abdomnal ducts, as applied to the common duct* with
   P. D. McMaster, J. exp. Med., 37: 11–19, Jan. 1923
MIXTURE—blood-dextrose-citrate.
   *The preservation of living red blood cells in vitro: I.
   Methods of preservation* with J. R. Turner, Ibid., 23:
   219–239, Feb. 1916
SARCOMA—
   *A transmissible avian neoplasm (sarcoma of the com-
   mon fowl).* Ibid., 12: 696–705, Sept. 1910
   *A sarcoma of the fowl transmissible by an agent sepa-
   rable from the tumor cells.* Ibid., 13: 397–410, 1911
TEST—for hemolysis.
   A rapid simple method of testing donors for transfusion
   with J. R. Turner, J. A. M. A., 64: 1980–1982, June
   12, 1915
Roussy, G. See F. J. Darier, J. J. Déjérine
Routier, Daniel. French physician. 1887–
SIGN—third sound in diastole.
   *Étude critique sur les dissociations auriculo-ventricu-
   laires.* Paris, 1915. 72 pp.
Roux, Dr. Lausanne surgeon
OPERATION—for slipping patella.
   Luxation habituelle de la rotule: traitement opératoire.
   Rev. de Chir., 8: 682–689, 1888

SIGN—in appendicitis.
   Traitement chirurgical de la perityphilite suppurée.
   Rev. méd. de la Suisse Romande, 10: 201–239, Apr.
   20; 289–331, May 20, 1890
Roux, Jean Charles. French surgeon
OPERATION—modification of Billroth II.
   *De la gastro-entérostomie. Étude basée sur les opéra-
   tions pratiquées du 21 Juin 1888 au 1er Septembre
   1896* Rev. de gyn. et de chir. abd., Paris, 1: 67–122,
   Feb. 10, 1897
OPERATION—for stricture of esophagus.
   *L'oesophago-jéjuno-gastrostomose, nouvelle opération
   pour rétrécissement infranchissable de l'oesophage.*
   Semaine méd., 27: 37–40, Jan. 23, 1907
Roux, Gabriel. French physician. 1853–1914
AGAR—peptone; culture medium.
   Précis de microbie et de technique bactérioscopique
   with A. Rochaix, Paris, Maloine, Éditeur, 1911.
   p. 115
Roux, Philibert Joseph. Paris surgeon. 1780–1854
   Performed staphylorrhaphy.
   *Mémoire sur la staphyloraphie, ou la suture du voile du
   palais.* Arch. gén. de méd., Paris, 7: 516–538, Apr.
   1825
   Performed suture of ruptured female perineum.
   *Mémoire sur la restauration du périnée chez la femme
   dans les cas de division ou de rupture complète de cette
   partie.* Gaz. méd. de Paris, 2 s., 2: 17–22, Jan. 11,
   1834
Roux, Pierre Paul Émile. French bacteriologist.
   1853–1933
METHOD—
   Sur la culture des microbes anaérobies. Ann. Inst.
   Pasteur, 1: 49–62, Feb. 1887
SERUM—antidiphtheric.
   Contribution à l'étude de la diphthérie with A. Yersin,
   Ibid., 2: 629–661, Dec. 1888
   Contribution à l'étude de la diphthérie (serum thérapie),
   with A. L. F. J. Martin, Ibid., 8: 609–639, 1894
STAIN—for B. diphtheriae.
   Contribution à l'étude de la diphthérie with A. Yersin,
   Ibid., 4: 385–426 (387), July 1890
   See also E. I. I. Metchnikoff, E. I. E. Nocard, L.
   Pasteur
Roux, Wilhelm. German physician. 1850–1924
THEORY—pressure stimulates, while tension in-
   hibits bone production.
   In his: *Gesammelte Abhandlungen über Entwickelungs-
   mechanik der Organismen.* Leipzig, Engelmann, 1895.
   2 vols. vol. 1, p. 357
   Wrote on heredity. Garrison and Morton
   Der Kampf der Theile im Organismus. Leipzig, 1881
Rovenstine, E. A. See J. A. Stiles
Rovida, Carlo Leopoldo. Italian physician. 1844–1877
   Used term silicosis and proved presence of silica in
   lung.
   Un caso di silicosi del polmone, con analisi chimica.
   Ann. di chim. applica. med., Milano, 3 s., 53, 1871
Rovsing, Niels Thorkild. Copenhagen surgeon. 1862–
   1927
OPERATION—for gastrocoloptosis.
   *Die sog. Enteroptosis und ihre chirurgische Behand-
   lung.* Samml. klin. Vortr., n. F. 15, No· 431, 1906,
   (Chir., No. 120, pp. 515–542)
SIGN—in acute appendicitis.
   Indirektes Hervorrufen des typischen Schmerzes an

McBurney's Punkt. Zbl. Chir., 34: 1257–1259, Oct. 26, 1907

Rowbotham, Edgar Stanley. English surgeon
Introduced endotracheal inhalation method of anesthesization. Garrison and Morton
Anaesthetics in the plastic surgery of the face and jaws with I. Magill, Proc. R. Soc. Med., London, 14, Sect. Anaest.: 17–27, 1921

Rowden, L. A. English obstetrician
PUBIC SCALE PRINCIPLE—
A simple and accurate method of radiographic pelvimetry. Brit. J. Radiol., n. s., 4: 432–439, Sept. 1931

Rowe, Carter Redd. American surgeon. 1906–
APPROACH—
A posterior approach to the shoulder joint with L. B. K. Yee, J. Bone and Joint Surg., 26: 580–584, July 1944

Rowe, L. W. See O. Kamm

Rowland, Russell Sturgis. Detroit physician. 1874–1938
Described—
Xanthomatosis and the reticulo-endothelial system: correlation of an unidentified group of cases described as defects in membranous bones, exophthalmos and diabetes insipidus (Christian's syndrome). Arch. intern. Med., 42: 611–674, Nov. 1928

Rowland, V. C. See E. E. Woldman

Rowlette, A. P. See D. O. Weiner

Rowntree, Leonard George. American physician. 1883–
TEST—
An experimental and clinical study of the functional activity of the kidneys by means of phenolsulfonephthalein with J. T. Geraghty, J. Pharmacol., 1: 579–661, June 1910
The phthalein test: an experimental and clinical study of phenolsulphonephthalein in relation to renal function in health and disease with J. T. Geraghty, Arch intern. Med., 9: 284–338, Mar. 1912
Introduced—
An experimental and clinical study of the value of phenoltetrachlorphthalein as a test for hepatic function with S. H. Hurwitz and A. L. Bloomfield, Johns Hopk. Hosp. Bull., 24: 327–342, Nov. 1913
See also J. J. Abel, A. W. Adson, N. M. Keith, R. L. Levy, E. D. Osborne

Roy, Charles Smart. Scottish physiologist. 1854–1897
Introduced—
Note on a method of measuring specific gravity of the blood for clinical use. J. Physiol., 5: ix–xi, 1884
Wrote—
Remarks on failure of the heart from overstrain with J. G. Adami, Brit. med. J., 2: 1321–1326, Dec. 15, 1888

Royle, Norman Dawson. Sydney surgeon
INCISION and OPERATION—
A new operative procedure in the treatment of spastic paralysis and its experimental basis. Med. J. Australia, 1: 77–86, Jan. 26, 1924
The operations of sympathetic ramisection. Ibid., 1: 587–590, June 14, 1924
The treatment of spastic paralysis by ramisection: experimental basis and clinical results. S. G. O., 39: 701–720, Dec. 1924

Rubaschkin, Vladimir Iakovlovitch. St. Petersburg physician. 1876–1925
METHOD—
Eine neue Methode zur Herstellung von Celloidinserien. Anat. Anz., 31: 30–31, July 1, 1907

Rubin, Isador Clinton. New York gynecologist. 1883–
TEST—
The nonoperative determination of patency of fallopian tubes by means of intra-uterine inflation with oxygen and the production of an artificial pneumoperitoneum. J. A. M. A., 75: 661–666, Sept. 4, 1920
Twelve years' experience with utero-tubal insufflation; diagnostic and therapeutic. Amer. J. Obstet. and Gynec., 24: 566–573, Oct. 1932

Rubner, Max. Berlin physiologist. 1854–1932
LAW—of constant growth quotient.
Introduced term "specific dynamic action of the foodstuffs."
Die Gesetze des Energieverbrauchs bei der Ernährung. Leipzig, Deuticke, 1902
TEST—for carbon monoxid in blood.
Eine Reaction des Kohlenoxydblutes. Arch. Hyg., 10: 397–398, 1891
TEST—for glucose.
Ueber die Einwirkung von Bleiacetat auf Trauben- und Milchzucker. Z. Biologie, 20: 397–418, 1884
Discovered that metabolism is proportional to surface area of body. Garrison
Die Vertretungswerthe der hauptsächlichsten organischen Nahrungsstoffe im Thierkörper. Ibid., 19: 313–396, 1883
One of the first to investigate metabolic changes in terms of heat and energy units by means of calorimeter. Garrison
Ueber den Einfluss der Körpergrösse auf Stoff- und Kraftwechsel. Ibid., 19: 535–562, 1883
Calorimetrische Methodik. Festschr. Carl Ludwig, Marburg, Elwert, 1891. 36 pp.

Rudbeck, Olof. Swedish physician. 1630–1702
Discovered intestinal lymphatics and their connection with thoracic duct, 1651. Garrison
Nova excercitation anatomica, exhibens ductus hepaticos aquosos, et vasa glandularum serosa, nunc primum inventa, aeneisque figuris delineata. Västeras, Lauringer, 1653
Also, transl. by A. E. Nielsen in: Bull. Hist. Med., 11: 312–337, Mar. 1942

Ruddock, John Carroll. Los Angeles physician. 1891–
TECHNIC—of
Peritoneoscopy. Western J. Surg., 42: 392–405, July 1934
Peritoneoscopy. S. G. O., 65: 623–639, Nov. 1937

Rudisch, Julius. New York physician. 1847–
TEST—for uric acid in urine.
A new method for the approximate determination of uric acid in urine with L. Boroschek, J. Amer. Chem. Soc., 24: 562–569, June 1902
Volumetric determination of the purin bodies (uric acid and the purin bases) in urine with K. Kleeberg, Amer. J. med. Sci., 128: 899–909, Nov. 1904

Rudnick, D. F. See R. T. Vaughan

Rudolf, Robert Dawson. Canadian physician. 1865–1941
METHOD—
A clinical method of estimating the coagulation time of

the blood. Amer. J. med. Sci., 140: 807–815, Dec. 1910

Rudolphi, Karl Asmund. Dutch physician. 1771–1832

Wrote system of helminthology and gave name "echinococcus." Garrison and Morton

Entozoorum, sive verminum intestinalium, historia naturalis. Amstelodami, 1800–10. 2 vols.

Ruediger, Ernest Henry. Bismarck, N. D. physician. 1875–

AGAR—blood.

Exclusion of air in the cultivation of the gonococcus. J. infect. Dis., 24: 376–377, Apr. 1919

Ruediger, Gustav Ferdinand. American pathologist. 1876–1935

AGAR—inulin ascitic fluid.

A method of isolating the pneumococcus in mixed cultures, such as throat cultures. J. infect. Dis., 3: 183–186, Apr. 6, 1906

Ruelens, G. See J. J. B. V. Bordet

Ruffini, Angelo. Italian anatomist. 1864–1929

CORPUSCLES or END-ORGAN—of nerve endings in skin.

Di un nuovo organo nervoso terminale. . . . Atti d. r. Accad. d. Lincei. Cl. di sc. fis., matemat. e nat., Roma, 4 s., 7, 1893

Ruggi, Gieuseppe. Italian surgeon. 1844–1925

OPERATION—

Del metodo inguinale nelle cura radicale dell'ernia crurale. Bologna, Zanichelli, 1893. 94 pp.

Operated for relief of pelvic pain.

La simpatectomia abdominale utero-ovarica come mezzo di cura di alcune lesioni interne negli organi genitali della donna. Bologna, Zanichelli, 1899. 49 pp.

Ruhlin, C. W. See A. Steindler

Ruigh, William L(ivingston). American chemist. 1905–

Prepared vinethene.

The preparation and properties of pure divinyl ether with R. T. Major, J. Amer. Chem. Soc., 53: 2662–2671, July 1931

Rukstinat, G. J. See L. Hektoen

Rule, Anna M. See J. A. Kolmer

Rummo, Gaetano. Palermo physician. 1852–1918

DISEASE—downward displacement of heart.

Sulla cardioptosi; primo abbozzo anatomo-clinico. Arch. di med. int. Palermo, 1: 161–183, 1898

Rumpel, Theodor. Hamburg surgeon. 1862–1923

OPERATION—excision of cardia followed by esophagogastrostomy.

Die klinische Diagnose der spindelförmigen Speiseröhrenerweiterung. Münch. med. Wschr., 44: 383–386, Apr. 13; 420–421, Apr. 20, 1897

PHENOMENON, TEST or SIGN—minute hemorrhages caused by constriction of arm in scarlet fever.

Photographien von Scharlachkranken mit multiplen Hautblutungen. Abstr.: Dtsch. med. Wschr., 35: 2297 (only), Dec. 23, 1909

Runeberg, Johan Wilhelm. Helsingfors physician. 1843–1918

ANEMIA—

Zur Kenntnis der sogenannten progressiven perniciösen Anämie. Dtsch. Arch. f. klin. Med., 28: 499–520, May 25, 1881

Runge, Friedlieb Ferdinand. German chemist. 1795–1867

First prepared carbolic acid from coal-tar. Garrison and Morton

Ueber einige Produkte der Steinkohlendestillation. Ann. Phys. u. Chem., Leipzig, 31: 65–78; 513–524; 32: 308–333, 1834

Rupel, Ernest. Indianapolis urologist. 1892–

BLADDER IRRIGATOR—

A simple automatic bladder irrigator with C. G. Culbertson, J. Urol., 50: 446–448, Oct. 1943

Rupp, P. See S. H. Ayers

Ruschig, H. See K. H. Slotta

Rush, Benjamin. Philadelphia physician. 1745–1813

Wrote early American contribution to anthropology. Garrison

An enquiry into the natural history of medicine among the Indians in North-America, and a comparative view of their diseases and remedies, with those of civilized nations. Philadelphia, Crukshank, (1774). 118 pp.

Described dengue.

In his: *Medical observations and inquiries.* Philadelphia, Prichard, and Hall, 1789. 206 pp. pp. 104–121

Wrote first general treatise on psychiatry in America. *Medical inquiries and observations upon the diseases of the mind.* Philadelphia, Kimber and Richardson, 1812. 367 pp.

Rush, Leslie Vaughan. Meridian, Miss. surgeon. 1905–

OPERATION—

A reconstruction operation for diastasis recti with H. L. Rush, Surgery, 3: 200–202, Feb. 1938

Russ, S. See Helen Chambers, B. H. Wedd

Russ, V. K. See R. Doerr

Russell, A. E. See T. G. Brodie

Russell, Frederick Fuller. American pathologist. 1870–

MEDIUM—

The isolation of typhoid bacilli from urine and feces with the description of a new double sugar tube medium. J. med. Res., 25: 217–229, Sept. 1911

See also P. H. Hiss, Jr.

Russell, J. P. See H. D. Evans

Russell, Josiah Cox. English physician

TREATMENT—of cardiospasm by a bag.

Diagnosis and treatment of spasmodic stricture of the esophagus. Brit. med. J., 1: 1450–1451, June 4, 1898

Russell, James Samuel Risien. London physician. 1863–1939

Wrote—

Subacute combined degeneration of the spinal cord with F. E. Batten and J. Collier, Brain, 23: 39–110, 1900

Russell, M. See L. Loewe

Russell, R. Hamilton. Melbourne surgeon

OPERATION—

Operation for severe hypospadias. Brit. med. J., 2: 1432–1435, Nov. 17, 1900

TECHNIC—

Inguinal herniae: their varieties, modes of origin, and classification. Brit. J. Surg., 9: 502–508, Apr. 1922

Inguinal hernia and operative procedure. S. G. O., 41: 605–608, Nov. 1925

TRACTION—

Fracture of the femur: a clinical study. Brit. J. Surg., 11: 491–502, Jan. 1924

Russell, Richard. London physician. 1700?–1771

Demonstrated value of sea water in relieving goiter. *De tabe glandulari, sive de usu aquae marinae in morbis*

glandularum dissertatio. (Oxoniae), Fletcher et al., 1750. 235 pp.
Also, in English. London, Owen and Goadby, 1752. 204 pp.

Russell, William. Edinburgh physician. 1852–1940
BODIES—fuchsin b.
An address on a characteristic organism of cancer. Brit. med. J., 2: 1356–1360, Dec. 13, 1890

Russo, Mario. Italian physician. 1866–
REACTION—for urine, in typhoid fever.
La bleumetilenereazione, suo valore clinico. Riv. med., 2: 507–509, May 13, 1905
Ueber den Ersatz der Ehrlichschen Diazoreaktion durch die Methylenblaureaktion. (Brief note) Münch. med. Wschr., 52: 1990 (only), Oct. 10, 1905

Rust, Johann Nepomuk. German surgeon. 1775–1840
DISEASE—tuberculous spondylitis of cervical vertebrae.
Aufsätze und Abhandlungen aus dem Gebiete der Medizin, Chirurgie und Staatsarzneikunde. Berlin, Enslin, 1834. Vol. 1, p. 196

Rusznyák, Stephan. Szeged physician
Discovered vitamin P: ("citrin").
Vitamin P: flavonols as vitamins with A. Szent-Györgyi, Nature, London, 138: 27 (only), July 4, 1936
See also A. Szent-Györgyi

Ruth, Charles Edward. Iowa surgeon. 1861–1930
TREATMENT—of penetrating fracture of acetabulum.
Fractures of the femoral neck—anatomic treatment. Therapeutic Gaz., 23: 145–159, Mar. 15, 1907

Rutherford, Daniel. English scientist. 1749–1819
Discovered nitrogen in 1772.
De aëre fixo dicto, aut mephitico. Edinburgi, Balfour et Smellie, 1772. 25 pp.

Ruttan, Robert Fulford. Montreal physician. 1856–1930
TEST—
A new reagent for detecting occult blood with R. H. M. Hardisty, Canad. med. Ass. J., 2: 995–998, Nov. 1912

Rutty, John. Dublin physician. 1697–1775
Described relapsing fever. Garrison
A chronological history of the weather and seasons, and of the prevailing diseases in Dublin; with all their various periods, successions, and revolutions, during the space of forty years. London, Robinson and Roberts, 1770. 340 pp. p. 75

Ruysch, Fredericus. Dutch anatomist. 1638–1731
GLOMERULUS, MEMBRANE, MUSCLE, TUBE, VEIN—
Observationum anatomico-chirurgicarum centuriae. . . . Amstelodami, Boom, 1691. 138 pp.
Thesaurus anatomicus. i–x. Amstelaedami, Wolters, 1701–16
Gave excellent illustration of diverticulum of terminal ileum in 1707. (Meckel-1809). Ibid., Vol. 7, fig. 283, 1707
Discovered valves in lymphatics. Garrison
Dilucidatio valvularum in vasis lymphaticis et lacteis. Hagae-Com., Gael, 1665

Ruzicka, Leopold. Zurich chemist
Evolved process for commercial synthesis of androsterone and testosterone.
Über die Synthese des Testikelhormons (Androsteron) und Stereoisomerer desselben durch Abbau hydrierter Sterine with M. W. Goldberg, J. Meyer, H. Brügger and E. Eichenberger, Helvet. Chim. Acta, 17: 1395–1406, 1934
Sexualhormone: VIII. Darstellung von testosteron unter Anwendung gemischter Ester with A. Wettstein and H. Kägi, Ibid., 18: 1478–1482, Dec. 2, 1935

Ryan, Marjorie. See A. I. Kendall

Rydygier, Ludwig. German surgeon. 1850–
SPLENOPEXY—
Die Behandlung der Wandermilz durch Splenopexis. Wien. klin. Wschr., 8: 431–433, June 13, 1895
Also: Arch. f. klin. Chir., 50: 880–886, 1895
Performed pyloric resection.
Die erste Magenresection beim Magengeschwür. Berl. klin. Wschr., 19: 39–41, Jan. 16, 1882
Ueber Pylorusresection. Samml. klin. Vortr., Sept. 21, 1882, No. 220 (Inn. Med., No. 75, 1977–2016)

Ryerson, Edwin Warner. Chicago surgeon. 1872–
OPERATION—for stabilization of knee.
The lateral ligaments of the knee. Surg. Clin. North Amer., 17: 335–340, Apr. 1937

Ryffel, J. H. See T. Lewis

Rynd, Francis. Irish surgeon. 1801–1861
First employed hypodermic injections by a gravity device of his own invention for relief of pain. Garrison
Neuralgia: introduction of fluid to a nerve. Dublin Med. Press, 13: 167–168, Mar. 12, 1845
Description of an instrument for the subcutaneous introduction of fluids in affections of the nerves. Dublin Quart. J. Med. Sci., 32: 13 (only), Aug. 1861

Rynearson, E. H. See R. M. Wilder

S

Sabin, Albert Bruce. New York bacteriologist. 1906–
METHOD—of "blind passages."
Identification of the filtrable, transmissible neurolytic agent isolated from toxoplasma-infected tissue as a new pleuropneumonia-like microbe. Science, 88: 575–576, Dec. 16, 1938
TEST—
The "stained slide" microscopic agglutination test: application to (1) rapid typing of pneumococci; (2) determination of antibody. Proc. Soc. exp. Biol., N. Y., 26: 492–494, Mar. 1929
The microscopic agglutination test in pneumonia: its application to rapid typing and control of serum therapy. J. infect. Dis., 46: 469–484, June 1930

Proved existence of Toxoplasma in North America.
Toxoplasma and obligate intracellular parasitism with P. K. Olitsky, Science, 85: 336–338, Apr. 2, 1937

Sabin, Florence Rena. American anatomist. 1871–
METHOD—of supravital staining of leucocytes.
Studies of living human blood-cells. Johns Hopk. Hosp. Bull., 34: 277–288, Sept. 1923
Studies on the maturation of myeloblasts into myelocytes and on amitotic cell division in the peripheral blood in subacute myeloblastic leucemia with C. R. Austrian, R. S. Cunningham and C. A. Doan, J. exp. Med., 40: 845–871, Dec. 1, 1924
Wrote—
Studies on the origin of blood-vessels and of red blood-

corpuscles as seen in the living blastoderm of chicks during the second day of incubation. Carnegie Inst. Contrib. to Embryol., 9: 213–262, 1920

Sabouraud, Raymond Jacques Adrien. French dermatologist. 1864–1938
METHOD—of treating ringworm.
Sur la radiothérapie des teignes. Ann. de Dermat. et Syph., Paris, 4 s., 5: 577–587, 1904
Studied varieties of trichophyton.
Les trichophyties humaines. Paris, Thèse No. 227, 1894. 233 pp.
Cultivated acne bacillus.
La séborrhée grasse et la pelade. Ann. Inst. Pasteur, 6: 134–159, Feb. 1897

Sabrazès, Jean Emile. Bordeaux physician. 1867–
METHOD—for determination of coagulation time of blood.
Procédés pratiques pour déterminer, au lit du malade, le début de la coagulation du sang et pour faciliter, l'examen du caillot et du sérum. Folia Haemat., 1: 394–396, July 1904

Sacchi, E. See G. Vassale

Sachar, Leo Aaron. St. Louis physician. 1915–
METHOD—for measuring urinary nitrogen.
Studies on hypoalbuminemia produced by protein-deficient diets. I. Hypoalbuminemia as a quantitative measure of tissue protein depletion with A. Horvitz and R. Elman, J. exp. Med., 75: 453–459, Mar. 1, 1942

Sachs, Adolph. Omaha physician. 1885–
METHOD—
Copper and iron in human blood with V. E. Levine and A. A. Fabian, Arch. intern. Med., 55: 227–253, Feb. 1935

Sachs, B. See E. Libman

Sachs, Bernard Parney. New York neurologist. 1858–1944
DISEASE—amaurotic familial idiocy.
On arrested cerebral development, with special reference to its cortical pathology. J. nerv. ment. Dis., 14: 541–553, Sept.–Oct. 1887
A further contribution to the pathology of arrested cerebral development. Ibid., 17: 603–607, Aug. 1892

Sachs, Ernest. New York physician. 1879–
Wrote—
On the structure and functional relations of the optic thalamus. Brain, 32: 95–186, Aug. 1909

Sachs, Hans. Frankfurt a. M. physician. 1877–1945
METHOD—for preparation of alcoholic extract of antigen for Wassermann test.
Ueber den Einfluss des Cholesterins auf die Verwendbarkeit der Organextrakte zur Wassermann'schen Syphilisreaktion. Berl. klin. Wschr., 48: 2066–2067, Nov. 13, 1911
REACTION or TEST—for syphilis.
Zur Kritik des serologischen Luesnachweises mittels Ausflockung with F. Georgi, Münch. med. Wschr. 66: 440–442, Apr. 18, 1919

Sachs, Willy. Bern surgeon. 1864–1909
MODIFICATION—of Senn's plates, for suturing intestine.
Drei kleine Beiträge zur Darmchirurgie. Zbl. Chir. 17: 753–757, Oct. 4, 1890

Sackett, Guy E. Kansas City scientist
METHOD—
Modification of Bloor's method for the determination of

cholesterol in whole blood or blood serum. J. biol. Chem., 64: 203–205, May 1925

Sacquépée, E. French scientist
AGAR—egg albumin infusion.
Nouveau milieu de culture pour le méningocoque et les germes voisins with Delater, C. R. Soc. Biol., 77: 224–226, June 27, 1914

Saegesser, Max. Bern surgeon
SPLENIC POINT—pressure between sternocleido-mastoid and scalenus anticus muscles on left side is painful in rupture of spleen.
Der linksseitige Phrenicusdruckpunkt als diagnostisches Merkmal bei Milzverletzungen. Zbl. Chir., 65: 2179–2180, Sept. 24, 1938

Saemisch, Edwin Theodor. Bonn ophthalmologist. 1833–1909
OPERATION or SECTION—for cure of
ULCER—of cornea.
Das Ulcus corneae serpens und seine Therapie; eine klinische Studie. Bonn, Cohen, 1870. 45 pp.
Described vernal conjunctivitis.
Der Frühjahrskatarrh. In: Graefe und Saemisch's *Handbuch der gesammten Augenheilkunde.* Leipzig, 4, Theile 2, pp. 25–29, 1876

Sänger, Max. Prage gynecologist. 1853–1903
OPERATION—cesarean section.
Der Kaiserschnitt bei Uterusfibromen, nebst vergleichender Methodik der Sectio caesarea und der Porro-Operation. Kritiken, Studien und Vorschläge zur Verbesserung des Kaiserschnitts. Leipzig, Engelmann, 1882. 202 pp.
Described decidual sarcoma of uterus.
Ueber Sarcoma uteri deciduo-cellulare und andere deciduale Geschwülste. Arch. Gynaek., 44: 89–148, 1893

Šafŕ, Karl. Vienna ophthalmologist
METHOD—of treatment of retinal detachment.
Behandlung der Netzhautabhebung mit Elektroden für multiple diathermische Stichelung. Abstr.: Klin. Mbl. Augenheilk., 88: 814 (only), June 1932

Sahli, Hermann. Bern physician. 1856–1933
METHOD—for determination of hemoglobin.
Über ein einfaches und exactes Verfahren der klinischen Hämometrie. Verh. dtsch. Cong. inn. Med., 20: 230–234, 1902
METHOD—of estimating free acid (pH) in gastric juice.
Ueber die Bestimmung der freien Säure des Magensaftes durch "Titration der Indicatorlösung," insbesondere unter Verwendung von Methylviolett und Lackmus. Schweiz. med. Wschr., 54: 1–6, 1924
MODIFICATION—of Pavy's sugar titration.
Ueber die Verwendbarkeit der Pavyschen Zuckertitrationsmethode für die Klinik und den praktischen Artz und über einige technische Modifikationen derselben. Dtsch. med. Wschr., 31: 1417–1423, Sept. 7, 1905
REACTION or TEST—of functional activity of stomach.
Über eine neue Untersuchungsmethode der Verdauungsorgane. Cor.-Bl. f. schweiz. Aerzte, 21: 65–74, 1891
Ueber ein neues Verfahren zur Untersuchung der Magenfunctionen. Berl. klin. Wschr., 39: 349–352, Apr. 21, 1902
SOLUTION—borax methylene blue.
Ueber die Anwendung von Boraxmethylenblau für die Untersuchung des centralen Nervensystems und

für den Nachweis von Mikroorganismen, speciell zur bacteriologischen Untersuchung der nervösen Centralorgane. Z. wiss. Mikr., 2: 49–51, 1885
TEST—glutoid, for digestive function.
  Ueber Glutoidkapseln. Dtsch. med. Wschr., 23: 6–8, Jan. 1, 1897
Introduced a portable mercury manometer. Garrison
  Ueber kompendiöse, leicht transportable Taschenqueck-silbermanometer zu klinischen Zwecken, sepziell zur Sphygmomanometrie; nebst Bemerkungen über eine Verbesserung der Riva-Roccischen Manschette. Ibid., 30: 1745–1746, Nov. 24, 1904
Introduced pantopon. Garrison
  Über Pantopon, ein die Gesamtalkaloide des Opiums in leicht löslicher und auch zu subkutaner Injektion geeigneter Form anthaltendes Opiumpräparat. Therap. Mschr., 23: 1–6, Jan. 1909
Sahyun, Melville. California scientist. 1895–
METHOD—
  The determination of amino acid nitrogen in blood and urine: a rapid colorimetric method with M. Goodell, J. Lab. clin. Med., 24: 548–553, Feb. 1939
MODIFICATION—of Pflueger's method.
  Determination of glycogen in tissues. J. biol. Chem., 93: 227–234, Oct. 1931
Saillant, Charles Jacques. French physician. 1747–1804
Wrote on influenza.
  Tableau historique et raisonné des épidémies catharrales vulgairement dites la grippe; depuis 1510 jusques et y compris celle de 1780. Paris, Didot, 1780
St. John, J. H. See J. S. Simmons
Saint-Remy, G. See L. D. Baraban
St. Yves, Charles. French physician. 1667–1733
Reported removal of cataract "en masse."
  Nouveau traité des maladies des yeux. Paris, Le Mercier, 1722
Saissy, Jean Antoine. French physician. 1756–1822
Described Eustachian bougie and diseases of tympanum and Eustachian tube. Garrison and Morton
  Essai sur les maladies de l'oreille interne. Paris, Baillière, 1829
Sajous, Charles Euchariste de Médicis. American physician. 1852–1929
Wrote on endocrinology.
  The internal secretions and the principles of medicine. Philadelphia, Davis, 1903–07. 2 pts.
Sakel, Manfred. Vienna physician
TREATMENT—of schizophrenia by insulin shock.
  Schizophreniebehandlung mittels Insulin Hypoglykämie sowie hypoglykämischer Schocks. Wien. med. Wschr., 84: 1211–1214, Nov. 3, 1934, passim
  Neue Behandlung der Schizophrenie. Vienna, Perles, 1935
  A new treatment of schizophrenia. Amer. J. Psychiat. 93: 829–841, Jan. 1937
Sakurada, H. See S. I. Yoshimatsu
Sale, Llewellyn. St. Louis physician. 1881–
PHENOMENON—reflex spasticity of diaphragm in acute appendicitis.
  A study of diaphragmatic movements in acute abdominal inflammations. J. A. M. A., 71: 505–508, Aug. 17, 1918
Salgado, Marcos Jose. Mexico City physician. 1671–1740

Author of first book on physiology written and published in the New World.
  Cursus medicus mexicanus. Mexico City, Michael de Rivera, 1727. 344 pp.
Saliceto, Gulielmus de. (William of Salicet) Italian surgeon. circa 1201–1277
Described renal dropsy. Garrison and Morton
  De duritie in renibus. In: *Liber in scientia medicinali.* Cap. 140 (Placentiae, 1476)
Salimbeni. See E. G. Marchoux
von Salis, H. Wolfgang. Bern surgeon
Reported leiomyosarcoma of duodenum.
  Ueber das Sarcom des Duodenum insebesondere das Myosarkom. Dtsch. Z. f. Chir., 160: 180–204, Dec. 1920
Also, abstr.: J. A. M. A., 76: 972, Apr. 2, 1921
Salishehov, Ernst Gavrilovich. See Salistcheff
Salistcheff, Ernst Gavrilovich. Tomsk surgeon. 1851–
OPERATION—
  Exarticulatio interileo-abdominalis. Arch. klin. Chir., 60: 57–70, 1900
Salkowski, Ernest Leopold. Berlin chemist. 1844–1923
METHOD—for estimation of purin bases.
  Ueber die Bestimmung der Harnsäure und der Xanthinkörper im Harn. Zbl. med. Wiss., 32: 514–515, July 28, 1894
MODIFICATION—of Trommer test for grape-sugar in urine.
  Ueber die Verbindungen des Traubenzuckers mit Kupferoxydhydrat. Z. physiol. Chem., 3: 79–97, 1879
REACTION—for cholesterol.
  Kleinere Mittheilungen physiologisch-chemischen Inhalts II. 1. Die Reaction des Cholesterin mit Schwefelsäure, etc. Arch. d. Physiol., 6: 207–222 (207–209), 1872
REACTION—for creatinine and creatine.
  Zur Kenntniss des Kreatinins. Z. physiol. Chem., 4: 133 (only), 1880
TEST—for bile pigments.
  Demonstration von präformirtem Urobilin im Harn. Ibid., 4: 134–135, 1880
TEST—for carbon monoxide in blood.
  Eine Modification der Hoppe-Seyler'schen Natronprobe auf Kohlenoxydhämoglobin. Ibid., 12: 227–228. 1888
TEST—for glucose in urine.
  Ueber das Vorkommen von Pentosen im Harn. Ibid. 27: 507–539. 1899
TEST—for indican in urine.
  Zum Nachweis des Indikans im Harn. Ibid. 57: 519–521, 1908
TEST—for hematoporphyrin.
  Ueber Vorkommen und Nachweis des Hämatoporphyrins im Harn. Ibid. 15: 286–309, 1891
TEST—for peptone in urine.
  Ueber den Nachweis des Peptons im Harn. Zbl. med. Wiss., 32: 113–115. Feb. 17, 1894
TEST—for silicic acid in urine.
  Über den Nachweis der Kiesselsäure im Harn ohne Veraschung desselben. Z. physiol. Chem., 83: 143–169, 1913
TEST—for thiosulfate in urine.
  Ueber das Verhalten der Isäthionsäure im Organismus und den Nachweis der unterschwefligen Säure im Harn. Arch. ges. Physiol., 39: 209–222 (213), 1886

Described pentosuria. Garrison
Ueber die Pentosurie, eine neue Anomalie des Stoffwechsels. Berl. klin. Wschr., 32: 364–368, Apr. 29, 1895

Salmon, Daniel Elmer. American veterinarian. 1850–1914

SALMONELLA GROUP or paratyphoid, causing enteric fever.

HOG CHOLERA of—

SWINE PLAGUE of—

The bacterium of swine-plague. Am. Month. Microscop. J., 7: 204–205, Nov. 1886

Report on inoculation as a preventive of swine diseases. U. S. Dept. Agric., Bur. Animal Indust., Spec. Bull. 1890. 10 pp.

Performed first experiment in immunization, when he demonstrated that immunity from hog cholera can be secured by injection of filtered products of the specific organisms. Garrison

On a new method of producing immunity from contagious diseases with Theobald Smith, Proc. Biol. Soc., Washington, 3: 29–33, 1886

Salmon, Udall Jules. New York gynecologist. 1904–

SIGN—

A pupillary sign in ruptured ectopic pregnancy. Amer. J. Obstet. Gynaec., 28: 241–243, Aug. 1934

TECHNIC—of implantation of estrogen.

Prolonged therapeutic effect of subcutaneously implanted crystals of ovarian hormone in women with R. I. Walter and S. H. Geist, Science, 90: 162–163, Aug. 18, 1939

TEST—

A six-hour pregnancy test with S. H. Geist, A. A. Salmon and I. L. Frank, J. clin. Endocrinol., 2: 167–170, Mar. 1942

Salomon, Hugo. Vienna physician. 1872–

REACTION—for cancer.

Ueber einen Harnbefund bei Carcinomatösen; . . . Berlin, 1910. 36 pp.

Eine Schwefelreaktion in Harne Krebskranker with P. Saxl, Wien. klin. Wschr., 24: 449–451, Mar. 30 1911

See also P. Karrer

Salter, Henry Hyde. English physician. 1823–1871

Described asthma due to hypersensitiveness.

On asthma: its pathology and treatment. London, Churchill, 1860. 372 pp. pp. 340–341

Salter, Sir Samuel James Augustus. English dentist. 1825–1897

LINE—incremental 1. of dentin.

Dental pathology and surgery. London, Longmans, Green, 1874. 399 pp.

Salter, W. T. See F. H. Scharles

Salvin, Arthur A. New York surgeon. 1881–

OPERATION—

Surgical treatment of rectal prolapse: a new operation for its relief. Ann. Surg., 101: 1051–1061, Apr. 1935

Salzer, Fritz Adolf. Utrecht surgeon. 1858–

OPERATION—

Ein Vorschlag zur Radikalheilung grosser Cruralhernien. Zbl. Chir., 19: 665–669, Aug. 20, 1892

Salzmann, Maximilian. German ophthalmologist. 1862–

DEGENERATION—nodular, of cornea.

Ueber eine eigentümliche Form von Hornhautentzündung. Mitt. Verein. Aerzte Steiermark, 53: 194–198, 1916

Ueber eine Abart der knötchenförmigen Hornhautdystrophie. Z. Augenheilk., 57: 92–99, 1925

Sampson, John Albertson. Albany gynecologist. 1873–1946

IMPLANTATION THEORY—

Perforating hemorrhagic (chocolate) cysts of the ovary; their importance and especially their relation to pelvic adenomas of endometrial type ("adenomyoma" of the uterus, rectovaginal septum, sigmoid, etc.) Arch. Surg. 3: 245–323, Sept. 1921

The life history of ovarian hematomas (hemorrhagic cysts) of endometrial (Müllerian) type. Amer. J. Obstet. Gynaec., 4: 451–512, Nov. 1922

TECHNIC—for salpingectomy to preserve circulation of ovary.

The variations in the blood supply of the ovary and their possible operative importance. S. G. O., 24: 339–350, Mar. 1917

Described sheath investing ureter as it passes through broad ligament. H. A. Kelly

The efficiency of the periureteral arterial plexus, and the importance of its preservation in the more radical operations for carcinoma cervicis uteri. Johns Hopk. Hosp. Bull., 15: 39–46, Feb. 1904

Samuels, Saul Simon. New York surgeon. 1895–

OSCILLOMETER—

The value of oscillometry in the study of the circulatory disturbances of the extremities. J. A. M. A., 88: 1780–1782, June 4, 1927

Thrombo-angiitis obliterans (Buerger). III. Prognostic value of the oscillometer. By Samuel Silbert with S. S. Samuels, Ibid., 90: 831–832, Mar. 17, 1928

SIGN—plantar ischemia.

The early diagnosis of thrombo-angiitis obliterans: a new diagnostic sign. Ibid., 92: 1571–1572, May 11 1929

Sanarelli, Giuseppe. Rome physician. 1864–1940

BACILLUS—B. icteroides; found and isolated first bacteria of paratyphoid group. Garrison

Études sur la fièvre typhoide expérimentale. Ann. Inst. Pasteur, 8: 193–230, Apr. 1894

SERUM—

Étiologie et pathogénie de la fièvre jaune. Ibid., 11: 433–June 1897

Sanchez, Juan A. Buenos Aires chemist

REACTIONS—for cystine.

Estudio químico functional de dos nuevas reacciones de la cistina. Semana med., Buenos Aires, 37: 31–32, July 3, 1930

TEST—for choline.

Acerca de una nueva reacción de la colina y de la lecitina. Ibid., 1416 (only), June 5, 1930

TEST—for creatinine.

Nuevas reacciones de la creatina y de la creatinina. Ibid., 616–617, Aug. 28, 1930

Sanctorius, Santorius. Padua professor. 1561–1636

Founded physiology of metabolism. Garrison

Ars de statica medicina, aphorismorum sectionibus septem comprehensa. . . . Leipzig, Shürer et Götze, (1614)

Described a clinical thermometer and a pulsilogium or pulse-clock, of his own devising, in 1625. Garrison

Commentaria in primam fen primi libri canonis Avicennae. Venetiis, 1626

Sand, Knud. Danish physician. 1887–

TEST—for carbon monoxide in blood.

Metode til Paavisning af Kulilte i Bloder. Ugeskr. Laeg., 76: 1721, 1914
Also, abstr. in English in: J. A. M. A., 63: 1890, Nov. 21, 1914

Sander, E. Stuttgart ophthalmologist
PUPILLOSCOPE—
Ueber quantitative Messung der Pupillenreaktion und einen in der Praxis hiefür geeigneten einfachen Apparat. Klin. Mbl. Augenheilk., 83: 318–322, Aug.-Sept. 1929

Sander, Wilhelm. Dalldorf psychiatrist. 1838–1922
DISEASE—a form of paranoia.
Über eine spezielle Form der primären Verrücktheit. Arch. Psych., 1: 387–419, 1868

Sanders, A. G. See E. Chain

Sanders, Clarence Elmer. Kansas City, Kan. physician. 1885–
OSCILLATING BED—
Cardiovascular and peripheral vascular disease: treatment by a motorized oscillating bed. J. A. M. A., 106: 916–918, Mar. 14, 1936

Sanders, M. See H. S. Simms

Sanders, Robert Lee. Memphis, Tenn. surgeon. 1882–
INCISION—
Transverse incision in the upper abdomen: its anatomic and physiologic advantages. Ann. Surg., 104: 74–86, July 1936

Burdon-Sanderson, Sir John Scott. See Burdon-Sanderson

Sandiford, Irene. See W. M. Boothby

Sandifort, Eduard. Dutch physician. 1742–1814
Wrote on pathological anatomy. "His work is almost equal with that of Morgagni." Garrison and Morton
Observationes anatomicae-pathologicae. Lugduni Batavorum, Eyk & Vygh, 1777–81. 4 vols.

Sandström, Ivar Victor. Norwegian physician. 1852–1889
BODIES—parathyroids.
Om en ny Körtel hos menniskan och otskilliga däggdjur. Upsala Läkareförenings Förhandlingar, 15: 441–471, 1880
Also, English transl. by C. M. Seipel in: Bull. Inst. Hist. Med., 6: 192–222, Mar. 1938

Sanford, Arthur Hawley. Rochester, Minn. pathologist. 1882–
METHOD—
The determination of hemoglobin with the photoelectrometer with C. Sheard, J. Lab. clin. Med., 15: 483–489, Feb. 1930
The photoelometer and its use in the clinical laboratory with C. Sheard and A. E. Osterberg, Amer. J. clin. Path., 3: 405–420, Nov. 1933
MODIFICATION—of Haden hematocrit.
A new centrifuge tube for volume index determinations (modified Haden method) with T. B. Magath, J. Lab. clin. Med., 15: 172–173, 1929
See also H. Z. Giffin

Sanger, Margaret Higgins. American nurse. 1883–
Early worker for birth-control.
The case for birth control. New York, Modern Art Print, 1917. 251 pp.

Sano, Machteld E. Philadelphia pathologist
METHOD—
Skin grafting: a new method based on the principles of tissue culture. Amer. J. Surg., 61: 105–106, July 1943
A coagulum contact method of skin grafting as applied to human grafts. S. G. O., 77: 510–513, Nov. 1943

Sansum, William David. Chicago physician. 1880–
TEST—for determination of urinary glucose tolerance.
Studies on the theory of diabetes. VII. The intravenous tolerance limit for dl-glyceric aldehyde and the improbability that it is a chief intermediate in glucose catabolism with R. T. Woodyatt, J. biol. Chem., 24: 343–346, Mar. 1916
See also R. M. Wilder

Sante, Leroy. St. Louis radiologist. 1890–
Described pneumonic process in tularemia.
Pulmonary infection in tularemia: case report. Amer. J. Roentgenol., 25: 241–242, Feb. 1931

Santorini, Giovanni Domenico. Italian anatomist. 1681–1737
DUCT—of lesser pancreas.
Observationes anatomicae. Venetiis, Recurti, 1724. 250 pp.
Also: Lugduni Batavorum, Langerak, 1739. 246 pp.
Anatomici summi septemdecim tabulae. Parma, 1775. p. 150, tabulae XII and XIII

Santorio. See Sanctorius

Santos, Reynaldo dos. Spanish physician. 1880–
First used thorotrast in arteriography. Garrison and Morton
Les derives du thorium dans l'artériographie des membres with J. Caldas, Med. Contemp., Lisboa, 26: 234–236, 1931

Sapiejko, K. Kiew surgeon
OPERATION—for umbilical hernia.
Un nouveau procédé de cure radicale des grands hernies ombilicales avec diastase des muscles grands droits. Rev. Chir., 21: 241–261, Feb. 1900

Sappey, Marie Philibert Constant. French anatomist. 1810–1896
ACCESSORY PORTAL SYSTEM or VEINS—
Mémoire sur un point d'anatomie pathologique relatif à l'histoire de la cirrhose. Mém. Acad. de Méd., 23: 269–278, 1859

Sappington, S. W. See J. G. Wurtz

Sarbo, Arthur von. Hungarian neuropathologist. 1867–
SIGN—analgesia of peroneal nerve, in locomotor ataxia.
Der Achillessehnenreflex und seine klinische Bedeutung. Beitrag zur Frühdiagnose der Tabes und der progressiven Paralyse. Berlin, Karger, 1903. 44 pp.

Sargent, A. F. See W. R. MacAusland

Sargent, James Clyde. Milwaukee urologist. 1892–
OPERATION—for hydronephrosis.
Basic principles governing conservative surgery in hydronephrosis. J. Urol., 47: 323–343, Mar. 1942

Sargent, Sir Percy William George. See G. M. Holmes

Sargnon. See M. Vernet

Sartory, Auguste. French scientist
Discovered S. Lemonniere, a pathogenic fungus in bronchitis.
Contribution à l'étude d'un Oospora pathogéne nouveau, Oospora bronchialis n. sp. C. R. Acad. Sci., Paris 159: 758–759, Nov. 30, 1914

Sass, Louis. American laryngologist
APPARATUS—spray for throat.
Illustrated in F. H. Bosworth: *A treatise on diseases of the nose and throat.* New York, Wood, 1889. Vol. 1, p. 12; 36–39

Sato, Akira. Japanese physician. 1871–

METHOD or TECHNIC—

The peroxidase reaction in epidemic encephalitis: a new diagnostic and prognostic method with Sh. Yoshimatsu, Amer. J. Dis. Child., 29: 301–312, Mar. 1925

A simple method for differentiation of myeloic and lymphatic leucocytes of the human blood: a new peroxidase reaction (copper method) with S. Sekiya, Tohoku J. exp. Med., 7: 111–115, Apr. 30 1926

Counting chamber peroxidase method for blood: simultaneous rapid differential leucocyte count and total leucocyte count with K. Shoji, J. Lab. clin. Med., 13: 1058–1060, Aug. 1927

Saucerotte, Nicolas. French surgeon. 1741–1812

Described acromegaly.

Accroissement singulier en grosseur des os d'un homme âgé de 39 ans. In his: *Mélanges de chirurgie.* Paris, 1801. Vol. 1, pp. 407–411

Sauer, Louis Wendlin. Evanston, Ill. physician 1885–

AGAR—potato blood, for H. pertussis.

Whooping cough: early diagnosis by the cough plate method with Leonora Hambrecht, J. A. M. A., 95: 263–264, July 26, 1930

VACCINE—

Whooping cough: a study in immunization. Ibid., 100: 239–241, Jan. 28, 1933

Immunization with Bacillus pertussis vaccine. Ibid., 101: 1449–1453, Nov. 4, 1933

Sauerbruch, Ernst Ferdinand. Greifswald surgeon. 1875–

DIET—salt restricted, in treatment of tuberculosis.

Ueber Versuche, schwere Formen der Tuberkulose durch diätetische Behandlung zu beeinflussung with A. Herrmannsdorfer and M. Gerson, Münch. med. Wschr., 73: 47–51, Jan. 8, 1926

GLOVE PROSTHESIS—

Die willkürlich bewegbare künstliche Hand. Berlin, Springer, 1923. vol. 2

OPERATION—for carcinoma of esophagus.

Die Chirurgie des Brustteils der Speiseröhre. Beitr. klin. Chir., 46: 405–494, 1905

OPERATION—paravertebral thoracoplasty for chronic pulmonary tuberculosis.

Technik der Thoraxchirurgie with E. D. Schumacher, Berlin, Springer, 1911. 97 pp. p. 44

Also: *Thoracic surgery* with L. O'Shaughnessey, Baltimore, Williams & Wilkins, 1938. 336 pp.

Invented pneumatic chamber at reduced atmospheric (negative) pressure for prevention of pneumothorax. Garrison

Über die Ausschaltung der schädlichen Wirkung des Pneumothorax bei intrathorakalen Operationen. Zbl. Chir., 31: 146–149, Feb. 13, 1904

Über die physiologischen und physikalischen Grundlagen bei intrathorakalen Eingriffen in meiner pneumatischen Operationskammer. Verh. dtsch. Ges. f. Chir., 23, pr. 2: 105–115, 1904

Advocated phrenicotomy in treatment of pulmonary tuberculosis.

Die Beeinflussung von Lungenerkrankungen durch künstliche Lähmung des Zwerchfells (Phrenikotomie). Münch. med. Wschr., 60: 625–626, Mar. 25, 1913

First successfully intervened in cardiac aneurysm. Garrison and Morton

Erfolgreich operative Beseitigung eines Aneurysma der rechten Herzkammer. Arch. f. klin. Chir., 167: 586–588, 1931

Saul, J. E. London scientist

TEST—

Note on the detection of raw milk and formaldehyde. Brit. med. J., 1: 664 (only), Mar. 21, 1903

de Sauvagos de la Croix, François Boissier. 1706–1767

Classified 2400 diseases by botanical system of Linnaeus. Garrison and Morton

Nosolgia methodica, sistens morborum classes, genera et species. Amstelodami, Tournes, 1763. 5 vols.

Sauvineau, Charles. French ophthalmologist. 1862–

OPHTHALMOPLEGIA—

Un nouveau type de paralysie associée des mouvements horizontaux des yeux. Ann. d'Ocul., 113: 363–364, May 1895

Savage, William George. English bacteriologist. 1872–

BOUILLON—for detection of B. coli.

Neutral-red in the routine bacteriological examination of water. J. Hyg., Camb., 1: 437–450 (437), Oct. 1901

Proved that paratyphoid C organism is truly Salmonella suipestifer.

An investigation of the Salmonella group, with special reference to food poisoning with P. B. White, Med. Research Council, Special series report, No. 91, London, His Majesty's Station. Off., 1925. 59 pp.

Savariaud, Maurice. Paris surgeon. 1870–

OPERATION—

Un cas de désarticulation inter-ilio-abdominale: procédé a lambeau interne. Rev. de Chir., 26: 345–366, 1902

Savill, Thomas Dixon. London dermatologist. 1856–1910

DISEASE—dermatitis exfoliativa epidemica.

On an epidemic skin disease. Brit. med. J., 2: 1197–1202, Dec. 5, 1891

On an epidemic skin disease, resembling eczema and pityriasis rubra. . . London, Lewis, 1892. 64 pp.

Savini, Emil. Paris physician

BOUILLON—bacteria blood.

Zur Züchtung des Influenzabicillus with Therese Savini-Castano, Zbl. Bakt., 60: 493–497 (494), Oct. 21, 1911

See also F. de Gasperi

Sawin, Luther R. New York scientist

BROTH—glycocholate extract.

Pancreatin-bile salt medium for the detection of B. coli in water. Amer. J. Pub. Hyg., n. s., 6: 672–681, Aug. 1910

Sawyer, William Alfred. New York physician. 1884–

TEST—

The use of mice in tests of immunity against yellow fever with W. Lloyd, J. exp. Med., 54: 533–555, Oct. 1931

Vaccination against yellow fever with immune serum and virus fixed for mice with S. F. Kitchen and W. Lloyd, Ibid., 55: 945–969, June 1, 1932

Saxe, George Alexander De Santos. New York physician. 1876–1911

METHOD—

On determining the specific gravity of small volumes of urine: with a preliminary note on a special hydrometer (urino-pyknometer) designed to work with a few cubic centimeters of fluid. New York med. J., 78: 739–744, Oct. 17, 1903

Saxl, Paul. German physician. 1880–1932

TREATMENT—
Ueber die Behandlung von Typhus mit Milchinjektionen. Wien. klin. Wschr., 29: 1043–1045, Aug. 17, 1916
Injected mercurial compound (Novasurol), a powerful diuretic, for treatment of cardiac failure.
(No title) Abstr. in: Ibid., 33: 179–180, Feb. 19 1920
See also H. Salomon

Saxon, Gordon Joel. Philadelphia physician. 1879–
METHOD—
A method for the determination of the total fats of undried feces and other moist masses. J. biol. Chem., 17: 99–102, Mar. 1914

Sayers, Royd Ray. Washington, D. C. surgeon. 1885–
TEST—
The pyrotannic acid method for the quantitative determination of carbon monoxide in blood and air with W. P. Yant and G. W. Jones, Public Health Rep. 38: 2311–2320, Oct. 5, 1923
See also W. P. Yant

Saylor, H. L. See W. H. Robey

Sayre, Lewis Albert. American surgeon. 1820–1900
APPARATUS, JACKET, OPERATION—
Treatment of fractured ribs by extension and expansion of the thorax, and retention by plaster-of-Paris bandage. Trans. Amer. Med. Ass., Philadelphia, 28: 541–549, 1877
Spinal disease and spinal curvature, their treatment by suspension and the use of the plaster of Paris bandage. Philadelphia, Lippincott; London, Smith, Elder, 1877. 121 pp.
DRESSING—
A simple dressing for fracture of the clavicle. Amer. Practitioner, 4: 1–8, July 1871
RESECTION—
Exsection of the head of the femur and removal of the upper rim of the acetabulum, for morbus coxarius with perfect recovery. New York J. Med., s 2, 14: 70–82, Jan. 1855

Sazerac, R. French physician
TREATMENT—
Traitement de la syphilis par le bismuth with C. Levaditi, C. R. Acad. Sci., 173: 338–340, Aug. 1, 1921

Sborov, V. See S. Schwartz, C. J. Watson

Scannell, John Matthew. Brooklyn surgeon. 1881–
METHOD—
Blood transfusion simplified; blood grouping, blood matching and blood transfusion. Brocton, Mass., Hylen and Farnsworth, 1930. 50 pp.

Scanzoni, Friedrich Wilhelm von Lichtenfels. German obstetrician. 1821–1891
MANEUVER or OPERATION—
Die Geburtshilflichen Operationen. In his: *Lehrbuch der Geburtshilfe.* Wien, Seidel, 1849–50. 2 vols. in 1

Scarpa, Antonius. Italian anatomist and surgeon. 1747–1832
CANAL, FLUID, FORAMEN, GANGLION, HIATUS, LIQUOR, MEMBRANE, NERVE—
De structura fenestrae rotundae auris, et de tympano secundario anatomicae observationes. Mutinae, apud Soc. typog., 1772. 141 pp.
Anatomicae disquisitiones de auditu et olfactu. Ticini, Galeatii, 1789. 101 pp.
De penitiori ossium structura. Lipsiae, Hartknoch, 1799

FASCIA, SHEATH, TRIANGLE—
Sull'ernia. Memoire anatomico-chirurgiche. Milano, d. reale Stamperia, 1809
Same, in English. Edinburgh, Bryce, 1814. 548 pp.
Sull'ernia del perineo. Pavia, Bizzoni, 1821. 32 pp.
OPERATION—tying of femoral artery in Scarpa's triangle.
Memoria sulla legatura delle principali arterie degli arti. Pavia, Bizzoni, 1817
STAPHYLOMA—posterior.
"Father of Italian Ophthalmology." Garrison and Morton
Saggio di osservazioni e d'esperienze sulle principali malattie degli occhi. Pavia, Comino, 1801. 278 pp.
Gave first proper delineation of nerves of heart. Garrison
Tabulae neurologicae, ad illustrandam historiam cardiacorum nervorum. . . . Ticini, Comini, 1794. 44 pp.
Described congenital club foot.
Memoria chirurgica sui piedi torti congenita dei fanciulli. Pavia, Comini, 1803
Showed disease of media to be forerunner of aneurism.
Sull'aneurisma; riflessioni ed osservazioni anatomico-chirurgiche. Pavia, Bolzani, 1804. 114 pp.

Schaaffhausen, D. Bonn scientist. 1816–1893
Described Neanderthal skull.
Zur Kenntniss der ältesten Rassenschädel. Arch. Anat., Physiol. u. wiss. Med., Berlin, pp. 453–478 1858

Schaber, H. See J. S. Thannhauser

Schachmann, M. See V. C. Hanot

Schachowa, Seraphina. Russian histologist in Bern
TUBES—spiral, of uriniferous tubules.
Untersuchungen über die Nieren. Bern, Thesis, Stämpfli, 1876. 36 pp.

Schaefer, Arthur. Rathenow surgeon. 1886–
METHOD—of blood transfusion, by rectal drip.
Intravenöse, intramuskuläre und rektale Infusion körpereigenen Blutes nach schweren Blutungen. Münch. med. Wschr., 65: 908–909, Aug. 13, 1918

Schäfer, Sir Edward Albert Sharpey. Edinburgh physiologist. 1850–1935
METHOD—
Description of a simple and efficient method of performing artificial respiration in the human subject, especially in cases of drowning, to which is appended instructions for the treatment of the apparently drowned. Med.-chir. Trans., 87: 609–623, 1904
Artificial respiration in its physiologic aspects. J. A. M. A., 51: 801–803, Sept. 5, 1908
See also G. Oliver

Schaeffer, G. See P. F. Armand-Delille

Schaeffer, Max. Bremen surgeon
OPERATION—puncture of floor of sinus.
Zur Diagnose und Therapie der Erkrankungen der Nabenhöhlen der Nase, mit Ausnahme des Sinus maxillaris. Dtsch. med. Wschr., 16: 905–907, Oct. 9, 1890

Schällibaum, Huldreich. Strassburg scientist
SOLUTION—for attaching paraffin sections to slides.
Ueber ein Verfahren mikroskopische Schnitte auf dem Objektträger zu fixiren und daselbst zu färben. Arch. mikr. Anat., 22: 689–690, 1883

Schafer, P. W. See L. R. Dragstedt, H. P. Jenkins

Schaffer, Josef. Gras histologist

METHOD—for staining bone.
Die Färberei zum Studium der Knochenentwicklung.
Z. wiss. Mikr., 5: 1–19, 1888
Schaibéle. See M. Pellissier
Schamberg, Jay Frank. Philadelphia dermatologist. 1870–1934
DISEASE—
A peculiar progressive pigmentary disease of the skin.
Brit. J. Dermat., 13: 1–5, Jan. 1901
An epidemic of a peculiar and unfamiliar disease of the skin. Philadelphia med. J., 8: 5–6, July 6, 1901
Schanz, Alfred. Dresden surgeon. 1868–1931
DISEASE—traumatic tendinitis of Achilles tendon.
Eine typische Erkrankung der Achillessehne. Zbl. Chir., 32: 1289–1291, Dec. 2, 1905
OSTEOTOMY—in nonunion of fracture of neck of femur.
Zur Behandlung der Schenkelhalsbrüche. Arch. f. klin. Chir., 83: 336–339, 1907
Ueber die nach Schenkelhalsbrüchen zurückbleibenden Gehstörungen. Dtsch. med. Wschr., 51: 730–732, May 1, 1925
SYNDROME—
Die statischen Belastungsdeformitäten der Wirbelsäule mit besonderer Berücksichtigung der kindlichen Skoliose. Stuttgart, Enke, 1904. 210 pp.
Eine typische Erkrankung der Wirbelsäule (Insufficientia vertebrae). Berl. klin. Wschr., 44: 986–992, Aug. 5, 1907
Schaper, Alfred. Boston histologist. 1863–1905
Wrote—
Die frühesten Differenzirungsvorgänge im Centralnervensystem: Kritische Studie und Versuch einer Geschichte der Entwickelung nervöser Substanz. Arch. EntwMech. Org., Leipzig, 5: 81–132, May 25, 1897
Schardinger, Franz. Vienna scientist
TEST—for boiled and unboiled milk.
Ueber das Verhalten der Kuhmilch gegen Methylenblau und seine Verwendung zur Unterscheidung von ungekochter und gekochter Milch. Z. Untersuch. Nahr.- u. Genussm., 5: 1113–1121, Nov. 15, 1902
Scharles, Frederick Herman. American physician. 1904–
METHOD—glycogenic, to determine amylase activity.
Tumor amylase: general properties and estimation of activity with W. T. Salter, Amer. J. Cancer, 20: 613–624, Mar. 1934
Scharpff, W. See H. Weese
Schatz, A. See S. A. Waksman
Schatzki, Richard. Boston roentgenologist. 1901–
METHOD—
Small intestine enema. Amer. J. Roentgenol., 50: 743–751, Dec. 1943
Schaudinn, Fritz Richard. German scientist. 1871–1906
BACILLUS—Spirocheta pallida. On May 17, 1905, read paper before Berlin Medical Society announcing discovery of Spirocheta pallida as cause of syphilis.
Vorläufiger Bericht über das Vorkommen von Spirochaeten in syphilotischen Krankheitsprodukten und bei Papillomen with E. Hoffmann, Arb. a. d. k Gesundh., 22: 527–534, 1905
Zur Kenntnis den Spirochaete pallida. Dtsch. med. Wschr., 31: 1665–1667, Oct. 19, 1905
Essays on the occurrence of spirochaetes in syphilis. Transl. by T. G. Brodie, Hamburg, Voss, 1911

FLUID—
Untersuchungen über den Generationswechsel bei Coccidien. Zool. Jahrb., Abt. f. Anat., 13: 197–292, Jan. 22, 1900
Differentiated between harmless Entamoeba coli and pathogenic Entamoeba histolytica. Garrison
Untersuchungen über die Fortpflanzung einiger Rhizopoden. Arb. a. d. k. Gesundh., 19: 547–576, 1903
Schaumann, Jörgen. Stockholm dermatologist. 1879–
DISEASE—granuloma benignum of Besnier-Boeck-Schaumann.
Étude sur le lupus pernio et ses rapports avec les sarcoides et la tuberculose. Ann. de Dermat. et de Syphil., 5 s., 6: 357–373, 1917
Sarcoides sous-cutanées. Acta derm. vener., Stockholm, 3: 431, 1922
Schechter, Milton S. American scientist
METHOD—
Colorimetric tests for DDT and related compounds with H. L. Haller, J. Amer. Chem. Soc., 66: 2129–2130, Dec. 1944
Schede, Max. Bonn surgeon. 1844–1902
CLOT, OPERATION, TREATMENT—removal of necrotic bone and permitting cavity to fill with blood.
Ueber die Heilung von Wunden unter dem feuchten Blutschorf. Arch. f. klin. Chir., 34: 245–266, 1886
OPERATION—
Die Behandlung der Empyeme. Verh. d. Cong. f. inn. Med., 9: 41–100, 1890
OPERATION—for varicose veins.
Ueber die operative Behandlung der Unterschenkelvaricen. Berl. klin. Wschr., 14: 85–89, Feb. 12, 1877
Schedel, H. E. See L. T. Biett
Scheele, Carl William. Swedish chemist. 1742–1786
First to isolate uric acid from urine. Garrison and Morton
Undersökning om blasestenen. K. Schwed. Akad. d. Wissensch., Abhandl., Leipzig, 38, 1776
Scheerer, Richard. Tübingen ophthalmologist. 1887–
ENTOSCOPE—
Die entoptische Sichtbarkeit der Blutbewegung im Auge und ihre klinische Bedeutung. Klin. Mbl. Augenheilk., 73: 67–107, July-Aug. 1924
Scheffler, Wilhelm. Jena scientist
MEDIUM—for typhoid bacilli.
Das Neutralrot als Hilfsmittel zur Diagnose des Bacterium coli. Zbl. Bakt., 28: 199–205, Aug. 22, 1900
Scheiner, Christophorus. Jesuit astronomer and physicist in Vienna. 1575–1650
EXPERIMENT or TEST—to illustrate accommodation and refraction.
Oculus, hoc est; fundamentum opticum, in quo ex accurata oculi anatome. . . . Oeniponti, Agricolam, 1619. 254 pp.
Schemm, Ferdinand Ripley. Montana physician. 1899–
TREATMENT—of cardiac edema.
A high fluid intake in the management of edema, especially cardiac edema: I. The details and basis of the régime. Ann. intern. Med., 17: 952–969, Dec. 1942
Schenck, Benjamin Robinson. American pathologist. 1873–1920
DISEASE—sporotrichosis; discovered parasite of —.

On refractory subcutaneous abscesses caused by a fungus possibly related to the sporotricha. Johns Hopk. Hosp. Bull., 9: 286–290, Dec. 1898

Schenck, Johann von Grafenberg. 1530–1598
Wrote a pathology, "the easiest source-book for the pathological observations of Sylvius, Vesalius and Columbus. Garrison and Morton
Observationum medicarum, rararum. Francofurti, sumpt. J. Rhodii, 1600. 2 vols.

Scherer
The account of his experiences with cod-liver oil led to its general use on the Continent of Europe. Garrison and Morton
Erfahrungen über die grossen Heilkräfte des Leberthrans gegen chronische Rheumatismen und besonders gegen das Hüft- und Lenden-Weh. J. d. pract. Heilk., Berlin, 55, 6 St.: 31–58, 1822; 62, 3 St.: 3 -40, 1826

Schereschewsky, Jacob. Moscow bacteriologist 1884–
SERUM—gelatinized horse s.
Züchtung der Spirochaete pallida (Schaudinn). Dtsch med. Wschr., 35: 835 (only), May 13, 1909
STAIN—
Das Verhalten der Spirochaete pallida (Schaudinn) bei der Giemsafärbung. Zbl. Bakt., 45: 91–94, 1908

Scheuermann, Holger Werfel. Copenhagen orthopedist. 1877–
DISEASE—vertebral epiphysitis.
Kyphosis dorsalis juvenilis. Ugeskrift for Laeger, 82: 385–393, 1920
Also, abstr. in German in: Z. f. orthrop. Chir., 41: 305–317, 1921
Also, abstr. in English in: Acta chir. scand., 54: 29, 1922

Schiassi, Benedetto. Italian surgeon
OPERATION—omental anastomosis.
La deviazione chirurgica del sangue portale. Bologna, 1901. 18 pp.
Le développement chirurgical d'une double circulation complémentaire dans le traitement de quelques maladies hépato-spléniques. Semaine méd., 23: 169–172, May 27, 1903
OPERATION—for varicose veins.
La cure des varices du membre inférieur par l'injection intravenieuse d'une solution d'iode. Ibid., 28: 601–602, Dec. 16, 1908

Schick, Béla. American pediatrician. 1877–
REACTION or TEST—
Kutanreaktion bei Impfung mit Diphtherietoxin. Münch. med. Wschr., 55: 504–506, Mar. 10, 1908
Die Diphtherietoxin-Hautreaktion des Menschen als Vorprobe der prophylaktischen Diphtherieheilserum-injection. Ibid., 60: 2608–2610, Nov. 25, 1913
See also C. P. Pirquet

Schieck, Franz. Göttingen ophthalmologist
PERITHELIOMATA OF—of optic nerve.
Das Peritheliom der Netzhautzentralgefässe, ein bislang unbekanntes Krankheitsbild. Arch. f. Ophthal., 81: 328–339, Mar. 26, 1912

Schiess. Alexandria physician
SERUM—
Ueber die Resultate von 48 mit Tuberkulin behandelten Tuberkulösen with Kartulis, Z. Hyg. InfektKr., 15: 229–282, 1893

Schiff, A. See E. Nirenstein

Schiff, Ugo. German chemist. 1834–1915

REACTION—for urea.
Eine Harnstoffreaction. Ber. d. dtsch. chem. Ges., 10: 773–776, Apr. 23, 1877
REACTION—for uric acid.
Zur Nachweisung der Harnsäure. Ann. d. Chem., 109: 65–71 (67), 1859

Schiff, J. Moritz. German physiologist. 1823–1896
Studied effect of section of vagus on respiration.
Die Ursache der Lungenveränderung nach Durchschneidung der pneumogastrischen Nerven. Arch. f. physiol. Heilk., Stuttgart, 6: 690–721; 769–804, 1847
Ueber den Einfluss der Vagusdurchschneidung auf das Lungengewebe. Ibid., 9: 625–662, 1850
Worked on experimental diabetes.
Bericht über einige Versuche, um den Ursprung des Harnzuckers bei künstlichem Diabetes zu ermitteln. Nachr. v. d. Georg-Aug. Univ. u. d. k. Ges. d. Wiss. z. Göttingen, 243–247, 1856
Made mouth-making experiments on thyroid gland and replacement therapy. Garrison
Résumé d'une nouvelle série d'expériences sur les effets de l'ablation des corps thyroides. Rev. méd. de la Suisse romande, 4: 65–75, Feb. 15; 436–445, Aug. 15, 1884

Schiff, L. See R. S. Morris

Schild, H. See J. H. Gaddum

Schilder, Paul. German-American psychiatrist. 1886–1940
DISEASE—
Zur Kenntnis der sogenannten diffusen Sklerose: (Über Encephalitis periaxialis diffusa). Z. ges. Neurol. Psychiat., 10: 1–60, June 27, 1912

Schiller, Joachim. See Joachim Schyller

Schiller, Walter. Austrian gynecologist
TEST—
Ueber Frühstadiem des Portiocarcinoms und ihre Diagnose. Arch. Gynaek., 133: 211–283, 1928
Early diagnosis of carcinoma of the portio uteri. Amer. J. Surg., 26: 269–280, Nov. 1934

Schilling, Claus Karl. Berlin physician. 1871–1946
HEMOGRAM—
Versuche einer Verbesserung der Blutuntersuchung auf Leukozyten. Dtsch. med. Wschr., 48: 1337 (only), Oct. 6, 1922

Schilling, Victor Theodor Adolf Georg. German physician. 1883–
HEMOGRAM—
Das Blutbild. . . . Jena, Fischer, 1912. 105 pp.
Das Hämogramm in der Poliklinik. I. Biologische Kurven der Leukocytenbewegung als Grundlage der praktischen Bewertung einmaliger Blutuntersuchungen. Z. klin. Med., 99: 232–247, 1924

Schimmelbusch, Curt. German surgeon. 1860–1895
DISEASE—
Das Cystadenom der Mamma. Arch. f. klin. Chir. 44: 117–134, 1892

Schindler, Rudolf. German-American surgeon. 1888–
CLASSIFICATION—of gastritis.
Classification of chronic gastritis with special reference to gastroscopic method: study based on 1,200 cases with Marie Ortmayer, Arch. intern. Med., 57: 959–978, May 1936
GASTROSCOPE—
Die diagnostische Bedeutung der Gastroskopie. Münch. med. Wschr., 69: 535–537, Apr. 14, 1922
Probleme und Technik der Gastroskopie mit der Be-

schreibung eines neuen Gastroskops. Arch. f. VerdauKr., 30: 133–166, Oct. 1922

Ein völlig ungefährliches, flexibles Gastroskop. Münch. med. Wschr., 79: 1268–1269, Aug. 5, 1932

Diagnostic gastroscopy, with special reference to the flexible gastroscope. J. A. M. A., 105: 352–355, Aug. 3, 1935

Schiötz, H. See L. E. Javal

Schippers, J. C. Amsterdam pathologist

TEST—for bile pigments in urine.

Gallenfarbstoffreaktionen im Harne. Biochem. Z., 9: 241–243, 1908

Schirmer, Otto Wilhelm August. Greifswald ophthalmologist. 1864–1917

OPACITY—thread-like-filiform.

Ein Fall von Schimmelpilzkeratitis. Arch. f. Ophthal., 42 (3): 131–139, 1896

Schlagenhaufer, Friedrich. German physician

One of the first to call attention to relation of parathyroid tumor to osteitis fibrosa.

Zwei Fälle von Parathyreoideatumoren. Wien. klin. Wschr., 28: 1362 (only), Dec. 9, 1915

Parathyreoideatumoren. Abstr.: Münch. med. Wschr., 63: 56 (only), Jan. 11, 1916

See also E. A. F. Finger

Schlange, Hans. Hannover surgeon

METHOD and OPERATION—arthrotomy for fracture-dislocation of shoulder and elbow.

Die operative Bahandlung frischer irreponibler Luxationen und Fracturen. Arch. f. klin. Chir., 81: 9–32, 1906

Schlatter, Carl. Zurich surgeon. 1864–1934

DISEASE—

Verletzungen des schnabelförmigen Fortsatzes der oberen Tibiaepiphyse. Beitr. klin. Chir., 38: 874–887, 1903

Unvollständige Abrissfrakturen der Tuberositas tibiae oder Wachstumsanomalien? Ibid., 59: 518–546, 1908

OPERATION—total gastrectomy.

Ueber Ernährung und Verdauung nach vollständiger Entfernung des Magens—Oesophagoenterostomie—beim Menschen. Ibid., 19: 757–776, 1897

Schlecht, Heinrich. Breslau physician. 1881–

TEST—for trypsin in feces.

Ueber eine einfache Methode zur Prüfung der Pankreasfunktion beim gesunden und kranken Menschen. Münch. med. Wschr., 55: 725–727, Apr. 7, 1908

Schleich, Carl Ludwig. Berlin surgeon. 1859–1922

ANESTHESIA—general, by mixture of chloroform, sulphuric ether and petroleum ether.

Schmerzlose Operationen. Berlin, Springer, 1894. 256 pp.

ANESTHESIA—infiltration.

Zur Infiltrationsanästhesie. Therap. Mschr., 8: 429–436, Sept. 1894

A new method of local anaesthesia (infiltration anaesthesia). Internat. Clin., Philadelphia, s 5, 2: 177–192, July 1895

Schleiden, Matthias Jacob. Hamburg botanist. 1804–1881

Demonstrated cell structure of plants and emphasized significance of nucleus in vegetable histology. Garrison

Beiträge zur Phytogenesis. Arch. f. Anat., Physiol. u. wiss. Med., pp. 137–176, 1838

Also, English transl. London, Sydenham Soc. 1847

Schleifstein, Joseph Isaac. Albany physician. 1901–

METHOD—

A rapid method for demonstrating Negri bodies in tissue sections. Amer. J. Pub. Health, 27: 1283–1285, Dec. 1937

Schlesinger, Emmo. Berlin physician

TEST—for blood in feces.

Vergleichende Untersuchungen über den Nachweis von Minimalblutungen in den Faeces nebst einer neuen Modifikation der Benzidinprobe with F. Holst, Dtsch. med. Wschr., 32: 1444–1447, Sept. 6, 1906

Schlesinger, Hermann. Vienna physician. 1868–1934

SIGN—displacement of umbilicus.

Die „Nabelverziehung" bei Ulcus ventriculi und anderen Abdominalaffectionen. Wien. klin. Wschr., 34: 1 (only), Jan. 6, 1921

Schlesinger, Monroe Jacob. Boston physician. 1892–

METHOD—

An injection plus dissection study of coronary artery occlusions and anastomoses. Amer. Heart. J., 15: 528–568, May 1938

Schlodtmann, Walter. Königsberg i. Pr. ophthalmologist. 1870–

BRAWNY SCLERITIS—

Ueber sulzige Infiltration der Conjunctiva und Sklera. Arch. f. Ophthal., 43: 56–82, 1897

Schloesser, O. Munich surgeon. 1857–1925

METHOD or TREATMENT—of facial neuralgia.

Heilung peripherer Reisssustände sensibler und motorischer Nerven. Klin. Mbl. Augenheilk., 41: 244–245, Sept. 1903

Also in: Ber. ophthal. Ges. Heildelberg, 31–32: 84–90, Sept. 14, 1903

Erfahrungen in der Neuralgiebehandlung mit Alkoholeinspritzungen. Münch. med. Wschr., 54: 902–904, Apr. 30, 1907

Schloffer, Hermann. Vienna surgeon. 1868–1937

BOUILLON—urine.

Ueber die Verwendung des Harnagar zur Züchtung des Diphtheriebacillus. Zbl. Bakt., 14: 657–662 (659), Nov. 18, 1893

OPERATION—for pituitary tumor, by nasal route.

Zur Frage der Operationen an der Hypophyse. Beitr. klin. Chir., 50: 767–817, 1906

Erfolgreiche Operation eines Hypophysentumors auf nasalen Wege. Wien. klin. Wschr., 20: 621–624, May 23, 1907

Berichtigung zum Artikel: Ergolgreich Operation eines Hypophysentumors auf nasalem Wege. Ibid., 670–671, May 30, 1907

Weitere Bericht über den Fall von operiertem Hypophysentumor. (Plötzlicher Exitus lethalis 2½ Monate nach der Operation). Ibid., 1075–1078, Sept. 5, 1907

TUMOR—inflammatory swelling of abdomen after laparotomy.

Chronisch entzündliche Bauchdeckengeschwülst nach Bruchoperationen. Zbl. Chir., 35: 113–115, 1908

Schlomovitz, B. H. See A. S. Loevenhart

Schloss, E. M. See H. Shay

Schloss, Ernst. Strassburg physiochemist. 1882–

TEST—for glyoxalic acid in urine.

Über Nachweis und physiologisches Verhalten der Glyoxylsäure. Beitr. chem. Physiol. Path., 449–455, 1906

Schmalfuss, Hans. Hamburg chemist

TEST—for oxalic acid in urinary calculi.

Einfacher Nachweis von Oxalsäure in Harnsteinen.

with H. Werner and R. Kraul, Klin. Wschr., 11: 791 (only), Apr. 30, 1932

Schmaltz, Richard. Dresden physician
METHOD—for estimation of specific gravity of blood.
Die Untersuchung des specifischen Gewichtes des menschlichen Blutes. Dtsch. Arch. klin. Med., 47: 145-158, Oct. 21, 1890

Schmid, Hans Hermann. Prague surgeon. 1884–
OPERATION—
Vorschlag eines einfachen Operationsverfahrens zur Behandlung des Oesophagusdivertikels. Wien. klin Wschr., 25: 487-488, Mar. 28, 1912

Schmidt, Adolf. Breslau physician. 1865–1918
DIET—
Die Funkstionprufe des Darmes mittels der Probe-kost. Wiesbaden, Bergmann, 1908. 2 ed.
SYNDROME—hemoplegia affecting vocal cord, palate, trapezius and sternocleidomastoid muscle.
Casuistische Beiträge zur Nervenpathologie. II. Doppelseitige Accessoriuslähmung bei Syringomyelie. Dtsch. med. Wschr., 18: 606-608, June 30, 1892
TEST—nucleus for pancreatic function.
Ein neues diagnostisches Merkmal bei Pankreas-Erkrankungen. Verh. d. Kong. f. inn. Med., 21: 335-343, 1904

Schmidt, Alexander. German physiologist. 1831–1894
Developed ferment theory of coagulation of blood and applied name fibrin.
Weiteres über den Faserstoff und die Ursachen seiner Gerinnung. Arch. f. Anat., Physiol. u. wiss. Med., Leipzig, 428-469; 533-564, 1862
Zur Blutlehre. Leipzig, Vogel, 1892. 270 pp.
Weitere Beiträge zur Blutlehre. Wiesbaden, 1895

Schmidt, C. See F. H. Bidder

Schmidt, C. F. See K. K. Chen

Schmidt, E. See J. M. Fehr

Schmidt, Emil Gustabe. Baltimore biochemist. 1900–
METHOD—
The determination of sulfanilamide in tungstic acid blood filtrates by means of sodium B-naphthoquinone-4-sulfonate. J. biol. Chem., 122: 757-762, Feb. 1938

Schmidt, E. R. See J. L. Neller, R. M. Waters

Schmidt, H. See E. Abderhalden

Schmidt, Johann Adam. German ophthalmologist. 1759–1809
Described and coined term iritis. Garrison and Morton.
Über Nachstaar und Iritis nach Staaroperationen. Abhand. d. k. k. med.-chir. Josephs-Acad. zu Wien. 2: 209-292, 1801

Schmidt, Martin Benno. German physician. 1863–
Supported theory of hematogenous origin of carcinoma metastases. Garrison and Morton
Die Verbreitungswege der Karzinome und die Beziehung generalisierter Sarkome zu den leukämischen Neubildungen. Jena, Fischer, 1903

Schmidt, Rolf. Freiburg i. Br. ophthalmologist
KERATITIS—
Ueber die streifenförmige Keratitis superficialis herpetica. Klin. Mbl. Augenheilk., 91: 47-58, July 1933

Schmidt, W. See H. Langer

Schmidt-Rimpler, Hermann. German physician. 1838–1915
Wrote on relationship between eye diseases and general organic diseases and was advocate of routine

examination of eyes of school-children. Garrison and Morton
Die Erkrankungen des Auges im Zusammenhang mit anderen Krankheiten. Wien, Hölder, 1898

Schmiedeberg, Johann Ernst Oswald. German pharmacologist. 1838–1921
METHOD—for estimation of ammonia.
Erwiderung auf die vorstehenden Bemerkungen des Herrn Salkowski. Arch. f. exp. Path., 7: 424-428, Aug. 17, 1877
Investigated action of poisons on frog's heart.
Untersuchungen über einige Giftwirkungen am Froschherzen. Arb. a. d. Physiol. Anst. zu Leipzig, 1870, 5: 41-52, 1871

Schmiedeberg, O. See G. von Bunge

Schmieden, V. See K. G. A. Bier, F. Volhard

Schmiedt, Walther. German surgeon. 1886–
OPERATION—
Beitrag zur Daumenplastik. Dtsch. Z. f. Chir., 145: 420-423, 1918

Schmier, Adolph Albert. American surgeon. 1901–
METHOD—of treatment of dislocated humeral epicondyle into joint.
Fracture-dislocation of the elbow with ulnar nerve involvement: reduction by tension on the superficial flexor group of muscles. J. Bone and Joint Surg., 18: 1030-1035, Oct. 1936
Fracture dislocation of the elbow with displacement of the internal epicondyle into the joint. Amer. J. Surg. 45: 116-119, July 1939
The internal epicondylar epiphysis and elbow injuries. S. G. O., 80: 416-421, Apr. 1945

Schmilinsky, H. Hamburg surgeon
OPERATION—total intragastric regurgitation.
Die Einleitung der gesamten Duodenalsäfte in den Magen (inner Apotheke). Zbl. Chir., 45: 416-418, June 22, 1918

Schmincke, Alexander. Munich pathologist. 1877–
TUMOR—
Über lymphoepitheliale Geschwülste. Beitr. path Anat., 68: 161-169, 1921

Schmitz, Karl Eitel Friedrich. Griefswald physician 1889–
AGAR—nutrose blood clot infusion.
Ein neuer Elektionährboden für Typhusbacillen. Zbl. Bakt., 76: 306-319 (307; 315), June 28, 1915
BACILLUS—Bact. ambiguum, a cause of dysentery.
Ein neuer Typhus aus der Gruppe der Ruhrbazillen als Erreger einer grösseren Epidemie. Z. Hyg. In fektKr., 84: 449-516, Dec. 9, 1917

Schmorl, Christian Georg. German pathologist 1861–1932
DISEASE or NODULE—on vertebra; often confused with prolapse of nuclear pulp.
Die pathologische Anatomie der Wirbelsäule. Verh. dtsch. orthop. Ges., 21: 3-41, 1926
Ueber Dehnungs- und Zerreissungsvorgänge an den Bandscheiben und ihre Folgen. Abstr.: Zbl. allg. Path. u. path. Anat., 40: 244-246, Sept. 15, 1927
METHODS—1 and 2, for staining lacunae and canaliculi of bone. Mallory
In: *Die pathologischen-histologischen Untersuchungsmethoden.* Leipzig, Vogel, 1914. Ed. 7, p. 233; 236
METHOD—for chromaffin cells. Ibid., p. 293

Schneider, Conrad Victor. German physician. 1614–1680
MEMBRANE—mucous m. lining nose.

REFLEX—irritation of nasal mucosa induces facial contraction on same side. Overthrew, with Richard Lower, old Galenic idea that nasal secretions originate in pituitary body. Garrison
Liber primus de catarrhis. . . . Wittebergae, Mevii et al., 1660. 257 pp.
Liber de osse cribriformi, et sensu ac organo odoratus. . . . Wittebergae, Mevii et al., 1655. 531 pp.

Schneider, Edward Christian. Middletown, Conn. scientist. 1874–
INDEX—of physical condition.
A cardiovascular rating as a measure of physical fatigue and efficiency. J. A. M. A., 74: 1507–1510, May 29, 1920

Schnitker, M. T. See E. C. Cutler

Schnitzler, Julius. Vienna surgeon
OPERATION—
Zur Technik der Gastrostomie. Wien. klin. Rund., 10: 513–514, July 26, 1896

Schöbl, Jos. Prague ophthalmologist
HYPERPLASTIC SCLERITIS—
Ueber hyperplastische Entzündungen der Augenhäute. Arch. f. Augenheilk., 20: 98–122, June 1889

Schöler, Heinrich Leopold. German ophthalmologist. 1844–1918
TREATMENT—for detachment of retina.
Zur operativen Behandlung und Heilung der Netzhautablösung. Berlin, Leist, 1889. 98 pp.

Schoeller, W. See E. Steinach

Shoemaker, Jan. Holland surgeon. 1871–
CLAMP, OPERATION—modification of Billroth I gastroduodenostomy.
Some technical points in abdominal surgery. S. G. O., 33: 591–596, Dec. 1921

Schöndorff, Bernhard. Bonn physiologist
METHOD—for quantitative estimation of urea in urine.
Eine Methode der Harnstoffbestimmung in thierischen Organen und Flüssigkeiten. Arch. f. Phys., 62: 1–57, Oct. 8, 1895

Schoenheimer, Rudolf. New York physician. 1898–
METHOD—
A micromethod for the determination of free and combined cholesterol with W. M. Sperry, J. biol. Chem. 106: 745–760, Sept. 1934

Schönlein, Johann Lukas. German physician. 1793–1864
DISEASE—pupura rheumatica, or peliosis rheumatica.
In his: *Allgemeine und specielle Pathologie und Therapie.* . . . Zweiter Teil, IV Ed., (St. Gallen 1839), p. 42. (Published by some of his pupils.)
Discovered parasitic cause of favus (achorion Schönleinii).
Zur Pathogenie der Impetigines. Arch. f. Anat., Physiol. u. wiss. Med., p. 82 (only), 1839

Schoepff, Johann David. German army surgeon. 1752–1800
Wrote, from experience in American Revolution— (Garrison and Morton)
Materia medica Americana. Erlangae, Palmii, 1787

Scholl, A. J. See E. D. Osborne

Scholtz, Walther. Breslau physician. 1871–
AGAR—ascitic fluid.
Beiträge zur Biologie des Gonococcus. Cultur, Thierexperimente und klinische Beobachtungen über Gonococcenhaltige Abscesse im Bindegewebe. Arch. f. Derm. u. Syph., 49: 3–28 (5), 1899

Schoonover, Janetta W. Philadelphia scientist
METHOD—
Some refinements upon the calorimetric method of Hastings and Sendroy for the determination of the pL of the blood with Gladys E. Woodward, J. Lab clin. Med., 16: 621–624, Mar. 1931

Schorrer, E. H. See C. W. Duval

Schott, Edward. German physician
TEST—of heart function.
Die Erhöhung des Druckes im venösen System be Anstregung als Mass für die Funktionstüchtigkei des menschlichen Herzens. Dtsch. Arch. klin. Med. 108: 537–553, Nov. 22, 1912

Schott, Theodore. Nauheim physician. 1852–1920
BATH or TREATMENT—for heart disease.
Die Wirkung der Bäden auf das Herz. Berl. klin Wschr., 17: 357–359, June 21; 372–374, June 28 1880
Also, in English. Philadelphia, Blakiston, 1914 191 pp.

Schottmüller, Hugo. Hamburg physician. 1867–1936
DISEASE—paratyphoid.
Über eine das Bild des Typhus bietende Erkrankung hervorgerufen durch Typhus ähnliche Bacillen Dtsch. med. Wschr., 26: 511–512, Aug. 9, 1900
Isolated Strep. viridans in cases of bacterial endocarditis and named condition endocarditis lenta Garrison and Morton
Endocarditis lenta. Zugleich ein Beitrag zur Artunter scheidung der pathogenen Streptokokken. Münch. med Wschr., 57: 617–620, Mar. 22: 697–699, Mar. 29 1910
Isolated Streptothrix (Actinomyces) muris ratt from human patients bitten by rats. Garrison and Morton
Zur Ätiologie und Klinik der Bisskrankheit (Ratten-Katzen-, Eichhörnchen-Bisskrankheit). Dermat Wschr., 58, suppl., 77–103, 1914

Schreiber, Ernst. Göttingen physician
TEST—for kryofine in urine.
Ueber Kryofin. Dtsch. med. Wschr., 23: 73–74, Nov. 4, 1897

Schrenk, H. H. See W. P. Yant

Schreyer, Johann. German physician
First put to practical proof Swammerdam's discovery that fetal lungs will float on water after respiration; in the case of a fifteen year old peasant girl accused of infanticide, the sinking of the infant's lungs secured acquittal. Garrison
Erörterung und Erläuterung der Frage: Ob es ein gewiss Zeichen, wenn eines todten Kindes Lunge im Wasser untersincket, dass solches in Mutter-Leibe gestorben sey? Zeitz, Ammersbachen, 1690. 35 pp.

Schridde, Hermann Robert August. Freiburg i. Br. pathologist. 1875–
DISEASE—congenital generalized dropsy.
Die angeborene allgemeine Wassersucht. Münch. med Wschr., 57: 397–398, Feb. 22, 1910
GRANULES—chondroconia.
STAINING METHOD—for granulation of myelocytes and leukocytes in sections.
Die haematologische Technik with A. Naegeli, Jena, Fischer, 1910. 135 pp.
METHOD—of fixation.
Ueber gleichzeitige Fixierung und Durchfärbung von Gewebsstücken with A. Fricke, Zbl. allg. Path. u path. Anat., 17: 721–723, Sept. 30, 1906

hroeder van der Kolk, Jacob Ludwig Conrad
German physician. 1797–1862
Wrote important histological work on localization of
function. Garrison and Morton
*Bau und Functionen der Medulla spinalis und ob-
ongata und nächste Ursache und rationelle Behand-
ung der Epilepsie.* Braunschweig, Vieweg, 1859

hröder, Karl Ludwig Ernst. German gynecologist
838–1887
ERATION—
Ueber die Laparotomie bei Uterusmyomen. Zbk.
Gynäk., 2: 494–503, Oct. 12, 1878
NG—contraction r. of uterus.
Der schwahgere und kreissende Uterus. Bonn, Cohen
1886

hroeder, Waldemar von. German physician. 1850–
1898
ST—for urea.
Ueber die Bildungsstätte des Harnstoffs. Arch. exp.
Path. Pharmak., 15: 364–402, (372), May 22, 1882

hrötter, Leopold von. Vienna laryngologist. 1837–
1908
OREA—of larynx.
Über „Chorea laryngis." Allg. Wien. med. Zeitung,
24: 67–68, Feb. 18, 1879

hubert, Gotthard. German gynecologist
ERATION—for formation of artificial vagina.
*Über Scheidenbildung bei angeborenem Vaginalde-
fekt.* Zbl. Gynäk., 35: 1017–1022, July 15, 1911

hücking, Adrian. German gynecologist
ERATION—for prolapsed uterus.
*Bemerkungen zur vaginalen Ligatur des Uterus bei
Retroflexio und Prolapsus uteri.* Zbl. Gynäk., 15:
249–251, Mar. 28, 1891

hüffner, Wilhelm. German physician. 1867–
Introduced—(Garrison and Morton)
*Das Oleum chenopodii anthelmintici gegen Ankylo-
stomiasis im Vergleich zu anderen Wurmmitteln.*
Trans. Internat. Cong. Hyg. and Demog., 1912,
Washington, 1: 734–739, 1913

hüller, Artur. Vienna neurologist. 1874–
SEASE—Hand-Schüller-Christian; craniohypophyseal xanthomatosis.
Uber eigenartige Schädeldefekte im Jugendalter. Fort.
a. d. Geb. d. Röntgenstrahlen, 23: 12–18, 1915–16
Suggested section of pathways in spinal cord for
pain.
*Ueber operative Durchtrennung des Rückenmarks-
strange (Chordotomie).* Wien. med. Wschr., 40: 2292–
2296, Sept. 24, 1910

hütte, D. German physician
Reported value of cod-liver oil in treatment of rick-
ets. Garrison and Morton
*Beobachtungen über den Nutzen des Berger Leber-
thrans (Oleum jecoris Acelli, von Gadus asellus L.)*
Arch. f. med. Erfahr., Berlin, 2: 79–92, 1824

hütz. See F. A. J. Löffler

hüz, E. See M. Gänsslen

hukow, Ivan. Charkow physiologist
LUTION—basal ammonium phosphate.
Ueber den Säureverbrauch der Hefen. Zbl. f. Bakt.,
2 Abt., 2: 601–612 (607), Oct. 30, 1896

hultes, Johann. See Johann Schultetus

hultess, Ernst. Jena physician
ETHOD—for detection of albumoses.
Die Beziehungen zwischen Albumosurie und Fieber.
Dtsch. Arch. klin. Med., 58: 325–338, 1897

Schulte-Tigges, Hugo. German physician. 1885–
STAINING METHOD—
Zur Tuberkelbazillenfärbung. Dtsch. med. Wschr.,
46: 1225 (only), Oct. 28, 1920

Schultz, Arthur Rudolf Heinrich. Kiel physician.
1890–
METHOD—for demonstrating cholesterol.
*Eine Methode des mikrochemischen Cholesterinnach-
weises am Gewebsschnitt.* Zbl. allg. Path. u. path.
Anat., 35: 314–316, Dec. 1, 1924

Schultz, Victor. St. Petersburg gynecologist
THEORY—uterine hypoplasia is a cause of primary
dysmenorrhea.
*Ein Beitrag zur Aetiologie und Pathogenese der Dys-
menorrhoe.* Mschr. f. Geburtsh. u. Gynäk., 18:
854–873, Dec. 1903

Schultz, Werner. Berlin physician. 1878–
REACTION or SIGN—of scarlet fever; extinction r.
Serologische Beobachtungen am Scharlachexanthem
with W. Charlton, Z. Kinderheilk., 17: 328–333,
Mar. 15, 1918
Described granulocytopenia or agranulocytosis.
*Ueber einenartige Halserkrankungen. a. Monozy-
tenangina. b. Gangräneszierende Prozesse und Defekt
des Granulocytensystems.* Dtsch. med. Wschr., 48:
1495–1496, Nov. 3, 1922

Schultze, Friedrich. German physician. 1848–1934
ACROPARESTHESIA—
Über Akroparästhesie. Dtsch. Z. Nervenheilk., 3:
300–318, Feb. 1, 1893
See also W. H. Erb

Schultze, Maximilian Johann Sigismund. German
histologist. 1825–1874
CELLS—olfactory.
*Untersuchungen über den Bau der Nasenschleimhaut,
namentlich die Structur und Endigungsweise der
Geruchsnerven bei dem Menschen und den Wirbelthieren*
Abh. d. naturf. Ges. zu Halle, 7: 1–100, 1862
Wrote on nerve-endings in internal ear.
Über die Endigungsweise des Hörnerven im Labyrinth.
Arch. f. Anat., Physiol. u. wiss. Med., 343–381, 1858
Showed likeness between animal and vegetable
protoplasm, structural, chemical and physiologic.
Introduced term protoplasm. Garrison
*Über Muskelkörperchen und das, was man eine Zelle
zu nennen habe.* Ibid., 1–27, 1861
*Das Protoplasma der Rhizopoden und der Pflanzen-
zellen.* Leipzig, Engelmann, 1863. 68 pp.
Described segmentation furrowing of egg.
*De ovorum ranarum segmentatione, quae "Furshungs-
process" dicitur.* Bonn, 1863
Recognized blood platelets.
*Ein heizbarer Objecttisch und seine Verwendung bei
Untersuchungen des Blutes.* Arch. mikr. Anat., 1:
1–42, 1865
Described nerve-endings in retina.
Zur Anatomie und Physiologie der Retina. Bonn,
Cohen, 1866

Schultze, Walter Hans Gustav. Göttingen pathol-
ogist. 1880–
REACTION—oxidase.
Zur Differentialdiagnose der Leukämieen. Münch.
med. Wschr., 56: 167–169, Jan. 26, 1909
*Weitere Mitteilungen über Oxydasereaktionen an
Gewebschnitten.* Ibid., 57: 2171–2173, Oct. 18, 1910

Schumacher, E. D. See E. F. Sauerbruch

Schumm, Otto. German chemist

TEST—for blood.
Zum klinischen Nachweis von Blut in den Fäzes.
Münch. med. Wschr., 56: 612 (only), Mar. 23, 1909
Schuntermann, Carl Erich. German physician.
1901–
TEST—
Über eine neue Methode des Urochromogennachweises im Urin. Beitr. Klin. Tuberkul., 65: 773–776, Mar. 14, 1927
Schuschania, Platon. Kiel gynecologist
Noted increase of estrin in urine of patients with granulosa cell tumors of ovary.
Ergebnisse von Mengenbestimmungen des Sexualhormons. 5. Mitteilung: Sexualhormon im Harn und Kot bei a. Metropathia haemorrhagica juvenilis (glandulär-cystischer Hyperplasie), b. Granulosazelltumor des Ovars mit glandulär-cystischer Hyperplasie des Endometriums. Zbl. Gynäk., 54: 1924–1936, Aug. 2, 1930
Schwab, S. I. See N. Allison
Schwalbe, Marcus Walter. German physician. 1883–
Described torsion spasm, dystonia musculorum deformans: later called Ziehm-Oppenheim's disease. Garrison and Morton
Eine eigentümliche tonischen Krampfform mit hysterischen Symptomen. Berlin, Schade, 1908
Schwanda, M. German physician
TEST—for bile in urine.
(Staederler'sche Bilirubin aus ikterischem Harn.) Jbr. d. ges. Med., 1: 103 (only), 1867
Schwann, Theodor. German physiologist. 1810–1882
Demonstrated respiration in embryonic chick. Garrison
De necessitate aëris atmosphaerici ad evolutionem pulli in ovo incubito. Berlin, Nietackianis, 1834 32 pp.
Discovered pepsin in 1835. Garrison
Über das Wesen des Verdauungsprocesses. Müller's Arch., Berlin, 90–138, 1836
Proved in 1836 that putrefaction is caused by living bodies which are destroyed if surrounding air be heated or vitiated. Garrison
Vorläufige Mittheilung betreffend Versuche über die Weingährung und Fäulniss. Ann. d. Phys. u. Chem. Leipzig, 41: 184–193, 1837
Demonstrated cell structure of animals.
Mikroskopische Untersuchungen über die Uebereinstimmung in der Struktur und dem Wachsthum der Thiere und Pflanzen. Berlin, Sander, 1839. 270 pp. Also, English transl. London, New Sydenham Soc., 1847. 268 pp.
Showed, by means of an artificial biliary fistula in a dog, that bile is absolutely essential to digestion. Garrison
Versuche um auszumitteln, ob die Galle im Organismus eine für das Leben wesentliche Rolle spielt. Müller's Arch., Berlin, 127–159, 1844
Schwartz, C. See B. L. K. Hamilton
Schwartz, Edouard. Paris surgeon. 1852–
OPERATION—for inguinal hernia, using flap of rectus.
Sur un procédé de cure radicale des hernies et en particulier des hernies crurale et inguinale; myoplastie herniaire. Ass. franç. de Chir. Proc.-verb., Paris, 7: 689–693, 1893
TEST—for state of valves in varicose veins: same as McPheeters' test.

Du traitement des varices par la ligature multiple de veine saphene interne et l'expirpation. Rev. gén. clin. et de therap., 2: 65–68, Feb. 2, 1888
See also A. L. C. Souligoux
Schwartz, Henry Gerard. St. Louis surgeon. 1909
OPERATION—
Section of the spinothalamic tract in the medulla w observations on the pathway for pain with J. O'Leary, Surgery, 9: 183–193, Feb. 1941
Schwartz, Samuel. Minneapolis physician
METHOD—petroleum ether extraction, for quant tative urinary urobilinogen.
Studies of urobilinogen. IV. The quantitative dete mination of urobilinogen by means of the Evely photoelectric colorimeter with V. Sborov and C. Watson, Amer. J. clin. Path., 14: 598–604, De 1944
See also C. J. Watson
Schwartz, S. P. See G. I. Swetlow
Schwartz, W. See J. E. Moore
Schwartze, Hermann Hugo Rudolf. German oto ogist. 1837–1910
OPERATION—on mastoid.
Ueber die künstliche Eröffnung des Warzenfor satzes with A. Eysell, Arch. f. Ohrenheilk., 7 157 187, June 6, 1873
Schwarz, Fritz. Zurich physician
REAGENT—for blood
Eine Verschärfung der Benzidinreaktion. Z. ge gerichtl. Med., 12: 216–218, Aug. 27, 1928
Schwarz, Gottwald. German roentgenologist. 1880
SIGN—x-ray shadow of fat at apex of heart, ofte confused with cardiac enlargement.
Ueber einen typischen Röntgenbefund am Herze Fettleibiger und dessen anatomische Grundlage. Wier klin. Wschr., 23: 1850–1852, Dec. 22, 1910
Schweigger-Seidel, Franz. German scientist. 1834 1871–
Proved that spermatozoon possesses a nucleus an cytoplasm. Garrison and Morton
Ueber die Samenkörperchen und ihre Entwicklun Arch. mikr. Anat., 1: 309–335, 1865
Schwer, See Hirschbruck
Schwyzer, Arnold. St. Paul surgeon. 1864–
OPERATION—
A new pyelo-ureteral plastic for hydronephrosis. Surg Clin. No. Amer., 3: 1441–1448, Oct. 1923
Schylhans, See H. von Gersdorff
Schyller, Joachim. fl. 1529
Wrote on German epidemic of sweating sickness c 1528–30. Garrison and Morton
De peste Brittanica commentariolus vere aureus Basileae, Petrus, 1531
Sclavo, Achille. Rome bacteriologist. 1861–1930
SERUM—anti-anthrax.
Sulla preparazione del siero anticarbonchioso. Riv d'ig. e san. pubb., Roma, 6: 841–843, 1895
Ueber die Bereitung des Serums gegen den Milzbrand Zbl. Bakt., 1 Abt., 18: 744–745, Dec. 23, 1895
Scotch douche
So called by Despine of Aix les Bains in 1760: hy drotherapy with quick changes of temperature, ad vocated by William Cullen. Garrison
Scott, Arthur Carroll. Temple, Texas surgeon. 1865 1940

OPERATION—
The radical cure of inguinal hernia. Texas State J. Med., 15: 5–6, May 1919

Scott, Arthur Carroll, Jr. Temple, Texas surgeon. 1890–
CLAMP—
Intestinal anastomosis by rapid suture clamp. Texas State J. Med., 21: 303–306, Sept. 1925

Scott, D. A. Toronto scientist
METHOD—
Crystalline insulin. Endocrinology, 25: 437–448, Sept. 1939

Scott, Gladwys M. See H. Chambers

Scott, John. English surgeon. 1799–1846
DRESSING—
In his: Chronic inflammations and diseases of joints. 1828

Scott, S. F. See W. M. Dehn

Scott, William Justus Merle. Rochester, N. Y. surgeon. 1894–
Showed that general anesthesia produces complete generalized vasodilatation.
Obliteration of vasoconstrictor gradient in the extremities under nitrous oxide-oxygen, ether, and tribromethyl alcohol anesthesias. Proc. Soc. exp. Biol., N. Y., 27: 945–949, June 1930
See also J. J. Morton

Scott-Wilson, H. English scientist
REAGENT—for acetone.
A method for estimating acetone in animal liquids. J. Physiol., 42: 444–470, July 15, 1911

Scudder, Charles Locke. American surgeon. 1860–
TREATMENT—reduction of supracondylar fractures of femur.
In his: The treatment of fractures. Philadelphia, Saunders, 1928. 10 ed. p. 741

Scultetus, Johannes. German surgeon. 1595–1645
BANDAGE or BINDER—"many tailed."
POSITION—patient lying on an inclined place with head downward.
Armamentarium chirurgicum. Ulm, 1653

Scupham, G. W. See G. de Takats

Sears, J. B. See J. Thew

Sebelien, John. Danish chemist
REAGENT—for albumin and peptone.
Studien über die analytische Bestimmungsweise der Eiweisskörper mit besonderer Rücksicht auf die Milch. Z. physiol., Chem., 13: 135–186 (150), 1899
(Nach dem dänischen Original in Oversigt af det kgl. danske Videnskabernes Selskabs Forhandlinger, 1888)

Sébileau, Pierre. French surgeon. 1860–
BANDS—thickenings of Sibson's fascia.
L'appareil suspenseur de la plèvre. Bull. Soc. anat. de Paris, pp. 410–445, July 1891

Sedillot, Charles Emmanuel. French surgeon. 1804–1883
Performed gastrostomy.
De la gastrotomie fistuleuse. C. R. Acad. Sci., Paris, 23: 222–228, July 27, 1846
Des cas auxquels l'operation de la gastrostomie est applicable. Ibid., 907–909, Nov. 16, 1846

Seefelder, Richard. Leipzig ophthalmologist. 1875–
PECTINATE LIGAMENT OF—at angle of anterior chamber of eye.
Zur Entwicklung der vorderen Kammer und des Kammerwinkels beim Menschen, nebst Bemerkungen

über ihre Entstehung bei Tieren with Dr. Wolfrum, Arch. f. Ophthal., 63: 430–451, May 22, 1906

Seelig, Major Gabriel. St. Louis surgeon. 1874–
OPERATION—
The inguinal route operation for femoral hernia; with a supplementary note on Cooper s ligament with L. Tuholske, S. G. O., 18: 55–62, Jan. 1914

Seeligmüller, Otto Ludovicus Gustavus Adolphus German neurologist. 1837–1912
SIGN—mydriasis on side of face affected with neuralgia.
Über syphilitische Neuralgien. Dtsch. med. Wschr., 9: 624–625, Oct. 24, 1883

Seemann, H. Geman physician.
METHOD—for determination of quantity of hydrochloric acid in stomach content.
Ueber das Vorhandensein freier Salzsäure im Magen. Z. klin. Med., 5: 272–279, 1882

Ségalas, Pierre Salomon. French urologist. 1792–1875
Did early work on endoscope and cystoscope. Homans
Traité des rétentions d'urine et des maladies qu'elles produisent, suivi d'un grand nombre d'observations. Paris, Méquignon-Marvis, 1828

Segoud, Paul. French surgeon. 1851–1912
POSTULATE—of malignancy due to single trauma.
Le cancer et les accidents du travail. Ass. Franc. d. Chir., 20: 745–782, Oct. 11, 1907

Séguin, Armand. French chemist. 1765–1835
Measured metabolism of man (himself). Garrison and Morton
Premier mémoire sur la respiration des animaux with A. L. Lavoisier, Hist. Acad. d. Sci., 1789, Paris, 566–584, 1793
Discovered a crystalline substance in opium, 1804
Sur l'opium. Ann. d. Chim., 92: 225–247, Dec. 31, 1814

Séguin, P. See W. Weinberg

Sehrt, Ernst. Freiburg physician. 1879–
REACTION—chemical, for cancer.
Eine neue Sauerstoffbestimmung des menschlichen Blutes mittels Indophenolblaus und die mit dieser Methode erhobenen Befunde beim Krebskranken und Krebsdisponierten. Dtsch. med. Wschr., 55: 1666–1667, Oct. 4, 1929

Seibert, Florence Barbara. American chemist. 1897–
Discovered pyrogens.
Fever-producing substances found in some distilled waters. Amer. J. Physiol., 67: 90–104, Dec. 1, 1923

Seidell, A. See R. Hunt

Seidlitz powder
Named from a mineral spring in Bohemia.

Seiffert, Gustav. German physician
AGAR—chlorophyll bouillon; selective medium for cholera.
Der Chemismus elektiver Cholera-Nährböden with H. Bamberger, Arch. Hyg., Berl., 85: 265–298 (288), 1916

Seitz, Ernest. Bonn bacteriologist. 1885–
SOLUTION—lactose peptone; differential medium for colon-typhoid group.
Die Lackmusmolke als differentialdiagnostisches Hilfsmittel und ihr Ersatz durch eine kürstliche Lösung. Z. Hyg. InfektKr., 71: 405–438 (434), 1912

Sekiya, S. See A. Sato

Selig, Arthur. Prague physician

TEST—staircase t. for cardiac insufficiency.
Die funktionelle Herzdiagnostik. Prag. med. Wschr.,
30: 418–419; 432, July 27, 1905
Selinger, M. A. See J. W. Lindsay
Selivanoff, Feodor. Russian chemist. 1859–
TEST—for fructose or levulose in urine.
Notiz über eine Fruchtzuckerreaction. Ber. dtsch.
chem. Ges., 20: 181–182, Jan. 24, 1887
Sell, Mariana. See H. Steenbock
Sellards, Andrew Watson. American physician. 1884–
SOLUTION—liver digest blood.
Investigation of the virus of measles with G. H. Bige-
low, J. med. Res., 42: 241–259 (242), Mar.–May,
1921
TEST—for acidosis.
*The determination of the equilibrium in the human
body between acids and bases with especial reference to
acidosis and nephropathies.* Johns Hopk. Hosp. Bull.,
23: 289–302, Oct. 1912
*The essential features of acidosis and their occurrence
in chronic renal disease.* Ibid., 25: 141–153, May 1914
See also E. L. Walker
Sellheim, Hugo. German obstetrician. 1871–1936
OPERATION—cesarean section through space en-
closed by vesico-uterine reflection of peritoneum.
Der extraperitoneale Unterusschnitt. Zbl. Gynäk.,
32: 133–142, Feb. 1, 1908
Selling, Laurence. American pathologist. 1882–
Described—
*A preliminary report of some cases of purpura hemor-
rhagica due to benzol poisoning.* Johns Hopk. Hosp.
Bull., 21: 33–37, Feb. 1910
See also F. C. McLean
Semb, Carl Boye. Norwegian surgeon. 1895–
DISEASE—
*Pathologico-anatomical and clinical investigations of
fibro-adenomatosis cystica mammae and its relation to
other pathological conditions in the mamma, especially
cancer.* Acta chir. Scandinav., 64, Suppl. 10, 1–484,
1928
OPERATION—
Thoracoplasty with extrafascial apicolysis. Ibid.,
Suppl. 37, part. 2, 76: 1–85, 1935
Semken, George Henry. New York surgeon. 1875–
INCISION—for unilateral dissection of lymph nodes
of neck.
Surgery of the neck. In: *Nelson's Loose Leaf Living
Surgery,* New York, 1941. Vol. 2, Ch. 14, p. 763
Semmelweis, Ignaz Philipp. Vienna obstetrician.
1818–1865
Demonstrated that puerperal fever is contagious
and infectious.
*Höchst wichtige Erfahrungen über die Aetiologie der
in Gebäranstalten epidemischen Puerperalfieber.* Z. d.
k. k. Ges. d. Aerzte in Wien, 4, pt. 2: 242–244, 1847–
48; 5: 64–65, 1849
A Gyermkágyi lás Koroktana. Orvosi hetil., Budapest,
2: 1; 17; 65; 81; 305; 337; 353; 1858
*Die Aetiologie, der Begriff und die Prophylaxis des
Kindbettfiebers.* Pest, Wien u. Leipzig, Hartleben,
1861. 543 pp.
Also, English transl. by F. P. Murphy in: Medical
Classics, 5: 350–773, Jan., Feb., Mar., Apr. 1941
Semmes, R(aphael) Eustace. Memphis, Tenn.
surgeon. 1886–
OPERATION—

*Diagnosis of ruptured intervertebral disk without co[n-
tra]st myelography and comment upon recent experien[ce]
with modified hemilaminectomy for their remova[l.]*
Yale J. Biol. and Med., 11: 433–435, May 1939
Semon, Sir Felix. London laryngologist. 1849–1921
LAW—
*On the proclivity of the abductor fibers of the recurre[nt]
laryngeal nerve to become affected sooner that the a[b-]
ductor fibers, or even exclusively, in cases of undoubt[ed]
central or peripheral injury or disease of the roots [,]
trunks of the pneumogastric, spinal accessory, or r[e-]
current nerves.* Arch. Laryngol., 2: 197–222, July
1881
SIGN—
*Double stenosis of the upper air passages, i.e., bilater[al]
paralysis of the glottis-openers and compression of t[he]
trachea, in a case of malignant (?) tumor of the th[y-]
roid gland.* Trans. Path. Soc. London, 33: 38–4[2]
1882
Suggested that cretinism, myxedema and cachex[ia]
strumipriva are all due to loss of thyroid function.
(*Discussion on a case of myxedema presented befo[re]
the Clinical Society of London, Nov. 23, 1883.*) Bri[t.]
med. J., 2: 1072–1073, Dec. 1, 1883
Semple, D. See A. E. Wright
Sénac, Jean Baptiste De. French physician. 169[3?]
1770
Used quinine for palpitation; described pericarditi[s.]
*Traité de la structure du coeur, de son action et de s[es]
maladies.* Paris, Vincent, 1749. 2 vols. Vol. 2, 18,
524
Also, transl. by M. N. Walsh in: F. A. Willius a[nd]
T. E. Keys' *Cardiac classics.* St. Louis, Mosby, 194[1]
pp. 162–163
Senator, Hermann. German physician. 1834–1911
DISEASE—Banti-Senator.
*Über Anaemia splenica mit Ascites (Banti'sch[e]
Krankheit).* Berl. klin. Wschr., 38: 1145–1150, No[v.]
18, 1901
Sencert, Louis. Nancy surgeon. 1878–
APPROACH—to first and second portions of subcl[a-]
vian vessels.
Wounds of the vessels. London, Univ. London Pres[s]
1918. 270 pp.
Sendroy, J., Jr. See A. B. Hastings, D. D. Van Sly[ke]
Senear, Francis Eugene. Chicago dermatologi[st]
1889–
SYNDROME—
*An unusual type of pemphigus, combining featur[es]
of lupus erythematosus.* Arch. Derm. Syph., N. Y.,
761–781, June 1926
Senez, Ch. See A. Besson
Senn, Emanuel John. Chicago surgeon. 1869–
OPERATION—
Gastrostomy by a circular valve method. J. A. M. [A.]
27: 1142–1145, Nov. 28, 1896
Senn, M. J. E. See A. F. Hartmann
Senn, Nicholas. American surgeon. 1844–1908
OPERATION—intestinal anastomosis by use of bon[e]
plates.
*An experimental contribution to intestinal surge[ry]
with special reference to the treatment of intestinal o[b-]
struction.* Ann. Surg., 7: 1 et seq. (179), Jan.
seq., 1888
*Enterorrhaphy; its history, technique and prese[nt]
status.* J. A. M A., 21: 215–235, Aug. 12, 1893

PERATION—
Subcutaneous drainage in the surgical treatment of hydrocephalus internus. Alienist and Neurol., 24: 316–324, Aug. 1903

EST—
Rectal insufflation of hydrogen gas an infallible test in the diagnosis of visceral injury of the gastro-intestinal canal in penetrating wounds of the abdomen. J. A. M. A., 10: 767–777, June 23, 1888
First to use Roentgen rays in treatment of leukemia. Garrison
Case of splenomedullary leukaemia successfully treated by the use of the Röntgen ray. Med. Rec., 64: 281–282, Aug. 22, 1903

ennert, Daniel. German physician. 1572–1637
Wrote on scurvy.
De scorbuto tractatus. Wittebergae, Schurerum, 1624. 755 pp.
Wrote on dysentery.
De dysenteria tractatus. (Same) 1626. 162 pp.

epulveda, Bernardo. Rochester, Minn. physician
METHOD—
Serum bilirubin: a procedure for the determination of indirect and direct values with A. E. Osterberg, J. Lab. clin. Med., 28: 1359–1368, Aug. 1943
(Correction), Ibid., 1654, Oct. 1943

equeira, J. H. See W. Bulloch
erra, A. Bologna surgeon
PERATION—section of quintothalmic tract for trigeminal neuralgia.
Die elektro-chirurgische Unterbrechung der Zentralbahnen des V. Paares am lateralen ventralen Rand des Pons Varoli als erster Behandlungsversuch von hartnäckigen Neuralgien des Trigeminus durch Tumoren der Schädelbasis with V. Néri, Zbl. Chir., 63: 2248–2251, Sept. 19, 1936

errano, J. A. See R. Bettencourt
erres, Antoine Étienne Renaud Augustin. French physiologist. 1786–1868
LANDS—pearly masses of epithelial cells near surface of gum of an infant. Dorland
Essai sur l'anatomie et la physiologie des dents, ou nouvelle théorie de la dentition. Paris, Méquignon-Marvis, 1817. 183 pp.

ertürner, Friedrick Wilhelm Adam. Hannover pharmacist. 1783–1841
Isolated morphine.
Darstellung der reinen Mohnsäure (Opiumsäure); nebst einer chemischen Untersuchung des Opiums, mit vorzüglicher Hinsicht auf einen darin neu entdeckten Stoff (Morphium). J. d. Pharm., Leipzig, 14: 47–93, 1806
Ueber das Morphium, eine neue salzfähige Grundlage, und die Mekonsäure, als Hauptbestandteile des Opiums. Ann. d. Physik, Leipzig, 55: 56–89, 1817

érulas, Georges Simon. French chemist. 1774–1832
Discovered iodoform.
Mémoire sur l'iodure de potassium, l'acide hydriodique, et sur un composé nouveau de carbone, d'iode et d'hydrogène. Ann. Chim. (Phys.), Paris, 20: 163–168, 1822

ervetus, Michael. Spanish physician. 1509–1553
First described lesser circulation of blood. Garrison
Christianismi Restitutio. Vienne, Arnollet, 1553

etchenoff, Ivan Michailovich. Russian neurologist. 1829–1905

Discovered cerebral inhibition of spinal reflexes. Garrison
Physiologische Studien über die Hemmungsmechanismen für die Reflexthätigkeit des Rückenmarks im Gehirn des Frosches. Berlin, Hirschwald, 1863. 51 pp.

Sever, James Warren. Boston surgeon. 1878–
OPERATION—
Obstetrical paralysis—an orthopedic problem. Amer. J. Orthop. Surg., 14: 456–475, Aug. 1916
The results of a new operation for obstetrical paralysis. Ibid. 16: 248–257, Apr. 1918
TREATMENT—
Recurrent dislocation of the shoulder joint: a mechanical consideration of its treatment. J. A. M. A., 76: 925–927, Apr. 2, 1921

Sewall, Edward Cecil. San Francisco otolaryngologist. 1875–
OPERATION—
Operative control of progressive exophthalmos. Arch. Otolaryn., 24: 621–624, Nov. 1936

Seybold, E. G. See A. S. Lovenhart
Seyfarth, Carly. Leipzig surgeon. 1890–
TREPHINE—
Die Sternumtrepanation, eine einfache Methode zur diagnostischen Entnahme von Knochenmark bei Lebenden. Dtsch. med. Wschr., 49: 180–181, Feb. 9, 1923

Shackell, Leon Francis. American biochemist. 1887–
METHOD—for determination of total solids in urine.
An improved method of desiccation, with some applications to biological problems. Amer. J. Physiol., 24: 325–340, June 1909

Shaffer, M. F. See Clara M. McKee
Shaffer, Philip Anderson. American biochemist. 1881–
DIET—
Protein metabolism in typhoid fever with W. Coleman, Arch. intern. Med., 4: 538–600, Dec. 15, 1909
METHOD—
A method for the quantitative determination of B-oxybutyric acid in urine. J. biol. Chem., 5: 211–223, Oct. 1908
The determination of oxybutyric acid with W. McK. Marriott, Ibid., 16: 265–280, Nov. 1913
METHOD—
Observations on creatine and creatinine. Ibid., 18: 525–535, Aug. 1914
METHOD—
The iodometric determination of copper and its use in sugar analysis. I. Equilibria in the reaction between copper sulfate and potassium iodide with A. F. Hartmann, Ibid., 45: 349–364, Jan. 1921
(Same) *II. Methods for the determination of reducing sugars in blood, urine, milk, and other solutions* with A. F. Hartmann, Ibid., 365–390
METHOD—
Copper-iodometric reagents for sugar determination with M. Somogyi, Ibid., 100: 695–713, May 1933
See also O. K. O. Folin

Shambaugh, George Elmer, Jr. Chicago otolaryngologist. 1903–
OPERATION—
The surgical treatment of deafness. Illinois med. J., 81: 104–108, Feb. 1942
Surgical treatment of otosclerosis: comparative analysis of results using different technics. Ann. Otol., Rhinol. and Laryng., 51: 817–825, Sept. 1942

Shapiro, P. F. See A. C. Ivy
Shapiro, Shepard. New York physician. 1896–
METHOD—
Hyperprothrombinemia, a premonitory sign of thromboembolization (description of a method). Exper. Med. and Surg., 2: 103–109, May 1944
Sharlit, Herman. New York dermatologist. 1892–
METHOD—
A method for the quantitative estimation of indoxyl compounds in urine. J. biol. Chem., 99: 537–545, Jan. 1933
Sharp, Elwood Armstrong. Detroit physician. 1891–
Described—
An antianemic factor in dessicated stomach. J. A. M. A., 93: 749 (only), Sept. 7, 1929
Sharp, Samuel. English surgeon. 1700–1778
Operated for cataract.
A description of a new method of opening the cornea, in order to extract the crystalline humor. Philos. Trans., 1753, 48: 161–163; 322–331, 1754
Sharpe, J. S. Glasgow physiologist
TEST—
A clinical method for the estimation of calcium in the blood and urine. Edinburgh med. J., 33: 27–30, Jan. 1926
Sharpe, William. New York surgeon. 1882–
OPERATION—use of linen threads.
The operative treatment of hydrocephalus: a preliminary report on forty-one patients. Amer. J. med. Sci., 153: 563–571, Apr. 1917
Sharpey, William. English anatomist. 1802–1880
Wrote early important work on cilia and ciliary motion.
On a peculiar motion excited in fluids by the surfaces of certain animals. Edinburgh Med. and Surg. J., 34: 113–122, July 1, 1830
Sharpey-Schäfer. See Schäfer
Shattock, Samuel George. American physician. 1852–1924
Discovered, in same year but independently of Landsteiner, blood groups.
Chromocyte clumping in acute pneumonia and certain other diseases, and the significance of the buffy coat in the shed blood. J. Path. Bact., 6: 303–314, Feb. 1900
Shattuck, George Cheever. American physician. 1879–
Called attention to occurrence of beri-beri in persons with chronic alcoholism, syphilis, carcinoma and chronic debilitating diseases.
The relation of beri-beri to polyneuritis from other causes. Amer. J. Trop. Med., 8: 539–543, Nov. 1928
Shattuck, Lemuel. Boston schoolmaster. 1793–1859
First promulgated periodic health examinations in America. Garrison
Reported of a general plan for the promotion of public and personal health, devised, prepared, and recommended by the commissioners appointed under a resolve of the legislature of Massachusetts relating to a sanitary survey of the State with N. P. Banks and J. Abbott, Boston, Dutton and Wentworth, State Printers, 1850
Shaw, E(ugene) Clay. Miami, Fla. surgeon. 1896–
METHOD—
The venous spaces of the penis as an avenue for transfusion. J. A. M. A., 90: 446–447, Feb. 11, 1928
MODIFICATION—of phenolsulphonphthalein test.
A study of the curve of elimination of phenolsulphon-

phthalein by the normal and diseased kidneys. J. Urol 13: 575–591, June 1925
Shaw, L. A. See P. Drinker
Shaw-Mackenzie, John Alexander. London physician. 1857–
REACTION—
A study in the diagnosis of cancer by means of serum reactions. Lancet 2: 759–762, Oct. 7, 1922
Shay, Harry. Philadelphia physician. 1898–
TEST—
II. The galactose tolerance test in the differential diagnosis of jaundice with E. M. Schloss and I. Rodin Arch. intern. Med., 47: 650–659, Apr. 1931
Shea, John Joseph. Memphis otolaryngologist. 1889
OPERATON—for fracture of malar bone.
The management of fractures involving the paranasal sinuses. J. A. M. A., 96: 418–421, Feb. 7, 1931
Shear, Murray Jacob. American chemist. 1899–
TEST—
A color reaction associated with vitamin D. Proc. Soc exp. Biol., N. Y., 23: 546–549, Apr. 1926
Sheard, C. See G. M. Higgins, A. H. Sanford
Shedden, W. M. See C. A. Porter
Sheftel, Abraham G. New York physician. 1892–
CHART—
A combined qualitative and quantitative test for sugar in the urine. Med. J. and Rec., 126: 663–664, Dec 7, 1927
Shepherd, Francis J. London surgeon. 1851–1929
FRACTURE—
A hitherto undescribed fracture of the astragalus. J Anat. and Physiol., London, 17: 79–81, Oct. 1882
Sherman, C. P. See I. R. Trimble
Sherman, H. C. See E. C. Kendall
Sherman, J. E. See R. S. Morris
Sherman, Lillian. See A. R. Dochez
Sherren, James. English surgeon. 1872–
"APPENDIX TRIANGLE"—
On the occurrence and significance of cutaneous hyperalgesia in appendicitis. Lancet, 2: 816–821, Sept. 19 1903
TREATMENT—of Ochsner-Sherren.
The causation and treatment of appendicitis. Practitioner, 74: 833–844, June 1905
Sherrington, Charles Scott. English physiologist 1875–
Awarded Nobel prize in 1932, with E. D. Adrian for work on physiology of nerves.
The integrative action of the nervous system. New Haven, Yale Univ. Press, 1906. 411 pp.
LAW—every posterior spinal nerve-root supplies special region of skin. Dorland
Experiments in examination of the peripheral distribution of the fibers of the posterior roots of some spinal nerves. Proc. roy. Soc., 52: 333–337, Dec. 8, 1892
Described association of lateral horn cells with sympathetic outflow. Garrison and Morton
Notes on the arrangement of some motor fibers in the lumbo-sacral plexus. J. Physiol., 13: 621–772, 189
First to study phenomena of "reciprocal innervation." Garrison
Further experimental note on the correlation of action of antagonistic muscles. Proc. roy. Soc., 53: 407–420 May 4, 1893
First to investigate phenomena of "decerebrate rigidity" produced by transection between corpora quadrigemina and thalamus opticus. Garrison

Decerebrate rigidity, and reflex coordination of movements. J. Physiol., 22: 319–332, Feb. 17, 1898

Sherwell, Samuel. Brooklyn dermatologist. 1841–1927

TREATMENT—of cutaneous epitheliomata with acid nitrate of mercury.

Remarks on, and queries as to relative frequency of pathological changes in moles and other tumors on face and head. J. Cutan. and Gen.-Urin. Dis., 5: 9–12, Jan. 1887

Shevky, Marian C. San Francisco scientist

METHOD—

A clinical method for the estimation of protein in urine and other body fluids with D. D. Stafford, Arch. intern. Med., 32: 222–225, Aug. 1923

See also T. Addis

Shiga, Kiyoshi. Japanese physician. 1870–

AGAR—potato blood; culture medium.

Eine Modifikation von Bordet-Gengous Nährboden für die Keuchhustenbacillen nebst einigen Ergebnissen in serologischer Biziehung with N. Imai and Ch. Eguchi, Zbl. Bakt., 69: 104–107, May 3, 1913

BACILLUS—

Ueber den Erreger der Dysenterie in Japan. Ibid., 1 Abt., 23: 599–600, Apr. 12, 1898

Ueber den Dysenteriebacillus (Bacillus dysenteriae). Ibid., 24: 817–828, Dec. 15: 870–874, Dec. 19, 1898

Shipley, Arthur Marriott. Baltimore surgeon. 1878–

OPERATION—for incisional hernia.

Broken-down abdominal incisions: a method of closure. Ann. Surg., 82: 452–457, Sept. 1925

Shipley, Walter C. Hartford, Conn. psychiatrist. 1903–

TEST—Hartford Retreat t. for intellectual impairment.

A self-administering scale for measuring intellectual impairment and deterioration. J. Psychol., 9: 371–377, Apr. 1940

A convenient self-administering scale for measuring intellectual impairment in psychotics with C. C. Burlingham, Amer. J. Psychiat., 97: 1313–1325, May 1941

Shirer, John Wesley. Pittsburgh surgeon. 1899–

MODIFICATION—

Modification of the King operation for bilateral vocal cord paralysis. Ann. Surg., 120: 617–622, Oct. 1944

Shirozy, E. See G. M. Dorrance

Shlaer, Simon. New York biophysicist. 1902–

VISUAL ACUITY MEASUREMENTS—

The relation between visual acuity and illumination. J. gen. Physiol., 21: 165–188, Nov. 20, 1937

See also S. Hecht

Shmamine, Tohl. Tokio physician

BOUILLON—liver serum; for cultivation of spirochetes.

Ueber die Reinzüchtung der Spirochaeta pallida und der nadelförmigen Bakterien aus syphilitischem Material, mit besonderer Berücksichtigung der Reinkultur von Spirochaeta dentium und des Bac. fusiformis aus der Mundhöhle. Zbl. Bakt., 65: 311–337 (323), July 17, 1912

Shoemaker, William Toy. Philadelphia ophthalmologist. 1869–

OPERATION—for ptosis.

Observations on the Motais operation for ptosis: report of three cases. Ann. Ophthal., 16: 608–615, Oct. 1907

Shohl, Alfred Theodore. American pediatrician. 1889–

METHOD—

Determination of the acidity of gastric contents: II. The colorimetric determination of free hydrochloric acid with J. H. King, Johns Hopk. Hosp. Bull., 31: 158–162, May 1920

METHOD—

A rapid and accurate method for calcium in urine with F. G. Pedley, J. biol. Chem., 50: 537–544, Feb. 1922

Demonstrated—

The growth of bacillus coli in urine at varying hydrogen ion concentration with J. H. Janney, J. Urol., 1: 211–229, Apr. 1917

Shoji, K. See A. Sato

Shope, Richard Edwin. American physician. 1901–

PAPILLOMA VIRUS—

A transmissible tumor-like condition in rabbits. J. exp. Med., 56: 793–803, Dec. 1932

VIRUS—Haemophilus influenzae.

Swine influenza. I. Experimental transmission and pathology. Ibid., 54: 349–359, Sept. 1, 1931

Shorr, E. See R. R. Hannon, G. N. Papanicolaou

Shortt, Henry Edward. English physician

METHOD—rapid, for Heidenhein stain.

Note on iron haematoxylin staining. Ind. J. med. Res., 10: 836 (only), Jan. 1923

Cultivated virus of pappataci fever. Garrison and Morton

Cultivation of the viruses of sandfly fever and dengue fever on the chorio-allantoic membrane of the chick-embryo with R. S. Rao and C. S. Swaminath, Ibid., 23: 865–870, Apr. 1936

See also C. S. Swaminath

Shoulders, Harrison H. Nashville surgeon. 1886–

STITCH—

A new stitch for uses in partial gastrectomy. S. G. O., 79: 537–538, Nov. 1944

Shrady, George Frederick. New York surgeon. 1837–1907

SAW—

A new subcutaneous saw, knife, and bone rasp. Med. Rec., 15: 24 (only), Jan. 11, 1879

Shrapnell, Henry Jones. English anatomist

MEMBRANE—

On the form and structure of the membrana tympani. London med. Gaz., 10: 120–124, Apr. 28, 1832

Shunk, Ivan Vaughan. American bacteriologist. 1891–

METHOD—

A modification of Loeffler's flagella stain. J. Bact., 5: 181–187, Mar. 1920

Shute, Evan Vere. London, Ont. obstetrician. 1905–

TEST—

Resistance to proteolysis found in the blood-serum of aborting women. J. Obstet. Gynaec. Brit. Emp., 42: 1071–1084, Dec. 1935

Shwartzman, Gregory. New York physician. 1896–

REACTION or PHENOMENON—

Studies on Bacillus typhosus toxic substances: I. Phenomenon of local skin reactivity go B. typhous culture filtrate. J. exp. Med., 47: 247–268, Aug. 1928

Reactivity of malignant neoplasms to bacterial filtrates. II. Relation of mortality to hemorrhagic necrosis and regression elicited by certain bacterial filtrates. Arch. Path., 21: 509–523, Apr. 1936

Sibson, Francis. English surgeon. 1814–1876
FURROW or GROOVE—
On the external signs of the position of the lungs and heart. London med. Gaz., n. s. 6: 754–760, 1848

Sicard, Jean Athanese. French physician. 1872–1929
OPERATION—to repair defect in cranium.
Plasties du crane par os cranien humain stérilisé with C. Dambrin, Pr. méd., 25: 60–61, Jan. 25, 1917
Used lipiodol in x-ray.
Méthode radiographique d'exploration de la cavité épidurale par le lipiodol with J. Forestier, Rev. neurol., 28: 1264–1266, Dec. 1921
Méthode générale d'exploration radiologique par l'huile iodée (lipiodol) with J. Forestier, Bull. Soc. méd. Hop. Paris, 46: 463–469, Mar. 17, 1922
Advocated sodium salicylate injections for treatment of varicose veins.
Traitement des varices par les injections phlébo-sclérosantes du salicylate de soude with J. Paraf and J. Lermoyez, Gaz. de Hôp., Paris, 95: 1573–1575, Dec. 1922
See also P. E. Brissaud

Sicard, R. French neurologist
SPASM—of facial nerve.
Paralysie faciale provoquée et sympathectomie cervicale supérieure homologue dans l'hémispasme facial "essentiel" with Robineau and Haguenau, Rev. neurol., 34: 343–347, Mar. 3, 1927
Reported idiopathic glossopharyngeal neuralgia.
Olgie vélo-pharyngée essentielle. Traitement chirurgical with Robineau, Ibid., 36: 256–257, Mar. 1920

Sick, Paul. German physician
Reported symptoms of loss of thyroid function following thyroidectomy.
Ueber die totale Exstirpation einer kropfig entarteten Schilddrüse und über die Rückwirkung dieser Operation auf die Circulationsverhältnisse im Kopfe. Med. corresp.-blatt. Stuttgart, 37: 199–205, Aug. 14, 1867

Sicord, A. See G. F. I. Widal

Siddal, Alcines Clair. Cleveland physician. 1897–
TEST—
A suggested test for pregnancy, based on the action of gravid female blood serum on mouse uterus: preliminary report. J. A. M. A., 90: 380–381, Feb. 4, 1928
The hormone test for pregnancy: report II. Ibid., 91: 779–782, Sept. 15, 1928

Sidler-Huguenin, Ernst. Zürich ophthalmologist. 1869–1922
ENDOTHELIOMA—of optic nerve.
Ein Endotheliom am Sehnervenkopf. Arch. f. Ophthal., 101: 113–122, Apr. 13, 1920

Siebert, Conrad. Marburg physician
BROTH—horse meat infusion.
Zur Biologie der Tuberkelbacillen. Zbl. Bakt., 51: 305–320 (305), 1905

Siebold, Adam Elias von. German gynecologist. 1775–1826
Wrote classic account of cancer of uterus. Garrison and Morton
Über den Gebärmutterkrebs, dessen Entstehung und Verhütung. Berlin, Dummler, 1824

Siegel, S. A. See J. S. Diamond

Siegemundin, Justine. Brandenburg midwife. 1650–1705
Advocated puncturing of amniotin sac to arrest

hemorrhage in placenta praevia. Garrison and Morton
Die Chur-Brandenburgische Hoff-Wehe-Mutter. Cölln an der Spree, Liebperten, 1690

Sieur, C. French physician. 1860–
SIGN—same as coin-test.
De la percussion métallique combinée à l'auscultation dans le diagnostic des épanchements liquides de la plèvre. Bordeaux, 1883. 41 pp.

Sigault, Jean Réné. French surgeon. 1740–?
OPERATION—delivery of fetus by symphysiotomy in cases of contracted pelvic outlet. (First performed successfully on Mme. Souchot in 1777.) Garrison
Mémoire (sur la section de la symphyse des os pubis, pratiquée sur la femme Souchot). Paris, Quillau, 1777. 16 pp.

Signorelli, Agnelo. Italian physician. 1876–
SIGN—of renal colic.
Il dolore ritmico pulsante nella colica renale e la patogenesi del dolore in tale sindrome morbosa. Riv. crit. di clin. med., 5: 217–222, Apr. 2, 1904

Silberstein, Fritz. Vienna pathologist
METHOD—for determination of mannitol in plasma.
Bestimmung mehrwertiger alkohole (sorbit, mannit usw.) neben Zucker im Blute. with F. Rappaport and I. Reifer, Klin. Wschr., 16: 1506–1507, Oct. 23, 1937
Detected presence of estrin in tissue of mouse carcinoma and in certain gastro-intestinal cancers in man.
Ueber das Auftreten eines Brunstoffes in Blut und Geweben unter pathologischen Verhaeltnissen. III. Mittheilung with O. O. Fellner and P. Engel, Z. Krebsforsch., 35: 420–427, Feb. 20, 1932

Silbert, Samuel. New York physician. 1894–
TREATMENT—
The treatment of thrombo-angiitis obliterans by intravenous injection of hypertonic salt solution; preliminary report. J. A. M. A., 86: 1759–1761, June 5, 1926
Thrombo-angiitis obliterans (Buerger); XI. Treatment of 524 cases by repeated intravenous injections of hypertonic salt solution; experience of ten years. S. G. O., 61: 214–222, Aug. 1935
See also S. S. Samuels

Sillian, Pierre Marie. French physician
Showed contagious nature of relapsing fever. Garrison and Morton
Fièvre à rechutes. Paris, Thèse No. 205, 1869

Silva, Ferreira da, French physician
REACTION—
Sur une réaction caractéristique de la cocaine. C. R. Acad. Sci., 111: 348–349, 1890

Silvatico, Giambattista. Italian physician. 1550–1621
Wrote first treatise on feigned diseases. Garrison and Morton
De iis qui morborum simulant deprehendis liber. Mediolani, Pontii, 1595

Silver, David. Pittsburgh surgeon. 1873–
OPERATION—
The operative treatment of hallux valgus. J. Bone and Joint Surg., 5: 225–232, Apr. 1923

Silverman, Irving. Brooklyn surgeon. 1904–
NEEDLE—
New biopsy needle. Amer. J. Surg., 40: 671–672, June 1938

Silvester, Henry Robert. English physician. 1829–1908
METHOD—of artificial respiration.
A new method of resuscitating stillborn children and of restoring persons apparently drowned or dead. Brit. med. J., pp. 576–579, July 17, 1858

Simmonds, Morris. German physician. 1855–1925
DISEASE—atrophy of anterior lobe of pituitary gland.
Ueber Hypophysisschwund mit tödlichem Ausgang. Dtsch. med. Wschr., 40: 322–323, Feb. 12, 1914
Ueber Kachexie hypophysären Ursprungs. Ibid., 42: 190–191, Feb. 17, 1916

Simmons, James Stevens. American bacteriologist. 1890–
AGAR—citrate.
A culture medium for differentiating organisms of typhoid-colon aerogenes groups and for isolation of certain fungi. J. infect. Dis., 39: 209–214 (209), Sept. 1926
Proved that Aëdes albopictus is vector of dengue. Garrison and Morton
Experimental studies of dengue with J. H. St. John and F. H. K. Reynolds, Philippine J. Sci., Manila, 44: 1–251, 1931

Simmons, Samuel William. American medical entomologist. 1907–
CAGE—
Surgical maggots in the treatment of infected wounds: a convenient blowfly cage. J. Econ. Entomol., 25: 1191–1193, Dec. 1932
See also W. Robinson

Simms, Henry Swain. New York biochemist. 1896–
MEDIUM—
Use of serum ultrafiltrate in tissue cultures for studying deposition of fat and for propagation of viruses with M. Sanders, Arch. Path., 33: 619–635, May 1942

Simon, Friedrich. German physician
TEST—for free hydrochloric acid in gastric juice.
Eine neue Reaktion auf freie Salzsäure im Mageninhalte Berl. klin. Wschr., 43: 1431 (only), Oct. 29, 1906

Simon, Gustav. Heidelberg surgeon. 1824–1876
OPERATION—repair of lacerated perineum.
Ueber die Heilung der Blasen-Scheidenfisteln. Giessen, Heinemann, 1854
Fälle von Operationen bei Urinfisteln am Weibe. Beobachtung einer Harnleiterscheidenfistel. Dtsch. Klin., pp. 310–312, July 26, 1856
POSITION—
Ueber die Methoden, die weibliche Urinblase zugängig zu machen und über di Sondirung der Harnleiter beim Weibe. Samml. klin. Vortr., Leipzig, No. 88, (Gynäk. No. 28), 649–676, 1875
First in Europe to excise kidney. Garrison
Exstirpation einer Niere am Menschen. Dtsch. Klinik, 22: 137–138, Apr. 9, 1870
Chirurgie der Nieren. I Theil. Glückliche Exstirpation einer Niere zur Heilung einer Harnleiter-Bauchfistel. Erlangen, Enke, 1871. 89 pp.

Simon, O. German chemist
TEST—
Glykogennachweis im Harn. Pharm. Zentralh., n. F., 24: 478 (only), July 23, 1903

Simon, Theodor. French physician. 1873–
TEST—Binet-Simon t.
Documents relatifs à la corrélation entre le développe-

ment physique et la capacité intellectuelle. Paris, 1900. 69 pp.
See also Alfred Binet

Simond, P. L. See E. G. Marchoux

Simons, Arthur. Berlin physician. 1877–
DISEASE—progressive lipodystrophie.
Eine seltene Trophoneurose („Lipodystrophia progressiva"). Z. ges. Neurol. Psychiat., 5: 29–38, Apr. 29, 1911

Simons, Irving. New York urologist. 1884–
MICROCYSTOMETER—
The microcystometer. A portable instrument for cystometry and sphincterometry. J. Urol., 34: 493–498, Nov. 1935
Studies in bladder function II. The sphincterometer. Ibid., 35: 96–102, Jan. 1936

Simpson, Frank Edward. Chicago dermatologist. 1868–
Described—
Kératodermie blennorrhagique: with report of a case. J. A. M. A., 59: 607–612, Aug. 24, 1912

Simpson, Sir James Young. Edinburgh obstetrician. 1811–1870
FORCEPS—obstetrical.
On a suction-tractor, or new mechanical power, as a substitute for the forceps in tedious labours. Edinburgh Month. J. med. Sci., 9, 1848–49
SOUND—uterine.
Contributions to the pathology and treatment of diseases of the uterus. Part II. On the measurement of the cavity of the uterus as a means of diagnosis in some of the morbid states of that organ. Ibid., 3: 547; 701; 1009, 1843; 4; 208, 1844
Introduced chloroform in obstetrics.
Anesthetic and other therapeutic properties of chloroform. Ibid., 8, 1847–48
Also: Medico-Chir. Soc. of Edinburgh, Nov. 16, 1847
On a new anesthetic agent, more efficient than sulphuric ether. Lancet, 2: 549–550, Nov. 20, 1847
Discovery of a new anesthetic agent, more efficient than sulphuric ether. Lond. med. Gaz., n. s. 5: 934–937, Nov. 26, 1847
An account of a new anesthetic agent, as a substitute for sulphuric ether in surgery and midwifery. Edinburgh, Sutherland and Knox, 1847
Also: New York, Rushton, Clarke and Co., 1848
Also: Philadelphia, Lindsay and Blakiston, 1849
Also in: *Epoch-making contributions to medicine, surgery and the allied sciences.* By C. N. B. Camac, Phiadelphia, Saunders, 1909. pp. 377–389

Simpson, Mariam E. See H. McL. Evans

Simpson, Samuel Levy. English physician
TREATMENT—
The use of synthetic desoxycorticosterone acetate in Addison's disease. Lancet, 2: 557–558, Sept. 3, 1938

Simpson, William Kelly. New York laryngologist. 1855–1914
SPLINT—
The use of the Bernays asceptic sponge in the nose and nasopharynx, with special reference to its use as a pressure haemostatic. New York med. J., 68: 474–476, Oct. 1, 1898

Sims, J. Marion. American gynecologist. 1813–1883

METHOD—
Amputation of the cervix uteri. Trans. New York med. Soc., Albany, pp. 367–371, 1861
OPERATION—
Remarks on cholecystotomy in dropsy of the gallbladder. Brit. med. J., 1: 811–815, June 8, 1878
OPERATION—for vesico-vaginal fistula.
SPECULUM—
On the treatment of vesico-vaginal fistula. Amer. J. med. Sci., n. s. 23: 59–82, 1852
Also in: Medical classics, 2: 677–712, Mar. 1938
Introduced—
Silver sutures in surgery. New York, Wood, 1858
Sinding-Larsen, Christian Magnus Falsen. Norwegian physician
DISEASE—epiphysitis at accessory center of ossification at apex of patella.
Ein hittel ukjendt sygdom i patella. Norsk. Mag. f. Laegevidensk., 82: 856–858, Dec. 1921
Singer, J. J. See E. A. Graham
Singleton, Albert O. Galveston, Texas surgeon. 1882–1947
INCISION—
Improvement in the management of upper abdominal operations, stressing the advantages of an anatomical incision. South. med. J., 24: 200–206, Mar. 1931
OPERATION—
One-stage perineo-abdominal operation for cancer of the rectum. Surgery, 14: 691–701, Nov. 1943
Sinkler, Wharteon. Philadelphia neurologist. 1847–1910
Isolated great toe reflex. Garrison
The toe reflex. Med. News, 53: 611–612, Dec. 1, 1888
Sinton, John Alexander. English physician. 1884–
SOLUTION—glucose serum; culture medium.
A clinical method for the cultivation of the parasite of Indian relapsing fever (Spirochaeta carteri). Ind. J. med. Res., 11: 825–828 (826), Jan. 1924
Sippy, Bertram Welton. Chicago physician. 1866–1924
METHOD or TREATMENT—
Gastric and duodenal ulcer; medical cure by an efficient removal of gastric juice corrosion. J. A. M. A., 64: 1625–1630, May 15, 1915
Sistrunk, Walter Ellis. Rochester, Minn. surgeon. 1880–1933
MODIFICATION—
Further experiences with the Kondolean operation for elephantiasis. J. A. M. A., 71: 800–806, Sept. 7, 1918
OPERATION—
The surgical treatment of cysts of the thyroglossal tract. Ann. Surg., 71: 121–122, Jan. 1920
Sjögren, Henrik Samuel Conrad. Stockholm ophthalmologist. 1899–
SYNDROME—
Zur Kenntnis der Keratoconjunctivitis sicca (Keratitis filiformis bei hypofunktion der Tränendrüsen). Acta Ophth., Suppl. 2, 1933. 151 pp.
Zur Kenntnis der Keratoconjunctivitis sicca. IV. Mikroskopische Untersuchungen über das initialstadium der Drüsenveränderungen. Ibid., 16: 70–79, 1938
A new conception of keratoconjunctivitis sicca. Transl. into English by J. B. Hamilton, Sydney, Australasian Med. Pub. Co., 1943
Sjögren, Tage Anton Ultimus. Swedish physician. 1859–1939
First to use successfully Röntgen rays in treatment of cancer.

Fall af epitheliom behandladt med Röntgenstraler. Förhandl. vid Svenska Läkare-Sallskapets Sammankonister, Stockholm, 1899, 208
Sjöqvist, Carl Olof. Stockholm neurosurgeon. 1901–
OPERATION—tractotomy for trigeminal neuralgia.
Studies on pain conduction in the trigeminal nerve: a contribution to the surgical treatment of facial pain. Acta psychiat. et neurol., (supp.), 17: 1–139, 1938
Eine neue Operationsmethode bei Trigeminusneuralgie: Durchschneidung des Tractus spinalis trigemini. Zbl. Neurochir., 2: 274–281, Jan. 1938
Sjöqvist, John August. Swedish physician. 1863–
METHOD—for determination of combined hydrochloric acid in stomach contents.
Eine neue Methode, freie Salzsäure im Mageninhalte quantitativ zu bestimmen. Z. phys. Chem., 13: 1–11, 1887
See also C. A. H. Mörner
Sjöström, Per Magnus. Lund surgeon
TEST—
The citric acid content in blood serum in disease of the liver and bile ducts: a new test of the liver function. Acta chir. Scand., 78: 252–253, June 1936
Skelton, Ruth F. See R. H. A. Plimmer
Skene, Alexander Johnston Chalmers. New York gynecologist. 1837–1900
DUCT, GLANDS, TUBULES—
The anatomy and pathology of two important glands of the female urethra. Amer. J. Obstet., 13: 265–270, Apr. 1880
Also in: *Treatise on the diseases of women.* New York, Appleton, 1889. 966 pp. pp. 614–615
Skinner, R. C.
Wrote first American book on teeth.
A treatise on the human teeth. . . . New York, Wood, 1801. 26 pp.
Skoda, Joseph. Bohemian physician. 1805–1881
RESONANCE, RÂLE, SIGN, TYMPANY—
Abhandlung über Perkussion und Auskultation. Vienna, Mosle und Braumüller, 1839. 271 pp.
THEORY—of heart beat.
Über den Herzstoss und die durch die Herzbewegungen verursachten Töne. Med. Jahrb. d. k. k. österr. Staates, Wien, n. F. 13: 227–266, 1837
Skorczewski, W. Lemberg physician
REACTIONS—for cinchophen in urine.
Ueber einige im Atrophanharne auftretende charakteristische Reaktionen. Wien. klin. Wschr., 24: 1700 (only), Dec. 7, 1911
Slawyk, Dr. Berlin physician
Described influenzal meningitis.
Ein Fall von Allgemeininfection mit Influenzabacillen. Z. Hyg. InfektKr., 32: 443–448, 1899
Sloan, Guy Arthur. Bloomington, Ill. surgeon. 1889–
INCISION—transverse.
A new upper abdominal incision. S. G. O., 45: 678–687, Nov. 1927
Sloan, LeRoy Hendrick. Chicago physician. 1892–
Described first case of tularemia in which B. tularense was found in sputum.
Tularemic pneumonia with A. S. Freedberg and J. C. Ehrlich, J. A. M. A., 107: 117–119, July 11, 1936
Sloan, Louise Littig. Baltimore psychologist. 1898–
TESTS—
Instruments and technics for the clinical testing of light sense: III. An apparatus for studying regional

differences in light sense. Arch. Ophthal., 22: 233–251, Aug. 1939

Slotta, K. H. Breslau chemist
Prepared hormone progesterone in crystalline form.
Reindarstellung der Hormon aus dem Corpus luteum, III Mitteil.: Konstitution von Luteosteron C und D with H. Ruschig and E. Blanke, Ber. dtsch. chem. Ges., 67: 1947–1954, Nov. 7, 1934

Sluder, Greenfield. St. Louis laryngologist. 1865–1928
OPERATION—
A method of tonsillectomy by means of a guillotine and the alveolar eminence of the mandible. J. A. M. A., 56: 867–871, Mar. 25, 1911
SYNDROME—
The rôle of the sphenopalatine (or Meckel's) ganglion in nasal headaches. New York med. J., 87: 989–990, May 23, 1908
The syndrome of sphenopalatine-ganglion neurosis. Amer. J. med. Sci., 140: 868–878, Dec. 1910

Slye, Maude. Chicago pathologist. 1879–
Did important work on heredity of cancer.
The incidence and inheritability of spontaneous cancer in mice. (Preliminary report). Z. f. Krebsforsch., Berlin, 13: 500–504, 1913
The incidence and inheritability of spontaneous tumors in mice. (Second report). J. med. Res., 30: 281–285, July 1914
(Same) *(Third report).* Ibid., 32: 159–200, Mar. 1915

Smedley, Ralph D. English physician
AGAR—blood infusion.
The cultivation of trypanosomata. J. Hyg., 5: 24–47 (28), Jan. 1905

Smellie, William. British obstetrician. 1697–1763
SCISSORS—used in craniotomy. Introduced steel-lock forceps in 1744 and curved and double-curved forceps during 1751–1753; first differentiated contracted from normal pelves by actual measurement. Garrison
A treatise on the theory and practice of midwifery. London, Wilson and Durham, 1752. 454 pp.

Smith, A. H. See B. Cohen
Smith, Allen John. American pathologist. 1863–1926
SOLUTION—litmus milk; culture medium.
Lessons and laboratory exercises in bacteriology. Philadelphia, Blakiston, 1906. p. 106
Smith, C. D. See B. Haskell
Smith, Carl Henry. New York City pediatrician. 1895–
Described—
Infectious lymphocytosis. Amer. J. Dis. Child., 62: 231–261, Aug. 1941
Acute infectious lymphocytosis: specific infection. Report of four cases showing its communicability. J. A. M. A., 125: 342–349, June 3, 1944
Smith, Clinton Kitto. Kansas City urologist. 1883–
OPERATION—
Surgical procedure for correction of hypospadias. J. Urol., 40: 239–247, July 1938
Smith Papyrus, Edwin. Egyptian surgical work 2500 B. C.–1700 B. C.
Published with translation by J. H. Breasted. Chicago, Univ. Press, 1930. 2 vols.
Smith, Erwin Frink. Washington, D. C. pathologist. 1854–1927
AGAR—infusion; culture medium.

Pseudomonas campestris (Pammel). The cause of a brown rot in cruciferous plants. Zbl. Bakt., 2 Abt., 3: 478–486 (480), Sept. 10, 1897
SOLUTION—potato infusion; culture medium.
Bacteria in relation to plant diseases. Washington, D. C , Carnegie Inst., 1905. pp. 285
Smith, Eugene. Detroit ophthalmologist. 1845–1927
OPERATION—
Treatment of irido-dialysis from contusion, partial iridenkeisis, with or without suture. Trans. Sect. Ophth., Amer. Med. Ass., pp. 285–287, 1891
Smith, Eustace. London physician. 1835–1914
MURMUR or SIGN—
On the diagnosis of enlarged bronchial glands in children. Lancet, 2: 240–241, Aug. 14, 1875
Smith, F. J. See C. I. Allen
Smith, Harry Pratt. Iowa City physician. 1895–
TEST—for prothrombin.
Clinical and experimental studies on vitamin K with S. E. Ziffren, C. A. Owen and G. R. Hoffman. J. A. M. A., 113: 380–383, July 29, 1939
See also E. D. Warner, S. E. Ziffren
Smith, Henry. English surgeon in India. 1823–1894
OPERATION—for hemorrhoids.
In his: *The surgery of the rectum.* London, 1865. 127 pp. p. 92
OPERATION—
Extraction of cataract in the capsule. Indian Med. Gaz., Calcutta, 35: 240–246, 1900
Smith, Homer Erastus. Norwich, N. Y. ophthalmologist. 1856–1928
OPERATION—
The advantages of a preliminary capsulotomy especially in immature cataracts. Arch. Ophthal., 41: 1–7, July 1912
Smith, Homer William. New York physiologist. 1895–
TEST—diodrast clearance t. of—
The measurement of the tubular excretory mass, effective blood flow and filtration rate in the normal human kidney with W. Goldring and H. Chasis, J. clin. Invest., 17: 263–278, May 1938
Smith, J. Blackburn. Irish pathologist. 1865–1928
METHOD—
Note on the staining of flagella. Brit. med. J., 1: 205–206, Jan. 26, 1901
Smith, J(ames) Lorrain. Manchester physician. 1862–1931
STAIN—for lipoids.
On the simultaneous staining of neutral fat and fatty acid by oxazine dyes. J. Path. Bact., 12: 1–4, 1908
Smith, L. W. See T. S. Fay
Smith, Letchworth. American bacteriologist
METHOD—
Flagella staining with night blue. J. med. Res., 6: 341–343, Nov. 1901
Smith, Maurice Isadore. Washington, D. C. physician. 1887–
METHOD—of essaying ergonovine.
A quantitative colorimetric reaction for the ergot alkaloids and its application in the chemical standardization of ergot preparations. Publ. Health Rep., 45: 1466–1481, June 27, 1930
Smith, Millard. Boston scientist. 1895–
TEST—
A micro-modification of the method of Benedict for the quantitative determination of reducing sugar in urine. J. Lab. clin. Med., 7: 364–368, Feb. 1922

Smith-Petersen, Marius Nygaard. Boston surgeon. 1886–
INCISION—
A new supra-articular subperiosteal approach to the hip joint. Amer. J. Orthop. Surg., 15: 592–595, Aug. 1917
METHOD—use of vitallium cap.
Arthroplasty of the hip: a new method. J. Bone and. Joint Surg., 21: 269–288, Apr. 1939
NAIL—
Intracepsular fractures of the neck of the femur: treatment by internal fixation with E. F. Cave and G. W. Van Gorder, Arch. Surg., 23: 715–759, Nov. 1931
Treatment of fractures of the neck of the femur by internal fixation. S. G. O., 64: 287–295, Feb. 15, 1937
OPERATION—
Arthrodesis of the sacroiliac joint: a new method of approach. J. Ortbrop. Surg., 3: 400–405, Aug. 1921
Smithwick, Reginald Hammerick. Boston surgeon. 1899–
OPERATION—
A technic for splanchnic resection for hypertension: preliminary report. Surgery, 7: 1–8, Jan. 1940
Surgical treatment of hypertension: the effect of radical (lumbodorsal) splanchnicectomy on the hypertensive state of one hundred and fifty-six patients followed one to five years. Arch. Surg., 49: 180–193, Sept. 1944
OPERATION—
Modified dorsal sympathectomy for vascular spasm (Raynaud's disease) of the upper extremity: a preliminary report. Ann. Surg., 104: 339–350, Sept. 1936
TREATMENT—injections of alcohol.
Elimination of pain in obliterative vascular disease of the lower extremity with J. C. White, S. G. O., 51: 394–403, Sept. 1930
See also J. C. White
Smyth, Andrew Woods. New Orleans surgeon. 1832–1916
Reported—
Report of a successful operation in a case of subclavian aneurism. New Orleans, 1864. 15 pp.
Successful operation for subclanian aneurism. Amer. J. med. Sci., 52: 280–282, July 1866
First to successfully ligate innominate artery. Garrison
A case of successful ligature of the innominate artery. New Orleans J. Med., 22: 464–469, July 1869
Smyth, Henry Field. Pennsylvania physician. 1875–
AGAR—egg trypsinized peptone.
A new medium for the cultivation of chick tissues in vitro, with some additions to the technic. J. med. Res., 31: 255–259 (255), Nov. 1914
Snapper, Isidore. Groningen physician. 1889–
TEST—
Der spektroskopische Nachweis von Blut in den Fäces. Berl. klin. Wschr., 53: 975–977, Aug. 28, 1916
Snapper, J. See A. A. H. van den Bergh
Snell, Albert Markley. Rochester, Minn. physician. 1896–
METHOD—of reestablishing normal prothrombin clotting time by oral administration of antihemorrhagic substances.
Treatment of the hemorrhagic tendency in jaundice; with special reference to vitamin K with H. R. Butt

and A. E. Osterberg, Amer. J. Digest. Dis., 5: 590–596, Nov. 1938
See also H. R. Butt, W. Walters, R. M. Wilder
Snell, Esmond Emerson. Texas biochemist. 1914–
METHOD—for assay of avidin and biotin.
A quantitative test for biotin and observations regarding its occurrence and properties with R. E. Eakin and R. J. Williams, J. Amer. Chem. Soc. 62: 175–178, Jan. 1940
Snellen, Hermann. Utrecht ophthalmologist. 1834–1908
TEST-TYPE—for vision.
Probebuchstaben, zur Bestimmung der Sehschärfe. Utrecht, van de Weijer, 1862. 6 pp.
Snow, John. York physician. 1813–1858
ETHER APPARATUS—
On the inhalation of the vapour of ether in surgical operations; containing a description of the various stages of etherization, and a statement of the result of nearly eighty operations in which ether has been employed in St. George's and University College Hospitals. London, Churchill, 1847. 88 pp.
First stated theory that cholera is water-borne and is taken into system by the mouth. Garrison
On the mode of communication of cholera. London, Churchill, 1849. 31 pp.
Same, 2 ed., 1855
Same, 2 ed., reprinted. New York, Commonwealth Fund, 1936
Snow, William. New York City physician. 1898–
Introduced—
Roentgen visualization of the placenta with C. B. Powell, Amer. J. Roentgenol., 31: 37–40, Jan. 1934
Soames, Katherine M. See R. Robison
Sobel, Albert Edward. New York biochemist. 1906–
METHOD—
A convenient method of determining small amounts of ammonia and other bases by the use of boric acid with H. Yuska and J. Cohen, J. biol. Chem., 118: 443–446, Apr. 1937
Sobel, Leo Lucius. Basel bacteriologist
AGAR—lactose beer.
Praktische Nährböden zur Diagnose von Cholera, Typhus und Dysenterie. Dtsch. med. Wschr., 41: 1573 (only), Dec. 30, 1915
Soberheim, Joseph Friedrich. German physician. 1803–1846
Introduced term "myocarditis."
Akute idiopathische Herzentzündung. In his: *Praktische Diagnostik.* Berlin, 1837. pp. 118–120
Soboleff, L. W. See L. W. Ssobolew
Soden, John Smith. London surgeon. 1780–1863
Advocated—
Case of inguinal aneurism, cured by tying the external iliac artery. Med.-chir. Trans., 7: 536–540, 1816
Söhngen, N. L. Delft scientist
SOLUTION—basal.
Einfluss von Kolloiden auf mikrobiologische Prozesse. Zbl. Bakt., 2 Abt., 38: 621–647 (628), Sept. 20, 1913
See also P. E. Verkade
Soemmering, Samuel Thomas von. Frankfurt a. M. physician. 1755–1830
FORAMEN—fovea centralis.
SPOT—macula lutea.
Abbildungen des menschlichen Auges. Frankfurt a. M., Varrentrapp und Wenner, 1801. 110 pp.
Icones oculi humani. Francof. a. M., 1804. 94 pp.

NUMBERING—of cranial nerves.
De basi encephali et originibus nervorum cranio egredientium libri quinque. Goettingae, Thesis, April, 1778. 184 pp.
Described, independently, line of Gennari in cerebral cortex.
Vom Hirn- und Rückenmark. Mainz, Winkopp und Komp, 1788. 115 pp. pp. 18–20
Described achondroplasia. Garrison
Abbildungen und Beschreibungen einiger Misgeburten, die sich ehewals auf dem anatomischen Theater zu Cassel befanden. Mainz, 1791. 38 pp. p. 30, pl. XI

Sørensen, S. P. L. Copenhagen scientist
Investigated buffer salts and hydrogen-ion concentration. Garrison
Enzymstudien. II. Mitteilung. Über die Messung und die Bedeutung der Wasserstoffionenkonzentration bei enzymatischen Prozessen. Biochem. Z., 21: 131–304, 1909
See also V. Henriques

Soffer, L. J. See G. A. Harrop

Solis-Cohen, Jacob DaSilva. American surgeon. 1838–1927
Operated for cancer of larynx.
Removal of a fibrous polyp from the inferior anterior surface of the right vocal cord with the aid of the laryngoscope. Amer. J. med. Sci., n. s., 53: 403–407, Apr. 1867
Sequel to case of laryngeal polyp. Ibid., 54: 565–566, Oct. 1867

Soliterman, P. See B. Klein

Sollmann, Torald Hermann. Minnesota physician. 1874–
Described carotid sinus depressor reflex.
The blood pressure fall produced by traction on the carotid artery with E. D. Brown, Amer. J. Physiol., 30: 88–104, Apr. 1, 1912

Solms, Eugen. Berlin physician
METHOD—of determining peptic activity.
Ueber eine neue Methode der quantitativen Pepsinbestimmung und ihre klinische Verwendung. Z. f. klin. Med., 64: 159–169, 1907

Somma, Luigi. Italian pediatrician. 1834–1884
Reported cases of infantile splenic anemia (von Jaksch's disease).
Sull'anemia splenica infantile: patologia e clinica. Arch. di patol. inf., Napoli, 2: 21–29, 1884

Sommer, René. German surgeon. 1891–
OPERATION—for slipping patella.
Die traumatischen Verrenkungen der Gelenke. Neue deutsche Chirurgie. Stuttgart, 1928. V. 41

Sommer, Robert. German psychiatrist. 1864–1937
Introduced new methods in psychopathological investigation.
Lehrbuch der psychopathologischen Untersuchungsmethoden. Berlin, Wien, Urban und Schwarzenberg, 1899

Somogyi, Michael. St. Louis biochemist. 1883–
METHOD—of preparation of yeast suspension.
Reducing non-sugars and true sugar in human blood. J. biol. Chem., 75: 33–43, Oct. 1927
METHOD—for determination of reducing sugars in blood.
Notes on sugar determination. Ibid., 52: 599–612, Nov. 1926
A reagent for the copper-iodometric determination of very small amounts of sugar. Ibid., 117: 771–776, Feb. 1937

METHOD—of determination of amylolytic activity in serum.
TEST—for acute pancreatitis.
Micromethods for the estimation of diastase. Ibid., 125: 399–414, Sept. 1938
Diastatic activity of human serum. Arch. intern. Med., 67: 665–679, Mar. 1941
METHOD—for determination of serum amylase.
Blood diastase in health and diabetes. J. biol. Chem., 134: 315–318, June 1940
See also C. A. Good, P. A. Shaffer

Sonden, K. Scandinavian physiologist
RESPIRATION CALORIMETER—
Untersuchungen über die Respiraion und den Gesammstoffwechsel des Menschen with R. Tigerstedt, Skandin. Arch. f. Physiol., 6: 1–224, 1895

Sonne, Carl Olaf. Copenhagen physician. 1882–
BACILLUS—
Ueber die Bakteriologie der giftarmen Dysenteriebacillen (Paradysenteriebacillen). Zbl. Bakt., 75: 408–456, Feb. 15, 1915

Sonnenfeld, A. Berlin physician
TREPHINE—
Zur Technik der Sternalpunktion. Dtsch. med. Wschr., 1380 (only), Aug. 17, 1928

Sonnenschein, F. L. Berlin scientist
REACTION—for blood.
Ueber ein neues Reagens auf Blut und Anwendung desselben in der forensischen Chemie. Viertelj. f. gerich. Med., 17: 263–266, 1872

Sordelli, E. See H. H. Corelli

Soresi, Agnelo Louis. New York surgeon. 1877–
CANNULA, TRANSFUSION APPARATUS—
Transfusion directe du sang et anastomose provisoire des vaisseaux sanguins avec un nouvel instrument. 16 Cong. Internat. d. Med., Budapest, 1909, p. 458
A new method of direct transfusion of blood, with report of cases and remarks on transfusion in general. New York med. J., 93: 622–626, Apr. 1, 1911
A new instrument for transfusion of whole blood. J. A. M. A., 84: 591–592, Feb. 21, 1925
OPERATION—
Exteriorization and utilization of the sac and redundant peritoneum in the radical treatment of inguinal hernia. Amer. J. Surg., 10: 130–135, Oct. 1930
OPERATION—
Intramural gastrostomy. Ibid., 36: 668–671, June 1937

Soskin, Samuel. Chicago physiologist. 1904–
TEST—intravenous glucose tolerance t.
Endocrine disturbances in the regulation of the blood sugar. Clinics, 1: 1286–1309, Feb. 1943

Soto-Hall, Ralph. San Francisco surgeon. 1899–
REACTION—neck flexion with tension on ligamentum nuchae causes pain at site of fracture of any vertebral body.
A useful diagnostic sign in vertebral injuries with K. O. Haldeman, S. G. O., 61: 827–831, Dec. 1935

Sottas, J. See J. J. Déjérine

Sotteau, Augusté Joseph Henrí. French surgeon. 1802–1851
OPERATION—
De la cure radicale de la hernie inguinale réductible. Grand, Gyselynck, 1840. 45 pp.

Sottery, C. T. See L. P. Hammett

Soubeiran, Eugène. French chemist. 1793–1858
Discovered chloroform, independently, but in same year as von Liebig.

Recherches sur quelques combinaisons du chlore. Ann. de chim., Paris, 48: 113–157, 1831
Soule, S. D. See T. K. Brown
Souligoux, Antoine Léonce Charles. French surgeon. 1865–1929
METHOD—of gastrostomy.
Gastrostomie par la procédé de la torsion de Souligoux. By Ed. Schwartz, Bull. Soc. de Chir. de Paris, 28: 815–819, July 16, 1902
Gastrostomie par torsion. Ibid., 37: 818 (only), June 7, 1911
Souques, Achille. French neurologist. 1860–
Described camptocormy; bent back seen in soldiers. Garrison
La camptocormie; incurvation du tronc, consécutive aux traumatismes du dos et des lombes: considérations morphologiques with Mme. Rosenoff-Saloff, Rev. neurol., 28: 937–939, Nov.–Dec. 1915
Sourdille, Maurice Louis Joseph Marie. French otologist
OPERATION—tympanolabyrinthopexy.
The present position of the surgical treatment of otosclerosis. J. Laryng. and Otol., 53: 78–83, Jan. 1938
Southey, Reginald S. English physician. 1835–1899
TUBES—for relief of anasarca.
Chronic parenchymatous nephritis of right kidney. Left kidney small and atrophie. Old scrofulous pyelitis. Trans. Clin. Soc. London, 10: 152–157, 1877
Traitement de l'anasarque general par un drainage capillaire. C. R. Assn. franc. pour l'avancement d. sci., 6: 856, 1877
Southworth, Hamilton. New York physician. 1907–
SYMPTOM COMPLEX—
Hematuria, abdominal pain and nitrogen retention associated with sulfapyridine with C. Cooke, J. A. M. A., 112: 1820–1821, May 6, 1939
Souttar, Henry Sessions. London surgeon. 1875–
TREPHINE—
Hunterian lecture on new methods of surgical access to the brain. Brit. med. J., 1: 295–300, Feb. 25, 1928
TUBE—
A method of intubating the oesophagus for malignant stricture. Ibid., 1: 782–783, May 3, 1924
Soutter, Robert. Boston surgeon. 1870–1933
OPERATION—
A new operation for slipping patella. J. A. M. A., 82: 1261–1262, Apr. 19, 1924
Souza-Leite. See P. Marie
Soxhlet, Franz von. German chemist. 1848–1926
METHOD—for glucose estimation in urine.
Das Reductions-Verhältniss der Zuckerarten zu alkalischen Kupferlösungen. Chem. Zbl., 49: 218–224, Apr. 3; 236–240, Apr. 10, 1878
TEST—for fats in milk. Garrison
Beiträge zur physiologischen Chemie der Milch. Leipzig, Metzger u. Wittig., 1872. 54 pp.
Spalding, Alfred Baker. San Francisco gynecologist 1874–
OPERATION—for uterine prolapse.
A study of frozen sections of the pelvis with description of an operation for pelvic prolapse. S. G. O., 29: 529–536, Dec. 1919
Spallanzani, Lazaro. Italian anatomist. 1729–1799
One of first to dispute doctrine of spontaneous generation. Garrison and Morton
Saggio di osservazioni microscopiche relative al sistema della generazione. Modena, 1767
Founder of doctrine of regeneration of spinal cord;

one of the pioneers of experimental morphology. Garrison
Prodromi sulla riproduzione animale: riproduzione della coda del girino. Modena, 1768
Wrote "On the action of the heart. . . ."
Dell'azione del cuore ne'vasi sanguigni; nuove osservazioni. (Modena, Montanari, 1768). 71 pp.
Discovered digestive power of saliva, and reaffirmed solvent property of gastric juice, showing that it will act outside the body, and that it can not only prevent putrefaction but will inhibit it when once begun. Garrison
Della digestione degli animale. In his: *Fisica animale e veg. . . .* Venezia, 1782. 1: 1–312; 2: 1–83
First to note that tissues consume oxygen and produce carbon dioxide.
Memoirs on respiration. Published posthum. by Senebier, London, Robinson, 1804. 373 pp. p. 352
Sparkman, Robert Satterfield. Cincinnati physician. 1912–
TECHNIC—
Studies of urobilinogen. I. A simple and rapid method for quantitative determination of urobilinogen in stool and in urine. Arch. intern. Med., 63: 858–866; 872–883, May 1939
Spatz, H. See J. Hallervorden
Spaulding, Harry Van Ness. New York surgeon. 1885–
OPERATION—
The traumatic shoulder with special reference to rupture of the supraspinatus tendon. Amer. J. Surg., 43: 298–309, Feb. 1939
Spee, Ferdinand Graf von. German anatomist. 1855–
CENTRAL LAYER OF—
Ueber den Bau der Zonulafasern und ihre Anordnung im menschlichen Auge. Anat. Anz., 21, Erg., 236–242, 1902
Speed, James Spencer. Memphis, Tenn. surgeon. 1890–
OPERATION—fusion of ankle.
Operative reconstruction of malunited fractures about the ankle joint with H. B. Boyd, J. Bone and Joint Surg., 18: 270–286, Apr. 1936
Speed, Kellogg. Chicago surgeon. 1879–
OPERATION—
Recurrent anterior dislocation at the shoulder; operative cure by bone graft. S. G. O., 44: 468–477, Apr. 1927
Spemann, Hans. German biologist. 1869–
Awarded Nobel prize in 1935 for "discovery of the organizing effect during the development of the embryo."
Über Induktion von Medullarplatte durch Medullarplatte im jüngeren Keim, ein Beispiel homöogenetischer oder assimilatorischer Induktion. By O. Mangold and H. Speman, Arch. f. EntwMech. Org., 111: 341–422, Oct. 28, 1927
Neue Arbeiten über Organisatoren in der tierischen Entwicklung. Naturwissenschafter, 15: 946–951, Dec. 2, 1927
Organizers in animal development. Proc. roy. Soc., 102: 177–187, Dec. 1927
Über den Anteil von Implantat und Wirtskeim an der Orientlierung und Beschaffenheit der induzierten Embryonalanlage. Arch. f. AntwMech. Org., 123: 389–517, Feb. 20, 1931
Spencer, Walter. London dermatologist

DISEASE—
Spencer's disease: dermatitis multiformis exfoliativa.
London, Pewtress, 1899. 16 pp.
(Simply infection by Staphylococcus aureus; named
Spencer's disease by Spencer himself.)
Spencer, Walter George. English surgeon
OPERATION—
Plastic operations on the thumb. Med. Sc. Abst. and
Rev., 3: 29–35, Oct. 1920
Spencer, William H. Philadelphia physician. 1854–
1924
METHOD—
*Gastro-intestinal studies. VIII. A method for the
quantitative estimation of trypsin in the gastric con-
tents.* J. biol. Chem., 21: 165–167, May 1915
Spengler, Carl. Swiss physician. 1861–1937
AGAR—glycerol somatose, for cultivation of tubercle
bacilli.
*Tuberkelbacillenzüchtung aus Bakteriengemischen und
Formaldehyddesinfection.* Z. Hyg. InfektKr., 42:
90–114 (92), 1903
SERUM, TREATMENT—of pulmonary tuberculo-
sis.
*Einfluss der spezifischen ,,I. K." (Immunkörper)—
Therapie C. Spenglers auf die Zerstörung der Tuber-
kuloseerreger. Ein Beitrag zum Schicksal des Tuberkel-
bazillenproteins im tuberkulösen Organismus. II.* By
A. Kirchensten (From the Privatlaboratorium C.
Spengler), Z. f. Tuberk., 20: 521–581, Sept. 1913
Spens, Thomas. Edinburgh physician. 1769–1842
SYNDROME—bradycardia with syncopal attacks;
Adams-Stokes' disease.
*History of a case in which there took place a remarkable
slowness of the pulse.* Med. Commentaries, 1792,
Edinburgh, 7: 458–465, 1793
Sperry, Warren M. See R. Schoenheimer
Spiegelberg, Otto. German gynecologist. 1830–1881
SIGN—of malignancy of cervix; a feeling like that of
friction against wet india-rubber on palpation with
finger.
*Die Diagnose des ersten Stadium des Carcinoma colli
uteri; mit Bemerkungen zur Anatomie und Therapie.*
Arch. Gynaek., 3: 233–240, 1872
Spiegler, Eduard. Vienna dermatologist. 1860–1908
TEST—
Eine empfindliche Reaction auf Eiweiss im Harne.
Ber. dtsch. chem. Ges., 25: 375–378, 1892
Spielmeyer, Walther. German pathologist
METHOD—for myelin sheaths in frozen sections.
Mallory
*Technik der mikroskopischen Untersuchungen des
Nervensystems.* Berlin, Springer, 1930. 4 ed., p. 97
Spies, Tom Douglas. Cincinnati physician. 1902–
Noted that porphyrinuria accompanying pellagra
consists of coproporphyrin I and III.
The use of nicotinic acid in the treatment of pellagra
with C. Cooper and M. A. Blankenhorn, J. A. M. A.,
110: 622–627, Feb. 26, 1928
*The treatment of subclinical and classic pellagra: use
of nicotinic acid, nicotinic acid amide and sodium
nicotinate, with special reference to the vasodilator
action and the effect on mental symptoms* with W. B.
Bean and R. E. Stone, Ibid., 111: 584–592, Aug.
13, 1938
Spiller, William Gibson. Philadelphia neurologist.
1864–1940

OPERATION—
*The division of the sensory root of the trigeminus for
relief of tic douloureux; an experimental, pathological
and clinical study, with a preliminary report of one
surgically successful case* with C. H. Frazier, Phila-
delphia med. J., 8: 1039–1049, Dec. 14, 1901
Suggested—
*The treatment of cerebral palsies and athetosis by nerve
anastomosis and transplantation* with C. H. Frazier,
J. nerv. ment. Dis., 32: 310–317, May 1905
Advocated—
*The treatment of persistent pain of organic origin in
the lower part of the body by division of the antero-
lateral column of the spinal cord* with E. Martin,
J. A. M. A., 58: 1489–1490, May 18, 1912
See also C. H. Frazier
Spiro, H. S. See M. R. Moffatt
Spiro, Karl. Strassburg physiochemist. 1867–1932
REACTION—for hippuric acid.
Ueber Nachweis und Vorkommen des Glycocolls. Z.
physiol. Chem., 28: 174–191, Aug. 10, 1899
Noted that urea in strong solution is able to "dis-
solve" proteins.
*Ueber die Beeinflussung der Eiweisscoagulation durch
stickstoffhaltige Substanzen.* Ibid., 30: 182–199, Aug.
16, 1900
Isolated ergotamine.
Über die wirksamen Substanzen des Mutterkorns
with A. Stoll, Schweiz. med. Wschr., Basel, 2: 525–
529, 1921
Spitz, J. See J. L. M. Lignieres
Spitzer, Alexander. Vienna anatomist
THEORY—of incomplete torsion in causation of
cardiac defects.
*Ueber den Bauplan des normalen und missbildeten
Herzens. Versuch einer phylogenetischen Theorie.*
Arch. path. Anat., 243: 81–272, May 25, 1923
Spitzka, Edward Charles. New York neurologist.
1852–1914
BUNDLE, COLUMN, NUCLEUS, TRACT—
The comparative anatomy of the pyramid tract. J.
comp. Med. and Surg., 7: 1–61, Jan. 1886
Spitzy, Hans. Vienna surgeon. 1872–
OPERATION—
*Stabilization of the shoulder joint for habitual disloca-
tion.* S. G. O., 46: 256–257, Feb. 1928
Spivack, Julius L. Chicago surgeon. 1889–
METHOD—
Eine neue Methode der Gastrostomie. Beitr. z. klin.
Chir., 147: 308–318, Aug. 7, 1929
*Utilization of the posterior wall of the stomach in
valvulo-tubular gastrostomy in case of small and con-
tracted stomach.* Clin. Med. and Surg., 40: 212–213,
Apr. 1933
Spratt, Charles Nelson. Minneapolis ophthalmol-
ogist. 1874–
OPERATION—
The pocket flap in cataract extraction. Amer. J.
Ophthal., 11: 347–351, May 1928
Pocket-flap sclerecto-iridodialysis in glaucoma. J. A.
M. A., 101: 1615–1619, Nov. 18, 1933
Spray, Robb Spalding. Morgantown, W. Va. bac-
teriologist. 1890–
METHOD—for rapid identification of gas gangrene
anaerobes.

An example of anaerobic dissociation. J. Bact., 25: 51–52, Jan. 1933

SOLUTION—

A blood-clot digest medium for cultivation of hemophilic and other bacteria. Ibid., 13: 14 (only), Jan. 1927

Sprengel, Kurt Polykarp Joachim. Pomeranian botanist. 1766–1833

The greatest medical historian of the 18th century. Garrison

Versuch einer pragmatischen Geschichte der Arzneikunde. Halle, Gebauer, 1792–1803. 5 vols.

Sprengel, Otto Gerhard Karl. Dresden surgeon. 1852–1915

DEFORMITY—congenital upward displacement of scapula.

Die angeborene Verschiebung des Schulterblattes nach oben. Arch. f. klin. Chir., 42: 545–549, 1891

Spronck, C. H. H. Utrecht physician

SOLUTION—yeast infusion peptone.

Préparation de la toxine diphthérique; suppression de l'emploi de la viande. Ann. Inst. Pasteur, 12: 701–704, Oct. 1898

Sprunt, Thomas Peck. Baltimore physician. 1884–

Introduced term infectious mononucleosis.

Mononuclear leucocytosis in reaction to acute infections ("infectious mononucleosis)" with F. A. Evans, Johns Hopk. Hosp. Bull., 31: 410–417, Nov. 1920

Spurling, Roy Glenwood. Louisville, Ky. surgeon. 1894–

TECHNIC—

Spasmodic torticollis: notes upon its etiology and treatment with F. Jalsma, South. med. J., 26: 237–241, Mar. 1933

Spurzheim, Johann Caspar. French neurologist. 1776–1832

See F. J. Gall

Squier, John Bentley. New York surgeon. 1873–

OPERATION—

Supra-pubic intra-urethral enucleation of the prostate. Boston Med. and Surg. J., 164: 911–917, June 29, 1911

Squire, Peter. London physician

ETHER INHALER—

On the inhalation of the vapour of ether, and the apparatus used for the purpose. Pharm. J. and Trans., 6: 350–352, Feb. 1, 1847

Squire, Trumann Hoffman. American surgeon. 1823–1889

CATHETER—

Synopsis of some important improvements in the treatment of obstinate organic stricture of the urethra and urinary fistulae. Boston Med. and Surg. J., 77: 401–406, Dec. 19, 1867

Ssobolew, Leonid Wassilyevitch. St. Petersburg pathologist. 1876–

Found that ligation of pancreatic excretory ducts led to atrophy of acinous tissue, islands of Langerhans remaining intact.

Zur normalen und pathologischen Morphologie der inneren Secretion der Bauchspeicheldrüse. (Die Bedeutung der Langerhans'schen Inseln.) Arch. f. path. Anat., Berlin, 168: 91–128, May 3, 1902

Stack, J. K. See P. B. Magnuson

Stacke, Ludwig. German otologist. 1859–1918

OPERATION—removal of mastoid and contents of tympanum.

Indicationen, betreffend die Excision von Hammer und Amboss. Verh. d. internat. Med. Cong., Berlin, 4, 11 Abth., 43–46, 1890

Weitere Mittheilungen über die operative Freilegung der Mittelohrräume nach Ablösung der Ohrmuschel. Berl. klin. Wschr., 29: 68–71, Jan. 25, 1892

Stadelmann, Ernst. Königsberg physiochemist. 1855–

Studied B-oxybutyric acid in relation to diabetic coma. Garrison

Ueber die Ursachen der pathologischen Ammoniakausscheidung beim Diabetes mellitus und des Coma diabeticum. Arch. f. exper. Path. u. Pharm., Leipzig, 17: 419–444, Nov. 20, 1883

Worked out, with M. Afanassyeff, experimental pathology of toxemic and hemolytic jaundice. Garrison

Der Icterus und seine verschiedenen Formen. Nebst Beiträgen zur Physiologie und Pathologie der Gallensecretion. Stuttgart, Enke, 1891. 287 pp.

Stadnichenko, A. See H. C. Sweany

Stähli, Jean. Zürich ophthalmologist

LINE—

Ueber den Fleischerschen Ring beim Keratokonus und eine neue typische Epithelpigmentation der normalen Kornea. Klin. Mbl. Augenheilk., 60: 721–741, June 1918

Stafford, D. D. See M. C. Shevky

Stafford, Richard Anthony. English surgeon. 1801–

Described sarcoma of prostate.

• *A case of enlargement from melanoid tumour of the prostate gland, in a child of five years of age.* Med.-chir. Trans., 22: 218–221, 1839

Stahl, Friedrich Karl. German physician. 1811–1873

EAR—

Einige Skizzen über Missgestaltungen des äusseren Ohres. Allg. z. f. Psychiat., 16: 479–490, 1859

Stahl, Georg Ernst. Bavarian physician. 1660–1734

Wrote early work on diseases of portal system. Garrison

De vena portae, porta malorum. 1698

Wrote original account of lacrimal fistula. Garrison

De fistula lachrymali. Halle, 1702

Stainsby, W. J. See R. L. Cecil

Stallworthy, John. English surgeon

SPECULUM—modification of Graves'.

A useful speculum. Brit. med. J., 2: 696–697, Nov. 15, 1941

Stamm, Martin. Fremont, Ohio surgeon. 1847–1918

METHOD—

Gastrostomy by a new method. Med. News, 65: 324–326, Sept. 22, 1894

Stammler, D. German surgeon

REACTION—for cancer serum.

Ueber neuere Methoden der serologischen Krebsdiagnose. Verh. dtsch. Ges. f. Chir., 40: 558–580, (Abst. 136–141), 1911

Stanculeanu, Georges. Bucharest surgeon. 1874–

OPERATION—for cataract.

Intrakapsuläre Staroperationen. Klin. Mbl. Augenheilk., 527–537, May 1912

Standfuss, Richard. Berlin veterinarian

SOLUTION—bone jelly; culture medium.

Ein neuen Bakteriennährboden. Zbl. Bakt., 85: 223–224, Oct. 12, 1920

Stanford, R. V. English chemist
TEST—for indican in urine.
Indigobildende Substanzen im Harn (,,Harnindi-kan)". I. Mitteilung. Z. physiol. Chem., 87: 188–206, Sept. 11, 1913
(Same) *II. Mitteilung. Neue qualitative Proben.* Ibid., 88: 47–55, Oct. 14, 1913

Stanley, Edward. London surgeon. 1793–1862
Described—
A case of disease in the posterior columns of the spinal cord. Med.-chir. Trans., 23: 80–84, 1840

Stanley, Wendell Meredith. American chemist. 1904–
First to isolate a virus, the virus of tobacco mosaic disease, and demonstrated that it is a protein.
Isolation of a crystalline protein possessing the properties of tobacco-mosaic virus. Science, 81: 644–645, June 28, 1935
Properties of virus proteins with H. S. Loring, Cold Spring Harbor Symp. Quant. Biol., 6: 341–360, 1938

Stanley-Brown, Margaret. See F. W. Bancroft, A. J. Quick

Stannius, Herman Friedrich. German biologist. 1808–1883
LIGATURE OF—between sinus venosus and auricle, of frog's heart.
Versuche am Froschherzen. Arch. f. Anat., Physiol. u. wiss. Med., 85–100, 1852
Confirmed Bell's law with fish.
Das peripherische Nervensystem der Fische, anatomisch und physiologisch Untersucht. Rostock, Stiller, 1849. 156 pp.

Stannus, Hugh Stannus. English physician. 1877–
Described—
A sixth venereal disease: climatic bubo, lymphogranuloma inguinale, esthiomene, chronic ulcer and elephantiasis of the genito-ano-rectal region, inflammatory stricture of the rectum. London, Baillière, Tindall and Cox, 1933

Stanski, Pierre-Gáetan. French physician. 1807–1879
Described bone lesions in parathyroid overfunction.
Du ramollissement des os en général, et de celui du sieur Potiron en particulier. Paris Thesis, 1839. 72 pp.

Stanton, William B. American physician. 1872–
SPHYGMOMANOMETER—
A practical clinical method for determining blood pressure in man, with a discussion of the methods heretofore employed. Univ. Penn. Med. Bull., 15: 466–475, Feb. 1903

Starin, William Alfred. American bacteriologist. 1878–
BROTH—casein digest veal infusion.
Agglutination studies of Clostridium botulinum with Gail M. Dock, J. infect. Dis., 33: 169–183 (173), Aug. 1923

Starkey, Robert Lyman. New Jersey soil bacteriologist. 1899–
SOLUTION—basal ammonium sulphate.
Concerning the physiology of thiobacillus thiooxidans, an autotrophic bacterium oxidizing sulfur under acid conditions. J. Bact., 10: 135–163 (138), Mar. 1925

Starling, Ernest Henry. English physiologist. 1866–1927
LAW—of heart.
THEORY—mechanical, of edema.
Discovered functional significance of serum proteins.

The influence of mechanical factors on lymph production. J. Physiol., 16: 224–267, 1894
On the absorption of fluids from the connective tissue spaces. Ibid., 19: 312–326, May 5, 1896
The Linacre lecture on the law of the heart, given at Cambridge, 1915. London, Longmans, 1918. 27 pp.
Used term hormone.
On the chemical correlation of the functions of the body. Lancet, 2: 339–341, Aug. 5; 423–425, Aug. 12; 501–503, Aug. 19; 579–583, Aug. 26, 1905
Demonstrated that tubules of kidney re-absorb water.
The secretion of urine as studied on the isolated kidney with E. B. Verney, Proc. roy. Soc., S. B., 97: 321–363, Feb. 2, 1925
See also W. M. Bayliss, Janet E. Lane-Claypon

Starr, Isaac. Philadelphia physician. 1895–
TEST—
The value of the cutaneous histamine reaction in the prognosis of pedal lesions in diabetes mellitus. After-histories of 89 patients for five years. Amer. J. med. Sci., 188: 548–554, Oct. 1934

Starry, A. C. See A. S. Warthin

State, D. See M. Levine

Stead, E. A. See M. I. Gregersen

Stearns, John. Waterford, N. Y. physician. 1770–1848
Introduced use of ergot in obstetrics.
Account of the pulvis parturiens, a remedy for quickening childbirth. Med. Reposit., 5: 308–309, 1808

Steel, Matthew. New York chemist. 1879–
MODIFICATION—
An improvement of the Folin method for the determination of urinary ammonia nitrogen. J. biol. Chem., 8: 365–379, Nov. 1910

Steele, A. H. See N. S. Ferry

Steele, Graham. Manchester physician. 1851–1942
MURMUR—
The murmur of high-pressure in the pulmonary artery. Med. Chronicle, 9: 182–188, 1888
Also in: F. A. Willius and T. E. Keys' *Cardiac classics.* St. Louis, Mosby, 1941. pp. 680–685

Steenbock, Harry. Wisconsin chemist. 1886–
Separated vitamin A from vitamin D.
Fat-soluble vitamine. VII. The fat-soluble vitamine and yellow pigmentation in animal fats with some observations on its stability to saponification with Mariana Sell and Mary Van Buell, J. biol. Chem., 47: 89–109, June 1921

Steensma, F. A. Dutch pathologist
REAGENT—for hydrochloric acid in gastric juice.
Zum Nachweis der freien Salzsäure im Mageninhalt. Biochem. Z. 8: 210–211, 1908
TEST—for bile pigments.
Een vereenvoudiging van de reactie van Huppert-Salkowski voot het opsporen van galkleurstoffen in urine. Ned. Tijdschr. Geneesk., 45: 1567–1569, Nov. 20, 1909
TEST—for urobilogen in urine.
Kleine Mitteilungen aus der Praxis der pathologischen Chemie. Berl. klin. Wschr., 45: 177–178, Jan. 27, 1908

Steenstrup, Johannes Japetus Smith. Swedish physician. 1813–1897
THEORY—of alternation of generation.
Om Formplantning og Udvikling gjennem vexlende

Generationsraekker. Kjøbenahvn, Reitzel, 1842
Also, English transl. London, Roy. Soc., 1845
Steffenhagen. See Potjan
Stefko, P. L. See A. H. Blakemore
Stehle, Raymond Louis. American-Canadian pharmacologist. 1888–
METHOD—
Gasometric determination of nitrogen and its application to the estimation of the non-protein nitrogen of blood. J. biol. Chem., 45: 223–228, Dec. 1920
Steiger, Marguerite. Zurich scientist
Synthesized desoxy-corticosterone acetate, a steroid compound capable of preventing death from adrenal insufficiency.
Partial synthesis of a crystallized compound with the biological activity of the adrenal-cortical hormone with T. Reichstein, Nature, 139: 925–926, May 29, 1937
Desoxy-cortico-steron (21-Oxy-progesteron) aus Δ5-3-Oxy-ätio-cholensäure with T. Reichstein, Helvet. chim. acta, 20: 1164–1179, 1937
Steigmann, A. Heidelberg chemist
REACTION—
Reaktionen des bestrahlten Ergosterins (D-Vitamin). Kolloid-Zeit., 45: 165–166, June 1928
Stein, Harry Charles. New York surgeon. 1890–
OPERATION—
Hallux valgus. S. G. O., 66: 889–898, May 1938
Stein, Herbert Edward. New York surgeon. 1883–
OPERATION—
Inguinal hernioplasty: a new modification. Report of 107 cases. Surgery, 5: 398–404, Mar. 1939
Inguinal hernia; a new concept and operation. Amer. J. Surg., 56: 480–482, May 1942
Stein, L. See C. Berens
von Stein, Stanislav Aleksandr Fyodorovich. Russian otologist. 1855–
TEST—for disease of labyrinth.
Ucheniya o funktsiyakh otdielnikh chastel ushnavo labirinta. Moskva, 1892. 841 pp.
Die Lehre von den Funktionen der einzelnen Theilen des Ohrlabyrinths. Jena, Fischer, 1894
Steinach, Eugen. Vienna surgeon. 1861–1944
OPERATION—ligation of vas deferens for impotence.
Die Verjüngung durch experimentelle Neubelebung der alternden Pubertätsdrüsen. Berlin, Springer, 1920
Described effects of ovarian hormone.
Willkürliche Umwandlung von Säugetier-Männchen in Tiere mit ausgeprägt weiblichen Geschlechtscharakteren und weiblicher Psyche. Arch. ges. Physiol., 144: 71–108, Feb. 2, 1912
Über die biologischen Wirkungen des weiblichen Sexualhormones with M. Dohrn, W. Schoeller, W. Hohlweg and W. Faure. Ibid., 219: 306–324, Apr. 12, 1928
Steinberg, Bernhard. Toledo pathologist. 1897–
PREPARATIONS—preoperative.
An improved method of protecting the peritoneum of dogs against fatal colon bacillus infection. Proc. Soc. exp. Biol., N. Y., 29: 1018–1019,May 1932
The expermental background and the clinical application of the Escherichia coli and gum tragacanth mixture (coli-bactragen) in prevention of peritonitis. Amer. J. clin. Path., 6: 253–277, May 1936
Steinberg, I. See G. P. Robb
Steindler, Arthur. Iowa City surgeon. 1878–
OPERATION—transplantation of extensor hallucis tendon for paralysis of anterior tibial muscle.

Operative treatment of pes cavus. S. G. O., 24: 612–615, May 1917
OPERATION—arthrodesis of wrist.
Orthopedic operations on the hand. J. A. M. A., 71: 1288–1291, Oct. 19, 1918
OPERATION—
Flexor plasty of the thumb in thenar palsy. S. G. O., 50: 1005–1007, June 1930
POSTERIOR SYNDROME—of low back pain.
Differential diagnosis of pain low in the back: allocation of the source of pain by the procaine hydrochloride method with J. V. Luck, J. A. M. A., 110: 106–113, Jan. 8, 1938
TREATMENT—
The conservative compensation-derotation treatment of scoliosis with C. W. Ruhlin, J. Bone and Joint Surg., 23: 67–80, Jan. 1941
Steinert, Hans. Leipzig physician
DISEASE or TYPE—dystrophia myotonica, type Batten-Steinert-Curschmann.
Myopathologische Beiträge. I. Über das klinische und anatomische Bild des Muskelschwunds der Myotoniker. Dtsch. Z. Nervenheilk., 37: 58–104, July 25, 1909
Steinhardt, Edna. See A. Besredka
Steinheim, Soloman Levi. German physician. 1789–1866
Described parathyroid tetany.
Zwei seltene Formen von hitzigen Rheumatismus. Litt. Ann. d. ges. Heilk., Berlin, 17: 22–30, 1830
Steinhöwel, Heinrich. 1420–1482
Wrote famous book on pestilence. Garrison and Morton
Buchlein der Ordnung der Pestilenz. Ulm, Zainer, 1473
Steinle, John Vernon. Wisconsin chemist. 1898–
REACTION—
A new method for the identification and estimation o cholesterol and certain other compounds with L Kahlenberg, J. biol. Chem., 67: 425–467, Feb. 1926
Steinman, Fritz. Bern surgeon. 1872–1932
PIN—for skeletal traction in fracture treatment.
Eine neue Extensionsmethode in der Frakturenbehandlung. Zbl. Chir., 34: 938–942, Aug. 10, 1907
Steinschneider, Moriz. Breslau physician. 1816–1907
AGAR—hydrocele fluid.
Zur Differenzirung der Gonokokken. Berl. klin. Wschr., 27: 533–537, June 16, 1890
Steinthal, C. Stuttgart surgeon
CLASSIFICATION—of cancers of breast; I local, II with axillary metastasis, III entire breast.
Zur Dauerheilung des Brustkrebses. Arch. f. klin. Chir., 86: 775–785, 1908
Weitere Mitteilungen über operative Dauerheilungen beim Mammacarcinom. Beitr. z. klin. Chir., 78: 669–680, 1912
Stellwag, Carl. Austrian oculist. 1823–1904
SIGN or SYMPTOM—apparent widening of palpebral opening in exophthalmic goiter.
Ueber gewisse Innervationsstörungen bei der Basedow'schen Krankheit. Med. Jb., 17: 25–54, 1869
Stenbuck, J. B. See J. F. Connors
Stengel, Alfred, Jr. Philadelphia physician. 1910–
APPARATUS—
An apparatus for continuous intravenous injections in unanesthetized animals with H. M. Vars, J. Lab. clin. Med., 24: 525–529, Feb. 1939

METHOD—
The maintenance of nutrition in surgical patients, with a description of the orojejunal method of feeding with I. S. Ravdin, Surgery, 6: 511–519, Oct. 1939
Stensen, Niels. Danish anatomist. 1638–1686
DUCT or CANAL—excretory, of parotid gland.
Observationes anatomicae, quibus varia oris, oculorum, et narium vasa describuntur, novique salivae. . . . Lugduni Batavorum, Chouet, 1662. 108 pp.
Recognized muscular nature of heart. Garrison
Grasped significance of fibrillar structure of skeletal muscle. Fulton
De musculis et glandulis observationum specimen cum epistolis duabus anatomicis. Copenhagen. Godicchenii, 1664. 84 pp.
Also: Amstelodanum, Le Grand, 1664. 90 pp.
Also, in part, transl. by M. N. Walso in: F. A. Willius and T. E. Keys' *Cardiac Classics.* St. Louis, Mosby, 1941. p. 104 (only)
Stenvers, Hendrik Willem. German roentgenologist. 1889–
POSITION—for x-ray of skull.
Röntyenologie des Felsenbeines und des bitemporalen Schädelbildes. . . . Berlin, Springer, 1928. 278 pp.
Stephens, J. G. See J. Barcroft
Stephens, John William Watson. English physician. 1865–
Discovered T. rhodesiense. Garrison and Morton
On the peculiar morphology of a trypanosome from a case of sleeping sickness and the possibility of its being a new species (T. rhodesiense). Proc. roy. Soc., S. B., 83: 28–33, 1910
See also A. A. Kanthack
Stephenson, William. Scottish obstetrician. 1837–1908
WAVE—
On the menstrual wave. Amer. J. Obstet., 15: 287–294, Apr. 1882
Stepp, Wilhelm. Strassburg physiochemist. 1852–
Discovered existence of fat-soluble vitamins without fully realizing it. Garrison and Morton
Versuche über Fütterung mit lipoidfreier Nahrung. Biochem. Z., 22: 452–460, 1909
Stern, K. See R. Willheim
Stern, Margarete. German scientist
TEST—modification of Wassermann t.
Eine Vereinfachung und Verfeinerung der serodiagnostischen Syphilisreaktion. Z. ImmunForsch., 1: 422–438, Feb. 10, 1909
Ueber die Bewertung der unsicheren und „paradoxen" Reaktionen bei der serodiagnostischen Untersuchung der Syphilis. Ibid., 5: 201–235, Mar. 26, 1910
Stern, Maximilian. New York surgeon. 1877–
RESECTOSCOPE—
Minor surgery of the prostate gland—a new cystoscopic instrument employing a cutting current capable of operation via water medium. Internat. J. Med. and Surg., 39: 72–77, Feb. 1926
Stern, Suzanne. See E. H. Goodman
Stern, Walter Gustav. Cleveland surgeon. 1874–1941
TEST—
The intracutaneous salt solution wheal test: its value in disturbances of the circulation in the extremities with M. B. Cohen, J. A. M. A., 87: 1355–1358, Oct. 23, 1926
Stern, Wilhelm. German bacteriologist

BROTH—basal fuchsin sulphite.
Studien zur Differenzierung der Bakterien der Coli-Typhus-Gruppe mittels gefärbter, flüssiger Nährböden.
Beiträge zur Biologie der Bakteriengruppe Paratyphus B-Enteritidis. Zbl. Bakt., 78: 481–492 (483), Nov. 18, 1916
Sternberg, Carl. Vienna pathologist. 1872–1935
CELLS—in Hodgkin's disease.
Über eine eigenartige unter dem Bilde der Pseudoleukämie verlaufende Tuberculose des lymphatisches Apparates. Z. f. Heilkunde, 19: 21–90, 1898
Universelle Primärerkrankungen des lymphatischen Apparates. Zbl. f. d. Grenzg. d. Med. u. Chir., 2: 641–650, Aug. 15, 1899, et seq.
DISEASE—leukosarcoma.
Leukosarkomatose und Myeloblastenleukämie. Beitr. path. Anat., 61: 75–100, 1915
Sternberg, George Miller. American bacteriologist. 1838–1915
BACILLUS—micrococcus lanceolatus.
Discovered a pneumococcus in same year as Pasteur, and independently.
A fatal form of septicemia in the rabbit, produced by the subcutaneous injection of human saliva. Rep. Nat. Bd. Health, 1881, Washington, 3: 87–92, 1882
METHOD—of testing bacteria for thermal death-point.
The thermal death-point of pathogenic organisms. Amer. J. med. Sci., 187: 146–160, July 1887
Sternberg, Maximilian. Vienna physician. 1863–
TEST—for bile.
Zum Nachweis des Bilirubins. Biochem. Z., 171: 217 (only), Apr. 21, 1926
Suggested term—
Pericarditis epistenocardica. Wien. med. Wschr., 60: 14–23, Jan. 1, 1910
Sternberg, T. See J. E. Moore
Stetten, DeWitt. American surgeon. 1879–
INSTRUMENT—
An improved colostomy spur crusher. Amer. J. Surg., 5: 327–328, Oct. 1928
OPERATION—
Further observations on a modified inguinal herniaplasty technic, with completed utilization of the aponeurosis of the external oblique. Ann. Surg., 78: 48–60, July 1923
Steuart, W. South African physician
APPARATUS—
Demonstration of apparatus for inducing artificial respiration for long periods. Med. J. So. Africa, 13: 147–150, Mar. 1918
Steudel, H. See A. Kossel
Stevens, Albert Mason. New York pediatrician. 1884–
DISEASE or SYNDROME—
A new eruptive fever associated with stomatitis and ophthalmia; report of two cases in children with F. C. Johnson, Amer. J. Dis. Child., 24: 526–533, Dec. 1922
Stevens, Edward
First to isolate gastric juice and to perform in vitro digestion. Garrison and Morton
Dissertatio physiologica inauguralis de alimentorum concoctione. Edinburgi, Balfour et Smellie, 1777. 56 pp.
Also, English transl. in: Spallanzani's *Dissertation relating to the natural history of animals.* 1784

Stevens, George Thomas. New York ophthalmologist. 1832-1921
OPERATION—
Tendon resection and tendon contraction for shortening the recti muscles. New York med. J., 49: 345-348, Mar. 30, 1889
PHOROMETER, TROPOMETER—
Classified motor anomalies of eye.
A system of terms relating to the conditions of the ocular muscles known as "insufficienties." Ibid., 44: 624-627, Dec. 4, 1886
The anomalies of the ocular muscles. Arch. Ophthal., 16: 149-176, 1887
Treatise on the motor apparatus of the eyes, embracing an exposition of the anomalies of ocular adjustments and their treatment; . . . Philadelphia, Davis, 1906. 496 pp.

Stevens, H. W. See S. B. Wolbach

Stevens, William. Santa Cruz surgeon. 1786-1868
Tied internal iliac successfully, Dec. 27, 1812. Garrison and Morton
A case of aneurism of the gluteal artery, cured by tying the internal iliac. Med.-chir. Trans., London, 5: 422-434, 1814

Stewart, Alexander Patrick. Scottish physician. 1813-1883
Separated typhoid and typhus fevers. Garrison and Morton
Some considerations on the nature and pathology of typhus and typhoid fever, applied to the solution of the question of the identity or non-identity of the two diseases. Edinburgh Med. and Surg. J., 54: 289-339, 1840

Stewart, Charles. Archangel surgeon
Described paroxysmal hematuria. Garrison
Account of a singular periodical discharge of blood from the urethra, terminating successfully. Med. Comment., Edinburgh, 1794, 9: 332-336, 1795

Stewart, F(rances) Constance. Albany, N. Y. physician. 1891-
METHOD—
A note on Petroff's cultural method for the isolation of tubercle bacilli from sputum and its application to the examination of milk. J. exp. Med., 26: 755-761, Dec. 1, 1917
See also A. B. Wadsworth

Stewart, Francis Torrens. Philadelphia surgeon. 1874-1920
INCISION—
Amputation of the breast by a transverse incision. Ann. Surg., 62: 250-251, Aug. 1915
(Same title) Trans. Amer. Surg. Ass., 33: 363-368, 1915

Stewart, George Neil. Canadian-American scientist. 1860-1930
CALORIMETER, METHOD—for estimating quantity of blood circulating through a part.
Studies on the circulation in man: the blood flow in the hands and feet in normal and pathological cases. Harvey Lectures, Series 1912-13, pp. 86-149
ESTIMATION—of epinephrine.
So-called biological tests for adrenalin in blood, with some observations on arterial hypertonus. J. exp. Med., 14: 377-400, Oct. 1911
See also J. M. Rogoff

Stewart, J. D. See M. I. Gregersen

Stewart, Jeremiah Clark. Minneapolis surgeon. 1854-1914
OPERATION—
The radical treatment of epithelioma of the lip. J. A. M. A., 54: 175-178, Jan. 15, 1910

Stewart, Purves. London physician
SIGN—
Paralysis agitans: with an account of a new symptom. Lancet, 2: 1258-1260, Nov. 12, 1898

Stewart, R. M. British neurologist
SYNDROME—
Localized cranial hyperostosis in the insane. J. Neurol. Psychopath., 8: 321-331, Apr. 1928

Stewart, Ulmont P. U. S. Army surgeon
REAGENT—
A new contact test for albumin in urine. J. A. M. A., 71: 1050 (only), Sept. 28, 1918

Stewart, W. H. See H. L. Lynah

Steyrer, Anton. German physician
METHOD—for quantitative determination of ammonia in urine.
Über osmotische Analyse des Harns. Beitr. z. chem. Phys. u. Path., 2: 312-335, July 1902
Invented a calorimeter. Garrison
Ueber den Stoff- und Energieumsatz bei Fieber, Myxödem und Morbus Basedowii. Z. exp. Path. Ther., 4: 720-746, Dec. 21, 1907

Stickel, J. E. San Francisco bacteriologist
SOLUTION—blood clot digest; culture medium.
SOLUTION—tryptic digest; culture medium.
Peptic and tryptic digestive products as inexpensive culture mediums for routine bacteriological work with K. F. Meyer, J. infect. Dis., 23: 68-81, July 1918

Sticker, Georg. German physician. 1860-
DISEASE—
Die neue Kinderseuche in der Umgebung von Giessen (Erythema infectiosum). Z. f. prakt. Aerzte, Frankfurt a. M., 8: 353-358, June 1, 1899

Stieda, Alfred. Königsberg surgeon. 1869-
DISEASE—Pellegrini-Stieda's d.; calcification of tibial collateral ligament following injury.
Über eine typische Verletzung am unteren Femurende. Arch. f. klin. Chir., 85: 815-826, 1908

Stierlin, Eduard. German physician. 1878-1919
SIGN—ulceration of colon demonstrated by x-ray.
Die Radiographie in den Diagnostik der Ileozoekaltuberkulose und anderer Krankheiten des Dickdarms. Münch. med. Wschr., 58: 1231-1235, 1911

Stieve, Hermann D. Leipzig anatomist. 1886-
Described pyloric sphincter.
Der Sphincter antri pylori des menschlichen Magens. Anat. Anz., 51: 513-534, Mar. 10, 1919

Stiles, Charles Wardell. Washington, D. C. scientist. 1867-1941
Described—
A new species of hookworm (Uncinaria americana) parasitic in man. Amer. Med., 3: 777-778, May 10, 1902

Stiles, Sir Harold Jalland. British surgeon. 1863-
OPERATION—
Epispadias in the female and its surgical treatment, with a report of two cases. Trans. Amer. Surg. Ass., 29: 11-61, 1911
OPERATION—for flexion deformity of fingers due to interossei muscle paralysis. In his: *Treatment of injuries of the peripheral spinal nerves* with Maude

Frances Forrester-Brown, London, Oxford Univ. Press, 1922. 180 pp. pp. 167–171

Stiles, John Alden. Madison, Wis. physician. 1905–
Used cyclopropane (trimethylene) clinically.
Cyclopropane as an anesthetic agent: a preliminary clinical report with W. B. Neff, E. A. Rovenstine and R. M. Waters, Curr. Res. Anaesth. and Analg., 13: 56–60, Mar.–Apr. 1934

Still, Sir George Frederic. London physician. 1868–1941
DISEASE or SYNDROME—
On a form of chronic joint disease in children. Med.-chir. Trans., 80: 47–59, 1897

Stiller, Berthold. Budapest physician. 1837–1922
DISEASE—habitus asthenicus.
THEORY—gastroptosis is due to universal asthenia characterized by weakness and laxity of viscera.
Die asthenische Konstitutionskrankheit (Asthenia universalis congenita, Morbus asthenicus.) Stuttgart, Enke, 1907. 228 pp.

Stilling, Benedict. German anatomist. 1810–1879
BUNDLE—solitary fasciculus of oblongata.
Ueber die Medulla oblongata. Erlangen, Enke, 1843. 72 pp.

Stillman, E. See F. M. Allen, D. D. Van Slyke

Stillman, Ernest Goodrich. New York pathologist. 1884–
CLASSIFICATION—of pneumococcus.
A study of atypical type II pneumococci. J. exp. Med., 29: 251–258, Mar. 1919

Stimson, Arthur Marston. American physician. 1876–
Discovered a spirochaete which was later called Leptospira icterohaemorrhagiae.
Note on an organism found in yellow-fever tissue. U. S. Publ. Health Rep., Washington, 22: 541, 1907

Stimson, Lewis Atterbury. American surgeon. 1844–1917
APPARATUS—combined traction and suspension for fractures of femur.
In his: *A practical treatise on fractures and dislocations.* New York and Philadelphia, Lea and Febiger, 1910. 6 ed., pp. 100–101
METHOD—of reducing dislocation of hip.
Five cases of dislocation of the hip. New York med. J., 50: 118–121, Aug. 3, 1889
Early contributor to technic of total abdominal hysterectomy.
Ligation of the uterine arteries in their continuity as an early step in total or partial abdominal hysterectomy. Abstr.: New York med. J., 49: 277–278, Mar. 9, 1889
On some modifications in the technique of abdominal surgery, limiting the use of the ligature en masse. Med. News, 55: 93–96, July 27, 1889

Stirling, William. English physician. 1851–1932
GENTIAN VIOLET—
Some recent and some new histological methods. J. Anat. and Physiol., 24: 601–610, July 1890
Wrote on summation of electrical stimuli to skin.
Garrison and Morton
Über die Summation elektrischen Hautreize. Arb. a. d. Physiol. Anst. zu Leipzig, 1874, 9: 223–291, 1875

Stitt, Edward Rhodes. American bacteriologist. 1867–
AGAR—glycerol egg; for cultivation of tubercle bacilli.
In his: *Practical bacteriology, blood work and animal parasitology.* Philadelphia, Blakiston, 1920. p. 35

BOUILLON—carbonate; culture medium. Ibid., p. 32
SOLUTION—bile peptone, for enrichment of typhoid bacilli. Ibid., p. 42

Stockard, Charles Rupert. New York city biochemist. 1879–1939
TEST—for oestrus, by vaginal smear.
The existence of a typical oestrus cycle in the guinea-pig—with a study of its histological and physiological changes with G. N. Papanicolaou, Amer. J. Anat., 22: 225–283, Sept. 15, 1917

Stockhusen, Samuel.
Wrote on industrial diseases. Garrison and Morton
Libellus de lythargyrii fumo morbifico, Goslar, 1656
Also, French transl., 1776. 220 pp.

Stokis, E. Belgian scientist
TEST—for carbon monoxide in blood.
Nouvelle réaction chimique pour le recherche de l'oxyde de carbone dans le sang. C. R. Soc. Biol., 84: 743–745, Mar. 26, 1921

Stoddard, C. L. See E. B. Wolcott

Stoddard, James Leavitt. Boston pathologist. 1889–
METHOD—
Titration method for blood fat with Phoebe E. Drury, J. biol. Chem., 84: 741–748, Nov. 1929
Described clinical and pathological characteristics of torula infection in man.
Torula infection in man. A group of cases, characterized by chronic lesions of the central nervous system, with clinical symptoms suggestive of cerebral tumor, produced by an organism belonging to the torula group (Torula histolytica, N. Sp.) with E. C. Cutler, Rockefeller Inst. Med. Research, Monog. 6, 25: 1–98, Jan. 31, 1916

Stoeltzner, Wilhelm. Königsberg i. Pr. physician. 1872–
TEST—for vitamin D.
Eine chemische Reaktion auf antirachitisches Vitamin. Münch. med. Wschr., 75: 1584 (only), Sept. 14, 1928

Stoerk, O. See H. Eppinger

Stoffel, Adolf. Heidelberg surgeon
OPERATION—selective nerve resection to diminish motor nerve impulses permanently in spastic paralysis.
Eine neue Operation zur Beseitigung der spastischen Lähmungen. Münch. med. Wschr., 58: 2493–2498, Nov. 21, 1911
The treatment of spastic contractures. Amer. J. Orthop. Surg., 10: 611–644, May 1913

Stoke
TREATMENT—of bronchiectasis by continuous inhalation of oxygen.
Discussion on therapeutic uses of oxygen. By J. Barcroft, Dr. G. H. Hunt, Dr. Haldane, Dr. Pyle et al. From North Staffordshire Infirmary of Stoke-on-Trent, England. Proc. roy. Soc. (Sec. Therap. and Pharmacol.), 13: pt. 3, 59–95, 1920

Stoker, William. Irish physician. 1773–1848
LAW—sedimentation velocity of corpuscles in a suspension of globular elements in fluid, is proportionate to square of their radius.
Pathological observations. Part I. On dropsy, purpura and the influenza . . . and on the morbid changes in the blood. . . . Dublin, Hodges and McArthur, 1823. 244 pp. p. 45

Stokes, Adrian. Lagos, Nigeria physician. 1887–1927
Wrote, after experimenting on monkeys—
Experimental transmission of yellow fever to labora-

tory animals with J. H. Bauer and N. P. Hudson, Amer. J. trop. Med., 8: 103–164, Mar. 1928

Stokes, F. J. See E. W. Flosdorf

Stokes, Sir George Gabriel. English physician. 1819–1903

Removed oxygen from hemoglobin by reducing agents and proved that the latter is agent of combustion.

On the reduction and oxidation of the coloring matter of the blood. Proc. roy. Soc., 13: 355–364, June 16, 1864

Stokes, Whitley. Dublin physician. 1763–1845

First to describe ecthyma terebrans or "pemphigus gangrenosa." Garrison

On the eruptive disease of children. Dublin Med. and Phys. Essays, 1: 146–153, 1807

Stokes, William. Dublin physician. 1804–1878

COLLAR—of varicose veins of neck.

Researches on the diagnosis and pathology of aneurism. Dublin J. Med. and Chem. Sci., 5: 400–440, 1834

DISEASE—exophthalmic goiter.

The diseases of the heart and the aorta. Dublin, Hodges and Smith, 1854. 689 pp.

RESPIRATION—of Cheyne-Stokes.

Fatty degeneration of the heart. In Ibid., pp. 320–327

Also: Medical classics, 3: 739–746, Mar. 1929

Also in F. A. Willius and T. E. Keys' *Cardiac classics.* St. Louis, Mosby, 1941. pp. 484–489

SYNDROME—bradycardia with syncopal attacks.

Observations on some cases of permanently slow pulse. Dublin Quart. J. med. Sci., 2: 73–85, 1846

Also in: *The diseases of the heart and the aorta.* Dublin Hodges and Smith, 1854. p. 333

Also: Medical classics, 3: 727–738, Mar. 1939

Also in F. A. Willius and T. E. Keys' *Cardiac classics.* St. Louis, Mosby, 1941. pp. 462–469

Wrote earliest systematic work on stethoscope in English language.

An introduction to the use of the stethoscope; with its application to the diagnosis in disease of the thoracic viscera; including the pathology of these various affections. Edinburgh, Machlachlan and Stewart, 1825 226 pp.

Wrote first observation on beneficial effect of pneumothorax in phthisis; author of unsurpassed discussion of emphysema and bronchiectasis.

A treatise on the diagnosis and treatment of diseases of the chest. Dublin, Hodges and Smith, 1837. 557 pp.

Stokes, Sir William. Irish surgeon. 1839–1900

OPERATION—Gritti-Stokes o; amputation through articular end of femur.

Contributions to practical surgery. (*On the resection of joints and bones.*) Dublin Quart. J. med. Sci., 45: 1–19, Feb. 1, 1868

On supra-condyloid amputation of the thigh. Trans. Roy. Med. and Chir. Soc. London, 53: 175–186, 1870

(Same title) Dublin J. med. Sci., 60: 97–104, Aug 2, 1875

Stokvis, Barend Josephus E. Dutch physician. 1834–1902

Introduced term "enterogenous cyanosis."

Bijdrage tot de casuistiek der autotoxische enterogene cyanosen (methaemoglobinaemia (?) et enteritis parasitaria). Ned. Tijdschr. Geneesk., 2 R., 38: 678–693, 1902

Same, in German: Intern. Beitr. z. inn. Med., Berlin, 1, 1902

Stoll, A. See K. Spiro

Stone, Coy Smith. Hobbs, N. M. surgeon. 1903–

MODIFICATION—

A modification of the Gius-Racely portable suction apparatus with S. A. Roddenbery, Surgery, 18: 598–602, Nov. 1945

Stone, D. See H. D. Gillies

Stone, Harvey Brinton. Baltimore surgeon. 1882–

OPERATION—

Umbilical hernia: a method of operative treatment. Arch. Surg., 12: 494–500, Feb. 1926

OPERATION—

Plastic operation for anal incontinence. Ibid., 18: 845–851, Mar. 1929

OPERATION—

Imperforate anus with rectovaginal cloaca. Ann. Surg., 104: 651–661, Oct. 1936

OPERATION—

Method of intestinal anastomosis with a new clamp. S. G. O., 65: 383–384, Sept. 1937

Advocated use of alcohol by subcutaneous injection for pruritus ani.

A treatment for pruritus ani. Johns Hopk. Hosp. Bull., 27: 242–243, Aug. 1916

Pruritus ani; treatment by alcohol injection. S. G. O. 42: 565–566, Apr. 1926

Stone, James Savage. Boston surgeon. 1868–1929

OPERATION—for ununited fracture.

Partial loss of the tibia replaced by transfer of the fibula, with maintenance of both malleoli of the ankle. Ann. Surg., 46: 628–632, Oct. 1907

Stone, R. E. See T. D. Spies

Stone, Willard John. American physician. 1877–

FACTOR—cardiac overload f.

The clinical significance of high and low pulse-pressures with special reference to cardiac load and overload. J. A. M. A., 61: 1256–1259, Oct. 4, 1913

TEST—

An improved test for occult blood, especially in the urine with G. T. Burke, Ibid., 102: 1549–1550, May 12, 1934

Stookey, Byron Polk. New York surgeon. 1887–

INCISION—question-mark, for exposure of sciatic nerve.

The technic of nerve suture. J. A. M. A., 74: 1380–1385, May 15, 1920

METHOD—of reducing fracture-dislocation of cervical vertebra.

Air-cushion reduction of incomplete fracture dislocations associated with spinal cord injuries. Amer. J. Surg., 26: 513–515, Dec. 1934

OPERATION—

Differential section of the trigeminal root in the surgical treatment of trigeminal neuralgia. Ann. Surg., 87: 172–178, Feb. 1928

TECHNIC—of spinofacial and of hypoglossofacial anastomosis.

Surgical and mechanical treatment of peripheral nerves. Philadelphia, Saunders, 1922

Storch, Ernest. See H. Lissauer

Storm van Leeuwen, Willem. See Leeuwen

Stout, A. P. See C. D. Haagensen

Stowe, W. P. See G. D. Delprat

Strachan, John B. American surgeon

Reported—(by T. F. Gillian of Peterburg, Va.) *Case of successful excision of the cervix uteri in a scirrhous state.* Amer. J. med. Sci., 5: 307–309, Feb. 1830

Stradner, F. See F. Hamburger

Strakosch, E. A. See H. M. Tsuchiya
Strambio, Cajetan. Italian physician. 1752–1831
Wrote on pellagra. Garrison and Morton
De pellagra. Mediolani, Bianchi, 1786–89. 3 vols.
Strasburger, Eduard Adolf. German scientist. 1844–1912
Wrote pioneer work on formation and division of cells. Garrison and Morton
Über Zellbildung und Zelltheilung. Jena, Fischer, 1880. 3 Aufl. (1st ed., 1875)
Strasburger, Julius. Bonn physician. 1871–
METHOD—gravimetric, for determining quantity of fecal bacteria.
Untersuchungen über die Bakterienmenge in menschlichen Fäces. Z. klin. Med., 46: 413–444, 1902
Straschesko, N. D. See W. P. Obrastzow
Strassman, Fritz. Berlin physiologist. 1858–
METHOD—for quantitative detection of ethyl alcohol in human tissues.
Untersuchungen über den Nährwerth und die Ausscheidung des Alcohols. Arch. f. d. ges. Physiol., 49: 315–330, June 13, 1891
Straub, Walther. Freiburg i. B. pharmacologist. 1874–
Wrote important analysis of action of digitalis on isolated heart.
Digitaliswirkung am isolierten Vorhof des Frosches. Arch. exp. Path. Pharmak., 79: 19–29, Aug. 19, 1915
Straus, Isidore. French physician. 1845–1896
REACTION—for diagnosis of glanders.
Sur un moyen diagnostic rapide de la morve. Arch. de Méd. exper. et d Anat. path., Paris, 1: 460–462, 1889
SIGN—
Des modifications dans la sudation de la face provoquée à l'aide de la pilocarpine comme un nouveau signe pouvant servir au diagnostic différentiel des diverses formes de paralysie faciale. C. R. Soc. Biol., 7 s., 1: 85–97, 1880
Strauss, Alfred Adolph. Chicago surgeon. 1883–
METHOD—
Blood transfusion by the direct syringe-cannula needle method; its application in major surgery. S. G. O., 41: 678–682, Nov. 1925
Strauss, Hermann. Berlin physician. 1868–
METHOD—of provocative polyuria for renal function.
Ueber den Einfluss der verschiedenen Zuckerarten auf die Zuckerausscheidung beim Menschen. Berl. klin. Wschr., 35: 398–401, May 2, 1898, et seq.
TEST—for bismuth in urine.
Untersuchungen über die Ausscheidung des Bismogenol (Tosse). Dermat. Wschr., 76: 417–419, May 12, 1923
TEST—for indican.
Zur Methodik der quantitativen Indikanbestimmung. Dtsch. med. Wschr., 28: 299–300, Apr. 17, 1902
TEST—for lactic acid in stomach.
Ueber eine Modification der Uffelmann'schen Reaction zum Nachweis der Milchsäure im Mageninhalt. Berl. klin. Wschr., 32: 805–807, Sept. 16, 1895
TEST—levulose-tolerance, in estimating hepatic function.
Zur Funktionsprüfung der Leber. Dtsch. med. Wschr., 27: 757–759, Oct. 31; 786–787, Nov. 7, 1901
Described metastasis of gastric carcinoma to pouch of Douglas.

Ueber die Abhängigkeit der Milchsäuregährung vom HCl Gehalt des Magensaftes with F. Bialocour, Z. f. klin. Med., 28: 567–585, 1895
See also C. Neuberg
Strauss, I. See L. Loewe
Strauss, J. Henry. Baltimore scientist
MODIFICATION—
A microscopic slide modification of the Eagle and Kahn flocculation tests for syphilis. Amer. J. Syph., Gonor. and Ven. Dis., 25: 186–188, Mar. 1941
Strecker, Adolf. German chemist. 1822–1871
Performed early important work on bile. Garrison
Untersuchung der Oxengalle. Ann. d. Chem. u. Pharm., Heidelberg, 65: 1; 67: 1, 1848; 70: 149, 1849
Stricker, Solomon. German physician. 1834–1898
Described vasodilatation on stimulation of posterior nerve roots.
Untersuchungen über die Gefässnervenwurzeln des Ischiadicus. S. B. Akad. Wiss. Wien, Math.-nat. Classe, Abt. 3, 74: 173–185, 1876
Strohl, A. See G. Guillain
Stromeyer, Georg Frederich Ludwig. German surgeon. 1804–1876
Performed subcutaneous section of tendo Achilles, 1831. Garrison
Die Durchschneidung der Achillessehne, als Heilmethode des Klumpfusses, durch zwei Fälle erläutert (1831-32). Mag. f. d. ges. Heilk., Berlin, 39: 195–218, 1833
Strong, F. N. See C. A. Elvehjem
Strong, Nathan. American physician. 1781–1837
Wrote on cerebrospinal meningitis. Garrison and Morton
On the disease termed petechial or spotted fever. Hartford, Gleason, 1810
Stronganoff, Vasilii Vasilovich. Russian obstetrician. 1857–
TREATMENT—
Profilakticheskiy method liecheniya eklampsii i yevo rezultati. St. Petersburg, 1908. 7 pp.
The treatment of eclampsia; an improved conservative method. Proc. R. Soc. Med., 17: Sect. Obstet. and Gyn., 164–168, 1923–24
On an improved prophylactic method of treatment of eclampsia. Lancet, 2: 62–63, July 12, 1924
Strother, Edward. English physician. 1675–1737
Introduced term "puerperal fever" Garrison
Criticon febrium.... London, Rivington, 1716. 211 pp.
Strouse, Solomon. American physician. 1882–
Reported fructosuria.
Levulosuria; with a report of an unusual case with J. C. Friedman, Arch. intern. Med., 9: 99–107, Jan. 1912
Strümpell, Adolf Gustav Gottfried von. Leipzig neurologist. 1853–1925
DISEASE—hereditary spastic spinal paralysis.
Über eine bestimmte Form der primären kombinierten Systemerkrankungen des Rückenmarks.... Arch. f. Psych., 17: 217–238, 1868
DISEASE—polioencephalomyelitis.
Über die acute Encephalitis der Kinder (Polioencephalitis acuta, cerebrale Kinderlähmung). Jbl. f. Kinderh., 22: 173–178, 1885
DISEASE—Strümpell-Marie; rhizomelic spondylosis.
Mentioned in his *Lehrbuches,* 1 Aufl., 2: 152, 1884-
Bemerkung über die chronische ankylosirende Ent-

zündung der Wirbelsäule und der Hüftigelenke.
Dtsch. Z. f. Nerbenheilk., 11: 338-342, Nov. 30,
1897
ENCEPHALITIS—
Über primäre acute Encephalitis. Dtsch. Arch. f.
klin. Med., 47: 53-74, Oct. 21, 1890
PSEUDOSCLEROSIS OF BRAIN—
*Über die Westphal'sche Pseudosklerose und über diffuse
Hirnsklerose, insbesondere bei Kindern.* Dtsch. Z. f.
Nervenheilk., 12: 115-149, Mar. 3, 1898
SIGN—dorsal flexion of great toe in an extremity
affected with paresis.
Ueber Wesen und Behandlung der Tabes. Münch.
med. Wschr., 37: 667-671, Sept. 30, 1890
TYPE—
Ueber hereditäre spastische Spinalparalyse. Arch. f.
Psychiat., 34: 1044-1046, Aug. 1901
Struve, Heinrich. Tiflis physician
TEST—for blood in urine.
Ueber Blutfarbstoffe. Z. anal. Chem., 11: 150-153,
1872
Stryker, Laura M. New York scientist
BROTH—serum infusion.
*Variations in the pneumococcus induced by growth in
immune serum.* J. exp. Med., 24: 49-68 (50), July
1916
Strzyzowski, Casimir. Lausanne physiochemist.
1868-
METHOD—for production of haemin crystals.
*Ueber ein neues Reagens und dessen Empfindlichkeit
für den krystallographischen Blutnachweis.* Therap.
Mschr., 16: 459-463, Sept. 1902
TEST—for diabetes.
*Eine in der Praxis leicht ausführbare Reaktion des
Diabetesharnes.* Ibid., 19: 109 (only), Feb. 1905
Stuart, Charles Arthur. Providence, R. I. biologist.
1893-
AGAR—stomach-liver infusion.
*The effect of environmental changes on the growth,
morphology, physiology and immunological charac-
teristics of Bacterium typhosum.* J. Bact., 9: 581-602
(591), Nov. 1924
Stuart-Harris, C. H. See W. Smith
Stubenrauch, Ludwig von. Munich surgeon
OPERATION—choledochoenterostomy.
*Ueber plastische Anastomosen zwischen Gallenwegen
und Magendarmcanal zur Heilung der completen
äusseren Gallenfistel.* Arch. f. klin. Chir., 79: 1015-
1030, 1906
Reported ligation of splenic artery for treatment of
purpura hemorrhagica.
Die Ligatur der Arteria lienalis. Dtsch. Z. f. Chir.,
172: 374-384, July 1922
Stuck, W. See C. S. Venable
Studdiford, William Emery. New York gynecologist.
1867-1925
OPERATIONS—on pelvic floor.
In: Johnsons' *Operative therapeusis.* New York,
Appleton, 1915. Vol. 5, pp. 282-294
Stuertz, Carl Adolf Ernst. Cologne physician. 1870-
Suggested phrenicotomy for basal lung disease,
1911.
*Experimenteller Beitrag zur „Zwerchfellbewegung nach
einseitiger Phrenicusdurchtrennung.* Dtsch. med.
Wschr., 38: 897-900, May 9, 1912
Stumpf, Pleikart. Munich roentgenologist. 1888-

Devised multiple-slit grid and perfected mechani-
cally apparatus for roentgen kymography.
*Die Gestaltanderung des schlagenden Herzens im
Röntgenbild.* Fort. a. d. Geb. d. Röntgenstrahlen,
38: 1055-1067, Dec. 1928
*Das röntgenographische Bewegungsbild und seine
Anwendung (Flächenkymographie und Kymoscopie).*
Abstr., Ibid., 44: 413 (only), Sept. 1931
Stumpf. R. See M. F. Hofmeister
Sturgis, Cyrus Cressey. Ann Arbor physician. 1891-
Advocated—
*Desiccated stomach in the treatment of pernicious
anemia* with K. Isaacs, J. A. M. A., 93: 747-749,
Sept. 7, 1929
Sturli, A. See A. Von Decastello
Sturtevant, A. H. See T. H. Morgan
Stutzer, Albert. Bonn scientist
REAGENT—for separating proteins.
Ein Beitrag zur Kenntniss der Proteinstoffe. Ber. d.
dtsch. Chem. Ges., 13: 251 (only), Feb. 9, 1880
SOLUTION—whey; culture medium.
Das Bacterium der Mau-lund Klauenseuche with R.
Hartleb, Arch. Hyg., Berl., 30: 372-404 (403),
1897
Subbarow, Y. See C. H .Fiske
Subbotin, Victor Andreyevich. St. Petersburg phy-
sician. 1844-1898
METHOD—for quantitative detection of ethyl alco-
hol in human tissues.
*Ueber die physiologische Bedeutung des Alkohols für
den thierischen Organismus.* Z. f. Biol., 7: 361-378,
1871
Sudeck, Paul Hermann Martin. Hamburg surgeon.
1866-
ATROPHY or DISEASE—acute "reflex" bone
atrophy.
Uber die acute entzündliche Knochenatrophie. Arch.
f. klin. Chir., 62: 147-156, 1900
*Über die akute (reflektorische) Knochenatrophie nach
Entzündungen und Verletzungen an den Extremitäten
und ihre klinischen Erscheinungen.* Fort. a. d. Geb.
d. Roentgenstr., 5: 277-293, 1901-2
Suggs, Frank. U. S. Army surgeon. 1875-
SUTURE—INTESTINAL.
An interlocking suture. Ann. Surg., 49: 590-591, Apr.
1909
Sulkowitch, Hirsh Wolf. Boston urologist. 1906-
REAGENT and TEST—for excessive calcium in
urine; of value in diagnosis of bone tumors or hyper-
parathyroidism.
Progress in the management of urinary calculi. By
J. D. Barney and H. W. Sulkowitch, J. Urol., 37:
746-762 (751), June 1937
See also F. Albright
Sullivan, Michael Xavier. Providence, R. I. phy-
sician. 1875-
AGAR—ammonium lactate peptone; culture medium.
*Synthetic culture media and the biochemistry of bac-
terial pigments.* J. med. Res., 14: 109-160 (113), Nov.
1905
AGAR—glucose. Ibid., p. 117
AGAR—glycerol asparagin; culture medium. Ibid., p.
119
AGAR—glycerol nitrate asparagin; culture medium,
Ibid., p. 120
AGAR—salt asparagin. Ibid., p. 117

METHOD—
The estimation of cystine in finger nail clippings with hydrolysis for one hour with N. W. Howard and W. C. Hess, J. biol. Chem., 119: 721–724, July 1937
REACTION—
A colorimetric test for guanidine. Proc. Soc. exp. Biol., N. Y., 33: 106–108, Oct. 1935
TEST—
A new distinctive test for cysteine. J. biol. Chem., Sc. Proc., 59: 1, 1924
Sulzberger, Marion Baldur. Swiss-American dermatologist. 1895–
DISEASE—Bloch-Sulzberger's d.: incontinentia pigmenti.
Ueber eine bisher nicht beschriebene congenitale Pigmentanomalie (Incontinentia pigmenti). Arch. f. Dermat, u. Syph., 154: 19–32, Dec. 27, 1927
See also J. I. Wolf
Sulzer, R. See R. K. Cannon
Summerville, W. W. See H. Goldblatt
Sumner, James Batcheller. Ithaca, N. Y. chemist. 1887–
Awarded Nobel prize in chemistry in 1946 for pioneering in crystallizing of protein.
The isolation and crystallization of the enzyme urease. J. biol. Chem., 69: 435–441, Aug. 1926
REAGENT and TEST—
A new reagent for the estimation of sugar in normal and diabetic urine. Ibid., 46: xxi–xxii, 1921
Dinitrosalicylic acid: a reagent for the estimation of sugar in normal and diabetic urine. Ibid., 47: 5–9, June 1921
Susman, William. Manchester pathologist
SPONGIO-BLASTOMA—
Intra-ocular tumours. Brit. J. Ophthal., 22: 722–739, Dec. 1938
Sussmann, Martin. Berlin physician
Introduced a modified type of gastroscope.
Ein biegsames Gastroskop. Therap. d. Gegenw., 52: 433–441, Oct. 1911
Sutherland, C. G. See E. D. Osborne
Sutton, H. G. See W. W. Gull
Sutton, L. E. See Haverhill fever
Sutton, Thomas. English physician. 1767–1835
Wrote classic account of—
Tracts on delirium tremens. . . . London, Underwood, 1813. 272 pp.
Suzanne, Jean Georges. French physician. 1859–
GLAND—mucous g. of mouth.
Recherches anatomiques sur le plancher de la bouche, avec étude anatomique et pathogénique sur la grenouillette commune ou sublinguale. Bordeaux, 1887. 124 pp.
Suzuki, B. Japanese scientist
METHOD—
Eine einfache Schnittserienmethode bei der Celloidine-inbettung. Anat. Anz., 34: 358–361, May 6, 1909
Swaine, William Edward. English physician. 1805–
Reported correct antemortem diagnosis of dissecting aneurysm of aorta.
Dissecting aneurysm of the aorta. Trans. Path. Soc. London, 7: 106–111, 1856
Swaminath, C. S. Indian physician
Transmitted kala-azar to man by bite of Phlebotomus argentipes.
Transmission of Indian Kala-azar to man by the bites of Phlebotomus argentipes, ann. and brun with H. E.

Shortt and L. A. P. Anderson, Indian J. med. Res., 30: 473–477, July 1942
See also H. E. Shortt
Swammerdam, Jan. Dutch physician. 1637–1680
The first to discern and describe red blood-corpuscles (1658), discovered valves of lymphatics (1664), discovered medicolegal fact that fetal lungs will float after respiration (1667), and, in 1677, devised method of injecting blood-vessels with wax, which was afterward claimed by Ruysch. He was also no mean experimental physiologist, studying movements of heart, lungs, and muscles by plethysmographic methods which are almost modern. Garrison
Tractatus physico-anatomico medicus de respiratione usque pulmonum. . . . Lugduni Batavorum, Abraham et Gaasbeeck, 1667. 121 pp.
Swan, J. M. See J. Marshall
Swan, Joseph. English anatomist. 1791–1874
Noted relation of optic thalamus to opposite-sided sensation, especially in eye. Garrison
On the origins of the visual powers of the optic nerve. London, Longman, 1856. 45 pp.
Swank, Roy Laner. American anatomist. 1909–
TECHNIC—
Chlorate-osmic-formalin method for staining degenerating myelin with H. A. Davenport, Stain Technol., 10: 87–90, July 1935
Swanson, W. W. See F. B. Kingsbury
Swartz, Ernest Osborne. Baltimore urologist. 1880–
METHOD—
A new culture method for the gonococcus: report of experimental studies. J. Urol., 4: 325–345, Aug. 1920
See also H. H. Young
Sweany, Henry Claris. Chicago pathologist. 1890–
METHOD—
A system of sputum analysis for the presence of acid-fast bacilli with A. Stadnichenko, J. Lab. clin. Med., 14: 547–557, Mar. 1929
Sweet, J. E. See H. D. Dakin
Sweet, William Merrick. American ophthalmologist. 1860–1926
METHOD—of localizing foreign bodies in eyeball.
The röentgen-rays in ophthalmic surgery. Amer. J. med. Sci., 116: 190–201, Aug. 1898
Swensen, S. A. See H. N. Harkins
Swenson, P. C. See W. E. Caldwell
Swetlow, George Irving. Brooklyn physician. 1897–
METHOD—
Paravertebral alcohol block in cardiac pain. Amer. Heart J., 1: 393–412, Apr. 1926
The treatment of cardiac pain by paravertebral alcohol block with S. P. Schwartz, J. A. M. A., 86: 1679–1682, May 29, 1926
Swett, Paul Plummer. Hartford, Conn. surgeon. 1882–
OPERATION—
Synovectomy in chronic infectious arthritis. J. Bone and Joint Surg., 21: 110–121, Jan. 1923
A review of synovectomy. Ibid., 20: 68–76, Jan. 1938
Swick, Moses. German-New York urologist. 1900–
Introduced intravenous urography. See also A. von Lichtenberg
Darstellung der Niere und Harnwege im Roentgenbild durch intravenöse Einbringung eines neuen Kontraststoffes, des Uroselectans. Klin. Wschr., 8: 2087–2089, Nov. 5, 1929

Swieten, Gerald L. B. van. German physician. 1700–1772

Wrote on diseases of military camps.

Kurze Beschreibung und Heilungsart der Krankheiten welche am öftesten in dem Feldlager beobachtet werden. Wien, Trattnern, 1758

Swift, Homer Fordyce. New York physician. 1881–
THEORY—of chronic arthritis.

Bacterial allergy (hyperergy) to nonhemolytic streptococci with C. L. Derick and C. H. Hitchcock, J. A. M. A., 90: 906–908, Mar. 24, 1928

TREATMENT—of general paresis: autoserosalvarsan.

The intensive treatment of syphilis with A. W. M. Ellis, Ibid., 59: 1251–1254, Oct. 5, 1912

VIRUS—of human rheumatic fever.

Pathogenic pleuro pneumonia-like microorganisms from acute rheumatic exudates and tissues with T. M. Brown, Science, 89: 271–272, Mar. 24, 1939

Swift, Katharine. See T. P. Almy

Swingle, Wilbur Willis. Princeton, N. J. zoologist. 1891–
CORTICAL HORMONE—

An aqueous extract of the suprarenal cortex which maintains the life of bilaterally adrenalectomized cats with J. J. Pfiffner, Science, 71: 321–322, Mar. 21, 1920

The adrenal cortical hormone with J. J. Pfiffner, Medicine, 11: 371–433, Dec. 1932

See also J. J. Pfiffner

Sword, Brian Collins. New Haven anesthetist. 1889–
METHOD—

The closed circle method of administration of gas anesthesia. Anesth. and Analg., 9: 198–202, Sept.-Oct. 1930

Sydenham, Thomas. English physician. 1624–1689
CHOREA—

Schedula monitoria de novae febris ingressu. London, 1686

Also in all editions of *The entire works of.* . . . See edition of Philadelphia, Kite et al., 1815, pp. 417–418

He described articular and muscular pains of dysentery in 1672 and its seasonal aspects during 1669–72. He gave a full account of scarlatina as it prevailed in London (1661–75), separating the disease from measles and identifying it by its present name. Garrison

Observationes medicae circa morborum acutorum historiam et curationem. Londini, Kettilby, 1676. 425 pp.

Gave classic account of hysteria. Garrison

Dissertatio epistolaris ad Gulielmum Cole, de observationibus nuperis circa curationem variolarum confluentium, nec non de affectione hysterica. Londoni, Kettilby, 193 pp.

His treatise on gout is esteemed his masterwork. Garrison

Tractatus de podagra et hydrope. Londini, Kettilby, 1683. 201 pp.

For selections, see Medical classics, 4: 304–397, Dec. 1939

Sydenstricker, Virgil Preston Willis. American physician. 1889–
METHOD—

Transfusion of blood by the citrate method. J. A. M. A., 68: 1677–1680, June 4, 1917

Sydow, A. F. See D. M. Glover

Sylvest, Ejnar. Norwegian physician

Described Bornholm disease and applied name myositis acuta epidemica.

En Bornholmsk epidemi-myositis epidemica. Ugeskr. Laeg., 92: 798–801, Aug. 21, 1930

Myositis epidemica. Ibid., 982–984, Oct. 16, 1930

Myositis epidemica. Ibid., 93: 1155–1156, Nov. 19, 1931

(Sylvius), Franciscus de La Boë. Dutch physician. 1614–1672
ANGLE, AQUEDUCT, ARTERY—

He regarded digestion as a chemical fermentation, and recognized importance of saliva and pancreatic juice. Garrison

He recognized role of tubercles in phthisis. Major

Disputationum medicarum pars prima, primaris corporis humani functiones naturales ex anatomicis, practicis et chymicis experimentis deductas complecteus. Amstelodami, van den Bergh, 1663. 167 pp.

Praxeos medicae idea nova. Lugduni Batavorum, apud Le Carpentier, 1671

Syme, James. Scottish surgeon. 1799–1870
AMPUTATION—

(Amputation at the ankle-joint, Sept. 8, 1842.) London and Edinburgh Month. J. med. Sci., 3: 93–96, 1843

OPERATION—

On stricture of the urethra and fistula in perineo. Edinburgh, Sutherland and Knox, 1849. 72 pp.

On the treatment of stricture by external incision. London and Edinburgh Month. J. med. Sci., 12, 1851

Operated for—

Case of iliac aneurism. Med.-chir. Trans., London, 45: 381–387, 1862

Symmers, Douglas. American physician. 1879–
DISEASE—

Follicular lymphadenopathy with splenomegaly: a newly recognized disease of the lymphatic system. Arch. Path., 3: 816–820, May 1927

Giant follicular lymphadenopathy with or without splenomegaly. Ibid., 26: 603–647, Sept. 1938

See also C. L. Brown

Symmers, W. St. Clair. Belfast pathologist
BROTH—basal ascitic fluid extract, for studying fermentation by bacteria.

Some points bearing on the bacteriology of cerebrospinal meningitis with W. J. Wilson, J. Hyg., 9: 9–16, Apr. 1909

Symons, Claude Trevine. Celon scientist
TEST—for blood in urine.

A note on a modification of Teichmann's test for blood. Biochem. J., 7: 596–598, Dec. 1913

Syms, Parker. New York surgeon. 1860–1933
TRACTOR—tube with inflatable rubber bag at end.

Perineal prostatectomy. J. A. M. A., 37: 1154–1156, Nov. 2, 1901

Szabó, Dionys. Budapest medical student
TEST—for free hydrochloric acid in gastric juice.

Beiträge zur Kenntniss der freien Säure des menschlichen Magensaftes. Z. physiol. Chem., 1: 140–156, 1878

Szabóky, Johann von. Budapest bacteriologist
AGAR—glycerol lung.

Ein Beitrag zur Kenntnis der kulturellen Eigenschaften der Tuberkelbacillen. Zbl. Bakt., 43: 651–660 (652), Apr. 6, 1907

Szásy, Alfred. Budapest bacteriologist

SZÁSY, ALFRED

396

TALIAFERRO, VALENTINE H.

INFUSION—blood clot; culture medium.
Ein billiger Nährböden (Bouillon) aus Blutkucher.
Zbl. Bakt., 75: 489–495 (491), Feb. 15, 1915
Szelöczey, J. See O. S. Gibbs
Szent-Györgyi, Albert. Hungarian physician. 1893–
Awarded Nobel prize in 1937. He was the first to
obtain vitamin C in pure form, and to identify it
with hexuronic acid, now known as cevitamic (ascor-
bic) acid.
Vitamin C, Adrenalin und Nebenniere. Dtsch. med.
Wschr., 58: 852–854, May 27, 1932
Postulated vitamin P as regulator of vascular per-
meability.
*Über den Einfluss von Substanzen der Flavongruppe
auf die Permeabilität der Kapillaren. Vitamin P.*
By L. Armentano, A. Benthsáth, T. Béres, St.

Ruszuyák and A. Szent-Györgyi, Ibid., 62: 1325–
1328, Aug. 14, 1936
See also S. Rusznyák
Szily, Aurel von. German ophthalmologist. 1847–
1920
ANODAL—BIPOLAR ELECTROLYSIS—CHEMI-
CAL CAUTERIZATION OF CHOROID—
*Zur Behandlung der Netzhautablösung mittels Elek-
trolyse.* Klin. Mbl. Augenheilk., 93: 721–745, Dec.
1934
Investigated problem of sympathetic ophthalmia in
relation to a filterable virus.
*Experimentelle endogene Infektionsübertragung von
Bulbus zu Bulbus.* Ibid., 72: 593–602, May–June
1924
Szlapka, T. L. See H. Z. Giffin

T

Tabora, D. See F. Moritz
Taccone, Girolamo. Italian physician
TEST—protides of cerebrospinal fluid.
*A proposito del lavoro: prove e considerazioni sulla
reazione al bicromato di potassis sul L. C. R. (reazione
di Taccone) per il dott. E. Broggi.* Rass. di studi
psichiat., 19: 871–879, 1930
Taenzer, Paul Rudolf. German physician. 1858–
1919
DISEASE—
*Ueber das Ulerythema ophyrogenes, eine noch nicht
beschriebene Hautkrankheit.* Mschr. f. prakt. Dermat.,
Hamburg, 8: 197–208, 1889
Tagliacozzi, Gasparo. Italian surgeon. 1546–1599
Famous for his work on rhinoplasty. First described
in G. Mercuriali's *De decoratione.* 2 ed., Francofurti,
1586
Also: *De curtorum chirurgia per insitionem.* Venetiis,
apud G. Bindonum, 1597
**Taillefer, Louis Auguste Horace Sydney Time-
léon.** French physician. 1802–1868
VALVE—fold of mucous membrane of nasal duct.
*Dissertation médico-chirurgicale sur les maladies de
l'appareil excréteur des larmes, dans laquelle ou
propose l'emploi du nitrate d'argent pour le traitement
de la fistule lacrymale, d'après un procédé de l'auteur.*
Paris, 1826. 27 pp.
Tait, Robert Lawson. English gynecologist. 1845–
1899
KNOT—same as Staffordshire k., for tying pedicles, as
of ovary.
"*Tait's knot.*" Brit. med. J., 2: 813 (only), Nov. 22,
1879
LAW—in every case of pelvic or abdominal disease in
which life is endangered or health ruined, exploration
by celiotomy should be made, except when disease is
known to be malignant. Dorland
*On the treatment of pelvic suppuration by abdominal
section and drainage.* Med.-chir. Trans., 63: 307–
316, 1880
OPERATION—dilatation of cervix and replacement
of inverted uterus. 1879
(*Inversion of the uterus.*) In his: *Diseases of women
and abdominal surgery.* Philadelphia, Lea Bros.,
1889. Vol. 1, pp. 144–148
OPERATION—
A new method of operation for repair of the female

perineum. Obstet. J. Gr. Brit., 7: 585–588, Dec.
1879
*On the method of flap-splitting in certain plastic opera-
tions.* Brit. Gynec. J., 3: 367–376, Nov. 1887
Introduced hepatotomy.
Four cases of hepatotomy. Birmingham med. Rev.,
10: 343–351, Oct. 1881
Performed first successful operation for ruptured
tubal pregnancy, Jan. 17, 1883. Garrison
*Five cases of extra-uterine pregnancy operated upon at
the time of rupture.* Brit. med. J., 1: 1250–1251, June
28, 1884
Takahashi, D. See P. Rona
Takaki, F. See K. Futaki
Takaki, Kanehiro. Japanese physician. 1849–1915
Showed dietary origin of beri-beri. Garrison and
Morton
On the cause and prevention of kak'ke. Trans. Sei-I-
Kwai, Tokyo, 4: 29–37, 1885
Takamine, Jokichi. Japanese-American scientist.
1854–1922
Isolated adrenaline.
*The blood-pressure raising principle of the suprarenal
glands; a preliminary report.* Therap. Gaz., 26: 221–
224, Apr. 15, 1901
*Adrenalin the active principle of the suprarenal glands
and its mode of preparation.* Amer. J. Pharm., 73:
523–531, Nov. 1901
Takata, Maki. Japanese physician. 1892–
REACTION or TEST—for liver disease.
*Ueber eine neue kolloidchemische Liquorreaktion und
ihre practischen Ergebnisse.* Far Eastern A. Trop.
Med., Trans. 6th Congr., 1: 667–671, 1925
Takeuchi, Kiyoshi. Japanese scientist
TEST—for indican in urine.
Indican in the urine, demonstration by a new method.
Tokyo Igakukai Zasshi, 31, No. 19, 1917
Also, abstr. transl.: China med. J., 32: 571, 1918
Talbott, John Harold. New York City physician.
1902–
Demonstrated that loss of base, chlorides and water
in sweat is primary factor in cause of heat cramps.
Heat cramps. A clinical and chemical study with J.
Michelsen, J. clin. Invest., 12: 533–549, May 1933
Taliacotius, Gasparo. See Tagliacozzi
Taliaferro, Valentine H. American surgeon. 1831–
1888

Performed episiotomy, Dec. 2, 1851. Garrison and Morton
Rigidity of the soft parts—delivery effected by incision in the perineum. Stethoscope and Virginia Med. Gaz., Richmond, 2: 382, 1852

Tallerman, Kenneth Harry. London pediatrician. 1894–
TEST—
The laevulose test for liver efficiency and an investigation of the hepatic condition in pregnancy. Quart. J. Med., 17: 37–52, Oct. 1923

Tallerman, Lewis A. English scientist
APPARATUS—for enclosing an extremity of the body for purpose of applying to it dry hot air in treatment of rheumatism, etc. Dorland
The Tallerman treatment by superheated dry air. . . . Ed. by A. Shadwell, London, Baillière et al., 1898. 173 pp.

Tallqvist, Theodor Waldemar. Finnish physician. 1871–1927
SCALE—for hemoglobin.
Ein einfaches Verfahren zur directen Schätzung der Färbestärke des Blutes. Z. f. klin. Med., 40: 137–141, 1900

Talma, Sape. Dutch surgeon. 1847–1918
DISEASE—
Over myotonia acquisita. Ned Tijdschr. Geneesk., 2 R., 28, pt. 1: 321–328, 1892
Ueber Myotonia acquisita. Dtsch. Z. Nervenheilk., 2: 210–216, Apr. 12, 1892
OPERATION—omentopexy; also Morison's o.
Chirurgische Oeffnung neuer Seitenbahnen für das Blut der Vena porta. Berl. klin. Wschr., 35: 833–836, Sept. 9, 1898
(Same title) Ibid., 41: 893–897, Aug. 22, 1904
TEST-MEAL—
Zur Untersuchung der Säuresecretion des Magens. Ibid., 32: 777–778, Sept. 9, 1895

Talpade, Sakuntala N. See Lucy Wills

Tamura, Joseph T. Cincinnati scientist. 1903–
Worked on—
Cultivation of the virus of lymphogranuloma inguinale and its use in therapeutic inoculation: preliminary report. J. A. M. A., 103: 408–409, Aug. 11, 1934

Tandler, Julius. Vienna anatomist. 1869–
INJECTION—fluid gelatin.
Mikroskopische Injectionen mit kaltflüssiger Gelatine. Z. wiss. Mikr., 18: 22–24, July 15, 1901
See also J. von Halban

Taniguchi, T. See K. Futaki

Tanner, Ernest Ketchum. Brooklyn surgeon. 1876–
OPERATION—
The operative treatment of varicose veins with W. H. Field, Surg. Clin. No. Amer., 7: 1103–1108, Aug. 1927

Tanner, F(red) W(ilbur). Illinois chemist. 1888–
BOUILLON—basal carbonate, for studying fermentation by bacteria.
Bacteriology and mycology of foods. New York, Wiley, 1919. p. 47
SOLUTION—carrot infusion; culture medium. Ibid., p. 60
SOLUTION—pea flour infusion; a peptone substitute. Ibid., p. 57
SOLUTION—milk powder; culture medium.
A study of green fluorescent bacteria from water. J. Bact., 3: 63–101, (83), Jan. 1918

Tanner, William Edward. English surgeon. 1889–

INCISION—for resection of upper lip. In: *Modern operative surgery.* Ed. by G. G. Turner, London, Cassell, 1934. 2: 497–498

Tanquerel des Planches, L. French physician. 1809–1862
Described lead encephalopathy.
Traité des maladies de plomb ou saturnines. Paris, Ferra, 1839. Also, English transl., 1848

Tanret, Charles. French physician. 1847–1917
REACTION—
De l'ergotinine. Ann. Chim. (Phys.), 17: 493–512, 1879
Isolated ergotinine from crude ergot.
Sur la présence d'un nouvel alcaloïde, l'ergotinine, dans le seigle ergoté. C. R. Acad. Sci., 81: 896–897, Nov. 8, 1875

Tansini, Iginio. Italian surgeon. 1855–
OPERATION—
Nuovo processo per l'amputazione della mammella per cancro. Rif. med., Jan. 2, 1896

Tapia, Antonio Garcia. Spanish neurologist. 1875–
SYNDROME—palato-pharyngo-laryngeal hemiplegia.
Un caso de parálisis del lado derecho de la laringe y de la lengua, con parálisis del esterno-cleido-mastoidea y trapecio del mismo lado; acompanado de hemiplejia total temporal del lado izquierdo del cuerpo. Siglo méd., Madrid, 52: 211–213, 1905

Taras, M. H. See A. E. Pacini

Tarchanoff, Ivan Romanovich. Russian physician. 1848–1909
PSYCHO-GALVANIC REFLEX—
Ueber die galvanischen Erscheinungen in der Haut des Menschen bei Raizungen der Sinnesorgane und bei verschiedenen Formen der psychischen Thätigkeit. Arch. f. ges. Physiol., 46: 46–55, 1890

Tardi, Claude. French physician. 1607–1670
Gave account of technic of direct transfusion of blood from one man to another; probably in theory only.
Traitté de l'ecoulement du sang d'un homme dans les venes d'un autre. . . . Paris, 1667

Tardieu, Auguste Ambroise. French physician. 1818–1879
SPOTS—of ecchymosis under pleura following death by suffocation.
Étude médico-légale sur la strangulation. Paris, Baillière, 1859. 90 pp.
TEST—for infanticide.
Étude médico-légale sur l'infanticide. Paris, Baillière, 2 ed., 1880. 372 pp.

Tarlov, Isadore Max. Brooklyn surgeon. 1905–
METHOD and INSTRUMENTS—
Autologous plasma clot suture of nerves with B. Benjamin, Science, 95: 258 (only), Mar. 6, 1942
Plasma clot and silk suture of nerves. I. An experimental study of comparative tissue reaction. S. G. O., 76: 366–374, Mar. 1943
Autologous plasma clot suture of nerves: its use in clinical surgery. J. A. M. A., 126: 741–748, Nov. 18, 1944

Tarnier, Étienne Stéphne. French obstetrician. 1828–1897
FORCEPS—axis-traction.
Des cas dans lesquels l'extraction du foetus est nécessaire, et des procédés opératoires relatifs à cette extraction. Paris, Baillière, 1860. 228 pp.
First to employ carbolic acid in obstetrics. Garrison

(No title) Trans. Internat. Med. Cong., London, 4: 390, 1881
De l'asepsie et antisepsie en obstetrique. Paris, Steinheil, 1894

Tattersall, T. English chemist
REACTION—for morphine.
Notes on the alkaloids. Chem. News, 41: 63 (only), Feb. 6, 1880

Tatum, Arthur Lewis. Wisconsin pharmacologist. 1884–
Introduced mapharsen.
An experimental study of mapharsen (meta-amino para-hydroxy phenyl arsine oxide) as an antisyphilitic agent. J. Pharmacol., 50: 198–215, Feb. 1934

Tatum, Walter Low. Salisbury, N. C. surgeon. 1899–
METHOD—use of plasma in emergency treatment.
A technique for the preparation of a substitute for whole blood adaptable for use during war conditions with J. Elliott and N. Nesset, Mil. Surgeon, 85: 481–489, Dec. 1939

Taub, A. See H. V. Arny

Tauber, Henry. American biochemist. 1897–
REACTION—
A color test for thiamin (vitamin B_1). Science, 86: 594 (only), Dec. 24, 1937

Taussig, Frederick Joseph. St. Louis gynecologist. 1872–
OPERATION—
Iliac lymphadectomy with irridation in the treatment of cancer of the cervix. Amer. J. Obstet. Gynaec., 28: 650–667, Nov. 1934

Taussig, Helen B. See A. Blalock

Taveau, R. deM. See R. Hunt

Tavel, Ernst. Swiss surgeon. 1858–1912
OPERATION—ligation and injection of varicose veins.
Behandlung der Varicen durch die Ligatur und die künstliche Thrombose. Cor.-Bl. f. schweiz. Aerzte, 34: 617–623, Oct. 1, 1904
OPERATION—gastrostomy.
Nouvelle méthode de gastrostomie. Arch. prov. de Chir., 15: 317–319, June 1906
Eine neue Methode der Gastrostomie. Zbl. f. Chir., 33: 634–635, June 9, 1906

Tawara, Sunao. Japanese pathologist. 1873–
NODE—arterioventricular, of Aschoff and Tawara.
Das Reizleitungssystem des Säugetierherzens. Eine anatomisch-histologische Studie über das Atrioventrikularbündel und die Purkinjeschen Fäden. Jena, Fischer, 1906. 200 pp. pp. 183–184
See also K. A. L. Aschoff

Tay, Warren. British physician. 1843–1927
DISEASE—degeneration of choroid.
Symmetrical changes in the region of the yellow spot in each eye of an infant. Trans. opt. Soc. U. Kingdom, 1: 55–57, 1881

Taylor, Alfred Simpson. New York surgeon. 1868–1942
METHOD—
Fracture-dislocation of the neck; a method of treatment. Arch. Neurol. Psychiat., 12: 625–639, Dec. 1924
Fracture-dislocation of the cervical spine. Ann. Surg., 90: 321–340, Sept. 1929
OPERATION—
Sub-dural auto-drainage in internal hydrocephalus. J. nerv. ment. Dis., 36: 422–424, July 1909
TECHNIC—of operation for—
Brachial birth palsy. In: Lewis' *Practice of surgery.*

Hagerstown, Md., Prior Co., 1929, vol. 3, ch. 7, pp. 41–47

Taylor, Alonzo Englebert. American biochemist. 1871–
GELATIN—salt free: culture medium.
On the preparation of salt-free culture media and the growth of bacteria upon them. J. exp. Med., 7: 111–118 (114), Feb. 25, 1905
METHOD—
On the estimation of phosphorus in biological material with C. W. Miller, J. biol. Chem., 18: 215–224, July 1914

Taylor, Charles Fayette. New York surgeon. 1827–1899
APPARATUS or BRACE—
On the mechanical treatment of Pott's disease of the spine. Trans. Med. Soc. New York, pp. 67–87, 1863

Taylor, F. E. See A. Castellani

Taylor, Frederic William. Indianapolis pathologist. 1902–
METHOD—
A simple method of plasma protein estimation with Marjorie M. Gibbons, Ann. Surg., 116: 426–429, Sept. 1942

Taylor, George Douglas Lawrence. Montreal physician. 1903–
CLASSIFICATION—
A table for the degree of involvement in chronic arthritis. Canad. med. Ass. J., 36: 608–610, June 1937

Taylor, George Mosser. Los Angeles surgeon. 1897–
NEUFELD'S FEMORAL NAIL-PLATE—
Internal fixation for intertrochanteric fractures. By G. M. Taylor, A. J. Neufeld and J. Jansen, J. Bone and Joint Surg., 26: 707–712, Oct. 1944

Taylor, Herbert Douglas. New York physician. 1889–1918
Did important work on tumor growth.
Experiments on the role of lymphoid tissue in the resistance to experimental tuberculosis in mice. II. Effect of cancer immunity on resistance to tuberculosis with J. B. Murphy, J. exp. Med., 25: 609–617, May 1, 1917

Taylor, Hermon. London surgeon
GASTROSCOPE—
A new gastroscope with controllable flexibility. Lancet, 2: 276–277, Sept. 6, 1941

Taylor, J. See V. A. H. Horsley

Taylor, Kempton Potter Aiken. Guatemala surgeon. 1893–
TREATMENT—
Apparent cure of purpura hemorrhagica by Bothropic antivenin. Bull. Antivenin Inst., 3: 42–43, July 1929

Taylor, Margaret L. See L. C. Havens

Taylor, Robert William. American dermatologist. 1842–1908
Described—(Garrison)
On a rare form of idiopathic localized or partial atrophy of the skin. Arch. Dermat., 2: 114–121, Jan. 1876

Taylor, Walter Freeman. Dallas biochemist. 1891–
METHOD—
An improved method for the determination of blood urea nitrogen by direct nesslerization with W. M. Blair, J. Lab. clin. Med., 17: 1256–1263, Aug. 1932

Taylor, William Johnson. Philadelphia surgeon. 1861–1936
OPERATION—

Excision of the wrist by a modification of Mynter's method. Ann. Surg., 32: 360–363, Sept. 1900

Teacher, John Hammond. Glasgow embryologist. 1869–1930
OVUM—early form.
Contributions to the study of the early development and imbedding of the human ovum. Glasgow, 1908

Teague, Oscar. New York bacteriologist. 1878–1923
AGAR—eosin Bismark brown nutrose.
A new differential culture medium for the cholera vibrio with W. C. Travis, J. infect. Dis., 18: 601–605 (602), June 1916
AGAR—
An improved brilliant-green culture medium for the isolation of typhoid bacilli from stools with A. W. Clurman, Ibid., 18: 647–652, June 1916
AGAR—serum peptone; culture medium.
Some observations on the bacillus of Unna-Ducrey with O. Deibert, J. med. Res., 43: 61–75 (70), Jan.-Mar. 1922
AGAR—Victoria blue infusion.
The toxicity of Victoria blue 4 R. for B. paratyphosus A, B. paratyphosus B, and B. enteritidis. J. Bact., 3: 1–6, Jan. 1918
METHOD—
The value of the cultural method in the diagnosis of chancroid with O. Deibert, J. Urol., 4: 543–550, Dec. 1920
SOLUTION—glycerine sodium-chloride.
A method of preserving typhoid stools for delayed examination and a comparative study of the efficacy of eosin brilliant-green agar, eosin methylene-blue agar, and endo agar for the isolation of typhoid bacilli from stools with A. W. Clurman, J. infect. Dis., 18: 653–671, June 1916
See also Jennie G. Drennan, J. E. Holt-Harris

Teale, Thomas Pridgin. Leeds surgeon. 1801?–1868
AMPUTATION—
On amputation by a long and a short rectangular flap. London, Churchill, 1858. 72 pp.

Tedeschi, Ettore. Torin pathologist
PHENOMENON—pupillary reflex to light.
Di una singolare reazione pupillare alla luce (Riflesso pupillare esauribile ed inverso). Riv. di clin. med., 4: 420–422, July 3; 433–437, July 11, 1903

Teevan, William Frederic. English surgeon. 1834–1887
LAW—fractures occur in line of extension, and not in line of compression.
Experimental inquiries into certain wounds of the skull. Brit. and For. Med.-chir. Rev., 34: 205–214, July 1864

Teichmann, Ludwig T. German histologist. 1823–1895
CRYSTALS, TEST—for blood.
Ueber die Krystallisation der organischen Bestandtheile des Bluts. Z. f. rat. Med., n. F., 3: 375–388, 1853

Teitler, M. H. See E. Wolff

Telford, Evelyn Davison. Manchester surgeon. 1876–
OPERATION—preganglionic sympathectomy.
The technique of sympathectomy. Brit. J. Surg., 23: 448–450, Oct. 1935
Sympathetic denervation of the upper extremity. Lancet, 1: 70–72, Jan. 8, 1938

Tellyesniczky, Kalmar. Budapest histologist

FLUID—fixing solution.
Ueber die Fixirungs- (Härtungs-) Flüssigkeiten. Arch. mikr. Anat., 52: 202–247, 1898

TenBroeck, Carl. Princeton, N. J. physician. 1885–
Identified paratyphoid C bacillus as a member of Salmonella suipestifer family.
Bacilli of the hog-cholera group (Bacillus cholerae-suis) in man. J. exp. Med., 32: 33–40, July 1920

Tenenbero, D. J. See H. M. Tsuchiya

Tenschert, O. See O. Weltmann

Terč, F. Austrian physician
Used bee stings therapeutically.
Ueber eine merkwürdige Beziehung des Bienenstiches zum Rheumatismus. Wien. med. Pr., 29: 1261–1263, Aug. 26; 1295–1298, Sept. 2; 1326–1327, Sept. 9; 1359–1362, Sept. 16; 1393 (only), Sept. 23; 1423–1426, Sept. 30, 1888

Terman, Lewis Madison. American psychologist. 1877–
TESTS—for masculinity and femininity.
Sex and personality: studies in masculinity and femininity with Catharine C. Miles, New York, McGraw-Hill Book Co., 1936, 600 pp.

Terrell, Emmett Herman. Richmond, Va. surgeon. 1878–
OPERATION—for cryptitis.
Pruritus ani. South. med. J., 13: 123–125, Feb. 1920

Terroine, E. See P. F. Armand-Delille

Terry, Benjamin Taylor. American pathologist. 1876–
METHOD—
A new and rapid method of examining tissue microscopically for malignancy. J. Lab. clin. Med., 13: 550–565, Mar. 1928
Improvement in technic and results made in examining microscopically by the razor section method 2000 malignant tissues. Ibid., 14: 519–531, Mar. 1929

Terson, Alfred. French ophthalmologist. 1838–1925
KERATO-IRIDIC PARACENTESIS—
L'iridotomie préparatoire. Ann. d'Ocul., 159: 441–446, June 1922

Teruuchi, Y. Tokio physician
SOLUTION—trypsinized casein; culture medium.
Beitrag zur bakteriologischen Choleradiagnostik with O. Hida, Zbl. Bakt., 63: 570–575 (572), June 1, 1912

Thacher, James. American physician. 1754–1844
First American medical biographer. Garrison
American medical biography. Boston, Richardson, 1828. 2 vols.

Thacher, Thomas. 1620–1678
English doctor who settled in New England in 1635 and in 1669 became pastor of the Old South Church, at same time practicing medicine with success. Wrote only medical work published in New England colonies in 17th century. Garrison
A brief rule to guide the common people of New England how to order themselves and theirs in the small pocks or measles. Boston, Foster, 1677
Reprinted by H. E. Handerson in: Janus, Amst., 4: 540–547, 1899
Also, Facsimile. Baltimore, Johns Hopkins Press, 1937

Thankrah, Charles Turner. Leeds physician. 1795–1833
First investigated brass-founders' ague, dust dis-

eases, etc. Wrote first systematic publication in Great Britain on industrial diseases. Garrison

The effects of the principal arts, trades and professions and of the civic states and habits of living on health and longevity with a particular reference to the trades and manufactures of Leeds, and suggestions for the removal of many of the agents, which produce disease and shorten the duration of life. London, Longman, 1831. 126 pp. 2 ed., 1832

Thal, Prof. Copenhagen surgeon

SAW—
Rotation saw, newly invented by Prof. Thal of Copenhagen.
Communicated by Frederick Howitz, Professor of Medicine in the University of Copenhagen and Secretary of the Royal Medical Society. Edinburgh Med. and Surg. J., 19: 55–57, Jan. 1, 1823

Thannhauser, Josef Siegfried. German physician. 1885–

MODIFICATION—of van den Bergh test.
Methodik der quantitativen Bilirubinbestimmung im menschlichen Serum with E. Andersen, Dtsch. Arch. f. klin. Med., 137: 179–186, Aug. 30, 1921

TEST—for cholesterol and cholesterol-ester in blood.
Über die Beziehungen des gleichgewichtes Cholesterin und Cholestermester im Blut und Serum zur Leberfunktion with H. Schaber, Klin. Wschr., 5: 252–253, Feb. 12, 1926

Thayer, S. A. See E. A. Doisy, D. W. MacCorquodale, R. W. McKee

Thayer, William Sydney. Baltimore physician. 1864–1932

Found gonococci in—
Ulcerative endocarditis due to the gonococcus; gonorrheal septicemia with G. A. Blumer, Johns Hopk. Hosp. Bull., 7: 57–63, Apr. 1896
Studied, with T. R. Brown, eosinophilia in trichinosis.
Remarks on Dr. T. R. Brown's paper on Studies on trichinosis. Ibid., 8: 80–81, Apr. 1897
On the increase of the eosinophilic cells in the circulating blood in trichinosis. Lancet, 2: 787–788, Sept. 25, 1897
Made first clinical notation of third sound of heart. Garrison
The early diastolic heart sound. (Brief note) Med. Rec., 73: 624 (only), Apr. 11, 1908
On the early diastolic heart sound (the so-called third heart sound). Boston Med. and Surg. J., 158: 713–726, May 7, 1908

Thaysen, Thorvald Einar Hess. Copenhagen physician. 1883–

DISEASE—
The "coeliac affection"—idiopathic steatorrhoeas. Lancet, 1: 1086–1089, May 25, 1929

Thebesius, Adam Christian. German physician. 1686–1732

FORAMEN, VALVES, VEINS—
Disputatio medica inauguralis de circulo sanguinis in corde. Lugduni Batavorum, Elzevier, 1708. 19 pp.

Theiler, Max. Boston scientist

TEST—intracerebral protection t. in mice.
Studies on the action of yellow fever virus in mice. Ann. Trop. Med. and Parasitol., Liverpool, 24: 249–272, July 8, 1930
See W. D. M. Lloyd

Theis, Ruth C. New York scientist

TEST—
The determination of phenols in the blood with S. R. Benedict, J. biol. Chem., 61: 67–71, Aug. 1924
See also S. R. Benedict

Thevenon, M. L. French pharmacologist

REACTION—
Sur une nouvelle réaction de la saccharine. J. pharm. chim., 7 s., 22: 421–422, 1920

TEST—for blood.
Procédé de recherche du sang dans l'urine, les matières fécales et les liquides pathologiques with Rolland, Ibid., 16: 18–20, 1917

Thibault, Henry. Scott, Ark. physician. 1879–

Discovered, in using quinine hypodermically to treat malaria, prolonged local anesthetic properties.
A new local anesthetic. J. Arkansas med. Soc., 4: 149–153, Sept. 1907

Thiele, Friedrich Karl. Berlin physician. 1880–

TEST—for albumin in gastric juice.
Beitrag für die diagnostische Verwendbarkeit des Gehaltes an gelöstem Eiweiss bei Achylia gastrica. Berl. klin. Wschr., 49: 544–545, Mar. 18, 1912

Thiele, George Henry. Kansas City, Mo. proctologist. 1896–

TREATMENT—
Coccygodynia and pain in the superior gluteal region and down the back of the thigh: causation by tonic spasm of the levator ani, coccygeus and piriformis muscles and relief by massage of these muscles. J. A. M. A., 109: 1271–1275, Oct. 16, 1937

Thierfelder, H. See G. H. F. Nuttall

Thiérry, Francois. French physician. 1719–?

Published an account o pellagra in 1755, having obtained his second-hand information from Gaspar Casal (q.v.). Garrison
Description d'une maladie appelée mal de la rosa. J. de méd., chir. et pharm., Paris, 2: 337–346, 1755

Thiers, J. See E. C. Achard

Thiersch, Carl. German surgeon. 1822–1895

GRAFT—
Ueber die feineren anatomischen Veränderungen bei Aufheilung von Haut auf Granulationen. Arch. f. klin. Chir., 17: 318–324, 1874
Also: Verh. d. dtsch. Ges. f. Chir., 3: 69–75, 1874

OPERATION—
Ueber die Entstehungsweise und operative Behandlung der Epispadie. Arch. d. Heilk., 10: 20–35, 1869

OPERATION—evulsion of nerve for trigeminal neuralgia.
Ueber Extraction von Nerven, mit Vorzeigung von Präparaten. Verh. d. dtsch. Ges. f. Chir., 18: 44–52, Apr. 25, 1889
Proved epithelial origin of carcinoma.
Der Epithelialkrebs namentlich der Haut. Eine anatomisch-klinische Untersuchung. Leipzig, Engelmann, 1865. 310 pp.
Studied phosphoric necrosis of bones.
De maxillarum necrosi phosphorica. Lipsiae, Edelmannum, 1867. 15 pp.

Thin, George. English dermatologist. ?–1903

Described dermatitis maligna.
Malignant papillary dermatitis of the nipple and the breast-tumours with which it is found associated; ... Brit. med. J., 1: 760–763, May 14; 798–801, May 21, 1881

On cancerous affections of the skin. A treatise on epithelioma and rodent ulcer. London, Churchill, 1886. 87 pp.

Thiry, Ludwig. Belgian physician. 1817–1897
FISTULA—of Thiry-Vella; a form of intestinal fistula made usually on a dog for purpose of obtaining intestinal juice.
Über eine neue Methode den Dünndarm zu isolieren. S. B. Akad. Wiss. Wien, Math.-nat. Klasse, Abt. 1, 50: 77–96, 1865
See also C. F. W. Ludwig

Thönnessen, Josef. German bacteriologist
SOLUTION—asparagin peptone.
Darstellung des Anthrakase immunproteidin und dessen immunisierende Wirkung gegen Milzbrand. Zbl. Bakt., 32: 823–831 (824), Nov. 17, 1902

Thoinot, Leon Henri. French bacteriologist. 1858–1915
AGAR—glucose glycerol; culture medium. In his: *Précis de microbie* with E. J. Masselin, Paris, Masson, 1902. p. 35
BASAL BOUILLON—for studying fermentation by bacteria. Ibid., p. 24
SOLUTION—yeast infusion; culture medium. Ibid., p. 29

Thomas, Franz. Aachen physician. 1875–
METHOD—for determination of gastric digestion.
Neue Methode zur quantitativen Bestimmung der tryptischen und peptischen Enzymwirkung with W. Weber, Zbl. f. Stoffwechsel u. Verdauungskr., 2: 365–369, July 1901

Thomas, Hugh Owen. Liverpool surgeon. 1834–1891
COLLAR—for tuberculosis of cervical spine.
SIGN—of tuberculosis of hip; on extension of diseased leg, a compensatory curve of spine is formed.
SPLINT—posterior, for hip joint disease.
SPLINT—for removing weight of body from knee.
WRENCH—for forced rectification of fixed flat feet.
Diseases of the hip, knee and ankle joints, with their deformities, treated by a new and efficient method; (enforced, uninterrupted, and prolonged rest). Liverpool, Dobb, 1875 (very rare). 2 ed., 1876. 283 pp.
Used active and passive hyperemia as adjuvant in surgical therapy. Garrison
Ibid.

Thomas, James William Tudor. Cardiff ophthalmologist
Advocated—
Transplantation of cornea: a preliminary report on a series of experiments in rabbits, together with a demonstration of four rabbits with clear corneal grafts. Trans. Ophthal. Soc. U. Kingdom, London, 50: 127–141, 1931
Observations on some matters associated with experimental corneal grafting. Brit. J. Ophthal., 18: 129–142, Mar. 1934

Thomas, John Davies. English physician
Transmitted Taenia echinococcus to dog from human sources. Garrison and Morton
Notes upon the experimental breeding of Taenia echinococcus in the dog from the echinococci of man. Proc. roy. Soc., 38: 449–457, June 18, 1885

Thomas, Joseph. Paris physician. 1872–1934
TEST—oxido-reduction t.; a chemical t. for cancer.
Étude de la variation du pouvoir réducteur des sérums

normaux et cancéreux, en présence d'extraits de tumeurs with M. Binetti, C. R. Soc. Biol., 86: 29–30, Jan. 7, 1922
El diagnóstico del cáncer. Sem. med., B. Air., 29, pt. 2: 722–725, 1922
Le diagnostic précoce "vrai" du cancer et le moment opportun du traitement. Monde méd., 34: 406–413, June 1–15, 1924

Thomas, Theodore Gaillard. New York surgeon. 1832–1903
SPECULUM—vaginal. In his: *Diseases of women.* Philadelphia, 1878. 4 ed., p. 67
First to perform vaginal ovariotomy. Garrison
Vaginal ovariotomy. Amer. J. med. Sci., 59: 387–390, Apr. 1870

Thomas, T(homas) Turner. Philadelphia surgeon. 1866–
OPERATION—
Habitual or recurrent anterior dislocation of the shoulder. I. Etiology and pathology. Amer. J. med. Sci., 137: 229–246, Feb. 1909
(Same) *II. Treatment.* Ibid., 367–377, Mar. 1909
Recurrent dislocation of the shoulder joint. J. A. M. A., 85: 1202–1208, Oct. 17, 1925

Thomas, William Alexander. Chicago physician. 1890–
Reported—
Generalized edema occurring only at the menstrual period. J. A. M. A., 101: 1126–1127, Oct. 7, 1933

Thomayer, Josef. Prague surgeon. 1853–1927
SIGN—to distinguish inflammatory from non-inflammatory ascites.
Beitrag zur Diagnose der tuberculösen und carcinomatösen Erkrankungen des Bauchfells. Z. f. klin. Med., 7: 378–409, 1884

Thompson, Basil. Tucson, Ariz. surgeon. 1903–
CLAMP—
A new stitching device. Canad. med. Ass. J., 24: 101 (only), Jan. 1931

Thompson, D. English scientist
AGAR—glucose plasma.
A new culture medium for the gonococcus. Preliminary note. Brit. med. J., 1: 869–870, June 30, 1917

Thompson, Gershom Joseph. Rochester, Minn. urologist. 1901–
RESECTOSCOPE—"cold cutting."
A new direct vision resectoscope. Urol. and Cutan. Rev., 39: 545–546, Aug. 1935

Thompson, Sir Henry. English surgeon. 1820–1904
OPERATION—for tumors of bladder.
On tumours of the bladder, their nature, symptoms, and surgical treatment. . . . London, Churchill, 1884. 111 pp.

Thompson, James Edwin. Texas surgeon. 1863–1927
OPERATION—
A study of modern operations in hypospadias from an anatomical and functional standpoint. S. G. O., 25: 411–422, Oct. 1917

Thompson, Marvin Russell. Baltimore pharmacologist. 1905–
Isolated ergostetrin.
The active constituents of ergot: a pharmacological and chemical study. J. Amer. Pharm. Ass., 24: 24–38, Jan.; 185–196, Mar. 1935

Thompson, Silvanus Phillips. English physicist. 1851–1916

CIRCLES—motion after-images.
Optical illusions of motion. Brain, 3: 289–298, Oct. 1880
Thomsen, Asmus Julius Thomas. Danish physician. 1815–1896
DISEASE—myotonia congenita.
Tonische Krämpfe in willkürlich beweglichen Muskeln in Folge von ererbten psychischer Disposition (Ataxia muscularis?). Arch. f. Psychiat., 6: 702–718, 1876
Thomsen, Oluf. Copenhagen pathologist
PHENOMENON—(T-agent), blood groups.
Ein vermehrungsfähriges Agens als Veränderer des isoagglutinatorischen Verhaltens der roten Blutkörperchen, eine bisher unbekannte Quelle der Fehlbestimmung. Z. ImmunForsch., 52: 85–107, July 26, 1927
Thomson, Adam. American physician. ?–1767
Originator of American method of inoculation against smallpox. Garrison and Morton
A discourse on the preparation of the body for the smallpox, and the manner of receiving the infection. Philadelphia, B. Franklin and D. Hall, 1750
Thomson, D. L. See J. B. Collip
Thomson, Elihu. American engineer. 1853–
Invented Roentgen stereoscope.
Stereoscopic Röntgen pictures. Electrical World, New York, 27: 280 (only), Mar. 14, 1896
Thomson, J. D. See H. G. Plimmer
Thomson, J. G. See J. S. Anderson
Thomson, Sir St. Clair. English physician. 1859–1943
Noted association of chronic nasal sinus disease with bronchorrhea.
Some of the symptoms and complications of sinusitis. Practitioner, 92: 745–754, June 1914
Thomson-Walker, Sir John William. London urologist
OPERATION—
Lettsomian lectures on enlarged prostate and prostatectomy. Lancet, 1: 1163–1168, May 31; 1219–1225, June 7; 1273–1280, June 14, 1930
Thorek, Max. Chicago surgeon. 1880–
OPERATION—plastic on breast.
Possibilities in the reconstruction of the human form. New York Med. J. and Rec., 116: 572–575, Nov. 15, 1922
Plastic surgery of the breast and abdominal wall. Springfield, Ill., Thomas, 1942
Twenty-five years' experience with plastic reconstruction of the breast and transplantation of the nipple. Amer. J. Surg., 67: 445–466, Mar. 1945
Thorel, Christen. Nürnberg physician. 1880–
BUNDLE—connecting sino-auricular and auriculoventricular nodes.
Pathologie der Kreislauforgane. Ergebn. d. allg. Path. u. path. Anat. d. Mensch., 9: 561–1116, 1903; 11: 194–589, 1907
Thorn, George Widmer. Baltimore physician. 1906–
Advocated—
Treatment of adrenal insufficiency by means of subcutaneous implants of pellets of desoxycorticosterone acetate (a synthetic adrenal cortical hormone) with L. L. Engel and H. Eisenberg, Johns Hopk. Hosp. Bull., 64: 155–166, Mar. 1939
Treatment of Addison's disease with pellets of crystalline adrenal cortical hormone (synthetic desoxy-corticosterone acetate) implanted subcutaneously with R.

P. Howard, K. Emerson, Jr., and W. M. Firor, Ibid., 339–365, May 1939
Thorne, W. S. See E. Rixford
Thornton, Lawson. Atlanta, Ga. surgeon. 1884–
PLATE—
The treatment of trochanteric fractures femur: two new methods. Piedmont Hosp. Bull., 10: 21–28, Jan. 1, 1937
Thornwaldt. See Gustav Ludwig Tornwaldt
Throckmorton, Tom Bentley. American neurologist. 1885–
REFLEX—a variant of Babinski r.
The rôle of extensor toe reflexes in neurological diagnosis. New York med. J., 94: 786–787, Oct. 14, 1911
Thunberg, Torsten. Swedish physiologist
BAROSPIRATOR—
Der Barospirator: Ein Apparat für küunstliche Atmung nach einem neuen Prinzip.
In: *Abderhalden's Handbuch der biologischen Arbeitsmethoden.* 1927. Sect. 5, pt. 1, p. 561
MICRORESPIROMETER—for estimating oxygen usage.
Mikro-respirometrische Untersuchungen. Zbl. f. Physiol., Leipzig, 18: 553–556, 1904
Ein Mikrorespirometer. Ein neuer Respirationsapparat, um den respiratorischen Gasaustausch kleiner Organe und Organismen zu bestimmen. Skandin. Arch. f. Physiol., Leipzig, 17: 74–85, 1905
Thurzo, E. von: Thurzo, J. See L. Benedek
Tichy, V. L. See C. S. Beck
Tickle, Thomas Gooch. New York otolaryngologist. 1892–
TECHNIC—
Surgery of the facial nerve in 300 operated cases. Laryngoscope, 55: 191–195, May 1945
Tidy, Charles Meymott. English scientist. 1843–1892
TEST—
On a new test for albumen. Lancet, 1: 691 (only), May 14, 1870
Tiedemann, F. See L. Gmelin
Tietze, Alexander. Breslau physician
DISEASE—a non-suppurative and non-specific swelling of rib cartilage.
Ueber eine eigenartige Häufung von Fällen mit Dystrophie der Rippenknorpel. Berl. klin. Wschr., 58: 829–831, July 25, 1921
Tietze, H. Leipzig surgeon
METHOD—of reduction of old shoulder dislocations.
Unblutige Reposition veralteter Schulterluxationen mit Hilfe von Novocaininjektionen. Chirurg, 8: 647–649, Aug. 15, 1936
Tietz, J. See O. Lentz
Tiffany, Louis McLane. Baltimore surgeon. 1844–1916
OPERATION—
Intracranial operations for the cure of facial neuralgia. Ann. Surg., 24: 575–619; 736–748, 1896
Tigerstedt, Robert Adolf Armand. Finnish physiologist. 1853–1923
RESPIRATION CALORIMETER—
Der Respirationsapparat im neuen physiologischen Institut zu Helsingfors. Skandin. Arch. f. Physiol., 18: 298–305, 1906
Studied effects of mechanical stimulation of nerve. Garrison and Morton

Studien über mechanische Nervenreizung. Acta Soc. Scient. Fennicae, Helsingfors, 11: 569–660, 1880
Demonstrated pressor activity in crude kidney extract.
Niere und Kreislauf with P. G. Bergman, Skand. Arch. f. Physiol., 8: 223–271, 1898
See also K. Sonden

Tileston, Wilder. New Haven physician. 1875–
Reported—
Chronic family jaundice with W. A. Griffin, Amer. J. med. Sci., 139: 847–869, June 1910

Tillett, William Smith. Baltimore physician. 1892–
TEST OF—
The fibrinolytic activity of hemolytic streptococci with R. L. Garner, J. exp. Med., 58: 485–502, Oct. 1, 1933

Tillmans, Josef. Frankfurt a. M. chemist
REACTION—for albumin.
Über den Gehalt der wichtigsten Proteinarten der Lebersmittel an Tryptophan und ein neues Verfahren der Tryptophanbestimmung with A. Alt, Biochem. Z., 164: 135–162, Nov. 2, 1925

Tilney, Frederick. New York neurologist. 1876–1938
Wrote on evolution of central nervous system.
The form and functions of the central nervous system with H. A. Riley, New York, Hoeber, 1921
The brain from ape to man: with chapters on the reconstruction of the gray matter in the primate brain stem by H. A. Riley. New York, Hoeber, 1928. 2 vols.

Timme, Walter. American physician. 1874–
SYNDROME—
A new pluriglandular compensatory syndrome. Endocrinol., 2: 209–240, July–Sept. 1918

Timoni, Emmanuel. Constantinople. fl. 1741
Wrote on small pox to John Woodward of England. Garrison and Morton
An account, or history, of the procuring of the small pox by incision or inoculation, as it has for some time been practised at Constantinople. Philos. Trans., 1714–1716, 29: 72–82, 1717
Tractatus bini de nova variolas per transplantationem excitandi methodo. Lugduni Batavorum, apud Janssonois van der Aa, 1721

Tinel, Jules. French neurologist
SIGN—distal tingling on percussion over divided nerve.
Les blessures des nerfs. . . . Paris, Masson, 1916. 311 pp.
Nerve wounds. Symptomatology of peripheral nerve lesions caused by war wounds. Transl. by F. Rothwell, New York, Wood, 1917. 317 pp. pp. 34–35
See also E. M. Labbé

Tinker, Martin Buel. Ithaca, N. Y. surgeon. 1869–
Advocated thyroidectomy in stages.
Surgical treatment of exophthalmic goiter. Some internists' views and surgical experience. Med. Rec., 81: 989–991, May 25, 1912

Tisdall, Frederick Fitzgerald. Baltimore pediatrician. 1893–
MODIFICATION—of Folin-Denis method.
Estimation of the phenolic substances in urine. J. biol. Chem., 44: 409–427, Nov. 1920
See also B. Kramer

Tissot, Jules. French physician
SPIROMETER—
Nouvelle méthode de mesure et d'inscription du débit et des mouvements respiratoires de l'homme et des animaux. J. Physiol. Path. gén., Paris, 6: 688–700, 1904

Tixier, Louis. French surgeon. 1871–
TEST—
Nouveau procédé pour la recherche de l'acide picrique dans le sang des ictères simulés with A. Bernard, Progres méd., 44: 218–220, Nov. 20, 1916
See also E. Apert

Tobey, George Loring, Jr. Boston otolaryngologist. 1881–
TEST—for thrombosis of lateral sinus.
Dynamic studies on the cerebrospinal fluid in the differential diagnosis of lateral sinus thrombosis with J. B. Ayer, Arch. Otolaryng., 2: 50–57, July 1925

Tobold, Adelbert August Oscar. German laryngologist. 1827–
APPARATUS—an illuminating a. for use with a laryngoscope.
Lehrbuch der Laryngoskopie. . . . Berlin, Hirschwald, 1863. 148 pp.

Tocantins, Leonardo Maues. Philadelphia physician. 1901–
METHOD—
Rapid absorption of substances injected into the bone marrow. Proc. Soc. exp. Biol., N. Y., 45: 292–296, Oct. 1940
Infusion of blood and other fluids into the general circulation via the bone marrow; technic and results with J. F. O'Neill, S. G. O., 73: 281–287, Sept. 1941
Infusion of blood and other fluids via the bone marrow: application in pediatrics with J. F. O'Neill and H. W. Jones, J. A. M. A., 117: 1229–1234, Oct. 11, 1941
See also H. W. Jones

Todd, Alexander Robertus. London biochemist
Isolated—
Studies on vitamin E. II. The isolation of B-tocopherol from wheat germ oil with F. Bergel and T. S. Work, Biochem. J., 31: 2257–2263, Dec. 1937
See also G. Barger

Todd, David Duke. Chicago physician. 1883–
AGAR—lactose serum.
A new color medium for the isolation and differentiation of streptococci. J. infect. Dis., 7: 73–77, Jan. 15, 1910

Todd, Frank C. American ophthalmologist. 1869–1918
CAUTERY—
A simple and effective instrument for cauterizing corneal ulcers. Ophth. Rec., 17: 180 (only), Apr. 1908
OPERATION—
Extra-ocular tendon lengthening and shortening operations which enable the operator to regulate the effect. Ibid., 23: 628–642, Dec. 1914

Todd, J. L. See J. E. Dutton

Todd, T. W. See J. G. Kramer

Toepfer, Gustav. Vienna scientist
TEST—for hydrochloric acid in gastric juice.
Eine Methode zur titrimetrischen Bestimmung der hauptsächlichsten Factoren der Magenacidität. Z. physiol. Chem., 19: 104–122, 1894

Töpfer, Hans Willi. German physician. 1876–
Isolated Rickettsia quintana from lice found on patients suffering from "trench fever." Garrison and Morton
Zur Ursache und Übertragung des Wolhynischen

Fiebers. Münch. med. Wschr., 63: 1495–1496, Oct. 17, 1916

Tollens, Bernhard. German chemist. 1841–1918
TEST—for sugar.
Ueber die Xylose (Holzzucker) und das Holzgummi. By H. J. Wheeler and B. Tollens, Ber. d. dtsch. chem. Ges., 22: 1046 (only), 1889
Ueber den Nachweis der Pentosen mittels der Phloro-glucin-Salzsäure-Absatz-Methode. Ibid., 29: 1202–1209, Apr. 27, 1896

Tolstoi, E. See T. P. Almy

Tomita, M. Japanese physician
TEST—
Condensation of ninhydrin with indoxyl: (a new test for indican). J. Oriental Med., 2: 189–190, May 1924

Tompkins, Charles Archibald. Indianapolis pediatrician. 1910–
Advocated apple diet for diarrhea.
Infant diarrhea with special reference to apple therapy. J. Indiana med. Ass., 28: 278–280, June 1935

Tompkins, Edna H. See R. S. Cunningham

Toomey, John Augustus. Cleveland pediatrician. 1889–
PHENOMENON—
Reappearance of a positive Dick test. J. A. M. A., 87: 941 (only), Sept. 18, 1926

Tooth, Howard Henry. English physician. 1856–1926
DISEASE or TYPE—Charcot-Marie-Tooth d.
The peroneal type of progressive muscular atrophy. London, Lewis, 1886. 43 pp.

Toprower, G. S. Leningrad surgeon
METHOD—of gastrostomy.
Novy sposob gastrostomii. Vestnik khir., 34: 23–30, 1934
Eine neue Methode der Gastrostomie. Zbl. Chir., 61: 1919–1921, Aug. 18, 1934

Torday, A. von. Budapest physician
TEST—for bile in urine.
Ueber neue Gallenfarbstoffreaktionen im Urin. Dtsch. med. Wschr., 35: 1470–1471, Aug. 26, 1909

Torek, Franz. American surgeon. 1861–1938
MANEUVER—bring vas and vessels of cord out through new internal ring at separate points, to obtain firm closure.
The technique of orcheopexy. New York med. J., 90: 948–953, Nov. 13, 1909
OPERATION—for inguinal hernia.
Combined operation for the removal of the appendix and the cure of right inguinal hernia. Ann. Surg., 43: 665–667, May 1906
OPERATION—
Orchiopexy for undescended testicle. Ibid., 94: 97–110, July 1931
OPERATION—
The first successful case of resection of the thoracic portion of the esophagus for carcinoma. S. G. O., 16: 614–617, June 1913
Carcinoma of the thoracic portion of the esophagus: report of a case in which operation was done eleven years ago. Arch. Surg., 10: 353–360, Jan. 1925

Tornwaldt, Gustavus Ludovicus. German physician. 1843–1910
DISEASE or BURSITIS—inflammation of Luschka's tonsil.
Ueber die Bedeutung der Bursa pharyngea für die Erkennung und Behandlung gewisser Nasenrachen-

raum-Krankheiten. Wiesbaden, Bergmann, 1885. 119 pp.

Torre, A. A. See G. Bizzozero

Torrey, J. P. See I. F. Huddleson

Torrey, John Cutler. New York bacteriologist. 1876–
BROTH—basal ascitic fluid infusion; for studying fermentation by bacteria.
Cultural methods for the gonococcus with G. T. Buckell, J. infect. Dis., 31: 125–147 (142), Aug. 1922
MEDIA—for gonococcus. Ibid.

Torti, Francesco. Italian pharmacologist. 1658–1741
Wrote an important treatise on pernicious malarial fevers, which brought about employment of cinchona bark into Italian practice and introduced term malaria. Garrison
Therapeutice specialis, ad febres quasdam perniciosas inopinato. Mutinae, Soliani, 1712. 736 pp.

Toti, Addeo. Italian ophthalmologist
OPERATION—dacryocystorhinostomy.
Nuovo metodo conservatore di cura radicale delle suppurazione croniche del sacco lacrimale (dacriocistorinostomia). Clin. mod., Pisa, 10: 385–387, 1904

Tournay, Auguste. French ophthalmologist
SIGN—
Sur l'anisocorie normale dans le regard latéral extrème. Arch. d'ophthal., 44: 574–576, Sept. 1927

Towns, Charles Barnes. American insurance agent. 1862–1947
TREATMENT—of Towns-Lambert.
Help for the hard drinker; what can be done to save the man worthwhile. Century Mag., New York, 84: 290–297, June 1912

Toynbee, Joseph. English anatomist. 1815–1860
CORPUSCLES—corneal c.
Researches, tending to prove the non-vascularity and the peculiar uniform mode of organization and nutrition of certain animal tissues, viz. articular cartilage, and the cartilage of the different classes of fibro-cartilage; the cornea, the crystalline lens, and the vitreous humour; and the epidermoid appendages. Philos. Trans., 131: 159–192, 1841
OTOSCOPE—
On a new ear speculum. Lancet, 2: 390–391, Oct. 5, 1850

Tracy, S. J. London physician
ETHER INHALER—
Apparatus for respiration of ether vapour. London med. Gaz., 4: 167 (only), Jan. 22, 1847
A description of an apparatus for inhalation of ether vapour, with some remarks on its use. London, Ferguson, 1847. pp. 30

Transkeian
SCAB—Veldt sore; an ulceration on legs and forearms, occurring in South Africa.

Trantenroth, A. See R. Bunge

Trapani, Pietro. Italian physician
TEST—for bilirubin.
La recherche de la bilirubine par le cyanure de mercure en milieu alcalin. Semaine med., 25: 615 (only), Dec. 27, 1905

Traquair, Harry Moss. Edinburgh ophthalmologist. 1876–
JUNCTION SCOTOMA OR—
Bitemporal hemiopia: the later stages and the special features of the scotoma: with an examination of current theories of the mechanism of production of the field

defects. Brit. J. Ophthal., 1: 216–239, Apr.; 281–294, May; 337–352, June 1917

Traube, Ludwig. German physician. 1818–1876
CURVES—high, bold curves seen in tracings of sphygmograph when respiration has been completely arrested.
Über periodische Thätigkeits-Ausserungen des vasomotorischen und Hemmungs-Nervencentrums. Zbl. f. d. med. Wiss., Berlin, 3: 881–885, 1865
DYSPNEA—
Die Symptome der Krankheiten des Respirations- und Circulations-Apparats. Berlin, Hirschwald, 1867. 168 pp.
HEART—heart disease of nephropathic origin.
Ueber den Zusammenhang von Herz- und Nieren-Krankheiten. Berlin, Hirschwald, 1856. 81 pp.
MURMUR—cantering or gallop rhythm.
PULSUS ALTERNANS—
Ein Fall von Pulsus bigeminus nebst Bemerkungen über die Leberschwellungen bei Klappenfehlern und über acute Leberatrophie. Berl. klin. Wschr., 9: 185–188, Apr. 15; 221–224, May 6, 1872
Also, English transl. by F. A. Willius in: F. A. Willius and T. E. Keys' *Cardiac classics.* St. Louis, Mosby, 1941, pp. 590–599
SEMILUNAR SPACE—
Published from Traube's clinic by Dr. Fraentzel
Linke Lungs in ihrer ganzen Ausdehnung grau hepatisirt. Fibrino-seröses Exsudat im Pericardium. Bemerkungen über den halbmondförmigen Raum und über den Vocalfremitus. Berl. klin. Wschr., 5: 509–511, Dec. 14, 1868

Traube, Moritz. German scientist. 1826–1894
Investigated osmosis and permeability of membranes. Garrison and Morton
Experimente zur Theorie der Zellenbildung und Endosmose. Arch. f. Anat., Physiol. u. wiss. Med., Berlin, 87–165, 1867

Travers, Benjamin. London surgeon. 1783–1858
Described—
A case of aneurism by anastomosis in the orbit, cured by the ligature of the common carotid artery. Med.-chir. Trans., London, 2: 1–16, 1811
Wrote—
An inquiry into the process of nature in repairing injuries of the intestines. London, Longman, 1812
Introduced use of mercury in non-specific iritis. Garrison
A synopsis of the diseases of the eye. . . . London, Longman, 1820. 425 pp.

Travis, W. C. See O. Teague

Treitz, Wenzel. Austrian physician. 1819–1872
FOSSA—duodenojejunal f.
HERNIA—retroperitoneal, through fossa.
LIGAMENT—musculus duodeni suspensorius.
Hernia retroperitonealis; Ein Beitrag zur Geschichte innerer Hernien. Prag, Credner, 1857. 150 pp.

Trendelenburg, Friedrich. Leipzig surgeon. 1844–1924
CANULA or TAMPON—
Erfahrungen über die Tamponnade der Trachea. Arch. f. klin. Chir., 15: 352–368, 1873
OPERATION—ligation of great saphenous vein to prevent reflux into varicose veins.
Ueber die Unterbindung der Vena saphena magna bei Unterschenkelvaricen. Beitr. z. klin. Chir., 7: 195–210, 1890

Also, in German with English transl. in: Medical classics, 4: 989–1023, May 1940
OPERATION—removal of pulmonary embolus.
Ueber die operative Behandlung der Embolie der Lungenarterie. Arch. f. klin. Chir., 86: 686–700, 1908
POSITION—
Ueber Blasenscheidenfisteloperationen und über Beckenhochlagerung bei Operationen in der Bauchhöhle. Samml. klin. Vortr., 355, Chir. No. 109, pp. 3373–3392, Jan. 30, 1890
Also, in German with English transl. in: Medical classics, 4: 936–988, May 1940
SIGN and SYMPTOM—of congenital dislocation of hip.
Ueber den Gang bei angeborener Hüftgelenksluxation. Dtsch. med. Wschr., 21: 21–24, Jan. 10, 1895
TABLE—
Demonstration eines neuen Operationstisches. Verh. d. dtsch. Ges. f. Chir., 19: 53–54, Apr. 10, 1890
Trendelenburg's new operating table, designed for operations in the posture bearing his name. By Willy Meyer, Med. Rec., 38: 658–659, Dec. 13, 1890
TEST—for insufficiency of valves in varicose veins. See OPERATION

Trescher, J. H. See G. A. Harrop

Treves, Sir Frederick. English surgeon. 1853–1923
CLAMP—for intestinal resection.
Intestinal obstruction. London, Cassell, 1884
OPERATION—for Pott's disease.
The direct treatment of psoas abscess with caries of the spine. Med.-chir. Trans., 67: 113–126, 1884

Treves, Norman. New York surgeon. 1894–
RADIUM NEEDLE—
A small platinum needle designed for the use of various strengths of radium element interstitially. Amer. J. Roentgenol., 33: 537–544, Apr. 1935

Tribondeau, L. See J. Bergonié

Triboulet, Henri. French physician. 1864–1920
TEST—for urobilin.
Exploration clinique des voies biliaires et de l'intestin par la réaction du sublimé acétique dans les selles. Pr. méd., 17: 777–779, Nov. 3, 1909

Trimble, H. See O. K. O. Folin

Trimble, Isaac Ridgeway. Baltimore surgeon. 1900–
A one stage operation for the cure of carcinoma of the ampulla of Vater and of the head of the pancreas with J. W. Parsons and C. P. Sherman, S. G. O., 73: 711–722, Nov. 1941

Tröltsch, Anton Friedrich von. German aurist. 1829–1890
Invented modern otoscope.
Die Untersuchung des Gehörgangs und Trommelfells. Ihre Bedeutung. Kritik der bisherigen Untersuchungsmethoden und Angabe einer neuen. Dtsch. Klin., 12: 113–115, Mar. 24; 121–123, Mar. 31; 131–135, Apr. 7; 143–146, Apr. 14; 151–154, Apr. 21, 1860
Devised modern mastoid operation.
Ein Fall von Anbohrung des Warzenfortsatzes bei Otitis interna mit Bemerkungen über diese Operation. Arch. f. path. Anat., 21: 295–314, 1861

Trömner, Ernest L. O. Hamburg neurologist. 1868–
SIGN—of finger flexion in pyramidal tract disease.
Ueber Sehnen—resp. Muskelreflexe und die Merkmale ihrer Schwächung und Steigerung. Berl. klin. Wschr., 50: 1712–1715, Sept. 15, 1913

Troisier, Charles Émile. French physician. 1844–1919

GLAND or NODE—of Virchow-Troisier.
Les ganglions sus-claviculaires dans le cancer de l'esto-mac. Bull. Soc. méd. Hôp. Paris, 3 s., 3: 394–398, Oct. 8, 1886

Trolard, Paulin. French physician. 1842–1910
VEIN—
Recherches sur l'anatomie du système veineux de l'encéphale et du crâne. Paris, thesis, 1868. 32 pp.

Trommer, Carl August. German chemist. 1806–1879
TEST—for glucose in urine.
Unterscheidung von Gummi, Dextrin, Traubenzucker und Rohrzucker. (Abstr. of Trommer's work) Ann. d. Chem., 39: 360–362, 1841

Tronchin, Théodore. Geneva physician. 1709–1781
Described lead colic.
De colica pictonum. Geneva, Cramer, 1757. 82 pp.

Troncoso, Manuel Uribe y. New York ophthalmologist. 1867–
INSTRUMENT—gonioscope.
Gonioscopy and its clinical applications. Amer. J. Ophthal., 8: 433–449, June 1925
OPERATION—
Cyclodialysis with insertion of a metal implant in the treatment of glaucoma; a preliminary report. Arch. Ophthal., 23: 270–300, Feb. 1940

Trotman, F. E. See H. D. Haskins, E. E. Osgood

Trotter, Thomas. British physician. 1761–1832
Wrote—
Observations on the scurvy. Edinburgh, Eliot and Robinson, 1786
Medicina nautica. London, 1797–1803. 3 vols.

Trousseau, Armand. Paris physician. 1801–1867
DISEASE—of Hodgkin-Trousseau.
De l'adénie. Gaz. hebd. d. med. et d. chir., Paris, 2 s., 1: 837 (only), Dec. 16; 874–879, Dec. 30, 1864; 2: 5–9, Jan. 6, 1865
SIGN—of tetany.
In his: *Clinique médicale de l' Hotel Dieu de Paris,* 2: 112–114, 1862
Wrote a laryngological classic.
Traité pratique de la phthisie laryngée, de la laryngite chronique et des maladies de la voix with H. Belloc, Paris, Baillière, 1837
Wrote—
Du tubage de la glotte et de la trachéotomie. Paris, Baillière, 1859
Described hemochromatosis.
Glycosurie, diabete sucré. In his: *Clinique médicale de l' Hôtel-Dieu de Paris,* 2 ed., 2: 663–698, 1865

Truesdale, Philemon E. Fall River, Mass. surgeon. 1875–1945
OPERATION—
Diaphragmatic hernia: its varieties and surgical treatment of hiatus type. Amer. J. Surg., 32: 204–216, May 1936

Trueta, José. Spanish surgeon. 1897–
METHOD—
Treatment of war wounds and fractures, with special reference to the closed method as used in the war with Spain. London, Hamilton, 1939. 150 pp.
Also: New York, Hoeber, 1940. 150 pp.

Truhaut, R. See M. Peronnet

Truszkowski, Richard. American scientist
Demonstrated advantage of a diet having a low potassium component for Addison's disease.

Cortico-adrenal insufficiency and potassium metabolism with R. L. Zwemer, Biochem. J., 30: 1345–1353, 1936

Try, W. K. See H. D. Gillies

Tschamer, Anton. German physician
Described, acute infectious erythema, fifth disease or Stickers disease.
Über örtliche Rötheln. Jb. Kinderheilk., n. F., 29: 372–379, 1889

Tscherning, Marius Hans Erik. Copenhagen ophthalmologist. 1854–
PHOTOMETRIC GLASSES—
L'adaptation compensatrice de l'oeil. Ann. d'Ocul., 159: 625–637, Sept. 1922

Tsuchiya, Henry M. Minnesota bacteriologist
TECHNIC—of resensitization of bacteria.
In vitro effect of urea-sulfathiazole combination on sulfathiazole-resistant staphylococci with D. J. Tenenberg, E. A. Strakosch and W. G. Clark, Proc. Soc. exp. Biol., N. Y., 51: 245–247, Nov. 1942

Tsuchiya, I. Tokio physician
REAGENT—for albumin and peptone.
Eine neue volumetrische Eiweissbestimmung mittels der Phosphorwolframsäure. Zbl. f. inn. Med., 29: 105–115, Feb. 1, 1908

Tubbs, O. S. See R. H. Overholt

Tubby, Alfred Herbert. English surgeon. 1862–1930
OPERATION—for brachial palsy.
On a method of treating by operation paralysis of the upper root of the brachial plexus (Erb-Duchenne type). Brit. med. J., 2: 975–976, Oct. 17, 1903

Tucker, Gabriel. Philadelphia otolaryngologist. 1880–
TREATMENT—
Cicatricial stenosis of the esophagus, with particular reference to treatment by continuous string, retrograde bouginage with the author's bougie. Ann. Otology, Rhinol. and Laryngol., 23: 1181–1223, Dec. 1924

Tübingen. Germany
HEART—dilatation and hypertrophy of heart from excessive beer drinking.

Türck, Ludwig. Vienna neurologist. 1810–1868
Noted association of retinal hemorrhage with tumors of brain. Garrison
Ein Fall von Haemorrhagie der Netzhaut beider Augen (bei einem Gehirntumor). Z. d. k. k. Ges. d. Aerzte zu Wien, 1 Abt., 9: 214–218, 1853
Established examination of larynx by means of laryngoscope of Garcia.
Der Kehlkopfrachenspiegel und die Methode seines Gebrauches. Ibid., 14: 401–409, 1858
Investigated cutaneous distribution of separate pairs of spinal nerves. Garrison and Morton
Über die Haut-Sensibilitätsbezirke der einzelnen Rückenmarksnervenpaare. Denkschr. d. k. Akad. d. Wissensch., Math.-nat. Cl., Wien, 29: 299–326, 1868

Türk, Wilhelm. Vienna physician. 1871–1916
Reported complete agranulocytosis. Garrison and Morton
Septische Erkrankungen bei Verkümmerung des Granulozytensystems. Wien. klin. Wschr., 20: 157–162, Feb. 7, 1907

Tuffier, Theodore. French surgeon. 1857–1929
OPERATION—extrapleural pneumolysis.
Gangrène pulmonaire ouverte dans les bronches et traitée par décollement pleuro-pariétal, et greffe d'une masse lipomateuse entre la plèvre décollée et les espaces

intercostaux. Bull. Soc. chir. Paris, n. s., 36: 529–538, May 11, 1910
TEST—for adequate collateral circulation.
Sur un procédé permettant de prévoir que l'irrigation sanguine persistera dans un membre après ligature de son artère principale with Hallion, Soc. Biol., Paris, 73: 606–608, Dec. 7, 1912
Effectively transplanted ureter to bowel in cystectomy, 1895.
De l'extirpation totale de la vessie pour néoplasmes with Dujarier, Rev. de chir., 18: 277–289, 1898
Wrote on surgery of lungs.
Chirurgie du poumon, en particulier dans les cavernes tuberculeuses et la gangrène pulmonaire. Paris, Masson, 1897
Did early work on spinal anesthesia.
Analgésie chirurgicale par l'injection sous-arachnoidienne lombaire de cocaine. C. R. Soc. Biol., 51: 882–884, Nov. 11, 1899
Wrote—
Étude expérimentelle sur la chirurgie des valvules du coeur. Bull. Acad. Méd. Paris, 3 s., 71: 293–295, 1914

Tufnell, Thomas Jolliffe. English surgeon. 1819–1885
DIET and TREATMENT—absolute rest and starvation diet.
The successful treatment of internal aneurism by consolidation of the contents of the sac. London, Churchill, 1875. 2 ed. 71 pp.

Tuholske, L. See M. G. Seelig

Tullio, Pietro. Sardinian physician
ACOUSTIC REACTIONS—
I riflessi sonori (condimostrazioni cinematografiche). Abstr.: Internat. Physiol. Congr., 13. Congr., 272 (only), 1929
De reflexibus sonoris demonstratio. Otorinolar. ital., 5: 443–456, 1935

Tulloch, William John. Scottish bacteriologist
AGAR—ox heart infusion pea flour.
Serological examination of one hundred strains of the gonococcus. J. Path. Bact., 25: 346–365 (348), July 1922

Tulp, Nikolaas. Dutch physician. 1593–1674
Described beri-beri. Garrison and Morton
Observationes medicae. Amstelredami, apud L. Elzevirium, 1652. pp. 300–325

Tunnicliff, Ruth. Chicago bacteriologist. 1876–
Discovered a diplococcus in measles. Garrison
The cultivation of a micrococcus from blood in pre-eruptive and eruptive stages of measles. J. A. M. A., 68: 1028–1030, Apr. 7, 1917

Turck, Raymond Custer. Jacksonville, Fla. surgeon. 1874–
SUTURE—for intestine.
The interlocking suture. Ann. Surg., 48: 837–847, Dec. 1908

Turnbull, H. M. See D. Hunter

Turnbull, Lawrence. Philadelphia surgeon. 1821–1900
Performed mastoidectomy.
Report on three cases of otitis interna successfully treated. Med. and Surg. Reporter, 7: 463–466, Feb. 15–22, 1862

Turner, B. B. See J. J. Abel

Turner, G(eorge) Grey. English surgeon. 1877–

OPERATION—"pull through", for carcinoma of esophagus.
Discussion on recent advances in the treatment of carcinoma of the esophagus from the surgical and radiological aspects. Proc. roy. Soc. Med., Sect. Laryngol., 27: 355–365, Feb. 1934
SIGN—
Local discoloration of the abdominal wall as a sign of acute pancreatitis. Brit. J. Surg., 7: 394–395, Jan. 1920
TECHNIC—of immobilizing left lobe of liver.
Some experiences in the surgery of the esophagus. New Engl. J. Med., 205: 657–674, Oct. 1, 1931

Turner, Henry Hubert. Oklahoma City physician. 1892–
SYNDROME—
A syndrome of infantilism, congenital webbed neck, and cubitus valgus. Endocrinology, 23: 566–574, Nov. 1938

Turner, J. R. See F. P. Rous

Turner, Philip. London surgeon. 1873–
OPERATION—for inguinal hernia.
Inguinal hernia, the imperfectly descended testicle and varicocele. London, Churchill, 1919. 104 pp.
Hernioplasty. Guy's Hosp. Rep., 83: 233–251, Apr. 1933

Tutin, Frank. English biochemist
TEST—
A modification of Webster's test for the presence of T. N. T. in urine. Lancet, 2: 554 (only), Oct. 26, 1918

Tuttle, James P. New York surgeon. 1857–1913
OPERATION—
A modified technic for the combined operation of extirpation of the rectum. Amer. J. Surg., 24: 165–168, June 1910

Tuttle, Waid Wright. Iowa physiologist. 1893–
TEST—
A simplification of the pulse-ratio technique for rating physical efficiency and present condition with R. E. Dickinson, Amer. Ass. for Health and Phys. Education, Research Quarterly, 9, No. 2: 73–80, May 1938

Tweedy, Wilbur R. Chicago biochemist
METHOD—
A suggested modification of the Kramer-Tisdall method for the microchemical estimation of ionizable calcium in blood plasma with F. C. Koch, J. Lab. clin. Med., 14: 747–750, May 1929

Twiss, John Russell. New York physician. 1899–
TUBE—
A new type of duodenal tube tip. Amer. J. med. Sci., 185: 109–114, Jan. 1933

Twitchell, Amos. American surgeon. 1781–1850
Described—
Gun-shot wound of the face and neck—ligature of the carotid artery, Oct. 18, 1807. New Engl. Quart. J. Med. and Surg., 1: 188–193, 1843

Twombly, G. H. See Helen Q. Woodard

Twort, Frederick William. London scientist. 1877–
Investigated bacteriophage and filterable viruses.
An investigation of the nature of ultra-microscopic viruses. Lancet, 2: 1241–1243, Dec. 4, 1915

Tyler, D. A. See J. Knight

Tyndall, John. British physicist. 1820–1893
TYNDALLIZATION—fractional sterilization.
Essays on the floating-matter of the air in relation to

TYNDALL, JOHN 408 UNNA, PAUL GERSON

putrefaction and infection. London, Longmans, Green and Co., 1881
Tzoni, H. See W. Halden
Tyzzer, Ernest Edward. American pathologist. 1875–
Studied heredity of mouse cancer.

A study of heredity in relation to the development of tumors in mice. J. med. Res., 12: 199–211, Nov. 1907
Recognized inclusion bodies in varicella.
The histology of the skin lesions in varicella. Ibid., 14: 361–392, Jan. 1906

U

Ucko, H. French physician
TECHNIC—for modified Takata-Ara test.
Réaction de précipitation par le mercure dans le sérum des hépatiques. C. R. Soc. Biol., 118: 534–536, Feb. 9, 1935
A serum test for the diagnosis of liver disturbances. Guy's Hosp. Rep., 86: 166–174, 1936
Udenfriend, S. See B. B. Brodie
Udranszky, László v. Budapest physiologist. 1862–1914
TESTS—for cholesterol and sugars.
Ueber Furfurolreactionen. Z. physiol. Chem., 12: 355–395, 1888
Uffelmann, Julius August Christian. German physician. 1837–1894
TEST—for hydrochloric acid and lactic acid in gastric juice.
Ueber die Methode der Untersuchung des Mageninhalts auf freie Säuren. Versuche an einem Gastrotomirten. Dtsch. Arch. f. klin. Med., 26: 431–454, Sept. 16, 1880
Uhlenhuth, Paul Theodore. Berlin bacteriologist. 1870–
TEST—for human blood; Uhlenhuth-Bordet precipit.
Eine Methode zur Unterscheidung der verschiedenen Blutarten, im besonderen zum differentialdiagnostischen Nachweise des Menschenblutes. Dtsch. med. Wschr., 27: 82–83, 1901
Weitere Mittheilungen über meine Methode zum Nachweise von Menschenblut. Ibid., 260–261, 1901
Described Bact. paratyphosum C.
Weitere Mitteilungen über Schweinepest mit besonderer Berücksichtigung der Bakteriologie der Hogcholeragruppe with E. A. Hübener, Zbl. Bakt., 1 Abt., 127–138, 1908
Uhthoff, Wilhelm. Berlin ophthalmologist. 1853–1927
SIGN—nystagmus in multiple cerebrospinal sclerosis.
Untersuchungen über die bei der multiplen Herdsklerose vorkommenden Augenstörungen. Arch. f. Psychiat., 21: 55–116; 303–410, 1889
Ulin, Alexander Wesley. Cincinnati surgeon. 1913–
METHOD—
A new presumptive test for prothrombin determination with E. Barrows, J. A. M. A., 120: 826–827, Nov. 14, 1942
Ullmann, Emerich. Vienna surgeon
OPERATION—
Zur Technik der Gastrostomie. Wien. med. Wschr., 44: 1662–1664, Sept. 22, 1894
Ulrich, A. Zürich physician
METHOD—for determination of total halogens and bromides.
Die Halogenanalyse des Urins und ihr praktischer Wert in der Bromtherapie. Schweiz. Arch. Neurol Psychiat., 13: 622–630, 1923
Ultymann, Robert. German chemist. 1842–1889

TEST—for bile pigments.
Zum Nachweise von Gallenfarbstoffen im Harne. Wien. med. Pr., 18: 1033–1036, Aug. 12; 1065–1067, Aug. 19, 1877
Underhill, Frank Pell. New Haven, Conn. scientist. 1877–1932
Studied—
Blood concentration changes in extensive superficial burns, and their significance for systemic treatment with G. L. Carrington, R. Kapsinow and G. T. Pack, Arch. intern. Med., 32: 31–49, July 1923
Underwood, Michael. London pediatrician. 1736–1820
DISEASE—scleroma neonatorum.
In his: *A treatise on the diseases of children. . . .* London, 1784. p. 76
Described infantile paralysis. Garrison
Debility of the lower extremities. In: Ibid., new ed. London, Mathews, 1789, 2: 53–57
Unger, Ernst. Berlin surgeon
METHOD—of injection of varicose veins.
Zur Technik der Varicenbehandlung. Zbl. f. Chir., 54: 3273–3274, Dec. 17, 1927
Unger, Lester Jarecky. New York surgeon. 1888–
METHOD—
A new method of syringe transfusion. J. A. M. A., 64: 582–584, Feb. 13, 1915
Recent simplifications of the syringe method of transfusion. Ibid., 65: 1029 (only), Sept. 18, 1915
Unger, Max. New York otolaryngologist. 1885–
NASAL SPECULUM—
A new, double, self-retaining nasal speculum. J. A. M. A., 62: 1557 (only), May 16, 1914
Ungermann, Hr. Berlin physician
METHOD—for cultivation of Leptospira ictohaemorrhagiae.
Demonstration einer Kultur des Erregers der Weil'schen Krankheit. Berl. klin. Wschr., 53: 408–409, Apr. 10, 1916
Unna, Paul Gerson. Hamburg dermatologist. 1850–1929
DERMATOSIS or DISEASE—
Das seborrhoische Ekzem. Mschr. f. prakt. Dermat., 6: 827–846, Sept. 15, 1887
Seborrhoeal eczema. J. cutan. Dis., 5: 449–459, Dec. 1887
LAYER—stratum granulosum of skin.
Beiträge zur Histologie und Entwickelungsgeschichte der menschlichen Oberhaut und ihrer Anhangsgebilde. Arch. f. mikr. Anat., 12: 665–741, 1876
PILLS—coated for absorption in duodenum.
Eine neue Form medicamentöser Einverleibung. Fort. d. Med., 2: 507–509, 1884
Ueber Dünndarmpillen. Verh. d. Cong. f. inn. Med., 3 Congr., pp. 328–341, 1885
SOLUTION—polychrome methylene-blue.

Ueber die Reifung unserer Farbstoffe. Z. wiss. Mikr.,
8: 475–487, 1891
STAIN—for mast cell granules in sections.
STAIN—differential, for mast cells and plasma cells
in sections. Mallory
In: *Enzyklopädie der mikroskopischen Technik.* Berlin
und Wien, Urban und Schwarzenberg, 1910. 2 ed.,
vol. 2, p. 72
STAIN—for elastic fibers or tissue.
*Notiz, betreffend die Taenzersche Orceinfärbung des
elastischen Gewebes.* Mschr. f. prakt. Dermat., 12:
394–396, May 1, 1891
Die Färbung der Epithelfasern. Ibid., 19: 1–10, July
1; 277–283, Sept. 15, 1894
Introduced ichthyol and resorcin in treatment of
skin diseases. Garrison
*Ichthyol und Resorcin als Repräsentanten der Gruppe
reduzierender Heilmittel.* Hamburg und Leipzig,
Voss, 1886. 85 pp.
Also: *Ichthyol and resorcin as representatives of the
group of reducing remedies.* Philadelphia, Lippincott,
1890. 64 pp.
See also E. O. E. von Bälz
Unverricht, Heinrich. Jena physician. 1853–1912
DISEASE—
Die Myoklonie. Leipzig und Wien, Deuticke, 1891.
128 pp.
Ueber familiäre Myoclonie. Dtsch. Z. f. Nervenh.,
7: 32–67, July 18, 1895
Unzen, Johannes Augustus. Halle physiologist.
1727–1799
First differentiated between voluntary and involun-
tary movements; described some conditional re-

flexes without understanding their real value. Garri-
son
Prinzip der Physiologie. Leipzig, 1771
Also, transl. by T. Laycock, London, Sydenham Soc.,
1851
Updegraff, Howard Leighton. Hollywood, Cal.
surgeon. 1896–
OPERATION—
Reconstruction of the columella nasi. Amer. J. Surg.,
29: 29–31, July 1935
Urano, Fumihiko. Strassburg physician. 1870–
REACTION—
*Einwirkung von Säureanhydriden auf Kreatin und
Kreatinin.* Beitr. chem. Physiol. Path., 9: 183–184,
1907
Urbach, Erich. Vienna physician
LIPOID PROTEINOSIS—
Lipoidosis cutis et mucosae with C. Wiethe, Arch. f.
path. Anat., 273: 285–319, Sept. 6, 1929
Urechia, Constantin I. French physician. 1883–
REACTION—of cerebrospinal fluid.
*La réaction de la gomme-laque dans le liquide céphalo-
rachidien.* C. R. Soc. Biol., 89: 1250–1252, Oct. 25,
1923
Usami, Kanichi. Japanese physician
REAGENT—for blood.
*Ueber eine neue Leukofarbstoffprobe für den Nachweis
okkulter Blutungen in den Fäzes.* Wien. klin. Wschr.,
39: 786–789, July 1, 1926
Uschinsky, N. St. Petersburg bacteriologist
CULTURE MEDIUM or SOLUTION—protein free.
*Ueber eine eiweissfreie Nährlösung für pathogene
Bakterien nebst einigen Bemerkungen über Tetanus-
gift.* Zbl. Bakt., 14: 316–319, Sept. 9, 1893

V

Valdiguié, A. See J. F. Aloy
Valenti, E. See A. Ascoli
Valentin, G. G. See J. E. v. Purkinje
Valentine, E. See C. Krumwiede
Valentini, Michael Bernhard. German physician.
1657–1729
Published first book on forensic medicine. Garrison
Corpus juris medico-legale. . . . Francofurti a. M.,
Jungii, 1722. 570 pp.
Valk, W. L. See F. A. Coller
Valleix, Francois Louis Isidore. French physician.
1807–1855
POINT—pointes douloureux; tender points on course
of certain nerves in neuralgia, or points where inter-
costal nerves pierce rectus sheath.
*Traité des névralgies, ou affections douloureuses des
nerfs.* Paris, Baillière, 1841. 719 pp.
Valleti, Guido. Rome physician
AGAR—whey.
*Ueber einen neuen Nährböden zur sehr raschen Ent-
wicklung des Tuberkelbacillus.* Zbl. Bakt., 68: 239–
241, Mar. 1, 1913
Valsalva, Antonio Maria. Italian anatomist. 1666–
1723
LIGAMENT—connecting pinna of ear to temporal
bone.
MANEUVER—in chronic otitis media, when mouth
and nostrils are closed, and attempt is made to blow

out air, discharge will appear in auditory canal.
Divided organs of hearing into external, middle and
internal ear.
De aura humana tractatus. . . . Bologna, vande
Water, 1704. 184 pp.
Also, Utrecht, 1717. Also, Leyden, 1735
Valsuani, Emilio. Italian physician
DISEASE—progressive pernicious anemia in puerperal
and lactating women.
*Cachessia puerperale raccolta nella clinica ginecologica
dell'ospitale Maggiore di Milano.* Milano, Bernardoni.
1870. 16 pp.
Van Allen, Chester Montague. American physician.
1896–
TUBES—cell volume.
An hematocrit method. J. A. M. A., 84: 202–203,
Jan. 17, 1925
Van Arsdale, William Waldo. New York surgeon
BONE SAW—
*The technique of temporary resection of the skull, with
demonstration of a new set of instruments.* Ann. Surg.,
24: 465–480, 1896
Van Beneden, Édouard. Liege biologist
Discovered that associated male and female pro-
nuclei in fertilized egg each contain half as many
chromosomes as normal body cells in same species.
Garrison

Recherches sur la maturation de l'oeuf et la fécondation.
Arch. d. Biol., 4: 265–640, 1883
Van Buell, Mary. See H. Steenbock
van Buren, William Holme. American surgeon.
1819–1883
DISEASE—hardening of corpora cavernosa.
In his: *A practical treatise on the surgical diseases of the genito-urinary organs, including syphilis* with E. L. Keyes, New York, Appleton, 1874. 672 pp.
pp. 24–27
OPERATION—treatment of prolapsus ani with Pacquelin cautery. In his: *Lectures on diseases of the rectum and the surgery of the lower bowel.* New York, Appleton, 1881. 2 ed., 412 pp. pp. 81–83
Vance, R. W. See C. M. Jones
Vandergrift, H. N. See K. S. Grimson
Delden, A. van. Delft bacteriologist
SOLUTION—basal gypsum.
Beitrag zur Kenntnis der Sulfatreduktion durch Bakterien. Zbl. Bakt., 1 Abt., 11: 81–94 (83), Oct. 27, 1903
van den Bergh, A. A. Hymans. Utrecht physician
DISEASE—sulph-hemoglobinemia.
Enterogene Cyanose. Dtsch. Arch. f. klin. Med., 83: 86–106, May 18, 1905
Enterogene Cyanose. Zweite Mitteilung with A. Grutterink, Berl. klin. Wschr., 43: 7–10, Jan. 1, 1906
TEST—for bile pigments.
Die Farbstoffe des Blutserums with J. Snapper, Dtsch. Arch. f. klin. Med., 110: 540–561, May 16, 1913
Untersuchungen über den Icterus with J. Snapper, Berl. klin. Wschr., 51: 1109–1112, June 15; 1180–1182, June 22, 1914
Der Gallenfarbstoff im Blute. Leiden, 1918
La formation de la bilirubine dans le plasma sanguin par la méthode de la réaction diazoique: réaction prompte et réaction ralentie. Pr. méd., 29: 441–443, June 4, 1921
Van Deusen, Edwin Holmes. American physician.
1828–1909
Described mental manifestations of neurasthenia.
Observations on a form of nervous prostration (neurasthenia), culminating in insanity. Lansing, Mich., George, 1869. 19 pp.
Van de Velde, Honore. Louvain physician
Demonstrated a leucocidin produced by staphylococci.
Étude sur le mécanisme de la virulence du staphylocoque pyogène. Cellule, 10: 403–463, June 30, 1894
Vandorfy, J. Budapest physician
REAGENT—for blood.
Studien über die Guajakprobe. Arch. VerdauKr., 30: 1–7, May 1922
Vandremer, A. See L. Martin
Van Dyke, Harry Benjamin. American pharmacologist. 1895–
Wrote—
The physiology and pharmacology of the pituitary body. Chicago: Univ. Press, 1936–39. 2 vols.
Vanghette, Giuliano. Italian surgeon. 1861–1940
OPERATION—method of cineplastic treatment of amputation stumps. Garrison
Plastica e protesi cinematiche. Nuova teoria sulle amputazioni. Empoli, Traversari, 1906. 231 pp.
van Gieson, Ira. New York neuropathologist. 1865–1913

STAIN—for Negri bodies.
Eine sichere und einfache Methode für Nervensystemstudien, hauptsächlich ihre Anwendung in der Diagnose und Untersuchung der Negrischen Körperchen. Zbl. Bakt., 1 Abt., 43: 205–206, Jan. 17, 1907
STAINS—acid fuchsin and picric acid, for nerve tissue, collagen and reticulum.
Laboratory notes of technical methods for the nervous system. New York med. J., 1: 57–60, July 20, 1889
Van Gorder, G. W. See M. N. Smith-Petersen
van Hook, Weller. Chicago surgeon. 1862–1933
OPERATION—uretero-ureterostomy.
The surgery of the ureters: a clinical, literary, and experimental research. J. A. M. A., 21: 911–916, Dec. 16; 965–973, Dec. 23, 1893
van Millingen, Edwin. Constantinople surgeon
OPERATION—
The tarsocheiloplastic operation for the cure of trichiasis. Ophthal. Rev., 6: 309–314, Nov. 1887
van Prohaska, J. See L. R. Dragstedt
Van Slyke, D. V. See B. F. Miller
Van Slyke, Donald Dexter. New York biochemist.
1883–
INDEX—urea i. for determining renal function.
REAGENT—for urea.
A permanent preparation of urease, and its use in the determination of urea with G. E. Cullen, J. biol. Chem., 19: 211–228, Oct. 1914
METHOD—for determination of amino-groups.
A method for quantitative determination of aliphatic amino groups: application to the study of proteolysis and proteolytic products. Ibid., 9: 185–204, May 1911; 12: 275–284, Aug. 1912
METHOD—for determining of carbon dioxide combining power of blood plasma.
Studies on acidosis. I. The bicarbonate concentration of the blood plasma; its significance, and its determination as a measure of acidosis with G. E. Cullen, Ibid., 30: 289–368, June 1917
METHOD—for determination of acetone bodies in blood and urine.
Studies of acidosis. VII. The determination of B-hydroxybutyric acid, aceto-acetic acid, and acetone in urine. Ibid., 32: 455–493, Dec. 1917
(Same) *VIII. The determination of B-hydroxybutyric acid, acetoacetic acid, and acetone in blood* with R. Fitz, Ibid., 495–497
METHOD—for determination of oxygen and oxygen capacity (or hemoglobin) of blood.
Gasometric determination of the oxygen and hemoglobin of blood. Ibid., 33: 127–132, Jan. 1918
METHOD—for determination of plasma bicarbonate.
Studies of acidosis. XIII. A method for titrating the bicarbonate content of the plasma with E. Stillman and G. E. Cullen, Ibid., 38: 167–178, May 1919
METHOD—oxygen capacity m. for calibrating hemoglobinometer.
The determination of gases in blood and other solutions by vacuum extraction and manometric measurement with J. M. Neill, Ibid., 61: 523–573, Sept. 1924
METHOD—for determination of calcium in blood.
Gasometric determination of oxalic acid and calcium, and its application to serum analysis with J. Sendroy, Jr., Ibid., 84: 217–232, Oct. 1929
METHOD—for specific gravities of whole blood and plasma.

See R. A. Phillips
See also R. Fitz, E. Kirk, F. C. McLean, E. Möller, N. S. Moore, I. H. Page
Vansteenberge, Paul. French physician
SOLUTION—glucose tyrosine, for cultivation of B. coli.
L'autolyse de la levure et l'influence de ses produits de protéolyse sur le développement de la levure et des microbes lactiques. Ann. Inst. Pasteur, 31: 601-630 (609), Dec. 1917
Van Wagenen, William Perrine. Rochester, N. Y. surgeon. 1897–
OPERATION—
A surgical approach for the removal of certain pineal tumors. S. G. O., 53: 217-220, Aug. 1931
Van Zwaluwenburg. J. G. See A. W. Hewlett
Vaquez, Louis Henri. French physician. 1860-1936
DISEASE—Vaquez-Osler erythraemia.
Sur une forme spéciale de cyanose s'accompagnant d'hyperglobulie excessive et persistante. C. R. Soc. Biol., 44: 384-388, May 7, 1892
KYMOMETER—for studying peripheral pulsations.
La détermination des pressions minima et moyenne par la méthode oscillométrique with P. Gley and D. M. Gomez, Pr. méd., 39: 281-284, Feb. 25, 1931
Made clinical diagnosis of a pheochromocytoma.
Les crises d'hypertension artérielle paroxystique with E. Donzelot, Ibid., 34: 1329-1331, Oct. 23, 1926
Varco, Richard Lynn. Minneapolis surgeon. 1912–
METHOD—
A method of implanting the pancreatic duct into the jejunum in the Whipple operation for carcinoma of the pancreas: case report. Surgery, 18: 569-573, Nov. 1945
See also C. F. Code, C. Dennis
Vardon, A. C. Kasauli physician
AGAR—
Desiccated nutrient media. Ind. J. med. Res., 11: 429-432 (432), Oct. 1923
Variot, Gaston. French physician
TYPE—of dwarfism, senile.
Le "nanisme type sénile" (progeria de Gilford); (1) origine surrénale probable with Pironneau, Bull. Soc. Pédiat., Paris, 12: 431-443, Nov. 15, 1910
Varoli, Costanzo. Italian anatomist. 1543-1575
BRIDGE or PONS—
VALVE—ileocecal.
Anatomiae, sive de resolutione corporis humani ... Francofurti, 1591. 184 pp.
Vars, H. M. See A. Stengel, Jr.
Vassale, Giulio. Italian physician. 1862-1912
Explained fatal results following complete thyroidectomies in which parathyroids were also removed.
Sugli effetti dell'estirpazione delle ghiandole paratiroidee with F. Generali, Riv. di pat. nerv. e ment., Firenze, 1: 95-99, Feb.–Mar. 1896
Studied hypophysectomy.
Sulla distruzione della ghiandola pituitaria with E. Sacchi, Riv. sper. di freniat., Reggio-Emilia, 18: 525-561, 1892
Vastine, Jacob Hursh. Philadelphia roentgenologist. 1897–
METHOD—of localizing pineal gland.
The pineal shadow as an aid in the localization of brain tumors with K. K. Kinney, Amer. J. Roentgenol., 17: 320-324, Mar. 1927

Vater, Abraham. German anatomist. 1684-1751
AMPULLA, DIVERTICULUM or PAPILLA—
Dissertatio anatomica qua novum bilis diverticulum circa orificium ductus choledochi ut et valvulosam colli vesicae felleae constructionem ad disceptandum proponit. Wittenbergae, Gerdesianus, 1720
Vaughan, George Tully. Washington, D. C. surgeon. 1859–
Successfully ligated abdominal aorta.
Ligation (partial occlusion) of the abdominal aorta for aneurism: report of a recent case with a résumé of previous cases. Ann. Surg., 74: 308-312, Sept. 1921
Vaughan, H. N. See F. A. Coller
Vaughan, Roger Throop. Chicago surgeon. 1878–
SIGN or TEST—
A new and early sign of ruptured bladder with D. F. Rudnick, J. A. M. A., 83: 9-12, July 5, 1924
Vaughan, Victor Clarence, Jr. American pathologist. 1851-1929
PRODUCT—split p.; a protein which has been split into a poisonous and a non-poisonous part, the former soluble in the menstruum, the latter not. Garrison
Protein split products in relation to immunity and disease with J. W. Vaughan, Philadelphia, Lea and Febiger, 1913. 476 pp.
TEST—for
Thyrotoxicon; its presence in poisonous ice cream; its development in milk; and its probable relation to cholera infantum and kindred diseases. San. News, Chicago, 8: 155-156, July 24; 167-168, July 31, 1886
The chemistry of tyrotoxicon; its action upon lower animals; and its relation to the summer diarrheas of infancy. Rep. Bd. Health Mich., Lansing, 1887. pp. 177-185
Vaughan, Warren Taylor. Richmond, Va. physician. 1893-1944
INDEX—
Food allergens. III. The leucopenic index: preliminary report. J. Allergy, 5: 601-605, Sept. 1934
Vautrin, Alexis. Nancy surgeon. 1859-1927
OPERATION—on retroduodenal choledochus.
De l'obstruction calculeuse du cholédoque. Rev. d. Chir., 16: 446-479, June 1896
Veal, J(ames) Ross. New Orleans surgeon. 1901–
OPERATION—
Repair of direct inguinal hernia by osteoperiosteal graft to the pectineal line of the pubis with D. D. Baker, Surgery, 3: 585-592, Apr. 1938
Veale, Henry Richard Lobb. British Army surgeon. 1832-1908
Introduced term "rubelle" to describe German measles. Garrison and Morton
History of an epidemic of Rötheln, with observations on its pathology. Edinburgh Med. J., 12: 404-414, Nov. 1866
Vedder, Edward Bright. American physician. 1878–
STARCH MEDIUM—
Starch agar, a useful culture medium. J. infect. Dis., 16: 385-388, May 1915
Found that emetin destroys amoebae. Garrison
A preliminary account of some experiments undertaken to test the efficacy of the ipecacuanha treatment of dysentery. Bull. Manila Med. Soc., 3: 48-53, 1911
Also: J. Trop. Med., London, 14: 149-152, May 15, 1911

Wrote on—
Beriberi. New York, Wood, 1913
Veillon, Adrien. Paris bacteriologist. 1864–1931
AGAR—serum.
Le gonocoque. Ann. de Derm. et Syph., 9: 18–35 (22), 1898
BOUILLON—ascitic fluid. Ibid., p. 24.
Veit, Johann. Halle gynecologist. 1852–1917
OPERATION—Porro-Veit's cesarean section.
Der Kaiserschnitt in moderner Beleuchtung. Samml. klin. Vortr., n. F. No. 515. (Gynäk. No. 189), pp. 519–541, 1909
Von den Velden, Reinhard. German physician. 1880–
Introduced—
Die intrakardiale Injektion. Münch. med. Wschr., 66: 274–275, Mar. 7, 1919
Veler, C. D. See E. A. Doisy
Velicogna, A. Turin physician
TEST—for adrenaline.
Nouvelle réaction de sensibilisation de l'adrénaline. C. R. Soc. Biol., 115: 140–142, Jan. 13, 1934
Vella, Luigi. Italian physiologist. 1825–1886
FISTULA—of divided intestine, to obtain pure intestinal juice.
Nuovo metodo per avere il succo enterico puro e stabilirne le proprietà fisiologiche. Mem. Accad. d. sci. d. Ist. di Bologna, 4 s., 2: 513–538, 1881
Velpeau, Alfred Armand Louis Marie. Paris surgeon. 1795–1867
BANDAGE—to support arm in fracture of clavicle.
Nouveaux éléments de médecine opératoire. Paris, 1839. 2 ed. Vol. 1, p. 229
Operated for aneurism. Garrison and Morton
Mémoire sur la piqûre ou l'acupuncture des artères dans le traitement des anévrismes. Gaz. méd. de Paris, 2: 1–4, 1831
Wrote important book on breast tumors.
Traité des maladies du sein et de la region mammaire. Paris, Masson, 1854
Also, transl. by M. Henry, London, Sydenham Soc., 1856. 608 pp.
Velse, Cornelius Henrik. Dutch surgeon
Operated for intussusception in adult. Garrison and Morton
De mutuo intestinorum ingressu. Lugduni Batavorum, Luzac, 1742
Venable, Charles Scott. San Antonio surgeon. 1877–
Introduced vitallium.
The effects on bone of the presence of metals; based upon electrolysis: an experimental study with W. Stuck and A. Beach, Ann. Surg., 105: 917–938, June 1937
Venegas, Juan Manuel. Mexican physician
Author of first general medical treatise published in the Americas. Garrison and Morton
Compendio de la medicina: ó medicina practica. Mexico, F. de Zuñiga y Ontiveros, 1788
Venel, Jean Andre. Geneva surgeon. 1740–1791
The real originator of surgical orthopedics. Corrected lateral curvatures and torsion of spine by mechanical devices. Garrison
Description de plusieurs nouveaux moyens méchaniques propres à prevênir, borner et même corrigen dans certains cas les courbures latérales et la torsion de l'épine du dos. Lausanne, 1788
Verbrycke, J. Russell, Jr. Washington, D. C. surgeon. 1885–
Mentioned pneumonic process specific for tularemia.

Tularemia, with report of a fatal case simulating cholangeitis, with postmortem report. J. A. M. A., 82: 1577–1581, May 17, 1924
Verge, J. See Mlle. Le Sodier
Verhoeff, Frederick Herman. Boston ophthalmologist. 1874–
METHOD—of serial sections by celloidin method.
Obstruction of the central retinal vein. Arch. of Ophthal., 36: 1–36, Jan. 1907
METHOD—
Scleral puncture of expulsive sub-choroidal hemorrhage after sclerotomy—scleral puncture for post-operative separation of the chorioid. Ophthal. Rec., 24: 55–59, Feb. 1915
OPERATION—
A corneo-sclero-conjunctival suture in operations for cataract. Trans. Amer. Ophthal. Soc., 25: 48–53, 1927
A new operation for removing cataracts with their capsules. Ibid., 54–64
An instrument simplifying the insertion of corneo-sclero-conjunctival sutures in operations for cataract. Amer. J. Ophthal., 17: 53–57, Jan. 1934
SOLUTION—
An improved carbolfuchsin solution. J. A. M. A., 58: 1355 (only), May 4, 1912
STAIN—for elastic tissue.
Some new staining methods of wide applicability; including a rapid differential stain for elastic tissue. Ibid., 50: 876–877, Mar. 4, 1908
STAIN—for leptotriches.
Parinauds conjunctivitis; a mycotic disease due to a hitherto undescribed filamentous organism. Arch. Ophthal., 42: 345–351, July 1913
Verkade, P. E. Rotterdam bacteriologist
SOLUTION—basal ammonium sulphate.
Die Angreifbarkeit von cis-transisomeren ungesättigten Säuren durch Pilze with N. L. Söhngen, Zbl. Bakt., 2 Abt., 50: 81–87 (82), Feb. 26, 1920
Vernes, Arthur. Paris physician
TEST—for cancer; a blood test based on flocculation of blood serum, produced by addition of copper acetate solution.
Conditions expérimentales du diagnostic sérologique des cancers with R. Bricq and A. Gager, Arch. Inst. Prophylactique, Paris, 1: 43–57, Jan.–Mar. 1929
(Same title) with R. Bricq. A. Gager and H. Chauchard, Ibid., 2: 211–249, Apr.–June, 1930
TEST—for syphilis.
Les signes humoraux de la syphilis. Introduction à l'etude des conditions expérimentales du traitement de la syphilis. Paris, Thèse, 1913
Sur la precipitation de l'hydrate de fer colloidal par le serum humain, normal our syphilitique. C. R. Acad. Sci., 165: 769–772, Nov. 26, 1917; 166: 575–578, Apr. 8, 1918
Vernet, Maurice. French neurologist. 1887–
SYNDROMES—of foramen, lacerum posterius. Garrison
Les paralysies laryngées associées. Thèse de Lyon, Mar. 1916. 224 pp.
Sur le "syndrome total" des quatre derniers nerfs crâniens (deux observations nouvelles de Blessés de Guerre) with Sargnon and Vernet, Rev. beurol. Paris, 23: 943–948, May 4, 1916
Verneuil, Aristide August Stanislas. French surgeon. 1823–1895

CANALS—collateral veins of a venous trunk.
Le système veineux (anatomie et physiologie). Paris,
Germer-Baillière, 1853. 175 pp.
OPERATION—iliac colostomy.

*Des rétrécissements de la partie inférieure du rectum, et
de leur traitement curatif ou palliatif par la rectotomie
linéaire ou section longitudinale de l'intestin à l'aide
de l'ecraseur.* Gaz. d. Hôp., 45: 996–998, Oct. 26;
1002–1003, Oct. 29; 1028 (only), Nov. 7; 1034–1035,
Nov. 9; 1043–1044, Nov. 12; 1059–1060, Nov. 16;
1067 (only), Nov. 19, 1872
*Traitement palliatif du cancer du rectum au moyen de
la rectotomie linéaire.* Gaz. hebd. de Méd., Paris,
11: 196–198, Mar. 27, 1874
OPERATION—forcipressure in hemorrhage. Garrison
De la forcipressure. Bull. Soc. med. et chir. de Paris,
n. s., 17: 108; 273; 522; 646, 1875
Also, Paris, Masson, 1875. 126 pp.
OPERATION—
*Observation de gastrostomie pratiquée avec succès pour
un rétrécissement cicatriciel infranchissable de l'oesophage.* Bull. Acad. Méd. Paris, 25: 1023–1038, Oct.
31, 1876

Verney, E. B. See E. H. Starling
Verocay, José. Prague pathologist. 1876–1927
METHOD—of fixation.
*Beseitigung der „Formolniederschläge" aus mikro-
skopischen Schnitten.* Zbl. f. allg. Path. u. path. Anat.,
19: 769–774, Oct. 15, 1908
Described neurogenic tumors of abdomen and differ-
entiated them from neuromas on histologic grounds;
coined term "neurinoma."
Zur Kenntnis der „Neurofibrome." Beitr. z. path.
Anat., 48: 1–69, Mar. 23, 1910

Verrall, Paul Jenner. London surgeon. 1883–
OPERATION—
Three cases of reconstruction of the thumb. Brit. med.
J., 2: 775 (only), Dec. 13, 1919

Vesalius, Andreas. Belgian anatomist. 1514–1564
FORAMEN, LIGAMENT, VEIN—
De humani corporis fabrica libri septem. Basileae,
Oporini, 1543. 663 pp.

Vetch, John. English physician. 1783–1835
Described infectious forms of granular conjunctivitis.
Garrison
*An account of the ophthalmia which has appeared in
England since the return of the British army from
Egypt.* London, Longman, 1807. 141 pp.

Vetch, Robert M'Leod. Edinburgh physician
TECHNIC—
*A simple and rapid method of estimating the phago-
cytic power of different bloods.* J. Path. Bact., 12:
353–367, 1908

Vialleton, Louis. Lyon urologist. 1859–1929
THEORY—of exstrophy of bladder.
*Essai embryologique sur le mode de formation de
l'exstrophie de la vessie.* Arch. prov. de chir., 1: 233–
258, Sept. 1892

de Vianna, Oliveira Gaspar. Brazil physician. 1885–
1914
Discovered value of antimony tartrate against kala-
azar. Garrison
Preliminary announcement to Brazilian Derma-
tological Society in: Arch. Brasil. de Med., Rio de
Janeiro, 2: 426–428, 1912
Sobre o tratamento da leishmaniose tegumentar. Ann.
Paulist. de Med. e Cir., Sao Paulo, 2: 167–169, 1914

Victorson, Ruth. See E. O. Jordan
Vicz d'Azur, Félix. French anatomist. 1748–1794
BAND, BUNDLE, or STRIPE—a layer of cerebral
cortex.
*Sur la structure de cerveau, de cervelet, de la moelle
alongée, de la moelle épinière; et sur l'origine des nerfs
de l'homme et des animaux.* Hist. de l'acad. des sci.,
495–622 (511), 1781
Vidal de Cassis, Auguste Théodore. French surgeon.
1803–1856
OPERATION—subcutaneous ligation of veins for
varicocele.
*De la cure radicale du varicocèle par l'enroulement des
veines du cordon spermatique.* Paris, 1850. 2 ed.
Vidal, Jean Baptiste Émile. Paris dermatologist.
1825–1893
DISEASE—lichen chronicus simplex.
De lichen (lichen, prurigo, strophulus). Ann. de derm.
et syph., 2 s., 7: 133–154, 1886
TREATMENT—of lupus vulgaris by scarification.
Etude sur le mycosis fongoide with L. A. J. Brocq,
France méd., 2: 946–949, July 9, 1885, et seq.
Described keratosis blennorrhagica.
*Éruption généralisée et symétrique de croûtes cornées,
avec chute des ongles, d'origine blennorrhagique, co-
incidant avec une polyarthrite de même nature.—
Récidivi à la suite d'une nouvelle blennorrhagie, deux
ans après la guérison de la première maladie.* Ann. de
derm. et syph., 4: 2–11, Jan. 1893
Vidius, Guido. Italian physician. 1500–1569
CANAL, FORAMEN, NERVE—
De anatome corporis humani libri VII. . . . Edited
by Vidius' nephew, Guido Guidi Venetiis, apud
Juntas, 1611. 342 pp.
Viehover, Arno. Philadelphia pharmacologist
TEST—
Field tests for marihuana (cannabis). Amer. J. Pharm.,
109: 589–591, Dec. 1937
Vierling, Karl. Frankfurt a. M. physician. 1890–
SOLUTION—whey peptone; culture medium.
Lackmusmolke aus Magermilchpulver. Zbl. Bakt.,
88: 93–94, Mar. 14, 1922
Vierordt, Karl. German physician. 1818–1884
HEMOTACHOMETER—graphic method of investi-
gating pulse.
*Die bildliche Darstellung des menschlichen Arterien-
pulses.* Arch. f. physiol. Heilk., Stuttgart, 13: 284–
287, 1854
*Die Erscheinungen und Gesetzte der Stromgeschwindig-
keiten des Blutes.* Frankfurt a. M., Meidinger, Sohn
und Co., 1858
*Die Lehre vom Arterienpuls in gesunden und kranken
Zuständen.* Braunschweig, Vieweg, 1855. 271 pp.
METHOD—of enumerating blood corpuscles.
*Neue Methode der quantitativen mikroskopischen
Analyse des Blutes.* Arch. f. physiol. Heilk., 11: 26–46
1852
Zählungen der Blutkörperchen des Menschen. Ibid.,
327–331
Introduced spectral analyses of hemoglobin, bile
and urine. Garrison and Morton
*Die quantitative Spectralanalyse in ihrer Anwendung
auf Physiologie, Physik, Chemie and Technologie.*
Tübingen, Laupp'sche, 1876
Vierordt, Karl Hermann. Tübingen physician. 1853–
METHOD—for determination of coagulation time of
blood.

Die Gerinnungszeit des Blutes in gesunden und kranken Zuständen. Arch. der Heilk., 19: 193–221, 1878

Vieussens, Raymond de. French anatomist. 1641–1716

ANNULUS OVALIS, ANSA SUBCLAVA, ARTERY, CORPUS ALBUM SUBROTUNDUM, GANGLION, RING, VALVE, VEINS, VENTRICLE—

Nevrographia universalis. Lugduni, J. Certe, 1685

Novum vasorum corporis humani systema. Amstelodami, Marret, 1705. 260 pp.

Nouvelles découvertes sur le colur. Toulouse, 1706

Traité nouveau de la structure et des causes due mouvement naturel du coeur. Toulouse, Guillemette, 1715. 141 pp.

Vieusseux, Gaspard. Geneva physician. 1746–1814

Described cerebrospinal meningitis.

Mémoire sur la maladie qui a régné à Genève au printemps ae 1805. J. de méd., chir., pharm., Paris, 11: 163–182, 1805

Villalba, Joaquin de

Wrote history of epidemics in Spain to end of seventeenth century. Garrison and Morton

Epidemiologia española. Madrid, M. Repullés, 1802. 2 vols.

Villaret, Maurice. Paris physician. 1877–

SPACE—retroparotid.

SYNDROME—myosis, enophthalmos, sweating and combined paralyses.

Le syndrome nerveux de l'espace rétro-parotidien postérieur. Rev. neurol., 23: 188–190, Jan. 6, 1916

Le syndrome de l'espace rétro-parotidien postérieur. Paris méd., 21: 430–431, May 26, 1917

Ville, J. French chemist

REACTION—for cholic acid.

Sensibilisation de la réaction indiquée par Mylius pour caractériser l'acide cholalique et le distinguer des acides biliaires proprement dits. Bull. Soc. chim., 102: 866–868, July 2, 1913

Villemin, Jean Antoine. French army surgeon. 1827–1892

THEORY—of infectiousness and specificity of tuberculosis, propounded before discovery of bacillus by R. Koch.

Études sur la tuberculose; preuves rationelles et expérimentales de sa spécificité et de son inoculabilité. Paris, Baillière, 1868. 640 pp. p. 528

Villiger, V. See A. Baeyer

Vincent, Beth. Boston surgeon. 1876–

METHOD—

Blood transfusion in infants by means of glass tubes. Amer. J. Dis. Child., 1: 376–381, May 1911

TEST—

A rapid macroscopic agglutination test for blood groups, and its value in testing donors for transfusion. J. A. M. A., 70: 1219–1220, Apr. 27, 1918

See also R. I. Lee

Vincent, James G. Rochester, N. Y. scientist

METHOD—

Filter paper disc modification of the Oxford cup penicillin determination with Helen W. Vincent, Proc. Soc. exp. Biol., N. Y., 55: 162–164, Mar. 1944

Vincent, Jean Hyacinthe. French bacteriologist. 1862–

ANGINA—

Sur une forme particulière d'angine diphthéroide (angine à bacilles fusiformes). Bull. Soc. méd. Hôp. Paris, 3 s., 15: 244–250, Mar. 11, 1898

Recherches bactériologiques sur l'angine à bacilles fusiformes. Ann. Inst. Pasteur, 13: 609–620, Aug. 1899

BOUILLON—phenol.

Sur un nouveau procédé d'isolement du bacille typhique dans l'eau. C. R. Soc. Biol., 42: 62–64, Feb., 1, 1890

METHOD—for staining capsules.

Nouvelle méthode de coloration des micro-organismes dans le sang. Gaz. méd. de Paris, pp. 296–297, June 23, 1894

VACCINE—

Remarques sur la vaccination antityphique. Ann. Inst. Pasteur, 25: 455–460, June 1911

Isolated Streptothrix (Actinomyces) madurae. Garrison and Morton

Étude sur le parasite du "pied de Madura." Ibid., 8: 129–151, Mar. 1894

Vinson, Porter Paisley. American physician. 1890–

SYNDROME—of Plummer-Vinson; hypochromic anemia, achlorhydria, atrophic gastritis, dysphagia and glossitis.

A case of cardiospasm with dilatation and angulation of the esophagus. Med. Clin. N. Amer., 3: 623–627, Nov. 1919

Hysterical dysphagia. Minnesota Med., 5: 107–108, Feb. 1922

Marked dilatation of the esophagus in cardiospasm. Ohio State Med. J., 20: 147–148, Mar. 1924

See also W. McK. Craig

Virchow, Rudolf. German pathologist. 1821–1902

DISEASE—congenital interstitial encephalitis.

Zur pathologischen Anatomie des Gehirns. Arch. f. path. Anat., 38: 129–138, Jan. 1867

HYPOTHESIS—human gastric ulcers are vascular in origin.

Historisches, Kritisches und Positive zur Lehre der Unterleibsaffektionen. Ibid., 5: 281–375 (362–364), 1853

LAW—cell-elements of tumors are derived from normal and preexisting tissue-cells. Homans

Die krankhaften Geschwülste. Berlin, 1864–67. Vol. 1, pp. 57–72

Described leukemia.

Weisses Blut. Neue Notizen aus dem Gebiete der Natur-und Heilkunde (Froriep's Notizen), Weimar, 25: 151–155, 1845

Weisses Blut und Milztumor. Erster Artikel. Med. Zeitung von dem Vereine für Heilkunde in Preussen, No. 34, 35, 36, 1846

(Same) Zweiter Artikel. Ibid., No. 3, Jan. 20; No. 4, Jan. 27, 1847

Described pulmonary embolism.

Die Verstopfung der Lungenarteire und ihre Folgen. Beitr. z. exper. Path., 2: 227–380, 1846

Thrombose und Embolie. Gefässentzündung und septische Infektion. In his: *Gesammelte Abhandlungen zur wissenschaftlichen Medicin.* Frankfurt a. M., Meidinger, Sohn und Co., 1856. pp. 219–732

Discovered neurologia, 1846. Garrison

Ueber eine im Gerirn und Rückenmark des Menschen aufgefundene Substanz mit der chemischen Reaction der Cellulose. Arch. f. path. Anat., 6: 135–138, 1854

Noted relation between destructive lesions of bones and pathologic calcification.

Kalk-Metastasen. Ibid., 8: 103–113, Apr. 1855

Described "strawberry gallbladder."

Ueber das Epithel der Gallenblase und über einen

intermediären Stoffwechsel des Fettes. Ibid., 11: 574–578, June 1857
Described melanosarcoma of meninges.
Pigment und diffuse Melanose der Arachnoides. Ibid., 16: 180–182, Jan.–Feb. 1859
Originator of modern movement for hygiene and inspection of school-children.
Ueber gewisse die Gesundheit benachtheiligende Einflüsse der Schulen. Ibid., 46: 447–470, 1869
Visscher, John Paul. Cleveland biologist. 1895–
REACTION—
Chemical determination of pregnancy with D. E. Bowman, Proc. Soc. exp. Biol. N. Y., 31: 460–461, Jan. 1934
Viteri, L. E. See P. S. Pelouze
Voegtlin, C. See W. G. MacCallum
Voelcker, Friedrich. Heidelberg surgeon. 1872–
OPERATION—on bladder.
Erfahrungen über Harnblasenresektionen. Arch. f. klin. Chir., 167: 616–625, 1931
TEST—indigo-carmine, for kidney function.
Funktionelle Nierendiagnostik ohne Ureterenkatheter. Münch. med. Wschr., 50: 2081–2089, Dec. 1, 1903
Introduced pyelography.
Die Gestalt der menschlichen Harnblase im Röntgenbilde. Ibid., 52: 1576–1578, Aug. 15, 1905
Pyelographie. (Röntgenographie des nierenbeckens nach Kollargolfüllung). Ibid., 53: 105–107, Jan. 16, 1906
Performed esophagogastrostomy.
Über Extirpation der Cardia wegen Karzinom. Zbl. f. Chir., 35: 90–92, Dec. 19, 1908
Voge, Cecil I. B. Edinburgh scientist
TEST—
A simple chemical test for pregnancy. Brit. med. J., 2: 829–830, Nov. 2, 1929
Vogel. See M. Gerlach
Vogel, Karl M. New York physician. 1877–
METHOD—
Detection of mercury in the excretions with O. I. Lee, J. A. M. A., 62: 532–534, Feb. 14, 1914
TECHNIC—for vital staining.
Blood transfusion and regeneration in pernicious anemia with U. F. McCurdy, Arch. intern. Med., 12: 707–722, Dec. 1913
Vogl, Alfred. Vienna physician
TEST—
Eine einfache Methode zum Nachweise pathologischer Bilirubinämie with B. Zins, Med. Klin., 28: 667–668, May 21, 1922
Vogt, Alfred. Zurich ophthalmologist. 1879–
GLAUCOMA—
Ein neues Spaltlampenbild: Abschilferung der Linsenvorderkapsel als wahrscheinliche Ursache von senilem chronischem Glaukom. Schweiz. med. Wschr., 56: 413; 426, 1926
OPERATION—cyclodiathermy, for glaucoma.
Ergebnisse der Diathermiestichelung des Corpus ciliare (Zyklodiathermiestichelung) gegen Glaukom. Klin. Mbl. Augenheilk., 99: 9–15, July 30, 1937
Die Zyklodiathermiepunktur (Z. D. P.) gegen Glaukom. Ibid., 103: 591–599, 1939
Vogt, Cécile. German neurologist. 1875–
SYNDROME—corpus striatum s.
Zur Lehre der Erkrankungen des striären Systems

with O. Vogt, J. Psychol. Neurol., Lpz., 25: Ergnzngsheft iii, pp. 627–846, 1920
Sur l'état marbré du striatum. Arch. gen. neur. psichiat., Nap., 7: 33–37, 1926
Vogt, L. G. Kiel surgeon
Procedure—for mammoplasty.
Beitrag zur plastischen Operation der Gynäkomastie. Chirurg, 10: 322–324, May 15, 1941
Vogt, M. See H. H. Dale
Vogt, Paul F. I. German surgeon. 1844–1885
Described epiphysitis of tibial tubercle.
Ein Fall von Abreissung der Tuberositas tibiae durch willkürliche Muskelcontraction. Berl. klin. Wschr., 6: 225–227, May 31, 1869
Voigtlander. See G. Deycke
Voinitch-Sianojentsky. Russian surgeon
TRIANGLE OF SAFETY—area of uncovered pericardium for surgical approach to heart. Thèse de St. Petersbourg, 1897
La péricardotomie et ses bases anatomiques. Abstr.: Rev. de chir., Paris, 18: 993–1011, 1898
von Voit, C. See M. J. v. Pettenkofer
Volhard, Franz. Giessen physician. 1872–
METHOD—of estimation of enzyme content of gastric secretion.
Ueber eine neue Methode der quantitativen Pepsinbestimmung nebst Bemerkungen über die Tryptophanreaktion und das Plastein bildende Ferment. Münch. med. Wschr., 50: 2119–2131, Dec. 8, 1903
TEST—of renal injury or function.
Die Brightsche Nierenkrankheit; Klinik, Pathologie und Atlas with Th. Fahr, Berlin, J. Springer, 1914 292 pp.
Performed cardiectomy for constrictive pericarditis.
Über Erkennung und Behandlung der Umklammerung des Herzens durch schwielige Perikarditis with V. Schmieden, Klin. Wschr., 2: 5–9, 1923
Volk, Marie D. See D. R. Gilligan
Volkmann, Alfred Wilhelm. German physiologist. 1800–1877
CANALS—in bone.
Described by Alfred's son, Richard, in:
Zur Histologie der Caries und Osteitis. Arch. f. klin. Chir., 4: 437–474 (451), 1863
See also F. H. Bidder
von Volkmann, Richard. Leipzig surgeon. 1830–1889
DISEASE—
Einige Fälle von Cheilitis glandularis apostematosa (myxadenitis labialis). Arch. f. path. Anat., 1: 142–144, Apr. 16, 1870
DEFORMITY—congenital tibiotarsal dislocation.
Ein Fall von hereditärer congenitaler Luxation beider Sprunggelenke. Dtsch. Z. f. Chir., 2: 538–542, July 25, 1873
ISCHAEMIC CONTRACTURE or PARALYSIS—
Die ischämischen Muskellahmungen und Kontrakturen. Zbl. f. Chir., 8: 801–803, 1881
Reported industrial occurrence of tar and paraffin cancers.
Beiträge zur Chirurgie, anschliessend an einen Bericht über die Thätigkeit der chirurgischen Universitäts-Klinik zu Halle im Jahre 1873. Leipzig, Breitkopf und Härtel, 1875, 388 pp. pp. 370–381
Escised rectal cancer.
Ueber den Mastdarmkrebs und die Exstirpatio recti. Samml. klin. Vortr., No. 131 (Chir. No. 42), 1113–1128, 1878

Vollgnad, Heinrich. 1634–1682
Reported variolation. Garrison and Morton
Globus vitulinus. Misc. Curiosa sive Ephem. nat. cur.,
Jenae, 2: 181–182, 1671
Vollmer, Hermann. New York pediatrician. 1896–
TEST—
A new tuberculin patch test with Esther W. Gold-
berger, Amer. J. Dis. Child., 54: 1019–1024, Nov.
1937
Voltolini, Frederick Edward Rudolph. Breslau
otolaryngologist. 1819–1889
DISEASE—
*Die akute Entzündung des heutigen Labyrinthes,
gewöhnlich irrtümlich für Meningitis cerebro-spinalis
Gehalten.* Mschr. Ohrenheilk., 1: 9–14, 1867
Employed galvanocautery in laryngeal surgery.
Garrison
*Die Anwendung der Galvanokaustik im Innern des
Kehlkopfes und Schlundkopfes, nebst einer kurzen
Anleitung zur Laryngoskopie und Rhinoskopie.* Wien,
Braumüller, 1867. 73 pp.
Performed first laryngeal operation through mouth
with external illumination. Garrison
*Die ersten Operationen in der Kehlkopfshöhle vom
Munde aus, bei der Durchleuchtung des Kehlkopfes
von aussen.* Dtsch. med. Wschr., 15: 340–343, Apr.
25, 1889
Vonderahe, Alphonse Ralph. Cincinnati neurologist.
1896–
Demonstrated a portal circulation from pituitary to
tuber cinereum.
The representation of visceral function in the brain.
Ohio State Med. J., 31: 104–109, Feb. 1935

Voorhoeve, N. Amsterdam radiologist
DISEASE—longitudinal striation of metaphyses, due
to varying degrees of ossification.
*L'image radiologique non encore décrite d'une anomalie
du squelette: ses rapports avec la dyschondroplasie et
l'osteopathia condensans disseminata.* Acta Radiol.,
3: 407–427, Nov. 10, 1924
Vorhaus, M. G. See L. M. Gompertz
Voronoff, Serge. Paris surgeon. 1866–
Reported testicular transplants for rejuvenation in
1919.
Greffes testiculaires. Paris, Doin, 1923
Vorschuetz, Johannes. Hamburg surgeon. 1876–
OPERATION—for slipping patella.
*Die operative Behandlung der habituellen Knieschei-
benverrenkung.* Zbl. f. Chir., 54: 2627–2628, Oct. 15,
1927
Vosges, O. Berlin physician
REACTION—for proteins.
*Beitrag zur Ernährungsphysiologie und zur Differen-
tialdiagnose der Bakterien der hämorrhagischen
Septicämie* with B. Proskauer, Z. Hyg. InfektKr.,
28: 20–32, 1898
Vries, Hugo de. Amsterdam botanist. 1848–
THEORY—of heredity.
Die Mutationstheorie. Leipzig, Veit, 1901–03. 2 vols.
Also, in English, Chicago, 1909
Vulpian, Edme Felix Alfred. French physician.
1826–1887
REACTION—for adrenaline.
*Note sur les réactions propres au tissu des capsules
surrénales chez les reptiles.* C. R. Soc. Biol., 2 s., 3:
223–224, 1856

W

Wade, Herbert Windson. Manila physician. 1886–
BROTH—blood infusion.
*Fungous developmental growth forms of Bacillus in-
fluenza* with C. Manalang, J. exp. Med., 31: 95–103
(98), Jan. 1920
Wadsworth, Augustus Baldwin. Albany, N. Y.
bacteriologist. 1872–
COMPLEMENT FIXATION TECHNIC—
*Quantitative studies on the relation of complement fixa-
tion with syphilitic serum and tissue extract* with F.
Maltaner and Elizabeth Maltaner, J. Immunol.,
35: 105–115, Aug. 1938
METHOD—of staining for capsules.
*Studies on simple and differential methods of staining
encapsulated pneumococci in smear and section.* J.
infect. Dis., 3: 610–618, June 30, 1906
Reported first proved case of Weil's disease in United
States and introduced laboratory methods for its
diagnosis.
*Infectious jaundice occurring in New York State.
Preliminary report of an investigation, with report of a
case of accidental infection of the human subject with
Leptospira icterochalmorrhagiae from the rat* with H.
Virginia Langworth, F. Constance Stewart, Anna C.
Moore and Marion B. Coleman, J. A. M. A., 78:
1120–1121, Apr. 15, 1922
Wagener, Henry Patrick. Rochester, Minn. ophthal-
mologist. 1890–
GRADES—of hypertension.
Diffuse arteriolar disease with hypertension and the

associated retinal lesions with N. M. Keith, Medicine,
18: 317–430, 1939
RETINITIS—
*Cases of marked hypertension, adequate renal function
and neuroretinitis* with N. M. Keith, Arch. intern.
Med., 34: 374–387, Sept. 15, 1924
The retinitis of malignant hypertension. Trans. Amer.
Ophth. Soc., 25: 349–380, 1927
See N. M. Keith
Wagner, Arthur. Lübeck surgeon
MODIFICATION—slide, of benzidin test for blood in
feces.
Zum Nachweis okkulter Blutungen in den Fäces.
Zbl. f. Chir., 41: 1182–1184, July 11, 1914
Wagner, Ernst Leberecht. German physician. 1829–
1888
Wrote on uterine cancer.
Der Gebärmutterkrebs. Leipzig, Teubner, 1858
Described dermatomyositis.
Fall einer seltnen Muskelkrankheit. Arch. d. Heilk.,
Leipzig, 4: 282–283, 1863
Described—
Das Colloid-Milium der Haut. Ibid., 7: 463–464,
1866
Wagner, Esther A. Illinois bacteriologist
SOLUTION—lactose peptone.
Lactose broth for isolating Bacterium coli from water
with W. F. Monfort, Amer. J. Pub. Health, 11: 203–
208, Mar. 1921
Wagner, Lewis Clark. New York surgeon. 1895–

OPERATION—
Modified bone block (Campbell) of ankle from paralytic drop-foot, with report of 27 cases. J. Bone and Joint. Surg., 13: 142–148, Jan. 1931
Wagner, Wilhelm. Königshütte surgeon. 1848–1900
OPERATION—osteoplastic craniotomy.
Die temporäre Resektion der Schädeldaches an Stelle der Trepanation. Zbl. Chir., 16: 833–838, Nov. 23 1889
Wagner von Jauregg, Julius. Austrian neurologist. 1857–1940
Awarded Nobel prize in 1927 "for his discovery of the therapeutic value of malarial inoculation in the treatment of general paresis (dementia paralytica)."
Ueber die Einwirkung fieberhafter Erkrankungen auf Psychosen. Jb. Psychiat. Neurol., 7: 94–131, 1887
Über die Einwirkung der Malaria auf die progressive Paralyse. Psychiat.-neurol. Wschr., 20: 132–134, Aug. 31, 1918; 251–255, Jan. 4, 1919
Die Behandlung der progressiven Paralyse und Tabes. Wien. klin. Wschr., 34: 171–172, Apr. 14, 1921
The treatment of general paresis by inoculation of malaria. J. nerv. ment. Dis., 55: 369–375, May 1922
Wahl, C. von. German bacteriologist
BASAL SALT SOLUTION—
Ueber Verderber von Gemusekonserven. Zbl. f. Bakt., 2 Abt., 16: 489–511, 1906
Wahl, Eduard von. German surgeon. 1833–1890
SIGN—blowing sound at systole heard over an artery soon after its partial division by an injury.
Die Diagnose der Arterienverletzung. Samml. klin. Vortr., No. 258 (Chir., No. 81), 2239–2258, 1885
Wait, Rudolf. Riga pharmacologist
REACTION—
Nachweis der Vitamine A, C und D. Pharm. Zentralhalle, 78: 237–238, Apr. 22, 1937
Waksman, Selman Abraham. New Jersey chemist. 1888–
SOLUTION—basal albumin.
Studies in the metabolism of actinomycetes. III. Nitrogen metabolism. J. Bact., 5: 1–30 (3), Jan. 1920
SOLUTION—basal sulphur ammonium sulphate.
Microorganism concerned in the oxidation of sulfur in the soil. II. Thiobacillus thiooxidans, a new sulfuroxidizing organism isolated from the soil with J. S. Joffe, Ibid., 7: 239–256 (239), Mar. 1922
Introduced streptomycin.
Bactericidal action of antibiotic substances with H. Christine Reilly, J. infect. Dis., 75: 150–159, Sept.–Oct. 1944
Isolation of antibiotic substances from soil microorganisms, with special reference to streptothricin and streptomycin with Elizabeth Bugie and A. Schatz, Proc. Staff Meet., Mayo Clin., 19: 537–548, Nov. 15, 1944
Walcher, Gustav Adolf. Stuttgart gynecologist. 1856–1935
POSITION—patient on back with hips at edge of table and legs handing down. Dorland
Die Conjugata eines engen Beckens ist keine konstante Grösse, sondern lässt sich durch die Körperhattung der Trägerin verändern. Zbl. f. Gynäk., 13: 892–893, Dec. 21, 1889
The influence of the position of the woman on the form and dimensions of the pelvis. St. Louis Cour. Med., 21: 341–349, Nov. 1899
Waldenburg, Louis. German physician. 1837–1881

APPARATUS—for exhausting or compressing air which is inhaled by patient or into which patient exhales.
Die Inhalationen der zerstäubten Flüssigkeiten, sowie der Dämpfe und Gase in ihrer Wirkung auf die Krankheiten der Athmungsorgane. Berlin, Reimer, 1864. 567 pp.
APPARATUS—for differential pneumotherapy.
Die pneumatische Behandlung der Respirations- und Circulationskrankheiten im Anschluss an die Pneumatometrie, Spirometrie und Brustmessung. Berlin, Hirschwald, 1875. 470 pp.
Waldenström, Henning. Stockholm surgeon. 1877–
DISEASE—osteochondritis dissecans; same as Legg—Calvé—Perthes' d.
Der obere tuberkulöse Collumherd. Z. f. orthop. Chir., 24: 487–512, 1909
Waldenström, J. A. See A. F. Lindstedt
Waldenström, Jan Gösta. Upsala scientist. 1906–
PORPHYRIN—
Some observations on acute porphyria and other conditions with a change in the excretion of porphyrins. Acta med. Scand., 83: 281–316, 1934
Studien über Porphyrie. Ibid., Suppl. 82, 1937. 254 pp.
Waldeyer, Heinrich Wilhelm Gottfried. German anatomist. 1836–1921
FOSSA—two duodenal f.
Hernia retroperitonealis, nebst Bemerkungen zur Anatomie des Peritoneums. Breslau, Junfger, 1868. 16 pp.
LAYER—vascular l. of ovary.
LINE—boundary of insertion of mesovarium at hilum of ovary.
Eierstock und Ei. Ein Beitrag zur Anatomie und Entwicklungsgeschichte der Sexualorgane. Leipzig, Engelmann, 1870. 174 pp.
RING—tonsillar, of adenoid tissue.
Ueber den lymphatischen Apparat des Pharynx. Abstr. in: Dtsch. med. Wschr., 10: 313 (only), May 15, 1884
THEORY—neuron.
Ueber einige neuere Forschungen im Gebiete der Anatomie des Centralnervensystems. Ibid., 17: 1244–1246, Nov. 5; 1267–1269, Nov. 12; 1287–1289, Nov. 19; 1331–1333, Dec. 3, 1352–1356, Dec. 10, 1891
Discovered germinal epithelium of ovary, 1870. Garrison
See LAYER and LINE.
Described supravesical fossa.
See FOSSA. Also, same title in: Arch. f. path. Anat., 60: 66–92, Apr. 10, 1874
Made first reference to tumors derived from interstitial cells of testicle, plexiform angiosarcoma. Confirmed work of Thiersch on epithelial origin of cancer, thereby disproving Virchow's theory. Garrison and Morton
Die Entwickelung der Carcinome. Ibid., 55: 67–159, June 13, 1872
Waldschmidt-Leitz, Ernst. German physician. 1894–
TEST—clinical, for cancer.
Ueber sterische Auslese durch Peptidasen in normalen und carcinomatösen Seren with K. Mayer, Z. f. physiol. Chem., 262: iv–vi, Dec. 15, 1939
Walker, A. W. See A. I. Kendall
Walker, Arthur Earl. Chicago surgeon. 1907–
OPERATION—
Mesencephalic tractotomy; methods for relief of uni-

lateral intractable pain. Arch. Surg., 44: 953–962, May 1942

Walker, Clifford Black. American otolaryngologist. 1884–

INSTRUMENT—
A new instrument for deep sewing. J. A. M. A., 68: 707–708, Mar. 3, 1917

OPERATION—
Retinal detachment—technical observations and new devices for treatment, with a specially arranged diathermy unit for general ophthalmic service. Amer. J. Ophthal., 17: 1–17, Jan. 1934
Treatment of the flat type of separated retina and of macular hole with special devices and modifications. Ibid., 19: 392–399, May 1936

Walker, Ernest Linwood. Philippine scientist. 1870–
Worked on—
Experimental entamoebic dysentery with A. W. Sellards, Philippine J. Sci., Manila, B. 8: 253–331, 1913
See also T. Smith

Walker, Isaac Chandler. Boston physician. 1883–
REACTIONS—cutaneous protein, for hay-fever and asthma.
A clinical study of 400 patients with bronchial asthma. Boston Med. and Surg. J., 179: 288–300, Aug. 29, 1918

Walker, J. See M. J. Couret

Walker, Mary Broadfoot. English physician
Advocated—
Treatment of myasthenia gravis with physostigmine. Lancet, 1: 1200–1201, June 2, 1934
Case showing the effect of prostigmin on myasthenia gravis. Proc. R. Soc. Med., 28: 759–761, Apr. 1935

Walker, Phoebe H. See I. Davidsohn

Wallace, George Barclay. New York pharmacologist. 1874–
TEST—for urobilinogen.
The significance of urobilogen in the urine as a test for liver function with a description of a simple quantitative method for its estimation with J. S. Diamond, Arch. intern. Med., 35: 698–725, June 1925

Wallace, William. Dublin physician. 1791–1837
Introduced use of potassium iodide for syphilis and gave first description of lymphogranuloma venereum. Garrison and Morton
A treatise on the venereal disease and its varieties. London, Burgess and Hill, 1833. 382 pp. p. 371

Wallenberg, Adolf. Danzig neurologist. 1862–
SYNDROME—
Akute Bulbäraffection (Embolie der Art. cerebellar. post. inf. sinistr.?). Arch. f. Psychiat. Nervenkr., 23: 504–540, 1895

Waller, Augustus Désiré. English physician. 1856–1922
Did basic work on string cardiac galvanometer. Garrison
A demonstration on man of the electromotive changes accompanying the heart beat. J. Physiol., 8: 229–234, 1887
Also in: F. A. Willius and T. E. Keys' *Cardiac classics.* St. Louis, Mosby, 1941, pp. 656–661

Waller, Augustus Volney. English physician. 1816–1870
WALLERIAN DEGENERATION—cf nerve.
Experiments on the section of the glossopharyngeal and hypoglossal nerves of the frog, and observations of the

alterations produced thereby in the structure of their primitive fibers. Philos. Trans., pp. 423–429, 1850

Wallgren, Arvid Johan. Gothenburg pediatrician. 1889–
Wrote on lymphocytic choriomeningitis.
Considerations sur l'erytheme noueux. Acta paedricata, 5: 225–253, Mar. 6, 1925

Wallhauser, Andrew. Pittsburgh physician. 1892–
METHOD—
Method for the detection of acetone. J. A. M. A., 91: 21 (only), July 7, 1928

Walpole, G. Stanley. English scientist
DETERMINATION—
The direct determination of creatine in pathological urine. J. Physiol., 42: 301–308, May 22, 1911

Walsh, M. N. See J. G. Love

Walshe, Walter Hayle. English physician. 1812–1892
Recognized presystolic character of direct mitral murmur in mitral stenosis. Garrison and Morton
A practical treatise on the diseases of the heart and the great vessels. London, Taylor, Walton and Maberly, 1851

Walter, Ernst. Greifswald physician. 1882–
TEST—benzidine t. for blood.
Zur Vereinfachung des chemischen Blutnachweises mittels Benzidin. Abstr.: Dtsch. med. Wschr., 35: 130 (only), Jan. 21, 1909
Ueber die Verwendung des Benzidins für den Blutnachweis, im besonderen über seine Anwendungsweise in der gerichtsärztlichen Praxis. Ibid., 36: 309–311, Feb. 10, 1910

Walter, Johann Gottlieb. German physician. 1734–1818
Described peritonitis. Garrison and Morton
Von den Krankheiten des Bauchfells und dem Schlagfluss. Berlin, Decker, 1785

Walter, L. A.

Walter, R. I. See U. J. Salmon

Walter, William Grey. American scientist
Introduced—
The location of cerebral tumors by electro-encephalography. Lancet 2: 305–308, Aug. 8, 1936

Walters, Geoffrey Alexander Bagox. English surgeon
SPECULUM—
Illuminated sims's vaginal speculum. Brit. med. J., 1: 151 (only), Jan. 31, 1942

Walters, Waltman. American surgeon. 1895–
DIET—jejunostomy feeding formula.
Preoperative and postoperative care of patients with lesions of stomach and of duodenum with H. R. Hartman, Arch. Surg., 40: 1063–1082, June 1940
METHOD—of dilating ampulla of Vater by long, smooth, graduated scoops. In his: *Diseases of the gall bladder and bile ducts* with A. M. Snell, Philadelphia, Saunders, 1940. 645 pp. p. 425
SYNDROME—
The suprarenal cortical syndrome with presentation of ten cases with R. M. Wilder and E. J. Kepler, Ann. Surg., 100: 670–688, Oct. 1934
See also H. Cabot

Walther, Philipp Franz von. German physician. 1782–1849
Described corneal opacity. Garrison and Morton
Über die Hornhautflecken. J. d. Chir. u. Augenheilk., 34: 1–90, 1845

Walther, W. W. See L. P. E. Laurent

Walton, George Lincoln. American surgeon. 1854–1941

METHOD—

A new method of reducing dislocation of cervical vertebrae. N. nerv. ment. Dis., 20: 609–611, Sept. 1893

Further observations on cervical dislocation and its reduction. Boston Med. and Surg. J., 149: 445–447, Oct. 15, 1903

Walton, Sir James. English surgeon. 1881–

OPERATION—

Reconstruction of the common bile duct. S. G. O., 79: 57–70, July 1944

Wandless, Henry Weitzell. American ophthalmologist. ?–1934

OPERATION—

A new procedure in cataract extraction: subconjunctival-flap method of capsulotomy. Arch. Ophthal., 43: 494–500, Sept. 1914

Wang, Chung Yik. Chinese pathologist. 1888–1931

TEST—

A precipitation test for syphilis. Lancet, 1: 274–276, Feb. 11, 1922

Wang, Eyvin. Christiana scientist

TEST—for indican.

Ueber die quantitative Bestimmung des Harnindikans. Z. f. physiol. Chrm., 25: 406–410, Aug. 23, 1898

Wang, Y. L. English scientist

TEST—for avitaminosis.

Methods for assessing the level of nutrition of the human subject: estimation of vitamin Bi in urine by the thiochrome test with L. J. Harris, Biochem. J., 33: 1356–1369, Aug. 1939

Wangensteen, Owen Harding. Minneapolis surgeon. 1898–

APPARATUS or DRAINAGE or SUCTION—

The early diagnosis of acute intestinal obstruction with comments on pathology and treatment: with a report of successful decompression of three cases of mechanical bowel obstruction by nasal catheter suction siphonage. West. J. Surg. and Gynaec., 40: 1–17, Jan. 1932

The necessity for constant suction to inlying nasal tubes for effectual decompression or drainage of upper gastro-intestinal tract; with comments upon drainage of other body cavities. By J. R. Paine and O. H. Wangensteen, S. G. O., 57: 601–611, Nov. 1933

Treatment of acute intestinal obstruction by suction with the duodenal tube with J. R. Paine, J. A. M. A., 101: 1532–1539, Nov. 11, 1933

GRAFT—

The implantation method of skin grafting. S. G. O., 50: 634–638, Mar. 1930

METHOD—

Imperforate anus—a method of determining the surgical approach with C. O. Rice, Ann. Surg., 92: 77–81, July 1930

METHOD—of closure of duodenal stump.

The problem of surgical arrest of massive hemorrhage in duodenal ulcer: the technique of closing the duodenum. Surgery, 8: 275–288, Aug. 1940

OPERATION—

Repair of recurrent and difficult hernias and other large defects of the abdominal wall employing iliotibial tract of fascia lata as pedicled flap. S. G. O., 59: 766–780, Nov. 1934

OPERATION—for non-rotation of intestine.

New operative techniques in the management of bowel obstruction: (1) Aseptic decompression suction enterostomy, (2) Aseptic enterotomy for removal of obstructing gall stone, and (3) Operative correction of nonrotation. Ibid., 75: 675–692, Dec. 1942

TECHNIC—of intestinal anastomosis.

Aseptic gastric resection. I. A method of aseptic anastomosis adaptable to any segment of the alimentary canal (esophagus, stomach, small or large intestine); II. Including preliminary description of subtotal excision of the acid secreting area for ulcer. Ibid., 70: 58–70, Jan. 1940

Wanger, J. O. See S. N. Blackberg

Wani, H. See Y. Ido

Warburg, Otto Heinrich. Freiburg biochemist. 1883–

Awarded Nobel prize in 1931 "for his discovery of the nature and function of the respiratory ferment."

APPARATUS—

MADE charcoal model of cell respiration. Garrison

Ueber den Stoffwechsel der Tumoren. Berlin, Springer, 1926. 263 pp.

Ueber die katalytischen Wirkungen der lebendigen Substanz. Berlin, Springer, 1928

The metabolism of tumors. Transl. by F. Dickens, London, Constable, 1930. 327 pp. New York, R. R. Smith, Inc., 1931

Ward, George Gray. American gynecologist. 1868–

TECHNIC—of vaginal hysterectomy.

Reconstructive pelvic surgery for genital prolapse: an evaluation of principles. J. Obstet. Gynaec. Brit. Empire, 43: 667–690, Aug. 1936

Ward, H. K. See G. Dreyer

Ward, Robertson. San Francisco surgeon. 1896–

Advocated continuous suction to duodenal tubes.

An apparatus for continuous gastric or duodenal lavage. J. A. M. A., 84: 1114 (only), Apr. 11, 1925

Wardell, Emma L. See V. C. Myers

Warden, Carl Cleghorn. Michigan physician. 1868–1925

AGAR—blood veal.

Studies on the gonococcus, III. J. infect. Dis., 16: 426–440 (426), May 1915

AGAR—salt.

(Same title) I. Ibid., 12: 93–105 (94), Jan. 1913

BROTH—veal infusion, for cultivation of C. diphtheriae.

The nature of toxin. The antigens of Corynebacterium diphtheriae and Bacillus megatherium and their relation to toxin with J. T. Connell and L. E. Holly, J. Bact., 6: 103–126 (104), Jan. 1921

Wardill, W. E. M. English surgeon

OPERATION—

Cleft palate. Brit. J. Surg., 16: 127–148, July 1928

Wardrop, James. English surgeon. 1782–1869

DISEASE—onychia maligna.

An account of some diseases of the toes and fingers, with observations on their treatment. Med.-chir. Trans., 5: 129–143, 1814. pp. 135–138 has subtitle: Onichia maligna; ulceration at the root of the nail.

Ware, John. Massachusetts physician. 1795–1864

Wrote on delirium tremens.

Remarks on the history and treatment of delirium tremens. Boston. Hale, 1831. 61 pp.

Warfield, J. O., Jr. See H. H. Kerr

Waring, C. H. See J. Goldberger

Warner, Emory Dean. Iowa City pathologist. 1905–
METHOD—of determining plasma prothrombin.
A quantitative study on blood clotting: prothrombin fluctuations under experimental conditions with K. M. Brinkhous and H. P. Smith, Amer. J. Physiol., 114: 667–675, Feb. 1936

Warren, John Collins. Boston surgeon. 1778–1856
OPERATION—
On an operation for the cure of natural fissure of the soft palate. Amer. J. med. Sci., 3: 1–3, 1828
Performed first operation with ether anesthesia at Massachusetts General Hospital on October 16, 1846.
Inhalation of etheral vapor for the prevention of pain in surgical operations. Boston Med. and Surg., J., 35: 375–379, Dec. 9, 1846

Warren, John Collins. Boston surgeon. 1842–1927
COLUMNS—fat-c.
Note on the anatomy and pathology of the skin. Boston Med. and Surg. J., 96: 453–458, Apr. 19, 1877
Columnae adiposa. A newly-described structure of the cutis vera, with its pathological significance in carbuncle and other affections. Cambridge, Riverside Press, 1881. 28 pp.
INCISION—
The operative treatment of cancer of the breast. Ann. Surg., 40: 805–833, Dec. 1904
Plastic resection of the mammary gland. Ibid., 45: 801–809, June 1907
OPERATION—
Ruptured perineum. Boston Med. and Surg. J., 98: 25–28, Jan. 3, 1878
A new method of operation for the relief of rupture of the perineum through the sphincter and rectum. Trans. Amer. Gynaec. Soc., 7: 322–330, 1883

Warren, Jonathan Mason. Boston surgeon. 1811–1867
OPERATION—
Operations for fissure of the soft and hard palate: (Palatoplastie). New Engl. Quart. J. Med. and Surg., Boston, 1: 538–547, Apr. 1843
Reported pilonidal sinus. In his: *Surgical observations, with cases and observations.* Boston, Ticknor and Fields, 1867. 630 pp. p. 192

Warren, S. L. See F. W. Bishop

Warren, Shields. American physician. 1898–
THEORY—of spread of carcinoma of prostate.
Osseous metastasis of carcinoma of the prostate with special reference to perineural lymphatics with P. N. Harris and R. C. Graves, Arch. Path., 22: 139–160, Aug. 1936
Drew attention to—
The angle of the mitotic spindles in malignant cells. Amer. J. Path., Suppl., 9: 781–788, 1933

Warthen, Harry Justice, Jr. Richmond, Va. surgeon. 1901–
OPERATION—
Operative treatment for benign rectal stricture (lymphogranuloma venereum): preliminary report. Arch. Surg., 38: 617–624, Apr. 1939

Warthin, Aldred Scott. Indiana physician. 1866–1931
CONSTITUTION or SYNDROME—
The constitutional entity of exophthalmic goiter and so-called toxic adenoma. Ann. intern. Med., 2: 553–570, Dec. 1928

METHOD—
A more rapid and improved method of demonstrating of spirochetes in tissues. (Warthin and Starry's cover-glass method) with A. C. Starry, Amer. J. Syph., 4: 97–103, Jan. 1920
Second improved method for the demonstration of spirocheta pallida in tissues: Warthin and Starry's silver-agar cover-glass method with A. C. Starry, J. A. M. A., 76: 234–237, Jan. 22, 1921
The staining of spirochetes in cover-glass smears by the silver-agar method with A. C. Starry, J. infect. Dis., 30: 592–600, June 1922
TUMOR—
Papillary cystadenoma lymphomatosum: a rare teratoid of the parotid region. J. Cancer Res., 13: 116–125, July 1929
Described—
Traumatic lipaemia and fatty embolism. Internat. Clin., Philadelphia, s 23, 4: 171–227, 1913

Washburn, Alfred Hamlin. San Francisco pediatrician. 1895–
STAIN—
A combined peroxidase and Wright's stain for routine blood smears. J. Lab. clin. Med., 14: 246–250, Dec. 1928

Wassén, Erik. Copenhagen physician. 1901–
REACTION—
Studies of lymphogranuloma inguinale from etiologic and immunological points of view. Acta path. et microbiol. Scandinav., suppl. 23, pp. 1–181, 1935
See also S. C. A. Hellerström

Wassermann, August von. German bacteriologist. 1866–1925
AGAR—nutrose serum.
Weitere Mittheilungen über Gonokokkencultur und Gonokokkengift. Z. Hyg. InfektKr., 27: 298–314 (300), 1898
REACTION or TEST—
Eine serodiagnostische Reaktion bei Syphilis with A. Neisser and C. Bruck, Dtsch. med. Wschr., 32: 745–746, May 10, 1906
Ueber das Vorhandensein syphilitischer Antistoffe in der Cerebrospinalflüssigkeit von Paralytikern with F. Plaut, Ibid., 1769–1772, Nov. 1, 1906

Wassilieff, N. J. See T. V. I. Bogomoloff

Watabiki, Tomomitsu. Tokyo physician
AGAR—whey ascitic fluid.
The behavior of the gonococcus in carbohydrate media. J. med. Res., 20: 365–368, Apr. 1909

Watelle, T. J. J. See B. Pol

Waterhouse, Benjamin. Boston physician. 1754–1846
Made first vaccinations in United States, in July, 1800. Garrison
A prospect of exterminating the small-pox: being the history of the variolae vaccinae, or kine-pox, commonly called the cow-pox, as it has appeared in England, with an account of a series of inoculations performed for the kine-pox in Massachusetts. Boston, 1800. 40 pp.

Waterhouse, Rupert. English physician. 1873–
SYNDROME—malignant form of meningococcus meningitis with bilateral adrenal hemorrhage.
A case of suprarenal apoplexy. Lancet, 1: 577–578, Mar. 4, 1911

Waterman, R. E. See R. R. Williams

Waters, C. A. See H. H. Young

Waters, Edward Gilmay. Jersey City obstetrician. 1898–
TECHNIC—
Supravesical extraperitoneal cesarean section; presentation of a new technique. Amer. J. Obstet. Gynaec., 39: 423–434, Mar. 1940

Waters, Ralph Milton. Madison, Wis. anesthetist. 1883–
METHOD—closed circuit.
Cyclopropane anesthesia with E. R. Schmidt, J. A. M. A., 103: 975–983, Sept. 29, 1934
TECHNIC—
Clinical scope and utility of carbon dioxid filtration in inhalation anesthesia. Anesth. and Analg., 3: 20–22; 26, Feb. 1924
Carbon dioxide absorption from anesthetic mixtures. California and West. Med., 35: 342–351, Nov. 1931
See also J. A. Stiles

Wathen, Jonathan. English physician
Treated catarrhal deafness by means of injections into Eustachian tube through a catheter inserted in nose. Garrison.
A method proposed to restore the hearing, when injured from an obstruction of the tuba Eustachiana. Philos. Trans., 1755, London, 49: 213–222, 1756

Watkins, A. B. K. English surgeon
OPERATION—
Treatment of depressed fractures of the malar bone. Brit. med. J., 1: 326–327, Feb. 13, 1937

Watkins, J. A. See C. C. Bass

Watkins, Thomas James. Chicago gynecologist. 1863–1925
OPERATION—interposition.
The treatment of cystocele and uterine prolapse after the menopause. Amer. J. Obstet. Gynaec., 15: 420–423, Nov. 1899
Treatment of cases of extensive cystocele and uterine prolapse. S. G. O., 2: 659–667, June 1906

Wats, Rattan Chaud. Indian physician
TEST—
Quantitative and qualitative methods for detection of atebrin in urine. Records of Malaria Survey of India, 4: 367–370, 1934

Watson, Cecil James. Minneapolis physician. 1901–
METHOD—
The average daily elimination of urobilinogen in health and in disease, with special reference to pernicious anemia: standardization of method based on mesobilirubinogen (H. Fischer). Arch. intern. Med., 47: 698–726, May 1931
Studies of urobilinogen. I. An improved method for the quantitative estimation of urobilinogen in urine and feces. Amer. J. clin. Path., 6: 458–475, Sept. 1936
TEST—quantitative urobilinogen for liver function.
Studies of urobilinogen. V. A simple method for the quantitative recording of the Ehrlich reaction as carried out with urine and feces with S. Schwartz, V. Sborov and Elizabeth Bertie, Amer. J. clin. Path., 14: 605–615, Dec. 1944
See also S. Schwartz

Watson, Francis Sedgwick. Boston surgeon. 1853–1942
Performed median perineal prostatectomy in 1889. Garrison and Morton
Some anatomical points connected with the performance

of prostatectomy: with remarks upon the operative treatment of prostatic hypertrophy. Ann. Surg., 4: 507–519, Apr. 1905

Watson, John. New York surgeon. 1807–1863
Performed esophagotomy for stricture.
Practical observations on organic obstructions of the oesophagus; preceded by a case which called for oesophagotomy and subsequent opening of the trachea. Amer. J. med. Sci., n. s., 8: 309–331, Oct. 1844

Watson, Kenneth. English surgeon
TECHNIC—
Carcinoma of ampulla of Vater; successful radical resection. Brit. J. Surg., 31: 368–373, Apr. 1944

Watson, Leigh Festus. Los Angeles surgeon. 1884–
OPERATION—for inguinal hernia. In his: *Hernia.* . . . St. Louis, Mosby, 1938. 2 ed., pp. 167–181

Watson, Sir Patrick Heron. British surgeon. 1832–1907
Pioneer of thyroidectomy.
Excision of the thyroid gland. Edinburgh med. J., 19: 252–255, Sept. 1873
(Same title) Brit. med. J., 2: 386–388, Sept. 25, 1875

Watson, Thomas. Los Angeles chemist
MODIFICATION—
An improved apparatus for use in Folin and Wu's method for the estimation of urea in blood with H.L. White, J. biol. Chem., 45: 465–466, Feb. 1921

Watson, W. L. See H. E. Martin

Watson-Jones, Reginald. See R. W. Jones

Watt, James. English scientist. 1736–1819
Invented gasometer, 1790. Garrison
Considerations on the medicinal use of factitious airs. By T. Beddoes and J. Watt, Bristol, 1795

Watts, James Winston. American neurologist. 1904–
Described—
Effect of lesions of the hypothalamus on the gastrointestinal tract and heart in monkeys with J. F. Fulton. Arch. Neurol. Psychiat., Chicago, 33: 446 (only), Feb. 1935
See also W. J. Freeman

Waugh, George Ernest. London surgeon
OPERATION—colopexy.
The morbid consequences of a mobile ascending colon, with a record of 180 operations. Brit. J. Surg., 17: 343–383, Jan. 1920

Wawra, Cecil Z. California scientist
Isolated vitamin P (hesperidin chalcone).
The isolation of a new oxidation-reduction enzyme from lemon peel (vitamin P) with J. L. Webb, Science, 96: 302–303, Sept. 25, 1942

Wearn, Joseph Treloar. Pennsylvania pharmacologist. 1893–
Wrote—
Observations on the composition of glomerular urine, with particular reference to the problem of reabsorption in the renal tubules with A. N. Richards, Amer. J. Physiol., 71: 209–227, Dec. 1, 1924

Webb, J. L. See C. Z. Wawra

Weber, Adolph. Darmstadt ophthalmologist. 1829–1915
Described closing of Schlemm's canal as cause of glaucoma.
Die Ursache des Glaucoms. Arch. f. Ophthal., 23: 1–91, 1877

Weber, Eduard Friedrich. German physiologist. 1806–1871

Discovered inhibitory power of vagus nerve.

Experimenta, quibus probatur nervos vagos rotatione machinae galvano-magneticae irritatos motum cordis retardare et adeo intercipere with E. H. Weber, Ann. univ. de med., Milan, 3 s., 20: 227–233, 1845

Also in: Wagner's *Handwörterbuch der Physiologie,* 3: 45–51, 1846

Weber, Ernst Heinrich. German physiologist. 1795–1878

LAW—variation of stimulus which causes smallest appreciable change in sensation maintains an approximately fixed ratio to whole stimulus. Garrison

De pulsu, resorptione, auditu et tactu. Annotationes anatomicae et physiologicae. Lipsiae, Koehler, 1834

Der Tastsinn und das Gemeingefühl. In: Wagner's *Handwörterbuch der Physiologie,* 3, Abt. 2: 481–588, 1846

First, with his brother, Eduard Friedrich, to measure velocity of pulse-wave. Garrison

Wellenlehre. Leipzig, Engelmann, 1825

First to measure and compare velocity of blood and lymph corpuscles in capillaries. Garrison

Microscopische Beobachtungen über die sichtbare Fortbewegung der Lymphkörnchen in den Lymphgefässen der Froschlarven. Arch. f. Anat., Physiol. u. wiss. Med., pp. 267–272, 1837

First to show that sensation can be analyzed into its visceral and muscular components, and that these can be separated from tactile sensations. Garrison

See LAW—second reference.

Wrote important work on touch and temperature sense which was the starting point of the experimental psychophysics of Fechner and Wundt. Garrison. Ibid.

Weber, Frederick Parkes. London physician. 1863–

DISEASE—Rendu-Osler-Weber d.; familial telangiectasis.

A note on cutaneous telangiectases and their etiology: comparison with the etiology of haemorrhoids and ordinary varicose veins. Edinburgh med. J., n. s., 15: 346–349, Apr. 1904

Multiple hereditary developmental angiomata (telangiectases) of the skin and mucous membranes associated with recurring hemorrhages. Lancet, 2: 160–162, July 20, 1907

DISEASE—Weber-Dimitri d.; angioma of brain visible by roentgenogram.

Right-sided hemi-hypotrophy resulting from right-sided congenital spastic hemiplegia, with a morbid condition of the left side of the brain, revealed by radiograms. J. Neurol. Psychopath., 3: 134–139, Aug. 1922

DISEASE—Weber-Christian d.

A case of relapsing non-suppurative nodular panniculitis, showing phagocytosis of subcutaneous fat-cells by macrophages. Brit. J. Dermat. and Syph., 37: 301–311, July 1925

DISEASE—localized epidermolysis bullosa.

Recurrent bullous eruption on the feet in a child. Proc. Roy. Soc. Med. (Sect. Dermat.), 19: 72 (only), June 1926

Weber, H. Marburg physician

TEST—for blood in stomach contents.

Ueber den Nachweis des Blutes in dem Magen- und dem Darminhalt. Berl. klin. Wschr., pp. 441–444, May 8, 1893

Weber, Harry Matthew. Rochester, Minn. roentgenologist. 1899–

TECHNIC—

The roentgenologic demonstration of polypoid lesions and polyposis of the large intestine. Amer. J. Roentg. and Rad. Therapy, 25: 577–589, May 1931

See also J. A. Bargen, P. W. Brown

Weber, Sir Hermann David. London physician. 1823–1918

SIGN, SYMPTOM or SYNDROME—paralysis of limbs and hypoglossal nerve on one side, and of oculomotor nerves on the other.

A contribution to the pathology of the crura cerebri. Med.-chir. Trans., 46: 121–139, 1863

Weber, W. See F. Thomas

Weber, Wilhelm Eduard. German physiologist. 1804–1891

Wrote on physiology of motion and locomotion. Garrison and Morton

Mechanik der menschlichen Gehwerkzeuge with E. F. W. Weber, Göttingen, Dietrich, 1836. 1 vol. and atlas.

Weber, Wilhelm. German surgeon. 1872–1928

OPERATION—pyloroplasty.

Ueber eine technische Neuerung bei der Operation der Pylorusstenose des Säuglings. Berl. klin. Wschr., 47: 763–765, Apr. 25, 1910

Webster, George Van O'Linda, Jr. U. S. Navy surgeon. 1911–

KNIFE—

A simple skin graft knife for general use. Amer. J. Surg., 67: 569–571, Mar. 1945

Webster, Jerome Pierce. New York surgeon. 1888–

METHOD—of mammoplasty.

Mastectomy for gynecomastia through a semicircular intra-areolar incision. Ann. Surg., 124: 557–575, Sept. 1946

Webster, John Clarence. Chicago gynecologist. 1863–

OPERATION—Baldy-Webster o. for retrodisplacement of uterus.

A satisfactory operation for certain cases of retroversion of the uterus. J. A. M. A., 37: 913 (only), Oct. 5, 1901

Webster, R. W. See W. S. Haines

Wechselmann, Dr. Berlin physician

METHOD—barium sulphate treatment of syphilitic sera.

Ueber Verschleierung der Wassermannschen Reaktion durch Komplementoidverstopfung. Z. ImmunForsch., 3: 525–530, Sept. 25, 1909

Wecker, Louis de. French ophthalmologist. 1832–1906

OPERATION—

Traitement chirurgical du strabisme paralytique. Arch. d'ophth., 24: 421–425, 1904

OPERATION—iridocapsulectomy.

Chirurgie oculaire. . . . Paris, Doin, 1879. 419 pp.

Traité complet de l'ophthalmologie with E. Landolt, Paris, Delahaye, 1880–89. 4 vols.

Wedd, Bernard Harry. English physician. 1877–1924

Studied immunity to cancer.

The effect of Röntgen and radium radiations upon the vitality of the cells of mouse carcinoma with S. Russ, J. Path. Bact., 17: 1–11, July 1912

On the immunity conferred upon mice by radium-irradiated mouse carcinoma with A. C. Morson and S. Russ, Ibid., 18: 566–571, Apr. 1914

Wedenskii, Nikolai Igorevich. St. Petersburg physiologist. 1844–

Wrote on physiology of nerves. Garrison and Morton

Wie rasch ermüdet der Nerv? Zbl. f. d. med. Wiss., Berlin, 22: 65–68, Feb. 2, 1884

Weech, Alexander Ashley. New York pediatrician. 1895–

FORMULA—for determining total plasma protein.
The relationship between specific gravity and protein content in plasma, serum, and transudate from dogs with E. B. Reeves and E. Goettsch, J. biol. Chem., 113: 167–174, Feb. 1936

Weed, Lewis Hill. American neurologist. 1886–
Mapped out circulation of cerebrospinal fluid. Garrison
Studies on cerebro-spinal fluid. No. III. The pathways of escape from the subarachnoid spaces with particular reference to the arachnoid villi. J. med. Res., 31: 51–117, Sept. 1914
Advocated injection or ingestion of hypertonic salt solutions in lowering intracranial tension. Garrison
Pressure changes in the cerebro-spinal fluid following intravenous injection of solutions of various concentrations. Amer. J. Physiol., 48: 512 (only), Apr. 1. 1919
Experimental alteration of brain bulk with P. S. McKibben, Ibid., 48: 531–558

Weeks, John Elmer. American ophthalmologist. 1853–
BACILLUS—Koch-Weeks.
The bacillus of acute conjunctival catarrh, or "pink-eye." Arch. Ophthal., 15: 441–451, 1886
The pathogenic microbe of "acute catarrhal conjunctivitis." New York med. Rec., 26: 571–577, May 21, 1887
OPERATION—
Description of an operation for providing cul-de-sacs for the lodgment of an artificial eye in cases in which the conjunctival sacs have been obliterated from any cause. Internat. Cong. Ophthal., pp. 298–305, Sept. 13–18, 1904
TREATMENT—
Treatment of corneal infections. Amer. J. Ophthal., 16: 293–297, Apr. 1933

Weese, Helmut. German scientist. 1897–
Introduced Evipal and Evipal soluble.
Evipan, ein neuartiges Einschlafmittel with W. Scharpff, Dtsch. med. Wschr., 2: 1205–1207, July 29, 1932

Weglowski, Romuald J. Moscow surgeon
OPERATION—transplantation of cartilage in treatment of ankylosis.
Die Behandlung der Gelenkankylosen vermittels Überpflanzung von Knorpelplatten. Zbl. Chir., pp. 481–484, Apr. 27, 1907

Wegner, Frederick Rudolph Georg. German pathologist. 1843–
DISEASE—syphilicis osteochondritis.
SIGN—broadened, discolored epiphyseal line in infants dying from hereditary syphilis.
Über hereditäre Knochensyphilis bei jungen Kindern. Arch. f. path. Anat. u. Physiol., 50: 305–322, June 27, 1870

Weichardt, Julius Wolfgang. German pathologist. 1875–
REAGENT—
Über die Serodiagnostik der Syphilis mittels Ausflockung durch cholesterinierte Extrakte. Med. Klin., 15: 139–140, Feb. 9, 1919

Weichert, Charles Kipp. Ohio zoologist. 1902–

Demonstrated that progestin prepares endometrium for reception and nourishment of fertilized ovum subsequent to preliminary influence of estrogenic principle.
Production of placentomata in normal and ovariectomized guinea pigs and albino rats. Proc. Soc. exp. Biol., N. Y., 25: 490–491, Mar. 1928
See also F. L. Hisaw

Weichselbaum, Anton. Austrian pathologist. 1845–1920
DIPLOCOCCUS—D. intracellularis.
Ueber die Aetiologie der akuten meningitis cerebro-, spinalis. Fort. d. Med., 5: 573–583, Sept. 15; 620–626, Oct. 1, 1887
Established causal relation of pneumococcus to lobar pneumonia.
Ueber die Aetiologie der acuten Lungen- und Rippenfellentzündungen. Med. Jb., 1: 483–554, 1886
Ueber seltenere Localisationen des pneumonischen Virus (Diplococcus pneumoniae). Wien. klin. Wschr., 1: 573–575, Oct. 11; 595–597, Oct. 18; 620–622, Oct. 25; 642–643, Nov. 1; 659–661, Nov. 8, 1888

Weidenfeld, Stephan. Vienna physician. 1870–1917
RATIO—of surface-area in burns.
Über den Verbrennungstod. Arch. f. Dermat. u. Syph., 61: 301–356, 1902

Weidenreich, Franz. Strassburg anatomist. 1873–
METHOD—of staining spirochetes.
Eine neue einfache Methode zur Darstellung von Blut-Trockenpräparaten. Folia haematol., 3: 1–7, Jan. 1906

Weigert, Carl. German pathologist. 1843–1904
METHOD—Gram-Weigert, of staining bacteria in tissues.
Ueber eine neue Methode zur Färbung von Fibrin und von Microorganismen. Fort. d. Med., 5: 228–232, Apr. 15, 1887
METHOD—for nuclei.
Eine kleine Verbesserung der Hämatoxylin-van Gieson-Methode. Z. wiss. Mik., 21: 1–5, 1904
METHOD—for neuroglia fibers.
Zur Technik der mikroskopischen Bakterienuntersuchungen. Arch. d. path. Anat. u. Physiol., 84: 275–315, May 9, 1881
METHOD—of serial sections by celloidin.
Ueber Schnittserien von Celloidinpräparaten des Centralnervensystems zum Zwecke der Markscheidenfärbung. Z. wiss. Mikr., 2: 490–495, 1885
METHOD—for myelin sheaths. Mallory
Ausführliche Beschreibung der in No. 2 dieser Zeitschrift erwähnten neuen Färbungsmethode für das Centralnervensystem. Fort. d. Med., 2: 190–191, 1884
NEUROGLIA MORDANT—Mallory
Die histologische Technik des Centralnervensystems. II. 2. Die Markscheidenfärbung. Anat. Hefte., Abt. II, 6: 3–25, 1896
STAIN—iron hematoxylin.
See METHOD (2).
STAIN—differential, for fibrin.
See METHOD, 1887
STAIN—differential, for neuroglia fibers. Mallory
Beiträge zur Kenntnis der normalen menschlichen Neuroglia. Festschr. 50 jähr. Jub. ärztl. Ver. Frankfurt a. M., 192–209, 1895
STAIN—for actinomyces.
See METHOD—for neuroglia fibers. p. 303
STAIN—for elastic tissue.

Ueber eine Methode zur Färbung elastischer Fasern.
Zbl. f. all. Path. Anat., 9: 289–292, May 1, 1898
First to stain bacteria. Garrison
Ueber Bacterien in der Pockenhaut. Zbl. f. d. med.
Wiss., 9: 609–611, Sept. 30, 1871
Über eine Mykose beineinem neugeborenen Kinde (Bakterienfärbung mit Anilinfarben). Zb. d. schles.
Ges. f. vaterl. Cultur, 1875, Breslau, 53: 229, 1876
Wrote classical account of pathologic anatomy of
Bright's disease. Garrison and Morton
Die Bright'sche Nierenerkrankung vom pathologisch-anatomischen Standpunkte. Samml. klin. Vortr., No.
162–163, (Inn. Med. No. 55), 1411–1460, 1879
Described thymic tumor in association with myasthenia gravis.
Pathologisch-anatomischer Beitrag zur Erb'schen Krankheit (Myasthenia gravis). Neurol. Zbl., 20: 597–601,
July 1, 1901
Weil, Arthur. German-American neurologist. 1888–
METHOD—
A rapid method for staining myelin sheaths. Arch.
Neurol. Psychiat., Chicago, 20: 392–393, Aug. 1928
See E. Abderhalden, M. L. Mason
Weil, Edmund. Vienna physician. 1880–1922
BACILLUS—of proteus group isolated from urine and
feces of typhus patients.
REACTION—
Zur serologischen Diagnose des Fleckfiebers with A.
Felix, Wien klin. Wschr., 29: 33–35, Jan. 13, 1916
Untersuchungen über das Wesen der Fleckfieber-Agglutination. Ibid., 30: 393–399, Mar. 29, 1917
Weil, H. Adolph. Heidelberg physician. 1848–1916
DISEASE—epidemic catarrhal jaundice.
*Ueber eine eigenthümliche, mit Milztumor, Icterus
und Nephritis einhergehende acute Infectionskrankheit.* Dtsch. Arch. f. klin. Med., 39: 209–232, July
28, 1886
Weil, Prosper Émile. French physician. 1873–
SOLUTION—pleuritic serum peptone.
Essais de culture du bacille lépreaux. Ann. Inst. Pasteur, 19: 793–803 (798), Dec. 1905
Weil, Richard. New York physician. 1876–1917
TEST—for hemolysis.
Sodium citrate in the transfusion of blood. J. A. M. A.,
64: 425–426, Jan. 30, 1915
Weill, A. See L. Ambard
Weill, Edmond. French physician. 1858–1924
Described low capillary resistance, beneath a tourniquet, in purpura.
Purpura provoqué par hypertension veineuse with J.
Chalier, Lyon Méd., 116: 936–940, May 21, 1911
Weinbach, Ancel P. Baltimore scientist
METHOD—
A micromethod for the determination of sodium. J.
biol. Chem., 110: 95–99, June 1935
Weinberg. See V. M. von Bechterew
Weinberg, Michel. Paris physician. 1868–1940
REACTION—
Séro-diagnostic de l'echinococcose. Ann. Inst. Pasteur,
23: 472–502, June 1909
Isolated Cl. oedematiens.
Notes bactériologiques sur les infections gazeuses with
P. Séguin, C. R. Soc. Biol., 78: 274–279, May 29,
1915
Isolated Cl. histolyticum.
Contribution à l'étiologie de la gangrène gazeuse with

P. Séguin, C. R. Acad. Sci., 163: 449–451, Oct. 23,
1916
Weiner, David Otis. St. Louis physician. 1908–
Introduced plasma therapy for burns.
Significance of loss of serum protein in therapy of severe burns with A. P. Rowlette and R. Elman, Proc.
Soc. exp. Biol., N. Y., 34: 484–486, May 1936
Weinland, R. F. See K. Binder
Weinstein, A. See G. A. Harrop
Weir, Robert Fulton. New York surgeon. 1838–1927
INCISION—for nephrectomy.
*Remarks on extirpation of the kidney, with cases of
nephrectomy for pyonephrosis and nephrotomy for
rupture of the kidney.* New York med. J., 40: 721–726,
Dec. 27, 1884
OPERATION—appendicostomy.
*A new use for the useless appendix, in the surgical
treatment of obstinate colitis.* Med. Rec., 62: 201–202,
Aug. 9, 1902
Weir Mitchell, S. See S. W. Mitchell
Weismann, August Friedrich Leopold. German
biologist. 1834–1914
THEORY—non-inheritance of acquired characters;
weismannism.
Studien zur Descendenz-Theorie. Leipzig, Engelmann,
1875–6
Ueber die Vererbung. Jena, Fischer, 1883. 59 pp.
On heredity. Transl. by Poulton, Schönland and
Shipley, Oxford, Clarendon Press, 1889. 455 pp.
Weiss, A. G. Belgian physician
Introduced use of histidine hydrochloride in treatment of peptic ulcer.
*La carence en acides amines non synthetisables dans la
pathogenie de l'ulcere experimental: application au
traitement de l'ulcere humain* with E. Aron, J. belge
de gastro-enterol., 1: 327–338, June 26, 1933
Weiss, Arthur. New York physician. 1902–
TECHNIC—
The prognostic value of the sedimentation rate in arthritis: a modification of the technique. Amer. J. med.
Sci., 181: 379–392, Mar. 1931
Weiss, Charles. American bacteriologist. 1894–
SOLUTION—egg.
Study of cultural requirements of Spirochaeta pallida
with Dorothy Wilkes-Weiss, J. infect. Dis., 34: 212–
226 (222), 1924
Weiss, Nathan. Vienna physician. 1874–
SIGN—contraction of facial muscles when lightly percussed.
Ueber Tetanie. Samml. klin. Vortr., No. 189 (Inn.
med., No. 63), 1675–1704, Feb. 9, 1881
Weiss, Soma. Boston physician. 1898–1942
SYNDROME—carotid sinus s.
*The carotid sinus in health and disease: its role in the
causation of fainting and convulsions* with J. P. Baker,
Medicine, 12: 297–354, Sept. 1933
Discovered that cutaneous analgesia stops pain due
to visceral disease referred to that area of skin.
*The significance of the afferent impulses from the skin
in the mechanism of visceral pain: skin infiltration as a
useful therapeutic measure* with D. Davis, Amer. J.
med. Sci., 176: 517–536, Oct. 1928
Weissbecker, Dr. German physician
Used human serum obtained from an individual recently recovered from scarlet fever to give passive
immunity to another individual.

Heilserum gegen Typhus, Scharlach, Pneumonie. Z. f. klin. Med., 32: 188–206, 1897
Weissberger, A. See H. Graupner
Weisser, Dr. Berlin physician
BROTH—sucrose extract, for cultivation of cholera and typhoid group.
Ueber die Emmerich'schen sogenannten Neapler Cholerabacterien. Z. f. Hyg. InfektKr., 1: 315–362 (355; 339), 1886
Weisz, Moriz. Vienna physician
TEST—for urochromogen.
Ueber eine neue Harnreaktion und ihren Zusammenhang mit der Ehrlichschen Diazoreaktion. Med. Klin., 6: 1661–1662, Oct. 16, 1910
Die Bedeutung des Urochromogens für die Prognose und Therapie der Lungentuberkulose. Münch. med. Wschr., 58: 1348–1352, June 20, 1911
Welch, Francis Henry. English physician. 1840–1910
Described syphilitic aortitis and degenerative lesions of aorta.
On aortic aneurysm in the army, and the conditions associated with it. Med.-chir. Trans., 59: 59–79, 1876
Welch, William Henry. Baltimore pathologist. 1850–1934
BACILLUS—B. aërogenes capsulatus.
A gas-producing bacillus (Bacillus aerogenes capsulatus, nov. spec.). capable of rapid development in the blood-vessels after death with G. H. F. Nuttall, Johns Hopk. Hosp. Bull., 3: 81–91, July–Aug. 1892
Also: Medical classics, 5: 852–885, June 1941
Morbid conditions caused by Bacillus aerogenes capsulatus. Johns Hopk. Hosp. Bull., 11: 185–204, Sept. 1900
Also: Medical classics, 5: 886–939, June 1941
METHOD—of staining capsule of pneumococcus. Ibid., 1892. p. 84
Investigated acute edema of lungs. Garrison
Zur Pathologie des Lungenödems. Arch. f. path. Anat., 72: 375–412, Mar. 5, 1878
Demonstrated pathological changes produced by experimental injection of toxins of diphtheria, simultaneously with Behring. Garrison
The histological changes in experimental diphtheria: preliminary communication with S. Flexner, Johns Hopk. Hosp. Bull., 2: 107–110, Aug. 1891
The histological lesions produced by the tox-albumen of diphtheria with S. Flexner, Ibid., 3: 17–18, Mar. 1892
Discovered Staphylococcus epidermidis albus and its relation to wound infection. Garrison
Conditions underlying the infection of wounds; . . . Trans. Cong. Amer. Phys. and Surg., New Haven, 2: 1–28, 1892
Investigated embolism and thrombosis. Garrison
Thrombosis and embolism. In: Allbutt's *System of Surgery,* London, 6: 155–285, 1899
Welcker, Hermann. German physician. 1822–1897
METHOD—for determination of total blood volume.
Bestimmungen der Menge des Körperblutes und der Blutfärbekraft, sowie Bestimmungen von Zahl, Maass Oberfläche und Volum des einzelnen Blutkörperchens bei Thieren und bei Menschen. Z. f. rat. Med., Leipzig, 3 R., 4: 145–167, 1858
Grösse, Zahl, Volum, Oberfläche und Farbe der Blutkörperchen bei Menschen und bei Thieren. Ibid., 20: 257–307, 1863
Weld, Edward Howland. American urologist. 1881–

Advocated—
The use of sodium bromide in roentgenography. J. A. M. A., 71: 1111–1112, Oct. 5, 1918
Wells, Herbert Sessions. Nashville physiologist, 1899–
DETERMINATION—
A modified Krogh osmometer for the determination of the osmotic pressure of colloids in biological fluids (with directions for its use). J. Tennessee Acad. Sci., 8: 102–115, Apr. 1933
Wells, Horace. Hartford, Conn. dentist. 1815–1848
First to use nitrous oxide in dentistry, 1844.
A history of the discovery of the application of nitrous oxide gas, ether, and other vapors, to surgical operations. Hartford, Wells, 1847. 25 pp.
Wells, Sir Thomas Spencer. English gynecologist. 1818–1897
FACIES—facial expression of ovarian disease.
Diseases of the ovaries: their diagnosis and treatment. London, Churchill, 1865. 376 pp.
FORCEPS—
Remarks on forcipressure and the use of pressure-forceps in surgery. Brit. med. J., 1: 926–928, June 21, 1879, et seq.
Wells, William Charles. Charleston, S. C. physician. 1757–1817
Described cardiac complications of rheumatism.
On rheumatism of the heart. Trans. Soc. Improve. Med. and Chir. Knowledge, London, 3: 372–412, 1812
also in: F. A. Willius and T. E. Keys' *Cardiac classics.* St. Louis, Mosby, 1941. pp. 294–312
Developed theory of dew and dew-point; important to ventilation.
An essay on dew and several appearances connected with it. London, Taylor and Hessey, 1814. 146 pp.
Welsh, Gottfried. German physician. 1618–1690
Wrote important book on lethal wounds. Garrison
Rationale vulnerum lethalium judicium. . . . Lipsiae, Ritzschianis, 1660
Wrote on pleural births. Garrison
De gemellis et partu numeriori. Lipsiae, Ritzschianis, 1667
Welsh, David Arthur. Edinburgh pathologist
Wrote—
Concerning the parathyroid glands: a critical, anatomical, and experimental study. J. Anat. and Physiol., 32: 292–307, Jan. 1898
Weltmann, Oskar. Vienna physician. 1885–1934
REACTION—serum coagulation, to distinguish inflammatory from exudative processes.
Untersuchungen über die Serumkoagulation with C. V. Medvei, Z. f. klin. Med., 118: 670–687, 1931
TEST—for urea.
Über die Tagesschwankungen im Urobilinogengehalt des Harnes bei Gesunden und Kranken with O. Tenschert, Wien. med. Wschr., 72: 766–770, Apr. 29, 1922
Weltmer, Sydney A. American
SYSTEM—weltmerism; suggestive treatment seeking to bring mind and body into harmony.
The healing hand. Nevada, Mo., Weltmer, 1922. 2 ed.
Welzel, Alfons. German physician
TEST—for carbon monoxide in blood.
Ueber den Nachweis des Kohlenoxydhämoglobins. Verh. d. phys.-med. Ges. zu Würzb., 23, 1889

Wenckebach, Karl Frederik. Vienna physician.
1862–1940
THEORY—mechanical, of cardiac pain in coronary
occlusion.
Toter Punkt, "second Wind," und Angina pectoris.
Wien klin. Wschr., 41: 1–6, Jan. 5, 1928
Wendel, Walther. Sudenburg surgeon. 1872–
OPERATION—
Zur Chirurgie des Oesophagus. Arch. f. klin. Chir.,
93: 311–329, 1910
Wendt, A. See J. E. v. Purkinje
Wenglowski, Romuald. Moscow surgeon
THEORY—of formation of branchial fistulas or cysts.
Über die Halsfisteln und Cysten. Arch. f. klin. Chir.
98: 151–208, Apr. 29, 1912
(Same title) *Zweiter Theil.* Ibid., 100: 789–892, Jan.
30, 1913
Wenyon, C. See P. H. Manson-Bahr
Wenzel, Carl. German physician. 1769–1827
First employed artificial induction of premature
labor, 1804. Garrison
*Allgemeine geburtshülfliche Betrachtungen und über
die künstliche Frühgeburt.* Mainz, Kupferberg, 1818
Wepfer, Johann Jacobus. German physician. 1620–
1695
Wrote early account of hemorrhagic nature of
apoplexy. Garrison
*Observationes anatomicae, ex cadaveribus eorum, quos
sustulit apoplexia, cum exercitatione de ejus loco
affecto.* Shaffhusii, Suteri, 1658. 304 pp.
Described lead poisoning.
Historiae apoplecticorum.... Amstelaedami, Jans-
sonio-Waebergias, 1694
Werbitzki, F. W. Berlin physician
AGAR—china green infusion.
*Ein neuer Nährboden zum Nachweis der Typhus-
bazillen in Fäzes.* Arch. f. Hyg., 69: 191–206 (205),
1909
Werder, Xavier Oswald. American surgeon. 1858–
1919
OPERATION—
*A new operation for the radical treatment of cancer of
the cervix, consisting of the removal of the uterus and
vagina en masse by the suprapubic method; with re-
port of a case.* Amer. J. Obstet., 37: 289–293, Mar.
1898
Werdnig, Guido. Graz neurologist
DISEASE or SYNDROME—of Werdnig-Hoffman;
infantile progressive muscular atrophy.
*Zwei frühinfantile hereditäre Fälle von progressiver
Muskelatrophie unter dem Bilde der Dystrophie, ober
auf neurotischer Grundlage.* Arch. Psychiat. Nerv-
enkr., 22: 437–480, 1890
Werlhof, Paul Gottlieb. German physician. 1699–
1767
DISEASE—purpura hemorrhagica or thrombocyto-
penic purpura.
*Disquisitio medica et philologica de variolis et anthraci-
bus.* Hannoverae, Brunswick, 1735
Also in his: *Opera omnia.* Haanoverae, imp. fratrum
Helwingiorum, 1775–76, Vol. 2, p. 539; 615–636
Also, abstr. in: Major's *Classic descriptions of dis-
ease.* Springfield, Ill., Thomas, 1939. 2 ed., pp. 561–
562
Werner, C. W. German physician
SYNDROME—progeria in adult.

Ueber Katarakt in Verbindung mit Sklerodermie.
Inaug. Diss., Kiel, 1904
Werner, Heinrich. German physician. 1874–
DISEASE—Werner-His d.; trench fever.
*Über eine besondere Erkrankung, die er als Fünftage-
fieber bezeichnet.* Abstr.: Berl. klin. Wschr., 53: 204
(only), Feb. 21, 1916
See also H. Schmalfuss
Wernicke, Carl. German neurologist. 1848–1905
APHASIA—cortical sensory a.
*Der aphasische Symptomencomplex. Eine psycholo-
gische Studie auf anatomischer Basis.* Breslau, Cohn
und Weigert, 1874. 72 pp.
DISEASE—
Die acute, hämorrhagische Poliencephalitis superior.
In his: *Lehrbuch der Gehirnkrankheiten fur Aerzte
und Studirende.* Kassel und Berlin, 1881. vol. 2, pp.
229–242
REACTION, SIGN or TEST—
Ueber hemiopische Pupillenreaction. Fort. d. Med.,
1: 49–53, Jan. 15, 1883
TRIANGLE—posterior segment of internal capsule.
*Erkrankung der innern Kapsel. Ein Beitrag zur
Diagnose der Heerderkrankungen.* Breslau, Cohn und
Weigert, 1875. 24 pp.
TYPE—of paralysis.
Zur Kenntnis der cerebralen Hemiplegie. Berl. klin.
Wschr., 26: 969–970, Nov. 11, 1889
Wernicke, Robert Johann. Buenos Aires patholo-
gist. 1873–
Reported case of coccidiodal granuloma.
*Ueber einen Protozoenbefund bei Mycosis fungoides
(?).* Zbl. Bakt., 12: 859–861, Dec. 28, 1892
Werth, Richard. German gynecologist. 1850–1918
Studied extrauterine pregnancy.
*Beiträge zur Anatomie und zur operativen Behand-
lung der Extrauterinschwangerschaft.* Stuttgart, Enke,
1887. 162 pp.
Wertheim, Ernst. Vienna gynecologist. 1864–1920
OPERATION—radical hysterectomy.
Zur Frage der Radicaloperation beim Uteruskrebs.
Arch. f. Gynaek., 61: 627–668, 1900
*Ein neuer Beitrag zur Frage der Radikaloperation
beim Uteruskrebs.* Ibid., 65: 1–39, 1902
*The radical abdominal operation in carcinoma of
cervix uteri.* S. G. O., 4: 1–10, Jan. 1907
*Die erweiterte abdominale Operation bei Carcinoma
colli uteri (auf Grund von 500 Fällen).* Berlin, Urban
und Schwarzenberg, 1911. 223 pp.
Demonstrated gonococcus in acute cystitis.
*Ueber Blasengonorrhöe. Ein neuer Beitrag zum
Verhalten der Gonokokken im Gewebe: Nachweis von
Gonokokken in Blutgefässen.* Z. f. Geburt. u. Gynaek.,
35: 1–10, 1896
Wesbrook, Frank Fairchild. Minneapolis physician.
1868–1918
CLASSIFICATION—
Varieties of bacillus diphtheriae with L. B. Wilson
and O McDaniel, Trans. Ass. Amer. Phys., 198–
223, 1900
Westcott, Henry Heyward. Roanoke, Va. surgeon.
1895–
OPERATION—
*Preliminary report of a method of internal fixation of
transcervical fractures of the neck of the femur in the*

aged. Virginia Med. Monthly, 59: 197–204, July 1932
End-results after internal fixation of trans-cervical fractures of the femur. Ibid., 62: 446–448, Nov. 1935
Wesselow, O. L. de. See H. MacLean
Wessely, Karl. Würzburg ophthalmologist. 1874–
RECORDING APPARATUS—mercury manometer, for intraocular pressure.
Experimentelle Untersuchungen über den Augendruck, sowie über qualitative und quantitative Beeinflussung des intraokularen Flüssigkeitswechsels. Arch. f. Augenheilk., 60: 1–48, Apr. 1908
West, Charles. English physician. 1816–1898
Wrote early pediatric book. Garrison and Morton
Lectures on the diseases of infancy and childhood. London, Longman, 1848
West, John Montgomery. American otolaryngologist. 1876–
OPERATION—hypophysectomy.
The surgery of the hypophysis from the standpoint of the rhinologist. J. A. M. A., 54: 1132–1134, Apr. 2, 1910
OPERATION—
A window resection of the nasal duct in cases of stenosis. Trans. Amer. Ophthal. Soc., 12: 654–658, 1910
OPERATION—
The intranasal lacrimal sac operation: its advantages and its results. Arch. Ophthal., 55: 351–361, July 1926
West, Randolph. New York physician. 1890–
METHOD—of producing reticulo-cytic response in anemia.
Antianemic material of liver and stomach. J. A. M. A., 105: 432–437, Aug. 10, 1935
See also H. D. Dakin
Westberg, Friedrich. Hamburg dermatologist
DISEASE—
Ein Fall von mit weissen Flecken einhergehender, bisher nicht bekannter Dermatose. Mschr. f. prakt. Dermatol., 33: 355–362, Oct. 1, 1901
Westergren, Alf. Swedish physician. 1891–
TECHNIC—for determining sedimentation rate of erythrocytes.
Studies of the suspension stability of the blood in pulmonary tuberculosis. Acta med. Scandinav., 54: 247–282, 1921
Also, abstr.: Brit. J. Tuberc., 15: 72–76, Apr. 1921
Die Senkungreaktion. Allgemein-klinische Ergebnisse. Praktische Bedeutung bei Tuberkulose. Ergebn. d. inn. Med. u. Kinderh., 26: 577–732, 1924
The technic of the red cell sedimentation reaction. Amer. Rev. Tuberc., 14: 94–101, July 1926
Westphal, Alexander Karl Otto. German neurologist. 1863–1941
PHENOMENON—contraction of pupil, followed by dilatation, after vigorous closing of lids.
Ueber ein bisher nicht beschriebenes Pupillenphänomen. Neurol. Zbl., 18: 161–164, Feb. 15, 1899
Westphal, Carl Friedrich Otto. Berlin neurologist. 1833–1890
NEUROSIS—hysteria with symptoms that simulate multiple sclerosis.
Über einen merkwürdigen Fall von periodischer Lähmung aller vier Extremitäten mit gleichzeitigem Erlöschen der elektrischen Erregbarkeit während der Lähmung. Berl. klin. Wschr., 22: 489–491, Aug. 3; 509–511, Aug. 10, 1885

PSEUDOSCLEROSIS—
Über eine dem Bilde der cerebrospinalen grauen Degeneration ähnliche Erkrankung des centralen Nervensystems ohne anatomischen Befund, nebst einigen Bemerkungen über paradoxe Contraction. Arch. f. Psychiat., 14: 87–134; 767–769, 1883
Described agoraphobia. Garrison
Die Agoraphobie, eine neuropathische Erscheinung. Ibid., 3: 138–161, 1871
Described syndrome of pathologic sleep.
Zwei Krankheitsfälle . . . Eigenthümliche mit Einschlafen verbundene Anfälle. Ibid., 7: 622–635 (631–635), 1877
Westphal, U. See A. F. J. Butenandt
Weszprémi, Stephan. German physician. 1723–1799
Proposed preventive inoculations against plague. Garrison
Tentamen de inoculanda peste. Londini, Tuach, 1755. 30 pp.
Wettstein, A. See L. Ruzicka
Wetzel, Norman Carl. Cleveland pediatrician. 1897–
METHOD—
Physical fitness in terms of physique, development and basal metabolism: with a guide to individual progress from infancy to maturity: a new method for evaluation. J. A. M. A., 116: 1187–1195, Mar. 22, 1941
Weyer, Johann. 1515–1588
Founder of medical psychiatry. Zilboorg
De praestigiis daemonum. Basileae, per J. Oporinum, 1563
Weyl, Theodor. German chemist. 1851–1913
TEST—for carbon monoxide in blood.
Ueber Kohlenoxyd-Hämoglobin with B. von Anrep, Ber. dtsch. chem. Ges., 13: 1294–1296, June 28, 1880
TEST—for nitrate in urine.
Ueber die Nitrate des Thier- und Pflanzenkörpers. Arch. f. path. Anat., 96: 462–474 (467), June 6, 1884
Wharton, Lawrence Richardson. Baltimore gynecologist. 1887–
OPERATION—
A simple method of constructing a vagina; report of four cases. Ann. Surg., 107: 842–854, May 1938
Further experiences in construction of the vagina: report of twelve cases. Ibid., 111: 1010–1020, June 1940
Wharton, Thomas. English physician. 1614–1673
DUCT—of submaxillary gland.
Adenographia: sive glandularum totius corporis descriptio. Londini, 1656. 287 pp.
Gave name to thyroid gland.
Ibid. *De glandulis thyroidoeis.* Ch. 18
Wheatley, B. See J. W. McLeod
Wheaton, C. E. W. See N. R. Barrett
Wheeler, G. A. See J. Goldberger
Wheeler, H. J. See B. Tollens
Wheeler, John Martin. New York ophthalmologist. 1879–1938
OPERATION—
War injuries of eyelids; plastic operations for a few types: case reports with photographs and drawings. Arch. Ophthal., 49: 35–42, Jan. 1920
The use of the orbicularis palpebrarum muscle in surgery of the eyelids. Amer. J. Surg., 42: 7–9, Oct. 1938

OPERATION—
Secondary cataract opening by single straight incision.
Iridectomy by the same method. Amer. J. Ophthal.,
8: 179–183, Mar. 1925
OPERATION—
Advancement of the superior oblique and inferior ob-
lique ocular muscles. Trans. Amer. Ophthal. Soc.,
32: 237–244, 1934
OPERATION—
Iridectomy with cyclodialysis for the reduction of ocular
tension. Arch. Ophthal., 16: 569–577, Oct. 1936
OPERATION—
Spastic-entropion correction by orbicularis transplan-
tation. Amer. J. Ophthal., 22: 477–483, May 1939
Wheeler, Mary Waterbury. Albany bacteriologist.
1891–
METHOD—
Isolation of B. botulinus, type B, from feces by use of
blood agar plates in anaerobic jar with Eleanor M.
Humphreys, J. infect. Dis., 35: 305–310, Sept. 1924
Wheelhouse, Claudius Galen. Leeds surgeon. 1826–
1909
OPERATION—external urethrotomy for impermeable
stricture.
Extract from a clinical lecture on perineal section.
Brit. med. J., 1: 125 (only), Feb. 5, 1870
Perineal section, as performed at Leeds. Ibid., 1: 779–
780, June 24, 1876
Wherry, William Buchanan. American bacteriol-
ogist. 1874–1936
AGAR—glycerol blood.
The necessity of carbon dioxide for the growth of B.
tuberculosis with D. M. Ervin, J. infect. Dis., 22:
194–197, Mar. 1918
SOLUTION—B, basal ammonium chloride.
Some chemical conditions influencing acid-proofness
and non-acid-proofness in a saprophytic culture of B.
tuberculosis. Ibid., 13: 144–154 (146), July 1913
SOLUTION—levulose ammonium chloride. Ibid., p.
150
Isolated the organism of tularemia from a human
being.
Infection of man with Bacterium Tularense with
B. H. Lamb, Ibid., 15: 331–340, Sept. 1914
A new bacterial disease of rodents transmissible to
man. Publ. Health Rep., Washington, 29: 3387–
3390, Dec. 18, 1914
See also W. W. Oliver
Whipple, Allen Oldfather. New York surgeon. 1881–
OPERATION—
Treatment of carcinoma of the ampulla of Vater with
W. B. Parsons and C. R. Mullins, Ann. Surg., 102:
763–779, Oct. 1935
Surgical treatment of carcinoma of the ampullary
region and head of the pancreas. Amer. J. Surg., 40:
260–263, Apr. 1938
TRIAD—of symptoms of islet-cell tumor of pancreas.
Adenoma of the islet-cells with hyperinsulinism: a
review with V. K. Frantz, Ann. Surg., 101: 1299–
1335, June 1935
Whipple, George Chandler. Brooklyn physician.
1866–1924
BROTH—glucose extract.
On the practical value of presumptive tests for Bacillus
coli in water. Pub. Health, 28: 422–431, 1902
Whipple, George Hoyt. American physician. 1878–

Awarded Nobel prize in 1934, with G. R. Minot
and W. P. Murphy, for work on liver therapy in
anemia.
Blood regeneration following simple anemia. I. Mixed
diet reaction with C. W. Hooper and F. S. Robscheit,
Amer. J. Physiol., 53: 151–166, Sept. 1920, et seq.
Blood regeneration in severe anemia. I. Standard basal
ration bread and experimental methods with F. S.
Robscheit-Robbins, Ibid., 72: 395–407, May 1, 1925
DISEASE—intestinal lipodystrophy.
A hitherto undescribed disease characterized anatomi-
cally by deposits of fat and fatty acids in the intestinal
and mesenteric lymphatic tissues. Johns Hopk. Hosp.
Bull., 18: 382–391, Sept. 1907
TEST—for liver function.
Fibrinogen of the blood as influenced by the liver ne-
crosis of chloroform poisoning with S. H. Hurwitz,
J. exp. Med., 13: 136–161, Jan. 5, 1911
Tests for hepatic function and disease under experi-
mental conditions with V. R. Mason and T. C.
Peightal, Johns Hopk. Hosp. Bull., 24: 207–209,
July 1913
See also D. P. Foster
Whistler, Daniel. English physician. 1619-1684
His book on rickets is without originality and was
probably based upon information gained from
Glisson. Norman Moore, quoted by Garrison
Disputatio medica inauguralis de morbo puerili
Anglorum, quem patrio idiomate indigenae vocant the
Rickets. Lugduni Batavorium, Boxius, 1645
Whitby, Lionel Ernest Howard. London pathol-
ogist. 1895–
Introduced use of sulfapyridine for pneumonia.
Chemotherapy of pneumococcal and other infections
with z-(p. Aminobenzene-sulfonamido) pyridine. Lan-
cet, 1: 1210–1212, May 28, 1938
White, Anthony. English surgeon. 1782–1849
Described—
Excision of the head of the femur for disease of the
hip-joint. In: S. Cooper's A dictionary of practical
surgery. London, 1838. 7 ed., pp. 272–273
White, Charles. Manchester surgeon. 1728-1813
Introduced method of reducing dislocations of
shoulder by means of heel in axilla. Garrison
An account of a new method of reducing shoulders
(without the use of an ambe), which have been several
months dislocated, in cases where the common methods
have proved inefficient. Med. Obs. and Inq., London,
2: 373–381, 1762
Excised head of humerus, 1768. Garrison
An account of a case in which the upper head of the os
humeri was sawed off, a large portion of the bone after-
wards exfoliated, and yet the entire motion of the limb
was preserved. Philos. Trans., 1769, 59: 39–46, 1770
Wrote classic work on puerperal fever and aseptic
midwifery; advocated postural uterine drainage.
Garrison
A treatise on the management of pregnant and lying-in
women, and the means of curing, but more especially
preventing, the principal disorders to which they are
liable. . . . London, Dilly, 1773. 353 pp.
Gave account of phlegmasia alba dolens. Garrison
An inquiry into the nature and causes of that swelling
in one or both of the lower extremities, which sometimes
happens to lying-in women. Warrington, Dilly, 1784.
87 pp.

White, E. C. See S. M. Rosenthal, H. H. Young
White, Frank David. Canadian biochemist. 1892–
METHOD—
The estimation of serum carotin with Ethel M. Gordon,
J. Lab. clin. Med., 17: 53–59, Oct. 1931
White, H. J. See E. K. Marshall, Jr.
White, H. L. See T. Watson
White, Horace Powell Winsbury. English surgeon
METHOD—
A new method of implanting the ureters into the bowel.
Proc. roy. Soc., 26: 1214–1216, July 1933
White, James Clarke. Boston dermatologist. 1833–
1916
DISEASE—
A case of keratosis (ichthyosis) follicularis. Amer. J.
cutan. Dis., 7: 201–213, June 1889
*Keratosis follicularis (psorospermose folliculaire
végétante). A second case.* Ibid., 8: 13–20, Jan. 1890
Advocated use of iron salts in—
*On the action of Rhus venenata and Rhus toxicoden-
dron upon the human skin.* New York med. J., 17:
225–249, Mar. 1873
White, James Clarke. Boston surgeon. 1895–
INCISION, OPERATION—
*A new muscle splitting incision for resection of the
upper thoracic sympathetic ganglia* with R. H. Smith-
wick, A. W. Allen and W. J. Mixter, S. G. O., 56:
651–657, Mar. 1933
OPERATION—
*Spinothalamic tractotomy in medulla oblongata; an
operation for the relief of intractable neuralgias of the
occiput, neck and shoulder.* Arch. Surg., 43: 113–127,
July 1941
TREATMENT—
*Angina pectoris; treatment with paravertebral alcohol
injections* with P. D. White, J. A. M. A., 90: 1099–
1103, Apr. 7, 1928
White, Joseph Warren. Greenville, S. C. surgeon.
1892–
INSTRUMENT—
*An instrument facilitating use of the flanged nail in
treatment of fractures of the hip.* J. Bone and Joint
Surg., 17: 1065–1066, Oct. 1935
OPERATION—
Femoral shortening for equalization of leg length.
Ibid., 17: 597–604, July 1935
White, J. William. Philadelphia surgeon. 1850–1916
OPERATION—
Castration for the cure of hypertrophied prostate.
Med. News, 65: 664–665; 674, Dec. 15, 1894
White, P. B. See W. G. Savage
White, P. D. See H. H. Brittingham, R. I. Lee, J. C.
White, L. Wolff
Whitehead, Walter. English surgeon. 1840–1913
OPERATION—
Entire removal of tongue by scissors. Brit. med. J.,
2: 803 (only), Dec. 8, 1877
A hundred cases of entire excision of the tongue.
Ibid., 1: 961–964, May 2, 1891
OPERATION—
The surgical treatment of hemorrhoids. Ibid., 1: 148–
150, Feb. 4, 1882
Whitehead, William Riddick. New York surgeon.
1831–1902
GAG, OPERATION—
Remarks on a case of extensive cleft of the hard and

soft palate, closed at a single operation. Amer. J. med.
Sci., 62: 114–119, July 1871
Whitehorn, John Clare. American biochemist. 1894–
METHOD—
*A system of blood analysis. Supplement II. Simplified
method for the determination of chlorides in blood or
plasma.* J. biol. Chem., 45: 449–460, Feb. 1921
METHOD—
*A method for the determination of lipoid phosphorus in
blood and plasma.* Ibid., 62: 133–138, Nov. 1924
METHOD—
A chemical method for estimating epinephrine in blood.
Ibid., 108: 633–643, Mar. 1935
REAGENT—
"Permutit" as a reagent for amines. Ibid., 56: 751–
764, July 1923
Whitelocke, Richard Henry Anglin. English sur-
geon. 1861–1927
OPERATION—
*The operative treatment of outward dislocations of the
patella.* Brit. J. Surg., 2: 6–16, July 1914
Whitfield, Arthur. English dermatologist. 1868–1947
OINTMENT—benzoic and salicylic acids in lanolin.
A handbook of skin diseases and their treatment.
London, Arnold, 1907. 320 pp.
Whitman, Royal. New York surgeon. 1857–1946
OPERATION—a method of astragalectomy.
*The operative treatment of paralytic talipes of the
calcaneus type.* Amer. J. med. Sci., 122: 593–601,
Nov. 1901
OPERATION—
*The reconstruction operation for ununited fracture of
the neck of the femur.* Ann. Surg., 73: 245–247, Feb.
1921
Also, same title: S. G. O., 32: 479–486, June 1921
SUPPORT—arch.
*Observations on forty-five cases of flat-foot with par-
ticular reference to etiology and treatment.* Boston
Med. and Surg. J., 118: 598–601, June 14; 616–620,
June 21, 1888
TREATMENT—
*A new method of treatment of fracture of the neck of the
femur, together with remarks on coxa vara.* Ann. Surg.,
36: 746–761, Nov. 1902
*The abduction treatment of fracture of the neck of the
femur: an account of the evolution of a method adequate
to apply surgical principles and therefore the exponent
of radical reform of conventional teaching and practice.*
Ibid., 81: 374–391, Jan. 1925
Whitmore, Alfred. Indian physician. 1876–
First described melioidosis. Garrison and Morton
*An account of the discovery of a hitherto undescribed
infective disease occurring among the population of
Rangoon* with C. S. Krishnaswami, Indian med.
Gaz., Calcutta, 47: 262–267, 1912
Whitmore, Eugene Randolph. American pathol-
ogist. 1874–
VACCINE—
*An experimental investigation of lipovaccines: a pre-
liminary note* with E. A. Fennel and W. F. Petersen,
J. A. M. A., 70: 427–431, Feb. 16, 1918
*An experimental investigation of lipovaccines: an ad-
ditional note, with a note on triple dysentery lipovac-
cine* with E. A. Fennel, Ibid., 70: 902–905, Mar. 30,
1918

Whitney, Willis Rodney. Schenectady scientist. 1868–
Developed radiotherm.
Radiothermy.... General Electric Rev., 35: 410–412, Aug. 1932
Whittaker, Harold A. Minnesota scientist
SOLUTION—lactose caseinogen.
A synthetic milk medium. Amer. J. Pub. Health, 2: 162 (only), Mar. 1912
Whittemore, Wyman. Boston surgeon. 1879–
OPERATION—
The treatment of such cases of chronic suppurative bronchiectasis as are limited to one lobe of the lung. Ann. Surg., 86: 219–226, Aug. 1927
Whytt, Robert. Scottish physician. 1714–1766
DISEASE—acute hydrocephalus.
Observations on the dropsy in the brain.... Edinburgh, Balfour, 1768. 193 pp.
REFLEX—destruction of anterior optic lobe—anterior corpora quadrigemina—abolishes contraction of pupil to light. Garrison
Observations on the nature, causes and cures of those disorders which have been commonly called nervous, hypochondriac or hysteric; ... Edinburgh, Balfour, 1764. 2 ed., 1765
Observed that absolute integrity of spinal cord is not necessary for maintenance of reflex functions, but that only a small segment is necessary and sufficient for a reflex arc. Garrison
An essay on the vital and other involuntary motions of animals. Edinburgh, Hamilton et al., 1751. 392 pp.
First to describe tuberculous meningitis in children. Garrison
See DISEASE.
Wrote first important English treatise on neurology after Willis. Garrison
See REFLEX.
Wichmann, Johann Ernst. German physician. 1740–1802
Established parasitic etiology of scabies. Garrison
Aetiologie der Krätze. Hannover, Helwing, 1786. 140 pp.
Widal, Georges Fernand Isidore. Paris physician. 1862–1929
SYNDROME—
Ictères hémolytiques non congénitaux avec anémie. Recherche de la résistance globulaire par le procédé des hématies déplasmatisées with P. Abrami, Abstr.: Pr. méd., 15: 749 (only), Nov. 16, 1907
Types divers d'ictères hémolytiques non congénitaux, avec anémie. La recherche de la résistance globulaire par le procédé des hématies déplasmatisées with P. Abrami, Bull. Soc. méd. Hôp. Paris, 24: 1127–1169, Nov. 8, 1907
TEST—
Sérodiagnostic de la fièvre typhoïde. Ibid., 3 s., 13: 561–566, June 21, 1896
Recherches de la réaction agglutinante dans le sang et le sérum desséchés des typhiques et dans la sérosité des vésicatoires with A. Sicord, Ibid., 681–683, July 31, 1896
Recherches sur les propriétés agglutinative et bactéricide du sérum des convalescents de fièvre typhoïde with A. Sicord, Ibid., 683–688, Oct. 9, 1896
Described relationship between anaphylactic shock and asthma.

Les phénomènes l'ordre anaphylactique dans l'asthme; la crise hémoclasique initiale with M. Lermoyez, P. Abrami, E. Brissand, and E. Joltrain, Pr. méd., 22: 525–527, 1914
See also A. Chantemesse
Wiechowski, Wilhelm. Prague pharmacologist. 1873–1929
REACTION—for allantoin.
Die Bedeutung des Allantoins im Harnsäurestoffwechsel. Beitr. chem. Physiol. Path., 11: 109–131. (129), 1908
Wieder, L. M. See O. H. Foerster
Wien, S. van. See G. H. Leland
Wiener, Meyer. St. Louis ophthalmologist. 1876–
OPERATION—
Operation for keratoconus. Amer. J. Ophthal., 7: 197–198, Mar. 1924
OPERATION—
Surgical removal of corneal opacities. In: *Contributions to Ophthal. Sci.,* dedicated to Edward Jackson. Menasha, Wis., Banta, 1926. pp. 193–199
OPERATION—for ptosis.
Correction of defect due to third nerve paralysis. Arch. Ophthal., 57: 597–602, Nov. 1928
Wierus. See Johann Weyer
Wiesel, Josef. Austrian physician. 1876–1928
METHOD—for chromaffin cells. Mallory
Beiträge zur Anatomie und Entwicklung der menschlichen Nebenniere. Anat. Hefte, Abt. 1, 19: 481–522, 1902
Wiethe, C. See E. Urbach
Wieting, Julius Pascha. Constantinople surgeon. 1868–
OPERATION—
Die angiosklerotische Gangrän und ihre operative Behandlung durch arteriovenöse Intubation. Dtsch. med. Wschr., 34: 1217–1221, July 9, 1908
Wigand, Rudolf. Marburg physician. 1894–
TEST—for cancer.
Erfahrungen mit der "Serologischen Karzinomdiagnose." Zbl. f. inn. Med., 41: 786–789, Nov. 13, 1920
Wiggers, Carl John. American surgeon. 1883–
METHOD—electrocardiogram recorded simultaneously with optically recorded pulses from main arteries.
The pressure pulses in the cardiovascular system. London and New York, Longmans, Green and Co., 1928. p. 15
Wilander, O. See E. Hammersten
Wilbur, Ray Lyman. San Francisco physician. 1875–
DETERMINATION—of urobilin and urobilinogen in urine.
Urobilin: its clinical significance with T. Addis, Arch. intern. Med., 13: 235–286, Feb. 1914
Wilcox, Harriet Leslie. New York scientist
AGAR—veal infusion.
METHOD—for production of tetanus toxin.
A modification of the hygienic laboratory method for the production of tetanus toxin. J. Bact., 1: 333–338, May 1916
Wilcox, Whitman. Baton Rouge, La. physician
Described rat-bite fever. Garrison and Morton
Violent symptoms from the bite of a rat. Amer. J. med. Sci., 26: 245–246, May 1840
Wild, F. German scientist

Described perfusion of isolated heart. Garrison and Morton

Ueber die peristaltische Bewegung des Oesophagus, nebst einigen Bemerkungen über diejenigen des Darms with Cassel, Z. f. rat. Med., 5: 76–132, 1846

Wilde, Sir William Robert Wills. Irish surgeon. 1815–1876

Wrote important work on otology. Garrison

Practical observations on aural surgery and the nature and treatment of diseases of the ear. London, Churchill, 1853

Wilder, Helenor Campbell. Washington, D. C. scientist

METHOD—

An improved technique for silver impregnation of reticulum fibers. Amer. J. Path., 11: 817–819, Sept. 1935

Wilder, Russell Morse. American physician. 1885–

METHOD—

D-glucose tolerance in health and disease with W. D. Sansum, Arch. intern. Med., 19: 311–334, Feb. 1917

Reported—

Carcinoma of the islands of the pancreas; hyperinsulinism and hypoglycemia with F. N. Allen, M. H. Power and H. E. Robertson, J. A. M. A., 89: 348–355, July 30, 1927

Reported successful operation on a parathyroid gland tumor for osteitis fibrosa.

Hyperparathyroidism: tumor of the parathyroid glands associated with osteitis fibrosa. Endocrinology, 13: 231–244, May–June 1929

Reported—

Control of Addison's disease with a diet restricted in potassium: a clinical study with A. M. Snell, E. J. Kepler, E. H. Rynearson, M. Adams and E. C. Kendall, Proc. Staff Meet., Mayo Clinic, 11: 273–283, Apr. 29, 1936

See also G. M. Higgins, W. Walters

Wildholz, Hans. German physician. 1873–

REACTION—

Der biologische Nachweis aktiver Tuberkuloseherde des menschlichen Körpers durch die intrakutane Eigenharnreaktion. Cor.-Bl. f. schweiz. Aerzte, 49: 793–809, 1919

Wilensky, N. D. See W. S. Collens

Wilhelm, Mable M. See E. E. Osgood

Wilkes-Weiss, Dorothy. See C. Weiss

Wilkie, Sir David P. D. Edinburgh surgeon. 1882–1938

DISEASE—dilatation of duodenum.

The blood supply of the duodenum, with special reference to the supraduodenal artery. S. G. O., 13: 399–405, Oct. 1911

METHOD—

The treatment of fracture of the neck of the femur. Ibid., 44: 529–530, Apr. 1927

OPERATION—direct gastroduodenostomy.

Indications for surgical treatment in peptic ulcer. Brit. med. J., 1: 771–774, May 6, 1933

Wilkinson, Oscar. Washington, D. C. ophthalmologist. 1870–

OPERATION—

Surgical treatment of concomitant squint. Arch. Ophthal., 11: 423–432, Mar. 1934

Wilks, Sir Samuel. English physician. 1824–1911

One of first to study visceral syphilis. Garrison

Specimens of disease of the lung, larynx, and liver, supposed to be syphilitic. Trans. Path. Soc. London, 9: 55–58, 1858

On the syphilitic affections of internal organs. Guy's Hosp. Rep., 9: 1–64, 1863

Described lineae atrophicae.

Description of some new wax models, illustrating a peculiar atrophy of the skin, etc. Ibid., 22: 297–301, 1861

Described subcutaneous tuberculosis of Laennec, or dissecting-room warts.

Disease of the skin produced by post-mortem examination, or Verruca necrogenica. Ibid., 8: 263–265, 1862

Applied name Hodgkin's disease.

On disease of the supra-renal capsules; or morbus Addisonii. Ibid., 3 s., 8: 1–63, 1862

Wrote classic account of alcoholic paraplegia. Garrison

Med. Times and Gaz., 2: 470, 1868

Described osteitis deformans. Garrison

Case of osteoporosis, or spongy hypertrophy of the bones (calvaria, clavicle, os femoris, and rib), exhibited at the Society. Trans. Path. Soc. London, 20: 273–277, 1869

Described—

On markings or furrows on the nails as the result of illness. Lancet, 1: 5–6, Jan. 2, 1869

Described bacterial endocarditis.

Capillary embolism or arterial pyaemia. Guy's Hosp. Rep., 3 s., 15: 29–35, 1870

Also in: F. A. Willius and T. E. Keys' *Cardiac classics.* St. Louis, Mosby, 1941. pp. 579–584

Willan, Robert. English dermatologist. 1757–1812

LEPRA—psoriasis vulgaris. In his: *Description and treatment of cutaneous diseases.* London, Johnson, (1796)–1808. 4 vols. Vol. 1, pp. 152–188

Described prurigo mitis. Ibid., pp. 73–76

Described abdominal purpura. Ibid., 457

Willcock, Edith Gertrude. English scientist

REACTION—for indole.

Demonstrated importance of tryptophane in diet.

The importance of individual amino-acids in metabolism with F. G. Hopkins, J. Physiol., 35: 88–102, Dec. 29, 1906

Willebrand, E. A. Von. Helsingford physician

HEMORRHAGIC DIATHESIS—thromopathy.

(*Hereditary pseudohaemophilia.*) Fin. läk. säll. hand., 68: 87–112, 1926

Über hereditäre Pseudohämophilie. Acta med. Scand., 76: 521–550, 1931

Über eine neue Bluterkrankheit, die Konstitutionelle Thrombopathie with R. Jürgens, Klin. Wschr., 12: 414–417, Mar. 18, 1933

Willems, Charles. Belgium Army surgeon

TREATMENT—

Treatment of purulent arthritis by wide arthrotomy followed by immediate active mobilization. S. G. O., 28: 546–554, June 1919

Willets, D. G. See J. Goldberger

Willheim, Robert. Vienna biochemist

REACTION—a cytolytic test for cancer.

Eine chemische Methode zur Messung der Carcinolyse with K. Stern, Biochem. Z., 226: 315–324, Oct. 10, 1930

Williams, Anna Wessels. American bacteriologist. 1863–

AGAR—flour peptone.
Growth of B. influenza without the presence of hemoglobin with Olga R. Povitzky, J. med. Res., 42: 406–417 (407), June–Sept. 1921
AGAR—tissue infusion.
Pure cultures of amebae parasitic in mammals. Ibid., 25: 263–283, Dec. 1911
MODIFICATION—of van Giesen's method of demonstrating Negri bodies.
The etiology and diagnosis of hydrophobia with May M. Lowden, J. infect. Dis., 3: 452–483, May 18, 1906
See also W. H. Park
Williams, Byron G. R. Paris, Ill. physician. 1883–
STAIN—
The invariable blood-stain. J. A. M. A., 61: 1627–1628, Nov. 1, 1913
Williams, Charles James Blasius. English physician. 1805–1889
TRACHEAL TONE or SIGN—
On the theory and practice of percussion as a mode of diagnosis. London med. Gaz., 19: 609–614, Jan. 21, 1837
Williams, Daniel Hale. American surgeon. 1858–1931
Performed successful suture of pericardium for stab wound, July 9, 1893.
Stab wound of the heart and pericardium—suture of the pericardium—recovery—patient alive three years afterward. Med. Rec., 51: 437–439, Mar. 27, 1897
Williams, Francis Henry. Boston physician. 1852–1936
PHENOMENON—diaphragm lag and decrease in apical transparency are early signs of pulmonary tuberculosis.
The Röntgen rays in thoracic diseases. Amer. J. med. Sci., 114: 665–687, Dec. 1897
Introduced fluoroscopy of heart.
A method for more fully determining the outline of the heart by means of the fluoroscope together with other uses of this instrument in medicine. Boston Med. and Surg. J., 135: 335–337, 1896
Also in: F. A. Willius and T. E. Keys' *Cardiac classics.* St. Louis, Mosby, 1941. pp. 701–706
Williams, Gertrude. See F. B. Kingsbury
Williams, Henry Willard. American ophthalmologist. 1821–1895
METHOD—
Suture of the flap, after extraction of cataract. Trans. Amer. Ophthal. Soc., N. Y., pp. 45–46, 1865
Introduced treatment of iritis without mercury. Garrison
Iritis—non-mercurial treatment. Boston Med. and Surg. J., 55: 49–55, Aug. 21; 69–74, Aug. 28; 92–99, Sept. 4, 1856
Williams, Horatio Burt. American physiologist. 1877–
RESPIRATION CALORIMETER—
Animal calorimetry. First paper. A small respiration calorimeter. J. biol. Chem., 12: 317–347, Sept. 1912
Williams, John Ralston, Jr. Nashville physician. 1910–
PHTHYSMOGRAPH—
A simple method for determining the systolic blood pressure of the unanesthetized rat with T. R. Harrison and A. Grollman, J. clin. Invest., 18: 373–376, May 1939

Williams, John Whitridge. American obstetrician. 1866–1931
Described—
Contributions to the histogenesis of the papillary cystomata of the ovary. Johns Hopk. Hosp. Bull., 2: 149–157, Dec. 1891
Described—
Deciduoma malignum. Johns Hopk. Hosp. Rep., 4: 461–504, 1895
Williams, R. J. See E. E. Snell
Williams, Robert Runnels. American chemist. 1886–
Discovered vitamin B_2.
The tripartite nature of vitamin B with R. E. Waterman, J. biol. Chem., 78: 311–322, July 1928
Identified chemically vitamin B_1.
Structure of vitamin B. J. Amer. Chem. Soc., 57: 229–230, Jan. 1935
Synthesis of vitamin B_1 with J. K. Cline, Ibid., 58: 1504–1505, Aug. 1936
Williamson, C. S. See F. C. Mann
Willis, David Arthur. Chicago surgeon. 1900–
FORCEPS—for
Localization and removal of foreign (metallic) bodies. S. G. O., 65: 698–699, Nov. 1937
Willis, Thomas. English physician. 1621–1675
ASTHMA—
On the convulsive cough and asthma. In his: *Practice of physick.* London, Dring, 1684. pt. e, pp. 92–96
CIRCLE—
In his: *Cerebri anatome, cui accessit nervorum descriptio et usus.* London, Flesher, 1664. 456 pp. opp. p. 24
Described fermentation and putrefaction. Garrison and Morton
Diatribae duae medico-philosophicae quarum prior agit de fermentatione sive de motu intestino particularum in quovis corpore. Londini, Roycroft, 1659
Gave first account of epidemic typhoid fever as it occurred in troops of Parliamentary War of 1643. Garrison
De febribus pestilentibus. London, 1659. p. 171 et seq.
Reported epidemic of cerebrospinal fever. Garrison and Morton
A description of an epidemical fever. . . . 1661 In his: *Practice of physick.* London, Dring, 1684. pt. 3, pp. 46–54
Described hysteria. Garrison and Morton
Affectionum quae dicuntur hystericae et hypochondriae pathologia spasmodica vindicata. Lugduni Batavorum, Driehuysen and Lopez, 1671
Described general paralysis. Garrison
In his: *De anima brutorum.* Londini, Davis, 1672. Ch. IX
Also: *Pathologiae cerebri, et nervosi generis specimen in quo agitur de morbis convulsivis et de scorbuto.* Amstelodami, Elzevirium, 1668. 338 pp.
He made the best qualitative examination of the urine which was possible in his time, and was the first to notice the characteristic sweetish taste of diabetic urine. Garrison
Pharmaceutice rationalis sive diatribe de medicamentorum operationibus in humano corpore. London, Scott, 1674. Sect. 4, Cap. 3
Described whooping cough. Garrison and Morton
In Ibid., ed. of 1684. Pt. 2, p. 38

Described intercostal and spinal nerves. Garrison and Morton

In his: *Practice of physick.* London, Dring, 1684. pp. 128-155

Willner, O. See Haverhill fever

Wills, Lucy. English scientist

ANEMIA—

Showed that autolyzed yeast is as effective as liver in "pernicious anemia of tropics."

Studies in pernicious anaemia of pregnancy. Part II. A survey of dietetic and hygienic conditions of women in Bombay with Sakuntala N. Talpade, Ind. J. med. Res., 18: 283-306, July 1930

Treatment of "pernicious anemia of pregnancy" and "tropical anemia," with special reference to yeast extract as a curative agent. Brit. med.' J., 1: 1059-1064, June 20, 1931

Willstätter, Richard. German biochemist. 1872-

Did important work on enzymes, 1918-1924. Garrison

Untersuchungen über Enzyme. Berlin, Springer, 1928. 2 vols. 1775 pp.

Proposed tribromethanol.

Zur Kenntnis des Trichlor- und Tribromäthylalkohols with W. Duisberg, Ber. dtsch. chem. Ges., 56: 2283-2286, Nov. 7, 1923

Wilmer, Bradford. English surgeon

Described "Coventry treatment" of goitre, with burnt sponge. Garrison and Morton

Cases and remarks in surgery: to which is subjoined, an appendix, containing the method of curing the bronchocele in Coventry. London, Longman, 1779

Wilmer, William Holland. American ophthalmologist. 1863-1936

OPERATION—for glaucoma.

Three years' experience in sclerocorneal trephining in glaucoma. Arch. Ophthal., 45: 333-341, July 1916

OPERATION—for occluded pupil.

The Wilmer iridocapsulectomy By B. Rones, Ibid., 11: 976-981, June 1934

Wilmoth, Clifford Lee. Denver, Col. surgeon. 1894-

OPERATION—

Femoral hernia in the male. Ann. Surg., 105: 549-555, Apr. 1937

Wilms, Max. German surgeon. 1867-1918

OPERATION—ligation of veins of ileocolic angle to prevent spread of pyelephlebitis complicating appendicitis.

Venenunterbindung bei eitriger Pfortaderthrombose nach Appendicitis. Zbl. f. Chir., 36: 1041-1043, July 24, 1904

OPERATION—resection of ribs to produce depression of chest and compression of lungs.

Eine neue Methode zur Verengerung des Thorax bei Lungentuberkulose. Münch. med. Wschr., 58: 777-778, Apr. 11, 1911

OPERATION—for benign stricture of common bile duct.

Bildung eines kunstlichen Choledochus durch ein einfaches Drainrohr. Berl. klin. Wschr., 49: 536-537, Mar. 18, 1912

TUMOR—embryonal adenomyosarcoma (congenital mixed tumor) of urinary tract.

Die Mischgeschwülste. I. Die Mischgeschwülste der Niere. Leipzig, Georgi, 1899

Wilson, Armine Taylor. American physician. 1909-

METHOD—

Method for testing in vitro resistance of group A hemolytic streptococci to sulfonamides. Proc. Soc. exp. Biol., N. Y., 58: 130-133, Feb. 1945

Wilson, C. See P. Kimmelstiel

Wilson, Edmund Beecher. American scientist. 1856-1939

Studied influence of reproductive chromosomes on heredity. Garrison and Morton

The cell in development and inheritance. New York, Macmillan, 1896. 371 pp.

Wilson, Frederick Morse. American ophthalmologist. 1850-1918

OPERATION—

The conjunctival flap and the cataract wound with H. S. Miles, Trans. Amer. Ophthal. Soc., 9: 503-511, 1902

Wilson, George Ewart. Toronto surgeon. 1903-

OPERATION—

Benign strictures of the bile ducts with a new method of treatment. S. G. O., 68: 288-294, Feb. 15, 1939

Wilson, H. See L. R. Dragstedt

Wilson, Harold William. English surgeon. 1880-

Reported—

A case of haematoma of the ovary simulating an attack of appendicitis. Lancet, 1: 1196-1197, May 6, 1905

Wilson, James Cornelius. Hartford, Conn. surgeon. 1881-

OPERATION—

Silk ligament in habitual dislocation or slipping of the patella. Amer. J. Surg., 39: 144-145, June 1925

Wilson, John Cree. Los Angeles surgeon. 1888-

OPERATION—

Operative fixation of tuberculous hips in children: end-result study of thirty-three patients from the Orthopaedic Department of the Childrens' Hospital. J. Bone and Joint Surg., 15: 22-47, Jan. 1933

Wilson, John Gordon. Chicago otolaryngologist. 1866-

METHOD—

Intra vital staining with methylene blue. Anat. Rec., 4: 267-277, July 1910

Wilson, Louis Blanchard. Rochester, Minn. physician. 1866-1943

METHOD—

Staining sections of living tissue, unfixed. J. Lab. clin. Med., 1: 40-45, Oct. 1915

See also F. F. Wesbrook

Wilson, Philip Duncan. Boston surgeon. 1886-

TECHNIC—of tendoplastic amputation of lower end of humerus.

Amputations. In: Nelson's *Loose-leaf living surgery.* New York, Nelson, 1937. Vol. 3, Ch. 6, pp. 564-694 (629-630).

Wilson, R. J. See C. E. Dolman

Wilson, Samuel Alexander Kinnier. English neurologist. 1877-1937

DISEASE—

Progressive lenticular degeneration: a familial nervous disease associated with cirrhosis of the liver. Brain, 34: 295-509 (486-487), Mar. 1912

Showed that corpus striatum is site of degenerative lesions associated with rigidity and tremor, as paralysis agitans or Parkinson's disease. Harris Ibid.

Wilson, William James. Belfast physician. 1879-

AGAR—brilliant green bile salt.
Useful media for isolation and cultivation of meningococcus, enterococcus and B. typhosus with Georgina Darling, Lancet, 2: 105 (only), July 27, 1918
REACTION—of Wilson-Weil-Felix, in typhus fever.
On heterologous agglutinins more particularly those present in the blood serum of cerebrospinal fever and typhus fever cases. J. Hyg., 9: 316–340, Nov. 1909
The Wilson-Weil-Felix reaction in typhus fever. Ibid., 19: 115–130, July 1920
See also W. St. Clair Symmers

Wilson, William James Erasmus. English dermatologist. 1809–1884
DISEASE—
On dermatitis exfoliativa. Med. Times and Gaz., 1: 118–120, 1870
Described—
On lichen planus: the lichen ruber of Hebra. Brit. med. J., 2: 399–402, Oct. 13, 1866

Wimmer, G. Bernburg scientist
SOLUTION—ammonium sulphate.
Beitrag zur Kenntniss der Nitrificationsbakterien. Z. f. Hyg., 48: 135–174 (140), 1904

Winckel, Franz Karl Ludwig Wilhelm von. Munich physician. 1837–1911
DISEASE—cyanotic afebrile jaundice with hemoglobinuria in infants.
Über eine bisher nicht beschreibene endemisch aufgetretene Erkrankung Neugeborener. Dtsch. med. Wschr., 5: 303–307, June 14; 415–418, Aug. 16; 431–436, Aug. 23; 447–450, Aug. 30, 1879

Windaus, Adolf. Göttingen biochemist. 1876–
REACTION—
Ueber Cholesterin. Freiburg, 1903. 37 pp.
Über die Entgiftung der Saponine durch Cholesterin. Ber. dtsch. chem. Ges., 42: 238–246, 1909
Über die quantitative Bestimmung des Cholesterins und der Cholesterinester in einigen normalen und pathologischen Nieren. Z. physiol. Chem., 65: 110–117, Mar. 21, 1910

Windbolz, Hans. Bern physician
TEST—auto-urine t. for tuberculosis.
Der biologische Nachweis aktiver Tuberkuloseherde des menschlichen Körpers durch die intrakutane Eigenharnreaktion. Cor.-Bl. f. schweiz. Aerzte, 49: 793–809, May 31, 1919

Wingrave, Vitruvius Harold Wyatt. English laryngologist. 1858–1938
Described—
The pathological and clinical features of atrophic rhinitis. J. Laryngol., Rhinol. and Otol., 8: 96–110, Feb. 1894

Winiwärter, Alexander von. German surgeon. 1848–1916
OPERATION—cholecystenterostomy.
Ein Fall von Gallenretention bedingt durch Impermeabilität des Ductus Choledochus—Anlegung einer Gallenblasen-Darmfistel. Heilung. Prag. med. Wschr., 7: 201–207, May 24; 213–217, May 31, 1882

Winiwater, Felix von. Vienna surgeon
Described condition now known as thrombo-angiitis obliterans.
Ueber eine eigenthümliche Form von Endarteriitis und Endophlebitis mit Gangrän des Fusses. Arch. f. klin. Chir., 23: 202–226, 1879

Winkelstein, Asher. New York physician. 1894–

METHOD—of administering aluminum hydroxide.
A new therapy of peptic ulcer: continuous alkalinized milk drip into the stomach. Amer. J. med. Sci., 185: 695–703, May 1933

Winkler, Cornelis. Dutch surgeon. 1855–
Described relations of auditory nerve. Garrison
(The central course of the Nervous octavus and its influence on motility.) Verh. d. k. Akad. v. Wetenschappen, Amsterdam, 2 Sect., 14, No. 1, 1907. 202 pp.

Winkler, Ferdinand. Vienna physician
REACTION—oxidase.
Der Nachweis von Oxydase in den Leukozyten mittels der Dimethylparaphenylendiamin-Alphanaphthol-Reaktion. Folia haemat., 4: 323–328, May 1907
TEST—for free hydrochloric acid in gastric juice.
Der Nachweis freier Salzsäure im Mageninhalt mittels Alphanaphthol. Zbl. ges. inn. Med., 1009–1011, Oct. 2, 1897

Winkler, Max. Luzerne dermatologist
DISEASE—
Knötchenförmige Erkrankung am Helix. (Chondrodermatitis nodularis chronica helicis). Arch. f. Dermat., 121: 278–285, 1915

Winnick, Theodore. Detroit scientist
METHOD—
Microdiffusion methods based on the bisulfite reaction. II. Determination of lactic acid by oxidation with ceric sulfate. J. biol. Chem., 142: 451–459, Feb. 1942

Winogradsky, S. French scientist
SOLUTION—ammonium sulphate.
Recherches sur les organismes de la nitrification. 5 e. mémoire. Ann. Inst. Pasteur, 5: 577–616 (577), 1891

Winsbury-White, Horace Powell. See H. P. W. White

Winslow, Charles Edward Amory. New York scientist. 1877–
BROTH—basal extract, for studying fermentation by bacteria.
Notes on the classification of the white and orange staphylococci with W. Rothberg and Elizabeth I. Parsons, J. Bact., 5: 145–167 (151), Mar. 1923

Winslow, Jacques Benigue. Dutch anatomist. 1669–1760
FORAMEN—
Exposition anatomique de la structure du corps humain. Paris, Desprez, 1732. pp. 352–365.
Also, in English, transl. by G. Douglas London, 1734. Vol. 2, pp. 171–172

Winter. See G. Hayem

Winterbottom, Thomas Masterman. American physician. 1765–1859
SYMPTOM—cervical polyadenitis occurring in sleeping sickness.
Gave original description of "kondee" or sleeping sickness. Garrison
An account of the native Africans in the neighbourhood of Sierra Leone; to which is added an account of the present state of medicine among them. London, Hatchard and Mawman, 1803. 2 vols. Vol. 2, pp. 29–31

Winternitz, Rudolf. Prague physician
Described milkers' nodules.
Knotenbildungen bei Melkerinnen. Arch. f. Dermat. u. Syph., 49: 195–206, 1899

Wintersteiner, Oskar. New York biochemist. 1898–

METHOD—for preparation of
Crystalline progestin with W. M. Allen, J. biol. Chem.,
107: 321–336, Oct. 19, 1934
See also J. J. Abel, W. M. Allen
Wintrich, Anton. German physician. 1812–1882
PHENOMENON or SIGN—change in pitch of tympanitic note over superficially situated cavities.
Krankheiten der Respirations-organe. Virchow's *Handbuch der speciellen Pathologie und Therapie.* Erlangen, 1854. Vol. 5, Sect. 1
Wintrobe, Maxwell Myer. Canadian-American physician. 1901–
HAEMATOCRIT, METHOD—venous blood m. for determination of cell volume per cent.
Macroscopic examination of blood. Discussion of its value and description of the use of a single instrument for the determination of sedimentation rate, volume of packed red cells, leukocytes and platelets, and of icterus index. Amer. J. med. Sci., 185: 58–71, Jan. 1933
METHOD—
A standardized technique for the blood sedimentation test with J. W. Landsberg, Ibid., 189: 102–115, Jan. 1935
TUBE—for determination of blood volume.
Normal blood determinations in the South with M. W. Miller, Arch. intern. Med., 43: 96–113, Jan. 1929
Wirsung, Johann Georg. Bavarian anatomist. ?–1643
DUCT—"Next came the finding of the pancreatic duct in Vesling's dissecting-room at Padua by his prosector, Georg Wirsung (1642)." Garrison (Recorded on a single rare copper plate of 1642.)
Figura ductus cujusdam cum multiplicibus suis ramulis noviter in pancreate in diversis corporibus humani observatis. Padua, 1643
Wirtz, F. See F. Würtz
Wise, E. C. See J. T. Correll
Wise, Fred. New York dermatologist. 1881–
LICHENOID—morbus moniliformis lichenoides.
Lichen ruber moniliformis (morbus moniliformis lichenoides): report of a case and description of a hitherto unrecorded histologic structure with C. R. Rein, Arch. Derm. Syph., Chicago, 34: 830–849, Nov. 1936
Lichen ruber moniliformis; report of observations at necropsy with C. R. Rein, Ibid., 38: 251–252, Aug. 1938
Wiseman, Bruce Kenneth. Columbus, Ohio physician. 1898–
SYNDROME—
Primary splenic neutropenia; a newly recognized syndrome, closely related to congenital hemolytic icterus and essential thrombocytopenic purpura with C. A. Doan, Ann. intern. Med., 16: 1097–1117, June 1942
Wiseman, Richard. English surgeon. 1622–1676
Described tuberculosis of joints as tumor albus; gave early historical, clinical, pathologic and prognostic account of King's Evil; classified aneurysms.
Severall chirurgicall treatises. London, Royston, 1676
Wising, Per Johan. Swedish physician. 1842–1912
Reported case of primary carcinoma of ureter with microscopic diagnosis.
Fall af primär kancer i högra ureteren med sekundär kancer i mesenterialkörtlarne, rectum och lefvern samt hydronefros with C. Blix, Hygeia, 40: 468–476, Sept. 1878

Wistar, Caspar. Philadelphia anatomist. 1761–1818
Wrote important anatomical text-book, first to be published in America. Garrison
Wisteria vine is named after him. His name is also perpetuated in Wistar Institute of Anatomy and Biology in Philadelphia.
A system of anatomy for the use of students of medicine. Philadelphia, Dobson, 1811–14. 2 vols.
Withering, William. English physician. 1741–1799
Pioneer in correct use of digitalis. He learned from an old grandame in Shropshire that foxglove is good for dropsy. Garrison
Account of the fox-glove, and some of its medical uses; with practical remarks on dropsy, and other diseases. Birmingham, Robinson, 1785. 207 pp.
Also in German. Leipzig, 1786
Also in: Medical classics, 2: 305–443, Dec. 1937
Also in: F. A. Willius and T. E. Keys' *Cardiac classics.* St. Louis, Mosby, 1941. pp. 231–252
Wittmer, Phil. Ludovicus. German physician. 1752–1792
Published early periodical devoted to history of medicine. Garrison
Archiv für die Geschichte der Arzeneikunde in ihrem ganzen Umfang. Nüremberg, 1790
Witts, Leslie John. English physician
ANEMIA—simple achlorhydric.
Achlorhydria and anaemia. Practitioner, London, 124: 348–357, Mar. 1930
Simple achlorhydric anaemia. Guy's Hosp. Rep., 80: 253–296, July 1930
Witwer, E. R. See T. B. Cooley
Witzel, Oscar. German surgeon. 1856–1925
OPERATION—gastrostomy.
Zur Technik der Magenfistelanlegung. Zbl. f. Chir., 18: 601–604, Aug. 8, 1891
Wodstrup, I. See H. C. Hagedorn
Wöhler, Friedrich. German chemist. 1800–1882
In 1824, Wöhler made, and in 1842 confirmed, a discovery which became the starting-point of modern chemistry of metabolism, viz., that benzoic acid taken in with the food appears as hippuric acid in the urine. Garrison
Tiedemann's Z. f. Physiol., 1: 142, 1824
Ueber die im lebenden Organismus vor sich gehende Umwandlung der Benzoësäure in Hippursäure. Ann. Phys., Lpz., 56: 638–641, 1842
Made first synthesis of an organic compound (urea) from inorganic substances. Garrison
Ueber künstliche Bildung des Harnstoffs. Ibid., 12: 253–256, 1828
Wölfler, Anton. Bohemian surgeon. 1850–1917
OPERATION—gastroenterostomy.
Ueber die von Herrn Professor Billroth ausgeführten Resectionen des carcinomatösen Pylorus. Wien, Braumüller, 1881. 53 pp.
OPERATION—repair of inguinal hernia.
Zur Radikaloperation des freien Leistenbruches. Beitr. z. Chir., Billroth Festschrift, pp. 552–603, 1892
Classified thyroid tumors; coined term "fetal adenoma."
Ueber die Entwickelung und den Bau des Kropfes. Arch. f. klin. Chir., 29: 1–97 (40), 1883
See also T. Billroth
Wörner, E. Berlin chemist

METHOD—of uric acid estimation.
Ein einfaches Verfahren zur Bestimmung der Harnsäure auf Grund der Fällung als Ammonurat. Z. f. phys. Chem., 29: 70–77, Dec. 30, 1898

Wohlgemuth, Julius. German physician. 1874–
APPARATUS—for perfusion.
Zur Methodik der Herzdurchblutung im Langendorffschen Apparat. Zbl. f. Physiol., 21: 828–831, Mar. 7, 1908
METHOD—for quantitative determination of diastatic ferments in blood.
Ueber eine neue Methode zur quantitativen Bestimmung des diastatischen Ferments. Biochem. Z., 9: 1–9, 1908
Untersuchungen über die Diastasen. I. Die tierischen Diastasen. Ibid., 9: 10–43, 1908
METHOD—for determination of amylolytic content of feces.
Beitrag zur funktionellen Diagnostik des Pankreas. Berl. klin. Wschr., 47: 92–95, Jan. 17, 1910
REGIMEN—to lessen pancreatic secretion; an aid to closure of pancreatic fistula.
Zur Frage der Aktivierung des tryptischen Fermentes im menschlichen körper. Biochem. Z., 2: 264–270, 1907
(Part II) *Untersuchungen über das Pankreas des Menschen.* Berl. klin. Wschr., 44: 47–51, Jan. 14, 1907
(Part III, same title as Part I.) Biochem. Z., 2: 350–356, 1907
(Part IV, same title as Part II.) Ibid., 4: 271–280, 1907
Zur Therapie der Pankreasfistel nebst Bemerkungen über den Mechanismus der Pankreassekretion während der Verdauung. Berl. klin. Wschr., 45: 389–393, Feb. 24, 1908

Woillez, Eugène Joseph. French physician. 1811–1882
DISEASE—acute idiopathic congestion of lungs.
De la congestion pulmonaire, considérée comme élément habituel des maladies aiguës. Arch. gén. de méd., 5 s., 3: 385–400, Apr.; 566–579, May 1854
SPIROPHORE or RESPIRATOR—
Du spirophore, appareil de sauvetage pour le traitement de l'asphyxie, et principalement de l'asphyxie des noyés et des nouveau-nés. Bull. Acad. de méd., Paris, 2 s., 5: 611–627, June 20; 754–761, Aug. 1, 1876

Wolbach, Simeon Burt. Boston pathologist. 1880–
AGAR—citrated blood.
Concerning the filterability of trypanosomes with W. H. Chapman and H. W. Stevens, J. med. Res., 33: 107–117 (109), 1915
MODIFICATION—of Giemsa's stain.
Studies on Rocky Mountain spotted fever. J. med. Res., 41: 1–197, Nov. 1919

Wolcott, Erastus Bradley. American surgeon. 1804–1880
Performed first nephrectomy, 1861. Garrison
Case of encephaloid disease of the kidney, removal, etc. By C. L. Stoddard, Med. and Surg. Reporter, Philadelphia, 7: 126, 1861–62

Woldman, Edward Elbert. Cleveland physician. 1897–
TECHNIC—
A new technic for the continuous control of acidity in

peptic ulcer by the aluminum hydroxide drip with V. C. Rowland, Amer. J. Digest. Dis. and Nutrition, 2: 733–736, Feb. 1936

Wolf, Alexander. New York neurologist. 1907–
Introduced—
Quinine: an effective form of treatment for myotonia. Arch. Neurol. Psychiat., 36: 382–383, Aug. 1936
Experiments with quinine and prostigmin in treatment of myotonia and myasthenia. By F. Kennedy and A. Wolf, Ibid., 37: 68–74, Jan. 1937

Wolf, C. G. L. See T. Lewis, W. McK. Marriott

Wolf, George. Optical physicist
See Rudolf Schindler

Wolf, Harriet. See R. Elman

Wolf, Jacob Irving. New York physician. 1881–
Introduced term—
Lymphopathia venerea (lymphogranulomatosis inguinalis) and the Frei test with M. B. Sulzberger, Brit. J. Dermat. and Syph., 44: 192–198, Apr. 1932

Wolfe, Jack Morris. Albany, N. Y. anatomist. 1906–
Reported—
Cyclic histological variations in the anterior hypophysis of the albino rat with R. Cleveland, Anat. Rec., 55: 233–249, Feb. 25, 1933
Pregnancy changes in the anterior hypophysis of the albino rat with R. Cleveland, Ibid., 56: 33–45, Apr. 25, 1933
See also W. R. Bryan

Wolfe, John Reissberg. Glasgow ophthalmologist. 1824–1904
OPERATION—skin grafting, full thickness.
A new method of performing plastic operations. Brit. med. J., 2: 360–361, Sept. 18, 1875

Wolff, Caspar Friedrich. German embryonologist. 1733–1794
BODIES, CYST, DUCTS—
Theoria generationis. Halae ad Salam, lit. Hendelianis, (1759)
De formatione intestinorum praedipue. Novi Comment, Acad. Sci. Petropol., 12: 43; 403, 1768; 13: 44; 478, 1769
Also, German transl. by J. F. Meckel, 1812

Wolff, Ernst. San Francisco pediatrician. 1892–
TEST—
A tape test with tuberculin ointment with M. H. Teitler, Amer. Rev. Tuberc., 27: 308–310, Mar. 1933
Tuberculin ointment patch test. Amer. J. Dis. Child., 47: 764–770, Apr. 1934

Wolff, Julius. German anatomist. 1836–1902
LAW—all changes in function of a bone are attended by definite alterations in their internal structure.
Das Gesetz der Transformation der inneren Architektur der Knochen bei pathologischen Veränderungen der äusseren Knochenform. S. B. preuss. Akad. Wiss., Phys.-math. Cl., 22, 1884

Wolff, Louis. Boston physician. 1898–
SYNDROME—of Wolff-Parkinson-White; anomalous arterioventricular excitation.
Bundle-branch block with short P-R interval in healthy young people prone to paroxysmal tachycardia with J. Parkinson and P. D. White, Amer. Heart. J., 5: 685–704, Aug. 1930

Wolff, Max. German scientist. 1844–1923
Isolated Actinomyces bovis.
Ueber Reincultur des Actinomyces und seine Ueber-

tragbarkeit auf Thiere. Arch. f. path. Anat., 126: 11–59, Oct. 1, 1891

Wolff, Richard. Bethanien physician
HYPOTHESIS—carcinoma cells may become osteoblasts and form bone. (Obsolete)
Zur Kenntniss der metastatischen Erscheinungen der Prostatacarcinome und ihrer diagnostischen Bedeutung. Dtsch. Z. f. Chir., 52: 397–411, July 1899

Wolff, W. A. See J. R. Elkington

Wolff, Walter. German physician. 1878–
TECHNIC—for protein concentration of gastric contents.
TEST—for gastric cancer.
Ueber die quantitative Bestimmung gelöster Eiweisstoffe im Mageninhalt with P. Junghaus, Berl. klin. Wschr., 48: 978–980, May 29, 1911

Wolff-Eisner, Alfred. Berlin physician. 1877–
REACTION or TEST—
Die kutane und konjunktivale Tuberkulinreaktion, ihre Bedeutung für Diagnostik und Prognose der Tuberkulose. Z. f. Tuberk., 12: 21–25, 1908
Die Ophthalmo- und Kutan-Diagnose der Tuberkulose. . . . Beitr. z. Klin. d. Tuberk., 9, Hft. 1, 1–197, 1908

Wolfrum. See R. Seefelder

Wolfson, William Leon. Brooklyn surgeon. 1888–
METHOD—of intestinal anastomosis.
A new triplicate colon clamp after de Martel. Amer. J. Surg., 42: 437–442, Nov. 1938
MODIFICATION—of pyloric resection.
The surgical treatment of complicated duodenal ulcer with R. E. Rothenberg, Surgery, 3: 663–669, May 1938

Wollaston, William Hyde. English physician. 1766–1828
Discovered urates in gouty joints. Garrison
On gouty and urinary concretions. Philos. Trans., 87: 386–400, 1797
Investigated pathological chemistry of calculi.
On cystic oxide, a new species of urinary calculus. Ibid., 100: 223–230, 1810

Wollstein, Martha. See H. L. Amoss, H. G. Bugbee

Wolter, Otto. Rostock physiochemist
METHOD—for determination of iron in urine.
Über das Harneisen. I. Die Bestimmung des Eisens im Harn. Biochem. Z., 24: 108–124, 1910

Wolters, Max. Bonn anatomist
MODIFICATION—of Weigert method for myelin sheaths.
Drei neue Methoden zur Mark- und Achsencylinderfärbung mittels Hämatoxylin. Z. f. wiss. Mikr., 7: 466–473, 1890

Wong, San Yin. Chinese biochemist. 1894–
METHOD—for determination of iron in blood.
Colorimetric determination of iron and hemoglobin in blood. J. Biol. Chem., 55: 421–425, Mar. 1923
(Same title), II. Ibid., 77: 409–412, May 1928

Wood, Francis Carter. New York pathologist. 1869–
STAIN—
A simple and rapid chromatin stain for the malarial parasite. Med. News. 83: 248–250, Aug. 8, 1903

Wood, Horatio Charles. Philadelphia physician. 1841–1920
Made important investigation of sunstroke. Garrison
Thermic fever, or sunstroke. Philadelphia, Lippincott, 1872 .128 pp.

Wrote important treatise on therapeutics which contains standard classification of drugs. Garrison
A treatise on therapeutics. . . . Philadelphia, Lippincott, 1874. 578 pp.
Discovered physiological and therapeutic properties of hyoscine. Garrison
Hyoscine; its physiological and therapeutic action. Detroit, Davis, 1885. 10 pp.

Wood, James Edwin, Jr. Charlottesville, Va. physician. 1897–
Reported—
Ephedrine in Adams-Stokes' syndrome. J. A. M. A., 98: 1364–1367, Apr. 16, 1932

Wood, John. English surgeon. 1825–1891
OPERATION—closure of hernial sac by subcutaneous sutures.
On rupture, inguinal, crural, and umbilical; . . . London, Davies, 1863. 326 pp.

Wood, W. B. See J. E. Moore

Wood, William. Scottish physician. 1774–1857
Described neuroma. Garrison and Morton
Observations on neuroma. Trans. Med.-Chir. Soc. Edinburgh, 3: 367–434, 1828–29

Woodard, Helen Quincy. New York chemist. 1900–
MODIFICATION—of Bodansky test.
A study of the serum phosphatase in bone disease with G. H. Twombly and B. L. Coley, J. clin. Invest., 15: 193–201, Mar. 1936
MODIFICATION—of the Franseen test for tissue phosphatase.
The correlation between serum phosphatase and roentgenographic type in bone disease with N. L. Higinbotham, Amer. J. Cancer, 31: 221–237, Oct. 1937

Woodbury, F. See J. Pancoast

Woodland, J. C. See Bullis

Woodbridge, John Eliot. American physician. 1845–1901
TREATMENT—of typhoid fever.
Can typhoid fever be aborted? Second paper. J. A. M. A., 22: 182–187, Feb. 10; 331–335 (334), Mar. 10; 530–536, Apr. 10, 1894

Woodbridge, Philip Dudley. Boston anesthetist. 1895–
MODIFICATION—of W. H. Jones' technic of spinal anesthesia.
Metycaine spinal anesthesia: report of 1381 cases. Amer. J. Surg., 37: 191–204, Aug. 1937

Woodhall, Maurice Barnes. Durham, N. C. surgeon. 1905–
OPERATION—
Modified double enterostomy (Mikulicz) in radical surgical treatment of intussusception in children. Arch. Surg., 36: 989–997, June 1938

Woodhull, Alfred Alexander. American Army Surgeon. 1837–1921
Introduced Indian method of giving massive doses of ipecac in dysentery. Garrison
Clinical studies with large non-emetic doses of ipecacuanha. Atlanta Med. and Surg. J., 12, 1874–75; 13, 1875–76
Studies, chiefly clinical, in the non-emetic use of ipecacuanha. Philadelphia, Lippincott, 1876. 155 pp.

Woodruff, Harry W. Joliet, Ill. ophthalmologist. 1868–
OPERATION—
Tendon transplantation of the eye muscles. Trans.

Sect. Ophthal., Amer. Med. Ass., pp. 276–285, 1917
Woodward, Gladys E. See Janetta W. Schoonover
Woodward, Joseph Janvier, American physician.
1833–1884
Wrote on dysentery. Garrison and Morton
Diarrhoea and dysentery. In: U. S. War Dept. Medical and Surgical History of the War of the Rebellion. Washington, 1879. pt. 2, 1: 1–869
Woodyatt, R. T. See W. D. Sansum
Woolbridge, Leonard Charles. English physiologist.
1857–1889
TISSUE FIBRINOGEN—
On intravascular clotting. Proc. roy. Soc., 40: 134–135, Feb. 4, 1886
On the coagulation of the blood. Ibid., 320–321, Apr. 8, 1886
Woolley, D. W. See C. A. Elvehjem
Wootton, Herbert Wright. Alexandria, Va. ophthalmologist. 1867–1941
OPERATION—
Cyclodialysis combined with iridectomy in glaucoma simplex: a preliminary report. Trans. Amer. Ophthal. Soc., 30: 64–70, 1932
Wordley, E. London scientist
SOLUTION—blood cell peptone, for studying hemolysis by streptococci.
A new method for the isolation of organisms from faeces and sputum, with some observations on hemolytic streptococci in faeces obtained by this method. J. Hyg., 20: 60–68 (66), July 1921
Work, T. S. See A. R. Todd
Worster-Drought, Cecil Charles. English physician. 1888–
Reported jaundice due to cinchophen.
Atophan poisoning. Brit. med. J., 1: 148–149, Jan. 27, 1923
Wreden, Robert Robertovich. St. Petersburg otologist. 1837–1893
SIGN or TEST—
Die "Otitis media neonatorum" vom anatomisch-pathologischen Standpunkte; . . . Mschr. f. Ohrenh., 2, 1868
Described otomycosis or fungus disease of external ear.
Sechs Fälle von Myringomykosis (Aspergillus glaucus Lk.). Arch. f. Ohrenh., 2: 1–25, 1867
Wreden, R. R. Leningrad surgeon
OPERATION—
A method of reconstructing a voluntary sphincter ani. Arch. Surg., 18: 841–844, Mar. 1929
Wren, Sir Christopher. English scientist and architect. 1632–1723
First injected, with assistance of Boyle and Wilkins, opium and crocus metallorum into veins of dogs, in 1656. Garrison
(*An account of the rise and attempts, of a way to convey liquors immediately into the mass of blood.*) By H. Aldenburg, Philos. Trans., 1: 128–130, Dec. 4, 1665
Wright, Sir Almroth Edward. English bacteriologist. 1861–1947
COAGULATION TIME OF—
In his: *Technique of the teat and capillary glass tube, being a handbook for the medical research laboratory and the research world* with L. Colebrook, London, Constable, 1921. 2 ed., 384 pp. pp. 109–115

VACCINE—
Remarks on the results which have been obtained by the antityphoid inoculation with Sir W. B. Leishman, Brit. med. J., 1: 122–129, Jan. 20, 1900
A short treatise on anti-typhoid inoculation. . . . Westminister, Constable, 1904. 76 pp.
Pointed out role of calcium salts in coagulation of blood and devised a coagulometer for estimating coagulation time. Garrison
On the conditions which determine the distribution of the intra-vascular injection of a solution of Wooldridge's tissue fibrinogen. J. Physiol., 12: 184–191, 1891
Developed agglutination test for Micrococcus melitensis.
On the application of the serum test to the differential diagnosis of typhoid and Malta fever, and on the further application of the method of serum diagnosis to the elucidation of certain problems in connexion with the duration of immunity and the geographical distribution of disease with D. Semple, Lancet, 1: 656–659, Mar. 6, 1897
Originated general vaccinotherapy (1902–07), with superadded feature of measuring protective substances in blood by means of opsonic index. Garrison
An experimental investigation of the rôle of the blood fluids in connection with phagocytosis. with S. R. Douglas, Proc. roy. Soc., 72: 357–370, July 29, 1903
Further observations on the rôle of the blood fluids in connection with phagocytosis. Ibid., 73: 128–142, Jan. 11, 1904
Immunity: opsonines. Abstr.: Brit. med. J., 2: 582 (only), Sept. 10, 1904
Wright, Arthur W(illiam). Albany, N. Y. pathologist. 1894–
Described—
Hyaline degeneration of the Islands of Langerhans in non-diabetics. Amer. J. Path., 3: 461–481, Sept. 1927
Wright, George Arthur. Manchester surgeon. 1851–
OPERATION—for slipping patella. In: H. Ashby and G. A. Wright's
The diseases of children. London, Longmans, 1889. 2 ED., 1893. 773 pp. p. 711
Wright, Irving Sherwood. New York physician. 1901–
TEST—
Determination of vitamin C saturation: a five hour test after intravenous test dose with A. Lilienfeld and Elizabeth MacLenathen, Arch. intern. Med., 60: 264–271, Aug. 1937
See also A. W. Duryee
Wright, James Homer. Boston pathologist. 1871–1928
METHOD—
A simple method of cultivating anaerobic bacteria. J. Boston Soc. Med. Sci., 5: 114–115, Dec. 4, 1900
METHOD—
A new method of counting the blood-platelets for clinical purposes and some of the results obtained with it with R. Kinnicutt, J. A. M. A., 56: 1457–1459, May 20, 1911
STAIN—for megakaryocytes and blood platelets.
The histogenesis of the blood platelets. J. Morphol., 21: 262–278, July 1910
STAIN—for Treponema pallidum. In: Mallory and Wright's *Pathological technique.* 7 ed., 1918, p. 397

STAIN—
A rapid method for the differential staining of blood films and malarial parasites. J. med. Res., 7: 138–144, Jan. 1902
Found Leishmania tropica in Delhi sore. Garrison and Morton
Protozoa in a case of tropical ulcer ("Delhi sore"). Ibid., 10: 472–482, Dec. 1903
Showed that megakaryocytes are only source of true platelets.
The origin and nature of the blood plates. Boston M. and S. J., 144: 643–645, June 7, 1906
The histogenesis of the blood platelets. J. Morphol., 21: 262–278, July 1910
Established sympathetic neuroblastomas as distinct clinical entity.
Neurocytoma or neuroblastoma, a kind of tumor not generally recognized. J. exp. Med., 12: 556–561, July 23, 1910
Wright, John Westley. Columbus, Ohio ophthalmologist. 1842–
Advocated intracapsular enucleation of lens.
Cataract—improved operation. Columbus med. J., 2: 403–409, Mar. 1884
Wright, L. E. See O. K. O. Folin
Wright, L. T. See J. F. Connors
Wright, Marmaduke Burr. Ohio obstetrician. 1803–1879
Introduced combined cephalic version. Garrison
Difficult labors and their treatment. Cincinnati, Jackson, White and Co., 1854. 32 pp.
Wrigley, C. H. See L. S. Dudgeon
Wrisberg, Heinrich August. German anatomist. 1737–1808
CARTILAGE—cuneiform.
Observationes anatomico-medicae de nervis pharyngis. Comment. phys., Göttingae, 1785, pp. 135–160
CORPUSCLES, GANGLION, LIGAMENT, LINES—
Descriptio anatomica embryonis observationibus illustrata. Göttingae, Vanderhoek, 1764. 80 pp.
NERVE—pars intermedia facialis.
Observationes anatomicae de quinto pare nervorum encephali et de nervis qui ex eodam duram matrem ingredi falso dicuntur. Göttingen, Dieterich, 1777. 28 pp.
Wroblewski, Vincenz. Krakow bacteriologist
BROTH—suprarenal capsule infusion; culture medium.
Ueber das Wachstum einiger pathogener Spaltpilze auf dem Nebennierenextraktnährboden. Zbl. f. Bakt., 20: 528–535 (529), Oct. 10, 1896
Wu, H. See O. K. O. Folin
Würtz, Felix. Swiss surgeon. 1518–1574
Wrote on infant surgery.
Kinderbuchlein. In his: *Wund-Artzney.* Basel, Petrini, 1638
Wützer, Karl Wilhelm. German surgeon. 1789–1863
GANGLION—
De corporis humani gangliorum fabrica atque usu, monographia. Berolini, Nicolai, 1817. 136 pp.

OPERATION—for inguinal hernia.
Ueber radicale Heilung beweglicher Leistenbruche. Org. d. ges. Heilk., Bonn, 1, pt. 1, 1840
Wullstein, Dr. Halle a. S. surgeon
OPERATION—for congenital dislocation of patella.
Eine neue Operationsmethode der kongenitalen Luxation der Patella. Zbl. f. Chir., 33: Beilage, 136–138, 1906
OPERATION—for ventral hernia.
Zur Technik der Radikaloperationen grosser Nabel- und Bauchwandhernien. Ibid., 153–154, 1906
Wunderlich, Carl Reinhold August. German physician. 1815–1877
CURVE—of typhoid fever.
Das Verhalten der Eigenwärme in Krankheiten. Leipzig, 1868
Wundt, Wilhelm Max. German ophthalmologist. 1832–1920
SENSORY PRECEPTION—
Beiträge zur Theorie der Sinneswahrnehmung. Z. f. rat. Med., 4: 229–293, 1858
Founder of experimental psychology. Garrison and Morton
Grundzüge der physiologischen Psychologie. Leipzig, Engelmann, 1873–74
Wurster, Casimir. Berlin physiologist. 1856–1913
REACTION—for albumin.
Ueber Eiweiss- und Tyrosinreactionen. Zbl. Physiol., 1: 193–195, July 23, 1887
Wurtz, John G. Pittsburgh physician. 1885–
SOLUTION—diluted blood.
A simple method for blood culture with S. W. Sappington, J. med. Res., 38: 371–378 (373), July 1918
Wurtz, Robert Théodore. French bacteriologist. 1858–1919
AGAR—nutrient; general culture medium.
Technique bactériologique. Paris, Masson, 1897. p. 29
Wyatt, W. See T. Brushfield
Wyeth, George Austin. New York surgeon. 1877–
TEST—for cancer.
A serological test with hormone organ antigens. I. Complement fixation test in neoplastic diseases, pregnancy, and sex determination. Med. J. and Rec., 133: 469–472, May 20, 1931
Wyeth, John Allan. New York surgeon. 1845–1922
OPERATION—
Eine neue Methode zur Exartikulation des Oberschenkels ohne Blutverlust. Zbl. f. Chir., 19: 441–445, May 28, 1892
A fourth case of amputation at the hip joint by the author's bloodless method. Med. Rec., 45: 33–35, Jan. 13, 1894
Wyman, Morrill. Boston physician. 1812–1903
Described—
Autumnal catarrh (hay fever). New York, Hurd and Houghton, 1872. 173 pp.
Wyss, Fernand. French physician
DETERMINATION—of insulin.
Dosage biochimique de l'insuline. C. R. Acad. Sci., 181: 327–328, Aug. 31, 1925

Y

Yamagiwa, Katsusaburo. Tokyo physician. 1863–1930
Experimentally produced tar cancer by painting ears of rabbits with coal tar.
Experimentelle Studie über die Pathogenese der Epithelialgeschwülste with K. Ichikawa, Mitt. d. m. Fakultät d. k. Univ. z. Tokyo, 15: 295–344, Mar. 18, 1916

Yannet, H. See D. C. Darrow

Yant, William Parks. Pittsburgh chemist. 1894–
METHOD—
Urine sulfate determinations as a measure of benzene exposure with H. H. Schrenk, R. R. Sayers, A. A. Horvath and W. H. Reinhart, J. indust. Hyg. and Toxicol., 18: 69–88, Jan. 1936
See also R. R. Sayers

Yarbrough, N. See H. P. Barret

Yastomi, T. See Z. Inouye

Yee, L. B. K. See C. R. Rowe

Yeomanns, Frank Clark. New York proctologist. 1873–
DIATHERMY SNARE— In his: *Proctology....* New York, Appleton, 1929. 661 pp. pp. 451–452
PROCTOSCOPE— Ibid., p. 82
TECHNIC—for treatment of coccygodynia. Ibid., pp. 192–193

Yergason, Robert Moseley. Hartford, Conn. surgeon. 1885–
SIGN—pain in bicipital groove with tendinitis of long head of biceps.
Supination sign. J. Bone and Joint Surg., 13: 160 (only), Jan. 1931

Yerkes, Robert Mearns. American psychologist. 1876–
POINT SCALE and TEST—
A point scale for measuring mental ability with J. W. Bridges and Rose S. Hardwick, Warwick and York, 1915
A point scale for the measurement of intelligence in adolescent and adult individuals with C. S. Rossy, Bull. Massachusetts Comm. Ment. Dis., 2: 132–152, 1918–19

Yersin, A. See S. Kitasato, P. P. E. Roux

Yerson, Alexander Emil Jean. French physician. 1862–1943
BACILLUS—B. pestis bubonicae.
La peste bubonique à Hong-Kong. Ann. Inst. Pasteur, Paris, 8: 662–667, Sept. 1894

Yonge, James. English surgeon. 1646–1721
Performed amputation by means of a flap. Garrison
Currus triumphalis, e terebintho; wherein also, the common methods and medicaments, used to restrain hemorrhagies, are examined. London, Martyn, 1679. 120 pp.

Yoshimatsu, Shun-Ichi. Tokyo pediatrician
METHOD—
A simple colorimetric method for the determination of iodine in urine with H. Sakurada, Tohoku J. exp. Med., 8: 107–112, Nov. 4, 1926
See also A. Sato

Young, A. M. See B. S. Kline

Young, Charles Stephen. Los Angeles surgeon. 1892–

OPERATION—
An operation for the correction of hammer-toe and claw-toe. J. Bone and Joint Surg., 20: 715–719, July 1938

Young, Hugh Hampton. Baltimore urologist. 1870–1945
OPERATION—
Suprapubic retrocystic extraperitoneal resection of the seminal vesicles, vasa deferentia, and half of the bladder. Ann. Surg., 32: 557–566, Oct. 1900
Genital tuberculosis, with special reference to the seminal vesicles. Report of two cases of spermatocystectomy. Ibid., 34: 601–636, Nov. 1901
OPERATION—
The early diagnosis and radical cure of carcinoma of the prostate; ... Johns Hopk. Hosp. Bull., 16: 315–321, Oct. 1905
Cancer of the prostate: a clinical, pathological and post-operative analysis of 111 cases. Ann. Surg., 50: 1144–1233, Dec. 1909
The radical cure of cancer of the prostate. S. G. O., 64: 472–484, Feb. 15, 1937
OPERATION—
Suture of the urethral and vesical sphincters for the cure of incontinence of urine, with a report of a case. Trans. South. Surg. and Gynec. Ass., 20: 210–217, 1908
OPERATION—for hypospadias. In his: *Practice of urology.* Philadelphia, Saunders, 1926. Vol. 2, pp. 604–605
OPERATION—for hydronephrosis.
Obstructions to the ureter produced by aberrant blood vessels: a plastic repair without ligation of vessels or transplantation of ureters. S. G. O., 54: 26–38, Jan. 1932
OPERATION—
A technique for simultaneous exposure and operation of the adrenals. Ibid., 63: 178–188, Aug. 1936
PUNCH—
A new procedure (punch operation) for small prostatic bars and contracture of the prostatic orifice. J. A. M. A., 60: 253–257, Jan. 25, 1913
TABLE—
Demonstration of a new combined cystoscopic and x-ray table. Trans. Amer. Urol. Ass., 12: 344–347, 1920
Advocated two-stage prostatectomy.
The operative treatment of hypertrophied prostate. Amer. J. Dermat. and Genitourin. Dis., 4: 17–19, Jan. 1900
Conservative perineal prostatectomy: a presentation of new instruments and technic. J. A. M. A., 41: 999–1009, Oct. 24, 1903
Studied production of dyes as germicides; introduced mercurochrome.
A new germicide for use in the genito-urinary tract "*mercurochrome-220:*" *preliminary report of experimental and clinical studies* with E. C. White and E. O. Swartz, Ibid., 73: 1483–1491, Nov. 15, 1919
Demonstrated vesiculography.
X-ray studies of the seminal vesicles and vasa deferentia after urethroscopic injection of the ejaculatory ducts with thorium—a new diagnostic method with C. A. Waters, Amer. J. Röntgenol., n. s. 7: 16–22, Jan. 1920

Young, James L. Washington, D. C. chemist
TEST—
The detection of cocaine in the presence of novocaine by means of cobalt thiocyanate. Amer. J. Pharm., 103: 709–710, Dec. 1931
Young, James Kelly. Philadelphia surgeon. 1862–1923
OPERATION—
Recurrent dislocation of the shoulder-joint. Ann. Surg., 63: 375 (only), Mar. 1916
Young, John Richardson. Philadelphia physiologist. 1782–1804
Wrote book on digestion and recognized acid character of gastric juice. Garrison
An experimental inquiry into the principles of nutrition and the digestive process. Philadelphia, Eaken and Mecum, 1803. 48 pp.
Young, Thomas. English physician. 1773–1829
RULE—of amount of medicine for a child. (Modern expression, add twelve to the age and divide by the age.)
In his: An introduction to medical literature, including a system of practical nosology. London, Underwood and Blacks, 1813. 586 pp. p. 428
THEORY—of color vision and of light.
On the theory of light and colors. Nicholson's Philos. Jour., 1801

An account of some cases of the production of colors. Ibid., 1802
On the theory of light and colours. Philos. Trans., 92: 12–48, 1802
Described astigmatism. Garrison
On the mechanism of the eye. Ibid., 91: 23–88, 1801
Youngburg, Guy Edgar. Buffalo biochemist. 1884–
METHOD—for determination of lecithin.
Phosphorus metabolism. I. A system of blood phosphorus analysis with Mamie V. Youngburg, J. Lab. clin. Med., 16: 158–166, Nov. 1930
MODIFICATION—of Van Slyke and Cullen's method of determination of urea in urine.
The removal of ammonia from urine preparatory to the determination of urea. J. biol. Chem., 45: 391–394, Feb. 1921
Yudin, Sergey Sergeevich. Moscow physician. 1891–
Advocated—
La transfusion du sang de cadavre à l'homme. Paris, Masson, 1933
Transfusion of cadaver blood. J. A. M. A., 106: 997–999, Mar. 21, 1936
Transfusion of stored cadaver blood; practical considerations: the first thousand cases. Lancet, 2: 361–366, Aug. 14, 1937
Yule, G. U. See M. Greenwood
Yuska, H. See A. E. Sobel

Z

Zaaijer, Johannes Henricus. Holland surgeon. 1876–
OPERATION—for dilatation of esophagus.
Oesophagotomia thoracalis. Beitr. z. klin. Chir., 77: 497–502, Feb. 1912
Cardiospasm in the aged. Ann. Surg., 77: 615–617, May 1923
Zacchias, Paulus. Rome physician. 1584–1659
Wrote important treatise on medical jurisprudence. Garrison and Morton
Quaesationes medico-legales. . . . Romae, Amstelaedami, 1621–66. 9 vols.
Zahorsky, John. St. Louis pediatrician. 1871–
Described—
Roseola infantilis. Pediatrics, 22: 60–64, Jan. 1910
Zaleski, Stanuslaus. Dorpat pharmacologist
TEST—for carbon monoxide in blood.
Ueber eine neue Reaction auf Kohlenoxydhämoglobin. Z. phys. Chem., 9: 225–228, 1885
Zambeccari, Giuseppe. Italian surgeon. 1655–1728
Pioneer in experimental surgery. Garrison
Esperienze del Dottor Giuseppe Zambeccari intorno a diverse viscere tagliate a diversi animali viventi, e da lui scritte e dedicate all'illustrissimo Signore Francesco Redi. Firenze, Onofri, 1680
Zander, Jonas Gustav Wilhelm. Swedish physician. 1835–1917
APPARATUS—to give exercise and to apply manipulations.
Die Apparate für mechanische Heilgymnastik und deren Anwendung. Stockholm, Haeggström, 1886. 85 pp.
Also, in English. New York, 1891. 50 pp.
Zanfrognini, A. Modena obstetrician
REAGENT and TEST—for adrenaline.
Eine neue kolorimetrische Methode der Adrenalin-

bestimmung. Dtsch. med. Wschr., 35: 1752–1753, Oct. 7, 1909
Zaufal, Emanuel. Prague surgeon. 1833–1910
OPERATION—radical mastoidectomy.
Sinusthrombose in Folge von Otitis media; Tepanation des Proc. mastoid. mit Hammer und Meissel. Prag. med. Wschr., 9: 474, 1884
Zazeela, H. See D. I. Abramson
Zeckwer, Isolde Therese. American pathologist. 1892–
METHOD—
The sedimentation rate of erythrocytes with Helen Goodell, Amer. J. med. Sci., 169: 209–216, Feb. 1925
Zeiss, Carl. German optician
COUNTING CELL—
Illustrirter Katalog über Mikroscope und Nebenapparate. Jena, 1878
Zeller, Albert. Berlin surgeon
TEST—
Ueber Melanurie. Arch. klin. Chir., 29: 245–253, 1883
Zeller, Simon. Vienna surgeon. 1746–1816
OPERATION—for webbed fingers.
Abhandlung ueber die ersten Erscheinungen venerischer Lokal-Krankheits-Formen, die angebornen verwachsenen Finger. . . . Vienna, Binz, 1810. 379 pp. p. 109
Zenker, Friedrich Albert. German pathologist. 1825–1898
FLUID or SOLUTION—fixing.
Chromkali-Sublimat-Eissesig als Fixirungsmittel. Münch. med. Wschr., 41: 532–534, July 3, 1894
Described intestinal and muscular forms of trichiniasis. Garrison and Morton
Arch. f. path. Anat., 18: 561–572, 1860

Described pulmonary fat embolism. Garrison and Morton
Beiträge zur normalen und pathologischen Anatomie der Lungen. Dresden, Schönfeld's Buchhandlung, 1862
Zentmire, Zelma. See P. C. Jeans
Zeri, Agenore. Rome physician
PHENOMENON—
Di un nuovo fenomeno osservato in un case di malattia di Adams-Stokes. Rif. med., 19: 701-707, July 1, 1903
Zins, B. See A. Vogl
Zipperlen, E. See M. Gänsslen
Zironi, A. See G. M. Fasiani
Zettnow, Hugh Oscar Emil. Berlin physician. 1842-1927
AGAR—meat infusion.
Nährboden für Spirillum Undula majus. Zbl. Bakt., 19: 393-395, Mar. 21, 1896
STAIN—for flagella.
Romanowski's Färbung bei Bakterien. Z. Hyg. InfektKr., 30: 1-18, 1899
Ueber Geisselfärbung bei Bakterien. Ibid., pp. 95-106
STAIN—for chromatin. Ibid., pp. 1-18
Ziegler, Samuel Lewis. Philadelphia ophthalmologist. 1861-1926
OPERATION—
History of iridotomy: knife-needle vs. scissors—description of author's V-shaped method. J. A. M. A., 52: 539-542, Feb. 13, 1909
Complete discission of the lens by the V-shaped method. Ibid., 77: 1100-1102, Oct. 1, 1921
Ziehen, Georg Theodor. German neurologist. 1862-
DISEASE—Ziehen-Oppenheim d.; dystonia musculorum deformans.
(No title). Neurol. Zbl., 30: 109-112, Jan. 16, 1911
Ziehl, Franz. German bacteriologist. 1857-1926
SOLUTION and STAIN—carbolfuchsin.
Zur Färbung des Tuberkelbacillus. Dtsch. med. Wschr., 8: 451-453, Aug. 12, 1882
Zielleczky, Rudolf. Prague bacteriologist
BROTH—phenolphthalein infusion, for differentiation of coli and typhoid organisms.
Biochemische und differentialdiagnostische Untersuchungen einiger Bakterien mittels Phenolphthaleinnährboden. Zbl. Bakt., 32: 752-768, Nov. 5, 1902
Ziemann, Hans Richard Paul. German physician. 1865-
METHOD—of staining chromatin.
Eine Methode der Doppelfärbung bei Flagellaten, Pilzen, Spirillen und Bakterien, sowie bei einigen Amöben. Zbl. Bakt., 24: 944-955, Dec. 30, 1898
Ziemmsen, Hugo Wilhelm von. Munich physician. 1829-1902
METHOD—canula, of blood transfusion.
Ueber die subcutane Blutinjection und über eine neue einfache Methode der intravenösen Transfusion. Münch. med. Wschr., 39: 323-324, May 10, 1892
POINT—motor p., of election in therapeutic application of electricity to muscles.
Die Electricität in der Medicin. Berlin, Hirschwald, 1857. 82 pp.
TREATMENT—of anemia by subcutaneous injections of defibrinated human blood.
Ueber subcutane Blutinjection. . . . In: Klinische Vorträge. Leipzig, Vogel, 1887. Vol. 2, Abt. 2.

Also, transl. by W. G. Eggleston:
Lecture on subcutaneous blood-injections, salt-water infusion, and intravenous transfusion. J. A. M. A., 9: 35-39, July 9; 68-72, July 16, 1887
Zierold, Arthur Adalbert. Minneapolis surgeon. 1886-
MANEUVER—
A new method of reduction of dislocations at the shoulder joint. S. G. O., 61: 818-820, Dec. 1935
Ziffren, Sidney Edward. Iowa City pathologist. 1912-
TEST—for prothrombin.
Control of vitamin K therapy. Compensatory mechanisms at low prothrombin levels with C. A. Owen, G. R. Hoffman and H. P. Smith, Proc. Soc. exp. Biol., N. Y., 40: 595-597, Apr. 1939
See also H. P. Smith
Zimmermann, Johann Georg. German physician. 1728-1795
Wrote on bacillary dysentery. Garrison and Morton
Von der Ruhr unter dem Volke im Jahr 1765. Zürich, Fuessli, 1767
Zimmermann, Karl Wilhelm Bruno. Bern anatomist. 1900-
PERICYTES—cells wrapped tightly about capillaires (modified smooth muscle cells), with contractile properties.
Der feinere Bau der Blutcapillaren. Z. f. Anat. u. Entwickl., 68: 29-109, June 30, 1923
Zimmerman, Leo M. Chicago surgeon. 1898-
OPERATION—
Inguina hernia. II. The surgical treatment of direct inguinal hernia. S. G. O., 66: 192-198, Feb. 1, 1938
Zingher, A. See W. H. Park
Zinn, Johann Gottfried. German anatomist. 1727-1759
CENTRAL ARTERY, CIRCLET, CORONA, MEMBRANE—
Descriptio anatomica oculi humani, iconibus illustrata. . . . Göttingae, Vandenhoeck, 1755. 272 pp.
APONEUROSIS, LIGAMENT, ZONE or ZONULE—
De ligamentis ciliaribus. Göttingen, Schulzii, 1753
Zins, Berthold. Vienna physician
TEST—
Zur Methodik des Nachweises von Bilirubin in Harn. Klin. Wschr., 2: 978 (only), May 21, 1923
Zinsser, Hans. American bacteriologist. 1878-1940
MEDIUM—
A simple method for the plating of anaerobic organisms. J. exp. Med., 8: 542-546, Aug. 1, 1906
METHOD—
Notes on the cultivation of Treponema pallidum with J. G. Hopkins and Ruth Gilbert, Ibid., 21: 213-220, Mar. 1, 1915
THEORY—that allergy constitutes most important background for development of chronic arthritis.
On the significance of bacterial allergy in infectious diseases. Bull. New York Acad. Med., 4: 351-353, Mar. 1928
Prepared vaccine of killed Rickettsias which produced protective immunity against typhus.
Studies on typhus fever. XII. The passive immunization of guinea pigs, infected with European virus, with serum of a horse treated with killed Rickettsia of the Mexican type with M. R. Castaneda, J. exp. Med., 59: 471-478, Apr. 1934

Zoeller, C. See G. Ramon
Zoeppritz, Heinrich. Kiel physician
TEST—for blood in feces.
Bemerkungen zur Technik des Nachweises von okkultem Blut mittels der Guajakreaktion. Münch. med. Wschr., 59: 180–182, Jan. 23, 1912
Zondek, Bernhard. Jerusalem gynecologist. 1891–
REACTION—for pregnancy. See also S. Aschheim
Das Hormon des Hypophysenvorderlappens. I. Testobjekt zum Nachweis des Hormons. Klin. Wschr., 6: 248–252, Feb. 5, 1927
TREATMENT—
Simplified hormonal treatment of amenorrhea. J. A. M. A., 118: 705–707, Feb. 28, 1942
Zondek, Hermann. German physician. 1887–
SYNDROME—"myxoedema heart."
Das Myxödemherz. Münch. med. Wschr., 65: 1180–1182, Oct. 22, 1918
Zouchlos, Constantin. German physician
REAGENTS—for albumin.
Ueber einige Reaktionen zum Nachweis des Albumins im Harn. Erlangen, Jacob, 1888. 18 pp.
Zuck, F. N. See H. H. Hopkins
Zuelzer, Georg Ludwig. Berlin physician. 1870–
HEART HORMONE—eutonon.
Das Herzhormon „Eutonon". Med. Klin., 23: 1502–1503, Sept. 30, 1927
Zum gegenwärtigen Stand der Herzhormonfrage. Ibid., 24: 571–574, Apr. 13, 1928
Isolated a pancreatic extract but abandoned his work. Garrison and Morton

Ueber Versuche einer spezifischen Fermenttherapie des Diabetes. Z. exp. Path. Ther., 5: 307–318, Sept. 16, 1908
Zulkowsky, Karl. German chemist
REAGENT—starch, for iodine.
Verhalten der Stärke gegen Glycerin. Ber. dtsch. chem. Ges., 13: 1395–1398, July 12, 1880
Zuntz, Nathan. Berlin physician. 1847–1920
THEORY—of muscle contraction.
Die Ernährung des Herzens und ihre Beziehung zu seiner Arbeitsleistung. Dtsch. med. Wschr., 18: 109–111, Feb. 11, 1892
Studied blood gases and respiratory metabolism. Garrison
Beiträge zur Physiologie des Blutes. Bonn, Georgi, 1868. 42 pp.
Zwaardemaker, Hendrik. Dutch physician. 1857–1930
HEART HORMONE—automatine.
Radiation-substances and cardiac hormones. Proc. Akad. met. Amsterdam, 30: sect. sc., 184–188, 1927
Die Automative als Strahlungsstoffe im Herzen. Z. KreislForsch., 20: 121–131, 1928
Zwally, M. R. See J. F. Mahoney
Zweifel, Erwin. German obstetrician
FORCEPS—
Ein neues Zangenmodell. Zbl. Gynaek., 50: 604–605, Mar. 6, 1926
A new obstetric forceps. Amer. J. Obstet., 21: 138–139, Jan. 1931
Zwemer, R. L. See R. Truszkowski

INDEX